Textbook of Cancer Epidemiology

Second Edition

MONOGRAPHS IN EPIDEMIOLOGY AND BIOSTATISTICS

Edited by Albert Hofman, Michael Marmot, Jonathan M. Samet, David A. Savitz

Textbook of Cancer Epidemiology

Second Edition

Edited by
Hans-Olov Adami
David Hunter
Dimitrios Trichopoulos

With an introductory chapter by
Brian MacMahon

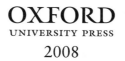

UNIVERSITY PRESS
2008

OXFORD
UNIVERSITY PRESS

Oxford University Press, Inc., publishes works that further
Oxford University's objective of excellence
in research, scholarship, and education.

Oxford   New York
Auckland   Cape Town   Dar es Salaam   Hong Kong   Karachi
Kuala Lumpur   Madrid   Melbourne   Mexico City   Nairobi
New Delhi   Shanghai   Taipei   Toronto

With offices in
Argentina   Austria   Brazil   Chile   Czech Republic   France   Greece
Guatemala   Hungary   Italy   Japan   Poland   Portugal   Singapore
South Korea   Switzerland   Thailand   Turkey   Ukraine   Vietnam

Published by Oxford University Press, Inc.
198 Madison Avenue, New York, New York 10016
www.oup.com

Oxford is a registered trademark of Oxford University Press

Library of Congress Cataloging-in-Publication Data
Textbook of cancer epidemiology /
edited by Hans-Olov Adami, David Hunter, Dimitrios Trichopoulos;
with an introductory chapter by Brian MacMahon.—2nd ed.
p. ; cm.
Includes bibliographical references and index.
ISBN 978-0-19-531117-4
1. Cancer—Epidemiology.
[DNLM: 1. Neoplasms—epidemiology. QZ 220.1 T355 2007]
I. Adami, Hans-Olov.
II. Hunter, David J. (David John)
III. Trichopoulos, Dimitrios.
RA645.C3T485 2008   614.5'9994—dc22   2007018120

9 8 7 6 5 4 3 2 1
Printed in the United States of America
on acid-free paper

To Barbro, Leona, and Antonia

We dedicate this second edition
to the late Brian MacMahon, MD,
who inspired, educated, and encouraged
several generations of cancer epidemiologists.

Preface to Second Edition

Little more than 5 years have elapsed since our *Textbook of Cancer Epidemiology* was first sent to print. As we hoped, and indeed predicted, the progress in our discipline has been substantial during these years. We therefore felt a growing need to update the text now, after the first edition has been printed three times. Without changing the overall disposition of the book or the uniform structure of site-specific chapters, this second edition has been thoroughly revised. We achieved this goal in many instances by inviting a new colleague to join the authors of the first edition. As a corollary, many chapters are now written by three rather than two authors, always with deep involvement of the editors.

Beside a thorough update—often with considerable expansion of genetic and molecular epidemiology—the second edition has some novel features too. Most importantly, the late Brian MacMahon, a towering Nestor in epidemiology, has written an extensive introductory chapter. This contribution provides a historical perspective on the evolution of cancer epidemiology. We hope this text will be particularly useful to younger colleagues who entered our field of scientific inquiry recently. We have also added a new chapter on the nasopharyngeal carcinoma. Although largely unknown in Western countries, this malignancy is endemic and has considerable public health consequences in some parts of Asia.

We are in debt to all colleagues who joined us in the effort to produce this second edition. But we are particularly grateful to Kristina Glimsjö. Without her insurpassable competence, exemplary coordination of the work, and meticulous technical editing of all chapters, it is hard to imagine how a timely finishing of this second edition would have been possible.

Boston and Stockholm	H.O.A
Boston	D.H.
Boston and Athens	D.T.

Preface to First Edition

We believe there are several reasons that familiarity with cancer epidemiology will become increasingly important for many health professionals besides those working in the traditional realm of epidemiology and public health. First, in the history of medicine, primary prevention has often, sooner or later, turned out to be the most successful and most cost-effective—sometimes the only possible—approach to disease control. Water sanitation and vaccination programs have saved more lives than antibiotics and intensive care. Second, now that the human genome has been sequenced, a gigantic challenge will be to understand how genes, environment, and lifestyle interact in the causation of human cancer. Epidemiologic approaches are needed to achieve this understanding. Third, therapeutic breakthroughs in oncology have certainly been important but few. If real progress ultimately occurs, as we all hope, it is not obvious that novel treatments will be available, or affordable, to the majority of the world's population.

Hence, primary prevention of cancer will likely be an increasingly important and integral part of any health professional's duties. The first step in preventing any disease is to understand its causes and the proportion of cases due to each cause. This is the background against which this book was written. It is intended for students of epidemiology, medicine, public health, biology, and the behavioral sciences, and for practitioners of medicine, public health, and other health professions. We assume no deep familiarity with epidemiologic theory, study design, biostatistics, and causal reasoning or any expertise in medicine, oncology, or biology.

Part 1 gives an introduction to basic concepts in epidemiology, a description of the global burden of cancer, definitions and characterizations of the various measures used, and approaches used to reveal genetic determinants of cancer risk and integrate biologic markers in the epidemiologic research process. Part 2 is devoted to specific cancer sites or types, each chapter starting with a brief synopsis that introduces the clinical characteristics of the specific cancer. The structure of these chapters is uniform. They all have three main sections: Descriptive Epidemiology, Genetic and Molecular Epidemiology, and Risk Factors. In order to facilitate reading, risk factors are discussed in the same order throughout all these chapters.

Admittedly, this short textbook does not cover all sites and types of cancer. Rare malignancies such as sarcomas have been omitted, as have some endocrine tumors, childhood cancers—accounting for less than 1% of the total—and certain anogenital cancers. It is worth emphasizing, though, that little is known about the etiology of the forms of cancer that we excluded.

Other volumes on cancer epidemiology are available—some larger and more detailed than ours, such as the important book by Schottenfeld and Fraumeni (1996), and others written by distinguished colleagues who have chosen approaches different from those we adopted. A range of book choices is beneficial to prospective readers, who will be able to choose on the basis of their particular objectives, orientation, or style.

Most of what we know about the causes of cancer in humans has been generated by epidemiologic research. Nevertheless, readers of this textbook may find the gaps in knowledge, the ambiguities, and the abundant contradictory findings frustrating. But a tidier picture would be unrealistic given the enormous challenges for the young discipline of cancer epidemiology in linking complex human characteristics and behavior, often during many decades of life, to the occurrence of cancer. We hope that the evidence put together in this book will leave the reader better equipped to follow the expansion of cancer epidemiology during the years to come.

Stockholm   H.O.A.
Boston   D.H.
Boston and Athens   D.T.

Contents

About the Authors

Hans-Olov Adami, MD, is Professor of Cancer Epidemiology and former Chairman of the Department of Medical Epidemiology and Biostatistics at the Karolinska Institutet, Sweden, Visiting Professor at the National University in Singapore, as well as Chairman of the Department of Epidemiology at the Harvard School of Public Health, Boston.

David Hunter, MBBS, is the Vincent L. Gregory Professor of Cancer Prevention at the Harvard School of Public Health, and Director of the Program in Genetic and Molecular Epidemiology.

Dimitrios Trichopoulos, MD, is the Vincent L. Gregory Professor of Cancer Prevention and Professor of Epidemiology, and the former Chairman of the Department of Epidemiology at the Harvard School of Public Health, Emeritus Professor and former Chairman of the department of Hygiene and Epidemiology at the University of Athens Medical School in Greece, and Adjunct Professor of Epidemiology at the Karolinska Institutet in Sweden.

Contributors

HANS-OLOV ADAMI, MD
Department of Epidemiology
Harvard School of Public Health
Boston, Massachusetts

JOHANNA ADAMI, MD
Clinical Epidemiology Unit
Department of Medicine
Karolinska Institutet
Stockholm, Sweden

PAOLO BOFFETTA, MD
Genetics and Epidemiology Cluster
International Agency for Research on
    Cancer
Lyon, France

PAUL BRENNAN, PhD
Genetic Epidemiology Group
International Agency for Research on
    Cancer
Lyon, France

ELLEN CHANG, ScD
Northern California Cancer Center
Fremont, California
Department of Health Research and Policy
Stanford University School of Medicine
Stanford, California

EUNYOUNG CHO, ScD
Department of Medicine
Brigham and Women's Hospital and
    Harvard Medical School
Boston, Massachusetts

IMMACULATA DE VIVO, PhD
Department of Medicine
Harvard Medical School
Boston, Massachusetts

JEFFREY ECSEDY, PhD
Department of Oncology
Millennium Pharmaceuticals
Cambridge, Massachusetts

ANDERS EKBOM, MD
Clinical Epidemiology Unit
Department of Medicine
Karolinska Institutet
Stockholm, Sweden

KARIN EKSTRÖM SMEDBY, MD
Department of Medical Epidemiology
    and Biostatistics
Karolinska Institutet
Stockholm, Sweden

MONTSERRAT GARCIA-CLOSAS, MD
Division of Cancer Epidemiology and
  Genetics
National Cancer Institute
Rockville, Maryland

DOROTA GERTIG, MBBS, PhD
Victorian Cytology Service
Carlton, Victorian Cytology Service
Australia

ADÈLE GREEN, MBBS
Queensland Institute of Medical Research
Brisbane, Queensland
Australia

CHRISTOPHER HAIMAN, ScD
Department of Preventive Medicine
University of Southern California
Los Angeles, California

PER HALL, MD
Department of Medical Epidemiology
  and Biostatistics
Karolinska Institutet
Stockholm, Sweden

SUSAN HANKINSON, ScD
Department of Medicine
Harvard Medical School
Boston, Massachusetts

HENRIK HJALGRIM, MD
Department of Epidemiology Research
Statens Serum Institut
Copenhagen, Denmark

DAVID HUNTER, ScD
Department of Epidemiology
Harvard School of Public Health
Boston, Massachusetts

MANOLIS KOGEVINAS, MD
Centre for Research in Environmental
  Epidemiology (CREAL)
Municipal Institute of Medical Research
  (IMIM)
Barcelona, Spain

PAGONA LAGIOU, MD
Department of Hygiene and
  Epidemiology
School of Medicine, University
  of Athens
Athens, Greece

PER LINDBLAD, MD
Department of Urology
Sundsvall Hospital
Sundsvall, Sweden

BRIAN MACMAHON
Professor Emeritus
Department of Epidemiology
Harvard School of Public Health
Boston, Massachusetts

MADS MELBYE, MD
Department of Epidemiology Research
Statens Serum Institut
Copenhagen, Denmark

LORELEI A. MUCCI, ScD
Department of Medicine
Harvard Medical School
Boston, Massachusetts

OLOF NYRÉN, MD
Department of Medical Epidemiology
  and Biostatistics
Karolinska Institutet
Stockholm, Sweden

INGEMAR PERSSON, MD
Department of Medical Epidemiology
  and Biostatistics
Karolinska Institutet
Stockholm, Sweden

ELENI PETRIDOU, MD
Department of Hygiene
  and Epidemiology
School of Medicine,
  University of Athens
Athens, Greece

APOSTOLOS POURTSIDIS, MD
Oncology Department
Children's Hospital Aglaia Kyriakou
Athens, Greece

JOHN D. POTTER, MBBS, PhD
Division of Public Health Sciences
Fred Hutchinson Cancer Research Center
Seattle, Washington

LORENZO RICHIARDI, MD
Unit of Cancer Epidemiology and Centre
  for Oncologic Prevention
University of Turin
Turin, Italy

DAVID A. SAVITZ, PhD
Department of Community
  and Preventive Medicine
Mount Sinai School of Medicine
New York, New York

LISA B.SIGNORELLO, ScD
International Epidemiology Institute
Rockville, Maryland
Department of Medicine
Vanderbilt University Medical Center
Nashville, Tennessee

SHERRI STUVER, ScD
Department of Epidemiology
Boston University School of
  Public Health
Boston, Massachusetts

RULLA TAMIMI, ScD
Department of Medicine
Harvard Medical School
Boston, Massachusetts

DIMITRIOS TRICHOPOULOS, MD
Department of Epidemiology
Harvard School of Public Health
Boston, Massachusetts

JOLIEKE VAN DER POLS, PhD
School of Population Health
University of Queensland
Brisbane, Queensland, Australia

PENELOPE WEBB, PhD
Queensland Institute of
  Medical Research
Brisbane, Queensland, Australia

NATHALIE YLITALO, MD
Department of Medical Epidemiology
  and Biostatistics
Karolinska Institutet
Stockholm, Sweden

I

BACKGROUND

1

Accomplishments in Cancer Epidemiology

BRIAN MACMAHON

The proper study of Mankind is Man
—(Alexander Pope, *An Essay on Man*)

Knowledge of the environmental causes of human cancer has come principally from study of the human experience. The roles of epidemiology have been to describe the distribution of cancer in populations and to seek deviations from randomness that offer clues as to their explanations, to assess the validity and strength of associations that are suspected causes, and to evaluate the effectiveness of preventive measures by continued monitoring of cancer incidence and mortality. Experiments on laboratory animals, inferences from the natural world outside man, biochemistry, and microbiology have all played important roles, but observation of human beings has often suggested lines of investigation and is essential in evaluating the efficacy of preventive measures. In this chapter we will review epidemiologic evidence on cigarette smoking, ionizing radiation, occupation, the physical and microbiologic environments, the reproductive experience of women, alcohol, and iatrogenic exposures as they bear on cancer risk in humans. In addition to accomplishments that identified specific cancer causes,

we will note some situations in which epidemiologic studies provided reassurance that an agent suspected of being carcinogenic has been demonstrated not to be so under the circumstance of human exposures—such findings are also accomplishments.

Had this chapter been written in 1930, barely 75 years ago, the list of accomplishments would have been modest. To summarize the progress that has been made in these 75 years requires economy of language and information—not to mention certain arrogance. We can present only in outline the main epidemiologic discoveries. Necessarily, the subject matter of this chapter cuts across that of the organ- and site-specific chapters that follow, but a review of accomplishments necessitates an approach that is more historical than state of the art. From a historical perspective, the classification based on exposures followed in this chapter seems more functional than one based on organs and sites as followed in later chapters, although, as with all classifications, one classification is in fact no more "natural" than the other.

In this chapter, risks reported in the original as "odds ratios," "standardized mortality ratios," or "hazard ratios" are identified as relative risks or risk ratios (R) when they are approximately equivalent.

THE CIGARETTE EPIDEMIC

In the early years of the twentieth century cancer of the lung was a rare disease. One hundred years later it is the most frequent fatal cancer in most of the Western World, accounting for 174 000 deaths annually in the United States (US) alone (Jemal et al, 2006). As shown in Chapter 2, in the US the epidemic struck early in the twentieth century, peaked during the 1990s, and then began slowly to decline. Between 1930 and 1990, the epidemic was responsible for about 4 million deaths from lung cancer in the US alone. In many parts of the world the epidemic has not yet peaked and promises to extend well into the 21st century. Epidemiology's place in cancer research was established by its role in investigating this epidemic: The discipline provided descriptive statistics to show that the epidemic existed, suggested its cause, proved the identity of that cause, and evaluated progress toward its control.

By 1930 several hypotheses were being offered to explain the increasing lung cancer rate: These included the introduction of cigarettes, the use of tar to pave roads, and air pollution from industry and coal fires in homes. In 1940 Muller reported a case-control study implicating cigarette smoking, and after a hiatus occupied by a world war this was followed by a handful of studies from Britain and the US, of which the most influential was that of Doll and Hill (1950). They established the extraordinarily high risk of lung cancer associated with cigarette smoking: Smoking of pipes and cigars were also shown to be associated with lung cancer but with risks much lower than that for cigarettes. Clearly, cigarette smoking was the cause of the epidemic: It had increased rapidly since the beginning of the century and its risks were much higher than those associated with any other suspected factor. In 1964, the Surgeon-General of the US recognized cigarette smoking as a cause of lung cancer.

While cigarettes were clearly shown to be causes of lung cancer in case-control studies, further evidence was needed for its general acceptance. Cohort (follow-up) studies are not undertaken lightly: They require that data on exposure be obtained on a large number of individuals (the cohort) and that a mechanism be available for ascertaining the occurrence of disease among the cohort members. Evidence from case-control studies was sufficient to stimulate two cohort studies: One based on British physicians (Doll & Hill, 1954) and one on the extensive network of volunteers for the American Cancer Society (ACS) (Hammond, 1966). The characteristics of the tobacco–lung cancer association were confirmed and refined in terms of amount and duration of smoking, effects of smoking-cessation, age, gender, and other variables.

The cohort studies also identified tobacco as causes of death other than lung cancer. The cohort of physicians, defined in 1951, was followed to its 50th anniversary in 2001, by which time 74% of the enrolled men had died (Doll et al, 2004). The age-adjusted death rate for smokers was almost double that of life-long nonsmokers, but only part of the excess could be attributed to lung cancer: 14% were attributed to lung cancer, 24% to ischemic heart disease, 21% to other cardiovascular disease, and 16% to nonmalignant respiratory disease, mostly chronic obstructive lung disease. Similar associations were reported from the study of the ACS cohort (Thun et al, 1995).

Cigarette smoking has been associated with several malignancies other than lung cancer (Doll et al, 2005). These are of less concern, either because they are less common or because it has not been established that their associations with tobacco are causal. They include cancers of the mouth, oral pharynx, larynx, esophagus, pancreas, liver, and bladder, and possibly kidney and myeloid leukemia (Boyle, 2005). Also relevant in considering the impact of the cigarette epidemic is the synergistic role that cigarette smoking plays with other known carcinogens such as asbestos, nickel, and radon.

In an illustration of the use of epidemiology in the evaluation of preventive measures, Rodu and Cole (2006), noting that the proportion of Americans who smoke had declined by 50% since 1965, estimated the number of deaths attributable to smoking in 1987 and 2002: between the 2 years smoking-attributable deaths had declined by 41% in males and 30% in females. It is likely that about half of this decline was attributable to reduction of deaths from malignant disease.

IONIZING RADIATION (IR)

IR is unique among carcinogens in the variety of tissues with which it comes in contact and in which it can induce neoplasia. Almost all our knowledge of its carcinogenic risks in humans comes from epidemiologic studies.

Skin Cancer

The earliest observations of cancer following IR were of skin cancers among pioneers in the discovery and investigation of radium and x-rays. The exposures were very large and irrelevant to current practices in the handling of radioactive material, but skin cancers are still being reported in survivors of the atomic bombs, after radiation therapy for benign skin conditions, and in a few occupations. Clinical observations rather than formal epidemiologic studies are responsible for most of these reports and estimates of risk are lacking.

Leukemia

Increased risk of leukemia associated with IR is the best documented of its neoplastic effects. Two bodies of data contributed importantly to the characterization of the relationship—patients with ankylosing spondylitis treated with x-rays between 1935 and 1954 (Smith and Doll, 1982) and the survivors of the atomic bombings in Nagasaki and Hiroshima (Little et al, 2004). They showed a linear relationship between level of exposure and risk of leukemia from the lowest levels for which reliable estimates can be made to the very high levels that cause cell death.

The role of age at exposure to IR came into prominence in 1958 with a study describing a doubling of risk of leukemia and solid tumors in childhood among children exposed to diagnostic x-rays *in utero* (Stewart et al, 1958): Many studies followed. Levels of IR exposure involved in pelvimetry (the most common reason for pelvic x-ray) are uncertain, but they were considerably lower than the levels at which carcinogenesis had been observed or predicted from studies of adults. A consensus emerged that the association probably existed, though at lower levels of risk than suggested in the 1958 study—the possibility of it being attributable to social or medical confounding factors calls for caution in its interpretation. Because x-rays have been replaced by other methods of pelvic and fetal imaging this controversy will probably never be resolved, but it played an important role in discouraging use of x-rays in pregnancy and in developing alternative methods of accomplishing its objectives.

Cancer of the Breast

Increased rates of breast cancer have been observed among women receiving multiple fluoroscopies in the treatment of tuberculosis, radiation treatment for benign skin lesions, enlargement of the thymus, or cancer of the cervix, and in women employed either as radiology technicians in the early years or as painters of watch dials using radium for its fluorescence. With regard to cancer of the breast IR has a dual effect: exposure of the ovary to levels sufficient to ablate ovarian function decreases breast cancer risk, but direct exposure of the breast increases it. Patients with cervical cancer whose IR exposure was sufficient to ablate the ovaries had reduced breast cancer risk, but women receiving 3.1 Gy to the breast had cancer risk three times as high as those receiving no radiation (Boice et al, 1989). Among women with Hodgkin's disease, those receiving the highest radiation exposures to the breast had an 8-fold increase in breast cancer incidence (Travis et al, 2003). Importantly, for young women treated with substantial radiation to the breast, risk increased with age: cumulative breast cancer frequencies at ages 35, 45, and 55, were 1, 7, and 29%, respectively (Travis et al, 2005).

Cancer of the Lung

The earliest known epidemic attributable to IR—though not recognized as such until late in its course—was the "mountain sickness" that killed thousands of workers in the mineral mines of Saxony and Czechoslovakia between the seventeenth and twentieth centuries. Lorenz (1944) recounts the history of these mines and the unique illness associated with them. Härting and Hesse recognized the disease as lung cancer in 1879, but it was not attributed to the presence of radon gas until the twentieth century when it developed among uranium miners in other areas.

Particularly well documented is the experience of uranium miners of the Colorado Plateau of the Western US, but large studies have also been undertaken and are continuing in several other countries. An analysis of the pooled data from 11 studies showed a linear relationship between lung cancer risk and accumulated underground mining experience (Lubin et al, 1995). The latent period between first exposure and death from cancer averaged 25 years (Samet, 1989): This fact and the disregard of the European experience were major factors in the failure to recognize this epidemic in the US at an earlier stage (Archer et al, 2004).

Several authors state that uranium miners are heavy smokers, but among nonsmoking uranium miners the risk of lung cancer associated with the highest level of cumulative exposure was 30 times as high as for those exposed at the lowest levels (Gilliland et al, 2000). However, there is clearly an interaction of some form between the two variables: Differences between studies in age at first exposure and length of follow-up may explain differences between studies

in suggestions as to whether the interaction is additive or more or less so (Archer, 1986).

There is no evidence of increased risk of any neoplasm other than lung cancer among uranium miners (Darby et al, 1995).

Cancer of the Thyroid

The thyroid gland is particularly sensitive to IR in childhood. In A-bomb survivors, the risk of thyroid cancer is limited to persons under 20 years of age at the time of exposure (see Chapter 25). Most of the other exposures that have been associated with increased risk have also involved young persons, including patients treated with IR for hemangiomas, enlarged thymus glands, or Hodgkin's disease. Concern for risk of thyroid cancer arose in the use of iodine-131 in the treatment of thyrotoxicosis, but follow-up studies have been null The epidemiologic studies of this topic are reviewed by UNSCEAR (2000).

Thorotrast

Thorotrast, an x-ray contrast medium introduced in 1928, was used extensively in Germany where it was developed, in some other European countries, and in Japan. An account of the development of thorotrast, its uses, and the early stages of understanding its complications is given by Abbatt (1979). The medium consisted of thorium dioxide and thorium-232 and was injected intravenously or intra-arterially: Its slow elimination from the body and its radioactive half-life of 400 years ensured that recipients would be exposed to alpha radiation for the remainder of their lives It had extensive use in visualizing vascular systems and exploring traumatic injuries. Abbatt estimates that sufficient thorotrast was produced for use in at least 2.5 million, and probably 10 million, examinations.

The first cases of angiosarcoma of the liver (ASL) in patients receiving thorotrast were reported in the 1940s. There have been follow-up studies totaling over 5 000 patients (van Kaick et al, 1999; Mori et al, 1999; Nyberg et al, 2002; dos Santos Silva et al, 2003). They showed exceedingly high incidence and mortality rates for cancer of the liver (around 40 times expected) and myelogenous leukemia (5–10 times expected). All types of liver tumor were involved but, because of the rarity of ASL, the relative risk (R) for this tumor was larger than for other types. Risks of both liver cancer and leukemia increased with the volume of thorotrast injected and with the time elapsed after exposure: Excess risks remained high more than 40 years after injection (dos Santos Silva et al, 2003).

Epidemiology documented the extent of the thorotrast tragedy, but it was an exercise in locking the barn door after the horses had fled. The potential of internalized radium and its daughters to produce fatal hematologic disorders and bone cancer were well known by the 1940s (Martland et al, 1925). The rapid accumulation of case reports (IAEA, 1965) gave ample warning of the toxic properties of thorotrast well before epidemiologic studies were under way. The tail of this epidemic has not yet passed.

Other Cancers

Other cancers seen in persons heavily exposed to IR include those of the brain, stomach, liver (Cologne et al, 1999), and bladder (in A-bomb survivors); cancers of the stomach and kidney (in patients with ankylosing spondylitis and radium dial painters); and the brain and ovary (in patients treated with IR for benign conditions). The potential of IR to induce neoplasia in most human tissues is well documented.

CANCER IN OCCUPATIONAL SETTINGS

Many cancer risks in occupations were first noted in reports from physicians or others familiar with working conditions, the seminal example being Percival Pott's 1775 description of scrotal cancer in chimney sweeps: Associations of cancer with arsenic, asbestos, chemical dyes, chromium, nickel, and vinyl chloride also came under suspicion in this way. Epidemiologic studies aimed to show that such observations re-

presented more than coincidence, to estimate the size of the risks, and to locate them to particular sections of the workplace or work processes. We note here only the numerically most important occupational carcinogens—a few other suspected carcinogens that have received some attention in occupational settings, such as dioxins, DDT, cadmium, and beryllium, are not included since the evidence of their occupational carcinogenicity is either null or inconclusive.

Acrylonitrile (AN)

AN is used in the manufacture of acrylic fibers and as a fumigant: Exposure is by inhalation of the volatile liquid. Beginning in the early 1980s reports of cases of cancer in exposed workers multiplied. A 1998 meta-analysis included 25 epidemiologic studies and suggested no increased risk associated with AN for cancer as a whole or for any specific neoplasm (Collins & Acquavella, 1998). A subsequent follow-up of workers potentially exposed to AN in eight US industries showed no increase in mortality for any neoplasm except cancer of the lung, which was somewhat elevated (R=1.4) only in the highest quintile of cumulative exposure (Blair et al, 1998). A small case-control study gave R for lung cancer of 2.9: The association is weaker than in that in the larger US study and is contrary to the bulk of evidence, chance variation cannot be excluded (Scélo et al, 2004).

Epidemiologic studies are reassuring with regard to the carcinogenicity of AN, limiting to concern for lung cancer, and then to the highest exposures experienced historically.

Arsenic

Occupational exposure to arsenic is primarily by inhalation of dust. Many metal ores are contaminated with arsenic and excess lung cancer has been found among miners or smelters of gold, tin, and copper. In a 50-year follow-up of workers in a Montana smelter, a 50% excess of deaths from lung cancer was found that was highest after time spent in areas with medium or high arsenic exposure: Among workers with 10 or more years work in such areas, observed deaths were three and four times, respectively, the number expected (Lubin et al, 2000). Other cancers were not in excess.

Exposure to arsenic compounds also occurs in the manufacture and use of wood preservatives, insecticides, and herbicides. The many reports of illness associated with these activities include cancers of the lung and other sites (International Agency for Research on Cancer [IARC], 1980), but the effects of arsenic have not been clearly differentiated from those of other known and suspected carcinogens in these compounds.

Asbestos

The name *asbestos* refers to a group of fibrous chemicals that can be spun into thread and woven into fabrics that are heat-resistant, light weight, and low cost. These "miracle fibers" were used in a wide variety of products during the twentieth century. Discovery of the dark sides of asbestos was a major epidemiologic accomplishment of the second half of the century: It led to a total ban on the use of asbestos in Britain and other European countries and heavy regulation with the prospect of a total ban in the US (Bartrip, 2004).

Three major health problems are associated with asbestos: pulmonary fibrosis and emphysema *(asbestosis)*, lung cancer, and mesothelioma. While our concern here is only with the last two, asbestosis was an important cause of morbidity and mortality and a major force in the call for control of the material.

The first epidemiologic study of asbestos and cancer was of workers in a small British asbestos plant (Doll, 1955). Over a period of 35 years, 11 died of lung cancer, whereas 0.8 would have been expected. A larger cohort was assembled from members of a New York Asbestos Workers Union. Observed and expected deaths from lung cancer were 45 and 6.6, from stomach cancer 12 and 4.3, and from cancers of the colon and rectum 17 and 5.4 (Selikoff et al, 1964). Larger numbers were reported on another cohort from the same source (Selikoff et al, 1965).

Subsequently, in studies of asbestos workers in many countries and different occupations the association with lung cancer was confirmed unequivocally, an exposure-risk relationship described, the induction period estimated, and the risks associated with specific types of asbestos clarified: Among the three major types of asbestos, crocidolite conveys the highest cancer risk and chrysotile the lowest. The association with stomach cancer has been found in other studies, although not all, and usually at levels of risk lower than that noted by Selikoff; and small excesses of cancers of the esophagus and kidney have also been reported (Enterline et al, 1987; Armstrong et al, 1988; Raffn et al, 1989; McDonald et al, 1993).

Mesothelioma, a highly malignant cancer of the pleura and peritoneum, was extremely rare prior to 1900, but during the next century rapidly became a signature for asbestos exposure. The first epidemiologic study was of cases from asbestos fields in South Africa (Wagner et al, 1960). Reports from North America and Europe followed. For six countries in Western Europe, annual deaths from mesothelioma increased from virtually zero at the beginning of the century to around 2500 in 1998 (Peto et al, 1999). In the United States during the period between 1973 to 2001, rates for males increased sharply until the mid-1990s but thereafter began to decline (Price & Ware, 2004).

As with lung cancer, crocidolite carries the highest risk of mesothelioma, and from a review of data from 71 studies Yarborough (2006) concluded there is little evidence that chrysotile, unless contaminated with other fibers, causes mesothelioma. As with lung cancer, latent periods between first exposure and appearance of disease are long—often many decades (Peto et al, 1982).

Benzene

Benzene is a solvent and starting material for the manufacture of other chemicals. It is also added to gasoline, of which it constitutes about 2%. The hemotoxicity of benzene has been known since the nineteenth century, but demonstration of its role in leukemia is credited to Aksoy et al (1974), who reported 26 cases of leukemia among 28 000 leather workers in Istanbul and estimated the "incidence" at $14/10^5$, which they believed to be a "significant" increase over that in the general population. Schnatter et al (2005) reviewed 22 published studies and concluded that there was an increase in risk of acute myeloid leukemia (AML) with benzene exposure and a positive relationship between level of exposure and risk. The risks were evident in the rubber, leather, and paint industries. Data on chronic myeloid leukemia and lymphoid leukemia were found to be sparse and inconclusive. R for workers at the highest levels of cumulative exposure have been around 10 (Yin et al, 1987; Glass et al, 2003), with earlier studies showing even higher risks (Rinsky et al, 1981). The exposure-risk relationship was evaluated by Hayes et al (2001) in a combination of information from two large cohorts, one from the US and one from China: There was progressive increase in risk of myeloid leukemia and its precursors with increasing cumulative benzene exposures over a 10-fold range of exposure.

Chemical Dyes

In the late nineteenth and early twentieth centuries there were many clinical reports of what came to be called "aniline tumors of the bladder" in workers engaged in the manufacture and use of chemical dyes. The progenitor of many retrospective cohort studies in occupations was the "field survey" of tumors of the urinary bladder conducted by Case et al (1954) in the British chemical industry. Among workers employed sinc 1920 for more than 6 months in the manufacture of aniline, benzidene, alpha-naphthylamine (ANA), or beta-naphthylamine (BNA), 341 cases of bladder cancer occurred, 298 (87%) of which were in workers who had had contact with one of the chemicals: 127 of the latter died of the disease, whereas 4 would have been expected based on national mortality data (R 32). There was no external source of data from which the expected

number of incidence cases could be computed.

Risk was highest (R 86) after exposure to BNA—among the highest risks ever reported for an occupational exposure; intermediate risks were associated with ANA and benzidene (45 and 62, respectively): ironically, there was no increase in risk among workers exposed only to aniline, although numbers were small. Risk increased with duration of exposure, but some increase was seen after exposures of less than 1 year. Some tumors appeared within 2 years of first exposure but others after more than 45 years: The average interval between first exposure and death was 18 years, presaging the long latent periods that came to be recognized as characteristic of occupational cancers. The authors estimated that by the time of the study bladder cancer had occurred in 10% of the exposed population, and that, even assuming no further exposure after 1951, given the estimated incubation periods, an additional 10% could be expected to be affected.

Chromium

The most common forms of chromium are trivalent (Cr-3) and hexavalent (Cr-6), of which Cr-3 is the more stable. Cr-6 has powerful oxidative properties and is thought to be most likely responsible for the metal's carcinogenic potential. In many studies the exposure is simply referred to as *chromium*.

Occupational exposure to chromium is primarily through inhalation of contaminated dust. Its association with lung cancer has been suspected for more than a century. Meta-analyses based on 49 epidemiologic studies published since 1950 showed an excess mortality (R 1.4) from lung cancer among chromium-exposed workers that became lower (1.1) when the analysis was limited to studies of better quality and adjusted for smoking (Cole and Rodu, 2005). R for stomach cancer in these analyses was also slightly elevated (1.1), but was lower (0.8) on adjustment for socioeconomic status. No other cancer showed higher than expected frequency. Increase in risk of lung cancer with increase in exposure has been noted in several studies, with risks in the highest categories of exposure being two to three times those in the lowest exposure groups (Park et al, 2004).

Clearly, risk of lung cancer is increased with exposure to occupational chromium but, even at the highest levels of exposure, chromium is a weak carcinogen.

Formaldehyde

Formaldehyde has been used as a disinfectant and preservative in industry, embalming, and medicine. Human exposure is primarily by inhalation of the gas, though skin absorption is possible with the use of the liquid formalin. Formaldehyde was reviewed by a Working Group of IARC in 2004(b) and judged "*sufficient*" to place the chemical in its Group 1 (*Carcinogenic to humans*). But, with the possible exceptions of nasopharyngeal cancers (NPC) and leukemia, the evidence of carcinogenicity in humans is weak.

Elevated risk of NPC has been found in many studies: In the largest cohort study, R in the most highly exposed subgroup was 1.7, based on six cases (Hauptmann et al, 2004). Collins et al (1997), in a summary of 47 epidemiologic studies of formaldehyde-exposed workers, found essentially no increased risk for any type of cancer other than leukemia. Leukemia mortality was found somewhat elevated in six of seven cohorts of persons exposed to formaldehyde in embalming or medical occupations (IARC, 2004b). Two recent US industrial cohort studies showed small excesses of leukemia, particularly myeloid leukemia, in the most heavily exposed groups (Hauptmann et al, 2003; Pinkerton et al, 2004).

Nickel

The main uses of nickel are as alloys in stainless steel and in the manufacture of batteries, but the principal studies of its health effects are of workers in mining and processing. Bradford Hill (1939) reported the first epidemiologic study of workers in a Welsh nickel refinery: Among workers during the years 1929–1938, there were 16 deaths from lung cancer when one would have been expected and 19 from cancer of the nose when the expected was less than one. There was no excess in deaths from other cancers. In a later study in the same refinery, there were 48 deaths from lung cancer (R 5) and 13 from nasal cancer (R 150) (Doll, 1958). Comparable results were obtained from early studies in refineries in Canada (Mastromatteo, 1967) and Norway (Pedersen et al, 1973). In later studies from the Welsh and Norwegian refineries smaller excess risks were found (Doll et al, 1977; Grimsrud et al, 2003). Grimsrud and Peto (2006) summarized the experience of the Welsh refinery, comparing the experience of workers first employed in three periods: 1902–1919, 1920–1929, and 1930–1969. R for lung cancer in the three periods was 6.2, 0.7, and 1.4, and for nasal cancer 380, 73, and 9, respectively—the last figure (for nasal cancer) being based on only two deaths. The analysis indicates that nickel is a potent carcinogen, and also illustrates the role of epidemiologic studies in evaluating the efficacy of control measures.

Exposures in nickel refineries include other agents besides nickel, some of which are also carcinogens—they include arsenic, sulphuric acid mists, cobalt, and sometimes asbestos. In an analysis of data from the Norwegian refinery in which individual assessments of these exposures were made, estimates of R for nickel exposure changed only slightly when adjusted for these variables alone or in combination (Grimsrud et al, 2005). Several authors have adjusted for smoking habits in the evaluation of nickel exposures, and it is clear that the risk associated with nickel is much greater in smokers than in nonsmokers (Andersen et al, 1996; Sorahan and Williams, 2005).

Polychorinated Biphenyls (PCBs)

Because of their persistence in the environment and biological fluids, PCBs have been suspected of producing a variety of health effects, including cancer. Reports in the last 2 decades have raised suspicions about association with specific neoplasms, but no clear pattern emerged. Bosetti et al (2003b) reviewed 6 cohort studies of workers occupationally exposed to PCBs, finding no excess cancer overall (0.9) and no excess mortality for any specific cancer. In 2006 the US National Institute for Occupational Health and Safety updated the follow-up of three cohorts of occupationally exposed workers assembled earlier (Prince et al, 2006; Ruder et al, 2006). (For analysis, data from two of the cohorts were combined.) Deaths from cancer overall were not elevated (0.8 and 1.0). Modest increases were seen for a few sites, but numbers were very small and there was no consistency, either between the cohorts or with sites suspected on the basis of earlier studies, and there was no convincing association with estimated levels of exposure.

Studies of cancer following exposure to PCBs are reassuring as to the chemicals' lack of carcinogenicity.

Vinyl Chloride (VC)

VC is a gas that is polymerized to produce polyvinyl chloride—a widely used plastic. Cleaning polymerization chambers exposes workers to residual VC monomer. Suspicion of the carcinogenicity of VC was raised in 1974 by a report of angiosarcoma of the liver (ASL)—a very rare tumor—in exposed workers. Within 2 years 40 such cases had been reported (Schlatter, 1976). In a literature review in 1999, McLaughlin and Lipworth (1999) concluded that, with the exception of ASL, no adverse outcomes (including cancers) could be conclusively linked to VC exposure. Bosetti et al (2003a) undertook an analysis of data from two meta-analyses of epidemiologic studies in Europe (Mundt et al, 2000) and North America (Ward et al, 2001). In total, there were data on more than 22 000 workers from 56 plants. There were 71 deaths from ASL in the cohorts: There were no external rates of this malignancy for comparison, but the tumor is rare. Deaths for cancer of the lung and larynx were lower than expected and mortality from soft tissue sarcoma, brain, and hematopoietic system were not higher than expected. A modest excess of non-ASL tumors of the liver (R 1.4) was considered likely to be due to misdiagnosis of ASL. A second analysis of the same material, with the addition of six smaller stud-

ies, found similar results for tumors of the liver, but a significant excess of soft tissue tumors (R 2.5) that was also suspected of being due to misdiagnosis of ASL (Boffetta et al, 2003). Two later, small studies gave conflicting evidence on whether lung cancer risk is increased in VC workers (Mastrangelo et al, 2003; Scélo et al, 2004).

The evidence suggests that ASL is the only cancer to be found in excess among VC workers.

Other Occupational Settings

With few exceptions, exposure to *poison gas* has largely been a problem of an occupation—soldiering. In the context of cancer, the most relevant is the mustard gas that was used extensively during the last years of World War I. Another seminal follow-up study was conducted by Case and Lea (1955). They identified deaths among veterans receiving disability pensions as a result of gas poisoning: 29 died of lung cancer, whereas 14 would have been expected. There was no excess of deaths from any cancer site other than lung. Not unexpectedly, given the date of this experience, cigarette smoking was not considered as a possible explanation of the excess.

Exposure to *wood dust* has been reported in several studies as a cause of NPC (Demers et al, 1998), but a multicenter case-control US study found only a modest association with wood dust that was explained by confounding by a stronger association with formaldehyde (Vaughan et al, 2000).

There is substantial literature on cancer risks on occupations in which chemical exposures are multiple and individual causes not identifiable—for example, agricultural workers, rubber workers, and metal welders. Such studies have relevance to the specific industries or plants identified and may have utility in suggesting avenues for more detailed investigation.

THE PHYSICAL ENVIRONMENT

Ultraviolet Radiation (UVR)

Exposure to UVR from the sun is the most frequent cause of the common basal and squamous cell carcinoma and melanoma of the skin cancer. Some evidence relating to the role of sun exposure in skin cancers, such as their greater frequency in fair-skinned people (they are about 10 times more frequent in whites than blacks) and their occurrence in areas of the skin most exposed to sunlight, comes from clinical observation, but other evidence of the relationship, such as their greater frequency in persons in outdoor occupations and in sunny geographic locations or areas in proximity to the equator, required epidemiologic studies (Oliveria et al, 2006).

The relationship of skin cancer risk to duration and intensity of sun exposure, continuous or repeated exposures, and skin-burning have all been explored, but there is no consensus on the influence of these parameters, except that they appear to differ between the pathologic types of cancer. The interrelationships of these features and the roles of genetic markers are complex: They are reviewed by Kricker et al (1994) and English et al (1997). There is evidence of association of risk with age, exposure in childhood being particularly harmful. In addition, lifetime alcohol consumption has been shown to be positively related to risk in high-risk areas (Le Marchand et al, 2006), but it seems possible that this is confounded by association with level or type of sun-exposure.

Arsenic

Some chemicals that have been shown to be carcinogenic in specific settings may have similar roles in the general environment. One of these is arsenic. Unlike its role in occupational cancer, the predominant general exposure to arsenic is by ingestion—in drinking water—and the principal tumors involved are not of the lung but of the bladder. The significance of this problem is that it may not be economically or politically feasible to reduce human exposure to a level below that at which carcinogenicity has been demonstrated. While the capacity of arsenic to induce cancer in humans is beyond question, no animal model has been found. This leaves epidemiology as the principal tool for investigating its carcinogenic potential at

low-exposure levels, although it is doubtful that epidemiological studies on a scale necessary to influence the debate will ever be conducted.

Drinking water was first associated with bladder cancer in areas of Taiwan in which "Blackfoot" disease—a serious constrictive disease of the peripheral arteries—was endemic (Tseng et al, 1968; Chen and Wang, 1990). The disease is due to high arsenic content of water from artesian wells. Correlations of cancer with arsenic content of drinking water have also been found in Chile, Argentina, Finland, and China: These correlations were most consistent and strongest for cancer of the bladder, but elevated risks for cancers of the stomach, lung, and skin were also reported. This evidence is ecological so that while the associations are strong they leave unclear whether arsenic is the sole factor that is responsible. In a cohort study in north Taiwan, in which each family had its own well, it was possible to obtain a more precise definition of exposure: There was a biologic gradient of risk of urinary tract cancer with level of exposure, with R for arsenic concentrations of less than 10, 10–49, 50–99, and 100 or more ug/liter of 1, 2, 8, and 15, respectively (Chiou et al, 2001).

The level of 50 ug/liter, suggested by Chen et al (2004) as a level at which arsenic in drinking water may cause observable increases in tumors, is the maximum currently permitted in US drinking water. In 2001 the Environmental Protection Agency proposed to reduce this standard to 10 ug/liter, but enforcement was delayed "for further study." Such study will require judicious balancing of the costs of compliance (which will be considerable, perhaps prohibitively so) with estimates of the reduction in the number of cancers prevented, the latter being determined primarily by the statistical model used to extrapolate the effect of exposures below the levels for which data are available (Frumkin and Thun, 2001).

Asbestos

Spreading of asbestos dust close in proximity to mining, processing, and distributing facilities, and in the removal or disintegration of asbestos insulation, brake linings and, other products, raises concern for the health of populations beyond production workers. These concerns are serious in the North Cape Provinces of South Africa where asbestos, including the highly carcinogenic crocidolite, was discovered in the 1880s and mined throughout the twentieth century. Although the mining was done by males, females and children were frequently involved in processing the ore (Wagner, 1991). Exploitive labor practices and living conditions, leaking distribution facilities, and careless disposal of incompletely extracted rock are described by Braun and Kisting (2006). Consequences to populations in terms of lung cancer, mesothelioma, and other asbestos diseases are documented by Bonn (1999), Mzileni et al (1999), Abratt et al (2004), and many others.

In the less dramatic conditions of North America, no excess of cancer was found in one Canadian town with asbestos deposits or another with asbestos processing facilities (Neuberger et al, 1984). A review of 13 epidemiologic studies of the roles of ingested asbestos showed no evidence of increased risk of cancer (Marsh, 1983). Detection of health effects of low-level asbestos exposure may become easier as the "background" of the occupational disease diminishes, but environmental exposures will also diminish, and the full consequences of the asbestos epidemic will never be known.

Benzene

Sources of benzene in the environment include gasoline, automobile exhaust, emissions from industrial processes, and cigarette smoke. However, because of the high volatility of the chemical, exposures to the general population—except for smokers—are likely to be transient and very low compared to those found in enclosed work spaces. Nevertheless, the issue has received some attention. In one study of gas station attendants, a small excess of deaths from AML was reported (Jacobsson et al, 1993), but in larger studies leukemia cases were below expectation (Lagorio et al, 1994; Lynge et al, 1997).

Most studies of this problem are ecological in nature. In a small area of Pennsylvania, gasoline leaked from underground storage tanks, exposing the population to chronic low levels of gasoline in the air and drinking water for several years. A study of affected households showed incidence rates of cancer to be in line with rates for the state as whole, but there were four cases of leukemia where only one was expected. The residences of two cases of AML were said to have "bordered the projected gasoline plume" (Patel et al, 2004).

Rates of lymphatic and hemopoietic cancers in an area in Italy that contained a major source of environmental benzene were compared with local areas with no such sources (Parodi et al, 2003). For leukemia, rates in males were about twice as high in the exposed as in the control areas, but among females, the reverse was the case. For non-Hodgkin's lymphoma rates were also higher in the exposed than in the control areas in males, but not in females. There is little reason to think that environmental exposures would affect males but not females, and if these differences are real, it would seem reasonable to seek their explanation elsewhere—perhaps in an occupational exposure. Comparisons have also been made of residents of areas believed to have had high benzene exposure because of proximity to traffic congestion (Crosignani et al, 2004; Raaschou-Nielsen et al, 2001). The findings are not striking and are inconsistent. In addition to the usual problems of interpreting ecologic associations, benzene is not the only possibly carcinogenic constituent of pollution from automobiles.

Overall, there is little evidence for a cancer effect from environmental contamination with benzene.

Chromium

As with arsenic, exposure to chromium in the general environment is not by inhalation but by ingestion and possibly from contact with water contaminated by discharges from industrial plants. After a review of 4 studies of environmentally exposed populations,

Proctor et al (2002) concluded that Cr-6 is not carcinogenic via the oral route of exposure from currently permitted concentrations of the compound in drinking water.

Cigarette Smoke

Cigarette smoke is inhaled not only by smokers but by others around them—in homes, work places, restaurants, and elsewhere. The terms *passive* and *involuntary-smoking* have been given to such exposures. In 1981, two studies of lung cancer in married women showed that women who did not smoke but were married to men who did had approximately twice the risk of women married to nonsmokers (Trichopoulos et al, 1981; Hirayama, 1981). An analysis of data from 37 studies of the issue suggested that lifetime nonsmokers who lived with a smoker had a risk of lung cancer 24% higher than those not living with a smoker (Hackshaw et al, 1997). There were positive exposure–risk relationships both with the amount smoked by the companion and with the duration of residence with a smoker. A later analysis based on 76 studies gave an excess risk of 29% (Taylor et al, 2001). The reality of the relationship between involuntary smoking and lung cancer was recognized by the IARC in 2004(a) and the Surgeon General of the US in 2006. The numerical impact of involuntary smoking is small relative to that of active smoking and it is likely to become smaller as the prevalence of smoking declines, but its recognition was important for the stimulation and acceptance of broad measures for cigarette control.

THE MICROBIOLOGIC ENVIRONMENT

The last 50 years have seen increasing recognition of roles for microorganisms in cancer etiology. In addition to the schistosome infestations that cause bladder cancer, the flukes related to liver cancer, and the HTLV viruses related to leukemia in certain parts of the world, there are more widespread human cancers, including those of the liver, cervix, and stomach, in which infectious agents are involved. In addition, epidemiologic studies have supported the prediction of Burnet (1965) that persons with compromised immune-response to infection are at increased risk of cancer. Parkin (2006) estimated that about 18% (1.9 million cases annually) of all world cancers can be attributed to infection and that prevention of these would lower cancer incidence by 8% in developed countries and 26% in developing areas. While credit for the identification of microbiologic agents as causes of cancer rests securely with the microbiologic sciences, epidemiologic studies have assisted in suggesting directions in which these sciences might be applied and in evaluating the effectiveness of vaccination programs.

Hepatitis Viruses

Hepatocellular carcinoma (HCC) is among the world's most common neoplasms and the discovery of hepatitis viruses as its principal cause rivals in public health importance the discovery of the carcinogenic effects of cigarette smoking. Microbiologic discoveries depended on the development of increasingly sensitive laboratory techniques: Epidemiologic evidence contributed by demonstrating a link to a known infectious disease, identifying the means of transmission of the responsible viruses and factors associated with their persistence in the host, evaluating the efficacy of vaccination programs, and exploring the roles of alcohol, tobacco, and aflatoxin.

HCC was known clinically to be a complication of chronic hepatitis and cirrhosis. During the 1960s it became evident that there are (at least) two forms of virus-related hepatitis—one of relatively short duration, transmitted by contagion with typical incubation periods of 20–30 days, and often called *infectious hepatitis*, and a second clinically more severe disease, with longer incubation periods and durations, prone to recurrence, often transmitted by blood products, and referred to as *serum hepatitis* (Krugman et al, 1967). Infectious hepatitis came to be known as hepatitis A, caused by the homonymous virus hepatitis (HAV), whereas serum hepatitis was distinguished as hepatitis B and C, again caused by homonymous viruses HBV and HCV, respectively. A previously unknown antigen found in an Australian Aborigine in 1966, and initially called *Australia antigen* (Blumberg et al, 1965), was subsequently identified as the surface antigen of HBV (HBsAg) and became a marker of infection.

The association of HBV with HCC was first observed ecologically: the high prevalence of chronic infections with HBV, as evidenced by high prevalence rates of serum HBsAg, in Asia and Central Africa and high prevalence in males corresponded to the epidemiologic features of HCC (Maupas and Melnick, 1981). Following Prince et al (1975), high prevalence of serum HBsAg-positivity was found in cases of HCC in many case-control studies. Follow-up studies followed, with R varying between more than 100 in Taiwan (Beasley et al, 1981) and 15 in Spain (Ribes et al, 2006). Risk of HCC was also found to be associated with the amount of HBV DNA in plasma: In a cohort of men known to be HBsAg positive, risk for men with estimated HBV DNA serum loads in the highest quintile were 7 times those of men in the lowest quintile (Yu et al, 2005).

A vaccine against HBV was developed and widely used in high-prevalence countries. In a disease with such devastating consequences, it is not surprising that evidence of the vaccine's efficacy came from observations in nonrandomized populations. In a prospective study of Korean males, of whom 13% had been vaccinated in the year prior to the observation period, the incidence of HCC was more than 50 times as high in unvaccinated as in vaccinated men (Lee et al, 1998). A nationwide vaccination in Taiwan began in 1984 with vaccination of newborns of HBsAg-positive mothers and was extended in stages to all newborns and then to all schoolchildren (Chien et al, 2006): Over a 10-year period the incidence of HCC in children declined by 50% (Chang et al, 1997).

HCV was also identified as an important cause of HCC, both as a cofactor with HBV and as an independent agent. Epidemiologic studies of this virus have followed closely the course of those for HBV, sometimes both viruses being evaluated in the same study. Risks associated with infection with HCV alone are of about the same order as those with HBV alone, and the risks associated with infection by the two viruses together appear to be additive (Sun et al, 2003; Yu et al, 2005).

High alcohol consumption, liver cirrhosis, and tobacco use are established causes of HCC; and, in countries with low prevalence of HCV and HBV, such as in Western Europe and North America, they may be responsible for the majority of liver cancers (Trichopoulos et al, 1987).

Human Papilloma Viruses (HPV)

Epidemiologic features of cancer of the cervix have long suggested that this disease is associated with early onset and variety of sexual activity (Jones et al, 1958; Beral, 1974). They include associations of high rates of the disease with early age at marriage or onset of sexual activity, frequency of intercourse, number of sexual partners including the number of sexual partners of the spouse as well as of the patient herself, and poor genital hygiene. Low rates were also seen among members of religious or social groups perceived as having low levels of sexual promiscuity (Brinton, 1992). Early hypotheses focused on possible chemical carcinogens transmitted from male partners in sperm or smegma or infection with herpes simplex virus type 2.

The evidence associating HPV infection with cervical cancer (as well as other genital cancers both in males and females) is reviewed by Bosch et al (2002). It is the result of the convergence of two distinct paths of inquiry: (1) clinical, pathologic, and epidemiologic studies demonstrating a seamless progression in cervical epithelial tissue from mild to severe dysplasias to carcinoma-in-situ (CIS) to infiltrating carcinoma, a progression recognized in the more recent designation of the premalignant stages as *cervical intraepithelial neoplasia* (CIN), and (2) development after the 1970s of sensitive microbiologic techniques for the identification of HPV DNA and its subtypes.

The largest cross-sectional study of the association is one sponsored by IARC in which more than 1000 specimens from patients with invasive cervical cancer in 22 countries were evaluated (Bosch et al, 1995). HPV DNA was detected in 93% of tumors. HPV types 16 and 18 predominated: Other HPV subtypes were also detected with high, though still lower, frequencies. R associated with any HPV type was 83 for squamous cell carcinomas and 69 for adenocarcinomas (Bosch et al, 2002).

In a study of cases of CIS with evaluation of HPV16 in specimens taken up to 26 years previously, women with high virus loads before age 25 were 30 times more likely to develop CIS, often when the original smears were cytologically normal (see chapter 17) (Ylitalo et al, 2000). In the same study, there was a strong relationship between the level of virus load and subsequent risk of CIS. Schiffman et al (2002) found that the natural history of HPV infection often includes periods before and after observable cytologic abnormality during which HPV DNA is a more sensitive indicator of subsequent malignant change than is cytology. The use of HPV assays as an adjunct to, or possibly replacement for, cytologic screening is a matter of current debate (Josefsson et al, 2000).

A vaccine—in lay terms a "cervical cancer vaccine"—was developed against HPV. Its effectiveness in terms of reduction of risk of cervical cancer remains to be demonstrated. The ethics and economics of use of the vaccine will depend in considerable part on the knowledge of the epidemiology of cervical cancer itself.

Helicobacter Pylori

The descriptive epidemiology of cancer of the stomach is challenging. For example, incidence rates vary over a fivefold range, with highest rates in Japan, Finland, and South America (Parkin et al, 2005). One contribution of epidemiology has been to recognize that the disease includes two entities that are pathologically and epidemiologically distinct. One of these occurs at the proximal (*cardiac*) end of the stomach, the other at the distal (*pyloric*) end. Both are more common in males than females, but the proximal by a factor of about five, the distal by about two. Distal tumors are more common in blacks than whites in the United States, while proximal tumors are twice as common in whites as blacks. In most western countries, rates for the disease as a whole have been declining (to about one-third of those seen around 1930), but proximal cancers have been increasing in recent years in Europe, Australia, and New Zealand (Crew and Neuget, 2006).

Despite these striking features of the disease, immediate prospects for prevention of stomach cancer come from the incidental discovery of a microorganism—Helicobacter *pylori*—that is strongly suspected as a cause of gastritis and duodenal ulceration (Marshall and Warren, 1984), and, less definitively, as a factor in cancer of the stomach. A review of five meta-analyses of the relationship of the organism to gastric cancer led to the conclusion that, while the data are conflicting, the consensus is that the frequency of gastric cancer is about doubled in the presence of H. *pylori* (Eslick, 2006). The main uncertainty is whether this represents a causal association or an opportunistic infection by the bacillus, either of the tumor itself or of one or more of its progenitors, such as chronic gastritis.

In the only randomized experiment reported to date, patients with helicobacter infection were assigned equally to receive either chemotherapeutic eradication therapy or placebo. After 7.5 years, 7 of the treatment and 11 of the placebo group developed gastric cancer (Wong et al, 2004). The significance of this finding has been criticized on the basis of the relatively short follow-up period (Parsonnet and Forman, 2004). Prospects for clarification of the role of this organism in gastric cancer depend on large-scale prospective studies, both observational and experimental. If a role for the agent is established it is evident from the high prevalence of the infection and the relatively low frequency of the disease that there are important modifiers of that role.

Immunodeficiency

Three recent developments have provided opportunities for investigation of the role of the immune system in protecting against cancer: the increased survival of infants with congenital immune deficiency, the epidemic of the acquired immunodeficiency syndrome (AIDS), and the use of artificial means of depressing patients' immunity prior to organ transplantation.

Congenital immunodeficiency is a feature of a few rare clinical syndromes, such as Wiskott-Aldrich syndrome, ataxia telangiectasia, and a few others. Estimates of risk of cancer associated with these syndromes are derived from clinical series rather than formal epidemiologic studies. They vary between syndromes and are heavily influenced by the duration of follow-up, the more important component of which is the duration of survival of immunocompromised infants. Overall risks of malignancy are low—generally less than 5%—but very much higher than in the general population of infants—in some instances by a factor of 1000 or more. A striking feature is the predominance of non-Hodgkin's lymphoma among the malignancies in these patients, generally constituting more than half of the tumors (Muller and Pizzo, 1995).

The association of the human immuno-deficiency virus (HIV), responsible for AIDS, with cancer has been demonstrated in clinical reports and in clinico-epidemiologic studies such as the cohorts of AIDS patients enrolled in Switzerland (Clifford et al, 2005), Italy (Nasti et al, 2003), England (Newnham et al, 2005), across Europe (Mocroft et al, 2000), and in the US (Kest et al, 2005). The dominant cancer seen in AIDS patients is Karposi's sarcoma—a previously uncommon tumor of lymphoid origin affecting principally the skin but also internal organs, seen mainly in tropical areas and formerly believed, often correctly as it developed, to be of venereal origin. The disease is estimated to be 10 000 times more common in HIV-infected than noninfected persons and is associated with infection by herpes virus, type 8. Other tumors associated with AIDS, but at lower levels of frequency (R 5–10), are non-Hodgkin's lymphoma and Hodgkin's disease, both associated with Epstein-Barr virus infections (Beral and Newton, 1998).

Patients undergoing organ transplant have a 3- 4-fold higher risk of cancer than the general population (Taioli et al, 2006), a phenomenon attributed to the immune suppression artificially induced prior to surgery. The pattern of posttransplant (predominantly renal transplant) cancers is similar to that seen in AIDS patients, with Kaposi's sarcoma predominating, tumors of lymphatic origin sharply increased, and a scattering of other cancers showing small increases (Penn, 2000; Pedotti et al, 2003; Serraino et al, 2005). The risks for posttransplant tumors appear to be lower than those for AIDS patients, but it is not clear whether this is a function of differences in survival of the two groups or of the nature of the immunosuppressant.

REPRODUCTION

The utility of studying variation in reproductive experience as a clue to cancer etiology became clear when early reports suggested that cancer of the breast is unusually frequent among nuns and single women. The first epidemiologic study was that of Lane-Claypon (1926) indicating, among other things, that breast-feeding protects a woman against breast cancer. The role of breast-feeding remains controversial, though it is not as significant as was thought for many years (MacMahon et al, 1970b; Collaborative Group, 2002b), but the role of childbearing itself has been more fully characterized. It is evident that the protective effect of childbirth is not primarily a function of the number of children borne but of the woman's age at the time she bears her first child (MacMahon et al, 1970a). If births after the first have an additional protective effect, it is small relative to that of the first (Trichopoulos et al, 1983).

The relationship has been further clarified in two respects: (1) while the risk of cancer increases with age at first birth up to about age 30, first births after that age are associated with *increased* risk relative to that for nulliparous women although, since most first births occur to mothers under 30 years of age, the overall effect is protection, and *(2)* the risk of cancer is actually increased in the first 10 years after a first birth—even a birth at a young age—but after 10 years it is decreased (Lambe et al, 1994). Since most of a woman's years of breast cancer risk occur more than 10 years after birth of her first child, the overall effect is protection. These observations are consistent with the idea that pregnancy stimulates replication and differentiation of breast cells, thus increasing in the short term the probability of a malignant mutation or expansion of an initiated clone but leading later to a population of cells at low risk of transformation—in line with a model suggested by Russo et al (1990) to account for similar observations in rats.

In a meta-analysis of 12 case-control studies, risk of cancer of the ovary was also found to be inversely associated with parity—women who had three to four full-term pregnancies had about half the risk of those who had none (Whittemore et al, 1992). La Vecchia et al (1984) suggested that, as with cancer of the breast, the association with high parity could largely be accounted for by an association with late age at first birth, but this observation has not been as fully investigated as has that with cancer of the breast.

As with cancers of the breast and ovary, risk of cancer of the uterine endometrium is also reduced by child-bearing (Henderson et al, 1983; Brinton et al, 1992), but specific patterns are different. From a large Swedish study it was estimated that, among parous women, each additional birth was associated with a 20% decrease in endometrial cancer risk (Lambe et al, 1999). There was no consistent association with age at first birth, but the older a woman was at the time of her last birth the lower her risk. It has been estimated that risk declines by 15% for each 5-year delay in a woman's age at last birth (Lambe et al, 1999).

The different patterns of reproductive experience preceding cancers of the breast, ovary, and endometrium, while suggesting agreement on the idea that childbearing promotes anticarcinogenesis, pose challenges to interpretation in terms of mechanisms.

ALCOHOL

Associations of some types of cancer with heavy and regular use of alcoholic beverages were first noted clinically Epidemiologic studies estimate the size of the risks involved. In addition, since alcohol use is associated with other variables, of which the most relevant is cigarette smoking, epidemiologic studies are needed to separate the contribution of alcohol to cancer rates following joint exposures. A recent and comprehensive review of the epidemiologic literature and of mechanisms that might underlie associations between alcohol use and cancer risk is that of Boffetta and Hashibe (2006). It is hardly necessary to note that assessments of alcohol intake, particularly intakes in the past, are approximations and quantitative estimates of risk are crude. With these limitations, Boffetta et al (2006) estimated that alcohol drinking accounts for 5.2% of world cancer in males and 1.7% in females.

Associations with high cancer risk have been noted for all organs with which unmetabolized alcohol comes in contact, with the exception of the stomach—that is, the mouth and pharynx, larynx, and esophagus. Corrao et al (2004), in a meta-analysis of 156 studies, estimated R associated with daily use of 25g of alcohol (estimated as two "drinks") for these three cancer sites were 1.9, 1.4, and 1.4; for daily use of 100g they were 6.5, 3.9, and 3.6, respectively.

The most direct evidence of an effect of alcohol-use independent of that due to smoking is by examination of its use among nonsmokers. With respect to oral and pharyngeal cancer, the results of such a study by Fioretti et al (1999) are generally consistent with those of earlier investigators. Among life-time nonsmokers, reported consumption of three or more drinks per day was associated with an R of 3. In a similar study of cancer of the larynx, while R for non-drinkers increased regularly with the number of cigarettes smoked daily to 14 for smokers of 25 daily, among nonsmokers increased risk was seen only for drinkers of eight or more drinks per day (R 2.5). The increase in larynx cancer risk associated with drinking among nonsmokers seems to occur only in parts of the larynx that are in direct contact with alcohol—an idea consistent with the early study of Tuyns et al (1988).

The effects of alcohol and tobacco in esophageal cancer were evaluated in a case-control study in high-risk areas of South America (Castellsagué et al, 1999). Supporting conclusions from earlier studies (Tuyns, 1983), this study showed independent effects of both alcohol and tobacco with multiplicative effects of the two exposures in combination: Heavy alcohol consumption combined with high use of so-called *black* tobacco was associated with a risk more than 100 times that of nondrinkers/nonsmokers. The associations were seen both in men and women. For cancer of the mouth and pharynx the combined and independent effects of alcohol and tobacco were clearly shown by Rothman and Keller in 1972.

Analyses specifying the effects of different types of alcoholic beverages generally show highest risk in the beverage most typical of the area in which the study was carried out, as for example calvados became the assigned culprit of the esophageal cancer epidemic in districts of Northern France. There is still much to be learned about the roles of alcohol concentration and adulterants in the carcinogenicity of alcoholic beverages to the upper respiratory-digestive tracts.

In light of the role of the liver in the metabolism of alcohol and the role of chronic alcohol abuse in hepatic cirrhosis, the association of alcohol use with HCC is hardly surprising. The meta-analysis of Corrao et al (2004) suggests R of 1.8 associated with the daily consumption of 100g of alcohol—perhaps smaller than clinical impressions and some studies would lead one to suppose. As noted earlier, life-styles associated with heavy alcohol consumption—including opportunities for multiple infections with hepatitis viruses—must be considered as at least partial explanations of the increased risk of HCC.

Small excesses of cancers of the colon and rectum (1.2 and 1.4, respectively, in Corrao et al, 2004) are more difficult to explain. Even more enigmatic is the association of alcohol use with cancer of the breast (2.4), possibly related to association of alcohol intake with estrogen levels (Reichman et al, 1993). It is difficult to identity other known epidemiologic features of breast cancer that explain the association that has been found consistently over the last 2 decades (Longnecker, 1994: Hamajima et al, 2002).

IATROGENIC EXPOSURE

Complications of therapy that appear immediately or within a short time are often recognized clinically, but those that develop after long intervals or require accumulation of exposure over time can usually be ascertained only by long-term follow-up studies in which epidemiologic principles are central. Such complications include neoplastic disease. The iatrogenic causes of cancer associated with IR and have already been referred to.

Diethylstilbestrol (DES)

Between 1940 and 1970 DES was prescribed for about 2 million pregnant women with a history of miscarriage or other complications of pregnancy. In 1970, Herbst and Scully reported seven cases of a very rare adenocarcinoma of the vagina in young women seen at one hospital, and in the next year Herbst et al (1971) published a study of eight cases and 32 normal infants delivered in the same institution: The mothers of seven cases but none of the controls had received DES during pregnancy. A registry for vaginal adenocarcinoma was established and in virtually all cases there were histories of maternal DES therapy (Ulfelder, 1973). The therapy was discontinued.

Whether prenatal exposures in general are associated with increased risk of cancer of the breast is currently an important area of investigation (Lagiou et al, 2006), and the experience of women exposed to DES prenatally, who are now in their middle and later years, is relevant. A large cohort of women exposed prenatally to DES and comparable unexposed women were identified from early studies and followed prospectively (Palmer et al, 2006). There was a small increase in risk (1.4) and a suggestion that the risk increased with age, although numbers were small in the older age groups. Continued follow-up of this group is important.

Oral Contraceptives (OC)

Introduction of OCs in the early 1960s raised fears that their use would increase risks of breast cancer and other hormone-dependent tumors. Combined analysis of 54 studies suggested a small increase in risk (1.2) of breast cancer for current users and an even smaller increase for women who had discontinued use within 10 years: Women who had discontinued use 10 or more years previously had no increase in risk. There was no evidence of increasing risk with duration of use (Collaborative Group, 1996). Another meta-analysis, based on 34 studies of premenopausal women, found a similar increase in breast cancer risk with OC use overall (R 1.2) and an indication that, while there was little difference in risk between parous and nonparous women, risk was somewhat higher among parous women who used OCs prior to their first full-term pregnancy. Among those with 4 or more years of use prior to their first birth R was 1.5 (Kahlenborn et al, 2006). The data do not permit an evaluation of whether the small increased risk among current and recently discontinued OC users represents an increased frequency of diagnosis of disease or a real increase, but an indication in the Collaborative Group study that the additional cancers were limited to tumors localized to the breast points in the direction of more frequent diagnosis.

Long-term use of OC is associated with decreased risk of ovarian cancer, a conclusion reached in a meta-analysis of 12 case-control studies (Whittemore et al, 1992). A later analysis of six studies showed reduction of risk (0.7) associated with any use of OC and a further reduction (to 0.5) with use for 5 years of more (Bosetti et al, 2002).

OC use is also associated with reduced risk of cancer of the endometrium. In a large Swedish case-control study, R for endometrial cancer risk was reduced to 0.5 after 3+ years of use and to 0.2 after 10 years of use (Weiderpass et al, 1999b). The decrease remained for at least 20 years after cessation of use—a matter of biologic as well as practical interest.

Evidence suggests a positive association of OC use with risk of cervical cancer, but while attempts were made in some studies to control for sexual activity it is not clear that this variable can be assessed with sufficient accuracy for its elimination as a source of confounding.

From a practical viewpoint, Schlesselman (1995) used available estimates of risk to compute additional or reduced annual tumors among 100 000 US women aged 20–54 that would be expected with use of OC for 8 years. They were for breast +151, cer-1, cervix +125, liver + 41, endometrium −197, and ovary −195. The net effect (+317, −392) is small though slightly favorable.

Exogenous Estrogens/progestins

Quite different conclusions come from studies of hormones prescribed for relief of symptoms in the menopausal years—initially estrogens and later progestins or a combination of the two. Increased risk of breast cancer was first demonstrated in a follow-up of patients taking premarin—a mixture of estrogens derived from the urine of pregnant mares. There was a 30% increase in risk of breast cancer in the group and among those taking the medication for 30 years or more the risk was doubled (Hoover et al, 1976). An extensive literature—both epidemiologic (Collaborative Group, 1997; Weiderpass et al, 1999a) and experimental (Roussouw et al, 2002)—generally supports these conclusions. Formulations combining progestin with estrogens are associated with higher risk than those containing estrogen alone (Newcomb et al, 2002).

In a randomized trial, women receiving estrogen alone (Anderson et al, 2004; Stefanick et al, 2006) had lower breast cancer risk (0.8) than those receiving no hormones, but participants had had prior hysterectomies (and probably oophorectomies) and consequently both trial groups were initially at low risk of breast cancer.

The association of endometrial cancer with exogenous estrogen is similar to that of breast cancer in that risk is elevated and increases with duration of use. A 1995 meta-analysis of 30 published studies estimated R as 2.3 for estrogen users and 10 after 10 or more years of use (Grady et al, 1995). However, the association differs from that of breast cancer in that addition of progestins reduces the increase associated with the use of estrogens alone (Persson et al, 1989; Beral et al, 2005). In a randomized trial, women given estrogen/progestagen combinations had slightly lower risk (0.8) than those given placebo (Anderson et al, 2003).

Analgesic Medications

Known for many years as a cause of renal nephropathy, *phenacetin* was banned or controlled in many jurisdictions. In a follow-up of analgesic abusers among males with chronic pyelonephritis, 11 developed urinary-tract tumors—all were using phenacetin-containing drugs (Bengtsson and Angervall, 1970). The induction times in these cases were long (6–35 years) and similar to those noted earlier for occupational bladder tumors. A larger study confirmed increased risk (R 12) of renal cancer following phenacetin use, but no increase with acetaminophen (McCredie et al, 1993). That acetaminophen is not associated with cancers, either of the renal pelvis or of the body of the kidney, was confirmed (McCredie et al, 1995; Rosenberg et al, 1998).

Other findings on the use of analgesics are less depressing—even positive. Thun et al (1991) found a reduction of close to 50% in risk of death from colon cancer among men and women reporting regular use of *aspirin* over a period of at least 1 year. This was confirmed for colorectal cancer both for men and women (Giovannucci

et al, 1994, 1995). The extensive literature that followed addressed primarily two questions: *(1)* is the apparently protective effect of aspirin shared with nonaspirin NSAIDs (NA-NSAIDs)? *(2)* does it extend to cancers in sites other than the large bowel?

On the first question, Garcia Rodriguez et al (2001) reviewed 18 studies published since 1988: There were 6 in which both aspirin and NA-NSAIDs were evaluated. The combined R from these was 0.6 both for aspirin and for NA-NSAIDs. In Garcia Rodriguez' own data 9 individual NSAIDs were evaluated and, although numbers were small, they did not show heterogeneity of the association between drugs. There is at present no reason to think that aspirin is different from other NSAIDS in its inverse association with colorectal cancer.

The second question was the subject of a review and meta-analysis of 47 published papers by Gonzales-Perez et al (2003). Aspirin use was found to be associated with reduced risk of cancer of the esophagus (0.5), stomach (0.5), and breast (0.8). Data for other NSAIDs gave similar results.

It is premature to suggest that NSAIDs be used for cancer prevention, but this has been considered a future possibility (Baron, 2003).

DIET

The contribution of diet to human cancer risk may be considerable. That this subject does not have a more prominent place in this chapter is because specific dietary constituents have not been established as being or not being causally related to cancer risk. However, epidemiologic studies have made considerable progress toward that end. The recent reviews of Willett (2001) and Lagiou et al (2002) are informative.

Suggestions of a role for some environmental factor in cancer etiology, among which diet seemed a likely candidate, came from studies of international variations in rates of specific neoplasms. These first became evident in mortality statistics compiled and published by the World Health Organization and brought to attention in a series of monographs by Mitsuo Segi (1962,

1964), and, with the development of cancer registries throughout the world, were much enhanced by incidence data compiled by IARC (Parkin et al, 2005). Studies of migrant populations showing that cancer rates of migrants and their descendents almost invariably move toward those of the host country, though at different rates, confirmed the environmental origin of the international differences: Studies of migrants to Hawaii (Haenszel and Kurihara, 1968) and Australia (McCredie et al, 1990) were early and influential in this regard. In the context of diet, hypotheses focused particularly on cancers of the breast and lower intestinal tract—sites in which international variation seemed less likely to be explained by difference in diagnostic or reporting practices. The high-caloric, high–fat, and low fiber diets of the developed countries came under particular suspicion.

Case-control studies showed moderate increases in risk for cancers of the breast and lower digestive tract associated with diets high in animal fat and low risk for colorectal cancer associated with high intake of fruits and vegetables, but these associations were generally not confirmed in prospective studies (Willett, 2001). In a combined analysis of 13 prospective studies, incorporating close to 726 000 men and women followed for between 6 month and 20 years, there was essentially no difference in risks of colon or rectal cancer between persons in the highest and the lowest quintiles of fiber intake, whether measured as reported intake of fruits and vegetables or all sources of dietary fiber (Park et al, 2005). In another analysis of the data from two large cohorts of health professionals, no relationship of cancer as a whole was found either for fruits and vegetable as a whole or for any of several subgroups (Hung et al, 2004).

Much was expected of the recent Women's Health Initiative trial in which 49 000 US women aged 50–79 were randomly assigned to one of two groups, to one of which dietary intervention, aimed toward reduction of total fat and increasing fruits and vegetables, was offered and encouraged. Both groups were followed, at latest report for an average of about 8 years (Prentice et al, 2006). Breast cancer incidence was slightly reduced in the intervention group relative to the comparison group (R 0.91) and secondary analyses suggested that the reduction was somewhat greater in women of initially higher risk and in those who had been most adherent to the study protocol. However, the secondary analyses do not carry the teleological advantages usually associated with randomization. Initial risk was not considered in the randomization and "adherence" carried different implications for the trial and comparison groups since women in the comparison group were not asked to make dietary modifications. For colorectal cancer rates were slightly higher in the intervention than the comparison group (R 1.08) and there was no difference relating to assessed adherence to study protocol (Beresford et al, 2006).

The results of this major undertaking are disappointing. When viewed against the 3- to 5-fold differences in disease rates that epidemiologic studies indicate need to be explained, the differences observed in the trial are small. However, they do not throw doubt on the possible significance of diet as an explanation of the epidemiologic observations. The populations in which major differences in cancer rates are noted experienced their diets for their entire lives whereas for the participants in this trial changes occurred over a relatively short period and, possibly more significantly, at a fairly late age. The most important lesson of this study may be that randomized trials are not the most effective way to investigate the role of dietary factors in cancer causation.

It is clear that obesity —a characteristic related at least in part to diet—is associated with increased cancer risk. In the ACS prospective study of over 900 000 US adults, death rates from cancer in the heaviest members of the cohort were, for men, 52% higher and, for women, 62% higher than for men and women of "normal" weight (Calle et al, 2003). The authors estimated that current patterns of overweight and obesity in the US account for 14% of cancer deaths in men and 20% of those in women.

While several cancers contribute to the excess rates associated with obesity, including cancers of the colon, rectum, gallbladder, pancreas, and kidney, cancer of the breast is the one site for which the observations are most consistent and that offers the greatest potential for fitting into the overall pattern of knowledge of the disease, stemming particularly from the positive correlation between endogenous sex hormones and breast cancer risk, at least in postmenopausal women (Key et al, 2002; Collaborative Group, 20002a), and the increased levels of plasma estrogens associated with body mass index (Hankinson et al, 1995). In a prospective study of 87 000 women age 30–55 years followed for 26 years, women who gained 25 kg or more of weight after age 18 and who did not take postmenopausal hormones had twice the breast cancer incidence of comparable women who maintained weight: Those who lost 10kg or more since menopause had less than half the risk of those who maintained postmenopausal weight (Eliassen et al, 2006).

An important area of investigation of the etiology of cancer of the breast was opened with accumulating evidence that the origins of the disease may be found in factors affecting breast growth and development in prenatal and early childhood: Among these must be considered both maternal and infant childhood diet (Trichopoulos, 1990; Lagiou et al, 2006). One of the first indications of prenatal influence was the association of breast cancer risk with the patient's birth weight. Unlikely as it seemed on first observation, this relationship is now well established (Ahlgren et al, 2003). In a classic illustration of the value of record linkage, Ahlgren et al (2004) combined information from birth certificates, school health records, and a national cancer registry to show positive associations between adult breast cancer risk and birth weight, height at ages 8 and 14 and body-mass-index, and growth rates around the time of puberty. The possibility that associations of birth weight and childhood growth rates with breast cancer risk may be influential in increasing rates of the disease among mi-

grants and yet be compatible with the weak or null associations between adult diets and breast cancer risk is explored by Lagiou et al (2003; 2006).

Additives to and contaminants of diet have frequently been suspected of carcinogenic potential and provoked much discussion and regulatory action. But most such concerns derive from extrapolations from experimental work rather than epidemiologic observations: They have rarely been evaluated epidemiologically, and lie outside the realm of this chapter.

CONCLUSION

That the past is prologue to the future is the *modus operandi* of academic admissions committees and other groups selecting candidates for advancement to new responsibilities. Exceptions to the success of such selections abound and are often highlighted, principally *because* they are exceptions, but the exceptions come about in divergent ways that are difficult to predict. What does the past offer in the way of predictive material in the field of cancer prevention? This chapter makes the case that epidemiology has made an effective contribution to the knowledge necessary for cancer prevention, both as an independent discipline and in partnership with other sciences.

Can specific areas of epidemiologic research be identified that on the basis of past contributions should be continued and strengthened? With increasing specificity, predictions become less reliable. But, again relying on the historical record, the following are suggested:

1. National and local statistics on causes of death and cancer registration and efforts to spread these resources to areas of the world that are not currently covered will continue to be productive. As in the past, the customs and diets of populations not now covered by death certification or cancer registration may reveal clues that have significance worldwide. Such statistics are also essential for the evaluation of the efficacy of preventive measures.

2. Facilities for maintenance and computerization of original medical and demographic records and statistical techniques for record linkage need continued development. The creation of the National Death Index in the United Sates and existing comparable facilities in Britain and the Nordic countries provide abundant examples of the value of such resources.

3. Multicenter studies, such as the collaborative case-control programs of the US National Cancer Institute and the EPIC prospective program in Europe are useful in expediting meaningful results and narrowing confidence intervals of observed risks. Another, and distinct, role for multicenter studies is the identification of unknown etiologic factors in diseases that show marked geographic variation or diseases associated with diets or customs that are limited in their geographic distribution. In this context centers would be selected for their heterogeneity, of either disease rate or environment, rather than their homogeneity.

4. Populations in which specific environmental and social characteristics are ascertained for linkage to later health outcomes need to be expanded. Groups of health practitioners established in Britain and the US and the population of American Cancer Society volunteers illustrate the productivity of such populations in the identification of possible cancer causes that are not recorded routinely.

5. The study of cancer in occupational settings has been highly productive. While such studies appear to be near the end of their potential for identifying unknown carcinogens, industry continues to develop new chemicals and processes of which the effects of long-term exposure have to be monitored. In addition, occupational studies will remain relevant for a long time to monitor the efficacy of preventive measures.

6. There is need for much stronger resources than now exist for detecting associations between use of medications and unexpected outcomes, including cancer—particularly for medications taken over long periods of time, and for diseases such as cancer that have long incubation periods.

It would be unfortunate if the recitation of accomplishments in this review were taken as an invitation to complacency. In the unlikely event that all of the advances described here were to come to full fruition—that is, if morbidity and mortality from cancers of the lung, ionizing radiation, known occupational carcinogens, and cancers of the oral cavity, pharynx, stomach, cervix, and liver were to be eliminated—the incidence of cancer would be reduced by about 20% and mortality by about 35% (Jemal et al, 2006). Cancers of the breast, endometrium, ovary, prostate, bowel, pancreas, and brain, as well as the leukemias and lymphomas, would remain as major causes of morbidity and mortality.

REFERENCES

Abbatt JD. History of the use and toxicity of thorotrast. Environ Res 1979;18:6–12.

Abratt RP, Vorobiof DA, White N. Asbestos and mesothelioma in South Africa. Lung Cancer 2004;45 Suppl 1:53–56.

Ahlgren M, Melbye M, Wohlfart J, Sorensen TI. Growth patterns and the risk of breast cancer in women, N Engl J Med 2004;351:1619–26.

Ahlgren M, Sorensen T, Wohlfart J, Hafldottir A, Holst C, Melbye M. Birth weight and risk of breast cancer in a cohort of 106,540 women. Int J Cancer 2003;107:997–1000.

Aksoy M, Erdem S, DinCol G. Leukemia in shoe workers exposed chronically to benzene. Blood 1974;44:837–41.

Andersen A, Berge SR, Engeland A, Norseth T. Exposure to nickel compounds and smoking in relation to incidence of lung and nasal cancer among nickel refinery workers. Occup Environ Med 1996;53:708–13.

Anderson GL, Judd Hl, Kaunitz AM, Barad DH, Beresford SA, Pettinger M. et al. Effects of estrogen plus progestin on gynecologic cancers and associated diagnostic procedures: the Women's Health Initiative randomized trial. JAMA 2003;290:1739–48.

Anderson GL, Limacher M, Assaf AR, Bassford T, Beresford SA, Black H. Effects of conjugated estrogen in postmenopausal women with hysterectomy; the Women's Health Initiative randomized controlled trial. JAMA 2004;291:1701–12.

Archer VE. Underground mining, smoking, and lung cancer. (Letter to the Editor) J Natl Cancer Inst 1986;76:553–54.

Archer VE, Coons T, Saccomanno G, Hong DY. Latency and the lung cancer epidemic among United States uranium miners. Health Phys 2004:87:480–89.

Armstrong BK, de Klerk NH, Musk AW, Hobbs MS. Mortality in miners and millers of crocidolite in Western Australia. Br J Ind Med 1988;45:5–13.

Baron JA. Epidemiology of non-steroidal anti-inflammatory drugs and cancer. Prog Exp Tumor Res 2003;37:1–24.

Bartrip PWS. History of asbestos related disease. Postgrad Med J 2004;80:72–76.

Beasley RP, Hwang LY, Lin CC, Chien CS. Hepatocelllar carcinoma and hepatitis B virus. A prospective study of 22,707 men in Taiwan, Lancet 1981;ii:1129–33.

Bengtsson U, Angervall L. Analgesic abuse and tumours of the renal pelvis. Lancet 1970; i:305. (Letter)

Beral V. Cancer of the cervix: a sexually transmitted disease? Lancet 1974;1037–40.

Beral V, Bull D, Reeves G; Million Women Study Collaborators. Endometrial cancer and hormone-replacement therapy in the Million Women Study. Lancet 2005;365:1543–51

Beral V, Newton R. Overview of the epidemiology of immunodeficiency-associated disorders. Natl Cancert Inst Mongr 1998;23:1–6.

Beresford SAA. Johnson KC, Ritenbaugh C, Lasser NL, Snetselaar LG, Black HR, et al. Low-fat diatary pattern and risk of colorectal cancer. The Women's Health Initiative randomized controlled dietary modification trial. JAMA 2006; 295:643–54.

Blair A, Stewart PA, Zaebst DD, Pottern L, Zey JN, Bloom TF, et al. Mortality of industrial workers exposed to acrylonitrile. Scand J Work Environ Heath 1998;24 Suppl 2:24–41.

Blumberg BS, Alter HJ, Visnich S. A "new" antigen in leukemia sera. JAMA 1965;191:541–46.

Boffetta P, Hashibe M. Alcohol and cancer. Lancet Oncology 2006;7:149–156.

Boffetta P, Hashibe M, La Vecchia C, Zatonski W. Rehm J. The burden of cancer attributable to alcohol drinking. Int J Cancer 2006; 11:884–87.

Boffetta P, Matisane L, Mundt KA, Dell LD. Meta-analysis of studies of occupational exposure to vinyl chloride in relation to cancer mortality. Scand J Work Environ Health 2003;29:220–29.

Boice JD Jr, Blettner M, Kleinerman RA, Engholm G, Stovall M, Lisco H, et al. Radiation dose and breast cancer risk for patients treated for cancer of the cervix. Int J Cancer 1989;44:7–16.

Bonn D. Asbestos—the legacy lives on. Lancet 1999;353:1336.

Bosch FX, Lorinez A, Muñoz N, Meijer CJLM, Shah KV. The causal relation between human papillomavirus and cervical cancer. J Clin Path 2002;55:244–265.

Bosch FX, Manos M, Muños N, Sherman M, Jansen AM, Peto J, et al. Prevalence of human papillomavirus cervical cancer: a worldwide perspective. J Natl Cancer Inst 1995; 87:796–802.

Bosetti C, La Vecchia C, Lipworth L, McLaughlin JK. Occupational exposure to vinyl chloride and cancer risk: a review of the epidemiologic literature. Eur J Cancer 2003a; 12:427–30.

Bosetti C, Negri E, Fattore E, La Vecclia C. Occupational exposure to polychlorinated biphenyls and cancer risk. Eur J Cancer Prev 2003b;12:251–55.

Bosetti C, Negri E, Trichopoulos D, Franceschi S, Beral V, Tzonou A, et al. Long-term effects of oral contraceptives on ovarian cancer risk. Int J Cancer 2002;102:262–65.

Boyle P. Tobacco smoking and the British doctors' cohort. (Editorial) Br J Cancer 2005; 92:419–20.

Braun L, Kisting S. Asbestos-related disease in South Africa. The social production of an invisible epidemic. Am J Pub Health 2006;96: 1386–96.

Bradford Hill A. Report to the Mond Nickel Company (1939). Quoted by Morgan (1958).

Brinton LA. Epidemiology of cervical cancer—overview. In The Epidemiology of Cervical Cancer and Human Papilloma Viruses. Eds. Muñoz N, Bosch FX, Shah KV, Meheus A. IARC Publ 119, Lyon, 1992. pp 3–23.

Brinton LA, Berman ML, Mortel R, Twiggs LB, Barrett RJ, Wilbanks GD, et al. Reproductive, menstrual, and medical factors for endometrial cancer: results from a case-control study. Am J Obstet Gynec 1992;167: 1317–25.

Burnet M. Somatic mutation and chronic disease. Br Med J 1965;i:338–42.

Calle EE, Rogriguez C, Walker-Thurmond K. Thun MJ. Overweight, obesity, and mortality from cancer in a prospectively studied cohort of U.S. adults. New Engl J Med 2003;348:1625–38.

Case RAM, Hosker ME, McDonald DB, Pearson JT. Tumours of the urinary bladder in workmen engaged in the manufacture and use of certain dyestuff intermediates in the British chemical industry. Br J Indust Med 1954;11:75–104.

Case RAM, Lea AJ. Mustard gas poisoning, chronic bronchitis and lung cancer. Br.J Prev Soc Med 1955;9:62–72.

Castellsagué X, Muñoz N, De Stefani E, Victora CG, Castelletto R, Rolón PA, et al. Independent and joint effects of tobacco smoking and alcohol drinking on the risk of esophageal cancer in men and women. Int J Cancer 1999;82:657–64.

Chang MH, Chen CJ, Lai MS, Hsu HM, Wu TC, Kong MS, et al. Universal hepatitis B vaccination in Taiwan and the incidence of hepatocellular carcinoma in children. Taiwan Childhood Hepatoma Study Group. N Engl J Med 1997;336:1855–59.

Chen CJ, Wang CJ. Ecological correlation between arsenic level and well water and age-adjusted mortality from malignant neoplasms. Cancer Res 1990;50:5470–74.

Chen CL, Hsu LI, Chiou HY, Hsueh YM, Chen SY, Wu MM, et al. Ingested arsenic, cigarette smoking, and lung cancer risk: a follow-up study in arseniasis-endemic areas in Taiwan, JAMA 2004;292:3026–29.

Chien YC, Jan CF, Kuo HS, Chen CJ. Nationwide hepatitis B vaccination program in Taiwan: effectiveness in the 20 years after it was launched. Epidemiol Rev 2006;28:126–35.

Chiou HY, Chiou ST, Hsu YH, Chou YL, Tseng CH, Wei ML et al. Incidence of transitional cell carcinoma and arsenic in drinking water: as study of 8,102 residents in an areniasis-endemic area in Northeastern Taiwan. Am J Epidemiol 2001;153:411–18.

Clifford GM, Polesel J, Rickenbach M, Maso LD, Keiser O, Kofler A, et al. Cancer risks in the Swiss HIV cohort study: associations with immunodeficiency, smoking, and highly active antiviral therapy. J Natl Cancer Inst 2005;97:425–32.

Cole P, Rodu B. Epidemiologic studies of chrome and cancer mortality: a series of meta-analyses. Reg Toxicol Pharmacol 2005;43: 225–31,

Collaborative Group. (The Endogenous Hormones and Breast Cancer Collaborative Group.) Endogenous sex hormones and breast cancer in postmenopausal women: reanalysis of nine prospective studies. J Natl Cancer Inst 2002a;94:606–16.

Collaborative Group on Hormonal Factors in Breast Cancer. Breast cancer and hormonal contraceptives: collaborative reanalysis of individual data on 53 297 women with breast cancer and 100 239 women without breast cancer from 54 epidemiologic studies. Lancet 1996;347:1713–27.

Collaborative Group on Hormonal Factors in Breast Cancer. Breast cancer and hormone replacement therapy: collaborative reanalysis of data from 51 epidemiological studies of 52,705 women with breast cancer and 108,411 women without breast cancer. Lancet 1997; 350:1047–59.

Collaborative Group on Hormonal Factors in Breast Cancer and Valerie Beral. Breast cancer and breast feeding: collaborative reanalysis of individual data for 47 epidemiological studies in 30 countries, including 50302 women with breast cancer and 93973 women without the disease. Lancet 2002b; 360:187–95.

Collins JJ, Acquavella JF, Review and meta-analysis of studies of acrylonitrile. Scand J Work Environ Health 1998; 24, Suppl 2: 671–80.

Collins JJ, Acquavella JF, Esmen NA. An updated meta-analysis of formaldehyde exposure and upper respiratory tract cancers. J Occup Environ Med 1997;39:639–51.

Cologne JB, Tokuoka S, Beebe GW, Fukuhara T, Mabuchi K. Effects of radiation on incidence of primary liver cancer among atomic bomb survivors. Radiat Res 1999;152:364–73.

Constantini A, Quinn M, Consonni D, Zappa M. Exposure to benzene and risk of leukemia among shoe factory workers. Scand J Work Environ Health 2003;29:51–59.

Corrao, G, Bagnardi V, Zambon A, La Vecchia C. A meta-analysis of alcohol consumption and the risk of 15 diseases. Prev Med 2004; 38:613–19.

Crew KD, Neugut AI. Epidemiology of gastric cancer. World J Gastroenterol 2006:12:354–62.

Crosignani P, Tittarelli A, Borgini A. Codazzi T, Rovelli A, Porro E, et al. Childhood leukemia and road traffic: a population-based case-control study. Int J Cancer 2004;108:596–99.

Darby SC, Whitley E, Howe GR, Hutchings SJ, Kusiak RA., Lubin JH, et al. Radon and cancers other than lung cancer in underground miners: a collaborative analysis of 11 studies. J Natl Cancer Inst 1995;87:378–84.

Demers PA, Boffetta P. Cancer Risk from Occupational Exposure to Wood Dust: a Pooled Analysis of Epidemiological Studies. (IARC Technical Report No.30) IARC, Lyon, France, 1998,

Doll R. Mortality from lung cancer in asbestos workers. Br J Indust Med 1955;12:81–86.

Doll R. Cancer of the lung and nose in nickel workers. Br J Indust Med 1958;15:217–23.

Doll R, Hill AB. Smoking and cancer of the lung. Preliminary report. Br Med J 1950;2:739–48.

Doll R, Hill AB. The mortality of doctors in relation to their smoking habits. A preliminary report. BMJ 1954;228:1451–55.

Doll R, Mathews JD, Morgan LG. Cancers of the lung and nasal sinuses in nickel workers:

a reassessment of the period of risk. Br J Ind Med 1977; 34:102–5.

Doll R, Peto R, Boreham J, Sutherland I. Mortality in relation to smoking: 50 years' observations on male British doctors. BMJ 2004; 438:1519–28.

Doll R, Peto R, Boreham J, Sutherland I. Mortality from cancer in relation to smoking: 50 years observations on British doctors. Br J Cancer 2005;92:426–29.

dos Santos Silva I, Malveiro F, Jones ME, Swerdlow AJ. Mortality after radiological investigation with radioactive Thorotrast: a follow-up study of up to 50 years in Portugal. Radiat Res 2003;159:521–34.

Eliassen AH, Colditz GA, Rosner B, Willett WC, Hankinson SE. . Adult weight change and risk of postmenopausal breast cancer. JAMA 2006;296:193–201.

English DR, Armstrong BK, Kricker A. Sunlight and cancer. Cancer Causes Control 1997;8: 271–83.

Enterline PE, Harley J, Henderson V. Asbestos and cancer: a cohort followed up to death. Br J Ind Med 1987;44:396–401.

Eslick GD. Helicobacter pylori infection causes gastric cancer? A review of the epidemiologic, meta-analytic, and experimental evidence. World J Gastroenterol 2006;12:2991–99.

Fioretti F, Bosetti C, Tavani A, Franceschi S, La Vecchi C. Risk factors for oral and pharyngeal cancer in never smokers. Oral Oncol 1999;35:375–78.

Frumkin H, Thun MJ. Arsenic. CA Cancer J Clinic 2001;51;254–62.

Garcia Rodriguez LA, Huerta-Alvarez. Reduced risk of colorectal cancer among long-term users of aspirin and nonaspirin and nonsteroidal antiinflammatory drugs. Epidemiology 2001;12:88–93.

Gilliland FD, Hunt WC, Archer VE, Saccomano G. Radon progeny exposure and lung cancer risk among non-smoking uranium miners. Health Phys 2000;79:365–72.

Giovannucci E, Egan KM, Hunter DJ, Stampfer MJ, Colditz GA, Willett WC, et al. Aspirin and the risk of colorectal cancer in women. N Engl J Med 1995;333:609–14.

Giovannucci E, Rimm EB, Stampfer MJ, Colditz GA, Asherio A, Willett WC. Aspirin use and the risk for colorectal cancer and adenoma in male health professionals. Ann Intern Med 1994;121:241–46.

Glass DC, Gray CN, Jolley DJ, Gibbons C, Sim MR, Fritschi L, et al. Leukemia risk associated with low-level benzene exposure. Epidemiology 2003;14:569–77.

Gonzales-Perez A, Garcia Rodriguez LA. Lopez-Ridaura R. Effects of non-steroidal antiinflammatory drugs on cancer sites other than the colon and rectum: a meta-analysis. BMC Cancer 2003;3:28.

Grady D, Gebretsadik T, Kerlikowske K, Ernster V, Petitti D. Hormone replacement therapy and endometrial cancer risk: a meta-analysis. Obstet Gynecol 1995;85:304–13.

Grimsrud TK, Berge SR, HaldorsenT, Andersen A. Can lung cancer risk among nickel refinery workers be explained by occupational exposures other than nickel? Epidemiology 2005;16:146–54.

Grimsrud TK, Berge SR, Martinsen JI, Andersen A. Lung cancer incidence among Norwegian nickel-refinery workers 1953–2000. J Environ Monit 2003;5:109–17.

Grimsrud TK, Peto J. Persisting risk of nickel-related lung cancer and nasal cancer among Clydach refiners. Occupat. Environ Med 2006;63:365–66.

Hackshaw AK, Law MR, Wald NJ. The accumulated evidence on lung cancer and environmental tobacco smoke. BMJ 1997:315:980–88.

Haenszel W, Kurihara M. Studies of Japanese migrants. I. Mortality from cancer and other diseases among Japanese in the United States. J Nat Cancer Inst 1968;40:43–68.

Hamajima N, Tajima HK, Rohan T, Calle EE, Heatth CW Jr, Coates RJ, et al. Alcohol, tobacco and breast cancer—collaborative analysis of individual data from 53 epidemiological studies, including 58,515 women with breast cancer and 95,067 without the disease, Br J Cancer 2002;87:1234–45.

Hammond EC. Smoking in relation to the death rates of one million men and women. Monogr Natl Cancer Inst 1966; 19:127–204.

Hankinson SE, Willett WC, Manson JE, Hunter DJ, Colditz GA, Stampfer MJ, et al. Alcohol, height, and adiposity in relation to estrogen and prolactin levels in postmenopausal women. J Natl Cancer Inst 1995;87:1297–303.

Harting FM, Hesse W. Der Lungenkrebs, die Bergkrankheit in den Schneeberger Gruben. Vjschr Geschrl Med Offendl Gesundheitswesen 1879; 31:102–32,313–37. (Quoted by Samet, 1989)

Hauptmann M, Lubin JH, Stewart PA, Hayes RB, Blair A. Morality from lymphohematopoietic malignancies among workers in formaldehyde industries. J Natl Cancer Inst 2003; 95:1615–23.

Hauptmann M, Lubin JH, Stewart PA, Hayes RB, Blair A. Mortality from solid cancers among workers in formaldehyde industries. Am J Epidemiol 2004;159:1117–30.

Hayes RB, Songnian Y, Dosemeci M, Linet M. Benzene and lymphohematopoietic malignancies in humans. Am J Ind Med 2001;40: 117–26.

Henderson BE, Casagrande JT, Pike MC, Mack T, Rosario I, Duke A. The epidemiology of endometrial cancer in young women. Br J Cancer 1983;47:749–56.

Herbst AL, Scully RE. Adenocarcinoma of the vagina in adolescence: a report of 7 cases including 6 clear cell carcinomas (so-called mesonephromas). Cancer 1970;25:745–57.

Herbst AL, Ulfelder H, Poskanzer DC. Adenocarcinoma of the vagina: association of maternal stilbestrol therapy with tumor appearance in young women. N Engl J Med 1971; 284:878–81.

Hirayama 1981, Non-smoking wives of heavy smokers have a higher risk of lung cancer: a study from Japan. BMJ 1981;282:183–85.

Hoover R, Gray LA, Cole P, MacMahon B. Menopausal estrogens and breast cancer. N Engl J Med 1976; 295:401–5.

Hung H-C, Joshipura KJ, Jiang R, Hu FB, Hunter D, Smith-Warner SA, et al. Fruit and vegetable intake and risk of major chronic disease. J Natl Cancer Inst 2004;96:1577–84.

IAEA. (International Atomic Energy Agency). Thorotrast: A Bibliography of its Diagnostic Use and Biological Effects. Monograph: IAEA. Vienna, 1965.

IARC (International Agency for Research on Cancer). Monographs on the Evaluation of Carcinogenic Risk of Chemicals to Humans. V01.23, 39–141: Arsenic and Arsenic Compounds. IARC, Lyon, 1980.

IARC. Monographs on the Evaluation of Carcinogenic Risks to Humans. Vol. 83: Tobacco Smoking and Involuntary Smoking. IARC, Lyon, 2004a.

IARC. Monographs on the Evaluation of Carcinogenic Risks to Humans. V01.88: Formaldehyde, 2-Butoxyethanol and I-tert-Butoxy-2-propanol. IARC, Lyon, 2004b.

Jacobsson R, Ahlbom A, Bellander T, Lundberg I. Acute myeloid leukemia among petrol station attendants. Arch Environ Health 1993; 48:255 59.

Jemal A, Siegel R, Ward E, Murray J, Xu J, Smigal C, Thun MJ. Cancer Statistics, 2006. CA:Cancer J Clin 2006; 56:106–30.

Jones EG, MacDonald I, Breslow L. A study of epidemiologic factors in carcinoma of the uterine cervix. Am J Obstet Gynecol 1958; 76:1–10.

Josefsson AM, Magnusson PK, Ylitalo N, Sorensen P. Quarforth-Tubbin P, Andersen PK. et al. Viral load of human papilloma virus 16 as a determinant for development of cervical carcinoma in situ: a nested case-control study. Lancet 2000; 355:2189–93.

Kahlenborn C, Modugno F, Potter DM, Severs WB. Oral contraceptive use as a risk factor for premenopausal breast cancer: a meta-analysis. Mayo Clin Proc 2006;81:1290–302.

Kest H, Brogly S, McSherry G, Dashefsky B, Oleske J, Seage GR 3rd. Malignancy in perinatally human immunodeficiency virus-infected children in the United Sates. Pediat Infect Dis J 2005;24:237–42.

Key T, Appleby P, Barnes I, Reeves G, Endogenous Hormones and Breast Cancer Collaborative Group. Endogenous sex hormones and breast cancer in postmenopausal women: reanalysis of nine prospective studies. J Natl Cancer Inst 2002;94:606–16.

Kricker A, Armstrong BK, English DR. Sun exposure and non-melanotic skin cancer. Cancer Causes Control 1994;5:367–92.

Krugman S, Giles JP, Hammond J. Infectious hepatitis: evidence for two distinctive clinical. epidemiological, and immunological types of infection. JAMA 1967;200:95–103.

La Vecchia C, Decarli A, Franceschi S, Regalio M, Tognoni H. Age at first birth and the risk of epithelial ovarian cancer. Int J Cancer 1984; 73:663–66.

Lagiou P, Adami HO, Trichopoulos D. Early life diet and the risk for adult breast cancer. Nutr Cancer 2006, in press.

Lagiou P, Hsieh CC, Trichopoulos D, Xu B, Wuu J, Mucci L, et al. Birthweight differences between USA and China and their relevance to breast cancer aetiology. Int J Epidemiol 2003;32:193–98.

Lagiou P, Trichopoulou A, Trichoroulos D. Nutritional epidemiology of cancer: accomplishments and prospects. Proc Nutr Soc 2002;61:217–22.

Lagorio S, Forastiere F, Iavarone I, Rapiti E, Vanacore N, Perucci CA, et al. Mortality of filling station attendants. Scand J Work Environ Health 1994;20:331–38.

Lambe M, Hsieh C-c, Trichopoulos D, Ekbom A, Pavia M, Adami HO Transient increase in the risk of breast cancer after giving birth. N Engl J Med 1994;331:5–9.

Lambe M, Wuu J, Weiderpass E, Hsieh CC. Childbearing at older age and endometrial cancer risk (Sweden). Cancer Causes Control 1999;10:43–49.

Lane-Claypon JE. A further report on cancer of the breast with special reference to its associated antecedent conditions. In Report on Public Health and Medical Subjects. No. 32. Ministry of Health, London, 1926.

Le Marchand L, Saltzman BS, Hankin JH, Wilkens LR, Franke AA, Morris SJ, et al. Sun exposure, diet, and melanoma in Hawaii Caucasians. Am J Epudemiol 2006;164: 232–45.

Lee MS, Kim DM, Kim H, Lee HS, Kim CY, Park TS, et al. Hepatitis B vaccination and reduced risk of primary liver cancer among male adults: a cohort study in Korea. Int J Epidemiol 1998;27:316–19.

Little MP, Blettner M, Boice RD Jr, Bridges BA, Cardis E, et al. Potential funding crises at the Radiation Effects Research Foundation. Lancet 2004;364:557–58.

Longnecker MP. Alcoholic beverage consumption in relation to risk of breast cancer: meta-analysis and review. Cancer Causes Control 1994;5:73–82.

Lorenz E. Radioactivity and lung cancer; a critical review of lung cancer in the miners of Schneeberg and Joachimsthal. J Natl Cancer Inst 1944;5:1–15.

Lubin JH, Boice JD Jr, Edling C, Hornung RW, Howe GR, Kunz E. et al. Lung cancer in radon-exposed miners and estimates of risk from indoor exposures. J Natl Cancer Inst 1995; 87: 817–27.

Lubin JH, Pottern LM, Stone BJ, Fraumeni JF Jr. Respiratory cancer in a cohort of copper smelter workers: results from more than 50 year of follow-up. Am J Epidemiol 2000;151: 554–65.

Lynge E, Andersen A, Nilsson R, Barlow L, Pukkala E, Nordlinder R, et al. Risk of cancer and exposure to gasoline vapors. Am J Epidemiol 1997;145:449–58.

MacMahon B, Cole P, Lin TM, Lowe CR, Mirra AP, Ravnihar B, et al. Age first birth and breast cancer risk. Bull World Health Organ 1970a;43:209–21

MacMahon B, Lin TM, Lowe CR, Mirra AP, Ravnihar B, Salber EJ. et al. Lactation and cancer of the breast. A summary of an international study. Bull World Health Organ 1970b; 42:185–94.

Marsh GM. Critical review of epidemiologic studies related to ingested asbestos. Environ Health Perspect 1983;53:49–56.

Marshall BJ, Warren RJ. Unidentified curved bacilli in the stomach of patients with gastritis and peptic ulceration. Lancet 1984;i: 1311–15.

Martland HS, Conlon P, Knef LF. Some unrecognized dangers in the use and handling of radioactive substances. JAMA 1925; 85:1769.

Mastrangelo G, Fedeli U, Fadda E, Milan G, Turato A, Pavanello S. Lung cancer risk in workers exposed to poly(vinyl chloride) dust: a nested case-referent study. Occupat Environ Med 2003;60:423–28.

Mastromatteo E. Nickel: a review of its occupational health aspects. J Occup Med 1967; 9:127–36

Maupas P, Melnick JL. Hepatitis B infection and primary liver cancer. Prog Med Virol 1981; 27:1–5.

McCredie M, Coated MS, Ford JM. Cancer incidence among migrants to New South Wales. Int J Cancer 1990;46:228–32.

McCredie M, Pommer W, McLaughlin JK, Stewart JH, Lindblad P, Mandel JS, et al. International renal-cell cancer study. II. Analgesics. Int J Cancer 1995;60:345–49.

McCredie M, Stewart JH, Day NE. Different roles for phenacetin and paracetamol in cancer of the kidney and renal pelvis. Int J Cancer 1993;53:245–49.

McDonald JC, Liddell FD, Dufresne A, McDonald AD. The 1891–1920 birth cohort of Quebec chrysotile miners and millers: mortality 1976–88. Br J Ind Med 1993;50:1073–81.

McLaughlin JK, Lipworth L. A critical review of the epidemiologic literaure on health effects of occupational exposure to vinyl chloride. J Epidemiol Biostat 1999;4:253–75.

Mocroft A, Katlama C, Johnson AM, Pradier C, Antunes F, Mulcahy F, et al. AIDS across Europe, 1994–98: the EUROSIDA study. Lancet 2000;356:291–96.

Morgan JG. Some observations on the incidence of respiratory cancer in nickel workers. Br J Indust Med 1958;15:224–34.

Mori MT, Kido C, Fukutomi K, Kato Y, Hatakeyama S, Machinami R, et al. Summary of the entire Japanese thorotrast follow-up study: updated 1998. Radiat Res 1999.152: S84–87.

Muller BU, Pizzo PA. Cancer in children with primary or secondary immunodeficiencies. J Pediat 1995;126:1–10.

Muller FH. Tabakmissbrauch und lungencarcinoma. Z. Krebsforsch 1940;49:57–85.

Mundt KA, Dell LD, Austin RP, Luippold RS, Noess R, Bigelow C. Historical cohort study to 31 December 1995 of 10,109 men in the North American vinyl chloride industry, 1842–72: update of cancer mortality. Occup Environ Med 2000; 57:774–81.

Mzileni O, Sitas F, Steyn K, Carrara H, Bekker P. Lung cancer, tobacco, and environmental factors in the African population of the Northern Province, South Africa. Tobacco Control 1999;8:398–401.

Nasti G, Talamini R, Antinori A, Martellotta F, Jacchetti G, Chiodo G. AIDS-related Kaposi's sarcoma: evaluation of potential new prognostic factors and assessment of the AIDS Clinical Trial Group Staging System in the Haart Era—the Italian Cooperative Group on AIDS and Tumors and the Italian cohort of patients naive from antiretrovirals. J Clin Oncol 2003;21:2876–82.

Neuberger M, Kundi M, Friedl HP. Environmental asbestos exposure and cancer mortality, Arch Environ Health 1984;39:261–65.

Newcomb PA, Titus-Ernstoff L, Egan KM, Trentham-Dietz A, Baron JA, Storer BE, et al. Postmenopausal estrogen and progestin use in relation to breast cancer risk. Cancer Epidemiol Biomarkers Prev 2002;11: 593–600.

Newnham A, Harris J, Evans HS, Evans BG, Moller H. The risk of cancer in HIV-infected people in southeast England: a cohort study. Br J Cancer 2005;92:194–200.

Nyberg U, Nilsson G, Travis LB, Holm LE. Hall P. Cancer incidence among Swedish patients exposed to radioactive thorotrast: a forty-year follow-up survey. Radiat Res 2002;157: 419–25.

Oliveria SA, Saraiya M, Geller AC, Heneghan MK, Jorgensen C. Sun exposure and risk of mesothelioma Arch Dis Child 2006 2006;91: 131–38.

Palmer JR, Wise, LA, Hatch EE, Troisi R, Titus-Ernstoph L, Strohsnitter W, et al. Prenatal diethylstilbestrol exposure and risk of breast cancer. Cancer Epidemiol Biomarkers Prev 2006;15:1509–14.

Park RM, Bena JF, Stayner LT, Smith RJ, Gibb HJ, Lees PS. Hexavalent chromium and lung cancer in the chromate industry: a quantitative risk assessment. Risk Anal 2004;24: 1099–108.

Park Y, Hunter DJ, Spiegelman D, Bergkvist L, Berrino F, van den Brandt PA, et al. Dietary fiber intake and risk of colorectal cancer: a pooled analysis of prospective cohort studies. JAMA 2005;294:2904–6.

Parkin DM. The global burden of infection-associated cancers in the year 2002. Int J Cancer 2006;118:3030–44.

Parkin DM, Whelan SL, Ferlay J, Storm H. Cancer Incidence in Five Continents. Vol. 1-VIII. CancerBase No. 7. IARC, Lyon, 2005.

Parodi S, Vercelli, M, Stella A, Stagnaro E, Valerio F. Lymphohaematopoietic system cancer incidence in an urban area near a coke oven plant; an ecologic investigation. Occupat Environ Med 2003; 60:187–93.

Parsonnet J, Forman D. Helicobacter pylori infection and gastric cancer—for want of more outcomes. JAMA 2004;291:244–45.

Patel AS, Talbott EO, Zborowski JV, Rychek JA, Dell D, Xu X, et al. Risk of cancer as a result of community exposure to gasoline vapors. Arch Environ Health 2004;59:497–503.

Pedersen E, Høgetveit AC, Andersen A. Cancer of respiratory organs among workers at a nickel refinery in Norway Int J Cancer 1973;12:32–41.

Pedotti P, Cardillo M, Rossini G, Arcuri V, Boschiero L, Caldara R, et al. Incidence of cancer after kidney transplant: results from the North Italy transplant program. Transplantation 2003;76:1448–51.

Penn I. Cancer in renal transplant recipients. Adv Ren Replace Ther 2000;7:147–56.

Persson I, Adami HO, Bergkvist L, Lindgren A, Pettersson B, Hoover R, et al. Risk of endo-metrial cancer after treatment with oestrogens alone or in conjunction with progestagens: results of a prospective study. BMJ 1989;298:147–51.

Peto J. Decarli A, La Vecchia C, Levi J, Jones JR. The European mesothelioma epidemic. Br J Cancer 1999;79:666–72.

Peto J, Seidman H, Selikoff IJ. Mesothelioma mortality in asbestos workers: implications for models of carcinogenesis and risk assessment. Br J Cancer 1982;45:124–35.

Pinkerton LE, Hein MJ, Stayner LT. Mortality among a cohort of garment workers exposed to formaldehyde: an update. Occup Environ Med 2004;61:193–200.

Pott P. Chirurgical Observations. Hawes, Clarke & Collings, London, 1775.

Prentice RL, Chlebowski RT, Patterson R, Kuller LH, Ockene JK, Margolis KL, et al. Low-fat dietary pattern and risk of invasive breast cancer. The Women's Health Initiative randomized controlled dietary modification trial. JAMA 2006;295:629–42.

Price B, Ware A. Mesothelioma trends in the United States: an update based on Surveillance, Epidemiology, and End Results Program data for 1973 through 2003. Am J Epidemiol 2004;159:107–12.

Prince MM, Hein MJ, Ruder AV, Waters MA, Laber PA, Whelan EA. Update: cohort mortality study of workers highly exposed to polychlorinated biophenyls (PCBs) during manufacture of electrical capacitors, 1940–1998. Environmental Health Global Access 2006;114:13–24.

Prince MM, Szmuness W, Micon J, Demaille J, Diebolt G. Linhard, J, et al. A case-control study of the association between primary liver cancer and hepatitis B infection in Senegal. Int J Cancer 1975;16:376–83.

Proctor DM, Otani JM, Finley BL, Paustenbach DJ, Bland JA, Speizer N, et al. Is hexavalent chromium carcinogenic via ingestion? A weight-of-evidence review. J Toxicol Environ Health A 2002,65;701–46.

Raaschou-Nielsen O, Hertel O, Thomsen BL, Olsen JH. Air pollution from traffic at the residences of children with cancer. Am J Epidemiol 2001;153:433–43.

Raffn E, Lynge E, Juel K, Korsgaard B. Incidence of cancer and mortality among employees in the asbestos cement industry in Denmark. Br J Ind Med 1989;46:90–96.

Reichman ME, Judd JT, Longcope C, Schatzkin A, Clevidence BA, Nair PP, et al. Effects of alcohol consumption on plasma and urinary hormone concentrations in premenopausal women. J Natl Cancer Inst 1993;85:722–27.

Ribes J, Clèries R, Rubió A, Hernández JM, Mazzara R, Madoz P et al. Cofactors associated with liver disease mortality in an HBsAg-positive Mediterranean cohort: 20 years of follow-up. Int J Cancer 2006;119: 687–94.

Rinsky RA, Young RJ, Smith AB. Leukemia in benzene workers. Am J Ind Med 1981;2: 217–45.

Rodu B, Cole P. Declining mortality from smoking in the United States. J Nicotine Tobacco Res 2006; in press.

Rosenberg L, Rao RS, Palmer JR, Strom BL, Zauber A, Warshauer ME, et al. Transitional cell cancer of the urinary tract and renal cell cancer in relation to acetaminophen use (United States). Cancer Causes Control 1998;9:83–88.

Rothman KJ, Keller A. The effect of joint exposure to alcohol and tobacco on risk of cancer of the mouth and pharynx. J Chronic Dis 1972;25:711–16.

Rossouw JE, Anderson GL, Prentice RL, LaCroix AZ, Kooperberg C, et al. Risks and benefits of estrogen plus progestins in healthy postmenopausal women: principal results from the Women's Health Initiative randomized controlled trial. JAMA 2002;288: 321–23.

Ruder AM, Hein MJ, Nilsen N, Waters MA, Laber P, Davis-King K., et al. Mortality among workers exposed to polychlorinated biphenyls (PCBs) in an electrical capacitor manufacturing plant in Indiana: an update. Environ Health Perspect.2006;114:18–23.

Russo J, Gusterson BA, Rogers AE, Russo IH, Welling SR, van Zweiten MJ. Comparative study of human and rat mammary carcinogenesis. Lab Invest 1990;62:224–78.

Samet JM. Radon and lung cancer. J Natl Cancer Inst 1989;81:745–57.

Scélo G, Constantinescu V, Csiki I, Zaridze D, Szeszenia-Dabrowska N, Rudnai P, et al. Occupational exposure to vinyl chloride, acrylonitrile and styrene and lung cancer risk (Europe). Cancer Causes Control 2004;15: 445–52.

Schiffman M, Wheeler CM, Castle PE. Human papillomavirus DNA remains detectable longer than related cervical abnormalities. J Infect Dis 2002;186:1169–72.

Schlatter C. Risks to consumers and PVC workers from vinyl chloride. Schweiz Med Wochenschr 1976;106:647–50.

Schlesselman JJ. Net effect of oral contraceptive use on the risk of cancer in women in the United States. Obstet Gynec 1995;85:793–801.

Schnatter AR, Rosamilia K, Wojcik NC. Review of literature on benzene exposure and leukemia subtypes. Chem Biol Interact 2005; 153–154:9–21.

Segi M. Cancer mortality for selected sites in 24 countries. 1950–7. With Kurihara M. 1958–59, 1960–61. Department of Public Health, Tohoku University School of Medicine. Sendai, Japan, 1962, 1964.

Selikoff IJ, Hammond EC, Churg J. Asbestos exposure and neoplasia. JAMA 1964;188: 22–26.

Selikoff IJ, Hammond EC, Churg J. Relation between exposure to asbestos and mesothelioma. N Engl J Med 1965;272:560–65.

Serraino D, Piselli P, Angeletti C, Minetti E, Pozzetto A, Civati G, et al. Risk of Kaposi's sarcoma and of other cancers in Italian renal transplant patients. Br J Cancer 2005;92: 572–75.

Smith PG, Doll R. Mortality from lung cancer and all causes among British radiologists. BMJ 1981;54:187–94.

Smith PG, Doll R. Mortality among patients with ankylosing spondylitis after a single treatment with x-rays. Br Med J 1982;284: 449–60.

Sorahan T, Williams SP. Mortality of workers at a nickel carbonyl refinery, 1958–2000. Occup Environ Med 2005;62:80–85.

Stefanick ML, Anderson GL, Margolis KL, Hendrix SL, Rodabough RJ, Paskett ED, et al. Effects of conjugated equine estrogens on breast cancer and mammography screening in postmenopausal women with hysterectomy. JAMA 2006;295;1647–57.

Stewart A, Webb J, Hewitt D. A survey of childhood malignancies. BMJ 1958;i:1495–508.

Sun CA, Wu DM, Lin CC, Lu SN, You SL, Wang LY, et al. Incidence and cofactors of hepatitis C virus-related hepatocellular carcinoma: a prospective study of 12,008 men in Taiwan. Am J Epidemiol 2003:57:674–82.

Surgeon-General. Smoking and Health. Report of the Advisory Committee to the Surgeon-General of the United States. Department of Health, Education and Welfare. Washington DC, Public Health Service Publication No. 1103. U.S.Government Printing Office 0–714–422, 1964.

Surgeon General. The Health Consequences of Involuntary Exposure to Tobacco Smoke. A Report of the Surgeon General. US Department of Health and Human Services. National Center for Chronic Disease and Health Promotion, Atlanta, GA, 2006. pp. 433–45.

Taioli E, Piselli P. Arbustini E. Boschiero L, Burra P, Busnach G, et al. Incidence of second primary cancer in transplanted patients. Transplantation 2006;81:982–85.

Taylor R, Cumming R, Woodward A, Black M. Passive smoking and lung cancer: a cumulative meta-analysis. Aust NZ J Public Health 2001;25:203–11.

Thun MJ, Day-Lally CA, Callee EE, Flander WD, Health CW Jr. Excess mortality among cigarette smokers: changes in a 20-year interval. Am J Public Health 1995;85:1223–30.

Thun MJ, Namboodiri MM, Heath CW. Aspirin use and reduced risk of fatal colon cancer. N Engl J Med 1991;325:1593–96.

Travis LB, Hill DA, Dores GM, Gospodarowicz M, van Leeuwen FE, Holowaty E, et al. Breast cancer following radiotherapy and chemotherapy among young women with Hodgkin's Disease. JAMA 2003;290:465–75.

Travis LB, Hill D, Dores GM, Gospodarowicz M, van Leewen FE, Holowaty E, et al. Cumulative absolute breast cancer risk for young women treated for Hodgkin's lymphoma. J Natl Cancer Inst 2005;97:1428–37.

Trichopoulos D. Hypothesis: Does breast cancer originate in utero? Lancet 1990;335:939–40.

Trichopoulos D, Hsieh C-c, MacMahon B, Lin T-m, Lowe CR, Ravnihar B, et al. Age at any birth and breast cancer risk. Int J Cancer 1983;31:701–4.

Trichopoulos D, Kalandidi A, Sparros L, MacMahon B. Lung cancer and passive smoking. Int J Cancer 1981;27:1–4.

Trichopoulos D, Day N, Kaklamani E, Tzonou A, Muñoz N, Zavitsanos X, et al. Hepatitis B virus, tobacco smoking and ethanol consumption in the etiology of hepatocellular carcinoma. Int J Cancer 1987;39:45–49.

Trichopoulos D, Kremastinou J, Tzonou A. Does hepatitis B cause hepatocellular carcinoma? *In* Host Factors in Carcinogenesis. *Eds.* Bartsch H, Armstrong B, Davis W. IARC Scientific Publication No. 39. IARC, Lyon, 1982.

Tseng WP, Chu HM, How SW. Prevalence of skin cancer in an endemic area of chronic arsenicism in Taiwan. J Natl Cancer Inst 1968;40:453–63.

Tuyns AJ. Oesophageal cancer in non-smoking drinkers and in non-drinking smokers. Int J Cancer 1983;32:443–44.

Tuyns AJ, Esteve J, Raymond L, Berrino F, Benhamou E, Blanchet F, et al. Cancer of the larynx/hypopharynx, tobacco and alcohol: IARC international case-control study in Turin and Varese (Italy), Zaragoza and Navarra (Spain), Geneva (Switzerland) and Calvados (France). Int J Cancer 1988;41:483–91.

Ulfelder H. Stilbestrol, adenosis, and adenocarcinoma. Am J Obstet Gynecol 1973;117:794–98.

UNSCEAR, 2000. United Nations Scientific Committee on the Effects of Ionizing Radiation. Sources and Effects of Ionizing Radiation, Report to the General Assembly, with Scientific Annexes. New York, United Nations, 2000.

Van Kaick G, Dalheimer A, Hornik S, Kaul A, Liebermann D, Luhrs H. et al. The German thorotrast study: recent results and assessment of risks. Radiat Res 1999;152(suppl.6):S64–71.

Vaughan TL, Stewart OA, Teschke K, Lynch CF, Swanson GM, Lyon JL, et al. Occupational exposure to formaldehyde and wood dust and nasopharyngeal carcinoma. Occup Environ Med 2000;57:376–84.

Voigt LF, Deng Q, Weiss NS. Recency, duration, and progestin content of oral contraceptives in relation to the incidence of endometrial cancer (Washington, USA). Cancer Causes Control 1994;5:227–33.

Wagner JC. The discovery of the association between blue asbestos and mesotheliomas and the aftermath. Br J Indust Med 1991;48:399–403.

Wagner JC, Sleggs CA, Marchand P. Diffuse pleural mesothelioma and asbestos exposure in the North Western Cape province. Br J Indust Med 1960;17:260–71.

Ward E, Boffetta P, Andersen A, Colin D, Comba P, Deddens JA, et al. Update of mortality and cancer incidence among European workers employed in the vinyl chloride industry. Epidemiology 2001;12:710–8.

Weiderpass E, Adami HO, Baron JA, Magnusson C, Bergstrom R, Lindgren A, et al. Risk of endometrial cancer following estrogen replacement with and without progestins. J Natl Cancer Inst 1999a;91:1131-37.

Weiderpass E, Adami HO, Baron JA, Magnusson C, Lindgren A, Persson I. Use of oral contraceptives and endometrial cancer risk (Sweden). Cancer Causes Control 1999b;10:277–78.

Whittemore AS, Harris R, Itnyre J. Characteristics relating to ovarian cancer risk: collaborative analysis of 12 case-control studies. II. Invasive epithelial ovarian cancer in white women. Collaborative Ovarian Cancer Group. Am J Epidemiol 1992;136:1184–203.

Willett WC. Diet and cancer: one view at the start of the millennium. Cancer Epidemiol Biomarkers Prev 2001:10:3–8.

Wong BC, Lam SK, Wong WM, Chen JS, Zheng TT, Feng RE, et al. Helicobacter pylori eradication to prevent gastric cancer in a high-risk region of China: a controlled trial. JAMA 2004;291;187–94.

Wong O, Raabe GK. Multiple myeloma and benzene exposure in a multinational cohort of more than 250,000 petroleum workers. Regul Toxicol Pharmacol 1997;26:188–99.

Yarborough, CM. Chrysotile as a cause of mesothelioma: an assessment based on epidemiology. Critical Rev Toxicology 2006;36: 165–87.

Yin SN, Li GL, Tain FD, Fu ZI, Jin C, Chen YJ, et al. Leukemia in benzene workers: a retrospective cohort study. Br J Ind Med 1987;44: 124–28.

Ylitalo N, Sorensen P, Josefsson AM, Magnusson PK, Andersen PK, Ponten J, et al. Consistent high viral load of human papillomavirus 16 and risk of carcinoma in situ: a nested case-control study. Lancet 2000;355: 2194–98.

Yu MW, Yeh SH, Chen PJ, Liaw YF, Lin CL, Liu CJ, et al. Hepatitis B virus-genotype and DNA level and hepatocellular carcinoma: a prospective study in men. J Natl Cancer Inst 2005;97:265–72.

Zanetti R, Rosso S, Martinez C, Nieto A, Miranda A, Mercier M, et al. Comparison of risk patterns in carcinoma and melanoma of the skin in men: a multi-centre case-control study. Br J Cancer 2006;94:743–51.

2

Measures and Estimates of Cancer Burden

PAGONA LAGIOU, JOHANNA ADAMI,
AND DIMITRIOS TRICHOPOULOS

Quantifying the burden of any disease is not an easy task. Indeed, no single measure can effectively capture the many dimensions of varying concerns and relevance to the individual, the health care system, and the society at large (Adami, 1993). Many would agree though that reducing mortality from cancer is an overriding goal in cancer control, and hence that mortality is the most relevant outcome. On the other hand, few would disagree that the cure of a young child with leukemia is a more important accomplishment than adding, say, 1 extra year of life to an 85-year-old patient with, for example, stomach cancer. Therefore, in this chapter, we want to address the complexity of the problem, by considering several complementary measures of disease burden with emphasis on cancer. These measures, summarized in Table 2–1, will first be discussed briefly. In the second part of this chapter, we will use some of these measures to outline the public health impact of cancer in different parts of the world.

MEASURES OF DISEASE BURDEN

Incidence

In theory, incidence rates provide the clearest measure of the burden of carcinogenic exposure(s) at the population level (Table 2–1). Incidence rates are the net effect of internal (genetic) and external (environmental) causal and preventive factors, weighted by their frequency and intensity. Synergistic and antagonistic effects between these exposures, whether genetic, environmental, or both, are integrated into the measure. Compared with mortality rates, incidence rates allow, in theory, a more meaningful comparison between populations, ethnic groups, countries, and time periods. This reflects the dependence of mortality rates on prognosis and, hence, treatment effectiveness. In addition, survival rates for many cancers depend markedly on stage at presentation, a function of both public and professional awareness, as well as access to health care.

Table 2–1. Measures of cancer burden, their determinants and limitations.

Measure	Definition	Determinants	Limitations
Incidence	Number of new cases, often per 10^5 person-years or absolute number of cases per year.	Burden of exposure to causes of cancer, weighted by the risk imparted by each cause.	Population-based cancer registration limited to a small proportion of global population. Affected by diagnostic intensity, screening, and autopsy rates.
Cumulative incidence	Proportion of people who develop cancer before a defined age.	Incidence.	Requires no loss to follow-up, no competing risks, same period of follow-up time for all study subjects and unchanged exposure status throughout follow-up.
Prevalence	Proportion of population with cancer.	Incidence, prognosis and mortality from other causes.	Requires population-based registration and follow-up. Cured patients cannot be readily identified.
Survival	Proportion of cancer patients surviving for a specified time after diagnosis.	Natural history of disease Stage at diagnosis Therapeutic efficacy	Requires long-term follow-up of large number of patients. Spurious patterns may arise due to lead-time bias Influenced by diagnostic intensity. Sometimes difficult to classify causes of death correctly.
Mortality	Number of cancer deaths, often per 10^5 person-years, or absolute number of deaths per year.	Incidence Prognosis	Influenced by adequacy of death certification, including autopsy rates.
Life-years lost	Number of years lost between age at death and expected (in the absence of this disease) age at death.	Incidence Age at diagnosis Prognosis	Requires reliable population life tables.
Disability adjusted life years (DALY)	Combines impact of cancer on both quality of life and survival.	Incidence Age at diagnosis Prognosis Expected longevity Residual disability	Requires reliable population life tables. Difficult to quantify disability adequately.

In practice, the use of incidence rates to measure the burden of cancer has numerous limitations. These limitations have been extensively discussed in the literature (Enstrom and Austin, 1977; Doll et al, 1994; Bailar and Gornik, 1997), although their impact may sometimes have been exaggerated. It is obvious, however, that reliable incidence data are available only for a small fraction of the global population (Parkin et al, 1999; 2005b). Beginning in 1966, the International Agency for Research on Cancer (IARC, World Health Organization) has compiled incidence data meeting acceptable standards in a series of informative volumes named *Cancer Incidence in Five Continents*. The eighth edition updates information on incidence rates until about 1997 (Parkin et al, 2003; 2005b).

The reasons why cancer incidence data are available for only a small proportion of the global population are obvious: Population-based cancer registration and calculation of incidence rates require a sophisticated infrastructure that exists only in a limited number of settings. Key prerequisites for reliability include census of the entire population by age and gender, access to adequate diagnostic facilities for everybody, ideally histologic confirmation for a high proportion of cancer cases, and complete, as well as timely, notification of all newly diagnosed (incident) cases to the registry.

Besides problems related to registration efficiency and reliability (which depend on numerous factors, such as proper and prompt diagnosis, coding, and reporting), incidence data may also suffer from more subtle limitations (Table 2–1). These limitations may entail both under- and overestimation of the "true" incidence, and may distort comparisons between population groups and across time periods. For example, increased diagnostic intensity (Helgesen et al, 1996) or introduction of new diagnostic technologies, such as computerized tomography, ultrasound, and magnetic resonance imaging, may advance the time of diagnosis, and may also entail detection of slow-growing nonlethal cancers that would have escaped attention without these technologies. Use of new screening tools—whether in organized or opportunistic settings—would have a similar effect on incidence. The introduction of testing for prostate specific antigen (PSA) to detect early prostate cancer is the preeminent example. Following its widespread use in the US, the reported incidence of prostate cancer increased sharply (Hankey et al, 1999; McDavid et al, 2004). This increase is interpreted as mostly, perhaps completely, artifactual, due to the introduction of new screening (Barry, 2001; McDavid et al, 2004). In contrast, declining autopsy rates may spuriously cause decreasing trends in cancer incidence because more cancers escape diagnosis (Burton et al, 1998).

These potential limitations should not mislead us to underestimate the value of incidence data. They convey unique information that cannot be derived easily from any other measure of disease burden. Indeed, every attempt should be made to increase the coverage of cancer registration, because no other source of data can reveal so directly and timely our successes or failures in cancer prevention. Issues of validity do always need attention, but they should not be carelessly generalized across registries, cancer sites, or time periods. The strengths and potential limitations should be carefully assessed for each specific issue that needs to be addressed. Biologic understanding and clinical experience are often needed to achieve this.

Age-standardization

Frequently, we are interested in comparing incidence rates (or mortality rates—see the following) between populations. A problem that arises when we try to compare crude incidence rates between two or more populations stems from differences in their age distributions, which makes the overall crude rates noncomparable. One way to address this problem is to standardize by age.

Standardization results in comparable weighted averages of the category-specific rates. Indeed, standardization yields the rates expected if the populations being compared had identical age distributions. A standard population with a known age distribution is used (Smith, 1992). In Tables 2–2A and 2–2B, the reported rates are standardized to the world population. Therefore, the rates are the summary rates that one would expect if each country had the same age distribution as the "world" standard. The age-standardized incidence rate of stomach cancer for white US women is 2.6 per 100 000 person-years, while it is 17.6 per 100 000 person-years for women in China. Because both rates have been standardized using the same population, the difference in rates can not be attributed to confounding due to age. Thus, rates, which are standardized to the same standard population, are comparable.

While standardization allows us to compare rates of cancer between different countries, the results we obtain will depend to a certain extent on the specific standard population used. Using one particular standard may occasionally rank country rates differently than if using an alternative population as the standard (Smith, 1992). The main reason for this is that cancer incidence varies strongly with age. In general, more-developed countries have a higher proportion of older people compared to less-developed ones. Moreover, the way in which cancer incidence changes with age can also vary. For example, the incidence rates for stomach cancer in Japan increase rapidly with age, whereas the increase in the corresponding incidence rates in most other countries is more modest (see relevant chapter).

Cumulative Incidence

Cumulative incidence, much like incidence rate, provides a measure of the burden of new disease (Table 2–1). Yet, unlike incidence rates, it is a more interpretable and intuitively appealing measure of disease frequency. Cumulative incidence is defined as the proportion of people who develop disease among those at risk over a specified period of time and is interpreted as the probability, or risk, that an individual will develop disease during that time period (Day, 1992). Tables 2–3A and 2–3B report

cumulative incidence data for the different cancers. For example, the cumulative incidence of an Australian woman developing skin melanoma by age 74 is 27 per 1 000, which can be interpreted as a 2.7% probability or risk of developing skin melanoma by the time she completes 74 years of age (Table 2–3A).

A number of assumptions are necessary in order for the cumulative incidence to be a valid measure (Table 2–1). It assumes that there is no loss to follow-up—the entire population at risk is followed for the same time period. In reality, this is difficult to accomplish over long periods of follow-up. In addition, cumulative incidence measures assume that there are no competing risks, meaning that individuals are not dying from other causes. Often times, assumptions required for cumulative incidence are not realistic and using incidence rates is a more appropriate measure of the disease (Parkin et al, 2003).

Prevalence

Cancer prevalence is defined as the proportion of the entire population, often by gender and age group, with a past or current diagnosis of cancer (Table 2–1). Many of these individuals may have been cured from their malignancy. To provide a more informative measure, one may choose to include only cancers diagnosed during the last 5 years in the prevalence measure. This approach, however, is arbitrary because for many cancers, including breast and prostate, an excess mortality exists for a much longer period following diagnosis and treatment. Prevalence conveys little information relevant to the study of cancer etiology. For example, prevalence may be relatively high for a rare malignancy such as testicular cancer that strikes young individuals and carries a favorable outlook. In contrast, prevalence rates may be low for common cancers with a poor prognosis. Cancers of the lung, liver, and pancreas are typical examples.

Cancer prevalence may, in contrast, provide information useful for the planning of health care resources. In particular, the need for patient care, regular checkups, treatment

Table 2–2A. Age-standardized, to the world population, incidence rates of cancer of various sites among women, per 100,000 person-years.

Cancer Registry	US-W[1]	US-B[2]	UK[3]	Japan[4]	China[5]	Sweden[6]	Netherlands[7]	Spain[8]	Poland[9]	Italy[10]	Uganda[11]	Australia[12]	Brazil[13]	Colombia[14]
Oral and Pharynx*	4.6	5.4	2.7	1.8	3.3	3.1	3.3	1.9	3.1	3.1	4.7	5.0	6.1	4.1
Esophageal	1.2	3.5	2.7	1.6	4.2	0.9	1.7	0.4	1.1	0.7	12.2	1.9	3.0	1.8
Stomach	2.6	5.3	4.4	23.8	17.6	4.4	6.0	7.4	6.6	13.6	5.5	4.0	9.4	18.8
Large Bowel	27.6	34.2	23.3	20.9	19.5	23.2	29.9	19.1	19.5	30.1	7.3	32.2	17.3	14.0
Liver	1.4	2.1	0.7	11.9	9.0	2.3	0.7	2.3	2.5	3.0	6.0	1.0	2.5	2.5
Biliary	1.5	1.5	1.6	5.3	4.1	3.0	2.2	3.1	6.2	2.5	0.1	2.0	3.1	6.6
Pancreas	5.5	9.1	4.5	5.5	4.8	5.3	3.8	3.6	5.4	5.3	1.1	5.0	2.4	4.4
Larynx	1.2	2.0	0.8	0.2	0.3	0.3	1.0	0.4	1.3	1.0	1.1	0.5	1.5	0.9
Lung	34.6	36.8	19.2	13.3	18.2	12.9	14.7	3.7	20.6	10.1	2.3	16.8	8.5	9.5
Skin Melanoma	11.6	0.5	7.1	0.3	0.3	11.9	12.3	3.3	4.1	9.0	2.0	25.9	3.8	2.7
Breast	92.1	83.1	73.9	27.9	27.2	76.5	85.3	51.8	53.7	72.3	20.7	80.7	49.1	37.3
Cervical	6.8	10.2	10.1	7.1	2.3	7.7	6.8	5.6	14.4	6.4	41.7	8.3	38.2	29.8
Endometrial	18.4	12.0	10.0	3.2	4.1	14.3	13.6	10.9	12.7	13.1	3.3	9.4	5.3	5.9
Ovarian	13.2	8.8	13.0	5.7	6.0	15.2	12.8	9.4	12.4	9.9	6.3	8.2	5.5	10.1
Bladder	6.2	4.2	5.8	1.7	1.9	4.8	5.8	3.4	3.5	2.9	1.2	3.3	2.7	2.1
Kidney	4.9	6.4	3.2	1.5	1.5	4.8	4.7	3.8	5.9	6.6	1.1	4.6	2.8	2.3
Brain	4.8	3.0	4.4	2.1	5.7	4.7	4.7	4.9	6.0	5.1	0.4	5.0	5.1	3.6
Thyroid	7.7	4.0	1.9	3.8	3.8	3.5	3.1	3.3	4.3	6.9	4.6	6.3	6.0	6.7
Hodgkins' Disease	2.6	2.0	1.6	0.2	0.2	1.7	1.6	2.2	1.7	3.2	0.7	1.6	1.6	0.8
Non-Hodgkins' Lymphoma	10.6	7.3	6.3	3.6	3.0	6.9	6.6	6.3	4.2	9.8	4.2	10.0	5.9	6.0
Leukemia	7.0	5.3	5.6	4.1	3.6	6.1	5.5	5.3	5.0	6.0	1.6	6.6	4.1	7.3
All cancers	284.6	273.5	240.9	154.6	153.7	235.3	245.4	167.7	211.9	238.7	169.9	259.8	205.2	199.2

*Including lip, tongue, mouth, tonsil, oropharynx, nasopharynx, hypopharynx and pharynx unspecified

[1]USA SEER: white, 1993–97.
[2]USA SEER: black, 1993–97.
[3]Birmingham and West Midlands Region, 1993–97.
[4]Osaka Prefecture, 1993–97.
[5]Shanghai, 1993–97.
[6]Sweden, 1993–97.
[7]Eindhoven, 1993–97.
[8]Zaragoza, 1991–95.
[9]Warsaw City, 1993–97.
[10]Florence, 1993–97.
[11]Kyadondo County, 1993–97.
[12]New South Wales, 1993–97.
[13]Goiania, 1995–98.
[14]Cali, 1992–96.

Table 2–2B. Age-standardized, to the world population, incidence rates of cancer of various sites among men, per 100,000 person-years.

Cancer Registry	US-W[1]	US-B[2]	UK[3]	Japan[4]	China[5]	Sweden[6]	Netherlands[7]	Spain[8]	Poland[9]	Italy[10]	Uganda[11]	Australia[12]	Brazil[13]	Colombia[14]
Oral and Pharynx*	11.6	18.0	5.8	6.3	6.4	6.8	8.5	18.0	9.9	8.3	6.2	15.6	16.0	6.0
Esophageal	4.7	10.7	8.5	10.0	8.2	3.1	4.1	5.2	4.7	2.2	13.2	4.5	10.8	3.9
Stomach	6.6	13.4	14.3	59.9	32.3	8.6	15.3	16.7	16.9	28.4	7.0	9.7	21.7	30.5
Large Bowel	38.4	44.2	38.4	35.8	20.5	30.3	43.2	29.4	29.4	46.2	7.7	47.9	16.5	12.2
Liver	3.8	7.1	2.0	44.5	23.3	4.1	1.4	6.1	4.1	9.3	6.5	3.7	3.7	3.0
Biliary	1.4	1.4	1.7	6.2	2.4	2.0	2.3	1.9	3.9	2.7	0.0	1.9	3.0	2.6
Pancreas	7.3	12.5	6.1	9.4	5.6	6.3	5.7	5.8	7.5	7.7	1.0	6.4	3.0	4.6
Larynx	5.3	9.6	4.3	3.2	2.3	2.2	6.3	18.0	10.2	11.2	1.3	4.7	6.4	5.0
Lung	54.4	85.9	50.6	44.6	44.4	22.0	73.0	50.3	64.4	57.7	3.9	42.0	22.3	22.3
Skin Melanoma	15.4	1.0	5.2	0.4	0.3	11.8	8.9	2.7	4.1	7.5	1.3	36.9	5.1	2.5
Breast	0.7	1.1	0.6	0.2	0.3	0.4	0.5	0.8	0.5	0.8	1.0	0.6	0.7	0.1
Prostate	107.8	185.4	39.9	9.0	3.0	63.0	52.1	30.7	22.2	35.1	37.1	90.1	92.4	42.2
Testis	5.6	1.0	5.3	1.2	0.7	5.0	4.4	2.2	4.2	3.3	0.5	5.1	0.5	1.9
Bladder	23.3	11.3	21.3	8.1	6.2	17.8	28.4	27.9	18.0	18.7	2.9	12.3	11.2	6.1
Kidney	9.6	12.1	7.0	4.4	2.6	7.8	8.2	6.5	12.2	13.7	1.0	8.7	3.9	2.9
Brain	7.0	4.0	6.3	2.7	5.4	6.6	6.2	8.1	7.7	6.0	0.8	6.9	8.0	5.0
Thyroid	2.8	1.4	0.8	1.2	1.1	1.3	0.8	0.9	1.4	2.5	0.6	2.2	2.1	1.6
Hodgkins' Disease	3.1	2.7	2.3	0.4	0.4	2.0	2.9	3.2	2.5	3.8	1.2	2.0	2.8	1.5
Non-Hodgkins' Lymphoma	16.8	15.4	9.8	6.3	4.3	10.1	9.8	8.9	6.5	12.9	5.8	14.2	6.8	7.3
Leukemia	11.2	8.8	8.1	6.0	5.0	8.7	8.9	7.4	6.2	9.1	0.9	10.6	5.2	8.6
All Cancers	364.5	485.5	275.3	272.4	188.7	243.7	322.6	273.9	259.4	313.2	158.1	359.0	268.9	192.2

*Including lip, tongue, mouth, tonsil, oropharynx, nasopharynx, hypopharynx and pharynx unspecified

[1] USA SEER: white, 1993–97.
[2] USA SEER: black, 1993–97.
[3] Birmingham and West Midlands Region, 1993–97.
[4] Osaka Prefecture, 1993–97.
[5] Shanghai, 1993–97.
[6] Sweden, 1993–97.
[7] Eindhoven, 1993–97.
[8] Zaragoza, 1991–95.
[9] Warsaw City, 1993–97.
[10] Florence, 1993–97.
[11] Kyadondo County, 1993–97.
[12] New South Wales, 1993–97.
[13] Goiania, 1995–98.
[14] Cali, 1992–96.

39

Table 2-3A. Cumulative incidence, per 1000 persons, of cancer of various sites among women by age 74.*

Cancer Registry	US-W[1]	US-B[2]	UK[3]	Japan[4]	China[5]	Sweden[6]	Netherlands[7]	Spain[8]	Poland[9]	Italy[10]	Uganda[11]	Australia[12]	Brazil[13]	Colombia[14]
Oral and Pharynx**	6	7	3	2	4	4	4	2	3	3	5	6	8	5
Esophageal	2	5	4	2	5	1	2	1	1	1	17	2	4	2
Stomach	3	6	6	26	21	5	6	7	7	14	7	4	12	22
Large Bowel	32	40	27	24	24	28	36	22	23	35	10	38	21	16
Liver	2	2	1	16	11	3	1	3	3	4	7	1	3	3
Biliary	2	2	2	6	5	4	3	4	7	3	0	2	4	9
Pancreas	6	11	5	6	6	7	5	4	6	6	2	6	3	5
Larynx	2	3	1	0	1	0	1	0	2	1	1	1	2	1
Lung	45	47	25	15	23	17	18	4	27	12	3	22	11	11
Skin Melanoma	12	1	7	0	0	12	11	3	5	9	3	27	4	3
Breast	107	95	81	30	30	87	96	57	66	81	22	91	57	43
Cervical	7	10	10	8	3	8	7	6	15	6	44	8	44	33
Endometrial	23	15	12	4	5	19	17	14	16	16	4	12	7	8
Ovarian	15	10	15	6	7	17	15	10	14	11	7	9	6	12
Bladder	8	5	7	2	2	6	7	4	4	3	2	4	4	2
Kidney	6	7	4	2	2	6	5	4	7	8	1	5	3	3
Brain	5	3	5	2	6	5	4	5	6	5	0	5	5	4
Thyroid	7	4	2	4	4	3	3	3	4	7	5	6	6	7
Hodgkins' Disease	2	2	1	0	0	1	1	2	1	3	1	1	1	1
Non-Hodgkins' Lymphoma	12	8	7	4	3	8	8	7	5	11	4	11	7	7
Leukemia	7	5	5	4	3	6	5	5	4	5	1	6	4	7
All Cancers	327	316	257	170	178	268	274	181	238	260	182	291	237	227

*Interpretable as probability

**Including lip, tongue, mouth, tonsil, oropharynx, nasopharynx, hypopharynx and pharynx unspecified

[1]USA SEER: white, 1993–97.
[2]USA SEER: black, 1993–97.
[3]Birmingham and West Midlands Region, 1993–97.
[4]Osaka Prefecture, 1993–97.
[5]Shanghai, 1993–97.
[6]Sweden, 1993–97.
[7]Eindhoven, 1993–97.
[8]Zaragoza, 1991–95.
[9]Warsaw City, 1993–97.
[10]Florence, 1993–97.
[11]Kyadondo County, 1993–97.
[12]New South Wales, 1993–97.
[13]Goiania, 1995–98.
[14]Cali, 1992–96.

Table 2–3B. Cumulative incidence, per 1000 persons, of cancer of various sites among men by age 74.*

Cancer	US-W[1]	US-B[2]	UK[3]	Japan[4]	China[5]	Sweden[6]	Netherlands[7]	Spain[8]	Poland[9]	Italy[10]	Uganda[11]	Australia[12]	Brazil[13]	Colombia[14]
Oral	14	22	7	8	7	8	10	21	12	10	7	20	19	8
Esophageal	6	14	10	13	10	4	5	6	6	2	16	5	14	5
Stomach	8	16	17	70	40	10	19	20	20	32	8	11	27	35
Large Bowel	46	53	45	43	26	36	53	35	35	56	8	58	18	14
Liver	5	8	2	59	27	5	2	8	5	12	8	5	5	4
Biliary	2	2	2	7	3	2	3	2	4	3	0	2	4	3
Pancreas	9	15	7	11	7	8	7	7	9	9	1	8	4	5
Larynx	7	13	6	4	3	3	8	22	13	14	2	6	8	6
Lung	70	111	63	52	60	29	92	65	83	75	5	54	27	27
Skin Melanoma	17	1	5	0	0	13	9	3	5	8	2	41	5	3
Breast	1	1	1	0	0	1	1	1	1	1	1	1	1	0
Prostate	146	253	43	9	4	78	63	37	27	41	45	115	118	51
Testis	4	1	4	1	1	4	4	2	3	3	1	4	0	2
Bladder	28	14	25	9	8	22	34	34	22	23	4	15	15	7
Kidney	12	14	8	5	3	9	10	7	15	16	1	11	4	4
Brain	7	4	7	2	6	6	6	8	8	7	1	7	8	5
Thyroid	3	2	1	1	1	1	1	1	2	2	1	2	2	2
Hodgkins' Disease	3	2	2	0	0	2	2	3	2	3	2	2	2	1
Non-Hodgkins' Lymphoma	18	16	11	7	5	11	11	10	7	13	5	15	8	8
Leukemia	11	10	8	5	4	9	9	7	6	9	1	10	5	8
All Cancers	445	612	309	319	231	286	384	323	308	368	175	426	326	219

*Interpretable as probability

**Including lip, tongue, mouth, tonsil, oropharynx, nasopharynx, hypopharynx and pharynx unspecified

[1] USA SEER: white, 1993–97.
[2] USA SEER: black, 1993–97.
[3] Birmingham and West Midlands Region, 1993–97.
[4] Osaka Prefecture, 1993–97.
[5] Shanghai, 1993–97.
[6] Sweden, 1993–97.
[7] Eindhoven, 1993–97.
[8] Zaragoza, 1991–95.
[9] Warsaw City, 1993–97.
[10] Florence, 1993–97.
[11] Kyadondo County, 1993–97.
[12] New South Wales, 1993–97.
[13] Goiania, 1995–98.
[14] Cali, 1992–96.

of long-term complications (whether due to the disease or the treatment), and resources for terminal care will depend critically on the number of subjects in the population with a cancer diagnosis. Prevalence may increase as a consequence of improved prognosis, even if incidence rates are stable. Advancement of the time of diagnosis (lead-time) following introduction of screening may further increase cancer prevalence. The impact of these factors may not be trivial, particularly in developed countries.

Notwithstanding its relevance to health care planning, cancer prevalence has been estimated only in a few settings. The reason is obvious: Prevalence is difficult to capture through population surveys because willingness to participate may differ between subjects with and without cancer. Reliable estimates of cancer prevalence require linkage between long-term cancer registration and survival databases, as well as updated population registers.

Survival

To affected patients and to clinicians, probability of survival is of paramount interest. In this book, survival data are provided chiefly in the clinical synopsis for each cancer site. Despite their intuitive appeal as a measure of prognosis and therapeutic efficacy, survival data have numerous determinants, limitations, and pitfalls, as indicated in Table 2–1. This is not to say that any other measure could replace survival data. Indeed, survival is the best available measure for evaluating the effectiveness of cancer care (the diagnosis and treatment of cancer). We need, however, to be aware of the different survival measures because they serve different purposes, and each has its limitations. These measures, though, have one prerequisite in common, namely the need for complete follow-up. If this cannot be achieved, we need to know the date when follow-up ended for each patient. The calculated survival probabilities would be correct only if losses to follow-up are unrelated to the outcome—that is, if we do not lose track preferentially of those with a good or bad prognosis.

The *observed survival* can be most readily calculated. This conveys the probability of surviving a specified time period, typically starting at the date of cancer diagnosis. Hence, all causes of death are taken into consideration, both those linked to the cancer of interest and those due to other diseases such as coronary heart disease, infections, or accidents. It is true that the malignancy is the predominant, often the overwhelming, cause of death, particularly during the early years of follow-up of a cancer patient. But as time goes by and the patients get older, these other causes are bound to play an increasingly important role. They create a "baseline" death rate to which the cancer-specific rate is added. If two groups with a similar baseline rate are compared, then the absolute difference in survival between the two groups may be relatively stable over time. As the baseline rate grows, however, the relative difference will be lower if all causes of death are considered than if only deaths caused by the malignant disease of interest are considered.

The cause-specific, sometimes-called *corrected*, survival provides a more valid estimate of the excess death rate attributable to the particular cancer under study. It does so by not counting deaths from other causes. Such patients are "censored" at their date of death from another cause, just as other subjects are "censored" at the end of follow-up, or when they are lost to follow-up. There is an important assumption when calculating corrected survival rates, namely that the cause of death is correctly classified. This cause may be obvious in a cancer patient who dies with disseminated advanced disease following a period with, for example, progressive fatigue, cachexia, jaundice, or organ failure. It is often also easy to correctly classify death in an apparently cancer-free patient who dies from a typical myocardial infarction. From time to time, however, attributing death to one specific cause may be complex or impossible, even if an autopsy is carried out. A gray zone exists, in which the malignancy may be a contributing cause of death. Residual disease, side effects of treatment, or other morbidity may act synergistically, making it difficult to assign one underlying cause of death. Fortunately, this gray zone is small in most instances and therefore corrected survival provides a reliable estimate of prognosis, uninfluenced by other causes. Corrected survival also allows more meaningful comparisons between patient groups with a different age distribution.

Calculation of the *relative survival* is based on a statistical methodology that allows the investigator to be independent of information about causes of death in the individual patients. It does so by relating the observed survival to that expected in a group from the general population with the same distribution of age and gender. Two basic assumptions must be met to assure valid estimates of relative survival. First, we need information about survival prospects in the absence of cancer. Reliable life tables from the general population must be available. Second, the group of cancer patients under study must have the same "baseline" risk of dying as the general population. For example, people who belong to a lower socioeconomic class or who smoke have a higher death rate than the general population at large. If such individuals are overrepresented in the group of cancer patients studied, then their baseline risk of dying will be underestimated. Hence, the relative survival will overestimate the excess death risk attributable to their cancers. In most situations, however, corrected and relative survival indices agree reasonably well, as they should, because their goal is the same.

Recently, attention has been drawn to the fact that the available estimates of survival are based on patients diagnosed several years in the past. For instance, in order to estimate 10-year survival, traditional methods require a cohort of patients in which at least some individuals are diagnosed more than 10 years in the past and all patients contribute to the survival proportion for the first year, including those diagnosed 10 or more years ago. It has been suggested that it might be more appropriate to estimate each of the successive conditional survival proportions using only the most recently diagnosed pa-

tients (Brenner et al, 2004; Dickman and Adami, 2006). For example, the conditional survival proportion for the first year would be based on patients diagnosed during the previous year; the conditional survival proportion for the second year would be based on patients diagnosed the year before that; and so on. Patients diagnosed many years in the past would only contribute to the estimates of conditional survival proportions for later intervals. This approach has been termed *period analysis* and allows for more accurate prediction of the survival of newly diagnosed groups of patients (Dickman and Adami, 2006).

Mortality

Because cancer mortality rates measure, at the population level, the rate of dying from specific, or from all, cancer(s), they are widely considered the single most important set of indicators of the burden of cancer (Table 2–1). Mortality is also the preferred measure for evaluating secondary prevention programs. However, individuals who are cured do not appear in the mortality statistics, thereby reducing the utility of mortality as a measure of the overall cancer burden. Nevertheless, reduction in mortality is the standard target for improvements in cancer control.

Mortality rates have several advantages. Foremost is their much wider availability than cancer incidence rates. Compilation of cancer mortality statistics is an easier task than obtaining any of the measures previously discussed. No follow-up is required, death is an unequivocal event (whereas definite histologic classification of malignancy is less trivial than generally perceived), and in many societies a death certificate is required before a funeral can take place. Indeed early attempts to collect death statistics began in the seventeenth century. Modern death registries were established in most developed countries by the middle of the twentieth century. In 1990, the coverage of mortality statistics ranged from only about 1% in the sub-Saharan Africa to around 40% in Latin America and close to 100% in economically developed countries (Murray and Lopez, 1996a).

Mortality rates have limitations too (Table 2–1), and these have sometimes been underestimated. The reliability of this measure depends critically on how accurately causes of death are classified. As already discussed, even in a patient with a known cancer diagnosis, it is not always easy to tell whether this disease was the underlying or a contributing cause of death, or whether it was irrelevant. In settings without public awareness of early cancer symptoms, poor access to health care, limited facilities for diagnostic work up, or low autopsy rates, opportunities for misclassification of causes of death are abundant.

Little information exists to enlighten us about the validity of mortality statistics and the comparability of rates across different populations and time periods (Murray and Lopez, 1996a, b). Moreover, mortality rates do not meaningfully reflect the burden of certain cancers with a favorable prognosis. Some cancers in that category are common, such as nonmelanoma skin cancer and endometrial cancer, whereas others with a high cure rate are rare, for example cancer of the thyroid and testis. At the other end of the spectrum, mortality rates approximate incidence rates for cancers that remain almost inevitably fatal, for example those of the lung, esophagus, liver, and pancreas.

Years of Life Lost

Though introduced relatively recently and not widely used, years of life lost (YLL) accommodate the fundamental differences between dying from cancer in childhood versus later in life (Table 2–1). This measure can also be obtained at the group level from computer programs that calculate relative survival rates. Ranking cancers by YLL rather than by incidence or mortality rates can dramatically influence the apparent impact of a specific form of cancer. For example, prostate cancer is by far the most common cancer in men in many western populations, sometimes accounting for 25% or more of all diagnosed cancers. However, age at diagnosis is typically high, often over 75 years. Therefore, if cancers are ranked by YLL at the population level, then, in the US, prostate cancer is reduced to the eighth most important malignancy. If, on the other hand, cancers are ranked by YLL per person dying of cancer, then the average for all cancers is 15.3 years, while for prostate cancer it is 9.2 years corresponding to a rank of 21 (Ries et al, 1997).

Disability-adjusted Life Years

By definition, one disability-adjusted life year (DALY) is one lost year of healthy life (Table 2–1). The attraction of DALY is that the impact of time and disability is integrated into one single measure. As a further development of an older concept, the quality-adjusted life year (QUALY), DALY uses as its reference the population of Japan, which has presently the world's longest life expectancy. Two parameters must be known to allow calculation of total DALYs in a defined population: the total number of life years lost due to the disease of interest, and the number of these years lived with a disability of known severity. For obvious reasons, assigning quantitative scores to disability is difficult or indeed arbitrary. Besides, the values involved in determining these scores may differ both within and between populations and they may undergo temporal changes.

Notwithstanding these limitations, DALY is a valuable tool. Few would disagree that life is a matter of both quality and quantity. Hence, rather than dismissing DALY, we should try to improve this measure through open discourse of our individual value systems and use DALY as a complement to other measures of disease burden. Although DALYs may convey limited biologic information, they may provide important guidance in developing public health priorities.

CANCER IN THE WORLD

Cancer and Other Causes of Death

Table 2–4 shows the 10 leading causes of death in low/middle- and high-income countries in 2001 (Lopez et al, 2006). In high-income countries, cancer mortality accounts for a considerable fraction of the deaths. Indeed, lung cancer is the third leading cause of death, with colorectal, breast, and stomach cancers also included in the list of 10 leading causes of death. These four cancers alone account for about 13% of all deaths in high-income countries. In contrast, cancer does not account for such a substantial fraction of mortality in low- and middle-income countries. It is expected, however, that in the coming years, as a result of the far-reaching and ever-increasing western influences of diet and tobacco, and changing age distributions in developing countries, cancer will account for a growing proportion of deaths in these countries.

The measures of disease burden described in the previous section can be used to determine the relative role of cancer to overall morbidity and mortality in any population throughout the world. As earlier indicated, however, incidence data are available only for a small proportion of the global population. Nationwide cancer registries exist in a small number of European countries, notably the Nordic ones. In the US, Japan, and most European countries, cancer registry coverage is far from complete, while in Africa and South America, it is quite limited. In developing countries, overall estimates are forced to rely primarily on extrapolation from the small number of available registries (Murray and Lopez, 1996a, b; Parkin et al, 2005b).

Cancer Burden by Site

It is estimated that close to 11 million new cases of cancer occurred throughout the world in the year 2002, excluding the rarely fatal nonmelanoma cases of skin cancer (Parkin et al, 2005a). There is considerable variation in the fatality of cancer depending on cancer site, histological type, and clinical stage. Whilst mortality is close to nil for an early diagnosed testicular or endometrial cancer, pancreatic cancer and hepatocellular carcinoma are almost invariably fatal. Life expectancy in the general population is reduced by an average of between 2 and 3 years depending on availability and utilization of health care.

Figures 2–1A (women) and 2–1B (men) provide age-standardized, to the world

Table 2–4. Leading causes of death in low/middle- and high-income countries in 2001.

	Low-and-middle-income countries			High-income countries	
Cause		Percent of total deaths	Cause		Percent of total deaths
1	Ischaemic heart disease	11.8	1	Ischaemic heart disease	17.3
2	Cerebrovascular disease	9.5	2	Cerebrovascular disease	9.9
3	Lower respiratory infections	7.0	3	Trachea, bronchus, lung cancers	5.8
4	HIV/AIDS	5.3	4	Lower respiratory infections	4.4
5	Perinatal conditions	5.1	5	Chronic obstructive pulmonary disease	3.8
6	Chronic obstructive pulmonary disease	4.9	6	Colon and rectum cancers	3.3
7	Diarrhoeal diseases	3.7	7	Alzheimer's disease and other dementias	2.6
8	Tuberculosis	3.3	8	Diabetes mellitus	2.6
9	Malaria	2.5	9	Breast cancer	2.0
10	Road traffic accidents	2.2	10	Stomach cancer	1.9
Total number of deaths		48.5 million	Total number of deaths		7.9 million

Source: Modified from Lopez et al, 2006.

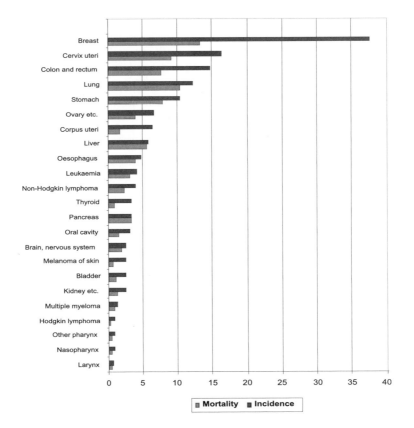

Figure 2–1A. Age-standardized, to the world population, Incidence and Mortality Rates, per 100,000 Women-Years, by Cancer Site, excluding non-melanoma skin cancer- Estimated world total, around 2000. (*Source*: Ferlay et al, 2004)

population, incidence and mortality rates, per 100 000 person per years, by cancer site in the world overall around 2000 (Ferlay et al, 2004). The comparison between mortality and incidence rates allows a crude assessment of the fatality of each type of cancer. Thus, mortality rates provide good approximation of incidence rates for liver or pancreatic cancer, but not for breast, prostate, or colorectal cancer. Among women, breast cancer is both the most common form of malignancy and the one causing the higher number of cancer deaths, although fewer than 50% of women with breast cancer die from this disease. Cancer of the uterine cervix is the second most common form of cancer among women around the world (always excluding nonmelanoma skin cancer), but it causes fewer deaths than

cancer of the lung, because of the higher fatality of the latter form of cancer.

Among men, lung cancer causes the higher number of new cases as well as deaths, whereas cancer of the stomach is in second place in terms of deaths, because of the high incidence in China and Japan and its high fatality. It is also notable that prostate cancer, on the global scale, causes fewer deaths than those caused by cancers of the stomach, large bowel, liver, or the esophagus, although its incidence is very high and increasing on account of expanding testing for the prostate specific antigen.

A comparison between Figures 2–1A and B reveals that, besides lung cancer, several other malignancies are substantially more common in men than in women. Foremost, this applies to the upper gastrointestinal tract

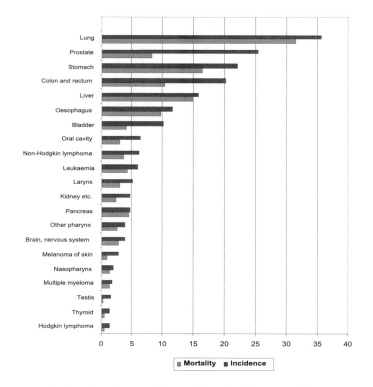

Figure 2–1B. Age-standardized, to the world population, Incidence and Mortality Rates, per 100,000 Men-Years, by Cancer Site, excluding non-melanoma skin cancer—Estimated world total, around 2000. (*Source*: Ferlay et al, 2004)

(oral-pharynx, esophagus, and stomach), liver, urinary bladder, and non-Hodgkin lymphomas. Only cancers of the gallbladder (not shown in Fig. 2–1) and thyroid are consistently more common in women.

Cancer Burden by Cause

At the beginning of the twenty-first century, the total number of cancer-related deaths in the world was estimated to be almost 7 million per year (Ferlay et al, 2004; Parkin et al, 2005a). Table 2–5 presents individual and joint contributions of specific causal factors to mortality from site-specific cancer (Danaei et al, 2005). A total number of 2.4 million (almost 35%) of all cancer deaths were attributable to the following risk factors: smoking, alcohol, low fruit and vegetable intake, overweight and obesity, physical inactivity, contaminated injections, indoor smoke from household use of solid fuels, urban air pollution, and unsafe sex.

Smoking alone is estimated to have caused 21% of deaths from cancer worldwide.

There are a number of interventions that can affect cancer incidence and mortality, such as hepatitis B vaccine for liver cancer, screening methods for cervical cancer, faecal occult blood test for colorectal cancer, mammography for breast cancer, and surgical prevention for those at high risk of colorectal cancer. Some other preventive interventions, such as sputum cytology and chest radiographs for lung cancer, have not been successful. Lastly, there are preventive interventions that warrant further investigation with respect to effectiveness, including vaccines for human papilloma virus to prevent anogenital cancers, and eradication of Helicobacter pylori infection in the stomach to prevent stomach cancer. Control of interventions that could affect cancer burden in the world is highly dependent on cost and health-system characteristics. This

Table 2–5. Individual and joint contributions of causal factors to mortality from site-specific cancers in the world, around 2000.

Cancer site	Total (in thousands per year)	PAF(%) and number of attributable cancer deaths (thousands) for individual risk factors	Due to joint hazards of risk factors
Mouth and oropharynx	312	Alcohol use (16%), smoking (42%)	52%
Oesophageal	438	Alcohol use (26%), smoking (42%), low fruit and vegetable intake (18%)	62%
Stomach	842	Smoking (13%), low fruit and vegetable intake (18%)	28%
Colon and rectum	614	Overweight and obesity (11%), physical inactivity (15%), low fruit and vegetable intake (2%)	13%
Liver	606	Smoking (14%), alcohol use (25%), contaminated injections in health-care settings (18%)	47%
Pancreatic	227	Smoking (22%)	22%
Trachea, bronchus, and lung	1227	Smoking (70%), low fruit and vegetable intake (11%), indoor smoke from household use of solid fuels (1%), urban air pollution (5%)	74%
Breast	472	Alcohol use (5%), overweight and obesity (9%), physical inactivity (10%)	21%
Cervix uteri	235	Smoking (2%), unsafe sex (100%)	100%
Corpus uteri	71	Overweight and obesity (40%)	40%
Bladder	175	Smoking (28%)	28%
Leukaemia	263	Smoking (9%)	9%
All other cancers	1538	Alcohol use (0.6%)	0.6%
All cancers	7020	Alcohol use (5%), smoking (21%), low fruit and vegetable intake (5%), indoor smoke from household use of solid fuels (<0.5%), urban air pollution (1%), overweight and obesity (2%), physical inactivity (2%), contaminated injections in health-care settings (2%), unsafe sex (3%)	35%

Source: Modified from Danaei et al, 2005.

reinforces the importance of primary prevention through lifestyle and environmental interventions when developing future policies and programs.

Trends in Mortality in the US

Figure 2–2 shows trends of mortality from cancer among women (2–2A) and men (2–2B) in the US (Jemal et al, 2006). Although trends vary around the world, the pattern in the US exemplifies the dynamic changes typical for many developed countries. The sharp increase in the mortality from lung cancer among both women and men during most of the twentieth century reflects the tobacco-smoking epidemic, whereas the decline in mortality during the last few years reflects the earlier abatement of that epidemic among men, but less so among women.

Among women, there are hopeful signs that mortality from breast cancer may have started to decline in several settings, including the United Kingdom (WHO, 2006). Mortality from cancer of the cervix has also declined, to a large extent because of Papanicolaou test screening entailing detection and removal of precursor lesions before they had progressed to invasive and therefore potentially lethal cancer. Among both women and men, mortality from stomach cancer is rapidly declining reflecting a similar decline in incidence. Reasons for this dramatic trend are not clear. However, improved hygienic conditions and patterns of food preservation and reduction or post-

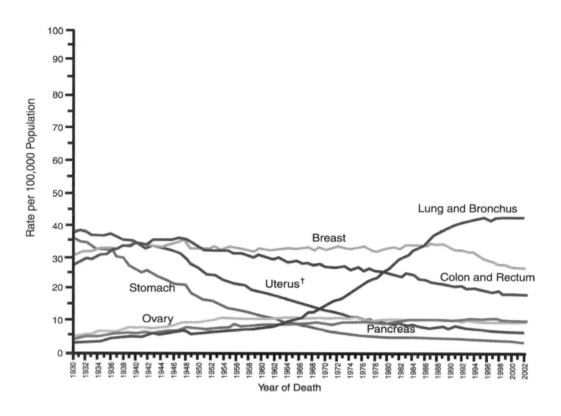

†Uterus includes uterine cervix and uterine corpus.

Figure 2–2A. Age- standardized, to the 2000 US standard population, cancer death rates (per 100,000 person-years) among women for selected cancers, US, 1930 to 2002. (*Source*: US Mortality Public Use Data Tapes, 1960 to 2002, US Mortality Volumes 1930 to 1959, National Center for Health Statistics, Centers for Disease Control and Prevention, 2005 [as reported by Jemal et al, 2006])

ponement of infection with Helicobacter pylori are probably important. Mortality from cancer of the large bowel initially increased, perhaps reflecting detrimental changes in dietary habits, but later declined, mostly among women, for reasons that are not obvious.

Two points need to be stressed. First, time and place mortality patterns mostly reflect concomitant incidence patterns. Exceptions include time trends of mortality from childhood leukemia, testicular cancer, and lymphomas, which declined because of improved treatment efficacy. And second, cancer mortality overall does not show, at least after 1950, an increasing trend with the ex-

ception of tobacco-related cancers, which shadow the tobacco epidemic. In fact, in several developed countries, there are hopeful indications of a decline (WHO, 2006).

Geographic Variability by Site

Table 2–2 shows age-adjusted incidence rates of several of the most important cancer sites per hundred thousand person years for women (1.2A) and men (1.2B) in selected registries around the world. The geographic variability is substantial even though it does not capture the variability within countries than can also be considerable. Thus, it is known, for example, that within Iran incidence of esophageal cancer

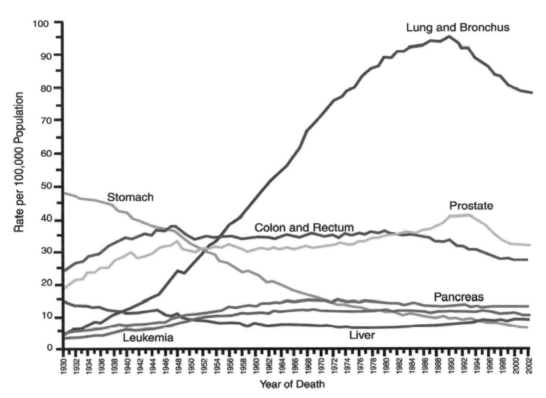

Figure 2–2B. Age- standardized, to the 2000 US standard population, cancer death rates (per 100,000 person-years) among men for selected cancers, US, 1930 to 2002. (*Source*: US Mortality Public Use Data Tapes, 1960 to 2002, US Mortality Volumes, 1930 to 1959, National Center for Health Statistics, Centers for Disease Control and Prevention, 2005 [as reported by Jemal et al, 2006])

varies more than 10-fold. Striking geographical variations exist also within large countries, such as China and India.

Figures 2–3A to 2–9 portray the geographical variability of major forms of cancer in selected registries. The indicated registries correspond to, although they do not necessarily represent, the six continents.

Stomach cancer is very common in Japan. Some researchers explain this in terms of the high salt consumption by the Japanese population. The disease is also common in Brazil and other countries of South America, particularly Colombia, possibly because of the low socioeconomic conditions in large fractions of the respective population. Such conditions facilitate early infection with Helicobacter pylori, an established cause for this malignancy. High consumption of food of plant origin may be responsible for

the relatively low incidence of stomach cancer in many African countries, notwithstanding the low socioeconomic status of the corresponding populations. Whilst it is obvious that the disease is twice as common among men as in women, the reason for the gender difference is not understood (Figs. 2–3A and 2–3B).

Cancer of the large bowel is uncommon in Uganda, where consumption of meat is low and intake of plant foods is high. The incidence of large bowel cancer has rapidly increased in Japan after World War II following the substantial dietary changes in that population during this period. Indeed, the speed of the change may indicate that the westernized diet increases risk of colorectal cancer at a late stage of the natural history of this disease. Cancer of the large bowel is common in both genders (Figs. 2–4A

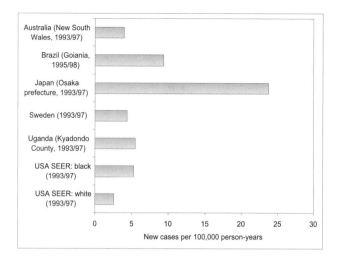

Figure 2–3A. Age-standardized, to the world population, incidence rates of stomach cancer among women. Data derived from cancer registries.

and 2–4B), although, for unknown reasons, men have generally higher incidence of rectal cancer.

Primary liver cancer is rare in western countries, but common in South East Asia and sub-Saharan Africa, reflecting the prev-alence pattern of the carcinogenic hepatitis B and C viruses. Primary liver cancer in Europe and North America is linked to alcoholic cirrhosis, other forms of cirrhosis, as well as tobacco smoking (Figs. 2–5A and 2–5B).

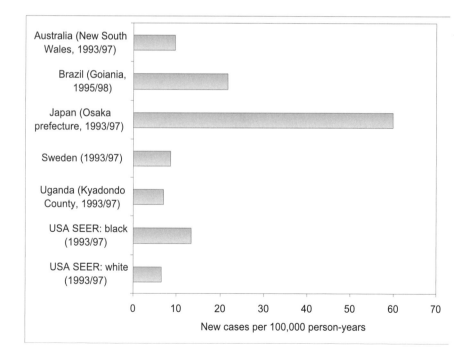

Figure 2–3B. Age-standardized, to the world population, incidence rates of stomach cancer among men. Data derived from cancer registries.

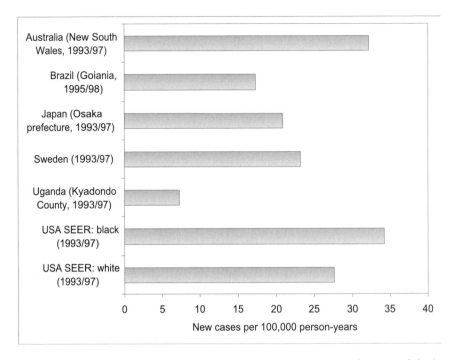

Figure 2–4A. Age-standardized, to the world population, incidence rates of cancer of the large bowel among women. Data derived from cancer registries.

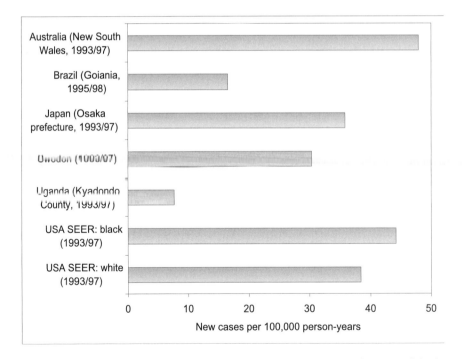

Figure 2–4B. Age-standardized, to the world population, incidence rates of cancer of the large bowel among men. Data derived from cancer registries.

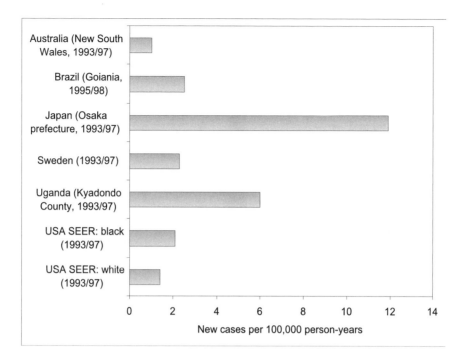

Figure 2–5A. Age-standardized, to the world population, incidence rates of liver cancer among women. Data derived from cancer registries.

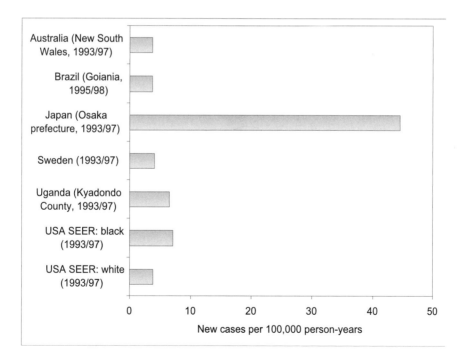

Figure 2–5B. Age-standardized, to the world population, incidence rates of liver cancer among men. Data derived from cancer registries.

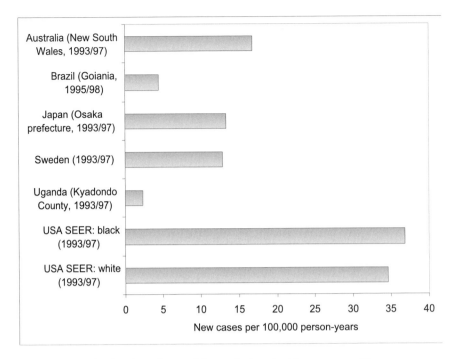

Figure 2–6A. Age-standardized, to the world population, incidence rates of lung cancer among women. Data derived from cancer registries.

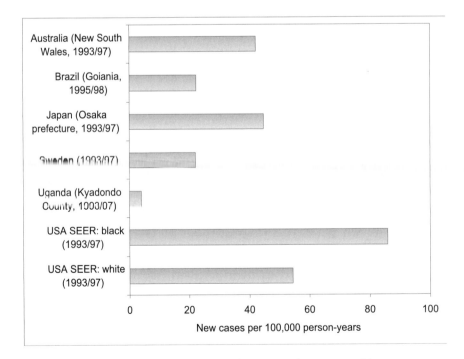

Figure 2–6B. Age-standardized, to the world population, incidence rates of lung cancer among men. Data derived from cancer registries.

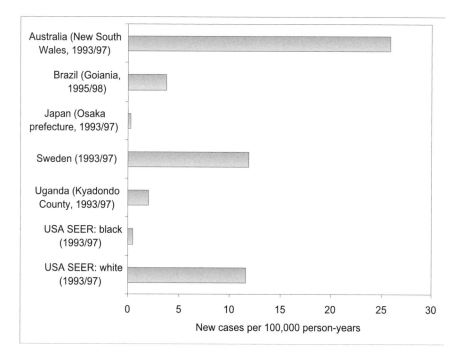

Figure 2–7A. Age-standardized, to the world population, incidence rates of melanoma among women. Data derived from cancer registries.

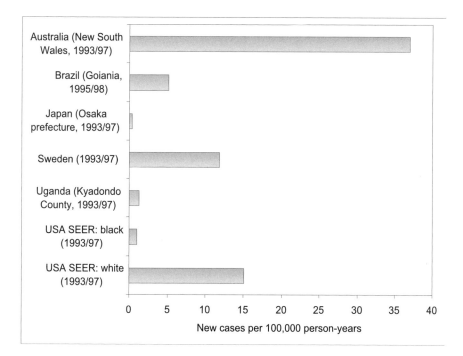

Figure 2–7B. Age-standardized, to the world population, incidence rates of melanoma among men. Data derived from cancer registries.

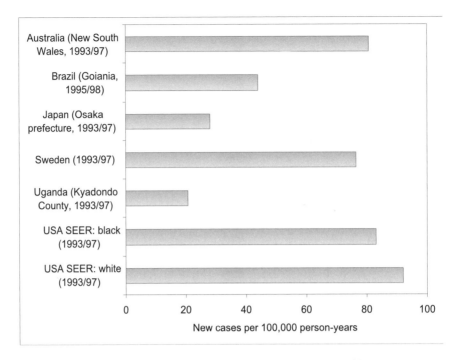

Figure 2–8. Age-standardized, to the world population, incidence rates of breast cancer among women. Data derived from cancer registries.

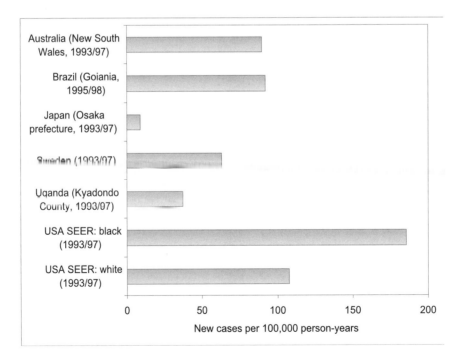

Figure 2–9. Age-standardized, to the world population, incidence rates of prostate cancer among men. Data derived from cancer registries.

Lung cancer is a world epidemic. Geographic and gender patterns reflect the stage of that epidemic. The incidence of the disease is higher among men than among women, due to the earlier spread of the smoking habit among men than among women. Poverty and tradition limit accessibility and utilization of cigarettes among Ugandans who are thus at low risk of lung cancer, whereas the lower rates in Sweden in comparison to the US reflect the earlier and more effective adoption of antismoking measures in the former country (Figs. 2–6A and 2–6B).

The incidence pattern of skin melanoma around the world could have immediately indicated to an uninitiated, but careful, person the principal causes of skin melanoma, sun exposure and skin color. Australians, who are mostly white and are intensely exposed to sunlight, have the highest incidence of melanoma in the world, whereas among US women and men, whites have much higher incidence in comparison to blacks (Figs. 2–7A and 2–7B).

Breast cancer is becoming a universal problem among women. Even in Japan and Uganda, where current rates are about one-third of the corresponding rates in US whites, the incidence is increasing. Nevertheless, the difference in breast cancer rates between Caucasian women in western countries and Asian women in China and Japan remains a challenging observation in the epidemiology of breast cancer (Fig. 2–8).

Among common cancers, few show such a striking international variability as prostate cancer, even though the excess cancer incidence in the US reflects to a substantial extent the wide-spread use of screening with the prostate specific antigen. Some researchers attribute the variability to different exposures to promoting or growth-enhancing rather than initiating agents, because the prevalence of subclinical prostate cancer detected at autopsy is fairly uniform around the world (Fig. 2–9).

The most important conclusion to be drawn from the large international variability of incidence around the world is that virtually all forms of cancer are largely preventable through environmental modifica-

tions (Doll and Peto, 1981). The rival explanation, that differences are due to different genetic constitution of the various populations, has been rejected when groups of migrants were found to acquire sooner or later the cancer pattern of their adopted country, rather than preserve the cancer pattern of their country of origin (Ziegler et al, 1993). Clearly, the genetic constitution of these migrants did not change during one or a few generations.

Tables 2–2A and 2–2B show age-adjusted incidence rates, which are directly comparable and some of them were compared in Figures 2–3A to 2–9. However, as indicated, rates have limited intuitive appeal and are difficult to interpret at the individual level. As a complement, Tables 2–3A and 2–3B show cumulative incidence among women and men for various forms of cancer on the basis of the rates in the various registries. These cumulative incidences can be interpreted as probabilities expressed per thousand. Thus, a white woman in the US has a probability of 285 per thousand to develop a cancer at any site by age 74, whereas a woman in Sweden has a corresponding probability of 235 per thousand. The probability for a black man to develop prostate cancer by age 74 in the US is 185 per thousand, whereas it is only 9 per thousand in Japan and 3 per thousand in China. Last, a woman in Australia has a probability of 26 per thousand to develop skin melanoma and a probability of 81 per thousand to develop breast cancer.

Overall Cancer Survival

As we have already indicated, the average cure rate for different cancer sites and types varies between close to 0% and almost 100% (Figs. 2–1A and 2–1B). Besides, cure rates differ substantially between groups of patients diagnosed with the same type of cancer, but at different clinical stages. Hence, any estimate of overall curability of cancer has limited applicability to individual patients. Such estimates, however, may be useful as we try to understand general progress in treatment and convey this information to the general public. We need to be aware,

Table 2–6. Trends in 5-year relative survival proportions (%) for selected cancers by year of diagnosis, US, 1974 to 2001.

Cancer site	5-year relative survival proportions (%)		
	1974 to 1976	1983 to 1985	1995 to 2001
Brain	22	27	33
Breast (female)	75	78	88
Colon	50	58	64
Esophagus	5	8	15
Hodgkin's lymphoma	71	79	85
Kidney	52	56	65
Larynx	66	67	66
Leukemia	34	41	48
Liver & bileduct	4	6	9
Lung & bronchus	12	14	15
Melanoma of the skin	80	85	92
Multiple myeloma	25	28	32
Non-Hodgkin's lymphoma	47	54	60
Oral cavity	54	54	59
Ovary	37	41	45
Pancreas	3	3	5
Prostate	67	75	100
Rectum	49	55	65
Stomach	15	17	23
Testis	79	91	96
Thyroid	92	93	97
Urinary bladder	73	78	82
Uterine cervix	69	69	73
Uterine corpus	88	83	84
All sites	50	53	65

Source: Ries LAG, Eisner MP, Kosary CL, et al (eds). SEER Cancer Statistics Review, 1975–2002. Bethesda, MD: National Cancer Institute. Available at: http://seer.cancer.gov/csr/1975_2002/ (as reported by Jemal et al, 2006).

though, that reliable estimates of the proportion of cancer patients that are cured exist mainly from developed countries. Indeed, prognostic outlook may be much worse in settings where access to and/or standards of health care are poor.

Based on data from all patients with invasive cancer diagnosed between 1995 and 2001 in the US, the estimated overall, relative 5-year survival was 65% (Table 2–6). Though corresponding overall estimates are not available for all European countries, the US rates are considered to be largely applicable for several of them. Over the world, however, even if therapeutic success is identical across settings for specific cancer sites, differences in overall survival can arise if the distribution of cancers differs. This is particularly true, if in one setting, cancers with a poor prognosis, such as those of the lung, esophagus, or liver, account for a larger proportion of the total.

Whilst 5-year survival is widely used as an estimate of cure, an excess death rate may continue for a much longer period of time, for example among patients with cancer of the breast or the prostate. Therefore, overall 10-year relative survival tends to be about 6% units lower than the 5-year estimates (Ries et al, 1997). Nevertheless, 5-year survival allows a valid and more timely assessment of overall therapeutic progress when patients diagnosed in different time periods are compared (Adami et al, 1989). Lastly, it is worth noting that women tend to have a more favorable prognosis than men.

CONCLUSION

Using different and complementary measures the burden of cancer can be assessed in considerable detail. Efforts to quantify the impact of cancer are limited primarily by the fact that only a small proportion of the global population is covered by cancer registries. Hence, any global estimate has to rely on extrapolation and on various statistical models. Moreover, any attempt to compare therapeutic success and progress between time periods and countries is hampered by difficulties to follow large, representative cohorts of patients over long periods of time.

Notwithstanding these limitations, the occurrence of cancer and its course following diagnosis and treatment show many salient and remarkable features. Foremost, the incidence of many types of cancer varies more than threefold between different geographic settings. Because migrating populations, sooner or later, adopt the cancer pattern of their adopted country, these geographic differences cannot be explained by variation in genetic susceptibility to cancer. The conclusion is dramatic: Cancer is, at least in theory, a highly preventable disease.

While in many settings most cancer types show fairly stable incidence over time, others undergo substantial temporal changes. The highly dynamic incidence rates of lung cancer are largely presaged by smoking patterns during the preceding decades, whereas increasing trends in malignant melanoma likely reflect changes in UV exposure from sunlight. In contrast, the precipitous decline in stomach cancer is incompletely understood. And the almost epidemic increases—on a relative scale—of non-Hodgkin's lymphomas, adenocarcinoma of the esophagus, and testicular cancer in many western countries remain enigmatic. These fascinating enigmas will be further discussed in the site-specific chapters.

In the coming decades, the global burden of cancer will likely change in several ways. As developing countries adopt a more western lifestyle, their cancer patterns are expected to approach that of the developed countries. More importantly, the total burden of cancer will increase substantially. Besides growing population size, this trend will have two main determinants, namely increasing longevity due to elimination of other causes of premature death, notably perinatal mortality and infections, and consequences of the tobacco epidemic already taking place in many developing countries.

REFERENCES

Adami HO. What is progress against cancer? Cancer Causes Control 1993;4:483–87.

Adami HO, Sparen P, Bergstrom R, Holmberg L, Krusemo UB, Ponten J. Increasing survival trend after cancer diagnosis in Sweden: 1960–1984. J Natl Cancer Inst 1989;81: 1640–47.

Bailar JC 3d, Gornik HL. Cancer undefeated. N Engl J Med 1997;336:1569–74.

Barry MJ. Prostate-specific antigen testing for early diagnosis of prostate cancer. N Engl J Med 2001;344:1373–77.

Brenner H, Gefeller O, Hakulinen T. Period analysis for 'up-to-date' cancer survival data: theory, empirical evaluation, computational realisation and applications. Eur J Cancer 2004; 40: 326–35.

Burton EC et al. Autopsy diagnoses of malignant neoplasms. JAMA 1998;280:1245–48.

Danaei G, Vander Hoorn S, Lopez AD, Murray CJL, Ezzati M, and the comparative risk assessment collaborating group (Cancers). Causes of cancer in the world: comparative risk assessment of nine behavioural and environmental risk factors. Lancet 2005; 366:1784–93.

Day N. Cumulative rate and cumulative risk. In: Cancer Incidence in Five Continents, Volume VI. Lyon, France: International Agency for Research Cancer, 1992, pp 862–64

Dickman PW, Adami HO. Interpreting trends in cancer patient survival. Journal of Internal Medicine 2006; 260: 103–17.

Doll R, Fraumeni JF, Muir CS (Eds): Trends in Cancer Incidence and Mortality. Volume 19/20. New York: Cold Spring Harbor Laboratory Press, 1994.

Doll R, Peto R. The causes of cancer: quantitative estimates of avoidable risks of cancer in the United States today. J Natl Cancer Inst 1981;66:1191–308.

Enstrom JE, Austin DF. Interpreting cancer survival rates. Science 1977; 195: 847–51.

Ferlay J, Bray F, Pisani P, Parkin DM. GLOBOCAN 2002. Cancer Incidence, Mortality and Prevalence Worldwide. IARC Cancer-Base No. 5, version 2.0. IARCPress, Lyon, 2004.

Hankey BF, Feuer EJ, Clegg LX, Hayes RB, Legler JM, Prorok PC, Ries LA, Merrill RM, Kaplan RS. Cancer surveillance series: interpreting trends in prostate cancer—part I: Evidence of the effects of screening in recent prostate cancer incidence, mortality, and survival rates. J Natl Cancer Inst 1999; 91:1017–24.

Helgesen F, Holmberg L, Johansson JE, Bergstrom R, Adami HO. Trends in prostate cancer survival in Sweden, 1960 through 1988: evidence of increasing diagnosis of nonlethal tumors. J Natl Cancer Inst 1996; 88:1216–21.

Jemal A, Siegel R, Ward E, Murray T, Xu J, Smigal C, Thun MJ. Cancer Statistics, 2006. CA Cancer J Clin 2006;56;106–30.

Lopez AD, Mathers CD, Ezzati M, Jrnison DT, Murray CJ. Global and regional burden of disease and risk factors, 2001: systematic analysis of population health data. Lancet 2006;367:1747–57.

McDavid K, Lee J, Fulton JP, Tonita J, Thompson TD. Prostate cancer incidence and mortality rates and trends in the United States and Canada. Public Health Reports 2004;119:174–86.

Murray CJL, Lopez AD (Eds): The Global Burden of Disease. Harvard University Press, 1996a.

Murray CJL, Lopez AD (Eds): Global Health Statistics. Harvard University Press, 1996b.

Parkin DM, Bray F, Ferlay J, Pisani P. Global cancer statistics, 2002. CA Cancer J Clin. 2005a;55:74–108.

Parkin DM, Pisani P, Ferlay J. Estimates of the worldwide incidence of 25 major cancers in 1990. Int J Cancer 1999;80:827–41.

Parkin DM, Whelan SL, Ferlay J, Teppo L (Eds): Cancer Incidence in Five Continents, Vol. VIII. IARC Scientific Publication No. 155. Lyon, France: International Agency for Research on Cancer 2003.

Parkin DM, Whelan SL, Ferlay J, and Storm H. Cancer Incidence in Five Continents, Vols. I to VIII. IARC CancerBase No. 7, Lyon, France 2005b.

Ries LAG, Kosary CL, Hankey BF, Miller BA, Harras A, Edwards BK (Eds): SEER Cancer Statistics Review, 1973–1994, National Cancer Institute. NIH Pub. No. 97–2789. Bethesda, MD, 1997.

Smith PG. Comparison between registries: Age-standardized rates. In: Cancer Incidence in Five Continents, Volume VI. Lyon, France: International Agency for Research Cancer, 1992, pp 862–64.

World Health Organization, Regional Office for Europe. European Health For All database (HFA-DB). WHO, Regional Office for Europe, 2006.

Ziegler RG, Hoover RN, Pike MC, Hildesheim A, Nomura AM, West DW, Wu-Williams AH, Kolonel LN, Horn-Ross PL, Rosenthal JF, et al. Migration patterns and breast cancer risk in Asian-American women. J Natl Cancer Inst 1993;85:1819–27.

3

The Origin of Cancer

JEFFREY ECSEDY AND DAVID HUNTER

An understanding of the origin of cancer is fundamental to cancer epidemiology. In order to evaluate risk factors and preventive behaviors in cancer, one must consider the complex and interwoven mechanisms that lead to the development of cancer. By understanding such mechanisms, an epidemiologist should be able to integrate biological plausibility into his or her research. This chapter covers more biological ground than is customary in epidemiology texts, but we deemed this desirable for three reasons: First, the rapid developments in molecular and cellular biology have created knowledge gaps for many midcareer epidemiologists, as well as for epidemiologists with statistical rather than biological backgrounds. Second, the natural history of cancer should be accounted for in epidemiologic research and often dictates conceptual and statistical approaches in different situations—for example, in studying factors that initiate rather than promote carcinogenesis. Third, this is an area where continued rapid expansion is expected, and epidemiologists should be in a position to follow developments. The intent of this chap-

ter is to convey basic molecular and cellular concepts essential to understanding cancer biology; it is not intended to give a complete overview of cancer biology. For a more comprehensive exposition on the origin and development of cancer, read *The Biology of Cancer* (Weinberg, 2006).

This chapter traces the evolution of cancer, beginning with the genetic alteration of a single cell, leading to the continuous proliferation and expansion of that cell's descendants, and culminating in an invasive mass that ultimately can kill the organism. For cancer to evolve along these lines, a multitude of barriers must be overcome, including cell-cycle control, limitations on replicative potential, absence of appropriate growth stimuli, programmed cell death, and immune-mediated eradication. In addition, transformed cells must alter the extracellular environment to favor continuous cellular propagation and tumor expansion. The factors that facilitate cancer initiation and progression are the same factors that regulate normal cell and tissue behavior. It is through progressive genetic changes that these regulatory mechanisms go awry, causing cells to gradually transform from a normal into a malignant state. Understanding how cancer arises is essential to all oncology fields, including the epidemiology of cancer. The genetic predispositions and external risk factors associated with increased cancer occurrence manifest themselves as molecular and cellular events, and it is these events that are ultimately responsible for the development of the cancerous state.

DEFINING CANCER

Cancer is a diverse family of diseases, consisting of over 100 forms, that spawn from almost every cell type in the body. Each cell type gives rise to distinct forms of cancer, and the diversity is greatly increased by the fact that multiple forms of cancer can develop from each cell type, depending on both the location of the cell and the genetic aberration. Despite broad diversity, several features are common to all cancers (Hanahan and Weinberg, 2000). These include:

- unrestricted cellular proliferation
- circumvention of cell-cycle control
- growth without appropriate signals
- escape from programmed cell death
- altered interactions between cells and the surrounding environment
- evasion of immune-mediated eradication
- invasiveness into normal tissue

The term *cancer* derives from the Greek word for crab, karkinoma, which the physician Hippocrates used to describe the radiating appendage-like projections extending from some breast tumors. Cancer manifests itself as either a solid tumor or a noncolid leukemia in the circulatory system. The term *tumor* is nonspecific for a lump or swelling, and tumors are characterized as either benign or malignant (Table 3–1). The hallmark of malignancy is the invasiveness of tumor cells into the surrounding normal tissue. Malignant tumor cells invade the surrounding tissue, whereas benign tumor cells remain clustered in a single mass and are often encapsulated. Benign tumors are usually not fatal, although at certain anatomic sites, such as in the skull, they can cause pressure on other organs and lead to substantial morbidity and, if untreated, death. Several categories are used to determine the degree of tumor malignancy, including rate of growth, degree of differentiation, extent of invasiveness, and metastatic potential. In most cases, metastasis characterizes the highest degree of tumor malignancy, as it is usually the cause of death in cancer patients.

Cancer Progression

Cancer progresses in distinct stages, often over long periods of time, whereby a prospective cancer cell progressively accumulates genetic aberrations resulting in increasing tumor malignancy (Weinberg, 1996). The early mutagenic events of cancer initiation overcome growth-restrictive mechanisms, thereby conferring a selective advantage to abnormal cells, allowing them to outgrow and displace their neighbors (Cairns, 1975). In addition, the accumulation of genetic aberrations detected in cancer may result from a mutator phenotype. Mutator phenotypes are caused by mutagenic events early in cancer development that subsequently jeopardize genomic stability and DNA integrity, thereby predisposing tumor cells to the accumulation of further mutations (Loeb, 1991; Jackson and Loeb, 1998; Loeb

Table 3–1. Comparison of benign and malignant tumors

	Benign tumor	Malignant tumor
Invasiveness	Noninvasive, often encapsulated	Invasive
Rate of Growth	Slow, often static	Rapid
Differentiation	Well differentiated; often resembles tissue of origin	Undifferentiated
Metastasis	Never	Often metastatic

and Loeb, 2000). Given the known mutation rate of normal cells, it is unlikely that cells would acquire sufficient mutations to become cancerous. In other words, the large number of genetic alterations present in many cancers cannot be accounted for by random mutagenic events (Loeb, 1991). Therefore, the mutator phenotype of premalignant cells causes them to be more susceptible to mutations than normal cells.

Most solid tumors originate from areas of hyperplasia, characterized by increased local tissue size due to abnormal cellular proliferation. Cells from hyperplastic tissue preserve their normal architecture and orientation. For example, hyperplastic glandular epithelial cells retain a normal polarized columnar shape. When normal cellular architecture and orientation are lost, the abnormal tissue displays dysplasia. Eventually the cytologic features of the abnormal cells progress to resemble fully developed cancer. However, if no abnormal cells invade the normal underlying tissue (the hallmark feature of malignancy), the abnormal tissue is defined as *carcinoma in situ*. Once cells invade the underlying tissue, the abnormal tissue is defined as cancer. Genetic aberrations can continue to accumulate in cancerous tissue and may alter the growth rate, the extent of invasiveness, and the metastatic potential. Progressive genetic changes may also influence the efficacy of various anticancer therapies, including surgical resection, radiation therapy, and chemotherapy.

It is not unreasonable to expect that genetic lesions that lead to the initial transformation of cells also increase proclivity toward cancer phenotypes characteristic of more advanced malignancies, including invasiveness and metastasis (Bernards and Weinberg, 2002). However, within the darwinian view of cancer progression, transformed cells with a predisposition for increased malignancy would still rely on further genetic alterations for these genetic lesions to manifest as advanced cancer.

Metastasis

Metastasis is defined as the migration of tumor cells from a primary mass to distant sites in the body, where the migrating cells take residence and eventually develop into secondary tumor masses. Tumors can metastasize to multiple regions of the same organ or to different organs, making complete eradication of metastatic cancers extremely difficult. In almost 50% of patients, surgical excision of the primary tumor does not cure the disease, as metastasis has already occurred (Fidler and Balch, 1987; Fidler and Ellis, 1994). Metastatic cancers have the potential to disrupt many organ systems. For these reasons, metastasis is considered the most severe and common life-threatening complication of cancer.

Many complex interdependent events need to occur in the tumor cells and in the surrounding stroma for metastasis. The tumor cells must first detach from neighboring cells and invade the surrounding stroma. This is mediated by altered cell–cell and cell–extracellular matrix (ECM) interactions. Some tumor cells decrease or alter the expression of cell–cell cohesive molecules, allowing them to detach from adjacent cells. In addition, tumor cells utilize specialized proteases to destroy the surrounding basement membranes (ECM substructures) that normally act as migration barriers. The tumor cells then adhere to and enter the endothelial-lined walls of vessels through a process known as *intravasation*. Tumor cells typically migrate to distant sites through lymphatic channels or blood vessels. The thin endothelial walls of capillaries and some lymphatic channels provide little resistance to tumor cell penetration. Tumor cells need to survive the mechanical stress and shearing forces of the circulatory flow. Those that survive then adhere to and exit vessel walls through a process known as *extravasation*. Finally, for the metastatic tumor cell to proliferate and develop into a secondary tumor mass, it must be able to adapt to a foreign environment, overcome the loss of survival and growth signals that were present in the primary tumor, and eventually develop its own vascular network. Although dissemination of cancer cells to distant sites is a frequent event in many tumors, few of these cells will evolve to form detectable tumors (macrometastases). Formation of macrometastases, a process known as *metastatic colonization*, is a rare event due to the absence of survival signals unique to the primary site that normally cultivate tumor growth and foreign inhibitory factors in the secondary site that suppress tumor growth.

Cellular Origin of Cancer

Two models address the cellular origins of cancer (Fig. 3–1). In the first model, cancer originates from a single cell, which undergoes a heritable alteration initiating continuous proliferation and expansion, ultimately resulting in the billions of cells often necessary for tumor detection. As the cells of the cancer originated from a single ancestor clone, it is said to have a monoclonal lineage. An alternative model suggests that multiple cells within a tissue simultaneously switch to a cancerous state, possibly as a result of an exogenous agent. As the cells of the cancer are descendants of many clones, the cancer is said to have a polyclonal lineage.

Most experimental evidence favors a monoclonal origin of cancer. For example, a normal female contains two classes of cells: those with either the maternal or paternal X-chromosome inactivated, an event that occurs in each cell early in development. Therefore, the descendants of each cell possess the same inactivated X-chromosome. The state of X-chromosome inactivation, either maternal or paternal, and the genes expressed by either chromosome can then be used as inherited markers to trace cell lineage. The X-chromosome encodes two isoforms of the glucose-6-phosphate dehydrogenase (*G6PD*) gene. Hematopoietic can-

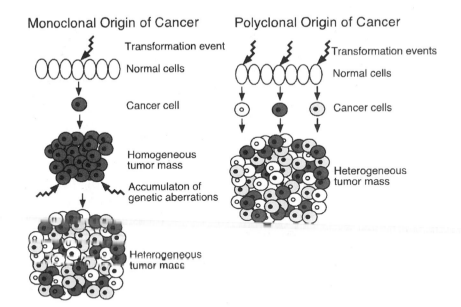

Figure 3–1. The cellular origin of cancer. Two models address the cellular origin of cancer, a monoclonal model and a polyclonal model. In the monoclonal model, a single normal cell is transformed into a cancerous cell through various mutagenic events. The cancer cell is then able to proliferate uncontrollably to form a homogeneous tumor mass. Subsequent genetic aberrations sustained by some of these cells result in the heterogeneous population of cancer cells characteristic of many tumors. Most experimental evidence favors a monoclonal origin of cancer. In the polyclonal model, multiple normal cells are simultaneously transformed into cancer cells. These cancer cells are then able to proliferate uncontrollably to form a heterogeneous tumor mass.

cers arising from females heterozygous for *G6PD* express only one isoform of the gene, suggesting that all of the cancer cells from individual patients derive from a single cell (Fialkow, 1976, 1979). In the majority of cases examined for X-chromosome inactivation in many forms of cancer, all of the cells from an individual tumor were found to have either the maternal or paternal copy of *G6PD* expressed, but not both. This evidence suggests that all the transformed cells from a tumor derive from a single clone and supports the theory of a monoclonal origin of cancer.

Another classic example demonstrating the monoclonal lineage of cancer comes from studying chronic myelogenous leukemia (CML), a disease that typically occurs in adults. Chronic myelogenous leukemia is associated with a specific chromosomal abnormality resulting from a translocation between the long arms of chromosomes 9 and 22 (Khouri, 1997). This translocation results in the formation of an aberrant oncogene, which has a role in CML pathogenesis. The site of the breakpoint and rejoining has been sequenced and can vary significantly when different patients are compared; however, the breakpoint site is the same for all the CML cells in a given patient (Zalcberg et al, 1986). It is unlikely that for a single patient several cells undergo identical translocations, and more likely that all the leukemia cells derive from a single ancestor clone and possess a monoclonal lineage.

Despite the monoclonal origin of cancer, tumors and leukemias frequently comprise heterogeneous populations of malignant cells (Fig. 3–1). As mentioned previously, tumor cells often continue to acquire genetic mutations after the initial entry into a transformed state and generally evolve into more aggressive forms, resulting in a worse prognosis for the patient. For example, the majority of glioblastomas (the most malignant grade of brain tumors) originate from less-malignant astrocytomas and anaplastic astrocytomas. After surgical resection and radiation of brain tumors, secondary tumors that arise from incomplete resection can have a higher grade of malignancy than

the original tumor. Tumors can continue to accumulate genetic mutations simply as a result of the rapid rate of cell division. It is a general rule that cells undergoing rapid turnover have a much greater chance of incurring mutations. This is due primarily to the increase in the likelihood of acquiring genetic mutations during DNA replication. Mutations are also amplified in tumors when there are lesions in DNA mutation detection or repair systems. These systems, which include cell-cycle checkpoint and DNA repair mechanisms, are discussed in greater detail later on in this chapter.

There is significant evidence supporting the hypothesis that cancer originates from the transformation of normal stem cells (Reya et al., 2001). Normal stem cells are undifferentiated, and undergo self-renewing cell division, whereby one daughter cell can proliferate into differentiated progeny, and the other daughter cell retains the original stem cell characteristics of being undifferentiated, and maintaining the capacity for unlimited replication. Similar to normal stem cells, cancer stem cells have the ability for unlimited self-renewing cell division. However, proliferation of normal stem cells is strictly regulated, whereas cancer stem cells have undergone mutations rendering these regulatory mechanisms ineffective. Pluripotent cancer stem cells can give rise to cancer cell heterogeneity. Despite their malignant state, these cells maintain the capacity to differentiate into their programmed fates. An example of this is multiple myeloma, a lymphoid stem cell leukemia. This disease is characterized by the presence of extremely high levels of B lymphocytes in all stages of development, ranging from the precursor stem cells to the fully differentiated antibody-secreting plasma cells (Slamon and Cassady, 1997). A major limitation of current cancer therapies is that they do not target cancer stem cells, which for unknown reasons are thought to have increased resistance to therapeutic intervention. Therefore, cancers often grow back after therapy, frequently in more aggressive forms as a result of continued cancer stem cell proliferation (Michor et al., 2005).

Clinical Behavior of Cancer

Several factors provide important clues in predicting the biological and clinical behavior of cancer, which may be necessary for directing appropriate therapy. Histogenesis (tissue origin) is the predictor of tumor behavior most commonly used by cancer pathologists. In simple terms, histogenesis is based on the concept that tumors derived from the same tissue generally behave in a similar way and tumors derived from different tissues behave differently. Another important prognosticator of tumor behavior is the histologic pattern of tissue differentiation. In general, the more tumors resemble the tissue from which they derived, the less malignant they are and the better the prognosis.

Tumors are often graded as well, moderately, or poorly differentiated. Poorly differentiated tumors do not resemble the tissue of origin and are generally highly malignant. To return to the example of brain tumors, astrocytomas can be subdivided into fibrillary, gemistocytic, and protoplasmic based on their morphologic similarity to normal and reactive astrocytes (Lopes et al., 1993). In contrast, glioblastoma cells retain no resemblance to astrocytes. The proliferative status, indicated by the number of cycling cells, and various molecular markers are also used to predict the behavior of cancers.

The stage of tumor development is another commonly used prognostic indicator. Tumor stage refers to the extent of tumor development at the time of presentation; the higher the stage, the worse the prognosis. Several factors contribute to tumor stage, including tumor size, extent of invasiveness in the surrounding normal tissue, presence of lymph nodes involved with metastatic spread, and presence of distant metastases.

A MOLECULAR APPROACH TO UNDERSTANDING CANCER

Cancer Genes

Some genes involved in the development and maintenance of normal cells and tissues may, in certain circumstances, be involved in cancer initiation and progression. These genes fall into three categories: proto-oncogenes, tumor-suppressor genes, and DNA repair genes (Vogelstein et al, 2000; Vogelstein and Kinzler, 2004). Mutations in proto-oncogenes, tumor-suppressor genes, and DNA repair genes cause cancer. These mutations can be acquired through germ-line transmission or by exogenous somatic damage.

Proto-oncogenes are nonmutated alleles of genes that contribute to cellular replication during normal growth and maintenance of tissues. When proto-oncogenes sustain mutations that impede their normal regulation, they become hyperactivated and uncontrollably stimulate cellular replication. Hyperactivated mutant alleles of proto-oncogenes are termed oncogenes.

Tumor-suppressor genes prevent cell growth in the absence of proper mitogenic (growth-stimulatory) signals. Although the name implies that tumor-suppressor genes function in suppressing cancer initiation, these genes also participate in regulating growth during normal development. Functional mutations in tumor-suppressor genes result in the loss of growth-inhibitory mechanisms. Restoration of tumor-suppressor gene function to a cancer cell should suppress its growth.

Unlike proto-oncogenes and tumor-suppressor genes, DNA repair genes do not stimulate or inhibit cellular replication. As their name implies, DNA repair genes function in sensing and repairing DNA mutations and therefore act as caretakers of the genome (Kinzler and Vogelstein, 1998). Functional mutations of DNA repair genes result in a mutator phenotype that accelerates accumulation of mutated proto-oncogenes and tumor-suppressor genes, thereby facilitating cancer initiation and progression (Jackson and Loeb, 1998; Loeb and Loeb, 2000). Restoration of DNA repair gene function to a repair-deficient cell will not affect its growth but will reduce the likelihood of progressive accumulation of mutations.

Much of what is known about cancer genes stems from studies of viruses in human tumors. Viral infection has served as a model of tumorigenesis in experimental systems and contributes directly to several human cancers. In fact, as many as 15% of all cancers have a viral etiology (Kuper et al, 2000). Viruses associated with human cancers include Epstein-Barr virus, hepatitis B and C viruses, human T-cell leukemia virus type 1, some human papilloma viruses[1], and several others. Tumor viruses contribute to cancers by expressing genes that mimic cellular oncogenes or interfere with the expression and activity of various proto-oncogenes and tumor-suppressor genes.

Genetic Carcinogenesis

Oncogenic mutations are dominant at the cellular level, as only one of the two proto-oncogene alleles needs to be mutated in a cell for the mutant gene product to influence downstream events that lead to cellular proliferation. Tumor-suppressor mutations are recessive at the cellular level, as both allele copies must be inactivated for cells to overcome the inhibitory mechanisms of the gene product. DNA repair mutations are also recessive. The successive mutagenic inactivation in both alleles of tumor-suppressor or DNA repair genes that facilitate cancer development is known as the *two-hit theory* of carcinogenesis (Fig. 3–2). Armitage and Doll first proposed this theory, suggesting that two successive mutagenic hits in the same growth-controlling region of homologous chromosomes are necessary for cellular transformation (Armitage and Doll, 1957). This concept was

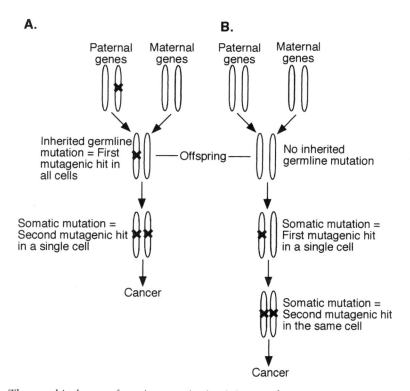

Figure 3–2. The two-hit theory of carcinogenesis. A minimum of two mutagenic events, one in each allele of a tumor-suppressor or DNA repair gene, is necessary to facilitate cancer development. A. The offspring inherits the first mutagenic hit in all cells from a germline mutation in the paternal genes. Therefore, only one somatic mutation in any cell is necessary for the second mutagenic hit, resulting in the inactivation of both alleles, thereby facilitating cancer development. B. The offspring inherits no mutagenic hits from the parents. Therefore, two successive somatic mutations in the same cell are necessary for the first and second mutagenic hits, resulting in the inactivation of both alleles.

elaborated by Knudson, who predicted that development of childhood retinoblastoma depended on two genetic hits, represented by mutations in both alleles of the tumor-suppressor gene Rb (Retinoblastoma gene) (Knudson et al., 1971).

Mutations resulting in the hyperactivation of a single proto-oncogene or the functional inactivation of a single tumor-suppressor gene are typically insufficient for cancer initiation. Cells utilize numerous checks and balances that prohibit uncontrolled growth in response to a single activating signal. Multiple genetic lesions in various signaling pathways are necessary for cancer to arise. The continuous accumulation of genetic lesions necessary for cancer genesis is termed *the multistep theory of carcinogenesis*. It is believed that multiple mutagenic hits are necessary for cancer development (Vogelstein and Kinzler, 1993; Hahn et al, 1999). The number of mutagenic hits necessary for cancer formation probably varies, depending on the signal pathways affected and the level of regulation. The accumulation of mutagenic hits results not only in the transformation of a cell from a normal into a cancerous state, but also in the increase of tumor malignancy after the initial transforming events.

Exogenous Mutagenesis

Many exogenous carcinogens cause genetic lesions. Several examples exist of exogenous carcinogens leading to somatic mutations, including chemicals such as polycyclic aromatic hydrocarbons, toxins, and physical agents such as ultraviolet radiation. Although exogenous carcinogens induce mutations by various mechanisms, one unifying outcome is the interference with DNA replication fidelity, resulting in a mutated genetic sequence. The risk of cancer occurrence is increased when these mutations occur in cancer genes.

Many chemicals that normally do not induce DNA damage are altered by metabolic pathways in the body, thereby inducing carcinogenic activity and resulting in genetic lesions. Various metabolic pathways are responsible for detoxifying or excreting chemical carcinogens. These outcomes engender the idea that differences in the sequence or abundance of activating or detoxifying enzymes may partially determine individual susceptibility to exogenous carcinogens. Therefore, much attention has been focused on endogenous compounds participating in these metabolic pathways and the role they play in DNA damage (Hussain and Harris, 2000).

Epigenetic Mechanisms of Gene Silencing

In addition to mutations in genes or loss of genetic material from chromosomes, recent work has indicated that genes may be silenced or turned off by nonmutational mechanisms. A silenced gene is still present in the genome, but is not expressed, and is thus functionally equivalent to a gene that expresses a mutant product or has been lost altogether. All genes have promoter sequences that determine the state of expression, and a common mechanism for silencing is the addition of methyl groups to key sites in these promoter sequences. For instance, hypermethylation of a tumor-suppressor gene causes the gene product to be absent. Therefore, a combination of an inherited or acquired somatic mutation in one copy of the gene, and a hypermethylated promoter in the other allele, would result in complete loss of the gene product in the cell. This is an example of the two-hit theory of carcinogenesis.

Hypermethylation is an example of an epigenetic phenomenon. Epigenetic changes influence gene expression without directly affecting the gene sequence (Jones and Laird, 1999). As a result, epigenetic changes are not inherited. For some genes in certain organs, promoter hypermethylation increases with age, perhaps providing part of the explanation of why many cancers are strongly age dependent. Understanding the environmental and endogenous causes of gene silencing will almost certainly prove valuable in elucidating the way epidemiologically determined risk factors cause cancer cells to arise.

Another endogenous epigenetic mechanism for gene silencing involves microRNAs. MicroRNAs, also known as miRNAs, are single-stranded RNA molecules of approximately 22 nucleotides in length. These molecules comprise a unique category of non-protein-coding regulators of gene expression (Esquela-Kerscher and Slack, 2006; Calin and Croce, 2006). miRNAs interfere with gene expression at the level of mRNA transcripts by two mechanisms: *(1)* they induce degradation of mRNAs containing complete or partial sequence complementarity through a mechanism known as RNA interference (RNAi), or *(2)* they suppress protein translation by binding to the 3' untranslated regions of target mRNAs. The number of miRNAs suspected to be present in the human genome ranges up to 1000. These molecules effect a diverse array of biological processes, including cell proliferation, differentiation, and death. Interestingly, variations in global miRNA signatures, specifically by downregulation in tumors relative to normal cells, have been implicated with tumorigenesis and cancer progression (Lu et al, 2005). Moreover, individual miRNAs have been shown to be significant regulators of specific tumor suppressor genes and oncogenes.

The Cell Cycle and Checkpoints

The division of a cell into two genetically equivalent daughter cells proceeds in an orderly fashion and is known as the *cell cycle*. The cell cycle is divided into four main phases: the mitotic phase (M), the postmitotic/presynthesis gap phase (G1), the DNA synthesis phase (S), and the postsynthesis/premitotic gap phase (G2) (Fig. 3–3). Cells that are not actively dividing may either be temporarily removed from the cycle by entering a resting state defined as G0, or be permanently removed from the cycle by terminal differentiation.

Proper orchestration of the cell cycle depends on the completion of all the steps in one phase before the next phase begins. Oscillating levels of cyclin/cyclin-dependent kinase (CDK) complexes regulate cell-cycle progression (Fig. 3–3). These complexes phosphorylate substrates required for DNA synthesis (S phase) or mitosis (M phase). Several different cyclin/CDK complexes participate in cell-cycle progression. Exogenous agents and events, including growth

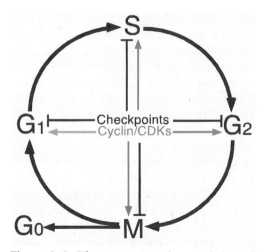

Figure 3–3. The successive phases of the cell cycle. The cell cycle is characterized by four main phases: a mitotic phase (M), a postmitotic/presynthetic phase (G1), a DNA synthetic phase (S), and a postsynthetic/premitotic phase (G2). The G1 phase marks the beginning of the cell cycle. This is followed by the S phase, which is characterized by the duplication of each chromosome into two sister chromotids. The G2 phase follows the S phase and precedes the M phase. The M phase is characterized by nuclear and cytoplasmic division of a parent cell into two genetically identical daughter cells. Cells that are not dividing may be temporarily removed from the cycle by entering a resting state, defined as G0, or permanently removed from the cycle by terminal differentiation. Cyclin/CDK complexes drive cell cycle progression. Checkpoints monitor the quality of DNA throughout the cell cycle and ensure proper orchestration of events.

factors, mitogens/antimitogens, differentiation inducers, cell–cell and cell–ECM interactions, oxygen pressure, and nutrients, ultimately control cyclin/CDK activity (Kastan, 1997). These agents/events utilize various signal transduction mechanisms to control cyclin/CDK activity by affecting expression levels, activity, and stability and by regulating specific inhibitors (CDK inhibitors) (Kastan, 1997).

The cell cycle is overseen by various checkpoints, quality controllers that monitor the condition of DNA throughout the cell cycle and ensure proper orchestration of cycle events, thus protecting genomic integrity (Fig. 3–3). In response to DNA damage or replicative stress, checkpoints perform diverse functions including activation of appropriate effectors necessary to repair the damage or alleviate the stress. Checkpoints arrest the cell cycle until the damage or stress is mended and activate DNA repair machinery. In extreme cases, they cause cells to commit suicide by initiating programmed cell death (Zhou and Elledge, 2000).

Checkpoints comprise a complex network of proteins that act as sensors, transducers, or effectors (Zhou and Elledge, 2000). The sensors identify genomic insults and initiate network activity. An example of a sensor is the ataxia-telangiectasia mutated protein (ATM), which participates in identifying DNA double-strand breaks. Once activated, sensor checkpoint proteins signal to transducer checkpoint proteins that in turn activate a variety of effector checkpoint proteins. As will be discussed in the following, ATM (a sensor) activates p53 (a transducer), which stimulates p21 (an effector). The p21 protein is associated with cell-cycle arrest at the G1/S transition.

The checkpoint network regulates phase transition at different points throughout the cell cycle, although the proteins involved and their activity vary, depending on the phase in which they are activated. The G1/S checkpoint ensures that damaged DNA is repaired prior to replication in the S phase. The S phase checkpoint is activated when DNA damage occurs in the early events of DNA synthesis. Any DNA damage sustained at the end of DNA synthesis or prior to mitosis activates the G2/M checkpoint. The mitotic spindle checkpoint ensures that all chromosomes are properly aligned on the mitotic spindle before anaphase begins. Defects in the mitotic spindle checkpoint result in aneuploidy, often leading to cancer.

The cell-cycle machinery is commonly targeted in tumorigenesis. Regulators of the cell cycle qualify as proto-oncogenes, tumor-suppressor genes, or DNA repair genes, according to their function in cell-cycle progression. For example, hyperacti-vating mutants of cyclin/CDK complexes, which facilitate cell-cycle progression, are classified as oncogenes. Functional mutations in p53 prevent its cell-cycle arrest activity (mediated through p21 and other proteins); therefore, *p53* is classified as a tumor-suppressor gene. Defects in some checkpoint mechanisms prevent proper orchestration of DNA replication or separation of chromosomes during mitosis. Defects in others result in impaired detection and repair of DNA damage. These checkpoints are therefore classified as DNA repair (caretaker) genes. Nevertheless, as DNA repair checkpoints ensure DNA integrity, functional defects in these checkpoints result in accelerated accumulation of mutated proto-oncogenes and tumor-suppressor genes.

Genomic Instability Disorders

Several human genetic disorders result from defects in DNA damage sensing and repair genes or in DNA recombination genes. These disorders result in gross chromosomal aberrations and are therefore characterized as genomic instability disorders. Genomic instability leads to many diverse developmental abnormalities in these patients, and a high cancer incidence is shared by all. Diseases characterized by these defects include ataxia-telangiectasia, Bloom's syndrome, Werner's syndrome, and Fanconi anemia, among several others. These diseases, which are inherited in a recessive manner, are very rare.

Ataxia-telangiectasia is characterized by cerebellar degeneration, immunodeficiency, radiation sensitivity, and cancer predisposition. Ataxia telangiectasia results from mutations in the *ATM* gene that encodes a protein involved in cell-cycle progression, and possibly in detection and repair of double-strand DNA breaks (Savitsky et al, 1995; Michelson and Weinert, 2000). Left unfixed, double-strand DNA breaks lead to high rates of chromosomal rearrangements.

Bloom's syndrome is characterized by prenatal and postnatal growth retardation, immunodeficiency, premature aging, and a high incidence of cancer. Werner's syndrome is characterized by premature aging and early onset of osteoporosis, artheosclerosis, type II diabetes mellitus, and cancer. Bloom's syndrome and Werner's syndrome arise from mutations in genes that encode DNA helicases (Ellis et al., 1995; Gray et al., 1997; Shen and Loeb, 2000). Loss of Bloom's or Werner's helicase activity can lead to entangled DNA, causing mutations to arise during DNA replication and chromosomal segregation (Watt and Hickson, 1996).

Fanconi anemia is characterized by growth retardation, skeletal malformations, and cancer predisposition. Unlike the other genomic instability disorders, Fanconi anemia arises from mutations in any one of several genes (Garcia-Higuera et al, 1999). Patients with defects in these genes demonstrate hypersensitivity to DNA cross-linking agents, suggesting that Fanconi anemia proteins function as part of this DNA repair process (Garcia-Higuera et al, 1999).

The p53 and Retinoblastoma Pathways

The Rb and p53 tumor pathways serve as paradigms for understanding cell-cycle regulation. Rb and p53 are components of two signal transduction pathways that negatively regulate cellular replication. In non-replicating cells, the Rb protein is normally "turned on," thus suppressing cell-cycle progression. In response to mitogenic signals, Rb is "turned off," allowing cells to proceed through the cell cycle. The p53 protein is normally "turned off" in cells. In response to DNA damage or oncogenic signals, p53 is "turned on," thus inducing cell-cycle arrest or programmed cell death.

Both Rb and p53 are tumor suppressors, as their functional inactivation results in the loss of cell-cycle control, leading to cellular transformation. Indeed, the *Rb* and *p53* genes are commonly mutated in human cancers. Other components of the Rb and p53 signal transduction pathways are also mutated in certain human cancers. These comprise various oncogenes and tumor-suppressor genes, depending on whether they stimulate or suppress Rb and p53 activity.

p53

The p53 protein was first described in 1979 through its association with the transforming simian virus 40 large T protein (Kress et al, 1979; Lane and Crawford, 1979; Linzer and Levine, 1979). Subsequently, p53 was identified as a tumor suppressor and became the most extensively studied gene in the field of cancer research (Prives and Hall, 1999). The attention focused on p53 is due in large part to its loss of function in many human cancers. Approximately one-half of all human cancers possess mutations in the *p53* gene that result in direct inactivation of the p53 protein (Hollstein et al, 1991; Greenblatt et al, 1994). Furthermore, many other cancers possess mutations in genes encoding p53 regulatory proteins that result in indirect inactivation of the p53 protein.

Under normal cellular conditions, wild-type p53 protein exists in an inactive state and is present in low levels. In response to various intracellular or extracellular stresses, including DNA damage or oncogenic signals, p53 switches to an active state and stabilizes (Fig. 3–4). Activated p53 serves as a sequence-specific transcription factor and promotes expression of target genes. The proteins expressed from the p53 target genes then initiate a variety of cellular events, most significantly cell-cycle arrest and apoptosis. Therefore, activation of p53 in response to genomic perturbations or oncogenic signals prevents potentially cancerous cells from attaining uncontrolled growth status and eventually developing into full-blown cancer.

Activation of the p53 protein requires both quantitative and qualitative changes. Quantitative changes result from a dramatic increase in the steady-state levels of cellular p53. This is due primarily to the removal of a p53-bound inhibitor, mdm2 (Fig. 3–4) (Bottger et al, 1997). The mdm2 protein binds to and promotes rapid degradation of p53. When mdm2 is removed, p53 is not targeted for rapid degradation and p53 protein levels increase. However, the increase in protein levels alone is not

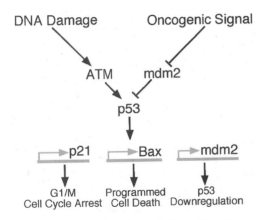

Figure 3–4. Signaling through the p53 pathway. The p53 protein is normally turned off in cells. In response to DNA damage or oncogenic signals, p53 undergoes both qualitative and quantitative changes and is subsequently turned on. ATM and other protein kinases phosphorylate p53 in response to DNA damage, altering p53 protein–protein interactions and increasing p53 DNA binding affinity. Oncogenic signals free p53 of mdm2, thereby stabilizing the protein and resulting in increased p53 levels. Activated p53 serves as a sequence-specific transcription factor and promotes expression of target genes, including p21, Bax, and mdm2. Activation of these genes results in cell cycle arrest, programmed cell death, and decreased p53 activity and stability, respectively.

adequate for p53 to become a transcriptional activator; qualitative changes that alter p53 conformation are also necessary (Prives and Hall, 1999).

The qualitative changes in p53 include posttranslational modifications, including phosphorylation and dephosphorylation events, among others. These changes alter the protein–protein interactions of p53 and increase the DNA binding affinity of p53, allowing it to act as a transcriptional activator. The protein kinase ATM and several other protein kinases phosphorylate p53 in response to DNA damage, leading to p53 activation (Fig. 3–4). The p53 protein is also activated in response to aberrant growth signals, such as overexpressing *Ras* oncogenes (Groth et al., 2000).

Once activated, p53 acts as a sequence-specific transcription factor, upregulating

expression of genes whose products induce cell-cycle arrest (either at the G1 or G2 phase) or programmed cell death (Fig. 3–4). One such target gene is *p21*, which is partly responsible for arresting the cell cycle in the G1 phase (Vogelstein et al, 2000). When p21 expression is elevated in response to p53 activation, it impedes cell-cycle progression at the G1 phase by interfering with the CDKs. The p53 target genes leading to programmed cell death include *Bax* and *Fas*, among others (Zhan et al, 1994; Owen-Schaub et al, 1995). The function of these two genes will be discussed in greater detail in the following. It is not clear why at times p53 induces genes whose products lead to cell-cycle arrest, and at other times induces genes whose products lead to programmed cell death. Interestingly, the *mdm2* gene is also a target for p53 transcriptional activation, thereby allowing p53 to negatively autoregulate its own activity (Barak et al., 1993).

Retinoblastoma

Individuals who inherit a mutant copy of the *Rb* gene are predisposed to the development of childhood retinoblastoma, characterized by multiple tumor foci in both eyes (Varmus and Weinberg, 1993). These individuals also are predisposed to other forms of malignancy later in life. The Rb protein functions as a tumor suppressor by inhibiting cell-cycle progression in the G1 phase. This activity is mediated by Rb interaction with E2F transcription factors, thereby inhibiting the expression of E2F target genes (Weintraub et al, 1992). E2F target genes facilitate progression of the cell cycle. In response to mitogenic signals, the Rb protein is phosphorylated by CDKs (Fig. 3–5). CDK-mediated phosphorylation of Rb disrupts Rb/E2F transcription factor complexes, resulting in E2F target genes expression (Adams and Kaelin, 1998).

Growth-Regulatory Signaling Pathways

The mediators of growth-regulatory signal transduction pathways are targets of deregulation in cancer. These mediators comprise an extremely diverse assortment of

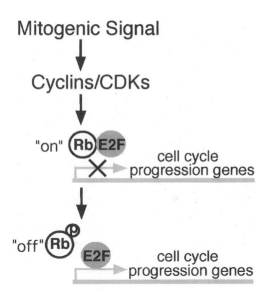

Figure 3–5. Signaling through the Retinoblastoma (Rb) pathway. In nonreplicating cells, Rb is turned on and interacts with E2F transcription factors, thereby repressing expression of genes involved in cell cycle progression. Rb is turned off by phosphorylation through cyclin/CDK complexes in response to mitogenic signals. Subsequently, E2F transcription factors are liberated from Rb and activate the expression of cell cycle progression genes.

membrane-spanning receptors, intracellular transducers, and effectors. Membrane-spanning receptors are normally activated in response to a multitude of growth-stimulatory signals, including growth factor polypeptides, hormones, and cell–cell and cell–ECM contacts. Activated receptors then relay signals to intracellular transducers, which elicit a diverse range of cellular responses and require complex effectors. Depending on whether they positively or negatively regulate growth signal transmission, mediators of these pathways are classified as proto-oncogenes or tumor-suppressor genes.

Unlike normal cells, cancer cells are able to divide in the absence of appropriate growth stimuli. Cancer cells circumvent dependency on these stimuli by generating their own growth signals (via oncogenic mutations) and by escaping growth-suppressive systems (via tumor-suppressor

mutations). In addition, some cancers secrete polypeptide growth factors that in an autocrine fashion stimulate their own growth. Importantly, specific mutations in growth regulatory genes can result in therapeutic resistance, making cancers refractory to certain types of drug therapy (Gorre et al, 2001; Michor et al, 2005). ErbB-2, Ras, and c-Myc serve as paradigms for cancer-deregulated membrane-spanning receptors, intracellular transducers, and effectors, respectively (Fig. 3–6).

ErbB-2
In many cancers, growth factor receptors are overexpressed or contain hyperactivating mutations resulting in their constitutive

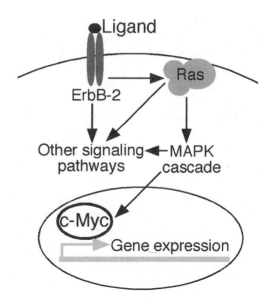

Figure 3–6. Growth-regulatory signaling pathways. ErbB-2 is a member of the membrane-spanning epidermal growth factor receptor family. In response to ligand-mediated activation, ErbB-2 initiates various signaling pathways, among them the mitogen-activated protein kinase (MAPK) cascade. Ras functions as an intracellular transducer of various signaling pathways. For example, Ras transduces ErbB-2 signals to the MAPK cascade. c-Myc functions as an effector by regulating expression of genes involved in a variety of cellular functions. The MAPK cascade and several other signaling pathways activate c-Myc. ErbB-2, Ras, and c-Myc expression are often deregulated in cancer.

activation. One such receptor, ErbB-2, is a member of a transmembrane tyrosine kinase receptor family known as the *epidermal growth factor receptors*. Deregulation of ErbB-2 activity in cancers is primarily due to gene amplification and overexpression or to structural mutations that result in hyperactivation of the tyrosine kinase domain. In either case, ErbB-2 signaling is activated independently of appropriate growth stimuli.

Several human cancers, including breast, lung, colon, and ovarian cancers, are associated with *ErbB-2* amplification or overexpression (Kapitanovic et al, 1994; Berchuck and Boyd, 1995; Giatromanolaki et al, 1996; Lupu et al, 1996). ErbB-2 serves as an ideal target for anti–breast cancer therapy, as it is expressed at high levels in approximately 30% of breast cancers and is correlated with a poor prognosis in breast cancer patients (Lupu et al, 1996). Herceptin, a monoclonal antibody that blocks the kinase activity of ErbB-2, is being used in the treatment of the majority of breast carcinomas that overexpress ErbB-2 (Pegram and Slamon, 2000).

Ras

One downstream intracellular transducer of ErbB-2 signaling is the *Ras* proto-oncogene, which is also a target for deregulation in tumorigenesis. The *Ras* gene encodes a G protein (guanine nucleotide binding protein) that localizes to the inner leaflet of the plasma membrane. Ras belongs to a large group of related proteins known as the Ras family of GTPases. After delivery of the appropriate signal, Ras binds to the guanine nucleotide GTP and undergoes conformational changes that activate the protein. Activated Ras then stimulates many diverse downstream pathways, the key signaling pathway being the mitogen-activated protein kinase (MAPK) cascade. Oncogenic Ras mutants fire continuously even without input from growth factor receptor signals.

Ras mutations have been implicated in up to 30% of all human cancers (Hernandez-Alcoceba et al, 2000). Ras and its family members also play a significant role in the intracellular changes associated with cellular migration in tumor invasion and metastasis (Hernandez-Alcoceba et al., 2000).

c-Myc

One downstream effector of many growth-regulatory signal transduction pathways is the proto-oncogene *c-Myc*. c-Myc is a transcription factor that regulates expression of many genes associated with a variety of cellular functions, including replication, growth, metabolism, differentiation, and apoptosis (Dang et al, 1999; Schmidt, 1999; Pelengaris et al, 2000). Regulation of these genes by c-Myc differs among cell types, suggesting that tissue-specific factors exist that modulate c-Myc expression. Many of these c-Myc mutants lose the ability to be shut down by normal mechanisms and thus remain constitutively active (Nesbit et al, 1999).

Mutations that disrupt c-Myc regulation are among the most common mutations found in human cancer. In fact, most human cancers display *c-Myc* amplification and/or overexpression (Nesbit et al, 1999). Almost all cases of Burkitt's lymphoma arise from chromosomal rearrangements that juxtapose the *c-Myc* gene located on chromosome 8 with regulatory elements of immunoglobulin genes located on other chromosomes (Spencer and Groudine, 1991; Nesbit et al., 1999).

Programmed Cell Death (Apoptosis)

Programmed cell death, or apoptosis, is a genetically regulated form of cell death characterized by a series of intracellular molecular events. Several changes in cellular morphology distinguish apoptosis from other forms of cell death (ie, necrosis or autophagy), including cell shrinkage, nuclear fragmentation, chromosomal condensation, and membrane blebbing. The removal of cells by apoptosis is an essential process in embryonic development and in homeostasis of adult tissues (Vaux and Korsmeyer, 1999). In developing embryos, for example, superfluous cells are removed during digit and brain formation by apoptosis. In adults, apoptosis participates in the postpartum involution of mammary glands and in homeostasis of cell number by balancing cell birth with cell death. In the context of cancer, apoptosis provides a means of eliminating cells that have sustained genetic aberrations from cytogenetic insults, thereby preventing damaged cells from attaining uncontrolled proliferation.

Genetic aberrations, such as DNA damage or oncogenic signals, can lead to apoptosis by p53 activation, for example, which induces expression of several pro-apoptotic genes. In addition, certain types of DNA damage also trigger apoptotic cell death by mechanisms that are independent of p53 (Clarke et al, 1993). For example, in response to certain types of DNA damage, some DNA repair mechanisms elicit cell death whether or not p53 is functionally active (Hickman et al, 1999). CD8+ (killer) T lymphocytes can also activate apoptosis in cells that present foreign antigens as a result of genetic aberrations. Therefore, the apoptotic process must fail for a cell to transform to a cancerous state.

The changes in cell morphology that distinguish the apoptotic phenotype reflect the activity of a family of proteases known as *caspases*. Caspases degrade specific intracellular polypeptides that ultimately result in cell death. Caspase activity is activated by two distinct pathways: one is triggered by receptor-mediated signaling at the cell surface, and the other is triggered by cytogenetic insults (Fig. 3–7) (Kaufmann and Gores, 2000). The receptor-mediated signaling pathway, often referred to as the *death receptor pathway*, is triggered when the extracellular domain of the membrane-spanning signaling molecule Fas contacts the Fas ligand. Fas then activates specific members of the caspase family, which initiate the proteolytic degradation characteristic of apoptosis.

Killer T lymphocytes utilize the death receptor pathway to destroy target cells.

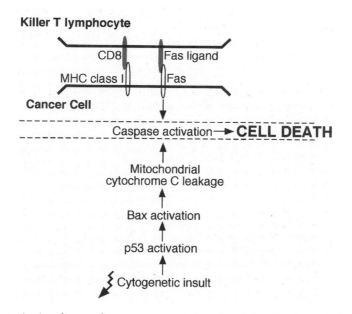

Figure 3–7. Apoptotic signaling pathways. Apoptosis is induced in cells through death receptor pathways or by cytogenetic insult. Killer T lymphocytes recognize foreign antigens presented on the cell surface through CD8–major histocompatibility complex (MHC) class I interactions. The death receptor pathway is then activated by Fas/Fas ligand contact and is mediated by intracellular caspase activity. Cytogenetic insult results in p53 activation, which in turn increases Bax expression. Bax stimulates leakage of mitochondrial cytochrome C, which eventually results in caspase activation and ultimately cell death.

Killer T lymphocytes trigger the death receptor pathways in target cells by expressing cell surface Fas ligand. In addition to Fas, several other death receptors exist that activate apoptosis by similar mechanisms. The other pathway for activating apoptosis is triggered when cytogenetic insults, by an unknown process, alter specific proapoptotic proteins, resulting in leakage of cytochrome c from mitochondria into the cytosol (Fig. 3–7). One such proapoptotic protein is Bax, whose expression is upregulated in response to p53 activation. Cytosolic cytochrome C induces conformational changes in the intermediary protein Apaf1, which subsequently activates the caspase cascade.

Elucidation of the cell death pathways has provided insight into the antiapoptotic changes that occur in tumor cells (Strand and Galle, 1998; Kaufmann and Gores, 2000). Many tumor cells express low levels of Fas or none at all, thereby evading killer T-lymphocyte recognition and subsequent death (Sikora et al, 1998; O'Connell et al, 2000). Tumor cells also secrete soluble polypeptides that act as decoy Fas receptors by binding surface Fas ligands (Pitti et al, 1998). Saturation of Fas ligands with decoy receptors prevents activation of Fas receptors. One gene encoding a decoy polypeptide was amplified in approximately 50% of lung and colon carcinomas examined (Pitti et al, 1998), suggesting that this may be a common mechanism of avoiding apoptosis by some cancers. Fas receptor signaling can also be blocked by reduced expression of downstream caspases.

Tumor cells also avoid apoptosis by overexpressing antiapoptotic proteins such as Bcl-2. Bcl-2 inhibits cell death by interfering with the activity of mitochondria-associated proapoptotic molecules such as Bax. Overexpression of Bcl-2 provided the first example of an oncogene that indirectly contributed to cell proliferation by inhibiting cell death (Vaux et al, 1988). Bcl-2 overexpression is detected in a variety of tumor types and is associated with a poor prognosis (Strand and Galle, 1998; Kaufmann and Gores, 2000).

In addition to evading killer T lymphocytes, suppression of death receptor pathways in certain circumstances may be important in tumor initiation and survival. Loss of essential growth factors, alterations in cell–ECM interactions, and other suboptimal growth conditions can induce Fas-mediated cell death (Le-Niculescu et al, 1999; Rytomaa et al, 1999). Therefore, evasion of the apoptotic process may allow tumors to survive and grow in environments that are restrictive to normal cells (Kaufmann and Gores, 2000). Such suboptimal growth conditions are common in tumor masses.

Many anticancer therapeutic agents act by inducing cytogenetic insults that subsequently lead to apoptotic death. Therefore, defects in apoptotic mechanisms circumvent the efficacy of many anticancer treatments. As a result, significant efforts have attempted to identify new methods that counteract antiapoptotic mechanisms. These methods may help to overcome drug resistance in some tumors, thereby increasing the efficacy of some standard anticancer therapies.

Unlimited Replicative Potential of Cancer

Normal somatic mammalian cells have a limited replicative potential, where, after continuous rounds of division, they lose their capacity to proliferate. This phenomenon is demonstrated in continuous in vitro cultures, where cells cease to replicate after a certain number of divisions (Hayflick and Moorhead, 1961). Viable cells no longer able to divide are said to be senescent. Senescence is an irreversible process, which distinguishes it from quiescence, the normal withdrawal from the cell cycle observed in many adult cells. Cells can reenter the cell cycle from a quiescent state, but not from a senescent state, upon treatment with appropriate growth stimuli. Despite an inability to divide, senescent cells can be maintained in culture for long periods of time.

Cells can evade senescence and attain a state of replicative immortality by undergoing specific genetic alterations. As an example, mouse embryonic fibroblasts containing homozygous deletions for some tumor-suppressor genes, including p53, divide continuously in culture (Jacks, 1996). Rodent cells can also spontaneously avoid senescence at a very low frequency when grown in culture, presumably through sporadically acquired genetic mutations. Interestingly, normal human cells grown in culture rarely give rise spontaneously to immortalized derivatives. The underlying mechanism for this species-specific difference is unclear. However, human cells treated with mutagens or infected by certain viruses can attain an immortalized state; although in certain circumstances, activation of oncogenic signaling in normal cells may also lead directly to senescence (Mooi and Peeper, 2006). The evasion of cellular senescence and entry into an immortalized state is one of the distinguishing features of cancer.

The mechanism(s) that forces cells to become senescent is often referred to as a molecular clock, which keeps track of cell divisions; at a critical point, an alarm signals and prevents further proliferation (Sedivy, 1998). The molecular clock is thought to exist in the form of telomeres, simple repeating DNA sequences located at chromosome ends that are capped by protein complexes. Telomeres prevent chromo-

somal erosion, fragmentation, and aberrant rearrangement (de Lange and Jacks, 1999). The DNA-protein complexes of telomeres oscillate stochastically between two states, capped and uncapped (Fig. 3–8) (Blackburn, 2000). Uncapping of telomeres occurs normally in dividing cells. With each successive round of cellular division, telomeres shorten due to the nature of the lagging strand during DNA replication of linear chromosomes (Watson, 1972).

As telomere length decreases, the stochastic oscillation of protein capping shifts toward the uncapped state. At a certain point, telomeres are uncapped for periods long enough to activate cell-cycle checkpoint mechanisms that initiate cell-cycle arrest, thereby inducing senescence (Blackburn, 2000). This limitation on the replicative potential of cells can be overcome by a specialized reverse transciptase known as *telomerase*. Telomerase extends the repeating telomeric sequence lost during each round of replication, thus preventing chromosomal shortening, stabilizing telomere protein caps, and conferring on cells unlimited replicative potential.

In humans, telomerase is not expressed in normal somatic cells but is expressed in germ cells and stem cells. Telomerases are also widely expressed in human cancers

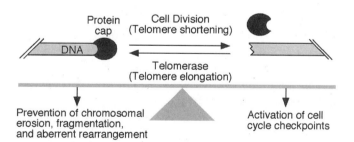

Figure 3–8. Telomeres regulate cell survival. Telomeres oscillate stochastically between capped and uncapped states. Telomere shortening favors the uncapped state, and telomere elongation favors the capped state. Capped telomeres prevent chromosomal erosion, fragmentation, and aberrant rearrangement. With each successive round of cellular division, telomeres shorten, shifting the balance toward the uncapped state. If telomeres are left in the uncapped state for long periods, cell cycle checkpoints are activated, resulting in cell cycle arrest and subsequent senescence. Telomerases extend telomeres, thereby shifting the balance toward the capped state and conferring on cells unlimited replicative potential.

(Counter et al, 1994; Chadeneau et al, 1995; Kolquist et al, 1998). For cancerous cells to avoid senescence and attain unlimited replicative potential, the progressive loss of telomeric sequence must be prevented, thus explaining the activation of telomerases in many tumors. Considering the fact that telomerases are activated in many tumors and not in normal somatic cells, they provide an ideal target for therapeutic intervention against cancer.

EXTRINSIC FACTORS INFLUENCE CANCER PROGRESSION

Although much cancer research focuses on cellulares intrinsic mechanisms of tumorigenesis, the extracellular environment plays a critical role in cancer initiation and progression. Bi-directional communication between extracellular and intracellular systems is requisite for tumorigenesis (Boudreau and Bissell, 1998; Park et al, 2000). Extracellular factors that influence tumor growth include ECM structural proteins, proteinases, growth factor/signaling molecules, and tumor-infiltrating host cells. These factors function in tissue growth and remodeling during normal development, tissue maintenance, and injury repair. In tumors, however, the activity of these extracellular factors is almost always irregular and facilitates tumor initiation, growth, invasiveness, and metastasis.

The Extracellular Matrix

The ECM comprises an organized meshwork of proteins and polysaccharides secreted locally into the extracellular space. These molecules communicate with membrane-spanning glycoproteins and glycolipids, and participate in normal cell and tissue dynamics including cell growth, shape, motility, and survival. Integrins and growth factor receptors are two groups of membrane-spanning glycoproteins that direct extracellular/intracellular communication. The membrane-spanning and ECM molecules expressed by tumors often differ quantitatively and qualitatively from the cell or tissue from which they are de-

rived. These differences can significantly affect tumor behavior. For example, some breast tumor epithelial cells express aberrant integrins that interact inappropriately with the ECM (Weaver et al, 1997; Boudreau and Bissell, 1998). Restoration of the appropriate integrins returns the malignant epithelial cells to a nonproliferating and differentiated state, regardless of the pre-existing genetic lesions. This finding highlights the critical role that extracellular/intracellular communication plays in tumorigenesis.

In addition to expressing different ECM and membrane-spanning proteins, tumors remodel preexisting ECM proteins using extracellular proteinases (Coussens and Werb, 1996; Bergers and Coussens, 2000; Johansson et al, 2000). Several classes of proteolytic enzymes degrade the ECM, including a class of metal-dependent endopeptidases known as *matrix metalloproteinases* (MMPs). Within tumors, both neoplastic tumor cells and infiltrating-host cells express ECM-degrading proteinases (Coussens et al, 2000). These proteinases normally participate in tissue growth, tissue maintenance, and injury repair. In tumors, however, MMPs are important regulators of ECM remodeling associated with growth, invasion, metastasis, and formation of new blood vessels. For example, MMPs and other extracellular proteinases participate in the regulation of polypeptide growth factor activity (Bergers and Coussens, 2000). Some growth factors are directed to the plasma membrane as latent precursors, and upon proteolytic cleavage, these factors are activated. Other growth factors are bound to ECM proteins that suppress their activity. Upon proteinase-mediated degradation of those ECM proteins, the growth factors are released and subsequently activated.

A positive correlation exists between increased MMP expression and increased tumor invasiveness and metastasis in many human cancers (Schoedel et al, 1996; Adachi et al, 1998, 1999; Nakayama et al, 1998). MMP expression is induced in response to cytokines, growth factors, and altered cell–cell or cell–ECM contacts, and is negatively regulated by a group of nonspecific inhibitors, including tissue inhibitors of metalloproteinases (TIMPs). The balance between MMP and TIMP activity is crucial in cancer progression, as tumor invasion and metastasis are inhibited by specific TIMPs (DeClerck et al, 1992; Testa, 1992; Blavier et al, 1999). Anticancer therapeutic approaches that interfere with MMP cancer-promoting activities may be useful in limiting tumor invasion and metastasis.

Tumor invasion and metastasis also require changes in cell surface adhesion molecules, including E-cadherin and CD44. Structural or expression changes in either of these molecules are associated with decreased cell–cell contact and cellular/tissue differentiation and with increased tumor invasiveness and metastasis (Shimoyama et al, 1989; Behrens et al, 1991; Gunthert et al, 1991; Oda et al, 1994; Umbas et al, 1994; Takeda et al, 1999; Herrlich et al, 2000). Activation of intracellular signaling cascades that affect cell shape and motility by causing cytoskeletal changes are also necessary for tumor invasion and metastasis (Liotta et al, 1991; Hernandez-Alcoceba et al, 2000).

Angiogenesis

Tumor expansion relies on adequate blood supplies for delivery of oxygen and nutrients. Therefore, proliferating tumor cells (and normal cells) must be located within 100 to 200 mm of blood vessels, a distance equal to the intratissue diffusion limit of oxygen (Carmeliet and Jain, 2000). Tumor cells become necrotic or apoptotic when not in close proximity to blood supplies (Holmgren et al, 1995; Parangi et al, 1996). Tumors access blood supplies by forming extensive vascular networks through the process of angiogenesis—the sprouting and expansion of blood vessels from preexisting vessels. Angiogenesis differs from vasculogenesis—the assembly of blood vessels from endothelial precursors—which is how blood vessels originate in developing embryos. In addition to causing tumor expansion, angiogenesis may be an important

step in tumor initiation, since this process can be visualized in transformed tissues prior to the appearance of solid tumors (Hanahan and Folkman, 1996). The sprouting of vascular networks in tumors also provides migrating tumor cells easy access to the circulatory system. Thus, angiogenesis also facilitates tumor metastasis (Fidler and Ellis, 1994; Holmgren et al, 1995).

Many endogenous pro- and antiangiogenic molecules exist, derived from cancer cells, endothelial cells, stromal cells, blood, and the ECM (Fukumura et al, 1998; Carmeliet and Jain, 2000). The relative contribution of each of these factors to the vascular density in tumors likely depends on tumor type, location, size, and stage of progression (Carmeliet and Jain, 2000). Variations in the microenvironment of tumors, such as the presence or absence of hypoxia (Helmlinger et al, 2000), may also influence vascular density. Proangiogenic molecules comprise mostly growth factors for vascular endothelial cells including members of the vascular endothelial growth factor (VEGf), angiopoietin, and fibroblast growth factor (FGf) families (Ferrara and Alitalo, 1999; Carmeliet and Jain, 2000).

These growth factors stimulate endothelial cell proliferation and migration by binding to transmembrane tyrosine kinase receptors, initiating signal cascades, and activating the cell proliferative and mobility machinery. Two prominent endogenous antiangiogenic molecules have also been identified—angiostatin and endostatin (O'Reilly et al, 1994, 1997). Angiostatin and endostatin derive from parent ECM molecules (Dong et al, 1997; Patterson and Sang, 1997; Lijnen et al, 1998). The exact biological activity of these molecules is uncertain, although it appears that they participate in suppressing endothelial cell proliferation and/or migration.

As angiogenesis is necessary for tumor growth and metastasis, inhibiting angiogenesis may be an effective approach to cancer therapy (Fidler and Ellis, 1994; Ferrara and Alitalo, 1999). The balance of proangiogenic and antiantigenic factors controls angiogenesis (Fig. 3–9) (Hanahan and Folkman, 1996). Tumors shift the balance in favor of the proangiogenic factors, thus allowing for the formation of extensive vascular networks and guaranteeing their survival. It may be possible, through clinical intervention, to shift the balance in favor of the antiangiogenic factors, thus depleting the tumor vasculature, resulting in decreased tumor growth and metastasis. One clinically successful approach for the treatment of cancer has been to interfere with the proangiogenic growth factor VEGF with the monoclonal antibody Avastin (Ferrara 2005).

Evasion of Immune-mediated Eradication

The genetic alterations that result in tumor transformation have the potential to be accompanied by the generation of tumor-specific antigens, in some if not all cancers (Klein and Klein, 2005). Theoretically, these antigens can elicit an immune response that ultimately can kill the tumor. Killer T lymphocytes are able to monitor the contents of cells by interacting with major histocompatability complex (MHC) class I molecules that present an array of cellular peptides on the cell surface. All cells in the body express MHC class I complexes that present antigens to killer T lymphocytes during immunosurveillance (Fig. 3–10). Cells that present foreign antigens to killer

T lymphocytes are destroyed by cytolytic perforin-granzyme mechanisms or by Fas receptor–induced apoptotic death.

The recognition and subsequent removal of foreign antigen by the immune system is known as immunosurveillance. In certain circumstances, immunosurveillance may eradicate tumors after early transforming events, thereby preventing development of full-blown cancer. However, no direct evidence for this exists (Strand and Galle, 1998). Indirect evidence for a role of immunosurveillance in cancer prevention comes from the fact that immunodeficient individuals have a greater incidence of some cancers than immunocompetent individuals (Beral and Newton, 1998). In addition, tumors elicit immune responses from their hosts that result in the infiltration of macrophages, lymphocytes, and polymorphonuclear granulocytes.

Despite the presentation of foreign antigens and often considerable immune infiltrates, tumors are able to evade immune recognition and cytotoxic activity by a number of mechanisms. For example, some tumor cells do not express MHC class I complexes or express them at greatly reduced levels (Ruiter et al, 1991; Garrido et al, 1993; Restifo and Wunderlich, 1997). Along this same line, tumor cells may fail

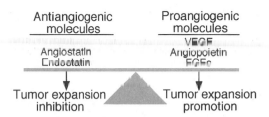

Figure 3–9. The balance of pro- and antiangiogenic molecules controls angiogenesis. Antiangiogenic molecules, including angiostatin and endostatin, impede vascular formation and subsequently inhibit tumor expansion. Proangiogenic molecules, including vascular endothelial growth factor (VEGF), angiopoietin, and fibroblast growth factors (FGFs), facilitate vascular formation and subsequently promote tumor expansion.

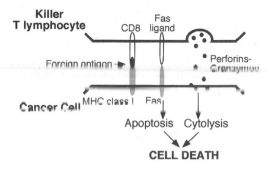

Figure 3–10. Killer T lymphocyte–mediated cell death. Killer T lymphocytes recognize foreign antigen through CD8—major histocompatibility complex (MHC) class I interactions. Killer T lymphocytes then destroy target (cancer) cells by inducing apoptosis through Fas/Fas ligand contacts or by inducing cytolysis through perforin-granzyme activity.

to process or present antigen that normally would be recognized by T lymphocytes. Tumors also utilize various methods to avoid T lymphocyte–induced apoptotic death. Some tumors may evade immune-mediated eradication by secreting cytokines that inhibit immune responses, for example protaglandin E2, transforming growth factor β, or interleukin 10 (Musiani et al, 1997). Lastly, the rapid growth of some highly malignant tumors may simply overcome the efforts of immune-system effectors.

Tumor immunosurveillance has stimulated a field of anticancer research known as *cancer immunotherapy*, which utilizes immunologic methods to target and kill cells containing tumor-specific or enriched antigens. In fact, antibodies have been developed that bind to tumor-specific or enriched antigens, which then elicit an immune response against the cancer, resulting in tumor regression (Pegram and Slamon, 2000; Ferrara 2005).

CONCLUSION

One of the major goals in cancer research is to elucidate the molecular and cellular events driving the progression of cells from a normal to a cancerous state. This transformation relies on the accumulation of mutations in various proto-oncogenes, tumor-suppressor genes, and DNA repair (caretaker) genes. Under normal circumstances, these genes participate in regulating cell and tissue behavior. However, progressive accumulation of mutations in these genes causes cells to transform to a malignant state. These mutations collaborate to overcome the numerous barriers and obstacles cells erect to prevent uncontrolled growth, including cell-cycle control, absence of appropriate growth stimuli, programmed cell death, limited replicative potential, and immune-mediated eradication. In addition, these mutations ultimately result in altered interactions with the extracellular environment, facilitating tumor initiation and progression.

An understanding of the molecular and cellular events associated with the origin of cancer is fundamental to cancer epidemiology. Cancer-related risk factors and genetic predispositions identified by epidemiologic methods manifest themselves as molecular and cellular events. Moreover, the complexity of cancer biology necessitates epidemiologic approaches to evaluate accurately basic research and therapeutic findings. The future of cancer research therefore lies in the collaborative efforts of epidemiologists, biologists, and clinicians. It is hoped that the collective efforts of these groups will translate into improved modalities of cancer-prevention programs and anticancer therapies.

REFERENCES

Adachi Y, Itoh F, Yamamoto H, Matsuno K, Arimura Y, Kusano M, et al. Matrix metalloproteinase matrilysin (MMP-7) participates in the progression of human gastric and esophageal cancers. Int J Oncol 1998;13:1031–35.

Adachi Y, Yamamoto H, Itoh F, Hinoda Y, Okada Y, Imai K. Contribution of matrilysin (MMP-7) to the metastatic pathway of human colorectal cancers. Gut 1999;45:252–58.

Adams PD, Kaelin WG Jr. Negative control elements of the cell cycle in human tumors. Curr Opin Cell Biol 1998;10:791–97.

Armitage P, Doll R. A two-stage theory of carcinogenesis in relation to the age distribution of human cancer. Br J Cancer 1957;11:161–69.

Barak Y, Juven T, Haffner R, Oren M. mdm2 expression is induced by wild type p53 activity. Embo J 1993;12:461–68.

Behrens J, Weidner KM, Frixen UH, Schipper JH, Sachs M, Arakaki N, et al. The role of E-cadherin and scatter factor in tumor invasion and cell motility. Exs 1991;59:109–26.

Beral V, Newton R. Overview of the epidemiology of immunodeficiency-associated cancers. J Natl Cancer Inst Monogr 1998;23:1–6.

Berchuck A, Boyd J. Molecular basis of endometrial cancer. Cancer 1995;76(10 Suppl):2034–40.

Bergers G, Coussens LM. Extrinsic regulators of epithelial tumor progression: metalloproteinases. Curr Opin Genet Dev 2000;10:120–27.

Bernards R, Weinberg RA. A progression puzzle. Nature 2002;418:823.

Blackburn EH. Telomere states and cell fates. Nature 2000;408:53–56.

Blavier L, Henriet P, Imren S, Declerck YA. Tissue inhibitors of matrix metalloproteinases in cancer. Ann NY Acad Sci 1999;878:108–19.

Bottger A, Bottger V, Sparks A, Liu WL, Howard SF, Lane DP. Design of a synthetic Mdm2-binding mini protein that activates the p53 response in vivo. Curr Biol 1997;7:860–69.

Boudreau N, Bissell MJ. Extracellular matrix signaling: integration of form and function in normal and malignant cells. Curr Opin Cell Biol 1998;10:640–46.

Cairns J. Mutation selection and the natural history of cancer. Nature 1975;255:197–200.

Calin GA, Croce CM. MicroRNA signatures in human cancers. Nat Rev Cancer 2006;6:857–66.

Carmeliet P, Jain RK. Angiogenesis in cancer and other diseases. Nature 2000;407:249–57.

Chadeneau C, Hay K, Hirte HW, Gallinger S, Bacchetti S. Telomerase activity associated with acquisition of malignancy in human colorectal cancer. Cancer Res 1995;55:2533–36.

Clarke AR, Purdie CA, Harrison DJ, Morris RG, Bird CC, Hooper ML, Wyllie AH. Thymocyte apoptosis induced by p53-dependent and independent pathways [see comments]. Nature 1993;362:849–52.

Counter CM, Hirte HW, Bacchetti S, Harley CB. Telomerase activity in human ovarian carcinoma [see comments]. Proc Natl Acad Sci USA 1994;91:2900–4.

Coussens LM, Tinkle CL, Hanahan D, Werb Z. MMP-9 supplied by bone marrow–derived cells contributes to skin carcinogenesis. Cell 2000;103:481–90.

Coussens LM, Werb Z. Matrix metalloproteinases and the development of cancer. Chem Biol 1996;3:895–904.

Dang CV, Resar LM, Emison E, Kim S, Li Q, Prescott JE, Wonsey D, Zeller K. Function of the c-Myc oncogenic transcription factor. Exp Cell Res 1999;253:63–77.

DeClerck YA, Perez N, Shimada H, Boone TC, Langley KE, Taylor SM. Inhibition of invasion and metastasis in cells transfected with an inhibitor of metalloproteinases. Cancer Res 1992;52:701–8.

de Lange T, Jacks T. For better or worse? Telomerase inhibition and cancer. Cell 1999;98:273–75.

Dong Z, Kumar R, Yang X, Fidler IJ. Macrophage-derived metalloelastase is responsible for the generation of angiostatin in Lewis lung carcinoma. Cell 1997;88:801–10.

Ellis NA, Groden J, Ye TZ, Straughen J, Lennon DJ, Ciocci S, et al. The Bloom's syndrome gene product is homologous to RecQ helicases. Cell 1995;83:655–66.

Esquela-Kerscher A, Slack FJ. Oncomirs-microRNAs with a role in cancer. Nat Rev Cancer 2006;6:259–68.

Ferrara N, Alitalo K. Clinical applications of angiogenic growth factors and their inhibitors. Nat Med 1999;5:1359–64.

Ferrara N. VEGF as a therapeutic target in cancer. Oncology 2005;69:11–16.

Fialkow PJ. Clonal origin of human tumors. Biochim Biophys Acta 1976;458:283–321.

Fialkow PJ. Clonal origin of human tumors. Annu Rev Med 1979;30:135–43.

Fidler IJ, Balch CM. The biology of cancer metastasis and implications for therapy. Curr Probl Surg 1987;24:129–209.

Fidler IJ, Ellis LM. The implications of angiogenesis for the biology and therapy of cancer metastasis [comment]. Cell 1994;79:185–88.

Fukumura D, Xavier R, Sugiura T, Chen Y, Park EC, Lu N, et al. Tumor induction of VEGF promoter activity in stromal cells. Cell 1998;94:715–25.

Garcia-Higuera I, Kuang Y, D'Andrea AD. The molecular and cellular biology of Fanconi anemia. Curr Opin Hematol 1999;6:83–88.

Garrido F, Cabrera T, Concha A, Glew S, Ruiz-Cabello F, Stern PL. Natural history of HLA expression during tumour development. Immunol Today 1993;14:491–99.

Giatromanolaki A, Koukourakis MI, O'Byrne K, Kaklamanis L, Dicoglou C, Trichia E, et al. Non–small cell lung cancer: c-erbB-2 overexpression correlates with low angiogenesis and poor prognosis. Anticancer Res 1996;16:3819–25.

Gorre ME, Mohammed M, Ellwood K, Hsu N, Paquette R, Rao PN, Sawyers CL. Clinical resistance to STI-571 cancer therapy caused by BCR-ABL gene mutation or amplification. Science 2001;293:876–80.

Gray MD, Shen JC, Kamath-Loeb AS, Blank A, Sopher BL, Martin GM, et al. The Werner syndrome protein is a DNA helicase. Nat Genet 1997;17:100–3.

Greenblatt MS, Bennett WP, Hollstein M, Harris CC. Mutations in the p53 tumor suppressor gene: clues to cancer etiology and molecular pathogenesis. Cancer Res 1994;54:4855–78.

Groth A, Weber JD, Willumsen BM, Sherr CJ, Roussel MF. Oncogenic Ras induces p19ARF and growth arrest in mouse embryo fibroblasts lacking p21Cip1 and p27Kip1 without activating cyclin D–dependent kinases. J Biol Chem 2000;275:27473–80.

Gunthert U, Hofmann M, Rudy W, Reber S, Zoller M, Haussmann I, et al. A new variant of glycoprotein CD44 confers metastatic potential to rat carcinoma cells. Cell 1991;65:13–24.

Hahn WC, Counter CM, Lundberg AS, Beijersbergen RL, Brooks MW, Weinberg RA. Creation of human tumor cells with defined genetic elements. Nature 1999;400:464–68.

Hanahan D, Folkman J. Patterns and emerging mechanisms of the angiogenic switch during tumorigenesis. Cell 1996;86:353–64.

Hanahan D, Weinberg RA. The hallmarks of cancer. Cell 2000;100:57–70.

Hayflick L, Moorhead PS. The serial cultivation of human diploid ccell strains. Exp Cell Res 1961;25:585–621.

Helmlinger G, Endo M, Ferrara N, Hlatky L, Jain RK. Formation of endothelial cell networks. Nature 2000;405:139–41.

Hernandez-Alcoceba R, del Peso L, Lacal JC. The Ras family of GTPases in cancer cell invasion. Cell Mol Life Sci 2000;57:65–76.

Herrlich P, Morrison H, Sleeman J, Orian-Rousseau V, Konig H, Weg-Remers S, et al. CD44 acts both as a growth- and invasiveness-promoting molecule and as a tumor-suppressing cofactor. Ann NY Acad Sci 2000;910:106–18; discussion 118–20.

Hickman MJ, Samson LD. Role of DNA mismatch repair and p53 in signaling induction of apoptosis by alkylating agents. Proc Natl Acad Sci USA 1999;96:10764–69.

Hollstein M, Sidransky D, Vogelstein B, Harris CC. p53 mutations in human cancers. Science 1991;253:49–53.

Holmgren L, O'Reilly MS, Folkman J. Dormancy of micrometastases: balanced proliferation and apoptosis in the presence of angiogenesis suppression [see comments]. Nat Med 1995;1:149–53.

Hussain SP, Harris CC. Molecular epidemiology and carcinogenesis: endogenous and exogenous carcinogens. Mutat Res 2000;462:311–22.

Jacks T. Lessons from the p53 mutant mouse. J Cancer Res Clin Oncol 1996;122:319–27.

Jackson AL, Loeb LA. On the origin of multiple mutations in human cancers. Semin Cancer Biol 1998;8:421–29.

Johansson N, Ahonen M, Kahari VM. Matrix metalloproteinases in tumor invasion. Cell Mol Life Sci 2000;57:5–15.

Jones PA, Laird PW. Cancer epigenetics comes of age. Nat Genet 1999;21:163–67.

Kapitanovic S, Spaventi R, Poljak L, Kapitanovic M, Pavelic ZP, Gluckman JL, et al. High c-erbB-2 protein level in colorectal adenocarcinomas correlates with clinical parameters. Cancer Detect Prev 1994;18:97–101.

Kastan MB. Molecular biology of cancer: the cell cycle. In: DeVita VT Jr, Hellman S, Rosenberg SA (Eds): Cancer: Principles and Practice of Oncology, 5th ed. Philadelphia, Lippincott-Raven, 1997, pp 121–134.

Kaufmann SH, Gores GJ. Apoptosis in cancer: cause and cure. Bioessays 2000;22:1007–17.

Khouri I. Molecular biology of leukemias. In: DeVita VR Jr, Hellman S, Rosenberg SA (Eds): Cancer: Principles and Practice of Oncology, 5th ed. Philadelphia, Lippincott-Raven, 1997, pp 2285–92.

Kinzler KW, Vogelstein B. Landscaping the cancer terrain [comment]. Science 1998;280:1036–37.

Klein G, Klein E. Surveillance against tumors–is it mainly immunological? Immunol Letters 2005; 100:29–33.

Knudson AG, DiFerrante N, Curtis JE. Mutation and cancer: statistical study of retinoblastoma. Proc Natl Acad Sci USA 1971;68:820–23.

Kolquist KA, Ellisen LW, Counter CM, Meyerson M, Tan LK, Weinberg RA, Haber DA, Gerald WL. Expression of TERT in early premalignant lesions and a subset of cells in normal tissues [see comments]. Nat Genet 1998;19:182–86.

Kress M, May E, Cassingena R, May P. Simian virus 40–transformed cells express new species of proteins precipitable by anti–simian virus 40 tumor serum. J Virol 1979;31:472–83.

Kuper H, Adami HO, Tricopoulos D. Infections as a major preventable cause of human cancer. J Int Med 2000;248:171–83.

Lane DP, Crawford LV. T antigen is bound to a host protein in SV40-transformed cells. Nature 1979;278:261–63.

Le-Niculescu H, Bonfoco E, Kasuya Y, Claret FX, Green DR, Karin M. Withdrawal of survival factors results in activation of the JNK pathway in neuronal cells leading to Fas ligand induction and cell death. Mol Cell Biol 1999;19:751–63.

Lijnen HR, Ugwu E, Bini A, Collen D. Generation of an angiostatin-like fragment from plasminogen by stromelysin-1 (MMP-3). Biochemistry 1998;37:4699–702.

Linzer DI, Levine AJ. Characterization of a 54K dalton cellular SV40 tumor antigen present in SV40-transformed cells and uninfected embryonal carcinoma cells. Cell 1979;17:43–52.

Liotta LA, Stracke ML, Aznavoorian SA, Beckner ME, Schiffmann E. Tumor cell motility. Semin Cancer Biol 1991;2:111–14.

Loeb KR, Loeb LA. Significance of multiple mutations in cancer. Carcinogenesis 2000;21:379–85.

Loeb LA. Mutator phenotype may be required for multistage carcinogenesis. Cancer Res 1991;51:3075–79.

Lopes MBS, VandenBerg SR, Scheithauer BW. The World Health Organization classification of nervous system tumors in experimental neuro-oncology. In: Levine AJ, Schmidek HM (Eds): Molecular Genetics of Nervous System Tumors. New York, Wiley-Liss, 1993, pp 1–36.

Lu J, Getz G, Miska EA, Alvarez-Saaverdra E, Lamb J, et al. MicroRNA expression profiles classify human cancers. Nature 2005;435: 834–38.

Lupu R, Cardillo M, Cho C, Harris L, Hijazi M, Perez C, Rosenberg K, Yang D, Tang C. The significance of heregulin in breast cancer tumor progression and drug resistance. Breast Cancer Res Treat 1996;38:57–66.

Michelson RJ, Weinert T. Closing the gaps among a web of DNA repair disorders. Bioessays 2000;22:966–69.

Michor F, Hughes TP, Iwasa Y, Branford S, Shah NP, Sawyers CL, Nowak MA. Dynamics of chronic myeloid leukaemia. Nature 2005;435:1267–70.

Mooi WJ, Peeper DS. Oncogene-induced cell senescence-halting on the road to cancer. NEJM 2006;355:1037–46.

Musiani P, Modesti A, Giovarelli M, Cavallo F, Colombo MP, Lollini PL, Forni G. Cytokines, tumour-cell death and immunogenicity: a question of choice. Immunol Today 1997; 18:32–36.

Nakayama Y, Okazaki K, Shibao K, Sako T, Hirata K, Nagata N, Kuwano M, Itoh H. Alternative expression of the collagenase and adhesion molecules in the highly metastatic clones of human colonic cancer cell lines. Clin Exp Metastasis 1998;16:461–69.

Nesbit CE, Tersak JM, Prochownik EV. MYC oncogenes and human neoplastic disease. Oncogene 1999;18:3004–16.

O'Connell J, Bennett MW, Nally K, Houston A, O'Sullivan GC, Shanahan F. Altered mechanisms of apoptosis in colon cancer: Fas resistance and counterattack in the tumor-immune conflict. Ann NY Acad Sci 2000; 910:178–92; discussion 193–95.

Oda T, Kanai Y, Oyama T, Yoshiura K, Shimoyama Y, Birchmeier W, et al. E-cadherin gene mutations in human gastric carcinoma cell lines. Proc Natl Acad Sci USA 1994; 91:1858–62.

O'Reilly MS, Boehm T, Shing Y, Fukai N, Vasios G, Lane WS. Endostatin: an endogenous inhibitor of angiogenesis and tumor growth. Cell 1997;88:277–85.

O'Reilly MS, Holmgren L, Shing Y, Chen C, Rosenthal RA, Moses M, et al. Angiostatin: a novel angiogenesis inhibitor that mediates the suppression of metastases by a Lewis lung carcinoma [see comments]. Cell 1994;79: 315–28.

Owen-Schaub LB, Zhang W, Cusack JC, Angelo LS, Santee SM, Fujiwara T, et al. Wild-type human p53 and a temperature-sensitive mutant induce Fas/APO-1 expression. Mol Cell Biol 1995;15:3032–40.

Parangi S, O'Reilly M, Christofori G, Holmgren L, Grosfeld J, Folkman J, et al. Antiangiogenic therapy of transgenic mice impairs de

novo tumor growth. Proc Natl Acad Sci USA 1996;93:2002–7.

Park CC, Bissell MJ, Barcellos-Hoff MH. The influence of the microenvironment on the malignant phenotype. Mol Med Today 2000; 6:324–29.

Patterson BC, Sang QA. Angiostatin-converting enzyme activities of human matrilysin (MMP-7) and gelatinase B/type IV collagenase (MMP-9). J Biol Chem 1997;272: 28823–25.

Pegram M, Slamon D. Biological rationale for HER2/neu (c-erbB2) as a target for monoclonal antibody therapy. Semin Oncol 2000; 27(5 Suppl 9):13–19.

Pelengaris S, Rudolph B, Littlewood T. Action of Myc in vivo—proliferation and apoptosis. Curr Opin Genet Dev 2000;10:100–5.

Pitti RM, Marsters SA, Lawrence DA, Roy M, Kischkel FC, Dowd P. Genomic amplification of a decoy receptor for Fas ligand in lung and colon cancer. Nature 1998;396:699–703.

Prives C, Hall PA. The p53 pathway. J Pathol 1999;187:112–26.

Restifo NP, Wunderlich JR. Essentials of immunology. In: DeVita VT Jr, Hellman S, Rosenberg SA (Eds): Cancer: Principles and Practice of Oncology, 5th ed. Philadelphia, Lippincott-Raven, 1997, pp 47–75.

Reya T, Morrison SJ, Clarke MF, Weissman IL. Stem cells, cancer, and cancer stem cells. Nature 2001;414:105–11.

Ruiter DJ, Mattijssen V, Broecker EB, Ferrone S. MHC antigens in human melanomas. Semin Cancer Biol 1991;2:35–45.

Rytomaa M, Martins LM, Downward J. Involvement of FADD and caspase-8 signalling in detachment-induced apoptosis. Curr Biol 1999; 9:1043–46.

Savitsky K, Bar-Shira A, Gilad S, Rotman G, Ziv Y, Vanagaite L, et al. A single ataxia telangiectasia gene with a product similar to PI-3 kinase [see comments]. Science 1995;268: 1749–53.

Schmidt EV. The role of c-myc in cellular growth control. Oncogene 1999;18:2988–96.

Schoedel KE, Greco MA, Stetler-Stevenson WG, Ohori NP, Goswami S, Present D, et al. Expression of metalloproteinases and tissue inhibitors of metalloproteinases in giant cell tumor of bone: an immunohistochemical study with clinical correlation. Hum Pathol 1996;27:1144–48.

Sedivy JM. Can ends justify the means? Telomeres and the mechanisms of replicative senescence and immortalization in mammalian cells. Proc Natl Acad Sci USA 1998;95: 9078–81.

Shen JC, Loeb LA. The Werner syndrome gene: the molecular basis of RecQ helicase-deficiency diseases. Trends Genet 2000;16: 213–20.

Shimoyama Y, Hirohashi S, Hirano S, Noguchi M, Shimosato Y, Takeichi M, et al. Cadherin cell-adhesion molecules in human epithelial tissues and carcinomas. Cancer Res 1989;49: 2128–33.

Sikora J, Dworacki G, Zeromski J. Expression of Fas and Fas ligand and apoptosis in tumor-associated lymphocytes and in tumor cells from malignant pleural effusions. Nat Immun 1998;16:244–55.

Slamon SE, Cassady JR. Plasma cell neoplasms. In: DeVita VR Jr, Hellman S, Rosenberg SA (Eds): Cancer: Principles and Practice of Oncology, 5th ed. Philadelphia, Lippincott-Raven, 1997, pp 2344–87.

Spencer CA, Groudine M. Control of c-myc regulation in normal and neoplastic cells. Adv Cancer Res 1991;56:1–48.

Strand S, Galle PR. Immune evasion by tumours: involvement of the CD95 (APO-1/Fas) system and its clinical implications. Mol Med Today 1998;4:63–68.

Takeda H, Shimoyama Y, Nagafuchi A, Hirohashi S. E-cadherin functions as a cis-dimer at the cell–cell adhesive interface in vivo. Nat Struct Biol 1999; 6:310–12.

Testa JE. Loss of the metastatic phenotype by a human epidermoid carcinoma cell line, HEp-3, is accompanied by increased expression of tissue inhibitor of metalloproteinase 2. Cancer Res 1992;52:5597–603.

Umbas R, Isaacs WB, Bringuier PP, Schaafsma HE, Karthaus HF, Oosterhof GO, et al. Decreased E-cadherin expression is associated with poor prognosis in patients with prostate cancer. Cancer Res 1994;54:3929–33.

Varmus H, Weinberg RA. Genes and the Biology of Cancer. New York, Scientific American Library, 1993.

Vaux DL, Cory S, Adams JM. Bcl-2 gene promotes haemopoietic cell survival and cooperates with c-myc to immortalize pre-B cells. Nature 1988;335:440–42.

Vaux DL, Korsmeyer SL. Cell death in development. Cell 1999;96:245–54.

Vogelstein B, Kinzler KW. The multistep nature of cancer. Trends Genet 1993;9:138–41.

Vogelstein B, Kinzler KW. Cancer genes and the pathways they control. Nature Med 2004; 10:789–99.

Vogelstein B, Lane D, Levine AJ. Surfing the p53 network. Nature 2000;408:307–10.

Watson JD. Origin of concatemeric T7 DNA. Nat New Biol 1972;239:197–201.

Watt PM, Hickson ID. Failure to unwind causes cancer. Genome stability. Curr Biol 1996;6: 265–67.

Weaver VM, Petersen OW, Wang F, Larabell CA, Briand P, Damsky C, et al. Reversion of the malignant phenotype of human breast cells in three-dimensional culture and in vivo by integrin blocking antibodies. J Cell Biol 1997;137:231–45.

Weinberg RA. How cancer arises. Sci Am 1996; 275:62–70.

Weinberg RA. The Biology of Cancer. New York, Garland Science, 2006, p 864.

Weintraub SJ, Prater CA, Dean DC. Retinoblastoma protein switches the E2F site from positive to negative element. Nature 1992; 358:259–61.

Zalcberg, JR, Friedlander ML, Minden MD. Molecular evidence for the clonal origin of blast crisis in chronic myeloid leukaemia. Br J Cancer 1986;53:459–64.

Zhan Q, Fan S, Bae I, Guillouf C, Liebermann DA, O'Connor PM, et al. Induction of bax by genotoxic stress in human cells correlates with normal p53 status and apoptosis [published erratum appears in Oncogene 1995; 16;10:1259]. Oncogene 1994;9:3743–51.

Zhou BB, Elledge SJ. The DNA damage response: putting checkpoints in perspective. Nature 2000;408:433–39.

4

Genetic Epidemiology of Cancer

CHRISTOPHER HAIMAN AND DAVID HUNTER

In this chapter we explore the genetic epidemiology of cancer: The identification and quantification of genetic factors and their interaction with the environment in the etiology of cancer in human populations. The availability of the complete DNA sequence of our genome, generated by the Human Genome Project, was followed by the creation of genome-wide databases of common genetic variation. This information, in addition to recent innovation in high-throughput genotyping technology, has provided researchers with the necessary tools to more comprehensively examine genetic variation in relation to cancer risk. These advances have revolutionized how we study inherited susceptibility to cancer and provide the framework for a more complete understanding of the role our genes play in the development and progression of human cancer. In addition to isolating and further characterizing specific genes that are likely to increase susceptibility to specific cancers, over the next few years researchers are likely to identify genes with modest effects that may interact with environmental factors. Our success in defining the underlying genetic etiology of cancer and the prediction of cancer risk in individuals will continue to rely on the integration of clinical genetics and genetic epidemiologic methods.

We also describe the techniques used to identify genes that contribute to cancer susceptibility. To facilitate the discussion, we have included a short glossary of genetic terms (*italicized*) at the end of the chapter. We will briefly describe the research methods for identifying the chromosomal localization of high-risk predisposing genes, such as linkage analysis within pedigrees and allele-sharing methods. We will also review the epidemiologic study designs that can be helpful in identifying low-risk alleles in candidate gene and genome-wide association studies, as well as gene–environment interactions. These concepts are further explored in Chapter 6. We will also describe some of the genotyping platforms commonly employed for high-throughout genome analysis and, in conclusion, we will discuss possible future directions in research on the genetic epidemiology of cancer.

CANCER GENES AND MECHANISMS OF GENE DISRUPTION

Discoveries in the field of molecular genetics have provided substantial insight into the genetic events required for the initiation and progression of cancer in humans. Genes involved in cellular growth, differentiation, apoptosis, and DNA repair have been directly implicated in cancer development. These genes were described in the previous chapter. Alterations that disrupt their normal activity have been identified, and include DNA mutation, loss of heterozygosity (LOH), gene amplification, chromosomal translocation, and silencing of transcription though DNA methylation. At the molecular level, cancer is complex; cell transformation and tumor growth result from the accumulation of multiple genetic and epigenetic alterations.

A distinction is made between DNA mutations originating in germline cells and those occurring in somatic cells. The former are inherited sequence variants passed on to progeny and found in the DNA of all cells of the body. Cancers resulting from inheritance of germline mutations are considered hereditary in origin, and approaches to identify these are the focus of this chapter. In contrast, mutations in somatic cells that arise during the process of carcinogenesis are limited to the cancerous tissue and are called somatic mutations. Sporadic cancers are generally attributed to somatic mutations.

Genetic Variation

A human gene is composed of coding (exons), noncoding (introns), and regulatory DNA sequences ranging in size from 1.5 to more than 2000 kilobases. Once the human gene sequence was available, the number of genes in the human genome was initially estimated to be approximately 30 000–40 000 (International Human Genome Sequencing Consortium, 2001), but later estimates are as low as 20 000 (International Human Genome Sequencing Consortium,

2004). An individual's complete genome, composed of the linear sequence of the four nucleotide bases (adenine, guanine, cytosine, and thymine), is unique (except for identical twins). This uniqueness contributes to the observed phenotypic diversity among individuals. Individual variation in one or more genes may explain differences in susceptibility to human diseases such as cancer. For instance, variations in the nucleotide sequence of genes encoding enzymes that detoxify carcinogenic environmental exposures have been identified. Such genes are now intensely studied as biomarkers of individual genetic susceptibility to various cancers (Vineis and Malats, 1999; Mucci et al, 2001).

Mutations and Polymorphisms

Aberrations in the DNA sequence of genes may alter the function of the encoded proteins. They may be present as germline mutations in individuals with a familial predisposition to cancer or may occur during life as somatic mutations in individual cells. These aberrations include nucleotide deletions, insertions, and substitutions (Fig. 4–1) Nucleotide insertions and deletions of fewer than three bases result in frameshift mutations—that is, they shift the three-base reading frame (the codon) in RNA that is translated into normal protein. Frameshift mutations either yield an incorrect string of amino acids or introduce a stop codon, which results in a shortened protein.

In coding regions, base pair substitutions may appear as either silent mutations that do not alter the encoded amino acid, missense mutations that result in an amino acid change, or nonsense mutations that give rise to a stop codon and the premature truncation of the protein during translation. Deletions, insertions, and noncoding single-base replacements may also influence the regulation of transcription and RNA splicing.

Some mutations are lethal, while others may be compatible with survival but are associated with a significant elevation in disease risk. Not all genetic alterations result in a change in phenotype. When mutations are identified within tumors or in the germline,

Deletion

>   Protein Truncation: BRCA1 185delAG

>>   Normal   5' - ...ATC TTA G*AG* TGT CCC... - 3'

>>   Mutant   5' - ...ATC TTA GTG TCC C...stop signal at codon 39

Insertion

>   Protein Truncation: BRCA1 5382insC

>>   Normal   5' - ...AAT CCC AGG ACA GA... - 3'

>>   Mutant   5' - ...AAT CCC *C*AG GAC AGA...stop signal at codon 1829

Single base pair substitution

>   Missense: Methylenetetrahydrofolate Reductase (MTHFR) 677Alanine → Valine

>>   Normal   5' - ...CGC GGA G*C*C GAT TTC... - 3'

>>   Mutant   5' - ...CGC GGA G*T*C GAT TTC... - 3'

>   Splice donor site: hMLH1 g → a leads to deletion of exon 15

>>   Normal   5' - ...A TCG *g*taagt... - 3'

>>   Mutant   5' - ...A TCG *a*taagt... - 3'

Figure 4–1. Examples of mutations in cancer-predisposition genes.

particularly if they do not truncate the protein, laboratory studies may be necessary to determine which ones are biologically relevant.

Mutations existing at a population allele frequency greater than 1% (ie, in 2% of individuals) are called polymorphisms (Khoury et al, 1993) and convey a range of biological phenotypes. Most polymorphisms have no functional consequence because they occur in a noncoding sequence, they do not alter the amino acid sequence of the protein, or the alteration does not affect the function of the protein. However, genetic polymorphisms are known to contribute to the phenotypic differences observed both within and between ethnic groups. As discussed later in this chapter, intense searches, both within candidate genes and genome-wide, are currently underway to identify polymorphic variants that are associated with complex multifactorial diseases including cancer.

STRATEGIES OF GENE IDENTIFICATION

Clustering of cancer within some families has been well documented for most cancer sites (Borch-Johnsen et al, 1994). Familial aggregation may be due to shared environmental exposures or lifestyle practices, such as dietary and reproductive histories among family members, or it may be due to the inheritance of one or more predisposing gene mutations. Mutations in single genes have been identified as the causal factors in many inherited cancers, and data suggest that genetic factors also make a substantial contribution to the causation of sporadic cancers (Lichtenstein et al, 2000; Pharoah et al, 2002). The degree of cancer risk associated with inheriting a mutation depends on gene penetrance—that is, the probability that an individual carrying a mutation will develop disease, which can be as great as 100%—and may be modified by a combination of genetic and environmental factors.

Familial clustering of cancer may also occur by chance. The common characteristics of truly inherited cancer that differentiate it from the sporadic form include a substantially increased risk of cancer in relatives from several generations, a Mendelian pattern of cancer inheritance in family pedigrees, an earlier age of cancer onset, and multiple or bilateral cancers among affected individuals.

Genetic epidemiologic methods developed to identify the chromosomal location of inherited cancer susceptibility genes in families include segregation analysis—to determine if there is an underlying Mendelian pattern of genetic inheritance, linkage analysis—to localize the chromosomal region coinherited with cancer that contains the cancer-causing gene—and allele-sharing methods—to identify cancer susceptibility loci. The latter two approaches use marker loci in genome-wide searches for DNA regions that cosegregate with a specific disease phenotype.

Segregation Analysis

Segregation analysis is a statistical technique initially carried out to identify and describe the underlying genetic mode of disease inheritance in families (Khoury et al, 1993). The goal of segregation analysis is to establish if a genetic model, such as Mendelian dominant or recessive inheritance, is compatible with the observed pattern of disease occurrence in pedigrees. Segregation analysis also provides gene penetrance and allele frequency parameter estimates required for classic linkage analysis methods. In addition to monogenic single-gene Mendelian models of inheritance, more complex models can be evaluated, thanks to advances in statistical techniques. These include polygenic models (the combination of many genes), the contribution of environmental factors, and the consideration of variable age at onset among family members (Khoury et al, 1993). Since the advent of techniques to directly analyze DNA in family members, segregation analysis is no

longer a mainstay of genetic epidemiology, as it has been substantially supplanted by these direct techniques.

Linkage Analysis

Once a pattern is established through segregation analysis, genetic linkage analysis (Ott, 1991) will localize the chromosomal region coinherited with cancer that contains the cancer-causing gene. This is based on the predicted model of disease transmission, and the analysis is conducted in cancer-prone pedigrees as a genome-wide search for chromosomal loci that occur more frequently in family members with cancer than in those without it. The ability to link marker loci and disease is contingent upon three factors: *(1)* a mode of inheritance is hypothesized for the disease (autosomal, X-linked, dominant, recessive);*(2)* gene penetrance has been estimated; and *(3)* allele frequencies of DNA markers are known. The theory behind this gene-identification approach is based on the understanding that genes are transmitted to offspring via inheritance of parental chromosomes. Chromosomes segregate independently during meiosis, and the inheritance of genes or DNA loci located on different chromosomes is consequently also independent. As a result, genes and markers on the same chromosome are more likely to be in coinherited (Botstein et al, 1980). This corrleation among alleles at nearby sites is known as *linkage disequilibrium*. The extent of linkage disequilibrium depends on the frequency of recombination between alleles, which is a function of their genetic distance and how recently they occurred. The distance between two genetic loci on the same chromosome influences the probability of being transmitted together. The farther apart they are, the greater the opportunity for genetic recombination or "crossing over" during meiosis with the same chromosomal region on the other parental chromosome. The closer together two loci are located on a chromosome, the more likely they will be genetically linked.

Multiple family pedigrees with available DNA specimens are normally required to conduct a genome-wide scan, in which typically 300 or more markers evenly spaced across the chromosomes are typed for each family member. Within families, regions of DNA serving as markers of disease susceptibility loci are identified. Markers used in linkage studies have included restriction fragment length polymorphisms (RFLPs) and highly variable DNA repeat sequences, and, more recently, informative panels of single nucleotide polymorphisms (SNPs). The power to detect linkage between two loci (the marker locus and the disease locus) depends on the distance between marker loci and the disease locus and the degree of polymorphism of the marker loci. Closely spaced, highly polymorphic markers are more informative for linkage studies, because they allow a more in-depth analysis of the genome.

The measure used to evaluate genetic linkage between genetic loci across families is the LOD score, which is calculated as a ratio of likelihoods on the log10 scale. The probability or likelihood of observing the inheritance pattern of two loci at a specified level of linkage or genetic recombination is divided by the likelihood of observing the data assuming no linkage between the two loci (Morton, 1955). A LOD score greater than 3 is conventionally used to indicate that the observed data are more likely to occur under the hypothesis of linkage between the marker and the causative gene and thus provides strong support for a further search for the causative gene in the neighborhood of the marker.

Positional Cloning

Once a chromosomal region has been observed to occur more frequently among cancer-affected family members, the molecular genetic technique known as *positional cloning* could then be applied to isolate and identify the disease gene (Watson et al, 1992). This strategy does not rely on the biological function of the genetic defect, but rather on "chromosome walking," carried out by using overlapping cloned DNA fragments that scan the DNA in the neighborhood of the marker locus. A comparison of the DNA sequences with those identified in other species may assist in determining conserved regions that are more likely to encode genes. The availability of the human gene sequence database now largely eliminates the need for constructing the DNA sequence, and a list of known and predicted genes in a chromosomal region can be rapidly downloaded.

The genes identified as potentially disease causing are then sequenced, seeking the mutation that is almost always carried by family members with cancer—and rarely or never in those without it. If the mutation has not led to an obvious alteration in protein function, such as a stop codon leading to protein truncation, in vitro analyses might make it possible to characterize how the genetic mutation disturbs the protein's normal biological function.

Examples of Linkage

A number of cancer susceptibility genes have been discovered by linkage analysis in family pedigrees. Examples of genes and the cancers to which they predispose (see Table 4–1) include *CDKN2A* (p16) on chromosome 9q21 and familial melanoma (Cannon-Albright et al, 1992); the *RET* oncogene on chromosome 10 and multiple endocrine neoplasia (types 2A and 2B) (Eng et al, 1996); Rb on chromosome 13q and retinoblastoma (Friend et al, 1986); *BRCA1* on chromosome 17q21 and early onset breast-ovarian cancer (Hall et al, 1990; Easton et al, 1993); *BRCA2* on chromosome 13q and early onset breast cancer (Stratton et al, 1994); *APC* on chromosome 5q and familial adenomatous polyposis (FAP) (Leppert et al, 1987); and *hMSH2*, *hMLH1*, *hPMS1*, and *hPMS2* on chromosomes 2p15–16, 3p21, 2q21, and 7q22, respectively, and hereditary nonpolyposis colorectal cancer (HNPCC) (Leppert et al, 1987; Peltomaki et al, 1993; Bronner et al, 1994; Nicolaides et al, 1994; Papadopoulos et al, 1994).

The study of families with early onset breast cancer serves as a paradigm for the use of genetic epidemiologic methods to identify genetic determinants underlying

Table 4–1. Examples of mutations in cancer-predisposition genes.

Gene	Syndrome
Oncogenes	
RET	Multiple endocrine neoplasia 2, familial medullary thyroid cancer
MET	Familial papillary renal carcinoma syndrome
Tumor Suppressors	
APC	Familial adenomatous polyposis
VHL	von Hippel-Lindau syndrome
WT1	Wilms' tumor syndrome
Rb	Hereditary retinoblastoma
NF1	Neurofibromatosis 1
NF2	Neurofibromatosis 2
p53	Li-Fraumeni syndrome
p16/CDKN2A	Hereditary melanoma syndrome
PTCH	Nevoid basal cell carcinoma syndrome
MEN1	Multiple endocrine syndrome (MEN1)
BRCA1	Hereditary breast-ovarian syndrome
BRCA2	Hereditary breast-ovarian syndrome
PTEN	Cowden syndrome
DNA Damage Response Genes	
hMSH2, hMLH1 hPMS1, hPMS2	Hereditary nonpolyposis colon cancer (HNPCC)
MYH	Colorectal cancer
ATM	Ataxia-telangiectasia
XP(A-G)	Xeroderma pigmentosum
BLM	Bloom syndrome

familial inheritance of cancer. Familial clusters of breast cancer are well established—the classic observations of Paul Broca in his wife's family being a well-known example (Broca, 1866). Women with one or more first-degree relatives with breast cancer have 1.5 to 3.5 times the risk of developing breast cancer compared with women without a family history (Pharoah et al, 1997). High-penetrance genes may account for 5%–10% of breast cancers in the general population (Claus et al, 1996). Segregation analyses in family pedigrees with multiple affected members with breast cancer alone or breast and ovarian cancers suggested a genetic component with an autosomal dominant mode of inheritance (Newman et al, 1988).

Linkage analysis was conducted as a genome-wide search among 23 families with multiple individuals affected with early onset breast cancer to identify genetic loci that may be associated with the disease (Hall et al, 1990). The initial discovery, later confirmed by others (Narod et al, 1991), linked a region on chromosome 17q21 with familial inheritance of early onset breast and ovarian cancers. Positional cloning was used to localize the BRCA1 gene in this region (Miki et al, 1994). BRCA1 is a large gene consisting of 22 coding exons, in which many hundreds of separate germline variants have been identified (see Breast Cancer Information Core Database: www.research.nhgri.nih.gov/bic/). Among women with early onset breast/ovarian cancer, approximately 95% of the variants are frameshift, nonsense, or splice-site mutations that lead to truncation of the encoded protein. Linkage to 17q21 was observed in only 45% of high-risk breast cancer families, suggesting that other high-penetrant susceptibility genes may explain the remaining portion of breast cancer within these families (Hall et al, 1990).

A second gene responsible for early onset breast cancer, designated *BRCA2*, was next identified on chromosome 13q12–13 in families in which linkage to the *BRCA1* locus was not observed (Wooster et al, 1994). From high-risk pedigrees, the cumulative probability of developing breast cancer for carriers of germline mutations in *BRCA1* or *BRCA2* was initially estimated at over 80% (Ford et al, 1994, 1998).

Gene penetrance estimates from linkage studies are generally overestimates because, by definition, they only include families with an unusually large number of affected members. In other words, families that do not show a striking excess of breast cancer, but may carry a mutated gene, are excluded from this ascertainment scheme. Results from a population-based kin-cohort study, a design employed to estimate the penetrance of an autosomal dominant gene, have set the estimate below 60% in Ashkenazi Jews (Struewing et al, 1997), although a later study in New York City sugggested a higher estimate (King et al, 2003). *BRCA1* and *BRCA2* are responsible for about 70%–80% of early onset breast cancer in high risk families; however they are estimated to only account for less than 20% of the excess risk of breast cancer associated with having a family history (Anglian Breast Cancer Study Group, 2000), suggesting the existence of other familial breast cancer susceptibility loci (Ford and Easton, 1995).

Epidemiologic studies have also identified geographic differences in the mutation frequencies of *BRCA1* and *BRCA2*. These differences are due to "founder" mutations in these genes originating throughout human evolution in subgroups of the population. For example, Ashkenazi Jews have a greater prevalence of specific mutations

in these genes than other subgroups. They have a combined prevalence of greater than 2% due to three common mutations: a two base-pair deletion (185delAG) and a one base-pair insertion (5382insC) in *BRCA1*, and a one base-pair deletion in *BRCA2* (6174delT) (Struewing et al, 1997). Similarly, a five base–pair deletion in *BRCA2* (999de15) among Icelanders is relatively common (0.6%) (Thorlacius et al, 1996). This deletion explains a large percentage of high-risk familial breast cancer in Iceland.

Limitations of Segregation and Linkage Analysis

The sample size required for sufficient power to provide a LOD score greater than 3 in a genome-wide linkage analysis depends on a number of factors. For many mutations in cancer susceptibility genes, the probability of a carrier developing cancer is much less than 100% (incomplete penetrance). Misspecification of gene penetrance and variable penetrance of different mutations may obscure the results of linkage studies (Ott, 1991). Penetrance is also age-dependent, with older individuals being more likely to develop disease. For instance, for a dominant gene with incomplete penetrance, it is difficult to determine whether a young, high-risk, nondiseased individual who carries the linked marker loci has in fact inherited the mutated gene, because disease has not yet occurred and may not occur. An age-dependent penetrance function can be used to assign a probability of having a susceptibility loci for those who are unaffected (Ott, 1991), but this will obviously misclassify some family members

A large number of family pedigrees may also be required to detect linkage if gene penetrance is low. An accurate case definition is also important for determining the genetic etiology of a disease. Labeling a family member who does not truly have the disease as a case can dramatically reduce the power of the pedigree approach. However, defining the case status may be difficult, as mutations in specific genes may result in variable degrees of the disease phenotype (variable expressivity). In addition, the inclusion of family members with disease not caused by the genetic factors (phenocopies) can decrease the power to detect linkage.

Genetic heterogeneity, that is, when a single disease is caused by mutations in independent genes at different loci, may also add complexity to linkage studies. Thus, when families are pooled to study linkage, a mixing of genetic effects from various chromosomal regions, such as the involvement of *BRCA1* and *BRCA2* with early onset breast cancer, may decrease the power to detect linkage with a specific genetic region. A larger number and closer spacing of highly informative (polymorphic) markers allow a more widespread evaluation of chromosomal regions and greater efficiency in locating disease loci.

Alternative Methods

Although the majority of familial cancer genes have been identified so far by linkage analysis and positional cloning, alternative strategies have also been employed. For instance, the strategy utilized to distinguish p53 as the gene responsible for Li-Fraumeni syndrome was based on information about the known biological function of this candidate gene. Li-Fraumeni syndrome is a rare autosomal dominantly inherited disorder characterized by a significantly elevated risk of developing early onset cancers, including soft tissue sarcomas, osteosarcomas, leukemias, and brain and breast tumors (Malkin et al, 1990).

Somatic mutations in the *TP53* gene were observed in many tumors of individuals with Li-Fraumeni syndrome (Hollstein et al, 1991). Previously, *TP53* had been located on the short arm of chromosome 17 (McBride et al, 1986), and experimental data showed that p53 was important in regulating cell growth (Hinds et al, 1989). Based on these observations, *TP53* was sequenced to search for mutations that might predispose to the cancer syndrome. It was shown that germline *TP53* mutations segregate with cancer in families with Li-Fraumeni syndrome (Malkin et al, 1990).

An additional gene discovery strategy is based on the knowledge of protein homol-ogy with lower organisms and is exemplified in studies of HNPCC (Table 4–1), the autosomal dominantly inherited disease characterized by an elevated risk of colon and rectal cancer (Aaltonen et al, 1993). Tumors in patients with HNPCC display insertions and deletions at repetitive DNA sequences, a condition described as "microsatellite instability" (MIN) or "replication error phenotype" (RER) (Aaltonen et al, 1993). Mutations in yeast mismatch repair genes (*PMS1, MLH, MSH2*) lead to MIN in yeast (Strand et al, 1993). Linkage studies mapped HNPCC loci to chromosomes 2p and 3p (Peltomaki et al, 1993; Bronner et al, 1994). Human mismatch repair homologs (hMSH1, hMLH) were discovered on the basis of similarity in sequence (homology) between the yeast and human genes, and the human genes were shown to map to chromosomes 2p and 3p. Germline mutations in these genes were later identified in the majority of individuals with HNPCC (Leach et al, 1993; Bronner et al, 1994; Nicolaides et al, 1994; Papadopoulos et al, 1994).

Allele-sharing Methods

An obvious Mendelian mode of disease inheritance will not usually be apparent for a common disease with a multigenic etiology or a strong environmental component, such as the majority of cancers that do not occur in high-risk families. Alternative study designs for evaluating genetic linkage that do not require the mode of disease inheritance to be specified (model-free) have been developed (Fishman et al, 1978). In general, these methods are more informative than classic linkage analysis studies when several genes with small to modest effects predispose an individual to the disease. Allele-sharing methods test for linkage using affected sib or relative pairs. Fundamental to these methods is the hypothesis that the two relatives who have the same type of cancer share more genetic loci than those who are discordant for this cancer. As in classic linkage analysis, marker loci are utilized and genotyped in family members. A higher frequency of marker transmission on specific chromosomes in diseased relatives suggests that predisposing genes may exist in the neighborhood of these markers.

Two types of allele-sharing measures are used: the number of alleles shared that are identical by state (IBS: alleles that are the same) and the number of alleles shared that are identical by descent (IBD: alleles inherited from a common ancestor). In general, incorporating alleles shared IBD in a study is more powerful than incorporating alleles shared IBS (Bishop and Williamson, 1990). However, IBD measures require parental marker genotypes to be known—which may not always be accessible, particularly if parents are deceased. Under normal Mendelian inheritance for a biallelic gene, the probability that two siblings share alleles is 25% for sharing none, 50% for sharing one, and 25% for sharing two. Any deviation from these expected distributions indicates potential linkage of a marker locus and a disease gene.

Issues similar to those encountered in family pedigree linkage analyses such as case definition, reduced gene penetrance, phenocopies, genetic heterogeneity, and the large number of highly variable markers necessary complicate the evaluation of genetic linkage using allele-sharing methods. In addition, the requirement for families with at least two affected individuals from which a DNA sample can be obtained is a potential limitation compared with association studies.

APPROACHES TO IDENTIFY COMMON, LOW-RISK DISEASE ALLELES

Generally, around 5% of most cancers can be explained by highly penetrant, rare mutations in cancer susceptibility genes transmitted in families with an established mode of inheritance. However, for many cancers, a more complex underlying etiology has been suggested, due to highly prevalent polymorphisms in multiple "candidate" genes in combination with exposures to nongenetic factors such as smoking, diet, and other lifestyle variables. Candidate cancer genes are usually chosen on the basis of their function in biological pathways thought to be important in the pathogenesis of cancer. Biologically functional polymorphisms in candidate genes may contribute to our understanding of the genetic etiology of cancer, serving as biomarkers of individual cancer susceptibility. These low-penetrance polymorphisms have been observed to convey only small excess risks. However, if they are common, then they may result in substantial population-attributable risks. If, in addition to categorizing individuals on the basis of genotype, we incorporate environmental and lifestyle exposure histories into epidemiologic studies, we will be better equipped to define population subgroups that are genetically susceptible or resistant to disease. This will consequently improve our ability to associate specific exposures with specific cancers.

Although the human species is 99.9% identical at the DNA sequence level, there is a remarkable spectrum of phenotypic diversity in the population. Most of this observed variation, including susceptibility to disease, is thought to stem from the 0.1% differences in our DNA. Genetic diversity is greater in noncoding than in coding regions, as noncoding variants are less likely to result in alterations in protein function and thus to be selected against. Nucleotide variation at codons that do not result in a change in the amino acid (synonymous sites) due to the redundancy of the genetic code (ie, more than one set of the three nucleotides may code for the same amino acid) are more frequent than base changes at nonsynonymous sites (Halushka et al, 1999). This further illustrates that genetic variation is constrained by the influence of each variant on protein function.

Nucleotide sequence variations occur and are maintained in different geographic populations over the course of human history. These variations include SNPs, one base-pair substitutions, sequence insertions and deletions, and highly variable repeating nucleotide segments. SNPs are the most common form of variation and exist every ~ 300 bp on average across the genome. SNPs with frequencies under 5% comprise roughly 50% of all SNPs, however, because they are rare they account for at most 10% of all heterozygous sites in an individual. SNPs with frequencies equal to or above 5% are estimated to account for ~90% of human heterozygosity meaning that most genetic variation is shared between any two individuals (International Hapmap Consortium, 2005). A central hypothesis regarding the underlying nature of genetic variation contributing to complex diseases such as cancer is the common-disease/common-variant hypothesis (CD/CV) (Lander, 1996; Chakravarti, 1999). The underlying premise of the CD/CV hypothesis is that alleles with appreciable frequencies in the population contribute to important variation in risk of disease. These causal variants are most likely to be old and predate the divergence of human populations and, thus, will be shared today across ethnically diverse populations. An increasing number of common variants have been reproducibly associated with risk of complex multifactorial diseases such as diabetes (Altshuler et al, 2000; Saxena et al, 2006), autoimmune diseases (Ueda et al, 2003; Criswell et al, 2005), and heart disease (Pennacchio, 2001). Over the last year, reproducible associations with common variants have also been reported for breast, prostate and colorectal cancer (Amundadottir et al, 2006; Easton et al, 2007; Freedman et al, 2006; Haiman et al, 2007; Haiman et al, 2007; Hunter et al, 2007; Stacey et al, 2007; Tomlinson et al, 2007; Yeager et al, 2007; Zanke et al, 2007).

LINKAGE DISEQUILIBRIUM AND TAGGING SNPS

The only comprehensive approach to test all variation (both common and rare) in a candidate gene or region of interest for association with disease risk is by resequencing. However, because of the high cost involved, routine resequencing in large numbers of subjects will not be practical in the immediate future, although some have predicted that whole genome sequencing will be affordable in epidemiologic studies

within 5 to 10 years. With recent advances in high-throughput genotyping technology (discussed in the following), it is now possible to survey the vast majority of human genetic variation due to common alleles. Genotyping large numbers of SNPs in different racial and ethnic population samples has revealed the genome to be comprised of discrete regions, or blocks, of linkage disequilibrium where nearby SNPs show strong correlation with one another (Gabriel et al, 2002). The size of LD block regions have been shown to be highly variable across the human genome yet their locations appear to be moderately conserved across populations. These observations have led to the development of linkage disequilibrium (LD)-based approaches to survey common genetic variation in a candidate gene or region, or genome-wide, for association with disease risk (Daly et al, 2001). Due to the high degree of correlation between SNPs in LD block regions, only a subset of SNPs, called tagging SNPs, are needed to comprehensively test human genetic variation (Johnson et al, 2001). Tagging SNPs serve as proxies for known and unknown common genetic variation and allow an indirect assessment of the association with a disease-causal allele. The utility of this approach has prompted efforts to characterize and catalogue polymorphisms across the genome, resulting in rich SNP databases to facilitate the exploration of genotype-phenotype associations.

POLYMORPHISM DATABASES

Large-scale efforts have been made to discover single nucleotide polymorphisms (SNPs) and identify variant alleles in candidate cancer susceptibility genes in the search for useful tools in population-based epidemiologic studies (Cargill et al, 1999). The SNP databases, established independently by research institutes in collaboration with governmental agencies and private industry, are publicly accessible to researchers over the internet. Table 4–2 includes a number of useful websites with access to such databases. The most comprehensive

Table 4–2. Websites of single nucleotide polymorphism (SNP) databases.

Organization	Website
National Human Genome Research Institute	http://www.ncbi.nlm.nih.gov/SNP
UCSC Genome Bioinformatics	http://genome.ucsc.edu/
University of Utah Genome Center	http://www.genome.utah.edu/genesnps
International Hapmap	http://www.hapmap.org
Wellcome Trust Case-Control Consortium	http://www.wtccc.org.uk/
NCI Breast & Prostate Cancer Cohort Consortium	http://epi.grants.cancer.gov/BPC3

variation database is dbSNP. This database was established by the National Center for Biotechnology Information (NCBI) in collaboration with the National Human Genome Research Institute and functions as a central public repository of genetic variation. The dbSNP database currently contains over 5.6 validated SNPs across the genome and is linked to other NCBI resources, such as Entrez Gene, which provides gene-specific information. The University of Santa Cruz Genome Browser is another database used to rapidly query genomic information for many species. This web-based tool allows for the visualization of genomic information, including the location of genes and polymorphisms.

Knowledge of LD patterns in the human genome provided the motivation for constructing a genome-wide SNP database of common variation. This effort, known as the International HapMap Project, was initiated in 2002 upon completion of the Human Genome Project. The HapMap database is a publicly available resource that provides information about LD patterns across the genome in multiple population samples. The HapMap project genotyped over three million SNPs (roughly 1 SNP per kb on average) in 269 samples from four populations (90 Utah Residents with Northern and Western European Ancestry; 45 Han Chinese from Beijing, China; 44 Japanese from Tokyo, Japan; and 90 Yorubans from Ibadan, Nigeria) (International Hapmap Consortium, 2005). The completion of this genome-wide variation database has provided an invaluable resource for researchers to use for selecting tagging SNPs across racial and ethnic populations. It is currently being used globally as a template for both LD-based candidate gene and genome-wide association studies.

In the United States, another SNP database has been established through the Environmental Genome Project developed by the University of Utah Genome Center, sponsored by the National Institute of Environmental Health Sciences. This project is aimed at identifying SNPs in environmental disease susceptibility genes in different population samples through gene resequencing (Livingston et al, 2004). All of these rapidly growing databases provide a rich source of information concerning genetic variation in human populations that can be utilized by genetic epidemiologists in association studies of specific diseases including cancer.

EPIDEMIOLOGIC STUDIES

In contrast to linkage analysis, used to localize disease loci, association studies quantify the effect of known genetic variants on disease in terms of relative risk. These methods have been shown to be more powerful than linkage analysis in identifying disease genes with modest effects (Risch and Merikangas, 1996). The term association studies is often used by geneticists to describe conventional epidemiologic studies designed to evaluate associations between genotypes and cancer, as well as their joint effects with environmental exposures. These include traditional case-control studies with unrelated controls, cohort studies, and alternative designs, including family based case-control, kin-cohort, and case-only designs.

Case-control Studies

The most common study design for assessing relationships between genotypes and cancer risk is the case-control study using unrelated controls. Comparisons of allele frequencies are initially made between individuals with cancer (cases) and those without it (controls). The measure of association computed between genotype and disease is the familiar odds ratio, which serves as a measure of relative risk. The usual procedures for proper design, conduct, and analysis of case-control studies also apply to case-control studies in which a gene variant is the exposure. They include the selection of an appropriate control group (Wacholder et al, 1992) and reduction/elimination of potential biases. Controls should be selected from, or be representative of, the population giving rise to the cases.

A critical potential bias is the selection of controls from populations with different ethnic backgrounds than the cases. Selection of cases from an ethnic population with a greater allele frequency than the controls will result in a positive association between genotype and disease even if there is no true underlying association in the population. This problem is often called *population stratification* by geneticists, and there are several studies in which it has led to spurious results (Knowler et al, 1988). In conventional epidemiologic parlance, population stratification can be seen as a form of selection bias, in that the controls do not represent a random sample of the population that gave rise to the cases.

Confounding is also of concern in any genetic studies if both genotype and disease are independently associated with a third variable. Ethnicity is a potential confounder in these studies because cancer incidence and allele frequencies vary among ethnic groups—. Confounding by ethnicity (also interpreted as *population stratification*) may be accounted for in the design of the study by matching on ethnicity or restricting the study population to a defined ethnic group. It can also be controlled for in the statistical analysis if information on this variable is available. However, simulation studies suggest that large differences in the prevalence of a genotype combined with substantial differences in ethnicity between cases and controls are required before serious confounding occurs due to population stratification (Wacholder et al, 2000). Recent empirical studies have confirmed that population stratification can be detected when very large numbers of SNPs are measured in cases and controls, even if controls are matched to the cases on self-reported ethnicity; however, the amount of spurious association introduced by this bias in well-designed studies tends to be small—in the range of relative risks of 0.8–1.25 (Campbell et al, 2005). If investigators are concerned that the small effects they observe may be due to population stratification, a variety of methods have been proposed to control for this source of confounding, mostly relying on stratification or multivariate techniques that control for a series of SNPs that identify the ancestral subpopulations that may give rise to confounding by differential ancestry between the cases and controls (Price et al, 2006).

The use of incident rather than prevalent cases is also preferable unless it can be shown that genotype does not influence the duration of survival. A "survivor bias" may occur if the prevalence of the gene variant is different in the prevalent cases compared with the original case group.

Genotype misclassification can also lead to erroneous conclusions regarding the relationship between genetic polymorphisms and disease. Often the biological function of the genetic polymorphism being studied is not known. In these studies, the polymorphic site may serve as a genetic marker of a nearby linked functional variant, either within or in proximity to the candidate gene. As a result, gene–disease associations may be underestimated if a high degree of linkage disequilibrium is not present between the nonfunctional marker and the true functional variant. On the other hand, a positive result between a nonfunctional polymorphism in a candidate gene and a specific cancer is far from conclusive evidence that the gene is causally associated with cancer, and should trigger a search to attempt to find the "true" functional variant in the gene or nearby on the chromosome.

Cohort Studies

Nested case-control studies within well-defined cohorts and case-cohort studies are the preferred method to evaluate associations between genes and disease if enough cases are available to provide adequate statistical power. In traditional case-control studies, the population giving rise to the cases is often difficult to define and control selection is therefore difficult. In nested studies, controls are selected from an explicitly defined source population—the original cohort (see Chapter 5). These studies may also provide prospective data free of recall bias about potential confounding and effect-modifying risk factors. However, these studies are still subject to some of the same potential biases that are specific to genetic studies—namely, confounding by ethnicity, genotype misclassification, and the potential problems of linkage disequilibrium, described previously. Moreover, these studies are expensive, as they require enrollment and long-term follow-up of an established cohort usually comprising tens of thousands of individuals. In addition, cohort participation rates must be high to minimize potential selection bias.

Family-based Association Studies

Case-control study designs using nontraditional controls have also been introduced to evaluate associations between genotype and disease (Gauderman et al, 1999). One approach is to select cases from identified probands and controls from unaffected siblings or cousins. This family based design has been proposed to eliminate biases caused by population stratification and confounding by environmental factors that may lead to spurious associations in traditional case-control study designs.

An alternative hybrid method is the case-parental-control design known as the *transmission disequilibrium test* (TDT) (Spielman et al, 1993). Alleles transmitted to affected offspring are compared with those of a fictitious control composed of nontransmitted parental alleles. One obvious limitation is the necessity of measuring the parental genotype, which may not be readily available. Similar methodologic issues, such as linkage disequilibrium, must also be considered in evaluating the results of nontraditional case-control study designs.

A novel kin-cohort design was developed to estimate mutation penetrance of autosomal dominant genes (Wacholder et al, 1998). A proband, with or without disease, is genotyped, and the history of disease in first-degree relatives is assessed from the participant. This protocol, which allows estimation of the cumulative probability of disease in mutation carriers, was used among Ashkenazi Jews to estimate the cumulative lifetime risk of breast cancer and other cancers associated with mutations in *BRCA1* and *BRCA2* (Struewing et al, 1997). The kin-cohort design is sensitive to biases, including selection bias, which may result if probands with a family history of disease are more likely to participate. Misclassification of disease status in relatives may also occur if the results are based solely on the probands' recollection.

Case-only Design

The case-only design is an efficient and valid approach designed specifically to evaluate gene environment interaction when there is independence between genotype and population exposure. This design avoids the potential problems of control selection as well as concern regarding systematic differences in the measurement of past exposures in cases and controls in case-control studies by employing cases only (Clayton and McKeigue, 2001). A comparison with regard to exposure prevalence is made between cases with and without the susceptibility genotype to provide an interaction parameter that could measure departure from a multiplicative genotype–exposure association. The joint effects of exposure and genotype are divided by the product of the individual genotype and exposure effects (Andrieu and Goldstein, 1998). Without controls, however, the prevalence of exposure and the genotype among nondiseased individuals is unknown. Thus, the independent effects of genotype and environmental exposure cannot be directly assessed in this design.

Gene–environment Interaction and Polygenic Models of Disease Risk

Variants in genes involved in carcinogen metabolism such as cytochrome P450s, N-acetyltransferases, and glutathione transferases have been widely studied with respect to environmental and dietary exposures and cancer susceptibility (Vineis and Malats, 1999). Indeed, they are the most common examples in the literature of gene–environment interaction. However, relatively few main effects of low penetrance alleles have been found to be reproducible (Ioannidis et al, 2001), and even fewer gene–environment interactions are clearly confirmed.

Establishing gene–environment interactions will always be more challenging than establishing the main effects of a genetic variant. To the issues discussed previously must be added the problems of measuring the relevant exposures, the fact that multiple statistical models of gene–environment interaction are possible, and the problem that gene–environment interactions may vary from study to study as a function of ethnic and geographic differences in both genotype and exposure prevalence, making the assessment of the reproducibility of interactions problematic (Hunter, 2005). Probably the largest single issue is that of sample size: Typically, studies of even a simple multiplicative interaction between two dichotomous variables need to be four or more times the size needed to detect the main effects. Relatively few studies in the literature have both exposures measured and DNA available from sufficient cases and controls to have subtantial power to

detect interactions, meaning that much of the literature to date is composed of underpowered studies in which the chances are higher that any statistically significant interaction is a false positive. Until multiple individual studies of adequate size are available, pooling data across consortia of studies may be the only way of obtaining adequate sample sizes (Kraft and Hunter, 2005).

Glutathione-S-transferase M1 (GSTM1) is an enzyme involved in detoxification of activated carcinogens (Strange and Fryer, 1999). The GSTM1 null genotype has been reported to interact with smoking in lung and other smoking-related cancers. In addition, gene–gene and gene–gene–environment interactions have been detected between these and other carcinogen-metabolizing genes and environmental exposures (Olshan et al, 2000). However, in a large meta-analysis of 43 studies with > 18 000 subjects, the relative risk for the GSTM1 deletion was reported to be 1.17 (95% CI 1.07–1.27), and in a subset of 21 studies with > 9 500 subjects for whom the authors had original primary data the relative risk for the main effect of genotype was nonsignificant, and no interaction with smoking was observed (Benhamou et al, 2002). Studies such as these demonstrate the sample sizes necessary to document the main effects of genetic low-penetrance alleles, and illustrate the dangers of relying on a small number of studies to document even biologically plausible gene–envirnoment interactions.

A functional polymorphism in the methylentetrahydrofolate reductase (MTHFR) gene illustrates some of these issues. Initial reports that the low activity variant of the C677T (A222V) was associated with modestly lower risk of colorectal cancer (Chen et al, 1996) have been confirmed in meta-analyses (Houlston and Tomlinson, 2001), although the effect size is modest (Relative Risk homozygous variant Val/Vall = 0.76, 95% CI 0.62–0.92). The initial report that this inverse association was abolished among persons with high alcohol consumption (alcohol is a folate antagonist) has been somewhat consistently replicated, although in other studies interactions have been reported with high folate consumption, or low consumption of methionine, another methyl group donor, or variables that combine alcohol, folate, and methionine intakes into a "methyl index" (Sharp and Little, 2004). This illustrates the difficulty of assessing gene–environment interactions in meta-analyses when the definition of the environmental variable changes between the published studies.

Polygenic models have also been proposed to explain the variation in cancer risk both within and between racial-ethnic groups (Ross et al, 1998; Henderson and Feigelson, 2000). These models focus on candidate genes that are selected based on the established role of the encoded protein in a pathway underlying the disease etiology, and on the possible presence of polymorphisms in the gene that may alter the normal biological activity of the protein. Examples include genes involved in steroid hormone biosynthesis, activation, transport, and metabolism, which are pathways that have been implicated in hormone-dependent cancers of the breast and prostate (Ross et al, 1998; Henderson and Feigelson, 2000). Large-scale collaborations, such as the NCI Breast and Prostate Cohort Consortium (Hunter et al, 2005), are currently underway to examine variation in genes in these and others pathways as well as gene–gene and gene–environment interaction in breast and prostate cancer. Gene–gene interactions will require large sample sizes, as do gene–environment interactions. If valid associations can be established for individual low-penetrance alleles or their combinations, then individuals with elevated susceptibility could be identified and targeted for specific cancer prevention strategies.

GENOTYPING METHODS USED IN EPIDEMIOLOGIC STUDIES

Many strategies are used to identify mutations and polymorphisms in cancer susceptibility genes, and the list is increasing rapidly with the advent of new laboratory techniques. The polymerase chain reaction (PCR), by which millions of copies of a specific area of the genome can be made from DNA present in a sample as small as a single cell, has been the most important single development (Mullis and Faloona, 1987). Genotyping methods have also evolved rapidly. In contrast to mutation-detection methods, they rely on prior knowledge of the exact location of the mutation. Following is a brief overview of some laboratory-based methods used for genotyping in genetic epidemiologic studies of cancer.

Epidemiologic studies will require large samples and automated, high-throughput genotyping techniques to detect the modest associations predicted between common alleles and cancer. Over the past decade, both the abundance of SNPs discovered in the human genome and the ease in which they can be detected have resulted in the development of a number of high-throughout SNP genotyping platforms (competition between the companies marketing these platforms has driven the per-SNP assay cost down by more than three orders of magnitude). In studies that require the analysis of a limited number of SNPs, such as missense or tagging SNPs in a handful of genes, but in a large numbers of subjects, the TaqMan method has been demonstrated to be most cost efficient. TaqMan is a single-plex fluorogenic 5' nuclease assay that allows for the analysis of one SNP at a time. Pyrosequencing is another platform that has been developed for interrogating small numbers of SNPs in large sample sizes. The Sequenom MassARRAY is a mid-level multiplexing platform that allows for the processing of up to 28 SNPs simultaneously. Fewer samples can be analyzed relative to single-plex platforms, however the per SNP cost is substantially lower. High-volume SNP genotyping platforms such as the Illumina BeadArray and the Affymetrix GeneChip array are capable of analyzing thousands of SNPs simultaneously and are most cost efficient in large studies. Recently, extreme high-throughput products have been released by Illumina and Affymetrix that allow for genotyping of 500K to 1,000,000

SNPs. SNPs on these chips "tag" a suitable amount of the common genetic variation in the human genome and are currently being used in genome-wide association studies (discussed in the following). We can expect the SNP density on these chips to surpass 1 000 000 in 2008 and the per SNP costs to drop well below $0.001.

WHOLE GENOME SCANS, COLLABORATION AND CONSORTIA

Genome-wide scans are currently underway for cancers of the breast and prostate. These efforts include the Cancer Genome Markers of Susceptibility (CGEMS) project, which is an NCI sponsored initiative (Yeager et al, 2007; Hunter et al, 2007), and scans sponsored by Cancer Research UK (Easton et al, 2007). These projects will employ the latest genotyping platforms (discussed previously) to genotype hundreds of thousands of SNPs spanning the genome. Because of the vast number of SNPs that can now be evaluated efficiently in association studies, concerns about multiple comparisons cannot be ignored. The more SNPs studied, the greater the chance of observing a false-positive association based on chance alone. In a study of 500 000 SNPs per sample, 25 000 would be expected to be statistically significant at the $p = 0.05$ level. Although a statistical "correction" for multiple comparisons is frequently suggested as the solution, it is far from ideal, as even in large studies many true associations will be modest and marginally significant at the $p = 0.05$ level. Demanding a more stringent level of significance may partially solve the false-positive problem, but at the price of creating false negatives and rejecting true associations. The high cost of whole genome scans per sample suggests that initial studies will have small numbers of cases and controls. The sobering prospect is that the literature is filled with contradictory reports from small independent studies, the vast majority of which are false-positive findings (Ioannidis et al, 2001). Incorporating an investigator-defined prior probability that

an association with a variant in a candidate gene is real has been suggested to help interpret nominally statistically significant findings (Wacholder et al, 2004). Regardless, replication of initial associations in multiple population samples will be crucial to rule out false-positive findings. With this in mind, Consortia of studies have been formed for some of the most common cancers—eg, the National Cancer Institute Breast & Prostate Cancer Cohort Consortium (http://epi.grants.cancer.gov/BPC3), and the Wellcome Trust Case Control Consortium (http://www.wtccc.org.uk)—but concern remains that currently available sample sets are simply too small, particularly for less common cancers, to permit epidemiologists to adequately capitalize on the new genomic and technical tools available.

CONCLUSION

Clarifying the complex etiologic role of environmental and genetic factors in carcinogenesis will be challenging but necessary to fully understand the causes of cancer and how it can be prevented. Experience gained in the past and present have raised many issues that must be addressed if we are to move forward in genetic epidemiology.

One concern is the potential risk to study subjects in epidemiologic studies. Guidelines must be established to minimize the potential risks to research participants while maximizing the benefits to society. Confidentiality regarding the results of genetic analyses, the potential for health insurance or employment discrimination, and the feedback, if any, to study participants are other concerns, as is, of course, the need for very large studies to evaluate gene–environment interaction.

The future of this discipline as an integrated part of cancer epidemiology will also rely on continued development of innovative molecular and statistical techniques as well as novel study designs. The object of these studies is to identify the genetic markers that will aid in assessing cancer risk. Such studies may also potentially provide clues for cancer therapy, and facilitate early detection and screening efforts in genetically susceptible subgroups of the population.

GLOSSARY

Allele One of the variant forms of a gene at a particular locus, or location, on a chromosome. Different alleles produce variation in inherited characteristics such as hair color or blood type. In an individual, one form of the allele (the dominant one) may be expressed more fully than another form (the recessive one).

Allele-sharing methods An approach used for studying complex traits. It examines marker allele-sharing between pairs of affected relatives. If relative pairs (or sib pairs) share marker alleles more often than would be expected by chance, this suggests that a susceptibility locus may be linked to the marker.

Apoptosis Programmed cell death—the body's normal method of disposing of damaged, unwanted, or unneeded cells.

Autosomal Pertaining to those chromosomes that are not sex chromosomes.

Chromosome One of the thread-like "packages" of genes and other DNA in the nucleus of a cell. Different kinds of organisms have different numbers of chromosomes. Humans have 23 pairs of chromosomes, 46 in all: 44 autosomes and 2 sex chromosomes. Each parent contributes one chromosome to each pair, so children get half of their chromosomes from their mothers and half from their fathers.

Codon Three bases in a DNA or RNA sequence that specify a single amino acid.

Deoxyribonucleic acid (DNA) The chemical inside the nucleus of a cell that carries the genetic instructions for making living organisms.

DNA chip technology A DNA chip (also called gene chip or DNA microarray) is a small, flat surface on which DNA strands are immobilized in distinct spots; each strand contains a unique DNA sequence. DNA chips use the same process of hybridization that is used in conventional Southern and Northern blots; the hybridization signals are detected and analyzed. DNA chips are more efficient than conventional methods and can be used for a wide array of biological experiments.

DNA repair A process that repairs DNA damage.

Dominant allele The allele that is phenotypically expressed despite the presence of other alleles of the same gene.

Enzyme A protein that encourages a biochemical reaction, usually speeding it up. Organisms could not function if they had no enzymes.

Epigenetic The term that refers to any factor that can affect the phenotype without a change in the genotype.

Exon The region of a gene that contains the code for producing the gene's protein. Each exon codes for a specific portion of the complete protein. In some species (including humans), a gene's exons are separated by long regions of DNA (called introns or sometimes junk DNA) that have no apparent function.

Frameshift mutation Nucleotide insertions and deletions that cause a shift in the three-base reading frame in RNA that is translated into normal protein. These mutations either yield an incorrect string of amino acids or introduce a stop codon, which will result in a shortened protein.

Gene The functional and physical unit of heredity passed from parent to offspring. Genes are pieces of DNA, and most genes contain the information for making a specific protein.

Gene amplification An increase in the number of copies of any particular piece of DNA. A tumor cell amplifies, or copies, DNA segments naturally as a result of cell signals and sometimes environmental events.

Genome All the DNA contained in an organism or a cell, which includes both the chromosomes within the nucleus and the DNA in mitochondria.

Genomic imprinting An epigenetic process resulting in the silencing of a gene. The functional genomic changes are not caused by inherited mistakes in the DNA sequence, but are believed to occur through the methylation of DNA in the regulatory regions of these genes.

Genotype The genetic identity of an individual that is not shown as outward characteristics.

Genotyping The process of determining an individual's genotype, or specific allelic composition for a certain gene or set of genes.

Germline The cell line from which gametes are derived.

Intron A segment of a gene that is initially transcribed into RNA but is then removed from the primary transcript by splicing together the exon sequences on either side of it. Intronic sequences are not found in mature mRNA.

Heterozygosity The presence of different alleles at one or more loci on homologous chromosomes.

Linkage Coinheritance of two or more nonallelic genes because their loci are in close proximity on the same chromosome, such that after meiosis they remain associated more often than the 50% expected for unlinked genes.

Loss of heterozygozity (LOH) Loss of the wild-type allele of a tumor-suppressor gene.

Meiosis A special type of cell division occurring in the germ cells of sexually reproducing organisms during which gametes containing the haploid chromosome number are produced from diploid cells. Two meiotic divisions occur, meiosis I and meiosis II; reduction in number takes place during meiosis I.

Mendelian inheritance The manner in which genes and traits are passed from parents to children. Examples of Mendelian inheritance include autosomal dominant, autosomal recessive, and sex-linked genes.

Microsatellite instability (MIN) Microsatellites are segments of DNA (usually located in noncoding regions) consisting of a segment of mono-, di-, or trinucleotide repeats (eg, CACACACACA). These microsatellites are highly susceptible to expansions or contractions when the machinery for DNA repair is somehow compromised.

Missense mutation A single DNA base substitution resulting in a codon specifying a different amino acid.

Mutation A permanent structural alteration in DNA. In most cases, such DNA changes either have no effect or cause harm, but occasionally a mutation can improve an organism's chance of surviving and passing on the beneficial change to its descendants.

Nonsense mutation A single DNA base substitution resulting in a stop (termination) codon.

Nucleotide One of the structural components, or building blocks, of DNA and RNA. A nucleotide consists of a base (one of four chemicals: adenine, thymine, guanine, and cytosine) plus a molecule of sugar and one of phosphoric acid.

Pedigree A simplified diagram of a family's genealogy that shows family members' relationships to each other and how a particular trait or disease has been inherited.

Penetrance An all-or-none phenomenon that refers to the observable expression, or lack of it, of the mutant gene. For a dominant disease, it is defined quantitatively by determining the proportion of obligate gene carriers (heterozygotes); for a mutant gene, it is defined by who express the phenotype.

Phenocopy A phenotype produced by environmental factors that mimics a genetically determined trait.

Phenotype The observable traits or characteristics of an organism, for example hair color, weight, or the presence or absence of a disease. Phenotypic traits are not necessarily genetic.

Polymerase chain reaction (PCR) A technique for amplifying a short stretch of DNA. The method depends on the use of two flanking oligonucleotide DNA primers and repeated cycles of primer extension using DNA polymerase.

Polymorphism A gene that exists in more than one version (allele) and where the rare allele can be found in more than 2% of the population.

Positional cloning A process that, through gene-mapping techniques, is able to locate a gene responsible for a disease when little or no information is known about the biochemical basis of the disease.

Recessive allele An allele that has no obvious phenotypic effect in a heterozygote; it produces a phenotypic effect only in the homozygous condition.

Restriction fragment length polymorphism (RFLP) A variation in DNA sequence that alters the length of a restriction fragment. These variations may be simple point mutations, which create or destroy a restriction site, or variable-length regions (so-called VNTRs, variable number of tandem repeats). RFLPs provide convenient markers for linkage analysis.

Ribonucleic acid (RNA) A chemical similar to a single strand of DNA. In RNA, the letter U, which stands for uracil, is substituted for T in the genetic code. RNA delivers DNA's genetic message to the cytoplasm of a cell where proteins are made.

Segregation In genetics, the separation of allelic genes at meiosis. Because allelic genes occupy the same locus on homologous chromosomes, they pass to different gametes—that is, they segregate.

Silent mutation A mutation that has no apparent effect on phenotype expression.

Somatic cell Any cell of an organism not involved in the germline.

Somatic mutation A mutation occurring in a somatic cell rather than in the germline.

Stop codon Any of three codons—UAA, UAG, or UGA—that signal the termination of the synthesis of a protein.

Transcription The synthesis of a single-stranded RNA molecule from a double-stranded DNA template in the cell nucleus, catalyzed by RNA polymerase.

Translation The process of synthesizing a polypeptide directed by the sequence of a specific mRNA.

Translocation Breakage and removal of a large segment of DNA from one chromosome, followed by the segment's attachment to a different chromosome.

Variant One that exhibits variation from a type, either the norm or a wild type.

X-linkage Genes on the X chromosome, or traits determined by such genes, are X-linked.

*Adapted from the Glossary at the National Human Genome Research Institute website (http:www.nhgri.gov).

REFERENCES

Aaltonen LA, Peltomaki P, Leach FS, Sistonen P, Pylkkanen L, Mecklin JP, et al. Clues to the pathogenesis of familial colorectal cancer. Science 1993;260:812–16.

Altshuler D, Hirschhorn JN, Klannemark M, Lingren CM, Vohl MC, Nemesh J, et al. The common PPARgamma polymorphism is associated with decreased risk of type 2 diabetes. Nat Genet 2000;26:76–80.

Amundadottir LT, Sulem P, Gudmundsson J, Helgason A, Baker A, Agnarsson BA, et al. A common variant associated with prostate cancer in European and African populations. Nat Genet 2006;38:652–58.

Andrieu N, Goldstein AM. Epidemiologic and genetic approaches in the study of gene–environment interaction: an overview of available methods. Epidemiol Rev 1998;20: 137–47.

Anglian Breast Cancer Study Group. Prevalence and penetrance of BRCA1 and BRCA2 mutations in a population-based series of breast cancer cases. Br J Cancer 2000;83:1301–8.

Benhamou S, Lee WJ, Alexandrie AK, Boffetta P, Bouchardy C, Butkiewicz D, Brockmoller J, Clapper ML, Daly A, Dolzan V, Ford J, Gaspari L, Haugen A, Hirvonen A, Husgafvel-Pursiainen K, Ingelman-Sundberg M, Kalina I, Kihara M, Kremers P, Le Marchand L, London SJ, Nazar-Stewart V, Onon-Kihara M, Rannug A, Romkes M, Ryberg D, Seidegard J, Shields P, Strange RC, Stucker I, To-Figueras J, Brennan P, Taioli E. Meta and pooled analyses of the effects of glutathione S-transferase M1 polymorphisms and smoking on lung cancer risk. Carcinogenesis 2002;23(8):1343–50.

Bishop DT, Williamson JA. The power of identity-by-state methods for linkage analysis. Am J Hum Genet 1990;46:254–65.

Borch-Johnsen K, Olsen JH, Sorensen TI. Genes and family environment in familial clustering of cancer. Theor Med 1994;15:377–86.

Botstein D, White RL, Skolnick M, Davis RW. Construction of a genetic linkage map in man using restriction fragment length polymorphism. Am J Hum Genet 1980;32: 314–31.

Broca P. Traite des tumeurs. Volume 1. Des tumeurs nen general. Paris, Asselin, 1866.

Bronner CE, Baker SM, Morrison PT, Warren G, Smith LG, Lescoe MK, et al. Mutation in the DNA mismatch repair gene homologue in hereditary non-polyposis colon cancer. Nature 1994;368:258–61.

Campbell CD, Ogburn EL, Lunetta KL, Lyon HN, Freedman ML, Groop LC, Altshuler D, Ardlie KG, Hirschhorn JN. Demonstrating stratification in a European American population. Nat Genet. 2005; 37(8):868–72.

Cannon-Albright LA, Goldgar DE, Meyer LJ, Lewis CM, Anderson DE, Fountain JW, et al. Assignment of a locus for familial melanoma, MLM, to chromosome 9p13-p22. Science 1992;258:1148–52.

Cargill M, Altshuler D, Ireland J, Sklar P, Ardlie K, Patil N, et al. Characterization of single-nucleotide polymorphisms in coding regions of human genes. Nat Genet1999;22: 231–8.

Chakravarti A. Population genetics—making sense out of sequence. Nat Genet 1999;21: 56–60.

Chen J, Giovannucci E, Kelsey K, Rimm EB, Stampfer MJ, Colditz GA, Spiegelman D, Willett WC, Hunter DJ. A methylenetetrahydrofolate reductase polymorphism and the risk of colorectal cancer. Cancer Res. 1996 Nov 1;56(21):4862–64.

Claus EB, Schildkraut JM, Thompson WD, Risch NJ. The genetic attributable risk of breast and ovarian cancer. Cancer 1996;77:2318–24.

Clayton D, McKeigue M. Epidemiological methods for studying genes and environmental factors in complex diseases. Lancet 2001; 358;1356–60.

Criswell LA, Pfeiffer KA, Lum RF, Gonzales B, Novitzke J, Kern M, et al. Analysis of families in the multiple autoimmune disease genetics consortium (MADGC) collection: the PTPN22 620W allele associates with multiple autoimmune phenotypes. Am J Hum Genet 2005;76:561–71.

Daly MJ, Rioux JD, Schaffner SF, Hudson TJ, Lander ES. High-resolution haplotype structure in the human genome. Nat Genet 2001; 29:229–32.

Easton DF, Bishop DT, Ford D, Crockford GP, and the Breast Cancer Linkage Consortium. Genetic linkage analysis in familial breast and ovarian cancer. Results from 214 families. Am J Hum Genet 1993;52:678–701.

Easton DF, Pooley KA, Dunning AM, Pharoah PD, Thompson D, Ballinger DG, et al. Genome-wide association study identifies novel breast cancer susceptibility loci. Nature 2007;447:1087–93.

Eng C, Clayton D, Schuffenecker I, Lenoir G, Cote G, Gagel RF, et al. The relationship between specific net protooncogene mutations and disease phenotype in multiple endocrine neoplasia type 2: International RET Mutation Consortium. JAMA 1996;276: 1575–79.

Fishman PM, Suarez B, Hodge SE, Reich T. A robust method for the detection of linkage in familial disease. Am J Hum Genet 1978;30: 308–21.

Ford D, Easton DF. The genetics of breast and ovarian cancer. Br J Cancer 1995;72:805–12.

Ford D, Easton DF, Bishop DT, Narod SA, Goldgar DE, et al. Risks of cancer in BRCA1-mutation carriers. Breast Cancer Linkage Consortium. Lancet 1994;343:692–95.

Ford D, Easton DF, Stratton M, Narod S, Goldgar D, et al. Genetic heterogeneity and penetrance analysis of BRCA1 and BRCA2 genes in breast cancer families. The Breast Cancer Linkage Consortium. Am J Hum Genet 1998;62:676–89.

Freedman Ml, Haiman CA, Patterson N, McDonald GJ, Tandon A, Waliszewska A, et al. Admixture mapping identifies 8q24 as a prostate cancer locus in African American men. Proc Natl Acad Sci USA 2006;103: 14068–73.

Friend SH, Bernards R, Rogelj S, Weinberg RA, Rapaport JM, Albert DM, et al. A human DNA segment with properties of the gene that predisposes to retinoblastoma and osteosarcoma. Nature 1986;323:643–46.

Gabriel SB, Schaffner SF, Nguyen H, Moore JM, Roy J, Blumenstiel B, et al. The structure of haplotype blocks in the human genome. Science 2002;296:2225–29.

Gauderman WJ, Witte JS, Thomas DC. Family-based association studies. Monogr Natl Cancer Inst 1999;26:31–37.

Haiman CA, Patterson N, Freedman ML, Myers SR, Pike MC, Waliszewska A, et al. Multiple regions within 8q24 independently affect risk for prostate cancer. Nat Genet 2007;39: 638–44.

Haiman CA, Le Marchand L, Yamamato J, Stram DO, Sheng X, Kolonel LN, et al. A common genetic risk factor for colorectal cancer and prostate cancer. Nat Genet 2007; 39:954–56.

Hall JM, Lee MK, Newman B, Morrow JE, Anderson LA, Huey B, et al. Linkage of early onset breast cancer to chromosome 17q21. Science 1990;250:1684–89.

Halushka MK, Fan J-B, Bentley K, Hsie L, Shen N, Weder A, Cooper R, Lipshutz R, Chakravarti A. Patterns of single-nucleotide polymorphism in candidate genes for blood pressure homeostasis. Nat Genet 1999;22: 239–47.

Henderson BE, Feigelson HS. Hormonal carcinogenesis. Carcinogenesis 2000;21:427–33.

Hinds PW, Finlay CA, Levine AJ. The p53 protooncogene can act as a suppressor of transformation. Cell 1989;57:1083–93.

Hollstein M, Sidransky D, Vogelstein B, Harris CC. P53 mutations and human cancers. Science 1991;253:49–53.

Houlston RS, Tomlinson IP. Polymorphisms and colorectal tumor risk. Gastroenterology. 2001; 121(2):282–301.

Hunter DJ. Gene-environment interactions in human diseases.Nat Rev Genet. 2005; 6(4): 287–98.

Hunter DJ, Riboli E, Haiman CA, Albanes D, Altshuler D, Chanock SJ, Haynes RB, Henderson BE, Kaaks R, Stram DO, Thomas G, Thun MJ, Blanche H, Buring JE, Burtt NP, Calle EE, Cann H, Canzian F, Chen YC, Colditz GA, Cox DG, Dunning AM, Feigelson HS, Freedman ML, Gaziano JM, Giovannucci E, Hankinson SE, Hirschhorn JN, Hoover RN, Key T, Kolonel LN, Kraft P, Le Marchand L, Liu S, Ma J, Melnick S, Pharoah P, Pike MC, Rodriguez C, Setiawan VW, Stampfer MJ, Trapido E, Travis R, Virtamo J, Wacholder S, Willett WC; National Cancer Institute Breast and Prostate Cancer Cohort Consortium. A candidate gene approach to searching for low-penetrance breast and prostate cancer genes. Nat Rev Cancer. 2005; 5(12):977–85.

Hunter DJ, Kraft P, Jacobs KB, Cox DG, Yeager M, Hankinson SE, et al. A genome-wide association study identifies alleles in FGFR2 associated with risk of sporadic postmenopausal breast cancer. Nat Genet 2007; 39: 870–74.

Ioannidis JP, Ntzani EE, Trikalinos TA, Contopoulos-Ioannidis DG. Replication validity of genetic association studies. Nat Genet 2001;29:306–9.

International Hapmap Consortium. A haplotype map of the human genome. Nature 2005 Oct 27;437:1299–320.

International Human Genome Sequencing Consortium. Initial sequencing and analysis of the human genome. Nat Genet 2001;409; 860–921.

International Human Genome Sequencing Consortium. Finishing the euchromatic sequence of the human genome. Nature 2004; 431: 931-45.

Johnson GC, Esposito L, Barratt BJ, Smith AN, Heward J, Di Genova G, et al. Haplotype tagging for the identification of common disease genes. Nat Genet 2001;29:233–37.

Khoury MJ, Beaty TH, Cohen BH. Fundamentals of Genetic Epidemiology. New York, Oxford University Press, 1993.

King M-C, Marks JH, Mandell JB. Breast and ovarian cancer risks due to inherited mutations in BRCA1 and BRCA2. Science 2003; 302:643–646.

Knowler WC, Williams RC, Pettitt DJ, Steinberg AG. Gm and type 2 diabetes mellitus: an association in American Indians with genetic admixture. Am J Hum Genet 1988;43: 5205–26.

Kraft P, Hunter D. Integrating epidemiology and genetic association: the challenge of gene-environment interaction. Philos Trans R Soc Lond B Biol Sci. 2005;360:1609–16.

Lander ES. The new genomics: global views of biology. Science 1996;274:536–39.

Leach FS, Nicolaides NC, Papadopoulos N, Liu B, Jen J, Parsons R, et al. Mutations of a mutS homologue in hereditary nonpolyposis colorectal cancer. Cell 1993;75:1215–25.

Leppert M, Dobbs M, Scambler P, O'Connell P, Nakamura Y, Stauffer D, et al. The gene for familial polyposis coli maps to long arm of chromosome 5. Science 1987;238:1411–13.

Lichtenstein P, Holm NV, Verkasalo PK, Iliadou A, Kaprio J, Koskenvuo M, et al. Environmental and heritable factors in the causation of cancer. N Engl J Med 2000;343:78–85.

Livingston RJ, von Niederhousern A, Jegga AG et al. Patterns of sequence variation across 213 environmental response genes. Genome Res 2004;141:1821–1831.

Malkin D, Li FP, Strong LC, Fraumeni JF Jr, Nelson CE, Kim DH, et al. Germline p53 mutations in a familial syndrome of breast cancer, sarcomas, and other neoplasms. Science 1990;250:1233–38.

McBride OW, Merry D, Givol D. The gene for human p53 cellular tumor antigen is located on chromosome 17 short arm (17q13). Proc Natl Acad Sci USA 1986;83:130–34.

Miki Y, Swenson J, Shattuck-Eidens D, Futreal PA, Harshman K, Tavtigian S, et al. A strong candidate for the breast and ovarian cancer susceptibility gene BRCA1. Science 1994; 266:66–71.

Morton NE. Sequential tests for the detection of linkage. Am J Hum Genet 1955;7:277–318.

Mucci LA, Wedrén S, Adami HO. Trichopoulos D. The role of gene environment interaction in the aetiology of human cancer: examples from cancers of the large bowel, lung and breast. J Intern Med 2001;249:477–93

Mullis KB, Faloona FA. Section II. In: Wu R (Ed): Methods of Enzymology. Vol 155, Part F. San Diego, CA, Academic Press, 1987, pp 335–50.

Narod SA, Feunteum J, Lynch HT, Watson P, Conway T, Lynch J, et al. Familial breast-ovarian cancer locus on chromosome 17q21-q23. Lancet 1991;338:82–83.

Newman B, Austin M, Lee M, King M-C. Inheritance of human breast cancer: evidence for autosomal dominant transmission in high risk families. Proc Natl Acad Sci USA 1988; 85:3044–48.

Nicolaides NC, Papadopoulos N, Liu B, Wei YF, Carter KC, et al. Mutations of two PMS homologues in hereditary nonpolyposis colon cancer. Nature 1994;371:75–80.

Olshan AF, Weissler MC, Watson MA, Bell DA. GSTM1, GSTT1, GSTP1, CYP1A1, and NAT1 polymorphisms, tobacco use, and the risk of head and neck cancer. Cancer Epidemiol Biomarkers Prev 2000;9:185–91.

Ott J. Analysis of Human Genetic Linkage, rev. ed. Baltimore: Johns Hopkins University Press, 1991.

Papadopoulos N, Nicolaides NC, Wei YF, Ruben SM, Carter KC, Rosen CA, et al. Mutation of the mutL homologues in hereditary colon cancer. Science 1994;263:1625–29.

Peltomaki P, Aalonen LA, Sistonen P, Pylkkanen L, Mecklin JR, Jarvinen H, et al. Genetic mapping of a locus predisposing to human colorectal cancer. Science 1993;260:810–12.

Pennacchio LA, Olivier M, Hubacek JA, Cohen JC, Cox DR, Fruchart JC, et al. An apolipoprotein influencing triglycerides in humans and mice revealed by comparative sequencing. Science 2001;294:169–73.

Pharoah PD, Day NE, Duffy S, Easton DF, Ponder BA. Family history and the risk of breast cancer: a systematic review and meta-analysis. Int J Cancer 1997;71:800–9.

Pharoah PD, Antoniou A, Bobrow M, Zimmern RL, Easton DF, Ponder BA. Polygenic susceptibility to breast cancer and implications for prevention. Nat Genet 2002;31:33–36.

Price AL, Patterson NJ, Plenge RM, Weinblatt ME, Shadick NA, Reich D. Principal components analysis corrects for stratification in genome-wide association studies. Nat Genet 2006 Aug;38(8):904–9.

Risch N, Merikangas K. The future of genetic studies of complex diseases. Science 1996;273:1516–17.

Ross RK, Pike MC, Coetzee GA, Reichardt JKV, Yu MC, Feigelson H, et al. Androgen metabolism and prostate cancer: establishing a model of genetic susceptibility. Cancer Res 1998;58:4497–504.

Saxena R, Gianniny L, Burtt NP, Giuducci C, Sjogren M, Florez JC, et al. Common single nucleotide polymorphisms in TCF7L2 are associated with type 2 diabetes and reduce insulin response to glucose in nondiabetic individuals. Diabetes 2006;55:2890–95.

Sharp L, Little J. Polymorphisms in genes involved in folate metabolism and colorectal neoplasia: a HuGE review. Am J Epidemiol 2004;159(5):423–43.

Spielman RS, McGinnis RE, Ewens WJ. Transmission test for linkage disequilibrium: the insulin gene region and insulin-dependent diabetes mellitus (IDDM). Am J Hum Genet 1993;52:506–16.

Stacey SN, Manolescu A, Sulem P, Rafnar T, Gudmundsson J, Masson G, et al. Common variants on chromosome 2q35 and 16q12 confer susceptibility to estrogen receptor-positive breast cancer. Nat Genet 2007;39:865-69.

Strand M, Prolla TA, Liskay RM, Petes TD. Destabilization of tracts of simple repetitive DNA in yeast by mutations affecting DNA mismatch repair. Nature 1993;365:274–76.

Strange RC, Fryer AA. Glutathione S-transferase: influence of polymorphism on cancer susceptibility. In: Vineis P, Malats N, Lang M, d'Errico A, Caporaso N, Cuzick J, et al. (Eds): Metabolic Polymorphisms and Susceptibility to Cancer. IARC Sci. Pub. No. 148. Lyon, International Agency for Research on Cancer, 1999, pp 251–70.

Stratton MR, Ford D, Neihausen S, Seal S, Wooster R, Friedman LS, et al. Familial male breast cancer is not linked to the BRCA1 locus on chromosome 17q. Nat Genet 1994;7:103–7.

Struewing JP, Hartge P, Wacholder S, Baker SM, Berlin M, McAdams M, et al. The risk of cancer associated with specific mutations of BRCA1 and BRCA2 among Ashkenazi Jews. N Engl J Med 1997;336:1401–8.

Thorlacius S, Olafsdottir G, Tryggvadottir L, Neuhausen S, Jonasson JG, Tavtigian SV, et al. A single BRCA2 mutation in male and female breast cancer families from Iceland with varied cancer phenotypes. Nat Genet 1996;13:117–19.

Tomlinson I., Webb E, Carvajal-Carmona L, Broderick P, Kemp Z, Spain S, et al. A genome-wide association scan of tag SNPs identifies a susceptibility variant for colorectal cancer at 8q24.21. Nat Genet 2007;39:984–88.

Vineis P, Malats N. Strategic issues in the design and interpretation of studies on metabolic polymorphisms and cancer. IARC Sci Publ 1999;148:51–61.

Wacholder S, Hartge P, Struewing JP, Pee D, McAdams M, Brody L, et al. The kin-cohort study for estimating penetrance. Am J Epidemiol 1998;148:623–30.

Wacholder S, McLaughlin JK, Silverman DT, Mandel JS. Selection of controls in case-control studies. Am J Epidemiol 1992;135:1019–28.

Wacholder S, Rothman N, Caporaso N. Population stratification in epidemiologic studies of common genetic variants and cancer: quantification of bias. J Natl Cancer Inst 2000;92:1151–58.

Wacholder S, Chanock S, Garcia-Closas M, El Ghormli L, Rothman N. Assessing the probability that a positive report is false: an approach for molcular epidemiology studies. J Natl Cancer Inst 2004;96:434–42.

Watson JD, Gilman M, Witkowski J, Zoller M. Mapping and cloning human disease genes. In: Watson JD, Gilman M, Witkowski J, Zoller M (Eds): Recombinant DNA, 2nd ed. New York: Scientific American Books, 1992, pp 511–37.

Wooster R, Neuhausen SL, Mangion J, Quirk Y, Ford D, Collins N, et al. Localization of a breast cancer susceptibility gene, BRCA2, to chromosome 13q12–13. Science 1994;265: 2088–90.

Yeager M, Orr N, Hayes RB, Jacobs KB, Kraft P, Wacholder S, et al. Genome-wide associations study of prostate cancer identifies a second risk locus at 8q24. Nat Genet 2007;39:645–49.

Zanke BW, Greenwood CM, Rangrei J, Kustra R, Tenesa A, Farrington SM, et al. Genome-wide association scan identified a colorectal cancer susceptibility locus on chromosome 8q24. Nat Genet 2007;39:989–94.

5

Biomarkers in Cancer Epidemiology

PAOLO BOFFETTA AND DIMITRIOS TRICHOPOULOS

Modern molecular methods are rapidly becoming an integral part of many epidemiological studies. While approaches to evaluate genetic factors were described in another chapter, this one deals with the use of molecular methods to measure exposure, early evidence of malignant transformation, and individual susceptibility. As we will see, such epidemiologic studies are subject to problems of design and analysis similar to those encountered in more traditional epidemiologic investigations.

The use of biological measurements to assess variables of interest in epidemiological studies is not new. In the areas of infectious and cardiovascular diseases, research that would nowadays be viewed in the context of biomarkers has been conducted for decades. As an example, Figure 5–1 shows the results linking elevated serum cholesterol levels to the risk of ischaemic heart disease in the Framingham prospective study (Truett et al, 1967). During the last decade, however, the use of biomarkers in cancer epidemiology has greatly increased.

Several reasons may explain this expansion. The search for carcinogens, characterized by complex exposure circumstances and possibly weak effects, has become increasingly difficult with traditional epidemiological approaches. An example is the investigation of the role of diet, in particular early in life, in breast carcinogenesis (Okasha et al, 2003). In parallel, increasing knowledge of mechanisms of carcinogenesis led to the proposal of models involving genetic and epigenetic events, as well as cellular and histological alterations. These models, which need to be tested in human studies, represent a theoretical framework for molecular epidemiological research. Furthermore, developments in molecular biology and genetics, such as the use of robots and the increasing throughput of automatic analytical equipments, allow the large-scale application of assays that would otherwise be very resource intensive.

It is useful to consider biomarkers in general and molecular epidemiology tools in particular within the larger framework of epidemiological studies. Epidemiology aims

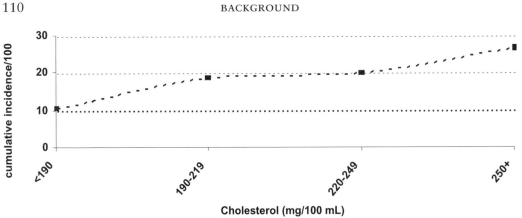

Figure 5–1. Incidence of ischaemic heart disease and serum cholesterol in Framingham cohort—12-year follow-up of men. (*Source*: Truett et al, 1967)

at identifying determinants of disease and quantifying their role, while taking into account sources of random and systematic error (bias and confounding), as well as factors that modify the effect of the determinant(s) of interest (Figure 5–2). To a large extent, biomarker-based epidemiological studies fit into the same framework: They represent epidemiological studies, in which risk factors, outcomes, confounders, or effect modifiers are measured with biomarkers. Similarly, the same arguments should be applied to the design, analysis, and interpretation of biomarker-based and more traditional epidemiological studies.

In practice, there is a continuum from the development of biomarkers to be applied in human studies, to their characterization in early field studies, to their application in full-scale epidemiological investigations (Garcia-Closas et al, 2006). However, these logical steps are often bypassed, with promising but yet unvalidated biomarkers being applied in human studies. While this pattern reflects the vivacity of a young discipline, a more cautious approach is needed in order to avoid misuse of research resources.

In the context of epidemiological studies, a biomarker has been defined as a substance, structure, or process that *(1)* can be measured in the human body or its products and *(2)* may influence the incidence or outcome of disease in human populations (Workshop Report, 1997). It is important to bear in mind the distinction between marker, assay, and measurement. While the marker is the variable to be measured, the assay is

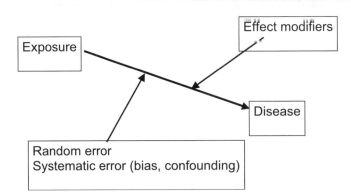

Figure 5–2. Identification of exposure-disease relations with epidemiology

the test used to measure the marker, and the measurement is an individual value of the marker.

A distinction has been made between biomarkers of exposure, intermediate events, disease, and susceptibility (Figure 5–3; Table 5–1). This distinction, however, is somewhat arbitrary. For example, chromosomal aberrations have been used for decades to monitor exposure to environmental carcinogens (Tucker et al, 1997). From this point of view, they can be classified as biomarkers of exposure. However, growing evidence points toward a role of chromosomal aberrations for prediction of cancer risk, irrespective of exposure (Norppa et al, 2006). In this respect, they can be seen as intermediate biomarkers. Furthermore, it is important to notice that any scheme, such as that represented in Figure 5–3, reflects our current understanding of the complex biological phenomenon of carcinogenesis and our ability to measure events that are considered relevant to it. In other words, the steps in the carcinogenic process depicted in Figure 5–3 represent "boxes" where we allocate available biomarkers: In fact, more emphasis is given in the scheme to the early steps (internal dose, biologically effective dose, etc) than to the later steps simply because of the larger availability of markers—and their more straightforward interpretation—to measure the former as compared to the latter events. The increase in the understanding of the late steps in carcinogenesis, and the development of relevant and valid biomarkers, represents a main challenge to molecular cancer epidemiology.

EXPOSURE BIOMARKERS

In many instances, epidemiologic research is hampered by misclassification of exposure ascertained, for example, by means of questionnaires, interviews, or job histories. The rationale for using biomarkers is to measure the biologically relevant exposure more precisely. In some instances, there is an obvious improvement in using an exposure biomarker. Aflatoxin provides a good example in which exposure biomarkers represent a step forward in the identification of the human cancer hazard. The fungus *Aspergillus flavus* is a contaminant of foodstuffs, in particular cereals and nuts. Exposure is common in West Africa and East Asia. Depending on storage conditions, *A. flavus* may produce a toxin, called aflatoxin, with strong hepatotoxic and carcinogenic properties in animal models. It is difficult to

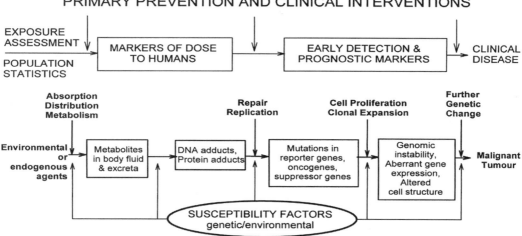

Figure 5–3. Schematic representation of application of biomarkers in molecular cancer epidemiology. (Derived from National Resource Council, 1987)

Table 5–1. Classes of biomarkers and examples of application to cancer epidemiology

Class	Biomarkers	Examples of application to cancer epidemiology (reference)
Exposure	Environmental pollutants	Dioxins and breast cancer risk (Warner et al, 2002)
	Nutrients	Folate and cancer risk (Rossi et al, 2006)
	Infectious agents	HPV infection and oral cancer risk (Mork et al, 2001)
	Endogenous compounds	Hormones and breast cancer risk (Kaaks et al, 2001)
	DNA adducts	Aflatoxin adducts and liver cancer risk (Ross et al., 1992)
	Protein adducts	Ethylene oxide adducts (Schulte et al, 1992)
Intermediate	Cytogenetic abnormalities	Chromosomal aberrations and cancer risk (Boffetta et al, 2007)
	DNA adducts	PAH-DNA adducts and lung cancer risk (Tang et al, 2001)
Disease	Gene mutation	TP53 mutations in lung cancer (Le Calvez et al, 2005)
	Epigenetic alteration	Promoter methylation and bladder cancer risk (Marsit et al, 2006)
	Genomic instability	Microsatellite instability in colorectal cancer (Slattery et al, 2000)
Susceptibility	Single nucleotide polymorphism	Polymorphisms in DNA repair genes and lung cancer risk (Hung et al, 2005)
	DNA repair capacity	DNA repair capacity and lung cancer risk (Wei et al, 2000)

know whether the food humans have consumed has been contaminated by aflatoxin. Studies on the carcinogenic effect of aflatoxin are therefore limited by the difficulty of determining exposure status at the individual level, although ecological analyses have indicated a higher incidence of hepatocellular carcinoma in areas with frequently contaminated food than in neighbouring areas with less frequent contamination.

The identification of serum and urine biomarkers of aflatoxin exposure—namely urinary metabolites of aflatoxin itself and of its adducts formed with DNA—paved the way for important developments. Table 5–2 reports an increased risk of hepatocellular carcinoma in the first study using exposure biomarkers in subjects with samples collected and stored prospectively. Individuals with any urinary marker of exposure had a 2.4-fold increased risk of liver cancer relative to individuals without markers; the relative risk was as high as 4.9 among individuals positive for the urinary adduct degradation product AFB_1-N^7 guanine (Ross et al, 1992). These results, replicated in

other populations, provide strong evidence of a causal association between aflatoxin and liver cancer in humans (IARC, 2002).

Exposure markers measure the presence or level of exogenous agents (eg, pollutants), agents formed endogenously (eg, hormones), the metabolites of exogenous and endogenous agents, the products of the interaction of the agents or the metabolites with macromolecules (eg, DNA adducts), and physiological responses elicited by the exposure (eg, antibodies).

The use of biomarkers to measure exposure is not a panacea; the performance of exposure biomarkers should be compared to that of other exposure-assessment methods, such as medical records, questionnaires, and environmental monitoring. Main concerns are the relevance of the biomarker to the exposure of interest, its specificity (eg, chemicals often share common metabolites), and the characteristics of the assay, including sensitivity, kinetics, source of variability, and effect modifiers (Rothman et al, 1995). For example, the half-life of blood and urine markers of exposure to chemicals varies

Table 5–2. Relative risk of hepatocellular carcinoma and biomarker of exposure to aflatoxin

Biomarker	Cases	Controls	Relative risk	95% confidence interval
No aflatoxin biomarker	9	87	1.0	Reference
Any aflatoxin biomarker	13	53	2.4	1.0-5.9
AFB_1-N^7-guanine	6	11	4.9	1.5-16

Source: Ross et al, 1992.

from a few hours (eg, chlorinated hydrocarbons) to years (eg, dioxins) (Coggon and Friesen, 1997).

Most biomarker-based studies, of both prospective and retrospective design, rely on a single biological sample. This represents a drawback as compared to traditional exposure assessment based on, for example, questionnaires or interviews. With the latter approaches, historical reconstruction of variations in exposure is—at least in some instances—feasible. An example is the assessment of tobacco smoking. Biomarker-based approaches, such as the measurement of nicotine or its metabolites in plasma, provide a precise indication of recent exposure. However, no biomarkers are currently available to assess cumulative tobacco consumption, or other time-related aspects of exposure that are important predictors of tobacco-related cancer risk.

Exposures in cancer epidemiology are often time-related variables. Moreover, both carcinogenesis models and empirical evidence strongly point toward the importance of induction and latency periods in cancer occurrence, the importance to evaluate both duration and intensity of exposure, and the need to assess changes in disease risk after cessation of exposure. The goal of exposure assessment is the reconstruction of a full history of exposure during relevant time periods. Different methods for exposure assessment (eg, biomarker-based versus questionnaire-based) should be evaluated on how well they accomplish this objective and on how well they complement each other.

While most biomarkers measure recent exposure, there are ways to use them to assess temporal changes. One approach is to collect repeated samples from subjects enrolled in prospective studies. While theoretically excellent, this option is often financially and logistically prohibitive. A compromise is the collection of repeated biologic samples from a fraction of the original cohort. If the sample is representative and large enough, it becomes possible to identify predictors of temporal changes in the biomarker and apply them to the whole study population. A more serious problem exists in retrospective studies, in which measurement of exposure biomarkers at the biologically relevant time (eg, several years before onset of the disease) is generally not possible.

When biological samples are available on a subset of the study population, it is possible to model exposure in a way similar to that described previously for repeated samples. For example, in a study assessing cancer risk from dioxin exposure among 1167 chemical workers from the Netherlands, recent serum dioxin measurements were available for 144 individuals, while a detailed occupational history was available for all workers (Hooiveld et al, 1998). In an analysis of the results from 144 workers, three factors—namely years in main production, employment before 1970, and exposure during an industrial accident—explained 85% of the variance in serum dioxin level. The application of these factors to the occupational histories, and the incorporation of terms accounting for the kinetics of dioxin accumulation during exposure and release after cessation of exposure, generated an estimated maximum level of exposure for all workers. In other instances, a biomarker can be used on a subset of the study population to validate exposures estimated by other means.

A special group of exposure markers are adducts formed by carcinogens with DNA and proteins (Farmer, 2004). DNA adducts are directly relevant to carcinogenesis, since they reflect the interaction of the active compound with the relevant cellular target. They also integrate internal dose and repair capacity, thus providing a relevant indicator of biologically active dose (Rundle, 2006). However, the drawbacks in their use in epidemiology are the low levels detected in most exposure circumstances and the relatively short half-life. Some techniques to measure adducts are more sensitive, although this is often obtained by losing specificity. The half-life of white blood cells, which are often used to measure DNA adducts, is variable, but in general rather short. On the other hand, the detection of adducts to proteins—mainly albumin and hemoglobin—allows a measure of internal dose integrated over several weeks or months. In general, DNA and protein adducts represents a useful complement to other approaches of exposure assessment, but in very few circumstances have they provided critical novel information, in either qualitative or quantitative terms, to epidemiological research.

The use of exposure biomarkers poses additional methodological problems. As discussed in the following, epidemiological results based on exposure biomarkers are potentially subject to bias and confounding, as are other types of observational studies. An additional problem exists when exposure markers are used in retrospective case-control studies: their possible dependence on the disease process. For example, lipid metabolism might be altered in breast cancer and other hormone-dependent neoplasms (Demark-Wahnefried et al, 2001), resulting in possible bias in the measurement of compounds stored in adipose tissue, such as many organic contaminants. Despite the potential limitations, exposure biomarkers represent an important tool in cancer epidemiology. Technological developments are rapid in the field, improving the accuracy, sensitivity, and precision of the assays and facilitating the application of the markers to large-scale population studies.

INTERMEDIATE BIOMARKERS

Intermediate biomarkers measure early—in general nonpersistent—biological events that take place in the continuum between exposure and cancer development. These events include measure of cellular or tissue toxicity; chromosomal alterations; changes in DNA, RNA, and protein expression; and alterations in functions relevant to carcinogenesis (eg, DNA repair, immunological response). Similar to exposure markers, these markers are generally measured in easily accessible biological samples, typically blood components. Several of these assays offer a potentially important contribution to molecular epidemiology, because of their direct relevance to carcinogenesis and the parallel development of intermediate- or large-throughput technical platforms (eg, microarrays).

The use of DNA and RNA expression arrays in large-scale population studies has started, and their contribution is expected in the next few years (Gunn and Smith, 2004). As proteins and peptides are more stable and relatively easier to measure than RNA and DNA, proteomics and metabolomics represent interesting new approaches to the investigation of intermediate events in molecular cancer epidemiology. Also in this instance, however, the application to large-scale population-based studies is only starting, and the characteristics and performances of the biomarkers are not fully understood. An additional challenge brought by microarray and proteomic analysis is the complexity of data, since several hundreds or even thousands of data points are generated for each sample, which poses novel statistical challenges, including an increased likelihood to produce false-positive results (see following).

Chromosomal alterations measured in peripheral lymphocytes have been used for monitoring exposure to mutagens and carcinogens. In recent years, several cohort

Table 5–3. Meta-analysis of studies of chromosomal aberrations and cancer risk

	Relative risk	95% Confidence interval	Test for heterogeneity p-value
Total chromosomal aberrations			
Low	1.0	Ref.	–
Medium	1.3	1.1, 1.6	0.4
High	1.4	1.2, 1.7	0.01
Chromatide-type aberrations			
Low	1.0	Ref.	
High	1.1	1.0, 1.3	0.2
Chromosome-type aberrations			
Low	1.0	Ref.	
High	1.3	1.1, 1.5	0.6

Meta-analysis of the studies by Hagmar et al, 1994; Bonassi et al 1995 (these two studies were combined in Hagmar et al, 2004); Rossner et al, 2005; Boffetta et al, 2007.

studies have been established by measuring the occurrence of cancer among individuals who underwent chromosomal aberration testing (Norppa et al, 2006). Four such cohort studies have been reported: A meta-analysis of their results suggests that higher levels of chromosomal aberrations are associated with a modest increase in cancer risk (Table 5–3)—the cancers with the highest excess risk were those of the digestive system.

Despite the fact that they are considered primarily biomarkers of exposure (see previous), DNA adducts have been used to predict cancer risk in several prospective studies (Phillips, 2005). Although the exact role of DNA adducts in predicting cancer risk has still to be elucidated, this is an additional example of the artificial distinction between "exposure" and "effect" biomarkers, and the need to study the exposure–disease relationship as a continuum.

DISEASE BIOMARKERS

As in the case of exposure markers, the use of biomarkers to measure the outcome of an epidemiological study (typically cancer) has the aim to increase the validity of the measurement—that is, to increase the specificity and the sensitivity in the definition of the outcome. For example, microarray-based techniques to measure the expression of a large number of genes has led to the discovery that cases of breast cancer indistinguishable according to traditional histological classifications may show profoundly different patterns of genetic expression (Sorlie, 2004).

Alterations (eg, mutations, deletions, epigenetic modifications) in genes with a role in carcinogenesis or a characteristic cytogenetic alteration, rather than the tumor itself, might become the outcome of a molecular epidemiological study. Studies based on biomarkers of disease are best suited in a prospective design, since the identification of early events relevant to carcinogenesis would hopefully impinge on preventive strategies. For example, mutations typical of tobacco-related cancers have been found in sputum samples of heavy smokers, suggesting that they can be used as markers of lung cancer (Kersting et al, 2000).

Disease biomarkers can also be used in retrospective designs, in which only diseased individuals are enrolled. In such case-only studies, comparisons are made among subgroups of cases with differences in the profile of genetic mutations (or other molecular characteristics). For example, different frequencies and patterns of mutations in *TP53* have been detected in lung cancer, in correlation with tobacco smoking and exposure to other carcinogens (Pfeifer et al, 2002).

As in the case of exposure markers, the time coordinates of early effect markers are crucial for their application in molecular epidemiology. While adequate knowledge of the natural history is lacking for most human neoplasms, models of carcinogenesis developed for various tumors, eg, colon cancer (Fearon and Vogelstein, 1990), stomach cancer (Correa, 1992), and head and neck cancer (Sidransky, 1997), provide a framework for the application of effect markers.

SUSCEPTIBILITY MARKERS

The broad interindividual variability at both the genetic and the epigenetic levels provides a framework to explain the inherited susceptibility to cancer. Susceptibility markers can be measured at the genotypic level and at the functional (phenotypic) level. The advantages of genotypic markers are their stability across tissues and time, and the growing throughput of genotyping technologies. Phenotypic markers, on the other hand, integrate the effect of multiple genes, epigenetic phenomena, and post-translational modifications with respect to given characteristics such as DNA repair: Their implementation in large-scale population studies, however, remains limited.

The most commonly studied genetic variants are single nucleotide polymorphisms (SNP); other types of variants include microsatellites, deletions, insertions, gene amplifications, and variations in the number of gene copies (Redon et al, 2006). Early studies of susceptibility markers considered only one or few variants in candidate genes; technological developments have later conferred the ability to look at hundreds or even thousands of variants in a panel of genes. In the last years, the analysis of a large number of variants has become possible (current microarrays include several hundreds of thousands of SNP, but this number is expected to grow in the near future). In such genome-wide association studies any effort to select variants and genes based on a priori functional knowledge has been abandoned.

While a detailed discussion of genetic cancer epidemiology is beyond the scope of this chapter, it should be stressed that few variants conferring modest, at most, increases in cancer risk have been consistently found. It is likely that most of the genetic susceptibility to cancer arises from a combination of deleterious variants in different genes, each providing only a marginal excess risk. Furthermore, it is plausible that most of the effect occurs from the combination of genetic make-up and exposure to endogenous or exogenous factors (so-called "gene–environment interactions"; see following) (Hunter, 2005). The high-throughput genotyping approaches developed in recent years have started to be applied to genetic cancer epidemiology. It is expected that they will contribute substantially to the understanding of mechanisms underlying genetic susceptibility, and eventually mechanisms of human carcinogenesis.

Epigenetic alterations, particularly changes in promoter methylation status, are increasingly used as markers of carcinogenesis. Methylation status in lymphocytes and other surrogate tissues may reflect inherited characteristics that are relevant to individual susceptibility, possibly in relation with lifestyle and environmental exposures.

Functional (phenotypic) markers can be used to complement the information provided by the analysis of genetic variations. In particular, the individual ability to repair DNA damage has been investigated using different types of assays—such as host-cell reactivation assay, mutagen sensitivity, Comet assay—in case-control settings (Spitz et al, 2003). In general, cancer cases have shown a decreased DNA repair capacity as compared to controls, but the interpretation of these results is hampered by the small sample size and the use of lymphocytes as surrogate cells. The technical complexity of these assays has so far prevented their application in large-scale prospective studies.

BIAS

Three main types of bias are recognized in epidemiology, and all three may operate in biomarker-based studies (Rothman and Greenland, 1996). Selection bias arises from lack of comparability of groups included in the study. For example, exposed cases might be more (or less) likely to participate in a study than exposed controls. Information bias involves differential or even nondifferential misclassification of participants with respect to disease or exposure status. In biomarker-based studies, information bias encompasses the issues of inherent validity, reproducibility, and stability of markers. Finally, confounding is a special form of bias, generated by co-exposure to causal factors other than those under study (see following).

Selection bias can be avoided by properly identifying the study population, and by optimizing the response rate. Furthermore, it can be controlled in the analysis by identifying factors that are related to selection and by controlling them as confounders. Unfortunately, many molecular epidemiological studies pay too little attention to the definition of source population and selection of participants. This is particularly common in studies of genetic factors, since it is considered that any selection of participants is unlikely to be associated with the genetic factors under study. In general, prospective studies are less prone to selection bias than retrospective studies.

BIOMARKER VARIATION

Sources of variation in biomarker-based measurements might arise from intergroup (eg, cases versus controls) variability: This is the very phenomenon molecular epidemiological studies usually aim to address. However, other sources of variation exist that generate misclassification. Interindividual variability might be due to genetic or environmental factors affecting the biomarker under study. Intraindividual variability refers to components of variation such as diurnal variation in hormonal level. Finally, measurement error might arise from sampling and laboratory variation. Table 5–4 provides some examples of sources of variation for selected biomarkers used in molecular cancer epidemiology (Vineis, 1997).

Proper precautions should be taken to minimize the sources of variation other than intergroup variability. Such sources are numerous: the circumstances under which biological samples are taken, processed, stored, and analysed; the technical aspects of the assays; etc. It is important to ensure that, if all sources of variation cannot be controlled (as it is often the case), they should apply equally to the groups being compared. Therefore, if long-term storage of samples might affect the measurement, it is important to match cases and controls in the study by duration of sample storage. In this situation, misclassification is said to be "nondifferential" (ie, acting equally on the groups being compared). Nondifferential misclassification generally produces bias toward the null value—that is, it obscures an existing association, but it does not generate one when none exists, nor does it accentuate an existing positive or inverse one.

Table 5–4. Sources of variation for selected biomarkers used in cancer epidemiology (modified from Vineis, 1997)

Biomarker	Inter-individual	Intra-individual	Laboratory
Hormones	+	+	(−)
Organochlorine compounds	+	−	+
DNA adducts in white blood cells	+	+	+
Chromosomal aberrations	+	−	+
SNP (genotyping)	−	−	(−)
DNA repair capacity	+	+	+

+ More important source of variation

− Less important source of variation

(−) No or few data

On the other hand, a misclassification that is "differential" with respect to case/control (or exposed/unexposed) status generates a bias in an unpredictable direction. For example, if there is substantial interbatch (or interreader) variability in the measurement, the inclusion of samples of cases and controls in different batches would generate differential misclassification, while a proper mix of samples in each batch would at worst result in nondifferential misclassification.

TRANSITIONAL STUDIES

The issue of variation in biomarker-based measurements impinges on the need to validate biomarkers before application to large-scale studies. This is the domain of so-called transitional studies, which aim to characterize the biomarker itself rather than the underlying biological phenomenon. The aspects assessed by transitional studies include intra- and intersubject variability, feasibility of application of a biomarker in field conditions (and optimization of its use), identification of determinants with confounding and effect-modifying potential, and exploration of biological mechanisms underlying the variation of the marker.

Transitional studies may involve healthy individuals, patients, or subjects with specific exposures (eg, groups of workers). Three types of transitional studies have been described in the continuum between development of a new assay and its large-scale application to human populations (Table 5–5) (Schulte and Perera, 1997; Rothman et al, 1995).

Developmental transitional studies have several goals. They aim to identify the biological phenomena measured by the marker and their relevance to the exposure, the disease, or the host variables of interest. In addition, developmental studies address the reliability (reproducibility) of the newly developed marker, by blindly measuring replicate samples. These samples should be representative of the values likely to be found in populations that the marker has to be applied to (Rothman et al, 1995). Assessment of reliability encompasses both random laboratory variation and nonrandom (systematic) error. Principles for assessment of marker reliability have been proposed (Vineis et al, 1993; Droz, 1993). Developmental transitional studies should also address aspects of relevance to field applications such as kinetics and stability of the marker. They should contribute to the clarification of the temporal relevance of the biomarker in relation to the underlying biological phenomenon (Droz, 1993).

The main aim of characterization-type transitional studies is to assess interindividual variation in the marker and to reveal genetic and acquired factors that contribute to such variation. When applied in the field, interindividual variation of the marker will

Table 5–5. Types of transitional studies (modified from Schulte and Perera, 1997)

Type of study	Aims	Characteristics
Developmental	Development of biomarkers	- Build on experimental studies - Test assay in human samples. - Evaluate biologic sample collection, processing, storage - Evaluate assay accuracy, precision
Characterization	Validation	- Assessment of biomarker range in representative human populations - Evaluation of external (or internal) exposure-biomarker relationship, biomarker kinetics, and of potential confounders and effect modifiers
Applied	Use in cross-sectional, metabolic, panel studies	- Evaluation of exposure status of various populations and further validation of the biomarker

be studied in conjunction with the exposure or the outcome of interest. Sources of interindividual variation should then be known and, to a certain extent, controlled for. One particular aspect of interindividual variability is the difference in presence or level of the marker in different organs and tissues, since field studies often have to rely on samples of surrogate tissues, typically blood. The identification of factors affecting the level of a marker goes beyond the characterization of the marker and impinges on the interpretation of the results of molecular epidemiological studies. For example, the finding that a metabolic polymorphism is a modifying factor for a marker of exposure provides important information on the metabolic pathways relevant to the exposure of interest.

Applied transitional studies aim to assess the relationship between a marker and the phenomenon that it is considered to indicate, ie, the relationship between exposure and marker or between marker and disease. For example, the association between exposure to butadiene and several markers, including mutations in the *HRPT* gene, has been studied, in order to assess the usefulness of these markers in predicting cancer risk among exposed workers (Albertini et al, 2001).

CONFOUNDING

The use of biomarkers does not prevent confounding. For example, an association between tobacco smoking and cancer of the uterine cervix has been observed in many populations but it is likely to be confounded by infection with the human papilloma virus (HPV), a cause of cervical cancer. In many populations, smokers are more frequently positive for HPV than nonsmokers. Hence, HPV would be a confounder no matter how smoking, infection, and cervical cancer are assessed (via questionnaires, medical records, biochemical methods, or molecular techniques). Furthermore, to use biomarkers might introduce confounding. If, for example, workers occupationally exposed to polycyclic aromatic hydrocarbons (PAH) have a higher consumption of tobacco (an important source of PAH) than other workers, then the assessment of occupational exposure with a biomarker of PAH is confounded by tobacco smoking (Figure 5–4) (Pearce et al, 1995). This would have not been the case if occupational exposure were assessed without biomarker methods.

INTERACTION

Biomarkers have been widely applied to studies of gene–environment interactions and gene–gene interactions in the pathogenesis of cancer and other chronic diseases (Hunter, 2005). Table 5–6 provides an example from a lung cancer study that addressed dietary intake of cabbages and other cruciferous vegetables. Such vegetables

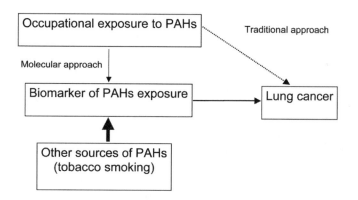

Figure 5–4. Example of confounding

Table 5–6. Example of gene-diet interaction: Relative risk of lung cancer for dietary intake of cruciferous vegetables, stratified by GSTM1 and GSTT1 polymorphism (Brennan et al., 2005)

	Dietary cruciferous vegetable intake - RR (95% CI)		
	High (reference)	Medium	Low
GSTM1+ and GSTTI+	1.00	0.87 (0.62, 1.22)	0.88 (0.65, 1.21)
GSTM1+ and GSTT1– or GSTM1– and GSTT1+	1.00	0.82 (0.60, 1.12)	0.80 (0.60,1.08)
GSTM1– and GSTT1–	1.00	0.26 (0.10,0.63)	0.28 (0.11, 0.67)

RR, relative risk; CI, confidence interval

contain the potentially chemopreventive iso-thiocyanates. Polymorphism for genes encoding for the enzymes glutathione-S-transferase (GST) M1 and T1, are implicated in the metabolism of isothiocyanates (Brennan et al, 2005). The apparent protective effect of high intake of iso-thiocyanate-rich diet was stronger among carriers of the null genotypes in the GST enzymes than in carriers of the wild-type genotype in one or both genes.

Molecular epidemiology studies addressing other types of interaction between two or more factors may be discussed following a similar approach. For example, in the study of aflatoxin exposure and liver cancer mentioned previously, the investigators addressed the possible interaction of aflatoxin with hepatitis B virus (HBV) (Ross et al, 1992). When compared to HBV-negative subjects exposed to aflatoxin, the relative risk in HBV-positive subjects also positive for aflatoxin markers was 60, which was greater than the product of the relative risks for the two factors separately (4.8 for HBV and 1.9 for aflatoxin). Thus a super-multiplicative synergism between aflatoxin and HBV in liver carcinogenesis is suggested. The wide confidence interval in the group with both exposures (6.4–560) precludes, however, rejections of the null hypothesis of no interaction according to a multiplicative model (4.8 x 1.9 = 9.1). This wide interval also stresses another methodological concern in molecular epidemiological studies, namely the need for a large sample size.

RANDOM ERROR

From several of the examples quoted previously it is clear that an important problem in biomarker-based epidemiological research is the insufficient number of subjects included in each study. The main reasons for a small study size are logistical and financial constraints. Indeed, any biomarker-based measure introduced in epidemiology should be compared with traditional measures, and the possible gain in sensitivity and specificity of the biomarker measure should be considered in the light of the possible decrease in the number of study subjects.

Authors have proposed formulas to calculate the sample size needed to detect main effects and interactions among risk factors (Garcia-Closas and Lubin, 1999). Molecular epidemiology studies often do not include a sufficient number of individuals, and this has been the reason for unstable and conflicting results. For example, many studies have been published on the possible association between slow acetylation polymorphism and bladder cancer risk. The biological rationale is that individuals with variants leading to reduced acetylation might have a reduced capacity to detoxify environmental bladder carcinogens, including aromatic amines. It is unlikely, however, that the relative risk would be higher than, say, 1.5, and, in fact, recent meta-analyses confirmed the presence of increased risk of the order of 40% (Garcia-Closas et al, 2005). Given that the frequency of the relevant polymorphic variant in Euro-

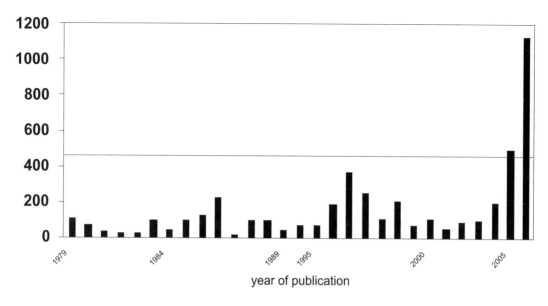

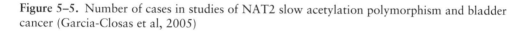

The line indicates the number of cases needed for 80% power to detect a statistically significant relative risk of 1.4 (prevalence of slow acetylation 0.5).

Figure 5–5. Number of cases in studies of NAT2 slow acetylation polymorphism and bladder cancer (Garcia-Closas et al, 2005)

pean populations is about 50%, 450 cases and the same number of controls are needed to achieve an 80% power to detect a statistically significant relative risk of 1.4. If the goal is to detect an interaction between the polymorphism and an environmental factor (eg, tobacco smoking or occupational exposure to aromatic amines), then the number of required cases and controls would be much larger (between 2- and 20-fold, depending on the expected strength of interaction).

As shown in Figure 5–5, only 2 out of the 29 studies of *NAT2* polymorphism and bladder cancer included in a recent meta-analysis had an adequate size to detect the main effect of the polymorphism, and only one had the power to document a strong interaction with an environmental exposure. In recent years, large-scale studies have been set up, in order to provide more robust results (eg, Slattery et al, 1998; Garcia-Closas et al, 2005; Hung et al, 2005). Another approach is the pooling of independently conducted studies (Ioannidis et al, 2005).

Since lack of statistical power is an important problem in molecular and genetic epidemiological studies aimed to detect weak associations, the independent conduct of small-scale studies that address several hypotheses is a reason for the generation of many false-positive results (Ioannidis et al, 2006a). This problem has been mainly addressed in the context of genetic association studies, and in particular as a consequence of the growing ability to measure a large number of genetic variants; but it may affect other areas of molecular epidemiological research. Guidelines for the reporting of results and the interpretation of "positive" associations have been proposed (Ioannidis, 2006).

PUBLICATION BIAS

A problem related to the generation of false-positive results is the tendency to selectively report significant results, in particular when they show an effect in the expected

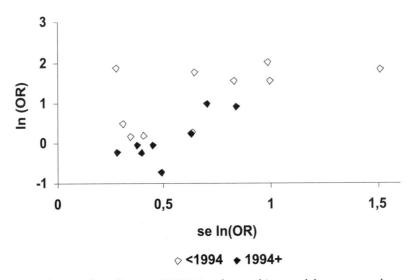

Figure 5–6. Funnel plot of studies on CYP2D6 polymorphism and lung cancer by year of publication

direction. The net result is a biased under-reporting of null results. As an example, several studies have been conducted on polymorphism of the *CYP2D6* gene, which encodes for an enzyme possibly involved in the activation of lung carcinogens, and lung cancer risk. Figure 5–6 shows the results of the 18 studies available for a meta-analysis (d'Errico et al, 1999) reported in terms of

the logarithm of the relative risk for high-risk *CYP2D6* polymorphism, and its standard error. Each study is identified by one dot, studies to the right of the figure are smaller than those to the left, and studies at the top are more positive than those at the bottom of the figure. If no publication bias existed, the pattern of such results should resemble a triangle (or a funnel), with larger

Table 5–7. Publication bias in studies of selected associations between polymorphisms in genes encoding for metabolic enzymes and cancer*

Gene	Cancer site	N of risk estimates	Publication bias, p-value
CYP1A1	Lung	18	0.0
CYP2D6	Lung	18	0.03
	Urinary bladder	7	0.8
	Breast	5	0.2
GSTM1	Lung	50	1.0
	Urinary bladder	28	0.3
NAT2	Lung	5	0.5
	Urinary bladder	29	0.9
	Colorectal	14	0.4
	Breast	9	0.03

* Based on d'Errico et al, 1999, except for GSTM1 and lung cancer (ad-hoc search), GSTM1 and bladder cancer (Garcia-Closas et al, 2005) and NAT2 and bladder cancer (Garcia-Closas et al, 2005).

Publication bias is assessed according to Begg and Mazumdar, 1994 studies converging on the left side around the central ("true") value, and smaller studies symmetrically dispersed on the right side. However, the empty side at the bottom right corner of the graph suggests that smaller studies were more likely to be reported if they showed a positive effect, and a formal analysis revealed publication bias for *CYP2D6* and lung cancer (Table 5–7), that was due to studies published before rather than after 1993.

It may be argued that such an initial report of false-positive results should be considered no major scientific problem, since subsequent studies, aimed to replicate the early positive results, will eventually establish the truth. However, this approach is inefficient and represents an important waste of resources, more so when it comes to expensive molecular epidemiological studies. A preferable approach is to critically evaluate and report results on the basis of criteria other than—or including but not limited to—statistical significance (Ioannidis, 2006). Biological plausibility, possible sources of bias and confounding, and numbers of tested associations are among such criteria. Statistical approaches have been proposed to take into account the possibility that significant results are generated by chance when many comparisons are made (Greenland, 1994). In addition, authors should be encouraged to systematically report their results, even those that are "negative" or "null."

CONCLUSIONS

Since the term *molecular epidemiology* was proposed in 1982 (Perera and Weinstein, 1982), molecular techniques have dominated biomarker research and have found an important and growing role in epidemiological studies. In several instances the application of a molecular approach has represented an important step beyond the evidence brought by traditional epidemiological methods. Assessment of exposure to aflatoxins, enhanced sensitivity and specificity of assessment of past viral infection, and detection of protein and DNA adducts in workers exposed to reactive chemicals such

as ethylene oxide, are among the examples in which molecular epidemiology has contributed to the understanding of human cancer. In many other cases, however, initial promising results have not been confirmed by subsequent, usually methodologically sounder, investigations. They include in particular the search for low-penetrance genetic variants leading to modest increases of cancer susceptibility (Ioannidis et al, 2006b).

If biomarkers are to offer new opportunities to overcome some of the limitations of epidemiology, then their added value over traditional approaches should be systematically assessed. Biomarkers should be validated and consideration of sources of bias and confounding should be no less stringent than in other types of epidemiological studies. Similarly, other aspects of the study such as determination of required sample size, statistical analysis, and reporting and interpretation of results should be approached with the same rigor as in epidemiology in general.

REFERENCES

Albertini RJ, Sram RJ, Vacek PM, Lynch J, Wright M, Nicklas JA, Rosenwald A, et al. Biomarkers for assessing occupational exposures to 1,3-butadiene. Chem Biol Interact 2001;135–136:429–53.

Begg CB and Mazumdar M. Operating characteristics of a rank correlation test for publication bias. Biometrics 1994;50:1088–101.

Boffetta P, van der Hel O, Norppa H, Fabianova E, Fucic A, Gundy S, et al. Chromosomal aberrations and cancer risk: results of a cohort study from Central Europe. Am J Epidemiol 2007;165: 36– 43.

Bonassi S, Abbondandolo A, Camurri L, Dal Pra L, De Ferrari M, Degrassi F, et al. Are chromosome aberrations in circulating lymphocytes predictive of future cancer onset in humans? Preliminary results of an Italian cohort study. Cancer Genet Cytogenet 1995;79:133–35.

Brennan P, Hsu CC, Moullan N, Szeszenia-Dabrowska N, Lissowska J, Zaridze D, Effect of cruciferous vegetables on lung cancer in patients stratified by genetic status: a mendelian randomisation approach. Lancet 2005;366:1558–60.

Coggon D, Friesen MD. Markers of internal dose: chemical agents. In: Toniolo P, Boffetta

P, Shuker DEG, Rothman N, Hulka B, Pearce N (Eds): Application of Biomarkers in Cancer Epidemiology. IARC Sci Publ No. 142. Lyon: IARC, 1997, pp 95–101.

Correa P. Human gastric carcinogenesis: a multistep and multifactorial process—First American Cancer Society Award Lecture on Cancer Epidemiology and Prevention. Cancer Res 1992;52: 6735–40.

Demark-Wahnefried W, Peterson BL, Winer EP, Marks L, Aziz N, Marcom PK, et al. Changes in weight, body composition, and factors influencing energy balance among premenopausal breast cancer patients receiving adjuvant chemotherapy. J Clin Oncol 2001;19: 2381–89.

d'Errico A, Malats N, Vineis P, Boffetta P. Review of studies of selected metabolic polymorphisms and cancer. In: Vineis P, Malats N, Lang M, d'Errico A, Caporaso N, Cuzick J, Boffetta P, eds, Metabolic Polymorphisms and Susceptibility to Cancer. IARC Sci Publ No. 148. Lyon: IARC; 1999, p. 323–93.

Droz PO. Biological monitroing and pharmacokinetic modeling for the assessment of exposure. In: Schulte PA, Perera FP (Eds): Molecular Epidemiology: Principles and Practices. San Diego: Academic Press. 1993, pp 137–57.

Farmer PB. Exposure biomarkers for the study of toxicological impact on carcinogenic processes. In: Buffler P, Rice J, Bird M, Boffetta P (Eds): Mechanisms of Carcinogenesis. Contributions of Molecular Epidemiology. IARC Sci Publ No. 157. Lyon: IARCPress; 2004, pp 71–90.

Fearon ER, Vogelstein B. A genetic model for colorectal tumorigenesis. Cell 1990; 61:759–67.

Garcia-Closas M, Lubin JH. Power and sample size calculations in case-control studies of gene-environment interactions: comments on different approaches. Am J Epidemiol 1999; 149;689–92.

Garcia-Closas M, Malats N, Silverman D, Dosemeci M, Kogevinas M, Hein DW, et al. NAT2 slow acetylation, GSTM1 null genotype, and risk of bladder cancer: results from the Spanish Bladder Cancer Study and meta-analyses. Lancet 2005;366:649–59.

Garcia-Closas M, Vermeulen R, Sherman ME, Moore LE, Smith MT, Rothman N. Application of biomarkers in Cancer Epidemiology. In: Schottenfeld D, Fraumeni JF. Cancer Epidemiology and Prevention, Third Edition. New York: Oxford University Press, 2006, pp70–88.

Greenland S. Hierarchical regression for epidemiologic analyses of multiple exposures. Environ Health Perspect 1994;102(Suppl 8):33–39.

Gunn L, Smith MT. Emerging biomarker technologies. In: Buffler P, Rice J, Bird M, Boffetta P, eds. Mechanisms of Carcinogenesis. Contributions of Molecular Epidemiology. IARC Sci Publ No. 157. Lyon: IARCPress; 2004, pp 437–50.

Hagmar L, Brogger A, Hansteen IL, Heim S, Hogstedt B, Knudsen L, et al. Cancer risk in humans predicted by increased levels of chromosomal aberrations in lymphocytes: Nordic study group on the health risk of chromosome damage. Cancer Res 1994;54: 2919–22.

Hagmar L, Stromberg U, Bonassi S, Hansteen IL, Knudsen LE, Lindholm C, et al. Impact of types of lymphocyte chromosomal aberrations on human cancer risk: results from Nordic and Italian cohorts. Cancer Res 2004;64:2258–63.

Hooiveld M, Heederik DJ, Kogevinas M, Boffetta P, Needham LL, Patterson DG Jr, et al. Second follow-up of a Dutch cohort occupationally exposed to phenoxy herbicides, chlorophenols, and contaminants. Am J Epidemiol 1998;147:891–901.

Hung RJ, Brennan P, Canzian F, Szeszenia-Dabrowska N, Zaridze D, Lissowska J, et al. Large-scale investigation of base excision repair genetic polymorphisms and lung cancer risk in a multicenter study. J Natl Cancer Inst 2005;97:567–76.

Hunter DJ. Gene-environment interactions in human diseases. Nat Rev Genet 2005;6: 287–98.

International Agency for Research on Cancer. Aflatoxins. IARC Monographs on the Evaluation of Carcinogenic Risks to Humans, Vol. 82. Some Traditional Herbal Medicines, Some Mycotoxins, Naphtalene and Styrene. Lyon: IARC, 2002;171–274.

Ioannidis JP, Bernstein J, Boffetta P, Danesh J, Dolan S, Hartge P, et al. A network of investigator networks in human genome epidemiology. Am J Epidemiol 2005;162:302–4.

Ioannidis JP. Commentary: grading the credibility of molecular evidence for complex diseases. Int J Epidemiol 2006;35:572–78

Ioannidis JP, Trikalinos TA, Khoury MJ. Implications of small effect sizes of individual genetic variants on the design and interpretation of genetic association studies of complex diseases. Am J Epidemiol 2006a;164: 609–14.

Ioannidis JP, Gwinn M, Little J, Higgins JP, Bernstein JL, Boffetta P, et al. A road map for efficient and reliable human genome epidemiology. Nat Genet 2006b;38:3–5.

Kaaks R, Berrino F, Key T, Rinaldi S, Dossus L, Biessy C, et al. Serum sex steroids in premenopausal women and breast cancer risk within the European Prospective Investigation into Cancer and Nutrition (EPIC). J Natl Cancer Inst 2005;97:755–65.

Kersting M, Friedl C, Kraus A, Behn M, Pankow W, Schuermann M. Differential frequencies of p16(INK4a) promoter hypermethylation, p53 mutation, and K-ras mutation in exfoliative material mark the development of lung cancer in symptomatic chronic smokers. J Clin Oncol 2000;18:3221–29.

Le Calvez F, Mukeria A, Hunt JD, Kelm O, Hung RJ, Taniere P, et al. TP53 and KRAS mutation load and types in lung cancers in relation to tobacco smoke: distinct patterns in never, former, and current smokers. Cancer Res 2005;65:5076–83.

Marsit CJ, Karagas MR, Danaee H, Liu M, Andrew A, Schned A, et al. Carcinogen exposure and gene promoter hypermethylation in bladder cancer. Carcinogenesis 2006;27: 112–16.

Mork J, Lie AK, Glattre E, Hallmans G, Jellum E, Koskela P, et al. Human papillomavirus infection as a risk factor for squamous-cell carcinoma of the head and neck. N Engl J Med 2001;344:1125–31.

National Resource Council. Biological markers in environmental health research. Environ Health Perspect 1987;74:3–9.

Norppa H, Bonassi S, Hansteen IL, Hagmar L, Stromberg U, Rossner P, et al. Chromosomal aberrations and SCEs as biomarkers of cancer risk. Mutat Res 2006;600:37–45.

Okasha M, McCarron P, Gunnell D, Smith GD. Exposures in childhood, adolescence and early adulthood and breast cancer risk: a systematic review of the literature. Breast Cancer Res Treat 2003;78:223–76.

Pearce N, de Sanjose S, Boffetta P, Kogevinas M, Saracci R, Savitz D. Limitations of biomarkers of exposure in cancer epidemiology. Epidemiology 1995;6:190–94.

Perera FP, Weinstein IB. Molecular epidemiology and carcinogen-DNA adduct detection: new approaches to studies of human cancer causation. J Chronic Dis 1982;35:581–600.

Pfeifer GP, Denissenko MF, Olivier M, Tretyakova N, Hecht SS, Hainaut P. Tobacco smoke carcinogens, DNA damage and p53 mutations in smoking-associated cancers. Oncogene 2002;21:7435–51.

Phillips DH. DNA adducts as markers of exposure and risk. Mutat Res 2005;577:284–92.

Redon R, Ishikawa S, Fitch KR, Feuk L, Perry GH, Andrews TD, et al. Global variation in copy number in the human genome. Nature 2006;444:444–54.

Ross RK, Yuan J-M, Yu MC, Wogan GN, Qian G-S, Tu J-T, Groopman JD, et al. Urinary aflatoxin biomarkers and risk of hepatocellular carcinoma. Lancet 1992;339:943–46.

Rossi E, Hung J, Beilby JP, Knuiman MW, Divitini ML, Bartholomew H. Folate levels and cancer morbidity and mortality: prospective cohort study from Busselton, Western Australia. Ann Epidemiol 2006;16:206–12.

Rossner P, Boffetta P, Ceppi M, Bonassi S, Smerhovsky Z, Landa K, et al. Chromosomal aberrations in lymphocytes of healthy subjects and risk of cancer. Environ Health Perspect 2005; 113:517–20.

Rothman KJ, Greenland S. Modern Epidemiology, 2nd edition. Philadelphia: Lippincott-Raven Publishers. 1996.

Rothman N, Stewart WF, Schulte PA. Incorporating biomarkers into cancer epidemiology: a matrix of biomarker and study design categories. Cancer Epidemiol Biomarkers Prev 1995;4:301–11.

Rundle A. Carcinogen-DNA adducts as a biomarker for cancer risk. Mutat Res 2006; 600:23–36.

Schulte PA, Perera, FP. Transitional studies. In: Toniolo P, Boffetta P, Shuker DEG, Rothman N, Hulka B, Pearce N (Eds): Application of Biomarkers in Cancer Epidemiology. IARC Sci Publ No. 142. Lyon: IARC, 1997, pp 19–29.

Schulte PA, Boeniger M, Walker JT, Schober SE, Pereira MA, Gulati DK, et al. Biologic markers in hospital workers exposed to low levels of ethylene oxide. Mutat Res 1992; 278:237–51.

Sidransky, D. Cancer of the head and neck. In: DeVita, VT, Jr, Hellman, S, Rosenberg, SA (Eds): Cancer: Principles and Practice of Oncology, 5th ed.. Lippincott-Raven Publishers, Philadelphia, 1997, pp 735–740.

Slattery ML, Potter JD, Samowitz W, Bigler J, Caan B, Leppert M. NAT2, GSTM-1, cigarette smoking, and risk of colon cancer. Cancer Epidemiol Biomarkers Prev 1998;7: 1097–84.

Slattery ML, Curtin K, Anderson K, Ma KN, Ballard L, Edwards S, et al. Associations between cigarette smoking, lifestyle factors, and microsatellite instability in colon tumors. J Natl Cancer Inst 2000;92:1831–36.

Sorlie T. Molecular portraits of breast cancer: tumour subtypes as distinct disease entities. Eur J Cancer 2004;40:2667–75.

Spitz MR, Wei Q, Dong Q, Amos CI, Wu X. Genetic susceptibility to lung cancer: the role of DNA damage and repair. Cancer Epidemiol Biomarkers Prev 2003;12:689–98.

Tang D, Phillips DH, Stampfer M, Mooney LA, Hsu Y, Cho S, et al. Association between carcinogen-DNA adducts in white blood cells and lung cancer risk in the physicians health study. Cancer Res 2001;61:6708–12.

Truett J, Cornfield J, Kannel W. A multivariate analysis of the risk of coronary heart disease in Framingham. J Chron Dis 1967;20:511–24.

Tucker JD, Eastmond DA, Littlefield LG. Cytogenetic end-points as biological dosimeters and predictors of risk in epidemiological studies. In: Toniolo P, Boffetta P, Shuker DEG, Rothman N, Hulka B, Pearce N (Eds): Application of Biomarkers in Cancer Epidemiology. IARC Sci Publ No. 142. Lyon: IARC, 1997, pp. 185–200.

Vineis P, Schulte PA, Vogt RF Jr. Technical variability in laboratory data. In: Schulte PA, Perera FP (Eds): Molecular Epidemiology: Principles and Practices. San Diego: Academic Press, 1993, pp 110–135.

Vineis P. Sources of variation in biomarkers. In: Toniolo P, Boffetta P, Shuker DEG, Rothman N, Hulka B, Pearce N (Eds): Application of Biomarkers in Cancer Epidemiology. IARC Sci Publ No. 142. Lyon: IARC, 1997, pp 59–71.

Warner M, Eskenazi B, Mocarelli P, Gerthoux PM, Samuels S, Needham L, et al. Serum dioxin concentrations and breast cancer risk in the Seveso Women's Health Study. Environ Health Perspect 2002;110:625–28.

Wei Q, Cheng L, Amos CI, Wang LE, Guo Z, Hong WK, et al. Repair of tobacco carcinogen-induced DNA adducts and lung cancer risk: a molecular epidemiologic study. J Natl Cancer Inst 2000;92:1764–72.

Workshop Report. In: Toniolo P, Boffetta P, Shuker DEG, Rothman N, Hulka B, Pearce N (Eds): Application of Biomarkers in Cancer Epidemiology. IARC Sci Publ No. 142. Lyon: IARC, 1997, pp 1–18.

6

Concepts in Cancer Epidemiology and Etiology

PAGONA LAGIOU, DIMITRIOS TRICHOPOULOS,
AND HANS-OLOV ADAMI

Epidemiology has been a powerful tool in the identification of causes of infectious diseases and the elucidation of the conditions underlying epidemic outbreaks that are frequently, but not always, of infectious etiology. Around the middle of the twentieth century, first in the United Kingdom (Doll and Hill, 1950) and later in the United States and the rest of the world (Wynder and Graham, 1950; Clemmesen and Nielsen, 1957; MacMahon, 1957), *epidemiology* expanded in scope by focusing also on the etiology of chronic diseases, irrespective of the nature of the causal agents. Since then, *epidemiology* has developed and matured to become a rich and powerful toolbox for the study of biologic phenomena in humans. With a number of fine textbooks nowadays available to students of epidemiology (for instance Miettinen, 1985; Hennekens and Buring, 1987; Walker, 1991; MacMahon and Trichopoulos, 1996; Rothman and Greenland, 1998; Rothman, 2002; and several others), this chapter is not intended to expand on methods or quantitative considerations. For the purpose of better

understanding the logic underlying cancer epidemiology, however, central concepts in epidemiology—the study of disease etiology—will be reviewed. We examine cohort and case–control studies (with special reference to studies of genetic epidemiology), we consider the impact of chance and systematic errors (*confounding* and bias), and we trace the process of causal reasoning. Familiarity with these concepts is essential for critical reading and understanding of the chapters on specific cancers. A glossary found at the end of the chapter provides a summary of definitions for words in italics.

ETIOLOGY

Causality

The definition of a *cause* should apply to all diseases, whether defined on the basis of a particular exposure, such as many infectious and occupational diseases, or documented by a constellation of clinical and/or laboratory findings—for example, malignant tumors, connective tissue disorders, or psychoses. In terms of a particular individual, exposure to a cause of a disease implies that the individual is now more likely to develop the disease, although there is no certainty that this will happen. The complexity of biological phenomena and our ignorance or limited understanding of many of the underlying processes hinder a deterministic, logically unassailable, explanation of disease causation. Hence, causation of disease can only be conceptualized in a probabilistic (stochastic) sense that involves statistical terms and procedures. For instance, while heavy smokers are much more likely to develop lung cancer than nonsmokers, most smokers never develop lung cancer and some nonsmokers do.

In epidemiology, there are several models of causality that have been applied to help clarify the role of various exposures in the etiology of disease. The causal pies presented by Rothman (1976) provide perhaps the most coherent approach to conceptualizing causality in a variety of epidemiologic settings (Rothman, 1986). Each of these pies describes a set of exposures that work together on the same pathway to cause disease (Fig. 6–1). Different exposures may occur within a short time span, or may happen decades apart. Once every exposure in a causal pie has occurred, that is

the pie is complete, disease is, in a deterministic context, inevitable. Table 6–1 provides a summary of the attributes of the causal pie model.

Causality is rarely, if ever, characterized by a simple one-to-one correspondence between a particular exposure and a specific disease. If so, the presence of the exposure would be both *necessary and sufficient* for the occurrence of the disease. By *necessary* we mean that the disease cannot occur without the presence of that exposure (although other exposures may be required for the occurrence of the disease). By *sufficient* we mean a set of exposures that inevitably produce disease. There may of course be different ways by which one could get disease, and thus sufficient causes may not be necessary.

In cancer epidemiology, the only known examples of exposures that are sufficient to cause disease refer to the genetic origin of some rare cancers due to dominant genes with complete penetrance. In this instance, the causal pie would require only one factor for the pie to be complete and this would be the way that carriers would get the specific cancer. Also rare is the existence of single factors that are in and by themselves sufficient (although not necessary) for the causation of a certain disease. Even powerful exogenous factors, such as life-long heavy

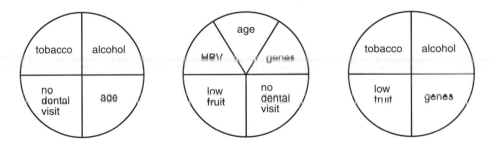

Figure 6.1. The causal pie model describes a set of exposures that work together in the same pathway to cause disease. These are hypothesized ways in which a series of exposures could interact biologically over time to cause disease. This figure provides an example of sufficient causes from cancer epidemiology. Tobacco is an established component cause in many cases of oral cancer. However, tobacco use by itself is not enough for the disease to occur; in addition, oral cancer can occur among people who have never used tobacco. In a given causal pie, the complementary exposures can occur simultaneously, or many years apart. If even one of the component causes did not occur, disease would be prevented by this pathway, although a person could develop the disease by another mechanism (a different causal pie).

Table 6–1. Attributes of the causal pie

ATTRIBUTE	DESCRIPTION
Inevitability	Completion of a sufficient cause (causal pie) is synonymous with eventual occurrence (though not necessarily diagnosis) of the disease.
Causality	A component cause (piece of a causal pie) can involve presence of a detrimental exposure or absence of a preventive exposure.
Burden of disease	The amount of disease caused by a sufficient cause depends on the prevalence of all complementary component causes.
Temporality	Component causes can act far apart in time
Interaction	Component causes in the same pie interact biologically to cause disease
Attributable fraction	Different component causes are responsible for more than 100 percent of disease cases.
Disease prevention	Blocking the action of any component cause prevents completion of the respective sufficient cause and therefore prevents disease by that pathway.

Source: Rothman, 1976.

smoking, and strong genetic influences, like those conveyed by dominant breast cancer genes, do not always cause disease in an individual.

Certain exposures are by definition necessary (although not sufficient) for the occurrence of a particular disease. For example, chronic lead disease cannot occur in the absence of lead exposure, and a motor vehicle injury requires the involvement of a motor vehicle (MacMahon et al, 1960; Hill, 1965; Rothman, 1976; Susser, 1991; MacMahon and Trichopoulos, 1996). Again, while these represent *necessary causes,* there are additional cofactors that must work in concert before disease is inevitable. Most human cancers can occur via several pathways, so it is hard to define any single necessary cause. Asbestos, in relation to mesothelioma (cancer of the pleura), and human papillomavirus infection, in relation to cervical squamous cell cancer, are close to being necessary. However, cases of these cancers do arise without the exposure being documentable, either because the exposure occurred but could not be identified, or because these exposures are not necessary for all cases.

For most diseases, there is no one necessary cause. Indeed there may be numerous causal pies by which disease can occur. Such an example is illustrated in Figure 6–1, with suggested sufficient causes of oral cancer. In the first example, exposure to tobacco and

alcohol over time are contributing factors (*component causes*) in the etiology of oral cancer. However, the oral cancer would not have occurred in the presence of a dental visit that could have treated precancerous lesions and might have prevented the disease. While smoking is a component cause in many causal pies for oral cancer, people can get oral cancer without smoking, as shown by the second causal pie in this figure.

Interventional Epidemiology

How do we design a scientific study to evaluate whether a particular exposure (for example, asbestos) is a cause of a specific disease (for example, lung cancer)? To understand the most appropriate design in practice, it is useful to begin by describing the ideal scientific study. Imagine for a moment that we have access to a time machine.

In an imaginary study, we follow a group of individuals from birth to death, where everyone is exposed to asbestos, and we observe whether they develop lung cancer. We then send everyone back in a time machine, to live the exact same lives they lived, except that we completely remove asbestos from the environment so that no one is exposed. We then compare whether there are changes in the frequency of occurrence of lung cancer before and after use of the time machine. Since the same people live identical lives but for the presence/absence of asbestos, any difference in the frequency may be attributed to alterations in the exposure to asbestos, which leads to the definition of cause.

How then can we develop the time machine analogy into a realistic epidemiologic approach? We could study two groups of people who are comparable on every characteristic, except that one group had exposure and one did not. The *randomized controlled trial* closely approximates this goal. By randomly allocating who receives an exposure, for example treatment, and who does not, the exposure occurs only because the investigator has assigned it. For example, an investigator randomly assigns one group of people to receive vitamin E supplements (exposed), while the other group receives a placebo (unexposed). Study participants are then followed forward in time to see whether they develop cancer. Whether someone receives vitamin E then does not depend on whether or not the subject, for example, smokes, drinks, eats a high-fat diet, or has a certain genetic susceptibility.

In this way, the randomization in a trial makes the two (or more) groups, those exposed and those unexposed, comparable on other study factors that might cause the disease. Hence, the unexposed group is a proxy of what would have happened to the exposed group if they had been unexposed—that is if we could have sent them back in the time machine. Comparability is essential in order to ascribe any changes in the frequency of disease to alterations in the exposure.

While some researchers describe the randomized controlled trial as the gold standard of scientific studies, this design is impractical in the majority of epidemiologic situations. For one thing, most exposures we study are detrimental. If we want to study the impact of asbestos on lung cancer, we cannot ethically randomize people to live in a house with asbestos. But even for exposures that are not necessarily detrimental, randomization may be difficult or impractical. For instance, it is very difficult and expensive to randomize a large group to eat a low-fat versus a normal diet, and have

everyone comply with this allocation over the course of many years. Most trials are thus only conducted for no more than a few years, an unrealistically short period to test the effect of most exposures because of the long latency between exposure and diagnosis of cancer. Furthermore, in many randomized trials, subjects become noncompliant over time—that is people allocated to the intervention arm stop taking the intervention, and those in the original placebo or usual care arm may adopt the intervention (a phenomenon called cross-over). This diminishes the contrast between the original randomized groups, reducing the power to detect a difference in disease rates between the groups.

Because of the limitations of the randomized controlled trial, the observational cohort and case–control designs are extensively utilized in epidemiology. As will be discussed later in the chapter, attention to both the design and analysis of these studies may allow us to approximate the standards of comparability, necessary to validly evaluate the effect of an exposure on the frequency of a disease.

Observational Epidemiology

The essence of observational epidemiology is the *noninterventional* investigation of disease causation in human population groups. The argument is that only by studying humans is it possible to draw confident conclusions about normal or pathological processes concerning humans (MacMahon, 1979; MacMahon and Trichopoulos, 1996). In vitro studies, such as those involving cell cultures, and studies in laboratory animals are valuable. They are indeed indispensable when toxic exposures or invasive procedures like repeated biopsies are needed for the study of physiologic or pathologic processes, such as carcinogenesis. However, in vitro systems are frequently artificial, and there are physiological and metabolic differences between humans and laboratory animals that hinder interspecies analogies. These analogies are further complicated by the unavoidably limited number of animals used in laboratory studies and the relatively short life span of these animals, both of which impose the administration of high doses of suspected agents in order to generate a sufficient number of outcomes. Consequently, questionable quantitative extrapolations to humans have to be undertaken.

Even when experimental studies, such as randomized controlled trials, in humans are ethical, they are, with few exceptions, impractical because most diseases are rare and their latent period, that is, the time between exposure to a cause and the appearance of a clinical disease, is long. This makes it necessary to enroll unrealistically large numbers of compliant volunteers for a very long period (Hennekens and Buring, 1987; MacMahon, 1979; MacMahon and Trichopoulos, 1996).

Observational, that is nonexperimental, studies represent the mainstream of modern epidemiology. Such studies seek to document causal relations on the basis of associations between particular exposures and cancer or other diseases. Inference of causation on the basis of association is easy when the association is both strong and biologically credible—smoking and lung cancer, or hepatitis B virus and liver cancer, are striking examples. It becomes more difficult when the association is biologically compelling but the epidemiologic experience weak—for example, in studies of low-level ionizing radiation and leukemia or passive smoking and lung cancer. Causal interpretation also becomes problematic when the epidemiologic association is fairly convincing but the biological rationale is uncertain, as it is with respect to red meat and colorectal cancer or alcohol and breast cancer. When an epidemiologic association is weak, is derived from a study with questionable quality, and floats in a biological vacuum, inferring causation is perilous.

STUDY DESIGN

Descriptive Studies

It is possible to distinguish observational epidemiological studies into descriptive and analytic. In descriptive studies the frequency of occurrence of a disease (incidence)—or of death from a disease (mortality)—is estimated in a population, by routinely available time, place, and/or group characteristics. Descriptive studies are essentially exploratory and hypothesis generating. For instance, descriptive studies that documented the increasing trend of lung cancer incidence among men, but not among women, in the early part of the twentieth century pointed to tobacco smoking as a likely cause of this disease. In contrast, the objective of analytic studies is to document causation from the pattern of association in individuals between one or more exposures on the one hand, and a particular disease on the other.

Ecologic Studies

Ecologic studies in epidemiology occupy an intermediate position between descriptive and analytic investigations, in that they share many characteristics with descriptive studies, but serve etiologic objectives. In ecologic studies, the exposure and the disease under investigation are ascertained not for individuals but for groups or even whole populations (Morgenstern, 1982). Thus the prevalence of hepatitis B virus (HBV) in several populations could be correlated with the incidence of liver cancer in these populations, even though no information could be obtained as to whether any particular individual in these populations was or was not an HBV carrier and has or has not developed liver cancer. Associations from ecologic studies are viewed with skepticism, because these studies are susceptible to unidentifiable and intractable confounding as well as to several other forms of bias (Morgenstern, 1982; Greenland and Robins, 1994).

When an exposure is fairly common, for example, smoking, or even prevalence of HBV carriers, ecologic studies can provide useful evidence on the possible effects of these exposures. For instance, following the increase in tobacco consumption, the incidence of lung cancer increased sharply over time, and the incidence of primary liver cancer is higher in populations with higher prevalence of HBV. As a corollary, lack of an association in ecologic studies between a widespread exposure that has rapidly increased over time and the incidence of a disease allegedly caused by this exposure, does not support a strong causal relation.

Analytic Studies

Analytic epidemiologic investigations ascertain exposure and disease outcome in individuals and are usually distinguished into cohort and case–control studies, although there are also several variants of these prototype designs (MacMahon and Trichopoulos, 1996; Rothman and Greenland, 1998). The objective of analytic epidemiologic studies is to ascertain whether a particular exposure, such as a physical, chemical, or biological agent, and a specific cancer or other disease are unrelated (independent) or associated. An association does not necessarily indicate causation. Chance, bias, and confounding (see following) can also generate associations, and they frequently do. Causation is unlikely when there is no association observed. Even if a causal relation does exist, however, it may sometimes be difficult to document it, particularly when the association is weak, the study has limited statistical power, or the exposure is seriously misclassified.

Person-time and Study Base

The concepts of *person-time* and *study base* are fundamental to the design and analysis of epidemiologic studies. As the name implies, there are two key components in our description of the person-time, namely the number of people and the time they are followed. To illustrate this, we could ask how many brain cancer cases we would expect if we followed one million people exposed to x-rays for zero seconds. Conversely, how many cases would we expect if we followed zero people for one million years? The answer in both instances is, of course, zero. Hence, neither people nor time alone provides adequate information about the disease experience of a population, and thus both should be taken into account. *Person-time* is the sum of all the time contributed in a study by subjects at risk of a disease.

Theoretically, an ambitious investigator might wish to include the entire world population in an epidemiologic study during many decades. Needless to say, such a study would provide marvelous opportunities to evaluate many different exposures in relation to many diseases. Millions of person-years would be generated even within a few weeks. In real life, however, any investigator has to restrict the person-time from which information is harvested. This specified person-time is called the *study base*. Defining the person-time to be included in the study base may include geographic restrictions, defined time periods, and certain age limits. Personal characteristics such as gender, ethnicity, and occupation may further specify the study base. For example, the study base may be comprised of all British doctors who answered a questionnaire in 1951 (Doll and Hill, 1956), or by all Swedish women who were aged 50 to 74 between 1994 and 1995 (Weiderpass et al, 1999), and who generated person-time until they died or until the follow-up was completed.

Thus, the study base is simply the person-time of a population of individuals at risk of a disease under study. Defining the study base is a crucial step in the design and conduct of an epidemiologic study. There are three central considerations. One is to accommodate realistic goals with regards to feasibility and resources, as certainly no investigator is independent of time and money. A second goal is to make the study efficient. For example, it would make little sense to study the association between smoking and cancer in a population where very few are smokers. Likewise, a study of diet and prostate cancer would be inefficient among men younger than 40, since virtually no cases arise among such young people. The final challenge is to identify a study base that allows valid inferences concerning associations between exposure(s) and a particular disease—that is, a study base that does not impose intractable confounding or raise insurmountable obstacles of other biases.

Person-time is the source of any event we want to investigate, for example the occurrence of cancer. To help set a foundation for better understanding *person-time* in a *study base,* we will use the example of x-rays and risk of brain cancer (Fig. 6–2). In this population, five people have been exposed to x-rays, and another five have not been exposed and remain unexposed during the study period. While in real life the study populations are much larger, we use this elementary example to illustrate the principles.

Among the people exposed to x-rays, persons 3 and 5 were followed from the time they were exposed to x-rays till the end of the study period—a total of 5 years each. Persons 1, 2, and 4, however, developed brain cancer at the end of years 1, 4, and 2, respectively. Once these individuals develop brain cancer, they are no longer at risk of the disease, and thus no longer contribute information to the study base. The person-time among those exposed to x-rays is estimated by summing up the person-time of all the individuals while at risk for the disease, that is:

$$(2 \text{ persons} \times 5 \text{ years}) + (1 \text{ person} \times 1 \text{ year}) \\ + (1 \text{ person} \times 4 \text{ years}) + (1 \text{ person} \\ \times 2 \text{ years}) = 17 \text{ person-years}$$

We can similarly sum up the person-time among the group of five individuals who were not exposed to x-rays:

$$(4 \text{ persons} \times 5 \text{ years}) + (1 \text{ person} \\ \times 2 \text{ years}) = 22 \text{ person-years}$$

Later on when we discuss analysis of epidemiologic studies, we will see how the

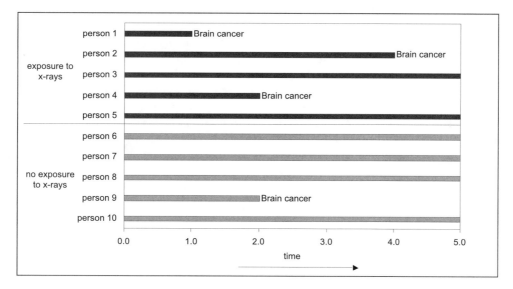

Figure 6.2. Experience of a theoretical study population over time. Five individuals who were exposed to x-rays and five individuals who are unexposed are followed over time to see if they develop brain cancer. Among those exposed to x-rays, persons 3 and 5 are followed for the duration of the study period, which in this case was five years. Person 1 develops brain cancer after 1 year, person 2 develops brain cancer after 4 years, while person 4 develops cancer after 2 years. Persons 1, 2 and 4 stop contributing person-time *after* they develop brain cancer, since they are no longer at risk for the disease. The total person-time in the exposed group is 17.0 person-years. Similarly, we can look at the population of people unexposed to x-rays over time. Of the five people who are unexposed, only one develops brain cancer during the study period (person 9). The remaining people are followed completely for five years. The experience of these ten individuals over time, that is the person-time that the subjects contributed, is the study-base.

person-time data will help us to compare disease incidence between exposed and unexposed people.

Cohort studies

The word *cohort* derives from the similar Latin word, which identified one of the ten divisions in a Roman legion. In epidemiology, cohorts are groups of individuals, which can be followed over time. In cohort studies, individuals are classified according to their exposure and are observed for ascertainment of the frequency of disease occurrence or death in the various exposure-defined categories (Fig. 6–3A). In each category the frequency of occurrence is calculated either as risk or as incidence rate. Risk describes the proportion of those who developed the disease under study among all individuals in this category. Rate describes the number of those who developed the disease divided by the person-time during which the individuals in this category have been under observation. Cohort studies have the following defining characteristics.

Cohort studies are exposure-based. The groups to be studied are selected on the basis of exposure. In special exposure cohorts, the groups are chosen on the basis of a particular exposure. In general population cohorts, groups offering logistical advantages for follow-up are initially chosen and the individuals are classified according to their exposure status. Special exposure cohorts may be necessary when rare exposures need to be studied, such as those encountered in the occupational setting. For example, to study efficiently the effect of vinyl chloride on liver angiosarcoma, or aromatic amines on bladder cancer, epidemiologic studies have been conducted in cohorts of workers in the plastic and dyestuff manufacturing industries, respectively.

The general population cohort is appropriate when the exposure under consideration is fairly common. Classical examples of general population cohorts, in which the profession facilitated accessibility of cohort members rather than being a study factor, include the British Doctors Study and the Nurses Health Study. The British Doctors cohort, established in 1951, consisted of more than 30 000 doctors from Great Britain. In this landmark study, Doll and colleagues prospectively followed the cohort and collected updated information on multiple exposures, particularly smoking, over several decades. Indeed, prospective data from the British doctors were among the first to demonstrate convincingly the role of tobacco in the etiology of lung cancer (Doll and Hill, 1956). More than four decades later, data from the British Doctors have continued to provide insight into the etiology of cancer (Doll et al, 2005).

Another notable cohort is the Nurses Health Study, which began in 1976 with over 120 000 US registered nurses. This cohort was assembled initially to evaluate prospectively the effect of oral contraceptives on the risk of breast cancer (Hennekens et al, 1984). Subsequently, diet and many other exposures have been studied in relation to the risk of cancer as well as other chronic conditions (Zhang et al, 2005). Information on these diverse exposures has been collected biennially through questionnaires. Moreover, blood samples have allowed researchers to explore biomarkers and genetic factors. For example, prospective data from the Nurses Health Study has provided insight into the role of both exogenous and endogenous estrogens in breast cancer etiology. A particular characteristic of these types of cohorts is that the individuals can be followed almost completely over time, due to their membership in groups with a high interest in health studies and registration requirements that facilitate initial contact and long-term follow-up.

Cohort studies are patently or conceptually longitudinal. The study groups are observed over a period of time to determine the frequency of disease occurrence among them. The distinction between retrospective and prospective cohort studies depends on whether the cases of disease occurred in the cohort at the time the study began. In a retrospective cohort study, exposures and health outcomes occurred before the investigation started. These are typically assembled from pre-existing records of a

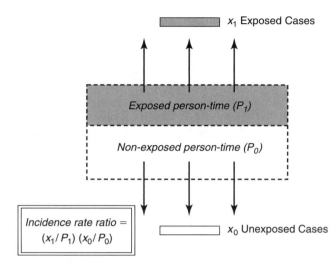

Figure 6.3A. A cohort study comprises individuals who are either exposed or unexposed to the factor(s) of interest. When these people are followed over time, they generate person time. Newly diagnosed cases of a particular disease, that occur while person-time is accumulated are recorded. The exposure status of a person can change. A person could be smoking high tar cigarettes for five years, then switch to light cigarettes for fifteen years, and then quit. Consequently, each person can contribute to person-time in different exposure groups. A case is considered exposed, if the disease occurred when the person who developed the disease was accumulating exposed person-time. A case is non-exposed if it occurred while the person was accumulating non-exposed person time. The example assumes, for simplicity, zero latency. The total amount of exposed and non-exposed person time and the number of exposed and non-exposed cases can be calculated. After that, one can determine whether more cases occurred in the exposed or non-exposed group per unit of person-time, that is, one can calculate the incidence rate ratio. This ratio will indicate whether there is a relationship between the exposure and the disease of interest.

population over time—for example, the employment histories of a factory can be linked to recorded health-outcome information of the workers. In a prospective cohort study, the relevant causes may or may not have acted and the cases of disease certainly have not yet occurred. Hence, following identification of the study cohort, the investigator must wait for the disease to appear among cohort members.

Methodologically, there are two types of cohort studies: closed or fixed cohorts, and open or dynamic cohorts. *Closed cohorts* are frequent in occupational epidemiology and the study of outbreaks, whereas *open cohorts* dominate cancer epidemiology and form the conceptual basis for most case–control studies. The key distinction between *open* and *closed* cohorts is how member-

ship in the cohort is determined. In a closed cohort, it is determined by a membership-defining event that occurs at a point in time. For example, people who were living in Hiroshima and Nagasaki when the atomic bombs were dropped in 1945 are part of a cohort whose membership began on the date of the bombing. These subjects remain in the cohort until they die.

Open cohorts are composed of individuals who contribute person-time to the cohort only as long as they meet the criteria for a membership-defining state (Fig. 6–3A). Examples of such criteria include place of residence, age, and health status. Once individuals can no longer be characterized by the defining state(s), they cease to contribute person-time to the open cohort and are no longer members. Open cohorts are used, for example, in cancer epidemiology studies based on registry data (Hansson et al, 1996). A person could be a member of the cohort, for example, only as long as he or she was a resident of Sweden and was not diagnosed with the cancer under study. If the person emigrated from Sweden to another country, he or she stopped contributing person-time to the cohort at that time. Similarly, if someone born outside of Sweden immigrates there later in life, he or she would begin contributing person-time to the cohort at that time. In studies based on open cohorts it is not possible to directly measure risk, otherwise referred to as *cumulative incidence*. Analyses are based on person-time using incidence rate measures.

As an example, assume that in a closed cohort among 5000 nonsmoking men followed for an average period of 10 years ($P_0 = 50\,000$ person-years), $x_0 = 25$ were diagnosed with lung cancer, and among 10 000 smoking men followed for an average period of 8 years ($P_1 = 80\,000$ person-years), $x_1 = 600$ were diagnosed with lung cancer. In this example the incidence rate among nonexposed would then be 50 per 10^5 person-years and among exposed 750 per 10^5 person-years. The *relative risk* (incidence rate ratio) would be $\frac{600/80,000}{25/50,000}$, or 15. The conclusion is that there is a 15-fold increase in lung cancer occurrence from smoking.

Case–control Studies

In case–control studies, patients diagnosed with the disease under consideration form the case series. As in cohort studies, their exposure to the factor under investigation is ascertained, for example, through questionnaires, interviews, examination of records, undertaking of laboratory tests in biological samples, and other means (Fig. 6–3B). Using the same methods, the pattern of exposure to the study factor(s) is then estimated in the population, or more strictly in the person-time from which the case series arose. This is done among control subjects selected as a sample of the study base from which the cases arose. If only two categories of exposure are relevant (exposed and unexposed), the relative risk can be estimated by dividing the odds of exposure among cases with the corresponding odds among the controls, the *odds ratio*.

Thus, if among 200 male patients diagnosed with lung cancer (cases), $a = 150$ were smokers and $b = 50$ nonsmokers, whereas among 300 men similar in age to the cases but without lung cancer (controls), $c = 50$ were smokers and $d = 250$ were nonsmokers, the odds ratio would be $\frac{a/b}{c/d} = \frac{ad}{bc} = \frac{150 \times 250}{50 \times 50}$ or 15. This measure is a good approximation to the relative risk (or risk ratio, or rate ratio). Hence, similar to the cohort study, these data from a case–control study show a 15-fold excess of lung cancer among smokers.

There are some features of case–control studies that make this design susceptible to bias (see following). A well-designed case–control study, however, is a valid and cost-efficient approach to the study of the etiology of cancer and other conditions.

Nested case–control studies

Some case–control designs are methodologically superior to others. The best example is the nested case–control design. The definition of this study design is still somewhat ambiguous (Walker, 1991; Rothman and Greenland, 1998). A definite requirement, however, is that controls are chosen from the clearly defined person-time from which all cases have arisen. In other words, if one of the controls had developed the disease under study, he or she would have definitely been included among the cases. Defining the underlying person-time from which a series of cases—for example, lung cancer cases presenting at a referral hospital—arose can be difficult. Sampling controls from a cohort different from the one that gave rise to the cases often results in *selection bias*.

According to a more strict definition, the term *nested case–control study* is used only when the underlying cohort and the corresponding person-time have been previously enumerated and the exposure information was collected prior to the diagnosis. In other words, the controls are selected from exactly the same person-time that gave rise to

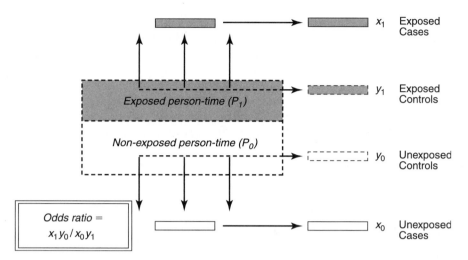

Figure 6.3B. It is not always practical or economical to evaluate the entire study person-time. The case–control study is a more efficient design. Instead of enumerating the total amount of exposed and unexposed person time that makes up the study person-time, the ratio of exposed to unexposed person-time is estimated. This is achieved by randomly selecting people (controls) without the disease of interest from the underlying study person-time and determining their exposure status. If a sufficient number of controls are selected, without regard for their exposure status, then the exposure distribution in the controls will estimate that in the total study person-time. The exposure distribution among the controls is then compared to that among the cases of the disease of interest that have arisen in the study person-time. An estimate can then be made of the odds of exposure among the cases compared to that among controls, or the odds ratio, which is an unbiased estimator of the incidence rate ratio and so indicates whether there is an association between the disease and the exposure of interest.

the cases, the study base. Unlike the traditional case–control design, which is liable to bias due to selective participation and differences in recall, this nested design preserves the validity of a prospective cohort study. Case–control studies nested in an existing cohort are being used increasingly for cost efficiency when analysis of all cohort members requires substantial resources.

Nested case–control studies have been frequently used in occupational epidemiology (Rothman and Greenland, 1998). The occupational cohort can often be readily defined whereas abstraction of detailed exposure information from existing records requires substantial work. Hence, it is more efficient to investigate only the cases of interest and a sample from the cohort that is the controls. Nowadays, nested case–control studies are used routinely when exposure information is derived, often through expensive laboratory procedures, from bio-

logic samples such as blood or blood products, tissue, urine, or nails.

One such example is a study of selenium status and breast cancer risk in the Nurses' Health Study (Hunter et al, 1990). On the basis of prior evidence that selenium intake may influence breast cancer risk and since selenium levels in toenails are a reliable source of selenium exposure over several months, the participating women were asked to provide toenail clippings in 1982. After 4 years of follow-up, there were 434 cases of breast cancer. It would have been very expensive and inefficient to get exposure information for all the 62 000 nurses who had returned toenail samples at the start of follow-up. Hence, 434 controls without breast cancer were sampled from the cohort. Using this design meant that only 868 rather than 62 000 samples had to be sent to the laboratory for selenium analyses (Hunter et al, 1990).

Matching in case–control studies

Occasionally, case–control studies are *matched*. This means that controls are chosen so as to match particular cases with respect to gender, age, race, or any other factor that is likely related to the disease under investigation but not intended to be analyzed in the particular study. Matching is not strictly necessary, nor does it increase the validity of results. But it improves statistical efficiency and, thus, the ability to substantiate a true association (Rothman and Greenland, 1998). What is necessary, however, is that, whenever matching has been used in the enrollment of cases and controls, the statistical analysis should accommodate the matching process. This can be done through either a matched analysis (for example, conditional modeling) or unmatched analysis with explicit control for the matching factors (proper application of unconditional modeling).

Studies of the Genetic Epidemiology of Cancer

Genetic epidemiology of cancer is considered in more detail in a distinct chapter (Chapter 4). Here, we refer briefly to such studies, to provide an integrated picture of epidemiologic designs available for the study of cancer etiology. Two main types of epidemiologic studies are used for the identification of genes predisposing to cancer: genetic linkage studies and genetic association studies.

Genetic linkage studies are generally undertaken in families with a high cancer burden and rely on the principle that two genetic loci, or a cancer and a particular locus, are linked when they are transmitted together from parent to offspring more often than expected by chance. Linkage extends over large regions of the genome and refers to a locus, rather than specific alleles in that locus, which can vary from study to study and from family to family (Teare and Barrett, 2005). Such studies have led to the identification of genes that have substantial impact on the occurrence of breast cancer and colorectal cancer, but these genes are generally rare, presumably because of natural selection pressure.

Genetic association studies can be of either cohort or, more frequently, case–control design. They are frequently undertaken in the general population, rather than in families, and are conceptually similar to traditional epidemiological investigations. The difference is, however, that instead of focusing on environmental factors, like smoking or diet, genetic association studies evaluate as "exposures" *specific* alleles (rather than loci) of genetic polymorphisms, usually single nucleotide polymorphisms (SNPs). The specific alleles may be etiologically related to cancer or, much more frequently, very closely linked to the truly etiological allele which may not be known. The actually investigated allele and the true etiological allele are said to be in linkage disequilibrium–that is, they are so closely linked that they tend to be inherited together. Two loci in linkage disequilibrium are obviously linked, but two linked loci may not be in linkage disequilibrium if they are sufficiently apart in the chromosome to be separated, sooner or later, by the frequent cross-over process in the meiosis phenomenon during the generation of gametes. In other words, linkage covers longer genetic regions than linkage disequilibrium (Cordell and Clayton, 2005; Teare and Barrett, 2005). The specific allele may be chosen to study because the corresponding locus is thought to be involved in the etiology of the cancer under investigation (eg, a candidate gene). Many SNPs over large parts of the genome, or even over the whole genome, may also be evaluated, with little or no prior evidence that most of them are etiologically relevant or are in linkage disequilibrium with etiologically relevant genes. In the latter situation, most statistically significant findings are likely to be false positive and special procedures are recommended to delineate which ones among the apparent associations are probably genuine (Wacholder et al, 2004). Genetic association studies have not been very successful to date in identifying genes or polymorphisms involved in cancer etiology, possibly because the respective relative risks deviate very little from the null value, but also because the tools to examine alleles across the genome simultaneously—rather than at a limited number usually selected on the basis of weak prior probabilities of being truly associated—are only just becoming available.

THE ROLE OF CHANCE

Before an epidemiologic association could be considered true and therefore deserve interpretation in causal terms, the role of chance and systematic errors should be considered.

The P-value

Our daily lives are full of highly unlikely events and coincidences. At the extremes, thousands of people have become wealthy from lotteries; many more have died in strange accidents, even though the probabilities for the respective events are extremely small—say one in 100 000 or smaller. The lesson is simple: Highly unlikely events happen by chance all the time. Chance does not operate differently in scientific research and everyday life. In science, however, proper quantification and judgment, relying on sound substantive knowledge, are necessary before considering chance as an unlikely explanation for a phenomenon.

Let us take, as an example, tossing a fair (unbiased) coin that has a 50% or 0.5 probability of turning up heads and an identical probability of turning up tails. Tossing the coin three times and getting three heads in a row is somewhat unusual but it can hardly be taken as an indication that the coin is systematically influenced (biased) toward tails. The *p-value* in this instance is 0.25 and is calculated by multiplying $0.5 \times 0.5 \times 0.5 = 0.125$, and then doubling 0.125, because the symmetrically opposite outcome, three tails in a row, is as extreme as three heads in a row. Getting five heads or tails in a row generates some suspicion $(p = [\frac{1}{2}]^5 \times 2 = 0.0625)$. But if 100 people have tossed a fair (unbiased) coin five times each, it should be expected

that about six (100×0.0625) among them would have obtained either five heads or five tails in a row.

It must be realized that stochastic (probabilistic), in contrast to deterministic, processes always have built-in uncertainty. In their research, all investigators want to reduce chance-related uncertainty as much as possible in order to allow more reliable conclusions. This can be achieved mainly by enrolling progressively larger numbers of individuals in a study. The remaining uncertainty can always be assessed by utilizing statistical procedures that generate a number of summary statistics, including the *p-value*.

The true meaning of the *p-value*, however, is poorly understood and the concept itself is widely misused. Surprisingly, this misunderstanding and misuse is quite common even in scientific research. Traditionally, *p-values* are expressed as numerical fractions of 1. For example, a *p-value* of 0.1 for a particular positive association (or difference) indicates that there is a 10% chance that such an association or a more extreme one (or a symmetrically opposite one—that is an inverse association) would appear by chance, even if there were in reality no association at all.

In essence, the *p-value* is interpretable as such when only one comparison or one test is performed. When multiple comparisons or multiple tests are carried out the set of the respective *p-values* loses its collective interpretability. Various procedures for adjusting *p-values* according to the number of comparisons undertaken or tests performed have been proposed (Wacholder et al, 2004).

A *p-value* of 0.05 or smaller is traditionally—and indeed arbitrarily—treated in medical research as evidence that an observed association may not have arisen by chance. For example, the proportion of long-term smokers is found to be larger among lung cancer patients than among individuals without the disease *and* the *p-value* for this difference is, say, 0.05. This implies that the probability of finding a difference of this magnitude or larger (in absolute terms) is 5% if smoking were unrelated to lung cancer. In this situation, chance is considered unlikely to explain the association. However, small *p-values*, including values considerably smaller than 0.05, do not guarantee that an association (or difference) is genuine—let alone causal.

Even when the *p-value* is very small and was generated from a carefully conducted study, it could still be dismissed when the relevant result makes no sense (Miettinen, 1985). Hence, a statistically significant association, linked by convention to a *p-value* of 0.05 or less, does not necessarily imply causation. Systematic errors, generated by confounding or bias (see following), cannot always be confidently discounted in observational epidemiology. Moreover, as indicated at the end of this chapter, the existence of a genuine association that can be confidently attributed to causation does not necessarily imply that someone who developed the disease following the exposure did so because of that exposure.

A common misconception (Miettinen, 1985) is that if a *p-value* (for example, $p = 0.03$) has been properly derived, then its complement (0.97 in our example) can be interpreted as the likelihood that the respective association is indeed causal. This misconception is rarely stated explicitly in the scientific literature, but it underlies the conclusions of many epidemiologic reports that are not securely anchored in methodological principles and biomedical substance.

Lastly, it must be recognized that the *p-value* itself does not convey any information about the strength of the respective association. A weak association may be statistically highly significant (very small *p*) when the study is large, and a strong association may be statistically nonsignificant (large *p*) when the study is small. Hence, all *p-values* are inherently dependent on the study size, because statistical power—the ability to detect an association (or a difference) when it exists—increases when a study is larger (Rothman and Greenland, 1998).

Confidence Intervals

In order to integrate information about the strength of an association (as reflected in the relative risk-effect measure, described later on) and its statistical significance, the concept of *confidence interval* has been developed. Most common are 95% confidence intervals. With a 95% confidence interval, one can be 95% confident that the interval covers the true measure of association (for example the relative risk). But in 5 times out of 100, the true measure is not included. The confidence interval is closely linked to the *p-value*. The width of the confidence interval is determined primarily by the desired level of confidence and the sample size. Hence, the interval is wider if it includes the true value with 95% confidence than with, for example, 80% confidence. Likewise, smaller studies create wider confidence intervals—that is, greater uncertainty about the true value—than larger studies.

SYSTEMATIC ERRORS

The Experimental Study

The chance-related issues apply to all types of studies, observational as well as experimental. As discussed earlier, *experimental studies* undertaken under optimal conditions are methodologically superior to observational studies. With randomization of exposure, complete follow-up of study subjects, and double-blind assessment of outcome, they are not as liable to the pitfalls of typical observational studies—that is confounding and bias (Miettinen, 1985; Hennekens and Buring, 1987; MacMahon and Trichopoulos, 1996; Rothman and Greenland, 1998; Rothman, 2002). Proper evaluation of the association between a particular exposure and a specific disease presupposes that every other factor that could influence disease occurrence is either constant among subjects studied or distributed equally between exposed and unexposed subjects.

In other words, an experimental study uses random allocation of study subjects into those who will be exposed and those who will not. Thus, the two or more groups will tend to be similar in distribution to known as well as unknown factors that may influence the results. In some studies, blinding of researchers and study subjects through the use of appropriate procedures and devices (for example, indistinguishable inert pills, the so-called placebos) may further assure that every factor that can affect disease occurrence, other than the exposure under study, is kept at about the same level between the exposed and unexposed groups.

Experimental studies aim to fulfill the Latin dictum *ceteris pariba* (other things being equal). However, in humans, the optimal conditions that completely eliminate confounding and bias are difficult to create even in randomized controlled trials. Moreover, as already indicated, there is no way to fully control the inherently unpredictable role of chance, except by the use of very large numbers of study subjects—an unrealistic objective in many studies.

The randomized controlled trial, with its methodological advantages, dominates experimental research in laboratory animals. In humans, however, the undertaking of experiments faces serious obstacles, the most important of which are ethical. It is obviously not acceptable to expose humans intentionally to a potentially carcinogenic agent in order to ascertain cancer causation. For this reason, most randomized controlled trials in humans have been performed to evaluate treatment effectiveness and occasionally to determine the preventive potential of vaccines, vitamins, or other supplements. In most instances, research on disease etiology has to rely either on animal models—with inherently dubious assumptions about interspecies similarities and exposure dose extrapolations—or on epidemiologic studies with an observational design.

Epidemiologic studies have indeed generated most of what is currently known about the etiology of human diseases in general, and cancer in particular. At the same time, however, epidemiologic studies have also generated conflicting results, unwarranted concern about everyday exposures, and considerable confusion over the rational ranking of public health priorities (Taubes, 1995). The problem arises because epidemiologic studies must confront not only the vagaries of chance but also the problems of systematic errors that undermine their validity.

Confounding

Confounding is the systematic error generated when another factor that causes the disease under study, or is otherwise related to it, is also related to the exposure under investigation (Fig. 6–4A). Thus, if one wishes to examine whether hepatitis C virus (HCV) causes liver cancer, hepatitis B virus (HBV) would be a likely confounder. Confounding arises because HBV causes liver cancer and carriers of HBV are more likely to also be carriers of HCV (because these two viruses are largely transmitted by the same routes). Hence, if the confounding influence of HBV is not accounted for in the design (by limiting the study to HBV-negative subjects) or in analyses of the data,

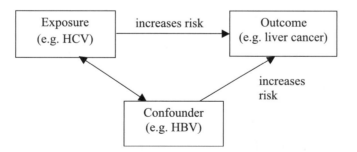

Figure 6.4A. Infection with hepatitis C virus (HCV), a cause of liver cancer, is (positively) confounded by hepatitis B virus (HBV) infection, another cause of liver cancer. If this confounding is disregarded, the strength of the association between HCV and liver cancer will be overestimated.

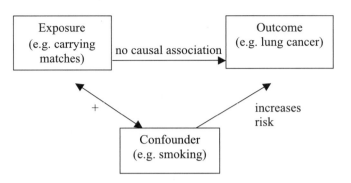

Figure 6.4B. An association between carrying matches and lung cancer would arise spuriously due to confounding by smoking—the major cause of lung cancer—unless this confounding is accounted for in the design or the analysis

then the strength of the association between HBC and liver cancer would be overestimated (Fig. 6–4A).

A more trivial example is the strong association between carrying matches or a cigarette lighter and developing lung cancer. Obviously, neither matches nor lighters cause lung cancer and their association to the disease is due entirely to *confounding* by cigarette smoking. The confounding factor, cigarette smoking, is the true cause of lung cancer and the dependence of cigarette lighting on matches or lighters generates the *confounded,* entirely spurious association of the latter two factors with the disease (Fig. 6–4B).

There are several ways to deal with confounding: some simple, others more complicated. They all assume that two conditions are satisfied: *(1)* that all the confounders have been identified or at least suspected, and *(2)* that the identified or suspected confounders can be adequately conceptualized and accurately measured. When the study is fairly large, it is always possible to evaluate all suspected confounders in the analysis. However, the ability to conceptualize and accurately measure all of them is frequently beyond the control of any investigator. The result is what has been termed *residual confounding,* that is, confounding left unaccounted for (Mac-Mahon and Trichopoulos, 1996; Rothman and Greenland, 1998).

Bias

Compounding the problems of epidemiologic studies is that the data are almost never of optimal quality. Data collection relies on the recollection of exposures and their accurate reporting by study participants, laboratory procedures, or existing records. These sources are rarely perfect. For example, studies on diet rely on individuals' imperfect recall on how frequently they eat specific foods, or on serum markers of nutrients that are far from perfect indicators of long-term consumption. Such misclassification, or *information bias,* can influence the relative risk in any direction and, thus, entails exaggeration, underestimation, or even reversal of the true associations.

In case–control studies, the ascertainment of exposure occurs after the occurrence of disease. Therefore, this study design is particularly subject to information bias. In particular, cases may be likely to remember their exposures differently than controls—a form of information bias called *recall bias.* For example, a reasonable concern is that cases, or their relatives, are inclined to ruminate about the disease and identify a particular exposure as the causative agent, either for conscious or subconscious reasons. Cases may also try harder than controls to recall relatives with the disease of interest, leading to a biased estimate of the effect of the family history (Chang et al, 2006).

A well thought-out protocol, standardized procedures, and built-in quality control measures can reduce bias and allow some quantification of its potential impact. However, complete assurance that bias has been eliminated can never be achieved. In addition, the reliance of case–control studies on a control series that simultaneously has to meet criteria of compliance, comparability to the case series, statistical efficiency, and general practicality makes them susceptible to *selection bias* of unpredictable direction and magnitude. Such biases arise when eligible controls are not representative of the population, or more strictly the person-time, that gave rise to the cases (Wacholder et al, 1992a; Wacholder et al, 1992b; Wacholder et al, 1992c).

Assume as in the same previous example that controls refuse to participate more often if they are smokers than if they are nonsmokers. We would then underestimate smoking in the control group and thereby overestimate both the difference between cases and controls and the excess risk. Hospital controls, neighborhood controls, and controls enrolled through searches of telephone lists have their own problems, and these have been extensively discussed (MacMahon and Trichopoulos, 1996).

In contrast to selection and information biases, issues of chance and confounding are equally relevant to cohort and case–control investigations (Hennekens and Buring, 1987; MacMahon and Trichopoulos, 1996; Rothman and Greenland, 1998).

ANALYSIS OF EPIDEMIOLOGIC STUDIES

Effect Measures

The underlying goal of epidemiology is to determine the magnitude of change in disease frequency caused by an exposure. How do we accomplish this? We could measure the cumulative incidence or incidence rate among those exposed to a factor. For example, we could observe that the incidence rate of breast cancer in a population of alcoholic women is 60/10 000 person-years. This information provides an estimate of the overall disease burden in this study base. However, we do not know how many cases would have arisen in the study base if all the women in this population had not been alcoholics. In epidemiology, the unexposed group stands in for the person-time experience of the exposed group had it not been exposed. Thus, we need to harvest information from both exposed and unexposed person-time.

There are several ways through which an association, or lack thereof, is assessed. Consider a population of women exposed to a high saturated fat diet and a group exposed to low saturated fat diets that are followed for 5 years to see if they develop breast cancer. The absolute effect of the high-fat diet would be the difference in the cumulative incidence between the two groups, or the difference in the incidence rates. Since the experience of the low saturated fat group should represent what would have happened to the high saturated fat group if they had not eaten the high saturated fat, and if the two groups are equivalent with respect to other breast cancer risk factors, the difference in risks or rates represents the excess risk or rate. These absolute-effect measures are called the *risk difference* and *rate difference*, respectively.

Although the absolute measures are easily interpreted, more common are effect measures that are taken as ratios and collectively known as the *relative risk*. This term includes the risk ratio, rate ratio, odds ratio, standardized mortality ratio, and standardized incidence ratio. The risk ratio is simply the cumulative incidence of disease among the exposed, divided by the cumulative incidence among the unexposed. The rate ratio is a ratio of the rates of disease among the exposed and unexposed. The odds ratio is the odds of disease among the exposed divided by the odds of disease among the unexposed. Lastly, the standardized mortality ratio or standardized incidence ratio is a ratio of the observed number of deaths or cases in a cohort, divided by the expected number of deaths or cases in the general population, usually stratified by age and gender.

A relative risk value of 1 implies that the exposure under study does not affect the incidence of the disease under consideration. Values below and above 1 indicate a negative (inverse) and a positive association, respectively. For example, a relative risk of 0.5 implies that the disease occurs only half as frequently among exposed as among unexposed individuals; the studied factor appears to be protective. In contrast, if the relative risk is 1.5, then the occurrence (usually the incidence) is 50% higher among exposed than among unexposed individuals.

Studies based on follow-up of closed cohorts may be analyzed by using either cumulative incidence (risk) measures or by counting person-time and calculating incidence rate measures. Analyses based on cumulative incidence measures are only useful under certain conditions, such as no *loss to follow-up,* no *competing risks,* and unchanged exposure status throughout follow-up. In addition, study subjects should be followed for the same period of time. Whether or not these conditions are met, it is always valid to conduct analyses based on person-time, using incidence rate measures.

Interaction

The term *interaction* has been used to describe different biological and statistical concepts. Indeed, even in the epidemiologic literature, statements about interaction are often ambiguous and inadequately specified. From a biological point of view, component causes within the same sufficient cause may be thought of as interacting (Fig. 6–1). In other words, the exposures act synergistically to produce disease, since in the absence of one factor, disease will not occur by that mechanism. From an epidemiologic point of view, interaction is frequently characterized as effect-modification: That is, a factor A and factor B alone have a certain relationship with a disease, but together the factors have an effect different than that expected on the basis of the magnitude of their individual effects. The expectation of the joint effect of factors A and B can be assessed in either an additive or a multiplicative way.

We can use the example in Table 6–2 to illustrate how interaction is assessed. When a multiplicative scale is assumed, there is statistical interaction if the relative risk among those exposed to both factors A and B (that is, RR_{AB}) is different than the product of the two individual relative risks (that is, $RR_A \times RR_B$). When an additive scale is assumed, there is interaction if the RR_{AB} is different than ($RR_A + RR_B - 1$). In this example, the expected relative risk for someone with both exposures is 6.0 ($6.0 = [4.0 + 3.0 - 1]$) under the additive-effect assumption (Table 6–2A), whereas it is 12.0 ($12.0 = 4.0 \times 3.0$) under the multiplicative-effect assumption (Table 6–2B).

Hence, interaction between two exposures is present when the relative risk is significantly different from what is expected according to a specified scale. Thus, for those with both exposures, we would have interaction on the additive scale if the relative risk is significantly different from 6.0 (Table 6–2A), and on the multiplicative scale if the relative risk is significantly different from 12.0 (Table 6–2B). If the relative risk following exposure to both factors compared to having neither is greater than the sum (minus the reference risk of 1, which should not be counted twice) or product of the individual risks, we call this interaction *super additive* or *super multiplicative,* respectively. If the relative risk is significantly lower, we refer to this as either *subadditive* or *submultiplicative.*

We can illustrate the concept of interaction using data from an epidemiological study of asbestos, smoking, and lung cancer risk. The source population for the data shown in Table 6–2C is a cohort of insulation workers from the United States and Canada (Hammond et al, 1979). The exposed person-time was the experience of over 12 000 male workers with at least 20 years of asbestos exposure. The comparison person-time came externally from the experience of more than 73 000 men of similar social class.

Table 6–2. Definitions of interaction. Relative risks of developing a certain disease among subjects exposed (+) or not exposed (−) to one or both factors denoted A and B. Subjects exposed to neither of these factors comprise the reference category and their relative risk is by definition 1.0.

Table 6–2A. Statistical interaction on the additive scale with examples of subadditive and superadditive factors.

Factor A	Factor B		
	−	+	
−	1.0 (reference)	3.0	
		2.0	Subadditive
+	4.0	6.0	Expected under additive effects assumption
		8.0	Superadditive

Table 6–2B. Statistical interaction on the multiplicative scale with examples of submultiplicative and supermultiplicative factors.

Factor A	Factor B		
	−	+	
−	1.0 (reference)	3.0	
		8.0	Submultiplicative
+	4.0	12.0	Expected under multiplicative effects assumption
		16.0	Supermultiplicative

Table 6–2C. Effects on lung cancer risk of smoking, asbestos, and both factors.

Smoking	Asbestos	
	−	+
−	1.0 (reference)	5.2
+	10.9	53.2

Source: Hammond et al, 1979.

Compared to men who had neither exposure, the relative risk of those who were smokers, but who were not exposed to asbestos occupationally was 10.9; the relative risk of those exposed to asbestos, but who were not smokers, was 5.2. For those exposed to both asbestos and smoking, the relative risk of lung cancer was 53.2 compared to those with neither factor. In this example, there appears to be interaction on the additive scale, since the $RR_{smoker\ and\ asbestos} = 53.2$ is substantially higher than the expected relative risk of 15.1 under the additive model ($RR_{smoker} + RR_{asbestos} - 1 = 10.9 + 5.2 - 1$). We do not, however, observe interaction on the multiplicative

scale, since the relative risk for both smoking and asbestos (53.2) does not represent a significant departure from what is expected under the multiplicative-effect assumption ($56.7 = RR_{smoker} \times RR_{asbestos} = 10.9 \times 5.2$).

There are not any clear-cut guidelines on whether to assess interaction in the additive or multiplicative setting for the various disease outcomes examined in epidemiology, although both approaches are used (Brennan, 1999).

Meta-analysis

Random variation per se in epidemiologic studies is not an insurmountable problem.

Larger studies and eventually quantitative summary analyses are increasingly used. Such systematic statistical evaluations of results of several independent investigations can effectively address genuine chance-related concerns. Quantitative summary analyses have been termed *meta-analyses* and *pooled analyses*. There is no completely accepted distinction between the two terms, although meta-analysis is used more frequently when published results are combined. By contrast, in pooled analysis primary individual-level data from different studies may be made available to an investigator who undertakes the task of combining them. This facilitates the use of uniform exposure categories and statistical analyses across studies and may permit analyses that were not in the original publications. For instance, analyses of effect modification for which each initial study may have been too small to be informative.

Meta-analyses and pooled analyses have been widely and effectively used for randomized controlled trials and intervention studies, because in properly undertaken investigations of this nature confounding and bias are nonissues (Sacks et al, 1987). For observational epidemiologic studies, however, the role of meta-analysis is not universally accepted (Shapiro, 1994; Feinstein, 1995). Some investigators are concerned that no statistical summarization can effectively address problems generated by residual confounding, unidentified bias, and the way investigators choose to present their results (legitimately, but occasionally selectively or arbitrarily). Nevertheless, meta-analyses have provided important, widely accepted data, even when derived from observational data.

CAUSAL INFERENCE IN EPIDEMIOLOGY

General Principles

Regulatory agencies and policy makers may recommend standards, set limits, or authorize action even when the scientific evidence is weak. These decisions serve public health objectives by introducing a wide safety margin, but they should not be confused with the establishment of causation based on scientific considerations alone.

When results of an observational epidemiologic study designed to address a specific hypothesis are striking, the study is large, and there is no evidence of overt confounding or major biases, it is legitimate to attempt etiologic inferences. In contrast, interpretation becomes problematic when a weak association turns out to be statistically significant—for example, in a large but imperfect data set. Although that association could reflect a weak—but genuine—causal association, it might also be the result of residual confounding, subtle unidentifiable bias, or chance, perhaps following a multiple testing process.

Repeated demonstration of an association of similar direction and magnitude in several studies, undertaken by different investigators in different population groups, increases confidence in a genuine causal basis but cannot conclusively establish this. Nor do meta-analyses establish causality. These techniques essentially address the issue of chance and provide no guarantee that a particular bias, unrecognized confounding, or selective reporting have not operated in the constituent studies. It is at this stage that both biologic and epidemiologic considerations should be taken into account in interpreting the results of empirical studies.

Criteria for inferring causation from epidemiologic investigations have been proposed, over the years, by several authors, including MacMahon et al (1960), the US Surgeon General (US Department of Health, 1964), Sir Austin Bradford Hill (Hill, 1965), the IARC (1987), and others. In spite of differences in emphasis, a similar set of principles have been invoked by most authors. Sir Austin Bradford Hill (1965) advocated the nine widely used criteria listed in Table 6–3, to distinguish causal from noncausal associations.

The Hill criteria, although sensible and useful, do not separately address the inherently different issues that are posed by the results of a single study, the results of several studies, and the likelihood of causation in a certain individual. In reality, the perceived likelihood of a causal association between a particular exposure and a specific disease moves forward or backward in a continuous spectrum as research results accumulate. The evidence for causality is declared as sufficient when a particular threshold has been reached, but on occasion requires reevalutation in the light of subsequent evidence (Cole, 1997).

The IARC Classification

The International Agency for Research on Cancer (IARC) evaluates the risk of specific agents to determine if they are carcinogenic in humans. In order to come to a conclusion, the IARC has implemented its own set of criteria for evaluating the carcinogenicity of agents. After considering all the evidence, the IARC working group assigns the agent to one of five categories, summarized

in Table 6–4. Group 1 indicates that there is sufficient evidence to conclude that the agent is carcinogenic to humans. A label of group 2A means that there are insufficient human data, but there is strong evidence that the agent is carcinogenic in animal models. Agents for which there is limited evidence in humans and insufficient evidence in experimental animals are assigned to group 2B. Group 3 is used when there is inadequate human and animal data to come to a conclusion. Group 4 indicates that the agent is most likely not a carcinogen in humans based on adequate evidence suggesting that it is not a carcinogen in both animal models and human studies.

The Process of Causal Inference

Criteria for causality can be invoked, explicitly or implicitly, in evaluating the results of a single epidemiologic study, although,

Table 6–3. The Hill criteria for inferring causation

Criteria	Definition
Strength	A strong association is more likely to be causal. The measure of strength of an association is the relative risk and not statistical significance.
Consistency	An association is more likely to be causal when it is observed in different population groups.
Specificity	When an exposure is associated with a specific outcome only (for example, a cancer site or even better a particular histological type of this cancer), then it is more likely to be causal. There are exceptions, however, for example, smoking causing several forms of cancer.
Temporality	A cause should not only precede the outcome (disease), but also the timing of the exposure should be compatible with the latency period (in non-infectious diseases) or the incubation period (in infectious diseases).
Gradient	This criterion refers to the presence of an exposure-response relationship. If the frequency or intensity of the outcome increases when an exposure is more intense or lasts longer, then it is more likely that the association is causal.
Plausibility	An association is more likely to be causal when it is biologically plausible.
Coherence	A cause and effect interpretation of an association should not conflict with what is known about the natural history and biology of the disease, or its distribution in time and place.
Experimental evidence	If experimental evidence exists, then the association is more likely to be causal. Such evidence, however, is seldom available in human populations.
Analogy	The existence of an analogy (for example, if a drug causes birth defects, then another drug could also have the same effect) could strengthen the belief that an association is causal.

Source: Hill, 1965.

Table 6–4. International Agency for Research on Cancer (IARC) classification of carcinogenicity of agents, mixtures or processes

Group 1	The agent is carcinogenic to humans
Group 2A	The agent is probably carcinogenic to humans
Group 2B	The agent is possibly carcinogenic to humans
Group 3	The agent is not classifiable in terms of its carcinogenicity
Group 4	The agent is not carcinogenic to humans

in this instance, a firm conclusion is all but impossible. In the approach introduced by Cole (1997), this situation is denoted as single study level, or level I. Criteria for causality are more frequently used for the assessment of evidence accumulated from several epidemiologic studies and other biomedical investigations. At this stage, the intellectual process is inductive, moving from the specifics to generalization (several studies level, or level II). Finally, when causation has been established at level II, then, and only then, can the cause of the disease in a particular individual be considered (specific person level, or level III). At this level, the intellectual process is deductive, moving from the general concept of disease causation to the examination of what might have caused disease in a particular individual.

The individual study (level I)
Causality can never be inferred on the basis of a single epidemiologic study, but the likelihood that an observed association is causal is strengthened when several of the following criteria are met: *(1)* minimal confounding; *(2)* minimal bias; *(3)* limited chance variation; *(4)* relatively strong association; *(5)* monotonic exposure-disease association, otherwise referred to as *exposure-response* or *dose-response association*; *(6)* internal consistency, exemplified by similarity of exposure-response patterns among various subgroups of study subjects; *(7)* compatibility of the temporal sequence of exposure and outcome with the known or presumed latency of the disease; and, lastly, *(8)* biologic plausibility, that is, a causal link between the exposure and the disease should be, at a minimum, biologically conceivable

(it should not contradict physical theory or biological principles).

The general case (several studies, level II)
Establishment of the etiologic role of a particular exposure on the occurrence of a disease ideally requires strong epidemiologic evidence, an appropriate and reproducible animal model, and documentation at the molecular or cellular level of the morphological or functional pathogenetic process. Sometimes, an intended or unintended change, or *natural experiment*, greatly facilitates etiologic inference: This happens when, for example, an occupational group is exposed to high levels of compounds rarely encountered in other settings, a religious group avoids an exposure that is otherwise widespread, or a vaccine that creates herd immunity against a particular virus turns out to reduce the incidence of a certain form of cancer.

These conditions, however, are rarely collectively satisfied. Instead investigators have to be guided by the best available biomedical evidence in order to interpret correctly epidemiologic data from several studies. The following criteria need to be considered: *(1)* consistency, that is similarity (lack of heterogeneity) of results obtained by different investigators using different study designs in different populations; *(2)* overwhelming biomedical evidence for weak associations, whereas for strong associations reliance on powerful biomedical knowledge is less critical; *(3)* compatibility of exposure-response patterns across different studies exploring the exposure-disease association in different exposure ranges; *(4)* coherence, which requires results from analytic epidemiologic studies to be compatible with ecologic patterns and time trends, such as the increasing incidence of lung cancer over time, following the increasing use of tobacco products by the population; *(5)* specificity, which exists when one type of disease is consistently linked with one type of exposure rather than several exposures all being associated with a certain disease, or one type of exposure being associated with several diseases; and *(6)* biological analogy, which exists when a similar exposure has been shown to cause a similar disease in another species or a different form of the disease in humans. For example, viruses have been shown to cause leukemia in several animal species and at least one rare form of leukemia in humans.

None of these criteria can be considered as absolutely necessary for causal inference—a sine qua non. But the evidence for causality is strengthened when most of them are met.

Disease in a specific person (level III)
Causality can be conclusively established between a particular exposure as an entity and a particular disease as an entity. In contrast, it is not possible to establish such a link conclusively between an exposure and a particular disease of a given individual—for example, smoking in a patient with lung cancer. It is possible, however, to infer deductively that the specific individual's illness was *more likely than not* caused by the specified exposure.

For this conclusion to be drawn, all the following criteria must be met (Cole, 1997): *(1)* The exposure under consideration, as an entity, must be an established cause of the disease under consideration, as an entity (level II). *(2)* The relevant exposure of the particular individual must have properties comparable (in terms of intensity, duration, associated latency, etc) to those that have been shown to cause the disease under consideration. *(3)* The disease of the specified person must be identical to, or within the symptomatological spectrum of, the disease that, as an entity, has been etiologically linked to the exposure. *(4)* The patient must not have been exposed to another established or likely cause of this disease. If the

patient has been exposed to both the factor under consideration (for example, smoking) *and* to another causal factor (for example, asbestos), individual attribution becomes a function of several relative risks, all versus the completely unexposed: *(a)* relative risk of those who only had the exposure under consideration, *(b)* relative risk of those who had only been exposed to the other causal factor(s), and, *(c)* relative risk of those who have had a combination of these exposures. *(5)* The relative risk should be reasonably elevated (eg, 2 or more).

The last criterion stems from the fact that the relative risk comprises a baseline component equal to 1, which characterizes the unexposed, plus another component that applies only to the exposed. When the relative risk is higher than 1 but less than 2 the individual who has been exposed and has developed the disease is more likely than not to have developed the disease for reasons not entirely due to the exposure. For instance, if the risk of a light-smoking 55-year-old man to suffer a first heart attack in the next five years is 6%, and that of a same-age non-smoking man is 4% (relative risk 1.5), then only 33% of the smoker's risk (that is, 1/3 of the total 6%) can be attributed to his smoking. When the relative risk is higher than 2, a particular individual who has been exposed and has developed the disease under consideration is more likely than not to have developed the disease because of the exposure.

CONCLUSION

Manipulation of exposures in humans, many of which may be harmful, is frequently unfeasible, unethical, or both. Therefore, epidemiologists have to base their inferences on experiments that humans subject themselves to intentionally, naturally, or even unconsciously. The study of risk for lung cancer among smokers compared with nonsmokers is one classic example of a natural experiment.

Because human life is characterized by myriad complex, often interrelated, behaviors and exposures—ranging from genetic traits and features of the intrauterine environment to growth rate; physical activity; sexual practices; use of tobacco, alcohol, and pharmaceutical compounds; dietary intake; exposure to infections, environmental pollutants, and occupational hazards; and so on—epidemiologic investigation is difficult and challenging. Given this complexity, it is not surprising that from time to time epidemiologic studies generate results that appear confusing, biologically absurd, or contradictory. However, it is reassuring that a wealth of new knowledge has been generated by epidemiologic studies over the last few decades. This knowledge now lays the scientific ground for primary prevention of many major cancers and other chronic diseases among humans globally.

A detailed study of epidemiologic methodology in any textbook (Hennekens and Buring, 1987; Miettinen, 1985; Walker, 1991; MacMahon and Trichopoulos, 1996; Rothman and Geenland, 1998; Rothman, 2002) can be fascinating and indeed necessary for those who want to pursue their own research. However, for the reader of this textbook, the general concepts introduced in this chapter should provide a sufficient basis. We have tried to convey that the sometimes esoteric theory of modern epidemiology can be condensed to a few central issues—namely *(1)* how to quantify and understand the impact of chance, *(2)* how to best harvest information on exposures and outcomes from a source population by using a cohort design, a case–control design, or variants thereof, *(3)* how to achieve valid results by minimizing the impact of confounding and bias, and, *(4)* how to address the central issue of causality in a structured way.

GLOSSARY

Cause A factor is a cause of a certain disease when alterations in the frequency or intensity of this factor—without concomitant alterations in other factors—are followed by changes in the frequency of occurrence of the disease, after the passage of a certain time period (latency, or induction period).

Closed cohort A closed cohort comprises a set of individuals who are followed for a defined period of time. After becoming a member of the cohort, an individual remains in the cohort until the end of the study, or development of the outcome.

Competing risks The risk of death from a certain disease competes with the risk of death from another disease by affecting time at risk. Competing risks generally bias risk ratios, but not rate ratios, since person-time allows for different follow-up time.

Component cause An exposure that acts in concert with other factors (component causes) to produce disease. None of these factors are sufficient in themselves to cause disease.

Confidence interval A statistical measure that provides range of possible values that include the true measure of association with a particular degree of certainty. For example, a 95% confidence interval provides a range of values that will include the true value 95% of the time.

Confounding A systematic error generated when another factor, that causes the disease under study or is otherwise related with it, is also related to the exposure under investigation, without being in the pathway that links exposure under investigation with the disease under study.

Ecologic study The study of exposure and the disease at the population level, rather than at the individual level.

Epidemiology The nonexperimental investigation of determinants of human disease.

Experimental study See randomized controlled trial

Information bias A random, or nonrandom, misclassification of information on either the exposure, outcome, or confounding variables that leads to a biased estimation of the true effect.

Loss to follow-up The inability to follow beyond a certain point in time and thus ascertain the ultimate fate of individuals in a cohort study.

Necessary cause A factor or exposure that is essential in the etiology of the disease and without which the disease cannot occur.

For example, the human immunodeficiency virus is a necessary cause of acquired immunodeficiency syndrome, although other factors may be involved in order for the disease to occur.

Nonexperimental study See observational study.

Observational study A study in which the investigator cannot control the circumstances of the exposure.

Odds ratio A relative measure of association, which is calculated as the ratio of the odds of disease among the exposed divided by the odds of disease among the unexposed.

Open cohort A cohort of individuals whose membership changes over time, with people entering or exiting based on defining criteria.

Person-time The sum of all time spent by each study participant at risk for a disease.

p-value A value that indicates the likelihood of observing an association as extreme as, or more extreme than, the one found between a particular exposure and a certain disease, if there were in fact no association.

Randomized controlled trial An experimental study design in which the researcher randomly allocates subjects to groups that will be subjected or not to a particular exposure.

Recall bias A misclassification of an exposure, common in case–control studies, that occurs when subjects with the disease remember or report their exposures differently than those without disease.

Relative risk A term that collectively describes the various relative measures of association, that is the risk ratio, the rate ratio, the odds ratio, and the standardized incidence or mortality ratio.

Selection bias A systematic error that results from the process of selecting participants for the study or on account of factors that influence participation in the study. Selection bias occurs when the relationship between the exposure and the disease is different for those in the study than for those not in the study.

Study base The person-time of a group of individuals at risk for a disease from which an investigator aims to harvest information about disease occurrence.

Sufficient cause A minimal set of factors or exposures that inevitably produce the disease after a certain period of time.

REFERENCES

Brennan P. Chapter 12: Design and analysis issues in case–control studies addressing genetic susceptibility. IARC Sci Publ 1999;148: 123–32.

Chang ET, Smedby KE, Hjalgrim H, Glimelius B, Adami HO. Reliability of self-reported family history of cancer in a large case-control study of lymphoma. J Natl Cancer Inst 2006; 98(1):61–68.

Clemmesen J, Nielsen A. Comparison of age-adjusted cancer incidence rates in Denmark and the United States. J Natl Cancer Inst 1957;19:989–98.

Cole P. Causality in epidemiology, health policy and law. Environmental Law Reporter 1997; 27:10279–85.

Cordell HJ, Clayton DG. Genetic Epidemiology 3—Genetic association studies. Lancet 2005; 366:1121–31.

Doll R, Hill AB. Smoking and lung cancer: preliminary report. Brit Med J 1950; 2:739–48.

Doll R, Hill AB. Lung cancer and other causes of death in relation to smoking. Brit Med J 1956; 2:1071–81.

Doll R, Peto R, Boreham J, Sutherland I. Mortality from cancer in relation to smoking: 50 years observations on British doctors. Br J Cancer. 2005;92:426–29.

Feinstein AR. Meta-analysis: statistical alchemy for the 21st century. J Clinical Epidemiology 1995;48:71–79.

Greenland S, Robins J. Invited commentary: ecologic studies—biases, misconceptions, and counterexamples. Am J Epidemiol 1994;139: 747–60.

Hammond EC, Seikoff IJ, Seidman H. Asbestos exposure, cigarette smoking and death rates. Ann NY Acad Sci 1979;330: 473–90.

Hansson LE, Nyren O, Hsing AW, Bergstrom R, Josefsson S, Chow WH, et al. The risk of stomach cacner in patients with gastric or duodenal ulcer disease. New Engl J Med 1996; 335:242–49.

Hennekens CH, Buring JE. Epidemiology in Medicine. Boston: Little, Brown, 1987.

Hennekens CH, Speizer FE, Lipnick RJ, Rosner, Bain C, Belanger C, et al. A case–control study of oral contraceptive use and breast cancer. J Natl Cancer Inst 1984;72:39–42.

Hill AB. The environment and disease: association or causation? Proc Roy Soc Med 1965; 58:295–300.

Hunter DJ, Morris JS, Stampfer MJ, Colditz GA, Speizer FE, Willet WC. A prospective study of selenium status and breast cancer risk. JAMA 1990;264:1128–31.

International Agency for Research on Cancer. IARC Monographs on the Evaluation of Carcinogenic Risks to Humans, Supplement 7, Overall Evaluations of Carcinogenicity: An Updating of IARC Monographs, Volumes 1 to 42, Lyon 1987.

MacMahon B. Epidemiological evidence on the nature of Hodgkin's disease. Cancer 1957; 10:1045–54.

MacMahon B. Strengths and limitations of epidemiology. In: The National Research Council in 1979. Current issues and studies. Washington, DC: National Academy of Sciences, 1979:91–104.

MacMahon B, Pugh TF, Ipsen J. Epidemiologic Methods. Boston: Little, Brown, 1960.

MacMahon B, Trichopoulos D. Epidemiology: Principles and Methods. Boston: Little, Brown, 1996.

Miettinen OS. Theoretical Epidemiology: Principles of Occurrence Research in Medicine. New York: Wiley, 1985.

Morgenstern H. Uses of ecologic analysis in epidemiologic research. Am J Public Health 1982;72:1336–44.

Rothman KJ. Causes. Am J Epidemiol 1976; 104:587–92.

Rothman KJ, Modern Epidemiology. Boston: Little, Brown, 1986.

Rothman KJ. Epidemiology: An Introduction. New York, Oxford University Press, 2002.

Rothman KJ, Greenland S. Modern Epidemiology—2nd Ed. Philadelphia: Lippincott-Raven, 1998.

Sacks HS, Berrier J, Reitman D. Meta-analysis of randomized controlled trials. N Engl J Med 1987;316:450–55.

Shapiro S. Meta-analysis/shmeta-analysis. Am J Epidemiol 1994;140:771–78.

Susser M. What is a cause and how do we know one? A grammar for pragmatic epi

demiology. Am J Epidemiol 1991;133: 635–48.

Taubes G. Epidemiology faces its limits. Science 1995;269:164–69.

Teare DM, Barrett JH. Genetic Epidemiology 2—Genetic linkage studies. Lancet 2005; 366:1036–44.

US Department of Health, Education and Welfare. Smoking and Health. Report of the Advisory Committee to the Surgeon General of the Public Health Service. Publication 1103. Washington, DC: US Government Printing Office; 1964.

Wacholder S, McLaughlin JK, Silverman DT, Mandel JS. Selection of controls in case–control studies: I. Principles. Am J Epidemiol 1992; 135:1019–28.

Wacholder S, Chanock S, Garcia-Closas M, El Ghormli L, Rothman N. Assessing the probability that a positive report is false: an approach for molecular epidemiology studies. J Natl Cancer Inst. 2004;96:434–42.

Wacholder S, Silverman DT, McLaughlin JK, Mandel JS. Selection of controls in case–control studies: II. Types of controls. Am J Epidemiol 1992;135:1029–41.

Wacholder S, Silverman DT, McLaughlin JK, Mandel JS. Selection of controls in case–control studies: III. Design options. Am J Epidemiol 1992;135:1042–50.

Walker AM. Observation and inference: an introduction to the methods of epidemiology. Newton Lower Falls, MA. Epidemiology Resources Inc, 1991.

Weiderpass E, Adami HO, Baron JA, Magnusson C, Bergstrom R, Lindgren A, et al. Risk of endometrial cancer following estrogen replacement with and without progestins. J Natl Cancer Inst 1999; 91:1131–37.

Wynder EL, Graham EA. Tobacco smoking as a possible etiologic factor in bronchiogenic carcinoma—a study of 684 proved cases. JAMA 1950;143:329–36.

Zhang SM, Hankinson SE, Hunter DJ, Giovannucci EL, Colditz GA, Willett WC. Folate intake and risk of breast cancer characterized by hormone receptor status. Cancer Epidemiol Biomarkers Prev. 2005;14:2004–8.

II

CANCER EPIDEMIOLOGY
BY SITE-SPECIFIC CANCERS

7

Oral and Pharyngeal Cancer

PAUL BRENNAN, LORELEI MUCCI,
AND HANS-OLOV ADAMI

We do not hear much about oral cancer publicly. Yet this cancer kills more people in the United States than either malignant melanoma or cervical cancer—two diseases that probably arouse much more concern. Moreover, in parts of Asia, notably India, oral cancer is one of the most common malignancies. Because the prognostic outlook following diagnosis is poor, much suffering and premature death could be avoided by a more dedicated preventive effort. At least in theory, public health initiatives might be effective in reducing the burden of oral cancer, since many predominant causes are well established.

Methodologically, epidemiologic research on oral and pharyngeal cancer is complicated by the many anatomic subsites, which include the lip, tongue, salivary gland, mouth, oropharynx, nasopharynx, and hypopharynx (ICD9 codes 140–148). While these sites are anatomically diverse, cancers occurring in the oral cavity and pharynx are for the most part homogeneous with respect to both the descriptive epidemiology and

risk factors. The major exception is cancer of the nasopharynx, which has a unique epidemiologic profile and therefore is described separately in Chapter 8. This chapter will deal mainly with oral and pharyngeal cancer, excluding nasopharyngeal cancer, and unless otherwise specified we will henceforth use the term *oral cancer*.

CLINICAL SYNOPSIS

Subgroups

Cancers of the oral cavity and pharynx, predominantly of a squamous cell type, are characterized chiefly by their various anatomic locations. While some risk factors appear to be uniquely linked with certain subsites, others play a causal role at many subsites, although the strength of the association may differ.

Symptoms

Early symptoms vary according to the subsite within the oral cavity and pharynx, but a sore or difficulty swallowing is typical. In some cases, metastases to lymph nodes in the neck bring the patient to medical attention.

Diagnosis

Cancers at these subsites are uniquely accessible for direct inspection that allows a biopsy for a definite histopathologic diagnosis. Computed tomography or magnetic resonance imaging is generally used for additional staging and planning of treatment.

Treatment

Primary treatment varies with the anatomic subsite and stage of disease. For most early cancers, surgical resection is the cornerstone of treatment. However, for certain anatomic sites such as the tonsils, the base of the tongue, and the floor of the mouth, as well as for all locally advanced cancers, radiotherapy is used, either alone or combined with surgery. Occasionally, chemotherapy may be used in addition to radiotherapy.

Prognosis

Following diagnosis of oral cavity and pharynx cancer, 5-year relative survival is close to 40% in the United States and in Europe, although it varies substantially among countries. Moreover, the prognosis is generally better for women and for malignancies of the oral cavity than for those arising in the hypopharynx.

Progress

In Europe, 5-year relative survival rates remained virtually identical from 1983 to 1994, suggesting that no major progress has been made (Coleman, 2003).

DESCRIPTIVE EPIDEMIOLOGY

An estimated 405 000 newly diagnosed cases of oral cancer occurred worldwide in 2002 (Ferlay et al, 2002). Oral cancer accounts for approximately 5% of total cancers among men and about 2.5% of total cancers among women. Mortality from oral cancer is quite high in both developed and developing countries, with approximately 211 000 deaths occurring in 2002 (Ferlay et al, 2002).

The incidence of oral cancer varies considerably worldwide (Figs. 7–1, 7–2). In India and areas within Southeast Asia, oral cancer is the most common malignancy among men. Some of the highest rates have been observed among men living in Hungary and France, with an age-standardized incidence of more than 52 per 100 000 person-years. Among women living in parts of India, oral cancer accounts for about two-thirds of all tumors.

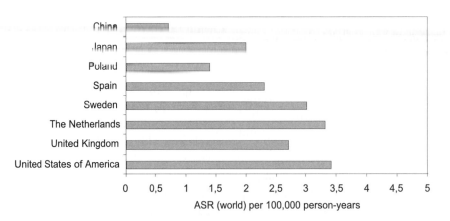

Figure 7–1. Age-standardized (to the world population) incidence rates of oral cancer among women. (*Source*: Ferlay et al, 2004)

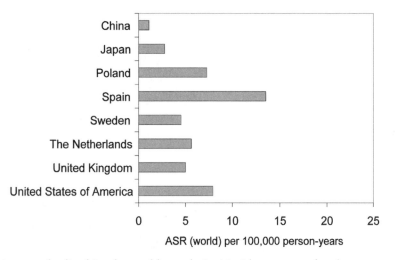

Figure 7–2. Age-standardized (to the world population) incidence rates of oral cancer among men. (*Source*: Ferlay et al, 2004)

Oral cancer is rare among both women and men younger than age 35 in most countries (Figs. 7–3, 7– 4). The age-specific rates are typical of many epithelial cancers; rates increase with increasing age. There are some exceptions to this pattern, for example among men in Bas-Rhin, France, where the rapid increases in oral cancer up to age 60 are followed by sharp decreases to age 85 and older. Although the shape of the

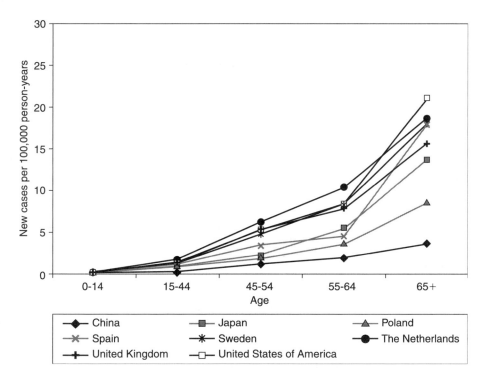

Figure 7–3. Age-specific incidence rates of oral cancer among women. (*Source*: Ferlay et al, 2004)

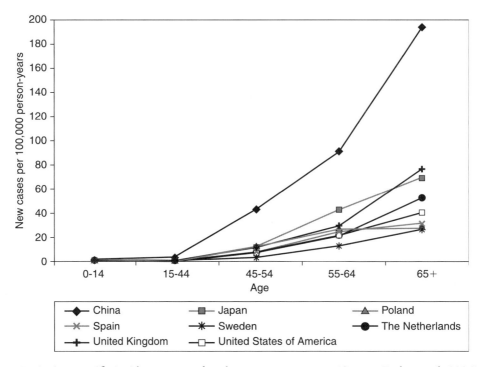

Figure 7–4. Age-specific incidence rates of oral cancer among men. (*Source*: Ferlay et al, 2004)

age-incidence curves is generally similar across countries, there are substantial differences in the absolute rates at every age (Figs. 7–3, 7–4).

In general, incidence rates are lower among women than among men (Figs. 7–1, 7–2). An extreme example of this is the almost sevenfold higher incidence of oral cancer among men in Spain compared to women. In most settings, however, rates are about twofold higher among men. Moreover, the current gender gap between men and women in the United States, for example, represents a notable decrease compared to 20 years ago due to increases in oral cancer rates for women in all age groups.

While the incidence of oral cancer has changed little over time in some populations, others have experienced marked increases or decreases. In the United States, age-adjusted incidence rates of oral cancer decreased among white men from 1973 to 1996, but increased among black men age 65 to 69 years and among young white men and women (Shiboski et al, 2000). During

the last few decades, the rate of oral cancer has increased over time across southern and eastern Europe (Franceschi et al, 2000). Indeed, the lifetime risk of developing oral cancer exceeds 2% in several European countries. Dramatic increases have been noted for both men and women in Japan, where this cancer was quite rare in the 1970s (< 1 per 100 000) and currently occurs at a rate of 2 per 100 000 and 6 per 100 000 for women and men, respectively. While the incidence of oral cancer remains high for men and women in India (10 per 100 000 and 10 per 100 000, respectively), consistent decreases have been observed, primarily due to fewer cancers of the oral cavity (Franceschi et al, 2000).

The morbidity and mortality associated with oral cancer are largely preventable. First, precancerous lesions precede the majority of tumors, and treatment leads to remission of the precancer and a decreased risk of malignant transformation. Second, invasive oral cancer exists in a preclinical detectable stage, and detection involves a simple examination and palpation of the oral cavity. Finally, with treatment at an early stage, the prognosis is good.

GENETIC AND MOLECULAR EPIDEMIOLOGY

Inherited Susceptibility

There appears to be a familial susceptibility to oral cancer. While the incidence is elevated among families with some, but not all, inherited cancer syndromes, such inherited mutations are rare and, taken together, account for a small proportion of cancer cases. Instead, there appears to be a role for common genetic alterations that by themselves may not substantially impact disease risk, but that in concert with environmental exposures may lead to the development of cancer. Primary candidates for gene–environment interaction studies in oral cancer have been genes encoding enzymes involved in the metabolism of established oral cancer risk factors: tobacco, alcohol, and certain components of diet.

High-penetrance gene mutations

A role for familial aggregation in the etiology of oral cancer is possible. First-degree relatives of cases may have up to a three- to fourfold increased risk of developing the disease (Prime et al, 2001). Moreover, familial susceptibility cannot be explained by a shared environment. Using a pedigree analysis, researchers found familial aggregation compatible with an autosomal dominant mode of inheritance in almost 1% of oral cancers in India (Ankathil et al, 1996).

The *p53* gene, in its normal capacity, acts as a gatekeeper by invoking cell-cycle arrest or cell death in response to genetic mutations. Germline mutations in *p53* have been implicated in the etiology of oral cancer. For example, the Li-Fraumeni syndrome, which is caused by inherited defects in the *p53* gene, results in an excess risk of multiple malignancies in affected family members, including oral cancer (Prime et al, 2001). An excess risk of oral cancer, however, has not been observed in other inherited cancer syndromes involving other gatekeeper genes, such as retinoblastoma, Wilms' tumor, or von Hippel-Lindau syndrome (Prime et al, 2001).

Caretaker genes are tumor-suppressor genes that maintain the integrity of the genome via DNA repair mechanisms. Several inherited cancer syndromes involving germline mutations in caretaker genes augment the oral cancer risk (Prime et al, 2001). For example, xeroderma pigmentosum is caused by inherited defects in nucleotide excision repair genes. These patients, who have extreme sensitivity to light, may be at elevated risk of early onset oral cancer.

Low-penetrance polymorphisms

A role for gene–environment interactions in the etiology of oral cancer is now emerging. Several epidemiologic studies suggest that polymorphisms in genes encoding enzymes involved in the metabolism of tobacco, alcohol, and other environmental factors may be linked to individual susceptibility to oral cancers. Carcinogen-metabolizing enzymes are expressed in the oral cavity (Peters et al, 1993; Dong et al, 1996), suggesting that metabolism of carcinogens could occur at this site. Differences in enzyme activity in the oral cavity could represent one mechanism by which oral cancer occurs.

Glutathione S-Transferase enzymes (GSTM1 and GSTT1). Glutathione S-transferase (GST) is a family of enzymes that play a significant role in the detoxification of activated metabolites of polycyclic aromatic hydrocarbons (PAHs) such as benzo(a)pyrene, found in tobacco smoke. In addition, the GSTM1 enzyme is involved in detoxifying ethanol and its metabolites. The GST enzymes are expressed in oral tissue (Peters et al, 1993). Thus, the null genotype may, in the presence of PAHs or ethanol, increase the risk of oral cancer through an inability to deactivate carcinogens. About 50% of Caucasian and Asian populations are homozygous for a null allele in which no GSTM1 enzyme activity is present (Strange and Fryer, 1999; Cotton et al, 2000).

A large number of studies have been conducted on the effect of *GST* genes and oral cancer. While no individual study has been able to provide conclusive evidence, taken together they do indicate a potentially important role for these genes. A pooled analysis of 42 published case-control studies on the effect of *GSTM1* and *T1* on head and neck cancer (ie, including cancer of the larynx) reported an increased risk for both GSTM1 deficiency (OR = 1.27, 95% CI 1.13–1.42) and GSTT1 deficiency (OR = 1.14, 95%CI 1.00–1.31), with evidence of a combined effect for deficiency to both genes (OR = 1.99, 95% CI 1.74–2.24) (Ye et al, 2004). When stratified by subsite, an increased risk among studies that included just oral cancer was still observed for *GSTM1* (OR = 1.56, 95% CI 1.35–1.80), although not for *GSTT1* (OR = 1.16, 95% CI 0.91–1.47).

A meta-analysis conducted reported similar effects for *GSTM1* (OR = 1.45, 95% CI 1.05–2.00) and *GSTT1* (OR = 1.15, 95% CI 0.82–1.63) for oral cancer, although it also reported an increased risk for *GSTP1* (OR = 1.52, 95% CI 1.05–2.20) (Hashibe et al, 2003). Based on a subset of studies that provided their data for a pooled analysis, an increased risk of head and neck cancer was found for individuals with all three risk *GST* genotypes (OR = 2.06, 95%CI 1.11–3.81), although results were not presented separately by cancer site.

Cytochrome P450 (CYP) enzymes. Other metabolizing genes that may be important for oral cancer include cytochrome P450 (CYP) enzymes. CYP1A1, of the CYP1 family, metabolizes PAHs, including benzo(a)pyrene and other constituents of tobacco smoke (Guengerich and Shimada, 1991). The CYP2E1 enzyme catalyzes the oxidation of several compounds found in cigarette smoke and betel quid, including N-nitrosamines and benzene, and is also involved in the metabolism of ethanol. While a large number of studies have been conducted for these variants, no conclusive findings have yet been identified. The only meta-analysis so far reported included CYP1A1, and, based on 5 studies, identified a potential increased risk of oral cancer

with the Va1462 allele (OR=1.48, 95% CI 0.77–2.83) (Hashibe et al, 2003).

N-acetyltransferases (NAT2). The NAT2 enzyme is involved in the metabolism of heterocyclic amines found in cooked and broiled meats, as well as in cigarette smoke to a lesser extent. Metabolism by NAT2 actually activates heterocyclic amines to an intermediate mutagenic substance, whereas it detoxifies aromatic amines such as those found in car exhaust and tobacco smoke. On the basis of these mechanisms, one would expect that the rapid acetylator genotype could augment oral cancer risk associated with dietary factors and decrease oral risk due to tobacco use. The four studies to date that have examined *NAT2* polymorphisms found no overall association with oral cancer risk, although the sample size of these studies has been limited (Katoh et al, 1998; Morita et al, 1999; Chen et al, 2001; Fronhoffs et al, 2001).

Alcohol dehydrogenase (ADH). Ethanol is primarily oxidized to acetaldehyde, its carcinogenic form, by alcohol dehydrogenase (ADH) (Bosron and Li, 1986). Although most ethanol metabolism occurs in the liver, ADH is also expressed in the oral cavity. Several phase I genes involved in metabolizing alcohol are prime candidates for influencing the risk of oral cancer. For example, the *ADH1B* and *ADH1C* genotypes are involved in metabolizing ethanol to acetaldehyde, a recognized animal carcinogen (IARC Monographs Vol. 71, 1999). The *ADH1C*1* and *ADH1B*2* alleles encode for enzymes, which results in the "fast" metabolism of ethanol.

In vitro studies have shown that the *ADH1C*1* allele increases ethanol oxidation by about 2.5-fold compared to *ADH1C*2*. In contrast the *ADH1B*1/1* genotype is associated with only 1% and 0.5% of the oxidation capability of the *ADH1B*1/2* and *ADH1B*2/2* genotypes, respectively.

ADH1B and *ADH1C* are located at only 16 kb of distance on chromosome 4, and linkage disequilibrium between *ADH1C*1* and *ADH1B*2* has been demonstrated in several populations (Brennan et al, 2004). *ADH1B* has not been previously studied for oral cancer, although studies in Asian populations have been reported that, even though they were of small sample size, have consistently shown that the *ADH1B*1* allele is associated with an increased risk of esophageal cancer (Brennan et al, 2004).

Studies in populations of European origin have focused on the gene *ADH1C*, although there is little evidence of a strong effect on oral cancer risk. In a pooled analysis of seven published case-control studies, including 1325 cases and 1760 controls, no increased risk of head and neck cancer (oral plus larynx) for the *ADH1C*1* allele was observed (Brennan et al, 2004). A recent study based in five countries of Central Europe, and also including larynx and esophageal cancer, reported an increased risk for the fast *ADH1C*1* allele (p = 0.05) and a strong protective effect for the fast *ADH1B*2* allele (p = 0.0002) (Hashibe et al, 2006). Similar results were observed among the subgroup of oral and pharynx cancer. These contradictory results appeared to be explained by a primary protective effect with the *ADH1B*2* fast allele, with the observed association with *ADH1C*1* being explained by linkage disequilibrium. While these studies do argue for a role of these genes in oral cancer, further studies in other populations will be required to elucidate the main effects.

Somatic Mutations

Oral carcinogenesis involves multiple molecular steps, with somatic mutations in tumor-suppressor genes and oncogenes on several chromosomes. Early changes are thought to include the loss of tumor-suppressor genes on chromosomes 17p and 9p (Scully et al, 2000). Although the specific genes involved on these chromosomes are still conjectural, *p16* and *p53* inactivation occurs in a high proportion of both oral precancer and invasive cancer cases (Scully et al, 2000).

The p53 gene, located on chromosome 17p, has multiple functions in controlling cellular replication, including acting as a G1 checkpoint control and as a trigger of apoptosis in response to cell damage. Mutations in *p53* have been demonstrated in approximately two-thirds of oral cancer cases, as well as in a significant proportion of oral precancerous lesions (Scully et al, 2000). The occurrence of *p53* mutations appears to be associated with exposure to specific risk factors indicating different causal pathways for oral cancer. Mutations have been found to be more strongly associated with alcohol- and tobacco-associated oral cancer, and less often with infection with HPV and also with betel quid chewing (Hafkamp et al, 2003; Dai et al, 2004; Thongsuksai et al, 2003). Oral cancers with *p53* mutations may also be less responsive to radiotherapy (Alsner et al, 2001).

A major role of the *p16* gene is to halt the progression of cell growth cycle at G1. Loss of the *p16* gene leads to loss of *p53* functions, and thereby loss of cell cycle control, contributing to unregulated cell growth. The loss of heterozygosity on chromosome 9p, where the *p16* gene is found, is the most commonly reported somatic mutation in oral cancer (Scully et al, 2000). In addition, *p16* inactivation can occur through mechanisms that block the promoter region and thus transcription. Changes in *p16* appear early in oral carcinogenesis and correlate with the use of tobacco and betel quid (Scully et al, 2000). *P16* alterations have also been associated with metastasis to lymph nodes (Tsai et al, 2001).

Mutations in the epidermal growth factor receptor-1 (*EGFR*) occur in about 7% of patients with squamous cell carcinoma of the head and neck and may have therapeutic implications (Willmore-Payne et al, 2006; Lee et al, 2005).

RISK FACTORS

Epidemiologic studies over the past several decades have elucidated several important risk factors for oral cancer, summarized in Table 7–1, and presented in detail in the following.

Table 7–1. Risk factors and preventive behaviors for oral cancer

Risk factor	Protective factor
Established	Established
Tobacco	
Alcohol	
HPV infection	
Possible	Possible
Mouthwash	Fruits and vegetables
Hot mate	Vitamin C, vitamin E,
	beta-carotene
Insufficient	Insufficient
HSV infection	Fiber intake
Fat intake	

HPV, human papillomavirus; HSV, herpes simplex virus

Tobacco

Tobacco is the most important risk factor for oral cancer, not only because of its strong association with the disease but also because of its prevalence in diverse populations. The form of tobacco used varies in different parts of the world. In Europe, the United States, Australia, and Japan, cigarettes, cigars, and pipes are the main types of smoked tobacco, while chewing tobacco and snuff are common smokeless forms. In India, Pakistan, China, and Southeast Asia, while cigarette consumption may be high, tobacco is also chewed as betel quid, paan, naswar, and nass (Gupta, 1996). Betel quid consists of the leaf of the betel vine wrapped around areca nut, lime, and tobacco. Paan is a mixture of areca nut, lime, spices, and sweeteners and may or may not include tobacco. Naswar is composed of tobacco and lime, while nass is an aqueous or oily mixture of tobacco, ash, and lime.

Almost 80% of all oral cancers are attributed to the use of tobacco (Rothman, 1978). Smoking tobacco as cigarettes exposes the oral cavity to several carcinogens including PAHs, aldehydes, and nitrosamines. A positive association between cigarette smoking and oral cancer has consistently been documented in numerous studies (IARC monographs on tobacco, Vol. 83, 2004). The risk increases substantially with duration of smoking and number of cigarettes smoked. In Italy, cigarette smokers had an 11-fold higher risk of oral cancer than nonsmokers (Franceschi et al, 1990). The risk increased with both the number of cigarettes smoked per day and the number of years that a person smoked. Moreover, high-tar cigarettes confer a greater risk than low-tar cigarettes (LaVecchia et al, 1990), while the use of mentholated cigarettes does not appear to affect the risk (Kabat and Hebert, 1994). Exclusive smoking in the form of cigars or pipes contributes to a twofold increased risk of oral cancer (Blot et al, 1988).

Quitting cigarette smoking dramatically reduces the risk of oral cancer (Blot et al, 1988; Franco et al, 1989; Merletti et al, 1989; Franceschi et al, 1990). The decline in oral cancer risk after quitting occurs quickly, so that former smokers who quit for more than 10 years approach the risk of never smokers. These findings have important public health implications and support smoking-cessation efforts as a means to reduce morbidity and mortality from oral cancer.

Snuff was introduced in countries as diverse as Sweden and Sudan almost 400 years ago (Idris et al, 1998). In western countries in the 1950s, the first epidemiologic studies examined a potential role for smokeless tobacco in the etiology of oral cancer. Chewing tobacco and snuff contain tobacco-specific N-nitrosamines that are carcinogenic and have been shown to cause oral cancer in mouse models (Hecht et al, 1986; Hecht and Hoffmann, 1988). Users of chewing tobacco and snuff are at higher risk of oral cancer, particularly cancers of the cheek and gum (Winn et al, 1981; Blot et al, 1988). However, in a large cohort study involving Swedish construction workers, a population in which snuff use is common, no excess risk of oral cancer at any site was observed for either current or former snuff users (Boffetta et al, 2005). The composition of snuff varies across different cultures, and this has been posited as one reason for the conflicting evidence on snuff use.

In India and other parts of Asia, smokeless tobacco in the form of betel quid, paan, or nass has long been suspected to be related to the elevated rates of oral cancer seen in these countries (Jayant and Deo, 1986). The use of betel quid (Ko et al, 1995; Hung et al, 1997) and paan (Chattopadhyay, 1989; Merchant et al, 2000) was repeatedly found to substantially increase the risk of oral cancer. While tobacco appears to be the key agent in the etiology of oral cancer, other components in these products may enhance the risk (Gupta et al, 1996). A recent evaluation of all epidemiological studies of betel quid concluded that betel quid both with and without tobacco was causally associated with oral cancer (IARC monograph Vol. 85, 2004).

The areca nut itself, a constituent of paan and betel quid, contains arecoline and other alkaloids, which can be converted into N-nitroso compounds. Even in the absence of tobacco, consumption of paan increased the risk of oral cancer (Merchant et al, 2000). The risk of oral cancer from chewing betel quid, paan, and naswar, however, is not well recognized among populations exposed to these risk factors. While 80% of participants in one study identified cigarette smoking as a risk factor for oral cancer, only 30% believed betel quid chewing would increase the risk (Ahmed et al, 1997).

The elevated rates of oral cancer in India, Southeast Asia, and other areas are strongly related to the prevalence and type of tobacco used there. In a large population-based survey in India, the prevalence of tobacco use was high among women (57%), almost solely in smokeless form as betel quid. Among men, 69% reported current tobacco use, and 24% were cigarette smokers (Gupta, 1996). In a survey of Bangladeshi living in London, the prevalence of betel quid chewing was over 80% among both men and women (Ahmed et al, 1997). In a large study of over 2000 oral cancers and 3000 controls from 2 centers in South India, chewing of tobacco emerged as the strongest risk factor for oral cancer, with highly significant risks also observed for smoking and chewing without tobacco (Znaor et al, 2003).

When considered by subsite, chewing was primarily a risk factor for cancer of the mouth, whereas smoking was the strongest risk factor for pharyngeal cancer.

Variations in the type of tobacco used across different populations may help explain the variability in the anatomic distribution of oral cancer. In Papua New Guinea, oral cancer is primarily located at the corner of the mouth and cheek, corresponding to the application of slaked lime and betel nut at this site (Thomas and Maclennan, 1992). The reverse smoking of Chutta cigars has been associated with an excess risk of cancer of the oral palate, which has been called *Chutta cancer* (van der Eb et al, 1993).

Black (air-cured) tobacco, traditionally used in Latin American and Mediterranean countries in preference to blond (flue-cured) tobacco, is now the predominant type in most industrialized countries. A potentially different risk of head and neck cancer for black and blond tobacco is plausible because the concentration of several carcinogens differs substantially between black and blond tobacco, notably a higher level of N-nitrosamines and aromatic amines in black tobacco smoke (Boffetta et al, 1993; Sancho-Garnier and Theobald, 1993; De Stefani et al, 1993). A hospital-based case-control study from Uruguay reported a threefold increased risk of both oral cancer and pharyngeal cancer (De Stefani et al, 1998). A case-control study in three areas of Brazil comprising cases of oral, pharyngeal, and laryngeal cancer found no difference between use of commercial cigarettes or hand-rolled black tobacco for oral cancer although the risk of pharyngeal cancer was approximately twice as high in black tobacco smokers (Schlecht et al, 1999). Finally, a study from Spain reported almost a fourfold increase in risk for smokers of black tobacco compared to those who smoked blond only (Castellsague et al, 2004). These results indicate a potentially important increased risk of oral cancers from the black tobacco type.

Diet

Fruit and vegetable intake

There is convincing evidence that a diet rich in fruits and vegetables provides protection against oral cancer. Studies conducted in the United States, Europe, South America, and China have repeatedly shown that a diet rich in fruits and vegetables reduces the risk of oral cancer by 50%–70% (McLaughlin et al, 1988; Franco et al, 1989; Zheng et al, 1992; La Vecchia et al, 1997; De Stefani et al, 1999). In particular, fresh fruit substantially reduces the risk of oral cancer (McLaughlin et al, 1988; Franco et al, 1989; La Vecchia et al, 1997). Strong protective effects of dark yellow vegetables (Zheng et al, 1992), citrus fruits, and carotene-rich foods such as carrots, pumpkins, and fresh tomatoes (Franco et al, 1989; La Vecchia et al, 1997) have also been found. In a prospective study, citrus fruits were associated with a significant reduction in risk of oral premalignant lesions (Maserejian et al, 2006). While there was no association of beta-carotene overall on premalignant lesions, among current smokers, higher intake was associated with an increased risk. The exact dietary pattern of fruits and vegetables that provides the greatest protection against oral cancer is still unclear.

Fruits and vegetables are rich in vitamins C and E, beta-carotene, and flavonoids. Many of these micronutrients have antioxidants or antitumor effects, which may help prevent oral cancer. Given the diversity of fruits and vegetables associated with a reduced oral cancer risk, it may be that a combination of several micronutrients in these foods decreases the likelihood of oral carcinogenesis. In a large comprehensive review of the role of fruits and vegetables on oral cancer, it was concluded that fruit and vegetable consumption may only "possibly" reduce risk (IARC Handbooks of cancer prevention, Vol. 8, 2003). This was because of the potential role of bias and confounding that could not be ruled out.

Micronutrient intake

Although it can be difficult to disentangle the role of individual micronutrients, observational and experimental studies indicate that beta-carotene and vitamins C and E may be effective in reducing oral cancer risk. A chemopreventive role of micronutrients in precancerous oral lesions has also become apparent. However, further studies must be undertaken to elucidate fully the role of micronutrients in the etiology of oral cancer.

Higher beta-carotene intake, measured through dietary assessment or serum levels, reduces the risk of oral cancer (La Vecchia et al, 1997; World Cancer Research Fund, 1997; Negri et al, 2000). A study in Italy and Switzerland found a relative risk of 0.6 for a one-standard-deviation increase in beta-carotene (Negri et al, 2000). Beta-carotene also appears to act in the chemoprevention of oral precancer. In Japan, men with 1 mmol/L higher serum beta-carotene had an 84% lower risk of developing the precancerous condition leukoplakia (Nagao et al, 2000). Intervention studies have shed some light on the effect of beta-carotene from other micronutrients found in fruits and vegetables. Patients with leukoplakia who were randomized to beta-carotene supplements showed sustained remission of the lesions compared to those on placebo (Garewal et al, 1999). Among betel quid chewers, those randomized to a cocktail of beta-carotene and retinol had a threefold decrease in the proportion of buccal cells with micronuclei (Stich et al, 1984). The chemopreventive nature of beta-carotene may be related to its role as an antioxidant, with the ability to quench oxygen-free radicals.

High vitamin C intake may also decrease the risk of oral cancer, as well as of oral precancerous lesions (Zheng et al, 1993; Marshall and Boyle, 1996; World Cancer Research Fund, 1997; Gupta et al, 1998; Negri et al, 2000). In Italy and Switzerland, oral cancer risk decreased 37% for a one-standard-deviation increase in vitamin C intake, controlling for energy intake as well as other potential confounders (Negri et al, 2000). In India, the risk of oral leukoplakia was halved among subjects in the highest quartile of vitamin C intake compared to those in the lowest quartile (Gupta et al, 1998). Because vitamin C is strongly correlated with fruit and vegetable intake, it is difficult to disentangle the effect of the nutrient in particular from that of the food in general. However, laboratory studies suggest that the antioxidant vitamin C may act as a chemopreventive agent, either alone or in concert with vitamin E, to prevent oral carcinogenesis (Sawant and Kandarkar, 2000).

Vitamin E, an antioxidant, may also protect against oral cancer. Dietary intake data have shown a decreasing risk of oral cancer with increasing vitamin E intake in most (Zheng et al, 1993; Marshall and Boyle, 1996; World Cancer Research Fund, 1997; Negri et al, 2000), although not all (World Cancer Research Fund, 1997), epidemiologic studies. Moreover, long-term use of vitamin E supplements may entail a 60% reduction in the risk of oral cancer (World Cancer Research Fund, 1997). Several clinical trials show that vitamin E, in concert with beta-carotene, produces regression of oral leukoplakia (Garewal and Schantz, 1995). Finally, in animal experiments, vitamin E has consistently inhibited oral carcinogenesis (World Cancer Research Fund, 1997).

A role of other micronutrients in protecting against oral cancer is becoming clearer. Folate, vitamin A, and iron have all been associated with a reduced risk of oral cancer. Additional epidemiologic evidence is required, however, before the contribu-

tion of these nutritional agents can be fully elucidated.

Fat intake

A potential role for dietary fat intake in the etiology of oral cancers has been examined only in a small number of studies. The evidence, however, appears converging. Increased consumption of butter (Fioretti et al, 1999; Franceschi et al, 1999a) or saturated fats (Franceschi, 1999a) was positively associated, and that of olive oil was negatively associated, with oral cancer risk (Franceschi, 1999a, 1999b). Further, a high proportion of calories from cholesterol may increase the risk of salivary gland cancer (Horn-Ross et al, 1997). However, while these findings suggest a role for fat intake in the etiology of oral cancer, the evidence is far from conclusive.

Fiber intake

A diet high in fiber may protect against both oral cancer (Gridley et al, 1990; Zheng et al, 1993; MacFarlane et al, 1995; Horn-Ross et al, 1997) and precancerous oral lesions (Gupta et al, 1998). In China, dietary fiber derived from fruits and vegetables was inversely associated with oral cancer risk, while fiber derived from other sources did not exhibit any protective effect (Zheng et al, 1993). Fiber from vegetables, fruits, or grains reduced oral cancer by 50% among an Italian population (Soler et al, 2001). Legumes, which are a rich source of dietary fiber, may also be protective against oral cancer (De Stefani et al, 1999). The link between oral cancer and fiber is not completely clear, however, since some studies found no association (McLaughlin et al, 1988).

Alcohol

Epidemiologic data collected over the past 30 years provide consistent evidence that alcohol elevates the risk of oral cancer. Evidence from US, European, Chinese, and Korean populations demonstrates an increased risk of oral cancer with increasing amounts of alcohol consumed or frequency of drinking (Blot et al, 1988; Kabat and

Wynder, 1989; Merletti et al, 1989; Franceschi et al, 1990; Zheng et al, 1990; Choi and Kahyo, 1991; Harty et al, 1997). For example, drinking up to 100 kg of alcohol over a lifetime increased the risk threefold compared to never drinking, while consuming more than 400 kg entailed a more than sevenfold excess risk (Franco et al, 1989). Investigators have tried to assess whether certain forms of alcohol have a stronger effect in the oral cavity (Blot et al, 1988; Merletti et al, 1989; Franco et al, 1989). While all types of alcohol contribute an excess risk, the most frequently used alcoholic beverage in each population tended to emerge as the strongest risk factor for oral cancer (La Vecchia et al, 1997).

Perhaps the most striking contribution of alcohol to the etiology of oral cancer is its consistently observed interaction with tobacco (Rothman and Keller, 1972). A positive effect of alcohol has been observed among nonsmokers; similarly, smoking increases oral cancer risk even among nondrinkers (Hashibe et al, 2007; Talamini et al, 1998). However, in concert, the effect of the two risk factors suggests a synergism between tobacco and alcohol, illustrated in Figure 7–5. While the relative risk of oral cancer among men who were intermediate cigarette smokers but who drank fewer than 35 drinks per week was 10.9, and was 2.3 for those who drank 60 or more alcoholic drinks per week but did not smoke, the risk for those who were both intermediate smokers and drinkers was more than 36-fold compared to that of men who did neither (Franceschi et al, 1990). The relative risk of 36.4 represents a departure from what we would expect under the additive model (see "Interaction" in Chapter 5).

The mechanism by which alcohol is a risk factor for head and neck cancer is unclear, especially as ethanol in its pure form does

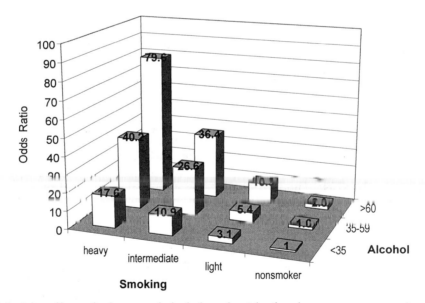

Figure 7–5. Joint effects of tobacco and alcohol on the risk of oral cancer among men in northern Italy. Relative risk estimates for categories of exposure. Light smoker: ex-smokers who quit more than 10 years ago or current smokers who smoked 1–14 cigarettes per day for less than 30 years. Intermediate smoker: smoked more than 14 cigarettes per day for less than 30 years or 15–24 cigarettes per day regardless of duration or for 30–39 years regardless of amount or 1–24 cigarettes for 40 years or more. Heavy smoker: smoked 25 or more cigarettes per day for 40 years or more. (*Source*: Data from Franceschi, 1990)

not act as a carcinogen in experimental models (IARC Monographs, Vol. 44, 1988). Potential reasons why alcoholic beverages are carcinogenic include it acting merely as a solvent for tobacco carcinogens (Seitz et al, 1998; Wight and Ogden, 1998). Similarly, impurities or contaminants in alcoholic drinks have been suggested to represent the main carcinogenic agent. For example, polycyclic aromatic hydrocarbons are found in dark strong liquors such as whiskey, and N-nitrosodiethylamine has been detected in some beers.

If contaminants in alcoholic beverages represent the primary risk factor this would suggest that type of alcohol beverage would be an important risk factor. A further possibility is that the primary metabolite of ethanol, acetaldehyde, is the cause of the carcinogenic effect of alcoholic beverages although, direct evidence linking acetaldehyde as a cause of head and neck cancers in humans is hard to establish.

Alcohol is not believed to be a carcinogen per se. However, when alcohol is metabolized by enzymes (ADH3, CYP2E1) for excretion, activated metabolites with a carcinogenic potential, such as acetaldehyde, are produced. Many of the metabolic enzymes are expressed at the oral mucosa (Peters et al, 1993; Dong et al, 1996), suggesting a mechanistic role for alcohol in oral cancer etiology. Alcohol may also contribute to carcinogenesis by direct irritation of the oral mucosa or through the nutritional deficiencies associated with heavy alcohol consumption (Lieber et al, 1979).

Reproductive Factors

There is limited evidence that menstrual and reproductive factors are associated with the risk of cancer of the salivary gland. No published studies have examined these factors in relation to oral cancer at other sites.

Anthropometric Measures

There is no evidence of a direct role for anthropometric measures in the etiology of oral cancer. However, few studies have examined this issue. Oral cancer cases have been observed to be leaner than controls, which may indicate a poor nutritional status (Kabat et al, 1994; D'Avanzo et al, 1996; Kreimer et al, 2006; IARC Publication No.154, 2001)

Infections

Human papillomaviruses (HPV) and perhaps herpes simplex viruses (HSV), in concert with other risk factors, may play a role in the etiology of oral cancer. Other infectious agents might also contribute to oral carcinogenesis through a chronic infectious mechanism.

Human papillomavirus

Human papilloma virus type 16 is now a recognized cause of some oral cancers (IARC monograph Vol. 90, in press). The evidence comes primarily from several large epidemiological studies that have shown a consistent presence of HPV DNA in tumor tissue, which is present in high copy numbers and is transcriptionally active. The largest such study, involving 1670 case patients and 1732 control subjects, reported a prevalence of HPV DNA in 3.9% of specimens from the oral cavity and 18.3% of specimens from the oropharynx (Herrero et al, 2003). Furthermore, when cases were compared to controls, a strong increased risk was observed for antibodies against HPV16 E6 and E7 proteins, for both cancers of the oral cavity (OR = 2.9, 95% CI 1.7 to 4.8) and oropharynx (OR = 9.2, 95% CI 4.8 to 17.7).

The presence of HPV infection may also alter the tumor profile and have implications for outcome. A higher prevalence of TP53 mutations has been observed in oral cancers that are negative for HPV, consistent with the disintegration of the TP53 protein by the E6 oncoprotein (Dai et al, 2004). Furthermore, individuals with HPV-associated oral cancer appear to have an increased survival rate, possibly due to enhanced radiation sensitivity. The exposure profile between HPV-positive and HPV-negative tumors may also differ, with an increased prevalence of never smokers and never drinkers among those who are HPV positive.

Other infections

Herpes simplex viruses 1 (HSV-1) and 2 (HSV-2) have also been associated with oral cancer. One study showed a threefold increased risk of oral cancer associated with HSV-1 overall, with a somewhat higher risk for cancer of the lip (Schildt et al, 1998); another study showed an almost twofold increased risk associated with HSV-2 (Maden et al, 1992). Data from an experimental model may help elucidate the mechanism by which HSV could impact oral cancer risk. The oral cavity of hamsters was exposed to snuff dipping and HSV infection (Park et al, 1986). While neither snuff dipping nor HSV infection alone induced malignant changes, HSV infection in combination with simulated snuff dipping substantially increased the risk of invasive oral cancer.

The increased incidence of oral cancer in general, and of cancer of the tongue in particular, among cohorts of patients with chronic syphilis (Michalek et al, 1994) provides some evidence for a role of this infection in the etiology of oral cancer (Binnie et al, 1983). Other chronic infections such as candidosis have also been suggested as risk factors for oral cancer (Binnie et al, 1983; Leigh et al, 2000).

Physical Activity

There is no evidence of a role for physical activity in the etiology of oral cancer.

Ionizing Radiation

There is no evidence of a role for ionizing radiation in the etiology of oral cancer.

Occupation

Much of the evidence on a role for occupational exposures in the etiology of oral cancer springs from the extensive follow-up of occupational cohorts in Scandinavia, Great Britain, and Germany. There are inherent difficulties in interpreting the results from these occupational cohorts due to lack of information on potential confounders such as smoking. Nevertheless, higher rates of oral cancer have been observed in some occupations. Workers exposed to compounds including aromatic amines and phenoxy herbicides have been reported to be at elevated risk of oral cancer in several cohort studies (Delzell and Monson, 1981; Sorahan et al, 1989; Merletti et al, 1991; Foppa and Minder, 1992; Straif et al, 2000), as well as in a case-control study that was able to adjust for potential confounders (Coble et al, 2003).

The rubber industry has some of the highest exposures to nitrosamines, produced in large part during salt bath curing and vulcanization processing. In a cohort of male rubber workers, those who had at least a year of high exposure—defined as working in these high-risk processing areas—had a three- to fourfold increased mortality from oral cancer (Straif et al, 2000). In addition, the risk of dying from the disease increased with increasing duration of high-risk exposure. An excess risk of oral cancer mortality has also been observed among workers in the US and British rubber industries (Delzell and Monson, 1981; Sorahan et al, 1989). Support for a role of nitrosamines in the etiology of oral cancer springs from experimental studies showing that nontobacco-specific nitrosamines result in the formation of DNA adducts in oral mucosa.

Occupational cohorts in Switzerland (Foppa and Minder, 1992) and Italy (Merletti et al, 1991) have shown elevated mortality from oral cancer among cooks. The elevated risk was pronounced among adults age 55 or younger, who experienced a more than sevenfold excess risk of death (Foppa and Minder, 1992). Interpretation of these findings is limited by the lack of information on potential confounding factors, since cooks may be more likely to use tobacco and alcohol than the general population. In fact, an excess mortality was seen for liver cirrhosis (SMR 53.4) and alcoholism (SMR 52.7) but not for lung cancer or bronchitis overall (Foppa and Minder, 1992).

Nevertheless, higher levels of volatile carcinogenic compounds, such as those formed from cooking meats, could constitute an occupational hazard to cooks (Rappaport et al, 1979; Teschke et al, 1989). Moreover, frequent tasting of hot foods could lead to chronic thermal irritation of the oral cavity. An increased risk of oral cancer was detected among butchers, which may also be at least partly due to confounding by tobacco smoking, alcohol drinking, and other lifestyle factors. However, exposures in the meat industry (eg, viruses, nitrosamines, polycyclic aromatic hydrocarbons) may contribute the elevated cancer risks (Boffetta et al, 2000).

Medical Conditions and Treatment

There is no evidence of a role for other medical conditions and treatment in the etiology of oral cancer.

Other Risk Factors

Mouthwash

Since the first report by Weaver and colleagues (1979), several researchers have sought to examine whether mouthwash increases the risk of oral cancer because it may contain up to 25% alcohol. A positive association has been observed among certain groups, for example nonsmoking women, as has an exposure–response trend with increasing daily frequency, years of use, or concentration of mouthwash (Blot et al, 1983). However, other investigators have been unable to replicate these findings with respect to both oral cancer and precancerous lesions (Wynder et al, 1983; Morse et al, 1997); thus, a role of mouthwash in the etiology of oral cancer remains equivocal.

Mate

Mate is an infusion commonly drunk in parts of South America, in particular southern Brazil, Uruguay, and northern Argentina. There are consistent reports of an association between esophageal cancer and consumption of mate when drunk at very hot temperatures, and it has been classified by the IARC monograph programme as being "probably carcinogenic," although only when drunk at hot temperatures (IARC monographs Vol. 51, 1991). Evidence for oral cancer is less consistent,

although a moderate increased risk has been reported from two studies in Uruguay and Brazil.

CONCLUSION

Many important risk factors for oral cancer have been elucidated in the epidemiologic literature. Tobacco in its many forms is perhaps the most important risk factor, both because of its strong relationship with the disease and because of its high prevalence in many populations around the world. Alcohol use alone may elevate the risk of oral cancer, although its predominant effect comes from interaction with tobacco. The epidemiologic evidence supporting an increased risk for HPV type 16 is also unequivocal. A protective effect with consumption of fruits and vegetables has been consistently shown, although it is difficult to interpret due to the potential for confounding and bias. Finally, there appears to be a role for common genetic polymorphisms that by themselves may not substantially impact the disease risk, but that in concert with environmental exposures may lead to development of oral cancer. The majority of oral cancers that occur globally are attributed to causes that are for the most part modifiable. Thus, minimizing the burden of oral cancer is possible.

REFERENCES

Ahmed S, Rahman A, Hull S. Use of betel quid and cigarettes among Bangladeshi patients in an inner-city proactive: prevalence and knowledge of health effects. Br J Gen Pract 1997;47:431–34.

Alsner J, Sorensen SB, Overgaard J. TP53 mutation is related to poor prognosis after radiotherapy, but not surgery, in squamous cell carcinoma of the head and neck. Radiother Oncol 2001;59(2):179–85.

Ankathil R, Mathew A, Joseph F, Nair MK. Is oral cancer susceptibility inherited? Report of five oral cancer families. Eur J Cancer B Oral Oncol 1996;32B:63–67.

Binnie WH, Rankin KV, Mackenzie IC. Etiology of oral squamous cell carcinoma. J Oral Pathol 1983;12:11–29.

Blot WJ, McLaughlin JK, Winn DM, Austin DF, Greenberg RS, Preston-Martin S, et al.

Smoking and drinking in relation to oral and pharyngeal cancer. Cancer Res 1988;48: 3282–87.

Blot WJ, Winn DM, Fraumeni JF. Oral cancer and mouthwash. J Natl Cancer Inst 1983; 70:251–53.

Boffetta P, La Vecchia C, Levi F, Lucchini F. Mortality patterns and trends for lung cancer and other tobacco-related cancers in the Americas, 1955–1989. Int J Epidemiol 1993; 22(3):377–84.

Boffetta P, Gridley G, Gustavsson P, Brennan P, Blair A, Ekstrom AM, Fraumeni JF Jr. Employment as butcher and cancer risk in a record-linkage study from Sweden. Cancer Causes Control 2000;11(7):627–33.

Boffetta P, Aagnes B, Weiderpass E, Andersen A. Smokeless tobacco use and risk of cancer of the pancreas and other organs. Int J Cancer. 2005;114(6):992–95.

Bosron WF, Li TK. Genetic polymorphism of human liver alcohol and aldehyde dehydrogenases, and their relationship to alcohol metabolism and alcoholism. Hepatology 1986;6:502–10.

Brennan P, Lewis S, Hashibe M, Bell DA, Boffetta P, Bouchardy C, Caporaso N, Chen C, Coutelle C, Diehl SR, Hayes RB, Olshan AF, Schwartz SM, Sturgis EM, Wei Q, Zavras AI, Benhamou S. Pooled analysis of alcohol dehydrogenase genotypes and head and neck cancer: a HuGE review. Am J Epidemiol 2004;159(1):1–16.

Castellsague X, Quintana MJ, Martinez MC, Nieto A, Sanchez MJ, Juan A, Monner A, Carrera M, Agudo A, Quer M, Munoz N, Herrero R, Franceschi S, Bosch FX. The role of type of tobacco and type of alcoholic beverage in oral carcinogenesis. Int J Cancer 2004;108(5):741–49.

Chattopadhyay A. Epidemiologic study of oral cancer in eastern India. Indian J Dermatol 1989;34:59–65.

Chen C, Ricks S, Doody DR, Fitzgibbons ED, Porter PL, Schwartz SM. N-Acetyltransferase 2 polymorphisms, cigarette smoking and alcohol consumption, and oral squamous cell cancer risk. Carcinogenesis 2001,22(12): 1993–99.

Choi SY, Kahyo H. Effect of cigarette smoking and alcohol consumption in the aetiology of cancer of the oral cavity, pharynx, and larynx. Int J Epidemiol 1991;20:878–85.

Coble JB, Brown LM, Hayes RB, Huang WY, Winn DM, Gridley G, Bravo-Otero E, Fraumeni JF Jr. Sugarcane farming, occupational solvent exposures, and the risk of oral cancer in Puerto Rico. J Occup Environ Med 2003;45(8):869–74.

Coleman MP, Gatta G, Verdecchia A, Esteve J, Sant M, Storm H, Allemani C, Ciccolallo L, Santaquilani M, Berrino F. EUROCARE Working Group. EUROCARE-3 summary: cancer survival in Europe at the end of the 20th century. Ann Oncol 2003;14 Suppl 5:v128–49

Cotton SC, Sharp L, Little J, Brockton N. Glutathione S-transferase polymorphisms and colorectal cancer: a HuGE review. Am J Epidemiol 2000;151:7–32.

Dai M, Clifford GM, le Calvez F, Castellsague X, Snijders PJ, Pawlita M, Herrero R, Hainaut P, Franceschi S; IARC Multicenter Oral Cancer Study Group. Human papillomavirus type 16 and TP53 mutation in oral cancer: matched analysis of the IARC multicenter study. Cancer Res 2004;64(2):468–71.

D'Avanzo B, La Vecchia C, Talamini R, Franceschi S. Anthropometric measures and risk of cancers of the upper digestive and respiratory tract. Nutr Cancer 1996;26: 219–27.

De Stefani E, Barrios E, Fierro L. Black (aircured) and blond (flue-cured) tobacco and cancer risk. III: Oesophageal cancer. Eur J Cancer 1993;29A(5):763–66.

De Stefani E, Boffetta P, Oreggia F, Mendilaharsu M, Deneo-Pellegrini H. Smoking patterns and cancer of the oral cavity and pharynx: a case-control study in Uruguay. Oral Oncol 1998;34(5):340–46.

De Stefani E, Deneo-Pellegrini H, Mendilaharsu M, Ronco A. Diet and risk of cancer of the upper aerodigestive tract—I. Foods. Oral Oncol 1999;35:17–21.

Delzell E, Monson RR. Mortality among rubber workers. III. Cause-specific mortality, 1940–1978. J Occup Med 1981;23:677–84.

Dong YJ, Peng TK, Yin SJ. Expression and activities of alcohol dehydrogenase in human mouth. Alcohol 1996;13:257–62.

Ferlay J, Bray F, Pisani P, Parkin DM. GLOBOCAN 2000—Updated version 2002: Cancer Incidence, Mortality and Prevalence Worldwide. International Agency for Research on Cancer, 2002.

Fioretti F, Bosetti C, Tavani A, Franceschi S, La Vecchia C. Risk factors for oral and pharyngeal cancer in never smokers. Oral Oncol 1999;35:375–78.

Foppa I, Minder CE. Oral, pharyngeal and laryngeal cancer as a cause of death among Swiss cooks. Scand J Work Environ Health 1992;18:287–92.

Franceschi S, Bidoli E, Herrero R, Munoz N. Comparison of cancers of the oral cavity and pharynx worldwide: etiological clues. Oral Oncol 2000;36:106–15.

Franceschi S, Favero A, Conti E, Talamini R, Volpe R, Negri E, et al. Food groups, oils and butter, and cancer of the oral cavity and pharynx. Br J Cancer 1999a;80:614–20.

Franceschi S, Levi F, Conti E, Talamini R, Negri E, Dal Maso L, et al. Energy intake and dietary pattern in cancer of the oral cavity and pharynx. Cancer Causes Control 1999b;10:439–44.

Franceschi S, Talamini R, Barra S, Baron AE, Negri E, Bidoli E, et al. Smoking and drinking in relation to cancers of the oral cavity, pharynx, larynx, and esophagus in northern Italy. Cancer Res 1990;50:6502–7.

Franco EL, Kowalski LP, Oliveira BV, Curado MP, Pereira RN, Silva ME, et al. Risk factors for oral cancer in Brazil: a case-control study. Int J Cancer 1989;43:992–1000.

Fronhoffs S, Bruning T, Ortiz-Pallardo E, Brode P, Koch B, Harth V, Sachinidis A, Bolt HM, Herberhold C, Vetter H, Ko Y. Real-time PCR analysis of the N-acetyltransferase *NAT1* allele *3, *4, *10, *11, *14 and *17 polymorphism in squamous cell cancer of head and neck. Carcinogenesis 2001;22(9):1405–12.

Garewal HS, Katz RV, Meyskens F, Pitcock J, Morse D, Friedman S, et al. Beta-carotene produces sustained remissions in patients with oral leukoplakia: results of a multicenter prospective trial. Arch Otolaryngol Head Neck Surg 1999;125:1305–10.

Garewal HS, Schantz S. Emerging role of beta-carotene and antioxidant nutrients in prevention of oral cancer. Arch Otolaryngol Head Neck Surg 1995;121:141–44.

Gridley G, McLaughlin JK, Block G, Blot WJ, Winn DM, Greenberg RS, et al. Diet and oral and pharyngeal cancer among blacks. Nutr Cancer 1990;14:219–25.

Guengerich FP, Shimada T. Oxidation of toxic and carcinogenic chemicals by human cytochrome P-450 enzymes. Chem Res Toxicol 1991;4:391–407.

Gupta PC. Survey of demographic characteristics of tobacco use among 99,598 individuals in Bombay, India using handheld computers. Tobacco Control 1996;5:114–20.

Gupta PC, Hebert JR, Bhonsle RB, Sinor PN, Mehta H, Mehta FS. Dietary factors in oral leukoplakia and submucous fibrosis in a population-based case control study in Gujarat, India. Oral Dis 1998;4:200–6.

Gupta PC, Murti PR, Bhonsle RB. Epidemiology of cancer by tobacco products and the significance of TSA. Crit Rev Toxicol 1996;26:183–98.

Hashibe M, Brennan P, Strange RC, Bhisey R, Cascorbi I, Lazarus P, Oude Ophuis MB, Benhamou S, Foulkes WD, Katoh T, Coutelle C, Romkes M, Gaspari L, Taioli E, Boffetta P. Meta- and pooled analyses of *GSTM1*, *GSTT1*, *GSTP1*, and *CYP1A1* genotypes and risk of head and neck cancer. Cancer Epidemiol Biomarkers Prev. 2003;12(12):1509–17.

Hashibe M, Boffetta P, Zaridze D, Shangina O, Szeszenia-Dabrowska N, Mates D, Janout V, Fabianova E, Bencko V, Moullan N, Chabrier A, Hung R, Hall J, Canzian F, Brennan P. Evidence for an important role of alcohol- and aldehyde-metabolizing genes in cancers of the upper aerodigestive tract. Cancer Epidemiol Biomarkers Prev 2006;15(4):696–703

Hashibe M, Brennan P, Benhamou S, Castellsague X, Chen C, Curado MP, Dal Maso L, Daudt AW, Fabianova E, Wunsch-Filho V, Franceschi S, Hayes RB, Herrero R, Koifman S, La Vecchia C, Lazarus P, Levi F, Mates D, Matos E, Menezes A, Muscat J, Eluf-Neto J, Olshan AF, Rudnai P, Schwartz SM, Smith E, Sturgis EM, Szeszenia-Dabrowska N, Talamini R, Wei Q, Winn DM, Zaridze D, Zatonski W, Zhang ZF, Berthiller J, Boffetta P. Alcohol drinking in never users of tobacco, cigarette smoking in never drinkers, and the risk of head and neck cancer: pooled analysis in the International Head and Neck Cancer Epidemiology Consortium. J Natl Cancer Inst. 2007;99:777–89.

Hafkamp HC, Speel EJ, Haesevoets A, Bot FJ, Dinjens WN, Ramaekers FC, Hopman AH, Manni JJ. A subset of head and neck squamous cell carcinomas exhibits integration of HPV 16/18 DNA and overexpression of p16INK4A and p53 in the absence of mutations in *p53* exons 5–8. Int J Cancer 2003;107(3):394–400.

Harty LC, Caporaso NE, Hayes RB, Winn DM, Bravo-Otero E, Blot WJ, et al. Alcohol dehydrogenase 3 genotype and risk of oral cavity and pharyngeal cancers. J Natl Cancer Inst 1997;89:1698–1705.

Hecht SS, Hoffman D. Tobacco specific nitrosamines, an important group of carcinogens in tobacco and tobacco smoke. Carcinogenesis 1988;9:875–84.

Hecht SS, Rivenson A, Braley J, DiBello J, Adams JD, Hoffmann D. Induction of oral cavity tumors in F344 rats by tobacco-specific nitrosamines and snuff. Cancer Res 1986;41:4162–66.

Herrero R, Castellsague X, Pawlita M, Lissowska J, Kee F, Balaram P, Rajkumar T, Sridhar H, Rose B, Pintos J, Fernandez L, Idris A, Sanchez MJ, Nieto A, Talamini R, Tavani A, Bosch FX, Reidel U, Snijders PJ, Meijer CJ, Viscidi R, Munoz N, Franceschi S; IARC Multicenter Oral Cancer Study Group. Human papillomavirus and oral cancer: the International Agency for Research on Cancer multicenter study. J Natl Cancer Inst 2003;95(23):1772–83.

Horn-Ross PL, Morrow M, Ljung BM. Diet and the risk of salivary gland cancer. Am J Epidemiol 1997;146:171–76.

Hung HC, Chuang J, Chien YC, Chern HD, Chiang CP, Kuo YS, et al. Genetic polymorphisms of CYP2E1, GSTM1, and GSTT1; environmental factors and risk of oral cancer. Cancer Epidemiol Biomarkers Prev 1997;6: 901–5.

IARC Monographs on the Evaluation of Carcinogenic Risks to Humans. Alcohol drinking. V01.44, 1988. IARCPublications, Lyon.

IARC Monographs on the Evaluation of Carcinogenic Risks to Humans. Coffee, Tea, Mate, Methylxanthines and Methylglyoxal. Vol 51, 1991. IARC Publications, Lyon.

IARC Monographs on the Evaluation of Carcinogenic Risks to Humans. Re-evaluation of Some Organic Chemicals, Hydrazine and Hydrogen Peroxide. Vol 71, 1999. IARC Publications, Lyon.

IARC Monographs on the Evaluation of Carcinogenic Risks to Humans. Tobacco smoke and involuntary smoking. Vol 83, 2004. IARC Publications, Lyon.

IARC Monographs on the Evaluation of Carcinogenic Risks to Humans. Betel-quid and Areca-nut Chewing and Some Areca-nut Related Nitrosamines. Vol 85, 2004. IARC Publications, Lyon.

IARC Monograph on the Evaluation of Carcinogenic Risks to Humans. Vol 90, in press. IARC Publications, Lyon.

IARC Handbooks of Cancer Prevention. Fruits and Vegetable. Vol 8, 2003. IARC Publications, Lyon.

IARC Scientific Publication No. 154. Biomarkers in Cancer Chemoprevention. Edited by Miller AB, Bartsch H, Boffetta P, Dragsted L, Vainio H, 2001.

Idris AM, Ibrahim SO, Vasstrand EN, Johannessen AC, Lillehaug JR, Magnusson B, et al. The Swedish snus and the Sudanese toombak: are they different? Oral Oncol 1998;34:558–66.

Jayant K, Deo MG. Oral cancer and cultural practices in relation to betel quid and tobacco chewing and smoking. Cancer Detect Prev 1986;9:207–13.

Kabat GC, Chanj CJ, Wynder EL. The role of tobacco, alcohol use, and body mass index in oral and pharyngeal cancer. Int J Epidemiol 1994;23:1137–44.

Kabat GC, Hebert JR. Use of mentholated cigarettes and oropharyngeal cancer. Epidemiology 1994;5:183–88.

Kabat GC, Wynder EL. Type of alcoholic beverage and oral cancer. Int J Cancer 1989; 43:190–94.

Katoh T, Kaneko S, Boissy R, Watson M, Ikemura K, Bell DA. A pilot study testing the association between N-acetyl transferases 1 and 2 and risk of oral squamous cell carcinoma in Japanese people. Carcinogenesis 1998;19:1803–7.

Ko YC, Huang YL, Lee CH, Chen MJ, Lin LM, Tsai CC. Betel quid chewing, cigarette smoking, and alcohol consumption related to oral cancer in Taiwan. J Oral Pathol Med 1995;24:450–53.

Kreimer AR, Randi G, Herrero R, Castellsague X, La Vecchia C, Franceschi S; IARC Multicenter Oral Cancer Study Group. Diet and body mass, and oral and oropharyngeal squamous cell carcinomas: analysis from the IARC multinational case-control study. Int J Cancer 2006;118(9):2293–97.

La Vecchia C, Bidoli E, Barra S, D'Avanzo B, Negri E, Talamini R, et al. Type of cigarettes and cancers of the upper digestive and respiratory tract. Cancer Causes Control 1990; 1:69–74.

La Vecchia C, Tavani A, Franceschi S, Levi F, Corrao G, Negri E. Epidemiology and prevention of oral cancer. Oral Oncol 1997; 33:302–12.

Lee JW, Soung YH, Kim SY, Nam HK, Park WS, Nam SW, Kim MS, Sun DI, Lee YS, Jang JJ, Lee JY, Yoo NJ, Lee SH. Somatic mutations of EGFR gene in squamous cell carcinoma of the head and neck. Clin Cancer Res 2005 Apr 15;11(8):2879–82.

Leigh IM, Breuer JA, Buchanan JAG, Harwood CA, Jackson S, McGregor JM, et al. Human papilloma viruses and cancers of the skin and oral mucosa. In: Goedert JJ (Ed): Infectious Causes of Cancer: Targets for Intervention. Totowa, NJ, Humana Press, 2000, pp 289–309.

Lieber CS, Seitz HK, Garro AJ, Worner TM. Alcohol-related diseases and carcinogenesis. Cancer Res 1979;39:2844–50.

MacFarlane GJ, Zheng T, Marshall JR, Boffetta P, Niu S, Brasure J, et al. Alcohol, tobacco, diet and the risk of oral cancer: a pooled analysis of three case-control studies. Oral Oncol Eur J Cancer 1995;31B:181–87.

Maden C, Beckmann AM, Thomas DB, McKnight B, Sherman KJ, Ashley RL, et al. Human papillomaviruses, herpes simplex viruses and the risk of oral cancer in men. Am J Epidemiol 1992;135:1093–1102.

Marshall JR, Boyle P. Nutrition and oral cancer. Cancer Causes Control 1996;7:101–11.

Maserejian NN, Giovannucci E, Rosner B, Zavras A, Joshipura K. Prospective study of fruits and vegetables and risk of oral premalignant lesions in men. Am J Epidemiol 2006;164(6):556–66. Epub 2006 Jul 17.

McLaughlin JK, Gridley G, Block G, Winn DM, Preston-Martin S, Schoenberg JB, et al. Dietary factors in oral and pharyngeal cancer. J Natl Cancer Inst 1988;80:1237–43.

Merchant A, Husain SS, Hosain M, Fikree FF, Pitiphat W, Siddiqui AR, et al. Paan without tobacco: an independent risk factor for oral cancer. Int J Cancer 2000;86:128–31.

Merletti F, Boffetta P, Ciccone G, Mashberg A, Terracini B. Role of tobacco and alcoholic beverages in the etiology of cancer of the oral cavity/oropharynx in Torino, Italy. Cancer Res 1989;49:4919–24.

Merletti F, Boffeta P, Ferro G, Pisani P, Terracini B. Occupation and cancer of the oral cavity or oropharynx in Turin, Italy. Scand J Work Environ Health 1991;17:248–54.

Michalek AM, Mahoney MC, McLaughlin CC, Murphy D, Metzger BB. Historical and contemporary correlates of syphilis and cancer. Int J Epidemiol 1994;23:381–85.

Morita S, Yano M, Tsujinaka T, Akiyama Y, Taniguchi M, Kaneko K, et al. Genetic polymorphisms of drug-metabolizing enzymes and susceptibility to head-and-neck squamous-cell carcinoma. Int J Cancer 1999;80:685–88.

Morse DE, Katz RV, Pendrys DG, Holford TR, Krutchkoff DJ, Eisenberg E, et al. Mouthwash use and dentures in relation to oral epithelial dysplasia. Oral Oncol 1997;33:338–43.

Nagao T, Ikeda N, Warnakulasuriya S, Fukano H, Yuasa H, Yano M, et al. Serum antioxidant micronutrients and the risk of oral leukoplakia among Japanese. Oral Oncol 2000;36:466–70.

Negri E, Franceschi S, Bosetti C, Levi F, Conti E, Parpinel M, et al. Selected micronutrients and oral and pharyngeal cancer. Int J Cancer 2000;86:122–27.

Park NH, Sapp JP, Herbosa EG. Oral cancer induced in hamsters with herpes simplex infection and simulated snuff dipping. Oral Surg Oral Med Oral Pathol 1986;62:164–68.

Peters WH, Wobbes T, Roelofs HM, Jansen JB. Glutathione S-transferases in esophageal cancer. Carcinogenesis 1993;14:1377–80.

Prime SS, Thakker NS, Pring M, Guest PG, Paterson IC. A review of inherited cancer syndromes and their relevance to oral squamous cell carcinoma. Oral Oncol 2001;37:1–16.

Rappaport SM, McCartney MC, Wei ET. Volatilization of mutagens from beef during cooking. Cancer Lett 1979;8:139–45.

Rothman K, Keller A. The effect of joint exposure to alcohol and tobacco on risk of cancer of the mouth and pharynx. J Chronic Dis 1972;25:711–16.

Rothman KJ. Epidemiology of head and neck cancer. Laryngoscope 1978;88:435–38.

Sancho-Garnier H, Theobald S. Black (air-cured) and blond (flue-cured) tobacco and cancer risk II: Pharynx and larynx cancer. Eur J Cancer 1993;29A(2):273–76.

Sawant SS, Kandarkar SV. Role of vitamins C and E as chemopreventive agents in the hamster cheek pouch treated with the oral carcinogen-DMBA. Oral Dis 2000;6:241–47.

Schildt EB, Eriksson M, Hardell L, Magnuson A. Oral infections and dental factors in relation to oral cancer: a Swedish case-control study. Eur J Cancer Prev 1998;7:201–6.

Schlecht NF, Franco EL, Pintos J, Kowalski LP. Effect of smoking cessation and tobacco type on the risk of cancers of the upper aerodigestive tract in Brazil. Epidemiology 1999; 10(4):412–18.

Scully C, Field JK, Tanzawa H. Genetic aberrations in oral or head and neck squamous cell carcinoma (SCCHN): 1. Carcinogen metabolism, DNA repair and cell cycle control. Oral Oncol 2000;36:256–63.

Seitz HK, Poschl G, Simanowski UA. Alcohol and cancer. Recent Dev Alcohol 1998;14: 67–95. Review.

Shiboski CH, Shiboski SC, Silverman S Jr. Trends in oral cancer rates in the United States, 1973–1996. Commun Dent Oral Epidemiol 2000; 28:249–56.

Soler M, Bosetti C, Franceschi S, Negri E, Zambon P, Talamini R, et al. Fiber intake and the risk of oral, pharyngeal and esophageal cancer. Int J Cancer 2001;91:283–87.

Sorahan T, Parkes HG, Veys CA, Waterhouse JA, Straughan JK, Nutt A. Mortality in the British rubber industry 1946–85. Br J Ind Med 1989;46:1–10.

Stich HF, Rosin MP, Vallejera MO. Reduction with vitamin A and beta-carotene administration of proportion of micronucleated buccal mucosal cells in Asian betal nut and tobacco chewers. Lancet 1984;1:1204–6.

Straif K, Weiland SK, Bungers M, Holthenrich D, Taeger D, Yi S, et al. Exposure to high concentrations of nitrosamines and cancer mortality among a cohort of rubber workers. Occup Environ Med 2000;57:180–87.

Strange RC, Fryer AA. The glutathione S-transferases: influence of polymorphism on cancer susceptibility. IARC Sci Pub No. 148. Vinei P, Malats N, Lang M, d'Errico A, Caporaso N, Cuzick J, BOffetta P, Metabolic Polymorphisms and Susceptibility to Cancer. Lyon, International Agency for Research on Cancer, 1999, pp 231–49.

Talamini R, La Vecchia C, Levi F, Conti E, Favero A, Franceschi S. Cancer of the oral cavity and pharynx in nonsmokers who drink alcohol and in nondrinkers who smoke tobacco. J Natl Cancer Inst 1998;90:1901–3.

Teschke K, Hertzman C, Van Netten C, Lee E, Morrison B, Cornista A, et al. Potential exposure of cooks to airborne mutagens and carcinogens. Environ Res 1989;50:296–308.

Thomas SJ, Maclennan R. Slaked lime and betel nut cancer in Papua New Guinea. Lancet 1992;5:577–78.

Thongsuksai P, Boonyaphiphat P, Sriplung H, Sudhikaran W. p53 mutations in betel-associated oral cancer from Thailand. Cancer Lett 2003;201(1):1–7.

Tsai CH, Yang CC, Chou LS, Chou MY. The correlation between alteration of p16 gene and clinical status in oral squamous cell carcinoma. J Oral Pathol Med 2001;30(9): 527–31.

van der Eb MM, Leyten EM, Gavarasana S, Vandenbroucke JP, Kahn PM, Cleton FJ. Reverse smoking as a risk factor for palatal cancer: a cross-sectional study in rural Andhra Pradesh, India. Int J Cancer 1993;54: 754–58.

Weaver A, Fleming SM, Smith DB. Mouthwash and oral cancer: carcinogen or coincidence? J Oral Surg 1979;37:250–53.

Wight AJ, Ogden GR. Possible mechanisms by which alcohol may influence the development of oral cancer—a review. Oral Oncol 1998;34:441–47.

Willmore-Payne C, Holden JA, Chadwick BE, Layfield LJ. Detection of c-kit exons 11- and 17-activating mutations in testicular seminomas by high-resolution melting amplicon analysis. Mod Pathol 2006;19(9):1164–69. Epub 2006 Jun 2.

Winn DM, Blot WJ, Shy CM, Pickle LW, Toledo A, Fraumeni JF. Snuff dipping and oral cancer among women in the southern United States. N Engl J Med 1981;304:745–49.

World Cancer Research Fund in association with American Institute for Cancer Research. Food, Nutrition and the Prevention of Cancer: A Global Perspective. Washington, DC, American Institute for Cancer Research, 1997, pp 96–106.

Wynder EL, Kabat G, Rosenberg S, Levenstein M. Oral cancer and mouthwash use. J Natl Cancer Inst 1983;70:255–60.

Ye Z, Song H, Guo Y. Glutathione S-transferase M1, T1 status and the risk of head and neck cancer: a meta-analysis. J Med Genet 2004; 41(5):360–65.

Zheng TZ, Boyle P, Willett WC, Hu H, Dan J, Evstifeeva TV, et al. A case-control study of oral cancer in Beijing, People's Republic of China. Associations with nutrient intakes, foods and food groups. Eur J Cancer B Oral Oncol 1993;29B:45–55.

Zheng W, Blot WJ, Shu XO, Diamond EL, Gao YT, Ji BT, et al. Risk factors for oral and pharyngeal cancer in Shanghai, with emphasis on diet. Cancer Epidemiol Biomarkers Prev 1992;1:441–48.

Znaor A, Brennan P, Gajalakshmi V, Mathew A, Shanta V, Varghese C, Boffetta P. Independent and combined effects of tobacco smoking, chewing and alcohol drinking on the risk of oral, pharyngeal and esophageal cancers in Indian men. Int J Cancer. 2003; 105:681–86.

8

Nasopharyngeal Carcinoma

ELLEN CHANG AND HANS-OLOV ADAMI

Autopsy records show that nasopharyngeal carcinoma (NPC) was prevalent in China by the early twentieth century, and ancient Chinese medical literature describes a disease resembling NPC in existence several hundred years ago (Ho, 1976). Studies of ancient Egyptian mummies (Wells, 1963) and Iranian skulls (Krogman, 1940) also show bone changes that have been attributed to NPC. Hence, genetic and/or stable environmental risk factors may have persisted for centuries in NPC-endemic regions and populations.

A review of ancient Chinese literature revealed that the development of NPC was originally attributed to a deficiency of qi (life force or vital energy), stagnation of liver qi or blood flow, coldness in circulatory channels, coagulation of phlegm, or other elemental imbalances (Zhou and Tian, 2001). Correspondingly, preventive measures included nourishing the qi, regulating the emotions, and harmonizing the nutrient qi. As this chapter will reveal, there has been some progress in etiologic understanding of NPC since then. However, many aspects of NPC remain enigmatic, making this malignancy a true challenge for further epidemiologic study.

CLINICAL SYNOPSIS

Subgroups

NPC, a carcinoma arising in the epithelial lining of the nasopharynx (Fig. 8–1), comprises the vast majority of cancers of the nasopharynx. The World Health Organization subclassifies NPC into three histologic types: keratinizing squamous cell carcinoma (type I) and nonkeratinizing carcinoma, which includes differentiated (type II) and undifferentiated (type III) carcinomas. In high-incidence areas, nearly all NPC is of type III histology, and most of the remainder is type II (Zong et al, 1983; Yu and Henderson, 1996), whereas in low-incidence areas, 30%–50% of tumors are of type I histology (Vaughan et al, 1996).

Symptoms

Most NPC patients present with a cervical neck mass after the tumor has reached a

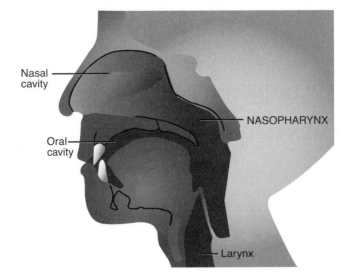

Figure 8–1. Anatomic location of the nasopharynx (Adapted from the Health Promotion Board, Singapore)

locally advanced disease stage with nodal involvement. Patients may also present with local symptoms such as nasal obstruction, bleeding, or discharge; serous otitis media; tinnitus; or conductive hearing loss. Symptoms of more advanced disease include cranial nerve palsy and neuropathies.

Diagnosis

Clinical examination is followed by computed tomography and magnetic resonance imaging of the head and neck area. An endoscopic examination and biopsy from the primary tumor are performed for definitive diagnosis; a chest radiograph, liver ultrasonograph, and bone scan are also indicated for evaluation of distant metastases.

Treatment

NPC is sensitive to both radiation therapy and chemotherapy. Early-stage NPC is currently treated with three-dimensional intensity-modulated radiotherapy, with a high probability of cure; locoregionally advanced disease is treated with combination chemotherapy and radiation therapy. Patients with distant metastases may be treated with chemotherapy alone or other palliative measures. Surgery is usually precluded by the tumor location in a deep anatomic location,

although surgery can be used for nodal dissection or excision in cases of persistent or recurrent regional nodal involvement.

Prognosis

In Hong Kong, 5-year relative survival for NPC at all stages is currently around 80% (Lee et al, 2005). Five-year relative survival is approximately 92% for stage I disease (based on the 1997 American Joint Committee on Cancer/International Union Against Cancer classification system), 87% for stage II, 81% for stage III, and 60% for stage IV. The 5-year relative survival rate for NPC in the US, based on data from 1992 through 2004, is 58% for all stages, and 80%, 60%, and 32% for localized, regional, and distant disease, respectively (SEER Program, 2007). Older age, male sex, type I (versus types II and III) histology, increased antibody titers against Epstein-Barr virus (EBV) antigens, and elevated circulating EBV DNA are also indicators of worse prognosis.

Progress

The responsiveness of NPC to both radiotherapy and chemotherapy distinguishes it from other head and neck cancers, which are typically insensitive to chemotherapy.

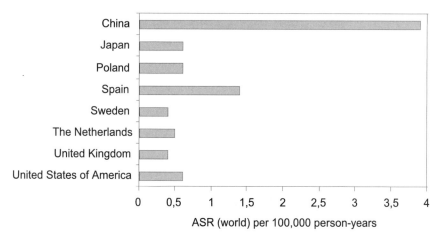

Figure 8–2. Age-standardized (to the 2000 world population) incidence rates of nasopharyngeal cancer among males. (*Source*: Ferlay et al, 2004)

Concomitant chemoradiotherapy has appreciably improved survival with NPC in recent years (Agulnik and Siu, 2005). Standardization of the staging system, as well as further clinical trials to evaluate the efficacy of newer chemotherapeutic agents and immunotherapy, will improve the precision of tailored therapy for different risk groups.

DESCRIPTIVE EPIDEMIOLOGY

Although NPC is a rare malignancy throughout most of the world, it is endemic in a few well-defined populations. In most regions, the age-standardized incidence rate of NPC for both males and females is below 1 per 100 000 person-years (Parkin et al, 2002) (Figs. 8–2 and 8–3). However, dramatically elevated rates are observed in the Cantonese population of southern China, and intermediate rates are observed in several indigenous populations in Southeast Asia, the Arctic region, North Africa, and the Middle East. Even within China, there is at least 50-fold variation in NPC incidence across regions, with rates generally increasing from northern China (eg, Beijing and Tianjin) to southern China (eg, Hong Kong) (Fig. 8–4). In 2002, approximately 80 000 incident cases of nasopharyngeal cancer were diagnosed worldwide and the estimated number of deaths exceeded 50 000, making it the 23rd most common new cancer in the world (Parkin et al, 2005); in contrast, NPC was the 4th most common new malignancy in Hong Kong.

In almost all populations surveyed, the incidence of NPC is two- to threefold higher in males than in females (Figs. 8–2 and 8–3). In most low-risk populations, NPC incidence rises monotonically with increasing age (Figs. 8–5 and 8–6). In contrast, in high-risk groups, the incidence peaks around ages 50–59 years and declines thereafter (Figs. 8–5 and 8–6), suggesting the involvement of exposure to carcinogenic agents early in life. Likewise, the minor incidence peak observed among adolescents and young adults in Southeast Asia, the Middle East/ North Africa, and the US is consistent with exposure to a common agent in early life.

Although geographic regions have generally been classified as high- or low-incidence areas, the racial/ethnic distribution of NPC within regions is far from uniform. In the southeastern Chinese province of Guangdong, where the overall NPC incidence rate is above 20 per 100 000 person-years among males, rates in Cantonese-speakers are double those in other dialect groups such as the Hakka, Hokkien, and Chiu Chau (Li et al, 1985). In Southeast Asia, NPC risk appears to vary with degree of racial and social admixture with southern Chinese. Incidence is low among Singapore Indians who have had practically no intermingling with Chinese,

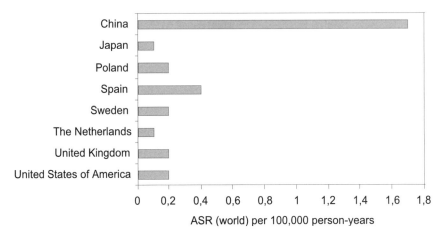

Figure 8–3. Age-standardized (to the 2000 world population) incidence rates of nasopharyngeal cancer among females. (*Source*: Ferlay et al, 2004)

but much higher in the Thai, Macaonese, and Malay indigenous populations, which have a history of intermarriage with Chinese ancestors (Ho, 1976). Close ties have existed between Japan and China for thousands of years—but mainly with northern China—and the incidence of NPC in Japan is low. NPC rates in the US are highest among Chinese Americans, followed distantly by Filipino Americans, then Japanese Americans, Blacks, Hispanics, and finally Whites (Burt et al, 1992).

Even when high- or intermediate-risk persons migrate to lower-risk countries, their incidence of NPC remains much higher than those of other races. Indeed, among southern Chinese living in Singapore, Malaysia, and Japan, NPC rates are comparable to those in natives of southern China (Sawaki et al, 1976; Devi et al, 2004; Seow et al, 2004). Likewise, NPC incidence is higher in North African migrants to Israel and their offspring than in native Israelis (Parkin and Iscovich, 1997). However, while the incidence of NPC among Chinese in the US remains 10 to 20 times higher than those among US Whites and Blacks, they are only about half as high as those observed in southern China (Parkin et al, 2002). A similar decline in risk has been described among Chinese migrants to the UK (Warnakulasuriya et al, 1999) and Australia (McCredie et al, 1999), where rates de-

crease with longer duration of residence. Conversely, risk of NPC increases among males of low-risk parentage born in China, the Philippines (Buell, 1973), or North Africa (Jeannel et al, 1993).

The apparent decline in NPC incidence among Chinese after migration to the West may be overestimated, since reported rates do not account for the inclusion of both high- and low-risk migrants in the source population. Because cancer registries generally do not record data on patients' ethnic subgroup, incidence rates of NPC in Chinese ethnic subgroups cannot be accurately estimated with existing data. Furthermore, migrants are a self-selected group and unlikely to be representative of the residents of their native country. Because certain aspects of a traditional Asian lifestyle are associated with elevated risk of NPC, individuals who migrate overseas may be an inherently lower-risk group. Thus, NPC incidence rates among migrants generally are not directly comparable to those among natives of their country of origin.

After several decades of high rates in Hong Kong, NPC incidence has declined steadily since the 1970s (Lee et al, 2003). A recent study found that the decrease was limited primarily to type I NPC, whereas the rates of types II and III NPC remained relatively stable between 1998 and 2002 (Tse et al, 2006). In Taiwan, NPC incidence has

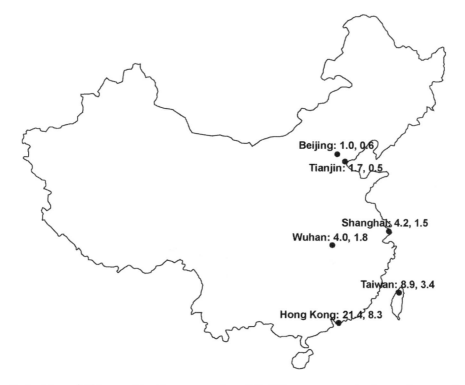

Figure 8–4. Map of China and incidence rates (per 100,000 person-years) of nasopharyngeal cancer among males and females, respectively, in selected areas, 1993–1997. (*Source*: Parkin et al, 2002)

decreased since the early 1980s (Hsu et al, 2006), and in Singapore Chinese it appears to be starting a downturn since the late 1990s (Seow et al, 2004). The lag in incidence trends may be attributable to differences in the timing of the onset of rapid economic development, which occurred in the mid-1940s in Hong Kong, the 1950s in Taiwan, and in the 1960s in Singapore. In contrast, the incidence rate of NPC was unchanged between 1978 and 2002 among males and females in the less developed county of Sihui in southeastern China, and increased slightly among males, while holding steady among females, in nearby Cangwu county between 1983 and 2002 (Jia et al, 2006). Between 1973 and 1999, the incidence rate of NPC in the US remained stable at around 0.7 per 100 000 person-years overall (Lee and Ko, 2005). However, in Chinese residents of California, the incidence of type I, but not types II or III, NPC

decreased significantly between 1992 and 2002 in males only (Sun et al, 2005). Of note, no increasing trend in NPC incidence has been noted in parallel with the onset of the HIV epidemic.

GENETIC AND MOLECULAR EPIDEMIOLOGY

Inherited Susceptibility

Familial susceptibility to NPC is well established. In epidemiologic studies, the excess risk of NPC is generally 4- to 10-fold among individuals with a first-degree relative with NPC, compared to those without such a family history (Zeng and Jia, 2002). However, inherited cancer syndromes are not presumed to account for a high proportion of cases. Rather, common genetic variation, particularly in genes that play a role in the immune response to EBV infection or the metabolism of environmental

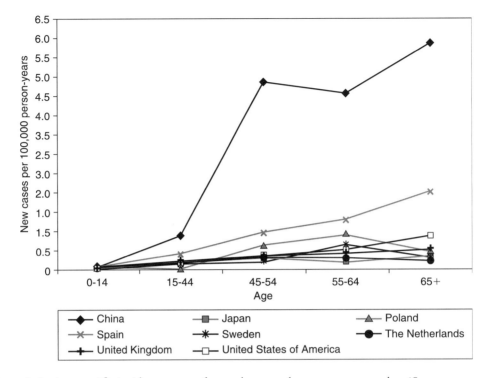

Figure 8–5. Age-specific incidence rates of nasopharyngeal cancer among males. (*Source*: Ferlay et al, 2004)

carcinogens, is likely to be an important factor in NPC development.

High-penetrance Gene Mutations

Familial aggregation of NPC has been widely documented in high-, intermediate-, and low-incidence populations (Zeng and Jia, 2002). For example, 15 of 109 family members across four generations of a southern Chinese family have developed NPC, and two cases of hepatocellular carcinoma and one case of breast cancer have also occurred (Zhang and Zhang, 1999). However, familial clustering does not explain the majority of cases, and a complex segregation analysis of familial NPC in southern China concluded that multiple genetic and environmental factors, rather than a single major susceptibility gene, are most likely to explain the observed pattern of inheritance (Jia et al, 2005). The increased risk of cancers of the salivary gland and uterine cervix in family members of NPC cases (Albeck et al, 1993; Friborg et al, 2005) suggests that relatives may share genetic susceptibility to virus-associated malignancies.

An excess of NPC has not been observed in any of the known inherited cancer syndromes (Garber and Offit, 2005). Some studies have detected an association between polymorphic variation in the *TP53* tumor-suppressor gene and risk of NPC (Birgander et al, 1996; Tsai et al, 2002; Tiwawech et al, 2003), although results are not entirely consistent (Yung et al, 1997).

Low-penetrance Gene Mutations

The human leukocyte antigen (*HLA*) genes encode proteins required for the presentation of foreign antigens, including viral peptides, to the immune system for targeted lysis. Since virtually all NPC tumors contain EBV, individuals who inherit *HLA* alleles with a reduced ability to present EBV antigens may have an increased risk of developing NPC, whereas individuals with

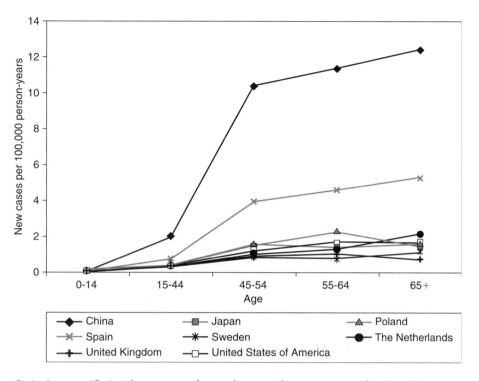

Figure 8–6. Age-specific incidence rates of nasopharyngeal cancer among females. (*Source*: Ferlay et al, 2004)

HLA alleles that present EBV efficiently may have a lower risk (Simons et al, 1975). Some *HLA* alleles have been consistently associated with NPC risk. In southern Chinese and other Asian populations, *HLA-A2-B46* and *B17* were generally associated with a two- to threefold increase in NPC risk (Simons et al, 1974; Simons et al, 1978). In contrast, 30%–50% lower risk of NPC was found in association with *HLA-A11* in both Chinese and Whites (Simons et al, 1978; Burt et al, 1996); *B13* in Chinese (Chan et al, 1983); and *A2* in Whites (Burt et al, 1994).

In a meta-analysis of studies in southern Chinese populations, the combined evidence suggested a positive association of NPC risk with *HLA-A2, B14,* and *B46,* and an inverse association with *HLA-A11, B13,* and *B22* (Goldsmith et al, 2002). In a linkage study, a gene closely linked to the *HLA* locus conferred a 21-fold excess risk of NPC (Lu et al, 1990); a separate study mapped an NPC susceptibility locus to a region near *HLA-A* (Lu et al, 2005). Reported associations between NPC risk and other *HLA* genes, including class II alleles, must be interpreted with caution due to the probability of chance findings due to multiple comparisons.

Genetic variation in genes involved in metabolism of nitrosamines, tobacco, and other contaminants may also influence NPC risk. Polymorphisms in cytochrome P450 2E1 (*CYP2E1*) (Hildesheim et al, 1995; Hildesheim et al, 1997; Kongruttanachok et al, 2001) and *CYP2A6* (Tiwawech et al, 2005) and the absence of glutathione S-transferase M1 (*GSTM1*) (Nazar-Stewart et al, 1999; Deng et al, 2004; Tiwawech et al, 2005) and/or *GSTT1* (Deng et al, 2004) were associated with two- to fivefold increased risk of NPC. In Taiwan, a variant of *CYP2E1* was evenly distributed between familial and nonfamilial NPC cases (Ung et al, 1999), with no association between NPC risk and genetic polymorphisms in *CYP1A1, GSTM1, GSTT1, GSTP1*, or N-acetyltransferase 2 (*NAT2*) (Cheng et al, 2003). Among Cantonese subjects, no association was found with genetic variation in *CYP2A13* (Jiang et al, 2004).

In Thailand (Hirunsatit et al, 2003) and China (Fan et al, 2005), polymorphisms in the polymeric immunoglobulin receptor (*PIGR*), a cell surface receptor proposed to mediate EBV entry into the nasal epithelium, were associated with two- to threefold increased risk of NPC. In addition, polymorphisms in the X-ray repair complementing gene 1 (*XRCC1*) were associated with 20%–50% lower risk of NPC in Taiwan (Cho et al, 2003) and southern China (Cao et al, 2006), whereas genetic variation in another DNA-repair gene, human 8-oxoguanine DNA glycosylase 1 (*hOGG1*), was associated with 60% increased NPC risk in Taiwan (Cho et al, 2003). Other genes in the DNA repair pathway, including protein kinase, DNA-activated, catalytic polypeptide (*PRKDC*), proliferating cell nuclear antigen (*PCNA*), and checkpoint kinase 1 (*CHEK1*), were also consistently overexpressed in NPC compared to normal nasopharyngeal tissue (Dodd et al, 2006). These results, and the additional finding of an enhanced inverse association of NPC risk with an *XRCC1* variant genotype among Cantonese smokers (Cao et al, 2006), invoke a possible role of these genes in repair of DNA damage caused by reactive intermediates during the metabolism of nitrosamines and other carcinogens in NPC development. Gene and protein expression profiling (Fung et al, 2000; Xie et al, 2000; Guo et al, 2002) and genome-wide scans in families with multiple NPC cases—approaches that identified putative susceptibility loci on chromosomes 4p15.1–q12 (Feng et al, 2002) and 3p21.31–21.2 (Xiong et al, 2004)—offer further means of identifying susceptibility genes or loci.

Somatic Mutations and Epigenetic Changes

Studies of loss of heterozygosity in NPC tumors detected a high frequency of allelic loss, especially on chromosomes 3p, 9p, 11q, 13q, and 14q (Mutirangura et al, 1997; Chen et al, 1999; Hui et al, 1999); such findings suggest that tumor-suppressor genes at these loci may be involved in NPC development. A recent meta-analysis of comparative genomic hybridization results revealed several genomic hot spots where chromosomal losses and gains have consistently been detected in NPC tumors (Li X et al, 2006).

Somatic mutations of tumor-suppressor genes, such as *TP53, pRb, p16*, and *VHL*, appear to be infrequent in NPC (Zeng and Jia, 2002). However, promoter hypermethylation of tumor-suppressor genes—such as Ras association domain family 1A (*RASSF1A*) (Lo et al, 2001; Chang et al, 2003), cyclin-dependent kinase inhibitor 2A (*CDKN2A, p16/INK4A*) (Lo et al, 1996; Chang et al, 2003), and immunoglobulin superfamily member 4 (*IGSF4, TSLC1*) (Hui et al, 2003; Lung et al, 2004)—appears to be another means of inactivating gatekeeper genes in NPC tumors.

RISK FACTORS

Tobacco and Other Smoke

The International Agency for Research on Cancer (IARC) panel concluded that there is sufficient evidence that tobacco smoking causes cancers of the nasopharynx in humans (IARC, 2004). However, it is unclear whether tobacco smoking affects the development of both endemic and nonendemic NPC. The majority of case-control studies examining cigarette smoking and risk of NPC in a variety of populations, especially those conducted more recently, reported an increased risk of two- to sixfold (Cheng et al, 1999; Armstrong et al, 2000; Yuan et al, 2000), although other studies found no association (Yu et al, 1986; Sriamporn et al, 1992; Zheng et al, 1994). Likewise, reports of a positive association between exposure to secondhand smoke at home and risk of NPC (Yu et al, 1988; Armstrong et al, 2000; Yuan et al, 2000) were countered by studies with null findings (Yu et al, 1990; Cheng et al, 1999). The discrepancy in findings may be due in part to differences in study design and/or exposure assessment, as well as study population; several of the studies reporting a positive association were conducted in low- or intermediate-incidence populations (Lanier et al, 1980; Nam et al, 1992; West et al, 1993; Vaughan et al, 1996).

In one US study, an estimated two-thirds of type I NPC was attributable to smoking, but risk of type II or III NPC was not associated with smoking (Vaughan et al, 1996). Thus, the declining prevalence of smoking may explain the recent decreasing trend in the incidence of type I NPC in the US (Sun et al, 2005) and Hong Kong (Tse et al, 2006). Nevertheless, any excess risk of NPC attributable to smoking would be an order of magnitude lower than the excess risk of lung cancer and other respiratory tract malignancies (IARC, 2004).

Some researchers have suggested that the high incidence of NPC in southern Chinese and North Africans is caused by smoke from wood fires in chimneyless homes (Dobson, 1924; Clifford, 1972). However, chimneyless homes are also found in northern China and other regions with a low incidence of NPC (Ho, 1972; Pandey et al, 1989). In two studies in China (Yao et al, 1987; Zheng et al, 1994), NPC cases were up to five times more likely to be exposed to domestic wood fire than controls, but others found no such association (Yu et al, 1986; Yu et al, 1988; Yu et al, 1990). Studies examining burning incense or antimosquito coils and risk of NPC have been similarly equivocal, with two studies finding up to a sixfold excess risk with use of antimosquito coils (Shanmugaratnam et al, 1978; West et al, 1993), and one finding a higher risk among individuals with religious altars at home (Geser et al, 1978), but most studies finding no association (Yu et al, 1986; Yu et al, 1988; Yu et al, 1990).

Diet

Dietary consumption of Chinese-style salted fish is an established cause of NPC, and intake of traditional Asian pickled vegetables is considered a possible cause (IARC, 1993). The early observation that Cantonese boat-dwelling fishermen and their families were at increased risk of NPC led to the hypothesis that their traditional diet, consisting heavily of dried, salted fish, was responsible for their excess risk (Ho, 1976). Although several studies have substantiated a positive association between consumption of salt-preserved fish and NPC risk, whereas intake of fresh fruits and vegetables appears to decrease NPC risk, other dietary factors—including other individual foods and food groups, macronutrients, and micronutrients—have not been well studied in relation to NPC risk.

Salt-preserved Fish and Other Foods

The exposure most consistently and strongly associated with risk of NPC is consumption of salt-preserved fish. In studies of Chinese populations, the relative risk of NPC associated with weekly consumption, compared to no or rare consumption, generally ranged from 1.4 to 3.2, while that for daily consumption ranged from 1.8 to 7.5 (Henderson and Louie, 1978; Yu et al, 1986; Yu et al, 1989). NPC risk is also elevated in association with other preserved food items, including meats, eggs, fruits, and vegetables, in southern Chinese, Southeast Asians, North Africans/Middle Easterners, and Arctic natives (Lanier et al, 1980; Jeannel et al, 1990; Armstrong et al, 1998; Yuan et al, 2000), as well as in low-incidence northern Chinese (Ning et al, 1990) and the US population (excluding type I NPC) (Farrow et al, 1998). A meta-analysis of studies in China, Southeast Asia, and North Africa found that high versus low preserved vegetable intake was associated with a twofold increase in NPC risk (Gallicchio et al, 2006). Salt-preserved foods are a dietary staple in all NPC-endemic populations; hence, this traditional dietary pattern may explain part of the international distribution of NPC incidence.

In southern China, intake of salted fish and other preserved foods is particularly high among boat-dwelling fishermen and their families, known as Tankas—the population subgroup at highest risk of developing NPC (Ho, 1976). Traditionally, the Tankas have used salt to preserve their fish during extended periods offshore, and prefer to eat salted fish while selling their more profitable fresh catch. Salted fish is also a traditional weaning food, resulting in early and frequent feeding of infants (Ho, 1976)—especially in the Cantonese population (Yu et al, 1989) and in families of lower socioeconomic status (Armstrong and Eng, 1983; Yu et al, 1986). Childhood exposure, especially at weaning, appears more strongly related to NPC risk than adulthood exposure. Furthermore, increasing duration and frequency of consumption are independently associated with elevated risk of NPC. Comparing persons who were weaned on salt-preserved fish to those who were not, the relative risk of NPC ranged from 1.7 to 7.5 (Armstrong et al, 1983; Yu et al, 1986; Chen et al, 1988; Yu et al, 1989).

The carcinogenic potential of salt-preserved fish is supported by experiments in rats, which develop malignant nasal and nasopharyngeal tumors after salted-fish consumption (Huang et al, 1978). The process of salt-preservation is inefficient, allowing fish and other foods to become partially putrefied (Ho, 1972). As a result, these foods accumulate significant levels of nitrosamines, which are demonstrated carcinogens in animals (IARC, 1993). Salt-preserved fish also contains bacterial mutagens, direct genotoxins, and EBV-reactivating substances, any or all of which could also contribute to the observed association.

Fresh Fruits and Vegetables

In contrast to preserved foods, frequent consumption of fresh fruits and/or vegetables, especially during childhood (Yu et al, 1989), has been associated with a lower risk of NPC (Armstrong et al, 1998; Ward et al, 2000; Yuan et al, 2000). In a meta-analysis of sixteen studies, high versus low fresh vegetable intake was associated with a 36% lower risk of NPC (Gallicchio et al, 2006). Some studies found inverse associations with intake of specific fruits or vegetables—including carrots (Ning et al, 1990; Arm-

strong et al, 1998), Chinese flowering cabbage (Armstrong et al, 1998), green leafy vegetables (Zheng YM et al, 1994), fresh soybean products (Ward et al, 2000), and citrus fruit, oranges, or tangerines (Armstrong et al, 1998; Farrow et al, 1998; Yuan et al, 2000)—or with dietary intake of vitamin E (Lee et al, 1994) or C (Farrow et al, 1998), or serum levels of carotene (Clifford, 1972). The apparent protective effect of fruits and vegetables has been attributed to antioxidant effects, prevention of nitrosamine formation, and other anticarcinogenic properties.

Alcohol

Alcohol consumption also appears not to be associated with NPC risk, since most (Chen et al, 1990; Sriamporn et al, 1992; Zheng et al, 1994; Cheng et al, 1999), but not all (Vaughan et al, 1996; Armstrong et al, 1998), case-control studies were negative.

Reproductive Factors

There is no evidence of a role for reproductive factors in the etiology of NPC.

Hormones and Hormone Receptors

There is no evidence of a role for hormones in the etiology of NPC, although the two- to threefold higher risk in men suggests a sex-based contribution to risk.

Anthropometric Measures

There is no evidence of a role for anthropometric measures in the etiology of NPC.

Infections

There is sufficient evidence that the Epstein-Barr virus (EBV) plays a causal role in NPC (IARC, 1997), while the etiologic role of other infectious agents is uncertain. The involvement of EBV in NPC has been postulated since 1966, when NPC patients were found to express antibodies against an antigen later identified as that of EBV (Old et al, 1966). This finding was confirmed in 1970, when anti-EBV antibodies were observed to be higher in NPC patients than in controls (Henle et al, 1970). Subsequently, a large body of laboratory, clinical, and epidemiologic research on the etiologic role of EBV in NPC has accumulated, although the precise role of the virus in NPC causation remains to be elucidated.

Epstein-Barr Virus

The ubiquitous EBV infects and persists latently in over 90% of the world's population, with infection usually occurring subclinically in childhood (Rickinson and Kieff, 2001). Because children in NPC-endemic areas are typically infected during infancy or early childhood (Kangro et al, 1994), very early infection with EBV may play a critical role in NPC development. NPC patients have elevated immunoglobulin G (IgG) and IgA antibody titers to the EBV viral capsid antigen (VCA) and early antigen (EA), as well as increased IgG against the latent viral nuclear antigens 1 and 2 (EBNA-1, EBNA-2) and neutralizing antibodies against EBV-specific DNase (Henderson et al, 1977; Lin et al, 1977; de Thé et al, 1978).

Moreover, these antibody titers, especially of IgA, precede tumor development by 1 to 2 years (Lanier et al, 1980; Levine et al, 1981; Chen et al, 1985) and are correlated with tumor burden, remission, and recurrence (Henle et al, 1973; de Schryver et al, 1974; Chan et al, 1979). Based on these patterns, anti-VCA IgA is now established as a screening test for NPC in high-risk populations (Zeng et al, 1985), particularly in combination with anti-EBV DNase antibodies (Chien et al, 2001). More recently, circulating cell-free EBV DNA has been detected in a higher proportion of NPC patients than controls, and levels are correlated with disease stage and prognosis (Nawroz et al, 1996; Mutirangura et al, 1998).

EBV is further linked to the development of NPC through EBV DNA, RNA, and/or gene products in tumor cells of virtually all cases, regardless of geographic origin (zur Hausen et al, 1970; Desgranges et al, 1975), although EBV detection in type I NPC has not always been consistent (Niedobitek et al, 1991). Because the EBV episome is identical in every tumor cell—as assessed by

the number of terminal repeats in the latent, circularized form of the virus in NPC tumors (Raab-Traub and Flynn, 1986)—NPC may originate from a single progenitor cell infected with EBV prior to clonal expansion. Clonal EBV has also been detected in severe dysplasia or carcinoma in situ of the nasopharynx (Pathmanathan et al, 1995), indicating a role for the virus in the early stages of tumor progression.

Considerable research has been directed toward determining whether at least part of the international pattern of NPC incidence can be explained by the distribution of different EBV strains. Compared to the prototype B95–8 EBV strain, consistent nucleotide variation in the amino terminus of the oncogenic viral latent membrane protein 1 (LMP1), including the loss of a *Xho*I restriction site, has been detected in EBV in NPC tumors from southern and northern Chinese, Malays, Alaska natives, and some US Caucasians, but not northern Africans (Tsao et al, 2002). Other types of sequence variation in the LMP1 carboxy terminus—including the number of copies of 33-base pair (bp) repeat element, a 15-bp insertion in the third repeat element, and a 30-bp deletion in the carboxy terminus—have repeatedly been detected in Chinese NPC tumors (Tsao et al, 2002).

The 30-bp deletion, detected also in a proportion of Alaska native, Caucasian, Malaysian, and North African NPC, appears to enhance the transforming potential of LMP1 in vitro, and may be present in more aggressive disease forms (Chen et al, 1992; Hu et al, 1993). However, there is no strong evidence that the deleted variant is associated with increased risk of NPC (Sandvej et al, 1997; Edwards et al, 1999), and large, well-designed epidemiologic studies of strain variation are lacking. Furthermore, the detection of specific LMP1 mutations in NPC tumors from high-, intermediate-, and low-incidence areas suggests that EBV strain variation is not geographically correlated with NPC incidence.

Infectious mononucleosis, a manifestation of late-childhood or young-adulthood infection with EBV, has not been well studied in relation to NPC, perhaps because late infection with EBV is rare in areas with high NPC incidence. One US study found that a history of infectious mononucleosis decreased the risk of NPC by 60%, although the association was not statistically significant (Vaughan et al, 1996). Another case-control study of US males also reported a nonsignificant 60% decrease in NPC risk among individuals with infectious mononucleosis at least 5 years before NPC diagnosis (or interview, for controls). In contrast, those diagnosed with infectious mononucleosis less than 5 years before the reference date had a nonsignificant increase in NPC risk of more than fourfold (Levine et al, 1998).

Other Infections

Human papillomavirus DNA has been detected in a minority of type I NPC tumors, but rarely in types II and III NPC (Hording et al, 1994; Giannoudis et al, 1995). There is no apparent excess of NPC incidence among AIDS patients (Melbye et al, 1996).

Most studies investigating prior chronic ear, nose, throat, and lower respiratory tract conditions found that they approximately doubled the risk of NPC (Yu et al, 1988; Yu et al, 1990; Yuan et al. 2000). These findings suggest that benign inflammation and infection of the respiratory tract may render the nasopharyngeal mucosa more susceptible to development of NPC. In addition, some bacteria can reduce nitrate to nitrite, which can then form carcinogenic N-nitroso compounds.

Physical Activity

There is no evidence of a role for physical activity in the etiology of NPC.

Ionizing Radiation

There is no evidence of a role for ionizing radiation in the etiology of NPC. A case-control study set in a high background-radiation area in China found that radiation exposure was not associated with NPC risk, and that risk factors for NPC were the same there as in other regions (Zou et al, 2000).

Occupation

The IARC panel found sufficient evidence to conclude that formaldehyde is a nasopharyngeal carcinogen in humans (Cogliano et al, 2005), whereas the evidence for wood dust is suggestive but inconclusive (IARC, 1995). Because specific occupational exposures tend to be uncommon in the general population, they are unlikely to account for a substantial proportion of NPC, especially in endemic areas.

Formaldehyde

Workplace exposure to formaldehyde has been examined in several studies of NPC, chiefly in low-incidence regions. An association with NPC is supported by experiments in rodents, which can develop squamous cell carcinomas of the nasal cavity after prolonged, high-level exposure to formaldehyde vapors (Swenberg et al, 1980; Albert et al, 1982). However, epidemiologic evidence in humans is limited, especially for endemic types II and III, and the majority of studies do not support a causal role of formaldehyde in NPC (Collins et al, 1997).

In a historical cohort of over 25 000 employees at 10 US facilities that produced or used formaldehyde, workers experienced a significant excess of NPC (Blair et al, 1986; Hauptmann et al, 2004). However, the positive association was driven by the findings at a single plant where five of the nine observed NPC deaths occurred, whereas there was no excess risk in the remaining nine plants (Marsh et al, 1996; Marsh et al, 2002, Marsh and Youk, 2005). Thus, occupational or nonoccupational exposures other than formaldehyde may have been responsible for the observed excess NPC mortality.

Dust

Specific types of dust have also been examined in association with NPC risk. Several studies, with some exceptions, found that risk of NPC was elevated among wood workers and other individuals potentially exposed to wood dust, with positive dose-response trends in accordance with longer duration and higher average or cumulative exposure to wood products (IARC, 1995). In three studies from China, textile workers, who typically have heavy exposure to cotton dust, were at significantly increased risk of NPC (Ng, 1986; Zheng et al, 1992; Li et al, 2006), especially with long-term employment or high estimated cumulative exposure. Like wood dust, cotton dust may promote NPC development through irritation and inflammation of the nasopharynx, either directly or via bacterial endotoxins in cotton dust (Lane et al, 2004). In contrast, investigators who found that NPC risk was 70% lower in workers exposed to cotton dust suggested that endotoxins could have a protective effect by potentiating an antitumor immune response (Yu et al, 1990)

Other exposures
Occupational exposure to industrial heat (Armstrong et al, 2000) or combustion products (Yu et al, 1990) more than doubled the risk of NPC, although these categories may encompass different exposures. Similarly, the excess of NPC incidence or mortality observed among welders (Lam and Tan, 1984; Zheng et al, 1992), furnacemen, boiler firemen, smiths and forging-press operators, bakers, metal workers (Zheng et al, 1992), and restaurant waitstaff (Yu et al, 2004) may be due to shared exposure to heat and fumes, or to disparate exposures. Three studies reported an excess risk of NPC among printing workers (Roush et al, 1987; Liu et al, 2002; Li et al, 2006), but did not identify specific inks, solvents, or other substances that could be responsible for the association. Although an excess risk of NPC has been observed among agricultural workers (Lam and Tan, 1984; Ng, 1986; Sriamporn et al, 1992), studies assessing overall use of pesticides found no association with NPC risk (West et al, 1993; Zou et al, 2000; Zhu et al, 2002; Li et al, 2006).

Medical Conditions and Treatment

Other than chronic ear, nose, throat, and lower respiratory tract conditions, there is no evidence of a role for other medical conditions in the etiology of NPC.

In Asian populations, several case-control studies reported a two- to fourfold excess risk of NPC in association with use of traditional herbal medicines (Shanmugaratnam et al, 1978; Hildesheim et al, 1992; West et al, 1993; Zheng et al, 1994, although others found no association (Yu et al, 1986; Yu et al, 1988; Yu et al, 1989). Any association with use of herbal drugs may be difficult to disentangle from other aspects of a traditional lifestyle, such as diet. A role of Chinese herbal plants in NPC development is, however, biologically plausible because several such commonly used plants can induce viral lytic antigen expression by activating EBV in vitro (Hirayama and Ito, 1981; Zeng et al, 1983).

In addition, EBV-inducers were detected in extracts of soils, as well as some vegetables grown in these soils, from areas in southern China where NPC is endemic (Zeng et al, 1984). Although use of certain EBV-inducing herbs of the Euphorbiaceae family was not associated with risk in southern China (Yu et al, 1986; Yu et al, 1988; Yu et al, 1990), use of other specific EBV-inducing herbal drugs has not been examined in relation to NPC risk. In the Philippines, use of any herbal medicines was associated with elevated NPC risk, especially among those who used herbal drugs and had high anti-EBNA antibody titers (Hildesheim et al, 1992), suggesting a direct proliferative effect of herbal medicines on EBV-transformed cells.

Other Risk Factors

Betel nut (*Areca catechu*) is an intoxicating stimulant commonly chewed in parts of Asia. In Taiwan, habitual chewing of betel nut for at least 20 years was associated with 70% higher risk of NPC in families with at least two affected members (West et al, 1993), whereas a study in the Philippines found no such association with overall NPC (Jeng et al, 2001). Although betel nut chewing is consistently associated with increased risk of oral cancer (Parkin et al, 2002), its role in NPC, if any, is unclear.

An ecologic study in southern China found two- to threefold higher trace levels

Table 8–1. Risk factors and preventive factors for nasopharyngeal carcinoma

Risk factor	Protective factor
Established	Established
Epstein-Barr virus	None
Salt-preserved fish	
Family history of NPC	
Human leukocyte antigen (*HLA*) class I genotypes	
Possible	Possible
Other preserved foods	Fresh fruits and vegetables
Tobacco smoke	Antioxidant micronutrients
Chronic respiratory tract conditions	*HLA* class I genotypes
Insufficient	
Other inhalants	
Herbal medicines	
Formaldehyde	
Occupational dusts	

HLA class II genotypes

of nickel in the rice, drinking water, and hairs of individuals living in a county with high NPC incidence, compared to those in a low-incidence county (Li et al, 1983). Furthermore, nickel levels were higher in NPC cases than controls in the high-incidence county. Likewise, nickel, zinc, and cadmium content in the drinking water of another high-incidence region was higher than that in the water of a low-incidence area, and nickel levels in drinking water were correlated with NPC mortality (Xia et al, 1988). A map-based ecologic study in China showed a geographical correlation between NPC mortality and low soil levels of the alkaline elements magnesium, calcium, and strontium (Bolviken et al, 1997), as well as high soil levels of radioactive thorium and uranium (Bolviken, 2000). All of these findings regarding a possible role of trace elements in NPC incidence or mortality remain to be confirmed in analytic epidemiologic studies.

CONCLUSION

The distinctive racial/ethnic and geographic distribution of NPC worldwide suggests that both environmental factors and genetic traits contribute to its development. Well-established risk factors for NPC include elevated antibody titers against the EBV,

consumption of salt-preserved fish, a family history of NPC, and certain *HLA* class I genotypes (Table 8–1). Consumption of other preserved foods, tobacco smoking, and a history of chronic respiratory tract conditions may be associated with elevated NPC risk, whereas consumption of fresh fruits and vegetables and other *HLA* genotypes may be associated with decreased risk. Evidence for a causal role of various inhalants, herbal medicines, and occupational exposures is inconsistent. Other than dietary modification, no concrete preventive measures for NPC exist. To date, there have been virtually no prospective studies of environmental risk factors, other than EBV, in NPC-endemic areas, nor have there been any large, strictly population-based case-control studies of gene-environment interactions in southern China. Comprehending how viral, genetic, and environmental factors interact to cause NPC will illuminate the pathways by which this malignancy—a model for a chronic disease caused by genes, environment, and an infectious agent—develops, as well as how it may be prevented.

REFERENCES

Agulnik M, Siu LL. State-of-the-art management of nasopharyngeal carcinoma: current and future directions. Br J Cancer 2005;92:799–806.

Albeck H, Bentzen J, et al. Familial clusters of nasopharyngeal carcinoma and salivary gland carcinomas in Greenland natives. Cancer 1993;72:196–200.

Albert RE, Sellakumar AR, et al. Gaseous formaldehyde and hydrogen chloride induction of nasal cancer in the rat. J Natl Cancer Inst 1982; 68:597–603.

Armstrong RW, Armstrong, MJ, et al. Salted fish and inhalants as risk factors for nasopharyngeal carcinoma in Malaysian Chinese. Cancer Res 1983; 43:2967–70.

Armstrong RW, Eng AC. Salted fish and nasopharyngeal carcinoma in Malaysia. Soc Sci Med 1983;17:1559–67.

Armstrong RW, Imrey PB, et al. Nasopharyngeal carcinoma in Malaysian Chinese: salted fish and other dietary exposures. Int J Cancer 1998;77:228–35.

Armstrong RW, Imrey PB, et al. Nasopharyngeal carcinoma in Malaysian Chinese: occupational exposures to particles, formaldehyde and heat. Int J Epidemiol 2000;29: 991–98.

Birgander R Sjalander A, et al. p53 polymorphisms and haplotypes in nasopharyngeal cancer. Hum Hered 1996;46:49–54.

Blair A, Stewart P, et al. Mortality among industrial workers exposed to formaldehyde. J Natl Cancer Inst 1986;76:1071–84.

Bolviken B. Relationships between nasopharyngeal carcinoma and radioactive elements in soils in China. Med Hypotheses 2000;55: 513–16.

Bolviken B, Flaten TP, et al. Relations between nasopharyngeal carcinoma and magnesium and other alkaline earth elements in soils in China. Med Hypotheses 1997;48:21–25.

Buell P. Race and place in the etiology of nasopharyngeal cancer: a study based on California death certificates. Int J Cancer 1973;11: 268–72.

Burt RD, Vaughan TL, et al. Descriptive epidemiology and survival analysis of nasopharyngeal carcinoma in the United States. Int J Cancer 1992; 52:549–56.

Burt RD, Vaughan TL, et al. Associations between human leukocyte antigen type and nasopharyngeal carcinoma in Caucasians in the United States. Cancer Epidemiol Biomarkers Prev 1996;5:879–87.

Burt RD, Vaughan TL, et al. A protective association between the HLA-A2 antigen and nasopharyngeal carcinoma in US Caucasians. Int J Cancer 1994; 56:465–67.

Cao YX, Miao XP, et al. Polymorphisms of XRCC1 genes and risk of nasopharyngeal carcinoma in the Cantonese population. BMC Cancer 2006;6:167.Chan SH, Day NE, et al. HLA and nasopharyngeal carcinoma in Chinese—a further study. Int J Cancer 1983; 32:171–76.

Chan SH, Levine PH, et al. A comparison of the prognostic value of antibody-dependent lymphocyte cytotoxicity and other EBV antibody assays in Chinese patients with nasopharyngeal carcinoma. Int J Cancer 1979;23: 181–85.

Chang HW, Chan A, et al. Evaluation of hypermethylated tumor suppressor genes as tumor markers in mouth and throat rinsing fluid, nasopharyngeal swab and peripheral blood of nasopharygeal carcinoma patient. Int J Cancer 2003;105:851–55.

Chen C-J, Chen J-Y, et al. Epidemiological characteristics and early detection of nasopharyngeal carcinoma in Taiwan. In: Wolf GT, Carey TE (Eds): Head and Neck Oncology Research. Amsterdam, Kugler Publications, 1988, pp 505–13.

Chen CJ, Liang KY, et al. Multiple risk factors of nasopharyngeal carcinoma: Epstein-Barr virus, malarial infection, cigarette smoking and familial tendency. Anticancer Res 1990; 10(2B):547–53.

Chen J. Y., Hwang LY, et al. Antibody response to Epstein-Barr-virus-specific DNase in 13 patients with nasopharyngeal carcinoma in Taiwan: a retrospective study. J Med Virol 1985;16:99–105.

Chen ML, Tsai CN, et al. Cloning and characterization of the latent membrane protein (LMP) of a specific Epstein-Barr virus variant derived from the nasopharyngeal carcinoma in the Taiwanese population. Oncogene 1992;7:2131–40.

Chen YJ, Ko JY, et al. Chromosomal aberrations in nasopharyngeal carcinoma analyzed by comparative genomic hybridization. Genes Chromosomes Cancer 1999;25:169–75.

Cheng YJ, Chien YC, et al. No association between genetic polymorphisms of CYP1A1, GSTM1, GSTT1, GSTP1, NAT2, and nasopharyngeal carcinoma in Taiwan. Cancer Epidemiol Biomarkers Prev 2003;12: 179–80.

Cheng YJ, Hildesheim A, et al. Cigarette smoking, alcohol consumption and risk of nasopharyngeal carcinoma in Taiwan. Cancer Causes Control 1999;10:201–7.

Chien YC, Chen JY, et al. Serologic markers of Epstein-Barr virus infection and nasopharyngeal carcinoma in Taiwanese men. New Eng J Med 2001;345:1877–82.

Cho EY, Hildesheim A, et al. Nasopharyngeal carcinoma and genetic polymorphisms of DNA repair enzymes XRCC1 and hOGG1. Cancer Epidemiol Biomarkers Prev 2003;12: 1100–4.Clifford P. Carcinogens in the nose and throat: nasopharyngeal carcinoma in Kenya. Proc R Soc Med 1972;65:682–86.

Cogliano VJ, Grosse Y et al. Meeting report: summary of IARC monographs on formaldehyde, 2-butoxyethanol, and 1-tert-butoxy-2-propanol. Environ Health Perspect 2005; 113:1205–8.

Collins JJ, Acquavella JF, et al. An updated meta-analysis of formaldehyde exposure and upper respiratory tract cancers. J Occup Environ Med 1997;39:639–51.

de Schryver A, Klein G, et al. EB virus-associated antibodies in Caucasian patients with carcinoma of the nasopharynx and in long-term survivors after treatment. Int J Cancer 1974; 13:319–25.

de Thé G, Lavoue MF, et al. Differences in EBV antibody titres of patients with nasopharyngeal carcinoma originating from high, intermediate and low incidence areas. IARC Sci Publ 1978;471–81.

Deng ZL, Wei YP, et al. [Frequent genetic deletion of detoxifying enzyme GSTM1 and GSTT1 genes in nasopharyngeal carcinoma patients in Guangxi Province, China]. Zhonghua Zhong Liu Za Zhi 2004;26:598–600.

Desgranges C, de-The G, et al. Further studies on the detection of the Epstein-Barr virus DNA in nasopharyngeal carcinoma biopsies from different parts of the world. IARC Sci Publ 1975;191–93.

Devi BC, Pisani P, et al. High incidence of nasopharyngeal carcinoma in native people of Sarawak, Borneo Island. Cancer Epidemiol Biomarkers Prev 2004;13:482–86.

Dobson WH. Cervical lympho-sarcoma. China Med J (Engl) 1924;38:786–87.

Dodd LE, Sengupta S, et al. Genes involved in DNA repair and nitrosamine metabolism and those located on chromosome 14q32 are dysregulated in nasopharyngeal carcinoma. Cancer Epidemiol Biomarkers Prev 2006;15: 2216–5.

Edwards RH, Seillier-Moiseiwitsch F, et al. Signature amino acid changes in latent membrane protein 1 distinguish Epstein-Barr virus strains. Virology 1999;261:79–95.

Fan Q, Jia WH, et al. [Correlation of polymeric immunoglobulin receptor gene polymorphisms to susceptibility of nasopharyngeal carcinoma]. Ai Zheng 2005;24:915–18.

Farrow DC, Vaughan TL, et al. Diet and nasopharyngeal cancer in a low-risk population. Int J Cancer 1998;78:675–79.

Feng BJ, Huang, W, et al. Genome-wide scan for familial nasopharyngeal carcinoma reveals evidence of linkage to chromosome 4. Nat Genet 2002;31:395–99.

Friborg J, Wohlfahrt J, et al. Cancer susceptibility in nasopharyngeal carcinoma families—a population-based cohort study. Cancer Res 2005;65:8567–72.

Fung LF, Lo AK, et al. Differential gene expression in nasopharyngeal carcinoma cells. Life Sci 2000;67:923–36.

Gallicchio LG, Matanoski G, et al. Adulthood consumption of preserved and nonpreserved vegetables and the risk of nasopharyngeal carcinoma: a systematic review. Int J Cancer 2006;119:1125–35.Garber JE, Offit K. Hereditary cancer predisposition syndromes. J Clin Oncol 2005;23:276–92.

Geser A, Charnay N, et al. Environmental factors in the etiology of nasopharyngeal carcinoma: report on a case-control study in Hong Kong. IARC Sci Publ 1978;213–29.

Giannoudis A, Ergazaki M, et al. Detection of Epstein-Barr virus and human papillomavirus in nasopharyngeal carcinoma by the polymerase chain reaction technique. Cancer Lett 1995;89:177–81.

Goldsmith DB, West TM, et al. HLA associations with nasopharyngeal carcinoma in Southern Chinese: a meta-analysis. Clinical Otolaryngol Allied Sciences 2002; 27:61–67.

Guo X, Lui WO, et al. Identifying cancer-related genes in nasopharyngeal carcinoma cell lines using DNA and mRNA expression profiling analyses. Int J Oncol 2002;21:1197–204.

Hauptmann M, Lubin JH, et al. (Mortality from solid cancers among workers in formaldehyde industries. Am J Epidemiol 2004;159:1117–30.

Henderson BE, Louie E. Discussion of risk factors for nasopharyngeal carcinoma. IARC Sci Publ 1978;251–60.

Henderson BE, Louie EW, et al. Epstein-Barr virus and nasopharyngeal carcinoma: is there an etiologic relationship? J Natl Cancer Inst 1977;59:1393–95.

Henle W, Henle G, et al. Antibodies to Epstein-Barr virus in nasopharyngeal carcinoma, other head and neck neoplasms, and control groups. J Natl Cancer Inst 1970;44:225–31.

Henle W, Ho HC, et al. Antibodies to Epstein-Barr virus-related antigens in nasopharyngeal carcinoma. Comparison of active cases with long-term survivors. J Natl Cancer Inst 1973;51:361–69.

Hildesheim A, Anderson LM, et al. CYP2E1 genetic polymorphisms and risk of nasopharyngeal carcinoma in Taiwan. J Natl Cancer Inst 1997;89:1207–12.

Hildesheim A, Chen CJ, et al. Cytochrome P4502E1 genetic polymorphisms and risk of nasopharyngeal carcinoma: results from a case-control study conducted in Taiwan. Cancer Epidemiol Biomarkers Prev. 1995;4: 607–10.

Hildesheim A, West S, et al. Herbal medicine use, Epstein-Barr virus, and risk of nasopharyngeal carcinoma. Cancer Res. 1992;52:3048–51.

Hirayama T, Ito Y. A new view of the etiology of nasopharyngeal carcinoma. Prev Med 1981; 10:614–22.

Hirunsatit R, Kongruttanachok N, et al. Polymeric immunoglobulin receptor polymorphisms and risk of nasopharyngeal cancer. BMC Genet 2003;4:3.

Ho HC. Current knowledge of the epidemiology of nasopharyngeal carcinoma—a review. IARC Sci Publ 1972;2:357–66.

Ho HC. Epidemiology of nasopharyngeal carcinoma. Cancer Asia. T. Hirayama. Baltimore, University Park Press: 1976;49–61.

Ho JH. Nasopharyngeal carcinoma (NPC). Adv Cancer Res 1972;15:57–92.

Hording U, Nielsen HW, et al. Human papillomavirus types 11 and 16 detected in nasopharyngeal carcinomas by the polymerase chain reaction. Laryngoscope 1994;104: 99–102.

Hsu C, Shen Y-C, et al. Difference in the incidence trend of nasopharyngeal and oropharyngeal carcinomas in Taiwan: implication from age-period-cohort analysis. Cancer Epidemiol Biomarkers Prev 2006;15:856–61.

Hu L F, Chen F, et al. Clonability and tumorigenicity of human epithelial cells expressing the EBV encoded membrane protein LMP1. Oncogene 1993;8:1575–83.

Huang DP, Ho JH, et al. Carcinoma of the nasal and paranasal regions in rats fed Cantonese salted marine fish. IARC Sci Publ 1978;315–28.

Hui AB, Lo KW, et al. Epigenetic inactivation of TSLC1 gene in nasopharyngeal carcinoma. Mol Carcinog 2003;38:170–78.

Hui AB, Lo KW, et al. Detection of recurrent chromosomal gains and losses in primary nasopharyngeal carcinoma by comparative genomic hybridisation. Int J Cancer 1999; 82:498–503.

International Agency for Research on Cancer (IARC) IARC Monographs on the Evaluation of Carcinogenic Risks to Humans. Volume 56: Some Naturally Occurring Substances: Food Items and Constituents, Heterocyclic Aromatic Amines and Mycotoxins. Lyon, IARC Press, 1993.

International Agency for Research on Cancer (IARC) IARC Monographs on the Evaluation of Carcinogenic Risks to Humans. Volume 62: Wood Dust and Formaldehyde. Lyon, IARC Press, 1995.

International Agency for Research on Cancer (IARC) IARC Monographs on the Evaluation of Carcinogenic Risks to Humans. Volume 70: Epstein-Barr Virus and Kaposi's Herpesvirus/Human Herpesvirus 8. Lyon, IARC Press, 1997.

International Agency for Research on Cancer (IARC) IARC Monographs on the Evaluation of Carcinogenic Risks to Humans. Volume 83: Tobacco Smoke and Involuntary Smoking. Lyon, France, IARC Press, 2004.

Jeannel D, Ghnassia M, et al. Increased risk of nasopharyngeal carcinoma among males of French origin born in Maghreb (north Africa). Int J Cancer 1993;54: 536–39.

Jeannel D, Hubert A, et al. Diet, living conditions and nasopharyngeal carcinoma in Tunisia—a case-control study. Int J Cancer. 1990;46:421–25.

Jeng JH, Chang MC, et al. Role of areca nut in betel quid-associated chemical carcinogenesis: current awareness and future perspectives. Oral Oncol 2001;37:477–92.

Jia WH, Collins A, et al. Complex segregation analysis of nasopharyngeal carcinoma in Guangdong, China: evidence for a multifactorial mode of inheritance (complex segregation analysis of NPC in China). Eur J Hum Genet 2005;13:248–52.

Jia WH, Huang QH, et al. Trends in incidence and mortality of nasopharyngeal carcinoma over a 20–25 year period (1978/1983–2002) in Sihui and Cangwu counties in southern China. BMC Cancer 2006;6:178.

Jiang JH, Jia WH, et al. Genetic polymorphisms of CYP2A13 and its relationship to nasopharyngeal carcinoma in the Cantonese population. J Transl Med 2004; 2:24.

Kangro HO, Osman HK, et al. Seroprevalence of antibodies to human herpesviruses in England and Hong Kong. J Med Virol 1994; 43:91–96.

Kongruttanachok N, Sukdikul S, et al. Cytochrome P450 2E1 polymorphism and nasopharyngeal carcinoma development in Thailand: a correlative study. BMC Cancer 2001; 1:4.

Krogman WM. Study of four skulls from Seleucia on the Tigris dating from 100 BC to 200 AD. Hum Biol 1940;12:313–22.

Lam Y. M. and T. C. Tan Mortality from nasopharyngeal carcinoma and occupation in men in Hong Kong from 1976–81. Ann Acad Med Singapore 1984; 13: 361–5.

Lane SR, Nicholls PJ, et al. The measurement and health impact of endotoxin contamination in organic dusts from multiple sources: focus on the cotton industry. Inhal Toxicol 2004;16:217–29.

Lanier A, Bender T, et al. Nasopharyngeal carcinoma in Alaskan Eskimos Indians, and Aleuts: a review of cases and study of Epstein-Barr virus, HLA, and environmental risk factors. Cancer 1980;46:2100–6.

Lanier AP, Henle W, et al. Epstein-Barr virus-specific antibody titers in seven Alaskan natives before and after diagnosis of naso-pharyngeal carcinoma. Int J Cancer 1980;26: 133–37.

Lee AW, Foo W, et al. Changing epidemiology of nasopharyngeal carcinoma in Hong Kong over a 20-year period (1980–99): an encouraging reduction in both incidence and mortality. Int J Cancer 2003;103:680–85.

Lee AW, Sze WM, et al. Treatment results for nasopharyngeal carcinoma in the modern era: the Hong Kong experience. Int J Radiat Oncol Biol Phys 2005;61:1107–16.

Lee HP, Gourley L, et al. Preserved foods and nasopharyngeal carcinoma: a case-control study among Singapore Chinese. Int J Cancer 1994;59:585–90.

Lee JT, Ko, CY. Has survival improved for nasopharyngeal carcinoma in the United States? Otolaryngol Head Neck Surg 2005; 132:303–8.

Levine PH, Pearson GR, et al. The reliability of IgA antibody to Epstein-Barr virus (EBV) capsid antigen as a test for the diagnosis of nasopharyngeal carcinoma (NPC). Cancer Detect Prev 1981;4:307–12.

Levine R, Zhu K, et al. Self-reported infectious mononucleosis and 6 cancers: a population-based, case-control study. Scand J Infect Dis 1998;30:211–14.

Li CC, Yu MC, et al. Some epidemiologic observations of nasopharyngeal carcinoma in Guangdong, People's Republic of China. Natl Cancer Inst Monogr 1985;69:49–52.

Li W, Ray RM, et al. Occupational risk factors for nasopharyngeal cancer among female textile workers in Shanghai, China. Occup Environ Med 2006;63:39–44.

Li X, Wang E, et al. Chromosomal imbalances in nasopharyngeal carcinoma: a meta-analysis of comparative genomic hybridization results. J Transl Med 2006;4:4.

Li ZQ, Pan QC, et al. Epidemiology of nasopharyngeal carcinoma. Nasopharyngeal carcinoma: Clinical and laboratory research. Li TQ, Pan QC, Chen JJ. Guangzhou, Guangdong Science and Technology Press 1983;1–68.

Lin TM, Yang CS, et al. Antibodies to Epstein-Barr virus capsid antigen and early antigen in nasopharyngeal carcinoma and comparison groups. Am J Epidemiol 1977;106:336–39.

Liu YH, Du CL, et al. (Increased morbidity from nasopharyngeal carcinoma and chronic pharyngitis or sinusitis among workers at a newspaper printing company. Occup Environ Med 2002;59:18–22.

Lo KW, Cheung ST, et al. Hypermethylation of the p16 gene in nasopharyngeal carcinoma. Cancer Res 1996;56:2721–25.

Lo KW, Kwong J, et al. High frequency of promoter hypermethylation of RASSF1A in na-sopharyngeal carcinoma. Cancer Res 2001; 61:3877–81.

Lu CC, Chen JC, et al. Nasopharyngeal carcinoma-susceptibility locus is localized to a 132 kb segment containing HLA-A using high-resolution microsatellite mapping. Int J Cancer 2005; 115:742–46.

Lu SJ, Day NE, et al. Linkage of a nasopharyngeal carcinoma susceptibility locus to the HLA region. Nature 1990;346:470–71.

Lung HL, Cheng Y, et al. Fine mapping of the 11q22–23 tumor suppressive region and involvement of TSLC1 in nasopharyngeal carcinoma. Int J Cancer 2004;112:628–35.

Marsh GM, Stone RA, et al. Mortality among chemical workers in a factory where formaldehyde was used. Occup Environ Med 1996;53:613–27.

Marsh GM, Youk AO. Reevaluation of mortality risks from nasopharyngeal cancer in the formaldehyde cohort study of the National Cancer Institute. Regul Toxicol Pharmacol 2005;42:275–83.

Marsh GM, Youk AO, et al. Pharyngeal cancer mortality among chemical plant workers exposed to formaldehyde. Toxicol Ind Health 2002;18:257–68.

McCredie M, Williams S, et al. Cancer mortality in East and Southeast Asian migrants to New South Wales, Australia, 1975–1995. Br J Cancer 1999;79:1277–82.

Melbye M, Cote TR, et al. Nasopharyngeal carcinoma: an EBV-associated tumour not significantly influenced by HIV-induced immunosuppression. The AIDS/Cancer Working Group. Br J Cancer 1996;73:995–97.

Mutirangura A, Pornthanakasem W, et al. Epstein-Barr viral DNA in serum of patients with nasopharyngeal carcinoma. Clin Cancer Res 1998;4:665–69.

Mutirangura A, Tanunyutthawongese C, et al. Genomic alterations in nasopharyngeal carcinoma: loss of heterozygosity and Epstein-Barr virus infection. Br J Cancer 1997;76:770–76.

Nam JM, McLaughlin JK, et al. Cigarette smoking, alcohol, and nasopharyngeal carcinoma: a case-control study among U.S. whites. J Natl Cancer Inst 1992;84:619–22.

Nawroz H, Koch W, et al. Microsatellite alterations in serum DNA of head and neck cancer patients. Nat Med 1996;2:1035–37.

Nazar-Stewart V, Vaughan TL, et al. Glutathione S-transferase M1 and susceptibility to nasopharyngeal carcinoma. Cancer Epidemiol Biomarkers Prev. 1999;8:547–51.

Ng TP. A case-referent study of cancer of the nasal cavity and sinuses in Hong Kong. Int J Epidemiol 1986;15:171–75.

Niedobitek G, Hansmann ML, et al. Epstein-Barr virus and carcinomas: undifferentiated carcinomas but not squamous cell carcinomas of the nasopharynx are regularly associated with the virus. J Pathol 1991;165:17–24.

Ning JP, Yu MC, et al. Consumption of salted fish and other risk factors for nasopharyngeal carcinoma (NPC) in Tianjin, a low-risk region for NPC in the People's Republic of China. J Natl Cancer Inst 1990;82:291–96.

Old LJ, Boyse EA, et al. Precipitating antibody in human serum to an antigen present in cultured Burkitt's lymphoma cells. Proc Natl Acad Sci 1966;56:1699–1704.

Pandey MR, Boleij JS, et al. Indoor air pollution in developing countries and acute respiratory infection in children. Lancet 1989;427–29.

Parkin DM, Bray F, et al. Global cancer statistics, 2002. CA Cancer J Clin 2005;55:74–108.

Parkin DM, Iscovich J. Risk of cancer in migrants and their descendants in Israel: II. Carcinomas and germ-cell tumours. Int J Cancer 1997;70:654–60.

Parkin DM, Whelan SL, et al. (Eds): Cancer Incidence in Five Continents Vol. VIII. IARC Scientific Publications No. 155. Lyon, International Agency for Research on Cancer, 2002.

Pathmanathan R, Prasad U, et al. Clonal proliferations of cells infected with Epstein-Barr virus in preinvasive lesions related to nasopharyngeal carcinoma. N Engl J Med 1995;333:693–98.

Pegtel DM, Subramanian A, et al. IFN-{alpha}-stimulated genes and Epstein-Barr virus gene expression distinguish WHO type II and III nasopharyngeal carcinomas. Cancer Res 2007;67:474–81.

Raab-Traub N, Flynn K. The structure of the termini of the Epstein-Barr virus as a marker of clonal cellular proliferation. Cell 1986;47: 883–89.

Rickinson AB, Kieff E. Epstein-Barr virus. In: Knipe DM, Howley PM (Eds): Field's Virology, 4th edition. Philadelphia, PA, Lippincott, Williams & Wilkins, 2001, pp 2575–2627.

Roush GC, Walrath J, et al. Nasopharyngeal cancer, sinonasal cancer, and occupations related to formaldehyde: a case-control study. J Natl Cancer Inst 1987;79:1221–24.

Sandvej K, Gratama JW, et al. Sequence analysis of the Epstein-Barr virus (EBV) latent membrane protein-1 gene and promoter region: identification of four variants among wild-type EBV isolates. Blood 1997;90:323–30.

Sawaki S, Hirayama T, et al. Studies on nasopharyngeal carcinoma in Japan. Cancer Asia. T. Hirayama. Baltimore, University Park Press, 1976, pp 63–74.

Seow A, Koh WP, et al. Cancer Incidence in Singapore 1968–2002, Singapore Cancer Registry Report No. 6, 2004

Shanmugaratnam K, Tye CY, et al. Etiological factors in nasopharyngeal carcinoma: a hospital-based, retrospective, case-control, questionnaire study. IARC Sci Publ 1978; 199–212.

Simons MJ, Chan SH, et al. Nasopharyngeal carcinoma and histocompatibility antigens. IARC Sci Publ 1978;271–82.

Simons MJ, Day NE, et al. Nasopharyngeal carcinoma V: immunogenetic studies of Southeast Asian ethnic groups with high and low risk for the tumor. Cancer Res 1974;34: 1192–95.

Simons MJ, Wee GB, et al. Immunogenetic aspects of nasopharyngeal carcinoma (NPC) III. HL-a type as a genetic marker of NPC predisposition to test the hypothesis that Epstein-Barr virus is an etiological factor in NPC. IARC Sci Publ 1975;249–58.

Sriamporn S, Vatanasapt V, et al. Environmental risk factors for nasopharyngeal carcinoma: a case-control study in northeastern Thailand. Cancer Epidemiol Biomarkers Prev 1992;1: 345–48.

Sun LM, Epplein M, et al. Trends in the incidence rates of nasopharyngeal carcinoma among Chinese Americans living in Los Angeles County and the San Francisco Metropolitan Area, 1992–2002. Am J Epidemiol 2005.

Surveillance, Epidemiology, and End Results (SEER) Program (www.seer.cancer.gov) SEER*Stat Database: Incidence - SEER 17 Regs Limited-Use, November 2006 Sub (1973–2004 varying) - Linked to County Attributes - Total U.S., 1969–2004 Counties, National Cancer Institute, DCCPS, Surveillance Research Program, Cancer Statistics Branch, released April 2007, based on the November 2006 submission.

Swenberg, JA, Kerns WD, et al. Induction of squamous cell carcinomas of the rat nasal cavity by inhalation exposure to formaldehyde vapor. Cancer Res 1980;40:3398–402.

Tiwawech D, Srivatanakul P, et al. Cytochrome P450 2A6 polymorphism in nasopharyngeal carcinoma. Cancer Lett 2006;241:135–41.

Tiwawech D, Srivatanakul P, et al. Glutathione S-transferase M1 gene polymorphism in Thai nasopharyngeal carcinoma. Asian Pac J Cancer Prev 2005;6:270–75.

Tiwawech D, Srivatanakul P, et al. The p53 codon 72 polymorphism in Thai nasopharyngeal carcinoma. Cancer Lett 2003;198: 69–75.

Tsai MH, Lin CD, et al. Prognostic significance of the proline form of p53 codon 72 polymorphism in nasopharyngeal carcinoma. Laryngoscope 2002;112:116–19.

Tsao SW, Tramoutanis G, et al. The significance of LMP1 expression in nasopharyngeal carcinoma. Semin Cancer Biol 2002;12: 473–87.

Tse LA, Yu IT, et al. Incidence rate trends of histological subtypes of nasopharyngeal carcinoma in Hong Kong. Br J Cancer 2006; 95:1269–73.

Ung A, Chen CJ, et al. Familial and sporadic cases of nasopharyngeal carcinoma in Taiwan. Anticancer Res 19 1999;661–65.

Vaughan TL, Shapiro JA, et al. Nasopharyngeal cancer in a low-risk population: defining risk factors by histological type. Cancer Epidemiol Biomarkers Prev 1996;5:587–93.

Ward MH, Pan WH, et al. Dietary exposure to nitrite and nitrosamines and risk of nasopharyngeal carcinoma in Taiwan. Int J Cancer. 2000;86:603–9.

Warnakulasuriya KA, Johnson NW, et al. Cancer of mouth, pharynx and nasopharynx in Asian and Chinese immigrants resident in Thames regions. Oral Oncol 1999;35:471–75.

Wells C. Chronic sinusitis with alveolar fistulae of medieval times. J Laryngol 1963;261:320–22.

West S, Hildesheim A, et al. Non-viral risk factors for nasopharyngeal carcinoma in the Philippines: results from a case-control study. Int J Cancer 1993;55:722–27.

Xia LW, Liang SX, et al. Trace element content in drinking water of nasopharyngeal carcinoma patients. Cancer Lett 1988;41:91–97.

Xie L, Xu L, et al. Identification of differentially expressed genes in nasopharyngeal carcinoma by means of the Atlas human cancer cDNA expression array. J Cancer Res Clin Oncol 2000;126:400–6.

Xiong W, Zeng ZY, et al. A susceptibility locus at chromosome 3p21 linked to familial nasopharyngeal carcinoma. Cancer Res 2004; 64:1972–74.

Yao KT, Wu PN, et al. The role of promotion in the carcinogenesis of nasopharyngeal carcinoma. Cancer of the Liver, Esophagus, and Nasopharynx G. Wagner and I. G. Zhang New York, Springer-Verlag, 1987, pp 187–93.

Yu IT, Chiu YL, et al. Deaths from nasopharyngeal cancer among waiters and waitresses in Chinese restaurants. Int Arch Occup Environ Health 2004;77:499–504.

Yu MC, Garabrant DH, et al. Occupational and other non-dietary risk factors for nasopharyngeal carcinoma in Guangzhou, China. Int J Cancer 1990;45:1033–39.

Yu MC, Henderson BE. Nasopharyngeal cancer. Cancer Epidemiology and Prevention, Second Ed. D. Schottenfeld and J. F. Fraumeni, Jr. New York, Oxford University Press, 1996, pp 603–18.

Yu MC, Ho JH, et al. Cantonese-style salted fish as a cause of nasopharyngeal carcinoma: report of a case-control study in Hong Kong. Cancer Res 1986;46:956–61.

Yu MC., Huang TB, et al. Diet and nasopharyngeal carcinoma: a case-control study in Guangzhou, China. Int J Cancer. 1989;43: 1077–82.

Yu MC, Mo C-C, et al. Preserved foods and nasopharyngeal carcinoma: a case-control study in Guangxi, China. Cancer Res 1988;48: 1954–59.

Yuan JM, Wang XL, et al. Non-dietary risk factors for nasopharyngeal carcinoma in Shanghai, China. Int J Cancer 2000;85:364–69.

Yuan JM, Wang XL, et al. Preserved foods in relation to risk of nasopharyngeal carcinoma in Shanghai, China. Int J Cancer. 2000;85: 358–63.

Yung WC, Ng MH, et al. p53 codon 72 polymorphism in nasopharyngeal carcinoma. Cancer Genet Cytogenet 1997;93:181–82.

Zeng Y, Miao XC, et al. Epstein-Barr virus activation in Raji cells with ether extracts of soil from different areas in China. Cancer Lett 1984;23:53–59.

Zeng Y, Zhang LG, et al. Prospective studies on nasopharyngeal carcinoma in Epstein-Barr virus IgA/VCA antibody-positive persons in Wuzhou City, China. Int J Cancer 1985;36: 545–47.

Zeng Y, Zhong JM, et al. Epstein-Barr virus early antigen induction in Raji cells by Chinese medicinal herbs. Intervirology 1983;19:201–4.

Zeng YX, Jia WH. Familial nasopharyngeal carcinoma. Semin Cancer Biol 2002;12:443–50.

Zhang F, Zhang J.Clinical hereditary characteristics in nasopharyngeal carcinoma through Ye-Liang's family cluster. Chin Med J (Engl) 1999;112:185–87.

Zheng W, McLaughlin JK, et al. Occupational risks for nasopharyngeal cancer in Shanghai. J Occup Med 1992;34:1004–7.

Zheng X, Tan L, et al. Epstein-Barr virus infection, salted fish and nasopharyngeal carcinoma. A case-control study in southern China. Acta Oncol 1994;33:867–72.

Zheng YM, Tuppin P, et al. Environmental and dietary risk factors for nasopharyngeal carcinoma: a case-control study in Zangwu County, Guangxi, China. Br J Cancer. 1994; 69:508–14.

Zhou X, Tian D. [A review on nasopharyngeal carcinoma in ancient Chinese literature]. Zhonghua Yi Shi Za Zhi 2001;31:115–18.

Zhu K, Levine RS, et al. Case-control study evaluating the homogeneity and heterogeneity of risk factors between sinonasal and nasopharyngeal cancers. Int J Cancer 2002;99: 119–23.

Zong YS, Zhang RF, et al. Histopathologic types and incidence of malignant nasopharyngeal tumors in Zhongshan County. Chin Med J (Engl) 1983;96:511–16.

Zou J, Sun Q, et al. A case-control study of nasopharyngeal carcinoma in the high background radiation areas of Yangjiang, China. J Radiat Res (Tokyo) 2000;41 Suppl:53–62.

zur Hausen H, Schulte-Holthausen H, et al. EBV DNA in biopsies of Burkitt tumours and anaplastic carcinomas of the nasopharynx. Nature 1970;228:1056–58.

9

Esophageal Cancer

OLOF NYRÉN AND HANS-OLOV ADAMI

An infamous "Asian esophageal cancer belt" stretches to the east from the Caspian Littoral in Iran via Turkmenistan, Uzbekistan, and Kazakhstan to the northern provinces of China. The Gonbad region in the northeastern section of Iran and the Linxian and Cixian provinces of China have the highest reported incidence rates in the world. In some of these areas, the incidence of squamous cell esophageal cancer exceeds by about 100-fold that in low-risk western countries including the United States. No plausible explanation exists for these amazing geographic differences. A new enigma in esophageal cancer epidemiology arose in the 1980s, when descriptive data from several western countries revealed an epidemic increase in adenocarcinomas.

The two histopathologic types of esophageal cancer, squamous cell carcinoma and adenocarcinoma, although differing histopathologically and etiologically, are not separated in this chapter. Specific comments on risk factors for adenocarcinoma, the less studied type of the two, are integrated in the text whenever relevant data are available.

CLINICAL SYNOPSIS

Subgroups

Esophageal cancer occurs mainly in two histologic types, squamous cell carcinoma and adenocarcinoma. Presently, the clinical management of these types is similar.

Symptoms

Dysphagia due to obstruction is the typical presenting symptom. As disease progresses, weight loss, bleeding, inability to swallow, regurgitation, pain, and fistulas contribute to the generally disastrous disease development.

Diagnosis

Esophago-gastroscopy with biopsy and cytology confirms the diagnosis. Various imaging techniques are used for staging and treatment planning.

Treatment

Radical surgical removal of a localized tumor, an extensive procedure, is the only curative treatment. The stomach or intestine is used to restore continuity. Most esophageal cancers are diagnosed in incurable and rapidly progressing stages. Various modalities including mechanical dilatation, application of self-expandable stents, radiotherapy, and chemotherapy are used to improve passage and achieve at least short-term palliation.

Prognosis

Esophageal cancer is one of the most deadly of all malignancies. No more than 16% of the cases in the United States, and 10% of those in Europe, survive for 5 years or more.

Progress

Despite the absence of any revolutionary breaktrough in diagnosis or treatment, there are hopeful signs of an ongoing improvement. In Sweden, the 5-year relative survival after an esophageal adenocarcinoma diagnosis increased from 5% between 1961 and 1989 to 13.7% between 1990 and 1996, while the corresponding survival after esophageal squamous cell carcinoma rose from 5% between 1961 and 1969 to 8.9% between 1990 and 1996. Similar observations have been made in the United States for adenocarcinoma as well as for squamous cell carcinoma.

DESCRIPTIVE EPIDEMIOLOGY

Geographic and Demographic Distribution

Worldwide, cancer of the esophagus ranks sixth among men and ninth among women (Parkin et al, 2005). With an esimated 462 000 new cases in 2002, it accounts for 4.2% of all cancers. Esophageal cancer is the sixth most common cause of cancer related death (5.7% of all cancer deaths). There is a wide variation in risk among geographic areas (Figs. 9–1 and 9–2). Among women, the age-standardized incidence rates in high-risk southern Africa and China are approximately 20-fold higher than those in low-risk southern Europe. In men the difference is about 15-fold between high-risk southern Africa and low-risk western Africa. In South Africa, esophageal cancer is the most common cause of cancer-related deaths among black men. Other areas of relatively high risk are eastern Africa, temperate South America, and South Central Asia (Parkin et al, 1999). Almost 80% of the cases occur in economically less-developed regions (Parkin et al, 1999). The age-standardized incidence rates among men and women in the extreme-risk Gonbad region of Iran were 206 and 262 per 100 000 person-years, respectively, in the 1970s (Hormozdiari et al, 1975); while still

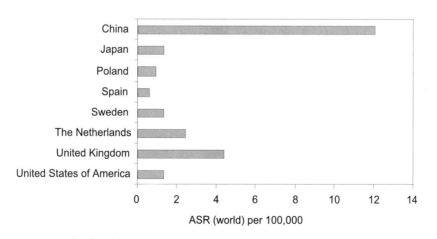

Figure 9–1. Age-*standardized* (to the world population) incidence rates of esophageal cancer among women. (*Source*: Ferlay et al, 2004).

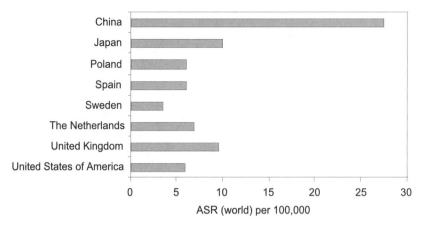

Figure 9–2. Age-standardized (to the world population) incidence rates of esophageal cancer among men. (*Source*: Ferlay et al, 2004).

being the most common cancer, the rates from 1996 to 2000 seem to have fallen to less than half (Semnani et al, 2006). The corresponding rates in Linxian, China, are 138 and 99 (Li and Rao, 2000), and in Cixian, China, 209 and 120 (He et al, 2005). In China overall, esophageal cancer ranks second in incidence, surpassed only by stomach cancer. Thus, China contributes almost half of all esophageal cancer cases occurring worldwide (Parkin et al, 1999).

People of Chinese descent seem to retain some of the excess risk also outside China. For example, the age-adjusted incidence rates among residents of Chinese ancestry in Singapore are threefold higher in women and eightfold higher in men than corresponding rates among Malays in the same small area (Parkin et al, 1997). If second-generation Chinese immigrants to Singapore are divided according to the area from which their parents originated, a threefold variation in esophageal cancer risk is observed among women and sevenfold among men (Munoz and Day, 1996). The offspring of parents from high-risk areas have the highest incidence. Among migrants who came from China to the United States, however, the rates declined rapidly in succeeding generations, leaving only a small residual excess risk in second-generation immigrants compared to white Americans (Thomas and Karagas, 1987).

A substantial variation in incidence is also observed in Europe (Figs. 9–3 and 9–4). In Sweden, a low-risk country, the age-adjusted incidence rates among men and women are 3.1 and 1.0, in England and Wales 7.6 and 3.2, in Scotland 9.4 and 5.0, and in Calvados, France, 22.3 and 1.1 per 100 000 person-years (Parkin et al, 1997). In the United States, incidence rates are about three times higher in blacks than in whites. The male/female ratio varies considerably among different populations, the extremes being almost 15:1 in Calvados, France, and 0.8:1 in the Gonbad region of Iran.

The age-specific incidence rates for women (Fig. 9–3) and men (Fig. 9– 4) show that esophageal cancer occurs rarely before the age of 45 years, although in China this diagnosis needs to be seriously considered already at ages 45 to 55. Noteworthy in Figure 9–3 is the very high incidence among elderly women in the United Kingdom.

Secular Trends by Histologic Types

The normal mucosa of the esophagus consists of squamous cell epithelium. Therefore, the dominant histologic type of esophageal cancer worldwide is squamous cell carcinoma. Although glandular columnar cell epithelium, typical of the rest of the gastrointestinal tract, is absent in the esophagus, adenocarcinoma may still oc-

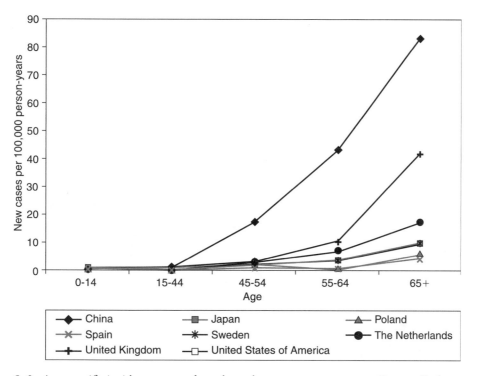

Figure 9–3. Age-specific incidence rates of esophageal cancer among women. (*Source*: Ferlay et al, 2004)

cur. Before the 1970s, this histologic type was considered a rarity (Hansen et al, 1997). Since then, however, the incidence of esophageal adenocarcinoma has increased rapidly in the United States and several other developed countries with western lifestyles, notably in North America, Europe, Australia, and New Zealand.

An analysis of 56 426 cases of esophageal cancer from registries in 12 countries revealed significant increases in the incidence of esophageal adenocarcinoma in both sexes in the United States (among whites and blacks), Canada, South Australia, and in six European countries (Scotland, Denmark, Iceland, Finland, Sweden, and Norway), while the increase was limited to men in France and to women in Switzerland (Vizcaino et al, 2002). An increasing trend could not be verified in either sex in the Netherlands (Botterweck et al, 2000; Vizcaino et al, 2002). In the other investigated western registries, the percentage increase per year among men varied between 2.3%

(Sweden) and 8.6% (US whites), while among women this range was between 3.1 (Sweden) and 18.6 (Iceland) (Vizcaino et al, 2002). Men had a 7- to 10-fold higher incidence compared to women.

While the age-standadized incidence of esophageal adenocarcinoma was well below 5 per 100 000 person-years in most of the studied registries, the occurrence of this cancer was markedly higher in Scotland, where it appears that the incidence among men is approaching 10 per 100 000 person-years (Pera et al, 2005). An incidence of 7 per 100 000 person-years has been reported from England and Wales (Newnham et al, 2003). As a comparison, the incidence rate among US white men in 2001, having increased sixfold since 1973 to 1975 and thereby being the most rapidly increasing cancer of all (Blot et al, 1991; Pohl and Welch, 2005), was no more than 2.3 per 100 000 person-years (Pohl and Welch, 2005).

Simultaneously, the incidence of esophageal squamous cell carcinoma, although

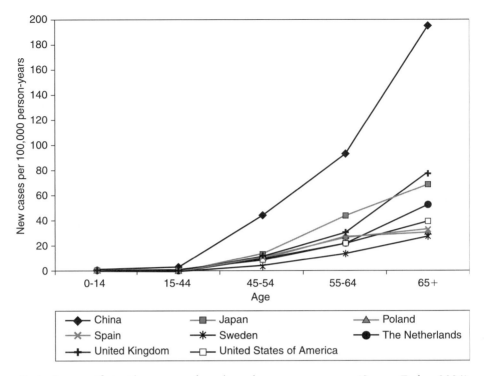

Figure 9–4. Age-specific incidence rates of esophageal cancer among men. (*Source*: Ferlay, 2004).

varying sevenfold across studied western registries, has been more stable over time (Vizcaino et al, 2002); increasing trends were observed in Denmark and the Netherlands among men and in Canada, Scotland, and Switzerland among women—but in most of the countries analyzed, the rates in men declined slowly. In contrast to the marked male predominance in adenocarcinoma, a less extreme male:female ratio (3–4:1) was observed for esophageal squamous cell carcinoma (Vizcaino et al, 2002). Adenocarcinoma has surpassed squamous cell carcinoma as the most common esophageal cancer type in US white men (Brown and Devesa, 2002; Vizcaino et al, 2002); Australian men (Vizcaino et al, 2002); English, Welsh, and Scottish men (Vizcaino et al, 2002; Newnham et al, 2003); and Swedish men (Ye, 2003; Ji and Hemminki, 2006).

Although changing classification practices might cloud the picture (Botterweck et al, 2000; Pohl and Welch, 2005; Lindblad, Ye et al, 2006), there is evidence that misclassification of esophageal and adjacent

adenocarcinomas leads to underestimation rather than overestimation of the esophageal adenocarcinoma incidence (Vizcaino et al, 2002; Lindblad, Ye et al, 2006). Moreover, there has has been little change in the proportion of patients found with in situ or localized disease, and the mortality has increased to the same extent or more than the incidence, strongly suggesting that overdiagnosis cannot explain the rise in incidence (Pohl and Welch, 2005). Therefore, there is wide consensus that we are witnessing a real and important increase in the occurrence of esophageal adenocarcinoma in western populations.

In contrast to the demographic pattern for squamous cell carcinoma in the United States, where incidence rates among African American men and women exceed those among whites by a factor of 3 or more, adenocarcinoma is more common in whites. The age-adjusted incidence of esophageal adenocarcinoma among white men during 1996 to 1998 was five times that among black men (Kubo and Corley, 2004; Wu, Chen et al,

2006). A similar gradient was observed in relation to Asians and Pacific Islanders. The trend in other areas, including the Central Asian populations at high risk for esophageal squamous cell carcinoma, is less clear, perhaps because many cancers in these populations are never confirmed histologically.

Recent efforts to correctly classify all incident cases in the high-risk Golestan province in Iran revealed that esophageal adenocarcinoma remains fairly rare; only 6% of investigated esophageal neoplasms were of this histological type (Islami et al, 2004). Similar conclusions are drawn also in Linxian, China (Islami et al, 2004) and Japan (Blaser and Saito, 2002), although there seems to be an increasing trend in esophageal adenocarcinoma mortality in the latter population (Hongo, 2004).

GENETIC AND MOLECULAR EPIDEMIOLOGY

Inherited Susceptibility

A positive family history was associated with an increased risk of esophageal cancer in several case-control and cohort studies in China. The excess risk among first-degree relatives varied between 70% and 500% (Li et al, 1989; Wang et al, 1992). Although one of the studies also included case patients with cancer of the gastric cardia, it must be assumed that most of the reported esophageal cancers were squamous cell carcinomas. The hypothesis that an autosomal recessive major gene influences the susceptibility to esophageal cancer found support in two pedigree surveys with segregation analyses—one in a high-risk area (Carter et al, 1992) and another in a moderate- to high-risk Chinese area (Zhang et al, 2000). The susceptibility-allele frequency was estimated at approximately 20%.

Familial aggregation also has been observed in Iran and Japan, where the excess pertained to other upper aerodigestive–tract cancers as well (Ghadirian, 1985; Morita, Kuwano et al, 1998; Akbari et al, 2006). The existence of such clustering remains controversial in low-risk populations; most studies based on self-reported family history

have been negative (Wynder and Bross, 1961; Brown et al, 1988), including the two case-control studies that analyzed family history by histologic type of esophageal cancer (Lagergren, Ye et al, 2000; Dhillon et al, 2001). However, positive findings of familial clustering in low-risk populations have been reported by some (Tavani et al, 1994; Ji and Hemminki, 2006). In a Swedish study based on the nationwide Swedish Family Cancer Database, with high-quality cancer data from the Swedish Cancer register and little risk of information bias, the standardized incidence ratio (SIR) for esophageal cancer in the offspring of parents with esophageal cancer was 2.6 (95% confidence interval 1.2–4.8) (Ji and Hemminki, 2006). Histology-specific concordance was also explored, but the number of observed cases was too small to allow firm conclusions.

Familial aggregation of esophageal adenocarcinoma would be biologically plausible since gastroesophageal reflux—a strong risk factor for esophageal adenocarcinoma (Lagergren, Bergström, Lindgren et al, 1999) and for Barrett's esophagus, an established precursor lesion for the same cancer type—seems to run in some families (Romero et al, 1997) and has a clear genetic component demonstrated in a twin study (Cameron et al, 2002). Although the scope for information bias is obvious, familial aggregation of Barrett's esophagus and adenocarcinoma of the esophagus or cardia has been reported by several investigators, albeit not by all. In a recent study, familial Barrett's esophagus could be confirmed through case record review in 7.3% of persons presenting with either of these conditions (Chak et al, 2006). Accrual of families with early onset or familial Barrett's esophagus and/or esophageal adenocarcinoma is ongoing with the aim of localizing and eventually identifying the putative susceptibility gene(s) (Drovdlic et al, 2003; Ochs-Balcom et al, 2007).

Tylosis, an autosomal dominant trait characterized by hyperkeratosis palmaris et plantaris, is associated with a substantial excess risk of esophageal squamous cell carcinoma. In a UK pedigree, more than 90% of the affected family members developed esophageal cancer before age 70 (Ellis et al, 1994). The susceptibility gene TOC (tylosis esophageal cancer) has been mapped to a 1-cM region on chromosome 17q25, but so far it has evaded cloning. Interestingly, loss of heterozygosity (LOH) in the TOC gene region of 17q25 is often seen in sporadic esophageal tumors (Iwaya et al, 1998). Apart from tylosis, there are no reports of esophageal cancer families with defined germline mutations.

Polymorphisms

ADH and ALDH. Genetic polymorphisms in enzymes involved in metabolism of carcinogens have attracted considerable attention in epidemiologic studies. Alcohol, a major risk factor for esophageal squamous cell carcinoma (IARC, 1988), is metabolized to acetaldehyde, which causes mutations and other DNA damage (IARC, 1985) while simultaneously inhibiting DNA repair. The oxidation of ethanol is catalyzed mainly (80%) by alcohol dehydrogenase (ADH) and to a lesser extent by CYP2E1. The acetaldehyde is then converted to acetate by aldehyde dehydrogenase (ALDH). Both ADH and ALDH are polymorphic. The presence of the mutant, inactive ALDH2*2 allele among Japanese alcohol drinkers is associated with a 7- to 12-fold increase in the risk of esophageal cancer relative to drinkers without this allele (Yokoyama et al, 1996). This allele, which is associated with a high concentration of blood acetaldehyde and flushing after alcohol consumption, is common among Asian Orientals but rare among Caucasians.

Several other studies from Japan and Taiwan confirmed the increased risk of esophageal cancer among drinkers with the ALDH2*2 allele (Itoga et al, 2002; Chen et al, 2006), but some others did not. According to the positive studies, these subjects are also prone to develop precursor lesions (Muto et al, 2000) or multiple cancers in the entire upper-aerodigestive tract (Yokoyama et al, 2001). Further, they are at increased risk of developing recurrent esophageal squamous cell carcinoma after mucosectomy of early esophageal cancer (Yokoyama et al, 1998). There are no data from Caucasian populations, in which the high-risk allele is rare.

Somewhat inconsistent with the notion that blood acetaldehyde levels are crucial for the risk of esophageal cancer among alcohol drinkers is the observation that alcoholics with the alcohol dehydrogenase-2 genotype ADH2*1/*1 (later termed ADH1B*1/*1), who have lower acetaldehyde levels, had a two- to fourfold increased risk of esophageal cancer compared to alcoholics who were hetero- or homozygous for the ADH2*2 allele (Yokoyama et al, 2001; Chen et al, 2006). The activity of the ADH2 enzyme in subjects who are homozygous for ADH2*1 (approximately 90% of Caucasians and 7% of Japanese) is only a small fraction of that in subjects who carry at least one ADH2*2 allele. This leads to slow oxidation of alcohol and prevents the formation of excessive amounts of acetaldehyde. Unexpectedly, the combination of ADH2*1/2*1 with ALDH2*1/2*2 was associated with a markedly increased (11–37 times) risk of esophageal cancer in these studies (Yokoyama et al, 1999; Yokoyama et al, 2001; Boonyaphiphat et al, 2002; Yokoyama et al, 2002; Wu et al, 2005).

Type 3 ADH (later termed ADH1C) is polymorphic in Caucasians. The enzymes encoded by the ADH3*1 allele metabolize ethanol to acetaldehyde 2.5 times faster than those encoded by the ADH3*2 allele. Data from Puerto Rico (Harty et al, 1997) suggest that alcohol drinkers with the ADH3*1/3*1 genotype are at increased risk of oral cancer compared to those with ADH3*1/3*2 or ADH3*2/3*2. However, Japanese findings do not support an important role of ADH type 3 polymorphism in esophageal carcinogenesis (Muto et al, 2000; Yokoyama et al, 2002).

CYP1A1. Tobacco smoking is the other major known risk factor for esophageal squamous cell carcinoma. Drug-metabolizing enzymes, which often display genetic polymorphism, convert many tobacco constituents into DNA-binding metabolites. Aromatic hydrocarbons, including benzo(a)pyrene, first require metabolic activation by phase I enzymes, notably the oxidative CYP-related enzymes. Subsequently, they are detoxified by phase II enzymes, including the glutathione-S-transferases (GSTs). Of the latter, one of the Mu class isozymes is considered to be most responsible for the detoxification of aromatic hydrocarbons in cigarette smoke.

Genetic polymorphisms occur in the coding region of the CYP1A1 gene. The variant *2C (KI nomenclature) allele is common in Asians but rare in Caucasians and associated with a twofold increase in microsomal enzyme activity. In China, heavy smokers homozygous for the *2C allele had a relative risk of esophageal cancer of 6.6 compared to heavy smokers who were not homozygous for the *2C allele (Nimura et al, 1997). Among heavy smokers who also lacked the Mu class GST (GSTM1 0/0 genotype), and in whom detoxification was impaired, the relative risk was 12.7, with a wide confidence interval. More recently, two case-control studies from Shaanxi Province (China) and Taiwan, respectively, confirmed the positive association between homozygous carriage of the CYP1A1 *2C variant allele and esophageal squamous cell carcinoma risk (odds ratio relative to homozygosity for the common allele was 2.5 in both studies) (Wang et al, 2002; Wu et al, 2002). There was a tendency for synergistic interaction with smoking, but no evidence of any interaction with the GSTM1 0/0 genotype.

In all, 10 case-control studies of variable epidemiologic rigorousness have addressed the relationship between the CYP1A1 *2C polymorphism and esophageal cancer, mostly squamous cell carcinoma but also adenocarcinoma. Nine of these studies were included in a meta-analysis (Yang, Matsuo, Wang et al, 2005). Although most studies failed to confirm a statistically significant association between presence of the variant *2C allele and an increased risk of esophageal cancer, all showed odds ratios above 1.0; the summary relative risk estimate in the meta-analysis was 1.44 (95% confidence interval 1.17–1.78) for hetero- or homzygous carriers of the variant allele with homozygous carriers of the wild-type allele as reference, and 2.52 (95% confidence interval 1.62–3.91) for homozygotes with the variant allele versus homozygotes with the wild-type allele. Subsequently published data from France (Abbas et al, 2004), despite a low frequency of the variant *2C allele and a small study, weakly support a role of the CYP1A1 *2C polymorphism with an odds ratio of 3 (albeit short of statistical significance) for esophageal squamous cell carcinoma among heterozygotes.

On the other hand, six studies that investigated the *2A polymophism of CYP1A1 yielded inconsistent results with point estimates among hetero- or homozygous carriers of the variant allele relative to homozygous carriers of the wild-type allele ranging between 0.4 and 2.8, and with a summary relative risk estimate of 1.07 (95% confidence interval 0.64–1.80) (Yang, Matsuo, Wang et al, 2005).

CYP2E1. The ethanol-inducible CYP2E1 metabolizes many known procarcinogens, including volatile nitrosamines found in tobacco smoke. Several polymorphic alleles occur at low frequency, but no relationship seems to exist between genotype and in vivo activity of the enzyme in Caucasians. While Japanese subjects carrying the variant c2 allele of the CYP2E1 (–1053 C>T) (*5) gene polymorphism exhibited a significant reduction in enzyme activity (Bartsch et al, 2000), there are also reports that this genotype is associated with enhancement of the CYP2E1 transcription rate.

Seven studies of varying epidemiological quality have investigated the relationship of the *5 polymorphism with esophageal squamous cell carcinoma; a marked and statistically significant risk reduction (odds ratio 0.2–0.3) among carriers of the variant allele was revealed in two Chinese studies emanating from the same group of investigators (Lin et al, 1998; Tan et al, 2000). A

Chinese population-based study, on the other hand, found no such protection (odds ratio 1.15) (Gao, Takezaki et al, 2002), nor did four studies conducted outside of China—two in Japan (Hori et al, 1997; Morita et al, 1997), one in South Africa (Li et al, 2005), and one in France (Lucas et al, 1996). In the South African study, however, there was a statistically nonsignificant trend toward low risk (odds ratio 0.58) among carriers of the rare variant allele. A recent meta-analysis of the five Asian studies showed a summary relative risk estimate of 0.63 (95% confidence interval 0.30–1.30) (Yang, Matsuo, Wang et al, 2005).

The *6 genetic polymorphism of CYP2E1 (-7632 T > A) was significantly associated with an increased risk (odds ratio 2.9) of esophageal squamous cell carcinoma in the South African study (Li et al, 2005), but not in the Chinese study that investigated this polymorphism (Lin et al, 1998).

A tandem repeat polymorphism in the CYP2E1 5'-flanking region (*1D) has also been investigated in relation to esophageal cancer; in a Japanese study, carriers of the A4/A4 genotype had a statistically significant risk elevation (odds ratio 4.0) compared to subjects who did not have this genotype (Itoga et al, 2002).

CYP3A. CYP3A, a CYP subfamily that metabolizes more than 50% of therapeutically used drugs, has also been investigated with regard to esophageal cancer risk. CYP3A5, the major CYP3A enzyme in the esophageal mucosa, is polymorphic; 10% of Caucasians lack CYP3A5 activity. Homozygous carriers of the variant alleles of the *3, *6, and *7 polymorphisms in the CYP3A5 gene have severely decreased enzyme activities. In one study (Dandara et al, 2005), individuals with such genetically determined reductions of the CYP3A5 enzyme activity who were also smokers or alcohol users exhibited a reduced risk of esophageal squamous cell carcinoma, compared to hetero- or homozygotes for the wild-type alleles. The crude odds ratio among smokers was 0.62 (95% confidence interval 0.38–1.01) and among alcohol us-

ers 0.54 (95% confidence interval 0.32–0.91). No protection was observed among nonsmokers or nondrinkers.

Microsomal epoxide hydrolase. Microsomal epoxide hydrolase (mEH) is another Phase I enzyme. It has dual roles in both activation and detoxification of environmental carcinogens. Two genetic polymorphisms of the EPHX1 gene, which encodes mEH, are associated with enzyme activity and have been implicated as risk factors for cancer. These polymorphisms have been examined in relation to esophageal squamous cell carcinoma in three studies and to esophageal adenocarcinoma in two. While presence of the variant allele in the polymorphism in exon 3 was positively linked to a 2.6-fold increased risk of esophageal squamous cell carcinoma in one Chinese study (Wang et al, 2003), none of the other studies was able to confirm any significant main effect of any of the two polymorphisms on either of the histological cancer types.

GSTs. The GSTs, multifunctional phase II enzymes, play a central role in the detoxification of toxic and carcinogenic electrophiles. The results of epidemiological investigations into the role of the Mu class GST, coded by the GSTM1 gene, are not convincing; among 15 published studies, the odds ratio among individuals with the 0/0 deletion genotype—associated with impaired detoxification—varied between 0.4 and 2.2. The summary odds ratio was 1.07 (95% confidence interval 0.76–1.51) among 12 studies included in a meta-analysis from 2005 (Yang, Matsuo, Wang et al, 2005). Similarly, nine studies of the importance of the GSTT1 0/0 deletion polymorphism were consistently negative and the summary relative risk estimate among six of these studies was 0.99 (95% confidence interval 0.80–1.22). Interestingly though, the 0/0 genotype was observed significantly less often in 27 French patients with esophageal adenocarcinoma than in 130 control subjects (odds ratio 0.1) (Abbas et al, 2004). Although this inverse association was not confirmed among 21 Dutch or

9 Indian patients with this histological type of esophageal cancer (Van Lieshout et al, 1999; Jain et al, 2006), more studies are needed in view of the scarcity of data about adenocarcinomas.

The *GSTP1* Ile104Val polymorphism, reportedly associated with higher levels of DNA adducts, implying an increased susceptibility to cancer induction, was evaluated in 11 studies. Results were highly variable with odds ratios ranging between 0.1 and 3.5 among hetero- or homozygous carriers of the variant Val allele, relative to homozygotes for the wild-type Ile allele. In a meta-analysis of seven of these studies the summary estimate of relative risk was 1.01 (95% confidence interval 0.60–1.70) (Yang, Matsuo, Wang et al. 2005). The highest odds ratio (4.6, 95% confidence interval 1.5–14.6) was noted for Dutch esophageal adenocarcinoma patients (Van Lieshout et al, 1999). The other studies that could evaluate adenocarinomas separately showed point estimates between 0.9 and 1.9 (Casson et al, 2003; Abbas et al, 2004; Casson et al, 2006; Jain et al, 2006; Murphy et al, 2007).

Sulfate conjugation. Sulfate conjugation is a key pathway in the detoxification and bioactivation of many dietary and environmental mutagens, including heterocyclic amines and polycyclic aromatic hydrocarbons. The SULT1A1 enzyme metabolizes or bioactivates a broad range of substrates and it is expressed in the esophagus. The variant *2 allele of a known single nucleotide polymorphism in the *SULT1A1* gene (638G > A) is associated with reduced SULT1A1 enzyme activity and stability. Two studies have shown that presence of the *2 allele is associated with a two- to threefold increased risk of esophageal squamous cell carcinoma (Wu, Wang et al, 2003; Dandara et al, 2006).

NAT 2. Two N-acetyltransferase isozymes, NAT1 and NAT2, are polymorphic and catalyze both N-acetylation (usually deactivation) and O-acetylation (usually activation) of aromatic and heterocyclic amine carcinogens. Epidemiologic studies have suggested an association between slow NAT2 acetylator genotypes and cancer of the head, neck, and urinary bladder. And rapid NAT2 acetylator genotypes have been implicated in colorectal cancer. A 2.5- to 4-fold increased risk of esophageal squamous cell carcinoma was found among subjects with the slow acetylator *NAT2* genotype compared with rapid acetylators in two Japanese investigations (Morita, Yano et al, 1998; Shibuta et al, 2001). However, in a study from Taiwan (Lee et al, 2000), no effect by this polymorphism could be verified.

NAD(P)H:quinone oxidoreductase 1. (NQO1), a cytosolic enzyme that catalyzes the two-electron reduction of quinone compounds, prevents the generation of semiquinone free radicals and reactive oxygen species. It also catalyzes the reductive activation of environmental carcinogens such as nitrosamines and heterocyclic amines. A C to T substitution polymorphism at nucleotide 609 of exon 6 of the *NQO1* gene causes a Pro187Ser amino acid change with reduced enzyme activity (a threefold reduction among hetrozygotes and complete lack of enzyme activity among homozygotes). The T/T genotype, relative to the C/T + C/C genotypes, was associated with significant, up to 4.6-fold, risk elevations for esophageal squamous cell carcinoma (Zhang, Schulz et al, 2003; Zhang, Li, Wang, Geddert et al, 2003). A two- to threefold increase also in adenocarcinoma risk was reported by one (Sarbia et al, 2003) but contested by another study (Von Rahden et al, 2005). A very strong inverse relationship (odds ratio 0.16) was revealed in a British study that compared esophageal adenocarcinoma patients to a control group of patients who underwent endoscopies for dyspepsia (many also with reflux symptoms) (Di Martino et al, 2007).

MTHFR. Adequate DNA methylation is of paramount importance for gene function. Both hyper- or hypomethylation states have been implicated in a wide array of cancers. Folate, in most human diets coming mainly from vegetables and fruits, is essential in the regeneration of methionine and the synthesis of S-adenosyl-L-methionine (SAM), the universal methyl donor for intracellular methylation reactions, including DNA methylation. Methylenetetrahydrofolate reductase (MTHFR) catlyzes the irreversible reduction of 5,10-methylene tetrahydrofolate (5,10-methylene THF) to 5-methyl tetrahydrofolate (5-methyl THF). Methionine synthase (MS), together with its co-enzyme B_{12}, catalyzes the transfer of a methyl group from 5-methyl THF to homocysteine, producing methionine, the precursor of SAM. Methionine synthase reductase (MTRR) maintains adequate concentrations of activated B_{12} for this reaction to occur. Thymidylate synthase (TS) is another important enzyme in the folate metabolism. With 5,10-methylene THF as substrate, TS catalyzes reductive methylation of deoxyuridylate (dUMP) to thymidylate (dTMP), which is an essential nucleotide for de novo DNA synthesis and repair.

Deficiencies in folate and B_{12} as well as alterations in MTHFR, MS, MTRR, or TS may contribute to carcinogenesis through altered DNA methylation (eg, DNA hypomethylation) and impeded thymidylate synthesis. These alterations may result in nucleotide imbalances, increased uracil misincorporation in DNA, DNA strand breaks, and impaired excision repair. All of the genes that encode these enzymes (*MTHFR, MTR*—coding for MS—*MTRR* and *TS*) have polymorphisms with known or suspected functional consequences. Two common polymorphisms in the *MTHFR* gene (C677T and A1298C) have been studied; in a first report from China, where the *MTHFR* 677T allele is more common than the 677C one, subjects with the *MTHFR* 677TT genotype had an odds ratio for esophageal squamous cell carcinoma of 6.2 (95% confidence interval 3.3–11.5) compared to those with the 677CC genotype (Song et al, 2001). Moreover, a significant allele-dose relationship was seen with an odds ratio of 3.1 (95% confidence interval 1.9–5.1) for the heterozygous 677CT genotype. In the same report, the variant *MTHFR* 1298CC genotype, although rare, was associated with an odds ratio of 4.4 (95% confidence interval 1.2–16.0), whereas heterozygous presence of the C allele did not confer any increased risk.

Subsequent reports have provided less striking results. One study noted a significant 2.6-fold risk for squamous cell carcinoma among homo- or heterozygous carriers of the 677T allele, relative to homozygotes with of the 677C allele (but the odds ratio for homozygous 677TT individuals relative to homo- or heterozygous carriers of 677C was no more than 0.94) (Zhang, Zotz et al, 2004). Four other Chinese studies showed nonimpressive risk elevations among heterozygous and/or homozygous carriers of the 677T allele, with odds ratios ranging between 1.25 and 2.0 (Stolzenberg-Solomon et al, 2003; Gao, Takezaki et al, 2004; Wang et al, 2005; Wang et al, 2007). Moreover, two studies conducted outside high-risk China showed no, or even a significant inverse, association between carriage of the 677TT genotype and risk of esophageal squamous cell carcinoma (Zhang, Zotz et al, 2004; Yang, Matsuo; Ito et al, 2005). Conceivably, the apparent inconsistencies may have to do with divergent folate intake in the different populations under study, but variable results need to be convincingly reconciled.

Two studies of the *MTHFR* A1298C polymorphism did not reveal any significant main effects on esophageal squamous cell carcinoma risk (Stolzenberg-Solomon et al, 2003; Gao, Toshiro et al, 2004). A Japanese study evaluated the importance of the *MTR* A2756T polymorphism in relation to esophageal cancer (mostly squamous cell carcinomas) and found a weak, nonsignificant positive trend with the variant genotype (Yang, Matsuo, Ito et al, 2005). On the other hand, a Chinese study of the *MTRR* A66G polymorphism reported a significant elevation in the risk of esophageal squamous cell carcinoma (odds ratio 1.59) among hetero- or homozygous carriers of the variant 66G allele, compared to subjects with the 66AA allele. A clear allele dose-risk trend was noted. Somewhat surprisingly, this association was confined to nondrinkers, among whom the risk gradient was 2.4-fold.

In the *TS* gene, there are several functional polymorphisms in the untranslated regions (UTRs). One of them is a unique tandem repeat sequence in the *TS* 5'UTR with two (2R), three (3R), or infrequently more 28-bp repeats. The rare 2R allele is associated with reduced *TS* mRNA transcription and protein expression. Nested within the 3R allele there is a G > C single nucleotide polymorphism; when 3R contains the C allele of this nested single nucleotide polymorphism ($3R_C$), the efficiency of translation is three to four times lower than when 3R contains the G allele ($3R_G$). Thus, $3R_G$ is associated with high TS expression while $3R_C$ and 2R are linked to a similarly reduced expression.

In one Chinese investigation, individuals with a "low TS expression genotype" (2R/2R, 2R/$3R_C$, or $3R_C$/$3R_C$), contrasted against those with "high" ($3R_G$/$3R_G$, $3R_G$/$3R_C$, or $3R_G$/2R), had a significant 47% increase in the odds of developing squamous cell carcinoma (Tan et al, 2005). This complex polymorphism interacted significantly with serum folate status so that the odds of esophageal sqamous cell carcinoma among individuals with the low TS expression genotype and a low serum folate concentration was more than 22 times higher (95% confidence interval 10.4–49) than among those with the high TS expression genotype and high serum folate concentration.

While the link between low TS expression genotype and increased esophageal squamous cell carcinoma risk gets some support from another study (Wang et al, 2005), a third study from China was unable to confirm any significant differences in the *TS* allelotype distributions among esophageal squamous cell carcinoma cases and controls (Zhang, Cui et al, 2004).

DNA repair genes. X-ray repair cross-complementing 1 (XRCC1) is an important protein in the DNA base excision repair (BER) pathway but is also thought to be involved in DNA single-strand break (SSB) repair. Three known single nucleotide polymorphisms in the *XRCC1* gene (Arg194Trp, Arg280His, and Arg399Gln) have been extensively studied, and an impaired DNA repair capacity has been substantiated for at least the latter. Despite the expected defective DNA repair, only one out of nine investigations of the *XRCC1* Arg399Gln polymorphism reported an increased risk (odds ratio 1.67, 95% confidence interval 1.08–2.59) of esophageal cancer among carriers of the variant allele. Of the other studies, all but two showed risk reductions, albeit nonsignificant, with odds ratios among Gln/Gln or Gln/Arg carriers, relative to Arg/Arg, ranging between 0.64 and 0.91 (crude odds ratios recalculated from exhibited raw data). The three studies that addressed risks for esophageal adenocarcinoma reported odds ratios between 0.75 and 1.19.

Five studies concerned with the *XRCC1* Arg194Trp and Arg280His polymorphisms were essentially negative, while one study noted a small (odds ratio 1.38) but significant positive association between the variant allele of the *XRCC1* 5'-UTR polymorphism T-77C and esophageal squamous cell carcinoma risk (Hao et al, 2004). In the latter study, this polymorphism interacted with a Val762Ala polymorphism in the *ADPRT* gene to yield an odds ratio of 7.9 (95% confidence interval 1.6–38.4) among homozygous carriers of the variant allele in both loci. The *ADPRT* gene product is ADP-ribosyltransferase, another enzyme involved in the BER DNA repair pathway.

Xeroderma pigmentosum complementary group C (XPC) and D (XPD) are two out of the more than 20 proteins that take part in the the nucleotide excision repair (NER) pathway. They repair bulky DNA adducts. The Lys939Gln and the poly (AT) insertion/deletion polymorphism (PAT) within the intron 9 of the *XPC* gene, as well as the Arg156Arg, Asp312Asn, and Lys751Gln polymorphisms of the *XPD* gene, have been examined in regard to their relations to esophageal sqamous cell carcinoma and adenocarcinoma. Positive findings have been reported for the *XPC* PAT and the *XPD* Lys751Gln polymorphisms, but unfortunately, the results lack consistency. Two studies—one Chinese (Yu et al, 2004) and one Swedish (Ye et al, 2006)—arrived at similar risk elevations (odds ratio around 2) for squamous cell carcinoma among homozygous or heterozygous carriers of the variant *XPD* 751Gln allele, but other studies from China reported null results (Xing et al, 2002; Xing et al, 2003). The Swedish investigation also revealed a positive association with esophageal adenocarcinoma (unadjusted odds ratio recalculated from raw data 1.85, 95% confidence interval 1.14–2.99), supported by results from a large American study (odds ratio 1.49, 95% confidence interval 1.02–2.14) (Liu et al, 2007) but not by Canadian findings (Casson, Zheng, Evans, Veugelers et al, 2005). In the latter study, carriers of the variant C allele had indeed a significantly reduced risk of esophageal adenocarcinoma (recalculated crude odds ratio 0.45, 95% confidence interval 0.23–0.88). This study also reported an almost fourfold risk elevation for esophageal adenocarcinoma among individuals who had the fairly common *XPC* PAT +/+ genotype, relative to those with the −/− genotype. More studies are needed to confirm this finding.

Recently, the homozygous presence of the variant allele of a polymorphism of the Xeroderma pigmentosum group G gene (*XPG* His1104Asp)—another important component of the NER pathway—was shown to be inversely and significantly (odds ratio 0.47, 95% confidence interval 0.27 0.82) associated with the risk of squamous cell carcinoma in the upperaerodigestive tract (oropharynx, larynx, and esophagus combined) (Cui et al, 2006). Too few cases prohibited a precise estimation of the specific relationship between the *XPG* His1104Asp polymorphism and esophageal squamous cell carcinoma, but the odds ratio point estimate (0.35) suggests that the protective effect conferred by homozygous carriage of the variant Asp allele may be present also for this particular neoplasm. Confirmatory studies are needed.

P53. The tumor-suppressor P53 pathway plays a crucial role in preventing carcinogenesis. The *P53* gene is polymorphic and among its single nucleotide polymorphisms a G > C change at codon 72 results in an Arg > Pro amino acid substitution. The Pro/Pro genotype appears to induce apoptosis with slower kinetics and to suppress transformation less efficiently than does the Arg/Arg genotype. The *P53* 72Pro/Pro genotype, compared to the 72Arg/Arg, was shown to be associated with an approximately doubled risk for esophageal squamous cell carcinoma in several studies from China and Taiwan (Lee et al, 2000; Li et al, 2002; Zhang, Li, Wang,Wen et al, 2003; Hong et al, 2005). However, this risk elevation could not be confirmed in a Japanese study (Hamajima et al, 2002).

One of the positive studies also found a gene-gene interaction with the *MDM2* T309G single nucleotide polymorphism. Subjects with the joint presence of *P53* 72Pro/Pro and *MDM2* 309GG, compared to those with the *P53* 72Arg/Arg or Arg/Pro and *MDM2* 309TT or TG haplotypes, had a more than threefold risk increase (Hong et al, 2005). The MDM2 protein regulates the P53 pathway by binding to the P53 protein, inhibiting its activity and mediating its degradation via the ubiquitination system. The *MDM2* 309GG genotype is associated with increased MDM2 expression and attenuation of the P53 pathway. This *MDM2* genotype alone, compared with the *MDM2* 309TT genotype, was in itself associated with a significant 50% elevation in the risk of esophageal squamous cell carcinoma (Hong et al, 2005).

Interestingly, homozygous carriers of the variant genotype of a compound polymorphism at positions 4 (G > A) and 14 (C > T) in the 5'UTR of exon 2 of the *P73* gene, a structural and functional homologue of *P53*, were found to have a ninefold reduced risk in an Irish study (Ryan et al, 2001).

This study included esophageal cancer cases of both histological types, but adenocarcinomas were in the majority. In fact, the risk reduction was essentially confined to adenocarcinomas, for which the relative risk was zero. In a Japanese case-control study of esophageal squamous cell carcinoma, the genotypes of this polymorphism were evenly distributed among cases and controls (Hamajima et al, 2002).

CCND1. Coding for cyclin D1 the *CCND1* gene is expressed in response to mitogenic signals. Cyclin D1 is a key protein in cell-cycle control, regulating the transition from G1-phase to S-phase. The *CCND1* G870A polymorphism creates a splice variant that lacks a phosphorylation site in the destruction box critical for ubiquitin-mediated proteolysis. This increases the stability or half-life of cyclin D1. It has been hypothesized that DNA-damaged cells in individuals with the A allele may bypass the G1/S checkpoint so that genetic alterations are allowed to accumulate.

One study in China reported a significant 2.7-fold risk elevation of squamos cell carcinoma among carriers of the *CCND1* 870A allele, relative to those with the 870GG genotype (Zhang, Li, Wang, Wen, Sarbia et al, 2003), but another found no such relationship (Yu et al, 2003). One Canadian (Casson, Zheng, Evans, Geldenhuys et al, 2005) and one German (Geddert et al, 2005) case-control study assessed this polymorphism in relation to esophageal adenocarcinoma. In the Canadian hospital-based study, individuals with the 870AA genotype had a risk that was six times higher than those who were homozygous with the wild-type 870G allele, whereas the German study found no differences in genotype distributions between cases and blood donor controls.

Inflammatory mediators. Given an undisputable link between esophageal adenocarcinoma and gastroesophageal reflux, esophagitis, and Barrett's esophagus (see following), polymorphic inflammatory mediators—strongly implicated in gastric

carcinogenesis—have been examined in relation to esophageal cancer risk. However, little evidence of any important roles has emerged. An American population-based case-control study (El-Omar et al, 2003) investigated single nucleotide polymorphisms in the *IL-1B* (−511 C/T), *IL-6* (−174 G/C), and *TNF-A* (−308 G/A), encoding the proinflammatory interleukins 1β, 6, and tumor necrosis factor-α, respectively, as well as *IL-4* (−590 C/T) and *IL-10* (−1082 G/A, −819 C/T, −592 C/A), coding for the anti-inflammatory interleukins 4 and 10, along with the variable number of tandem repeat (VNTR) polymorphism of *IL-1RN*, which encodes the endogenous interleukin-1 receptor antagonist IL-1ra, were investigated both in relation to risk of esophageal adenocarcinoma and to risk of esophageal squamous cell carcinoma. A few significant associations emerged, including a link between homozygous carriage of the *IL-1RN* *2 allele and risk of esophageal squamous cell carcinoma. However, the results were erratic and deemed to be insufficient evidence of any causal relationship.

In a more convoluted study comparing genoypes in patients with uncomplicated esophagitis and reflux patients with esophageal adenocarcinoma or dysplasia, the *2/*2 genotype of *IL-1RN* polymorphism was noted significantly more often in the adenocarcinoma/dysplasia group than in the uncomplicated esophagitis category (OR = 3.7, with borderline significance) (Gough et al, 2005). Similarly, the active G/G genotype of *IL-10* (−1082 G/A) was overrepresented in the adenocarcinoma/dysplasia group (OR = 2.05, 95% confidence interval 1.15–3.62). This is somewhat surprising in view of the immunoregulatory action of interleukin-10. No associations were seen with polymorphisms of the *IL-1B* (−511 C/T), *TNF-A* (−238G/A), and *IL-4R* (−1902 A/G) genes, the latter encoding the interleukin-4 receptor. Studies comparing different disease categories must be interpreted with much caution, though. The *IL-1RN* finding was subsequently challenged by

Dutch investigators, who found no association at all in a study of identical design (Moons et al, 2005).

The lack of importance of the *TNF-A* (−308 G/A) polymorphism in squamous cell carcinoma development was confirmed in a Chinese case-control study (Guo, Wang, Li et al, 2005). However, the latter study reported a significant excess risk among B1 hetero- and homozygotes relative to B2 homozygotes in the *TNF-B* (+252 G/A) polymorphism confined to subjects with a negative family history of upper gastrointestinal cancer. Since multiple significance testing in various substrata increases the risk of statistical type-I errors, it seems prudent to remain skeptical until this association has been confirmed in other studies.

Absence of association with esophageal squamous cell carcinoma risk was reported for the *IL-2* (−384 G/T), *IL-2* (+114 G/T), *IL-6* (−174 G/C), *IL-10* (−1082 G/A), *IL-10* (−819 T/C), and *IL-10* (−592 C/A) polymorphisms in a study from Linxian, China (Savage et al, 2004). The lack of a positive relationship between the *IL-10* (−1082 G/A) polymorphism and esophageal squamous cell carcinoma risk was further noted in northern China (Guo, Wang, Wang et al, 2005).

Cycloxygenases. Cyclozygenases (COXs) regulate many biologic processes such as inflammation, immune function, cell proliferation, and angiogenesis. Overexpression of COX-2 is associated with many steps of cancer development, including hyperproliferation, transformation, tumor growth, invasion, and metastasis. Recently, relationships have been reported between two single nucleotide polymorphisms of the *COX-2* gene (G765C and G1195A) and esophageal squamous cell carcinoma (Zhang et al, 2005). The *COX-2* G765C polymorphism appears to disrupt an Sp1-binding site and thus displays a lower promoter activity. In contrast, the *COX-2* G1195A creates a c-MYB binding site resulting in a higher promoter activity. Significant 1.72-fold and 2.24-fold excess risks of developing esophageal squamous cell carcinoma were found for the

COX-2–1195AA and −765CC carriers, respectively, compared with noncarriers. The same research group has also reported a 1.42-fold excess among homozygotes for the variant A allele of the Arg261Gln polymorphism in exon 6 of the *Platelet 12-lipoxygenase* gene (*12-LOX*) (Guo et al, 2007). The gene product converts arachidonic acid into 12-hydroxyeicosatetraenoate (12-HETE), which – like prostaglandins – is implicated in cancer development. Confirmatory studies are awaited.

Somatic Events

Squamous cell carcinoma

Like many other malignancies of epithelial cell origin, esophageal squamous cell carcinoma develops after the stepwise accumulation of genetic alterations. These alterations may represent molecular fingerprints of critical risk factors. It is therefore of interest to compare not only cancers of different histologic types or clinical expressions, but also cancers arising in geographic areas with different incidence patterns. This vast literature will not be reviewed in detail, but a brief general overview seems appropriate. Consistently observed genetic changes in the tumor cells, regardless of patient origin and suspected etiologic factors, are *(1)* mutation of the *P53* gene, *(2)* deregulation of cell-cycle control in G1 by disturbance of the cyclin-dependent kinase-Rb pathway, and *(3)* alteration of oncogenes, with ensuing deregulation of signal transduction (Mandard et al, 2000).

Cell cycling is controlled strictly through two major pathways—the p53 (p14–MDM2 p53 p21) and pRb (p16 cyclin D1–pRb) pathways. The prevalence of *P53* gene aberrations ranges between 10% and 85%—with a modal value of approximately 50% (Lam, 2000)—and appears higher in high-incidence than in low-incidence areas. Many of the aberrations are point mutations, of which G→T transversions have been associated with environmental chemical carcinogens like cigarette smoke and aflatoxin. In the United States and Europe, *P53* mutations are seen more frequently in smokers than in nonsmokers.

The most common site of the mutations varies with geographic area (Lam, 2000). In western and Japanese populations, the *P53* mutations are evenly distributed in exons 5, 6, and 8. In China, they tend to occur more often in exon 5, in Taiwan in exons 6 and 7, and in Hong Kong in exons 7 and 8. Moreover, in Hong Kong and mainland China, they are seen as often in nonsmokers as in smokers.

Mutations in the *P53* gene may be an early event in the development of esophageal squamous cell carcinoma because alterations in p53 protein expression are frequently observed in precursor lesions (Tian et al, 1998). Synchronous or metachronous cancers or precursor lesions at multiple sites is a prominent feature of esophageal cancers. This phenomenon can be explained by two theories of tumorigenesis. The field cancerization theory postulates that an area of tissue becomes genomically unstable and predisposed to multiple neoplasia, probably due to prolonged exposure to carcinogens (Strong et al, 1984). In contrast, the monoclonal theory postulates that cells originating from a single neoplastic parent cell may spread laterally to produce multiple tumors (Nowell, 1976) (see Chapter 2). While these theories are not mutually exclusive, there is relatively little histopathologic evidence for the latter. Studies of cell proliferative activity in tumors and surrounding mucosa seem to support the field cancerization theory. Data on the presence of predisposing mutations in esophageal cancer, notably *P53* mutations and p53 protein accumulation, are consistent with both theories. Absence of expression of p21 was noted in 15% to 73% of squamous cell carcinomas.

Inactivation of the *CDKN2A* (p16^{NK4a}) gene is common in esophageal squamous cell carcinoma. In the early stages of carcinogenesis, this occurs mainly through methylation or loss of heterozygosity (LOH), while homozygous deletion is a late event (Kuwano et al, 2005). The prevalence of *CDKN2A* mutations ranged between 0% and 68% in 12 studies. While the prevalence varied between 10% and 30% in most studies, it was highest (> 50%) among Chinese and Japanese patients. One study found that p15^{INK4a} alterations were common (50%) (Xing et al, 1999), while another found them to be rare (3%) (Suzuki et al, 1995). It appears that p15^{INK4a} is inactivated through abnormal methylation or homozygous deletion at the same time as *CDKN2A*. The simultaneous inactivation of these genes results in loss of the pRb-regulated restriction point, and plays an essential role in esophageal carcinogenesis.

Cyclin D1 and E maintain the G1-S checkpoint. Overexpression of the cyclin D1 protein or amplification of its encoding *CCND1* gene is found in one-fourth to three-fourths of esophageal squamous cell carcinomas (Lam, 2000; Kuwano et al, 2005). Cyclin D1 overexpression is commonly seen already in dysplasias and early cancers, indicating that it is an early event in esophageal carcinogenesis. Alterations of the retinoblastoma (*Rb*) gene varies between 0% and 100% but usually exist in one-third to one-half of the cases (Lam, 2000). As deletions or mutations of the *Rb* gene seem to be rare in esophageal squamous cell carcinoma, LOH appears to be the major mechanism (Kuwano et al, 2005).

Frequent deletions have been observed on chromosome arms 3p, 5q, 9p, 13q, and 17p. Data on the association between alterations in tumor-suppressor genes frequently involved in colon carcinogenesis (*MCC, APC, DCC*) are conflicting. Some investigators have reported mutations or LOH in up to 77% of the patients (Boynton et al, 1992; Miyake et al, 1994), while others found no such alterations (Shibagaki et al, 1994). Mutations in the *ras* oncogenes, common in colon cancer, are rare or absent in esophageal squamous cell carcinoma (Lam, 2000; Mandard et al, 2000). In one study, LOH in the region containing the *BRCA1* gene, involved in hereditary breast cancer, was seen in 62% of esophageal squamous cell carcinoma patients (Mori et al, 1994). *RASSF1A* is another candidate tumor-suppressor gene that is reportedly silenced through promoter hypermethylation in 34% to 52% of esophageal squamous cell carcinoma cases (Kuroki et al, 2003a; Wong et al, 2006).

There are insufficient clinical data to evaluate the importance of growth factors in the development of esophageal squamous cell carcinoma (Lam, 2000). Some members of the epidermal growth factor receptor gene family have been investigated. A significant proportion (29% to 92%) of all squamous cell carcinomas show erb-B-1 overexpression, while overproduction of erb-B-2 is less commonly seen in this histologic type of esophageal cancer (Lam, 2000). When it occurs, polysomy appears to be a more frequent mechanism than amplification (Bizari et al, 2006).

The fragile histidine triad gene (*FHIT*), a member of the histidine triad gene family, encodes a diadenosine 5,'5'''-P1,P3-triphosphate hydrolase involved in purine metabolism. Aberrant transcripts of the *FHIT* locus are found in about half of esophageal squamous cell carcinomas (Kuwano et al, 2005). Epigenetic silencing through hypermethylation was reported in close to half of the cases (Kuroki et al, 2003b). Since such aberreations can occur even in normal-appearing squamous epithelium in patients heavily exposed to environmental carcinogens, they are believed to represent early carcinogenic events. Similarly, epigenetic silencing of the retinoic acid receptor beta (*RAR*-β) gene through hypermethylation was observed in more than 50% of esophageal squamous cell carcinomas, with even higher rates among early stage tumors, again suggestive of an early event (Kuroki et al, 2003b).

Adenocarcinoma

Adenocarcinomas of the esophagus are thought to develop through a stepwise process termed the *metaplasia-dysplasia-carcinoma sequence* (Souza and Spechler, 2005). *Metaplasia* is the process whereby one adult cell type replaces another adult cell type. In the esophagus the squamous epithelium is replaced by metaplastic specialized intestinal-type columnar epithelium, termed *Barrett's esophagus*. This metaplasia constitutes a possibly obligatory precursor lesion for esophageal adenocarcinoma

(see following). As in squamous cell carcinoma, mutations of genes that control the cell cycle also occur frequently in esophageal adenocarcinoma. However, mutation of *Rb* is rarely seen in esophageal adenocarcinomas.

It appears that cell-cycle abnormalities are mainly caused by inactivation of genes that block Rb function, such as *P53* and *CDKN2A*. With a prevalence of up to 90%, mutations of *P53* appear to be more common in adenocarcinoma than in squamous cell carcinoma (Taniere et al, 2001). Such mutations have already been observed in Barrett's esophagus. The prevalence of p53 alterations increases with increasing severity of epithelial dysplasia from 5% to 10% in indeterminate dysplasia to 75% of cases with high-grade dysplasia (Younes et al, 1993). Further, the prevalence increases with increasing DNA ploidy abnormalities from 1% to 5% in diploid cell populations to almost 100% in aneuploid cells (Galipeau et al, 1996).

The pattern of *P53* mutations in esophageal adenocarcinoma differs markedly from that in squamous cell carcinoma (Montesano et al, 1996). Adenocarcinomas show one of the highest frequencies (up to 69%) of transition at CpG dinucleotides observed in any cancer, while those transitions are seen in only about 18% of squamous cell carcinomas. Other common aberrations of cell-cycle genes in esophageal adenocarcinoma, observable also in the Barrett precursor state, include mutations in *CDKN2A* and increased cyclin D1 expression. As opposed to the squamous cell carcinomas, promoter hypermethylation with loss of heterozygosity (LOH) appears to be the dominating mechanism behind the inactivation of *CDKN2A* in adenocarcinomas. Most likely contributing to this inactivation and the inactivation of *P53* is the LOH at 9p and 17p that is frequently seen in both Barrett's esophagus and esophageal adenocarcinoma (Galipeau et al, 1999). Inactivation of the adenomatous polyposis coli gene (*APC*) by promoter methylation and LOH of 5q21 have been found both in esophageal adenocarcinoma and in its precursor, Barrett's esophagus with and without high-grade dysplasia.

Increased expression of epidermal growth factor (EGF), the EGF recptor (EGFR or erb-β-1), and transforming growth factor-α (TGF-α) have been found in esophageal adenocarcinoma (Souza and Spechler, 2005). Because elevated levels of TGF-α and EGFR have been observed in nondysplastic Barrett's esophagus, these overexpressions are thought to be early events in the carcinogenic process. Ras proteins, identified as important human oncogenes, play important roles in the regulation of cell growth. *KRAS* mutations have been reported in 11% to 40% of esophageal adenocarcinomas.

Overexpression of COX-2 has been detected in esophageal adenocarcinoma, as well as in Barrett's esophagus (with increasing expression as the cells progress to dysplasia and adenocarcinoma). COX-2 blocks the apoptotic machinery that would otherwise protect the organism from accumulation of genetically damaged cells. Telomerase, the enzyme responsible for the synthesis and maintenance of telomeres and thus with the potential of making cells immortal, is normally supressed in somatic cells. However, high levels of telomerase expression have been found in esophageal adenocarcinomas. In contrast, low levels of telomerase have been found in nondysplastic specialized intestinal metaplasia, with a marked increase during the transition from low-grade to high-grade dysplasia (Souza and Spechler, 2005).

Another genetic alteration of uncertain significance is the frequent loss of the whole Y chromosome, which was observed in one study in 9% of cases with Barrett's metaplasia without dysplasia, in 38% of cases with indefinite dysplasia, and in 100% of cases with high-grade dysplasia (Barrett et al, 1996). *APC* tumor-suppressor gene mutations and β catenin accumulation are also common findings in esophageal adenocarcinoma (Wu et al, 1998), and they appear to occur late in the metaplasia-dysplasia-adenocarcinoma sequence (Ransford and Jankowski, 2000).

RISK FACTORS

Tobacco and Alcohol

Squamous cell carcinoma

The positive association between heavy alcohol use, tobacco smoking, and the risk of esophageal cancer is well established. A large number of studies, including nearly 60 with case-control designs, have addressed the association with esophageal squamous cell carcinoma or unspecified esophageal cancer, the latter presumably consisting mainly of squamous cell carcinoma. Although some variation does exist, the overall results are unusually consistent; even in the absence of the other (Tuyns, 1983; Tavani et al, 1994; Castellsague et al, 1999), both smoking and alcohol habits are strong and independent risk factors for esophageal squamous cell carcinoma (Fig. 9–5). In Western (including South America) and African populations, the relative risk among heavy smokers, relative to non-smokers, is typically on the order of four to seven (Wynder and Bross, 1961; Cheng, Day and Davies 1992; Parkin et al, 1994; Castellsague et al, 1999).

All quantitative aspects of tobacco use seem to be dose-dependently related to the risk (Launoy et al, 1997; Lagergren, Bergström et al, 2000). The risk increases throughout the whole dose range, possibly in a less than linear manner (Segal et al, 1988; Launoy et al, 1997). Since cohort studies yield results similar to those of case-control studies, the association cannot be attributed to recall bias. In a US case-control study, the population-attributable risk percent (PAR) for smoking vis-à-vis esophageal squamous cell carcinoma was estimated to be 56.9% (Engel et al, 2003). PAR expresses the percent of the studied outcome disease that can be attributed to the exposure under study, or, in other words, the percent of all cases that might be prevented by eliminating this risk factor.

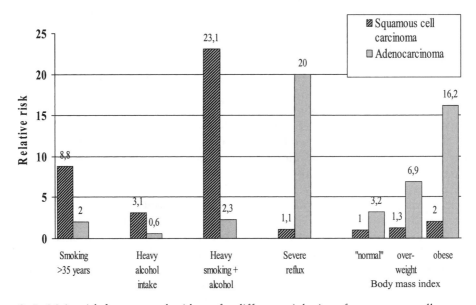

Figure 9–5. Major risk factors—and evidence for different etiologies—for squamous cell cancer and adenocarcinoma of the esophagus. (*Source*: Lagergren, 1999)

A review of 9 cohort and 11 case-control studies indicated that the risk of esophageal cancer remains elevated many years (at least 10) after cessation of smoking, to decline by about 40% only thereafter (Bosetti et al, 2006). After 10 years since cessation of smoking, ex-smokers still have a twofold increased risk as compared to never smokers.

There are consistent indications that the use of pipes, cigars, hand-rolled and/or high-tar cigarettes, bidi, dark, or black tobacco—all perceived as "strong" or unrefined tobacco products—is associated with steeper risk increases than is the use of commercially available cigarettes made from blond tobacco (Castellsague et al, 1999; Launoy et al, 2000). It is also reported that filter-tipped cigarettes confer less risk than nonfilter-tipped ones (Launoy et al, 2000).

Chewing of various local tobacco products like betel quid, paan, and nass was repeatedly associated with an increased esophageal cancer risk. Interestingly, for chewing betel quid without tobacco, excess risk was at least as great as for chewing betel quid with tobacco (Jussawalla and Deshpande, 1971; Nandakumar et al, 1996).

The dose–risk trend with alcohol consumption has been described as linear (Tuyns et al, 1979; Launoy et al, 1997) or more than linear (Tuyns et al, 1977; Segal et al, 1988; Graham et al, 1990). Substantial excesses in risk are generally seen only in the heavy consumption categories, where the relative risk in comparison with that of nonusers typically exceeds 10 and may approach 100. For alcohol, as opposed to tobacco, the current weekly or daily dose, and not the duration of the habit, appears to be the most important determinant of risk (Yu et al, 1988; Hu et al, 1994; Launoy et al, 1997; Castellsague et al, 1999). Moderate and heavy alcohol consumers can apparently reduce their risk of esophageal squamous cell carcinoma substantially by restricting their alcohol use (Cheng et al, 1995).

The results regarding the importance of type of beverage are contradictory. While many authors claim that the risk of squamous cell carcinoma is most strongly associated with hard liquor consumption (Brown et al, 1988; Gammon et al, 1997; Lagergren, Bergström et al, 2000), others report that wine and/or beer drinkers have the highest risks (Segal et al, 1988; Zambon et al, 2000). Most authors, however, find no important variation in risk with type of alcoholic beverage. But it has even been suggested that wine, compared to hard liquor, may be protective (Gronbaek et al, 1998); two population-based case-control studies provide some suggestive support for this hypothesis (Gammon et al, 1997; Lagergren, Bergström et al, 2000).

Early on, it was noted that the joint deleterious effects of alcohol and tobacco are not additive but act synergistically in a multiplicative manner (Tuyns et al, 1977). There is now abundant evidence to support this multiplicative relationship in most populations (Fig. 9–5). The risk among the heaviest users of both alcohol and tobacco, relative to nonusers of both, is typically increased 20- to 50-fold, but the excess may be more than 100-fold (Brown, Hoover et al, 1994; Zambon et al, 2000).

Some authors have tried to compare risk factor patterns for different tumor subsites within the esophagus, but the results are partly contradictory. In a study from Shanghai (Gao, McLaughlin, Blot, Ji, Benichou et al, 1994), the relation with smoking appeared stronger for tumors of the middle and lower thirds of the esophagus than for the upper third. An Indian study (Nandakumar et al, 1996) related drinking, smoking, and chewing habits to tumor site. Bidi smoking was associated with an increased risk of tumors in the entire esophagus, but the risk was highest for tumors in the upper third. The association with alcohol drinking was significant only for cancers of the middle third. Among men, tobacco chewing was associated with a significant excess risk only in the lower third, while nontobacco chewing conferred an increased risk only for tumors in the middle third. A Japanese study (Takezaki et al, 2000), on the other hand, found that alcohol drinking was associated with risk increases in all esophageal subsites, whereas cigarette smoking was associated with a significantly increased risk only in the middle part.

Even though the incidence of esophageal squamous cell carcinoma is considerably lower among women than among men in western populations, the combined literature seems to indicate that tobacco and alcohol are strong and important risk factors in both genders (Franceschi et al, 1994; Castellsague et al, 1999). However, the relative risk estimates are systematically lower among women than among men (Castellsague et al, 1999). In western Europe and North America, 90% or more of the risk of esophageal cancer can be attributed to alcohol and tobacco (Munoz and Day, 1996). Given that risk estimates seem to be lower in women than in men, and that the exposure prevalence for alcohol and tobacco smoke is generally lower among women, the estimated attributable fraction will be considerably lower in women than in men. In a large South American case-control study, the fraction of all cases that could be attributed to smoking and/or alcohol use was estimated at 90% among men and 29% among women (Castellsague et al, 1999).

The strong and multiplicative effects of smoking and drinking are not universal. The risks associated with these habits seem to be considerably lower or even absent in the high-incidence areas in the Asian esophageal cancer belt. But in low- to moderate-incidence areas in China, the "western" risk pattern prevails (Hu et al, 1994; Wu, Zhao et al, 2006). Moreover, unusually weak associations between smoking/drinking and the esophageal cancer risk were observed in Greece, a low-incidence country (Garidou et al, 1996). The causes of these discrepancies are unknown.

Adenocarcinoma
Compared with the esophageal squamous cell carcinomas, the esophageal adenocarcinomas are less strongly associated with alcohol and tobacco use (Fig. 9–5). The interpretation of published data on risk factors for the latter histologic type is complicated by the fact that some early studies have lumped adenocarcinomas of the esophagus and gastric cardia into one category. Subsequent studies strongly suggest that these two tumor types represent different disease entities with distinct

risk factor patterns (Lagergren, 1999; Ekström, 2000). This complication notwithstanding, relative risk estimates associated with smoking cluster around 1.5–2.5 in the studies published to date, all with a hospital-based or population-based case-control design (Kabat et al, 1993; Gammon et al, 1997; Lagergren, Bergström et al, 2000; Wu et al, 2001; Lindblad et al, 2005). Yet, in the US, population-attributable risk percent (PAR) pertaining to esophageal adenocarcinoma was estimated at 39.7% (Engel et al, 2003). A review paper with a combined evaluation of the effect of smoking cessation did not unveil a clear reduction of risk (Bosetti et al, 2006).

It also appears that alcohol use is not a risk factor for these tumors; all but one (Brown, Silverman et al, 1994) of the large studies were negative. Interestingly, wine even tended to be protective, as was the case with squamous cell carcinoma, in two studies from the United States (Gammon et al, 1997) and Sweden (Lagergren, Bergström et al, 2000).

Diet

Squamous cell carcinoma

Dietary factors have been addressed in numerous etiologic studies of esophageal cancer. Because the fraction of all esophageal cancers that can be attributed to genetic predisposition, smoking, and alcohol use appears to be small in the Asian high-incidence areas, dietary peculiarities have come into focus. The picture emerging from ecologic studies in these areas is not consistent. However, a common denominator in high-risk areas is poverty and lack of variation in the diet, which is mainly vegetarian, with a relatively small contribution from animal products (Hormozdiari et al, 1975; Thurnham et al, 1985; Jaskiewicz et al, 1988). Corn (Van Rensburg, 1981), wheat (Thurnham et al, 1985), or maize (Thurnham et al, 1985), is the chief staple, and cereals and bread dominate the diet.

Consumption of fruit and vegetables is typically low in areas with the highest incidence of esophageal cancer (Hormozdiari et al, 1975; Jaskiewicz et al, 1988). However, studies in Linxian, China, found that vegetable consumption was higher in high-risk populations than in low-risk comparison areas (Thurnham et al, 1985), but the common practice of sun-drying may have reduced the contents of anticarcinogenic substances. Analyses of food samples in high-incidence areas in Iran (Hormozdiari et al, 1975) did not reveal remarkably high levels of aflatoxin, polycyclic aromatic hydrocarbons (PAH), or nitrosamines.

Vitamins and micronutrients. The corn- or wheat-based diet has been estimated to be marginal or deficient in vitamins A and C, riboflavin, nicotinic acid, magnesium, and zinc (Hormozdiari et al, 1975; Van Rensburg, 1981). Deficiency of vitamin A (retinol), essential for growth, development, and differentiation of all tissues, has been associated with cancers of epithelial origin, and riboflavin (vitamin B_2) is essential for maintaining the integrity of the skin and the squamous epithelium of the esophagus. Zinc, which protects against free-radical formation and peroxidation, is also critical for the maintenance of normal bioactive retinol levels in blood. Zinc deficiency further increases the CYP2E1-dependent microsomal metabolism of nitrosamines and enhances the carcinogenicity of methylbenzylnitrosamine in animal models (Barch, 1989).

Deficiencies in vitamin or microelement levels have, indeed, been documented in high-risk countries like China (Yang et al, 1984; Thurnham et al, 1985) and South Africa (Jaskiewicz et al, 1988). The most striking and consistent finding in China and Uzbekistan is the high (up to 97%) prevalence of riboflavin deficiency. This prevalence seems to be lower (about 40%) in South Africa. Vitamin A deficiences were common (20% to 40%) in some but not all high-risk areas in China, while the vitamin A levels were generally acceptable in South Africa. Zinc deficiences were common (about 25%) in a few areas in both China and South Africa but less common in others. Data regarding carotenoids, vitamin C, and vitamin E were patchy and variable. Low levels were noted in some but not all high-risk areas. Other deficiencies reported in single studies include vitamin B_{12}, folic acid, magnesium, calcium, and selenium. Noteworthy is the nicotinic acid deficiences observed in about three out of four subjects in high-risk Transkei, South Africa. In an ecological study from China (Chen et al, 1992), dietary intake of a long list of trace elements was associated with esophageal cancer mortality, and zinc, in particular, emerged as inversely related to mortality risk. Further, copper intake was inversely and calcium intake positively related to this risk.

Data on individual intake, derived from case-control studies, indicate that a low intake of vitamins A, C, and B_2 is associated with an increased risk in both high- and low-risk populations. On the other hand, foods containing retinol were positively associated with a risk in several studies from Europe and the United States. Thus, the combined evidence from observational studies concerned with vitamin and mineral intake is fairly strong with regard to the protective effect of vitamins B_2 and C, but less convincing for vitamin A and most trace elements. Folate intake was consistently inversely associated with risk for both squamous cell carcinoma and adenocarcinoma of the esophagus in several studies in Western populations (Mayne et al, 2001; Bollschweiler et al, 2002; Chen, Tucker et al, 2002a; Galeone et al, 2006). Morover, Chinese cases with esophageal squamous cell carcinoma reported a significantly lower selenium intake in the past than did controls (Cai et al, 2006).

Endoscopic surveys conducted in high-incidence northern Iran and in Linxian, China, unveiled a remarkably high prevalence (> 80%) of chronic esophagitis of cryptic etiology (Munoz et al, 1982). It is typically located in the lower and middle thirds of the esophagus, accompanied by atrophy (about 10%) and dysplasia (4% to 8%), and clinically as well as histologically distinct from the reflux-related esophagitis seen in western populations. The prevalence of this presumed precancerous lesion is considerably higher in high-risk than in low-risk areas for esophageal cancer (Crespi et al, 1984). Three main hypotheses have been formulated regarding its etiology: (1) thermal injury resulting from the drinking of very hot beverages; (2) physical injury caused by ingesting very coarse food; and (3) nutritional deficiencies, notably of riboflavin, vitamin A, and zinc.

The nutritional hypotheses led to the launching of three randomized, placebo-controlled intervention trials among high-risk subjects in China. In one, 610 subjects aged 35 to 64 were treated with a combination of retinol, riboflavin, and zinc (Munoz et al, 1985). This regimen had no visible impact on the mysterious esophagitis after 13.5 months, but it did reduce the prevalence of micronuclei in the esophageal cells (Munoz et al, 1987). Another intervention trial in Linxian, China, used a factorial design to compare four combinations of vitamin/mineral supplements in 29584 subjects aged between 40 and 69 (Blot et al, 1993). In the group receiving a combination of β-carotene, vitamin E, and selenium daily for about 5 years, subjects experienced significantly lower total mortality and overall cancer mortality, but an observed 4% decline in esophageal cancer mortality was not statistically significant. A borderline reduction in esophageal cancer incidence was found in the group receiving riboflavin and niacin. No significant reduction in the prevalence of esophageal dysplasia was noted (Wang et al, 1994).

The third intervention trial compared daily supplementation consisting of 14 vitamins and 12 minerals with placebo among 3318 persons with cytologic diagnosis of esophageal dysplasia (Li et al, 1993). No difference was found in the cumulative incidence of esophageal cancer between the two treatment groups. A small, nonsignificant reduction in the occurrence of esophageal dysplasia (Dawsey et al, 1994) and a modest reduction in squamous cell proliferation (Rao et al, 1994) were noted, though. Although it is impossible to tell what would have happened if other doses had been used, or if the supplements had been given earlier, these intervention trials did not provide the critical evidence that would definitely establish the vitamin/mineral deficiency hypothesis in esophageal carcinogenesis.

Recently a fourth intervention study was conducted among subjects in Linxian with mild or moderate dysplasia (Limburg et al, 2005); in a randomized controlled trial with factorial design, participants were given selenomethionine 200 μg daily and/or celecoxib 200 mg twice daily for 10 months. Endoscopies were performed before and after the treatment period. Although selenomethionine treatment resulted in a trend toward increased dysplasia regression (43% versus 32% among subjects who did not receive this treatment), and a trend toward decreased progression (14% versus 19%), the overall effect was nonsignificant. However, the effect was greater (and statistically significant) among subjects with mild dysplasia at baseline, compared to those with moderate dysplasia. Since the latter stratification was an unplanned ad hoc analysis, this result has to be interpreted with caution.

Fruits and vegetables. The most consistent finding in the numerous case-control and cohort studies of dietary factors is a strong inverse relationship between fruit and/or vegetable intake and the risk of esophageal cancer. This literature has been reviewed repeatedly (Cheng and Day, 1996; Steinmetz and Potter, 1996; WCRF, 1997). Most of more than 50 cohort and case control studies have corroborated this inverse association, and the more recent additions constitute no exceptions; the overwhelming majority have demonstrated a protective effect of fruits and/or vegetables, or of their microconstituents (Kjaerheim et al, 1998; Launoy et al, 1998; Castellsague et al, 2000; Franceschi et al, 2000; Takezaki et al, 2000; Brown et al, 2001; Mayne et al, 2001; Terry, Lagergren, Hansen et al, 2001; Chen, Ward et al, 2002; De Stefani et al, 2003; Boeing et al, 2006).

In a case-control study from Uruguay, De Stefani et al (De Stefani et al, 2005) tried to dissect the association further; while the inverse overall association was impressive (odds ratio 0.31, 95% confidence interval 0.18–0.51), fruit intake was more protective than vegetable intake, and among various fruit categories, citrus fruits were particularly linked to a low risk. Based on data from a US case-control study, population-attributable risk percent (PAR) for low fruit and vegetable consumtion was estimated to be 28.7% when esophageal squamous cell carcinoma was the outcome (Engel et al, 2003).

However, exceptions exist among studies from high-risk countries in the Asian esophageal cancer belt; Li et al (1989) reported an increased risk with consumption of fresh vegetables and corn in a large case-control study in Linxian, China, and Wang et al (1992) associated intake of boiled vegetables with a considerable excess risk. Others were unable to confirm any positive or negative association between fruit/vegetable intake and esophageal cancer risk (Guo et al, 1994; Takezaki et al, 2001; Gao, Takezaki et al, 2002; Wu, Zhao et al, 2006) or found only a weak inverse association (Yu et al, 1993).

A recent meta-analysis included 13 studies—1 cohort and 12 case control (Riboli and Norat, 2003). On average, there was a significant protective effect of fruit and vegetables (summary odds ratio 0.89, 95% confidence interval 0.82–0.97) that seemed to be more important for fruit than for vegetables. The results were statistically heterogeneous. Contrary to the intuitive impression, subgroup analyses showed that the protective effect was not statistically different by geographical area (P > 0.05). European and North American studies, however, had more consistent results, while the heterogeneity persisted in Asian and South American studies.

Other food groups. The overall evidence regarding the association with food groups other than fruits and vegetables is inconsistent and thus less persuasive. One reason might be that dietary habits are closely linked to ethnic, cultural, and socioeconomic factors that are difficult to measure. If these factors are independently related to the esophageal cancer risk, confounding is unavoidable. While meat and fish were seemingly protective in some studies (Launoy et al, 1998)—but not invariably so (Bosetti et al, 2000)—and red meat was associated with a moderate risk increase in others (Bosetti et al, 2000; Castellsague et al, 2000; De Stefani et al, 2003), several studies showed no relationship with meat intake (Cheng and Day, 1996; Tavani et al, 2000).

Consumption of wheat and maize was a risk factor in some studies (Li et al, 1989); cereal or fiber intake, on the other hand, was inversely related to risk in others (Tzonou et al, 1996; Mayne et al, 2001; Chen, Tucker et al, 2002). High bread intake was associated with a sizable risk reduction in a Norwegian cohort study (Kjaerheim et al, 1998), as was the preference for whole-grain bread or whole-grain cereals in two studies that also linked high consumption of white bread (Yu et al, 1988) or refined fiber (Levi et al, 2000) to a high risk.

Butter consumption has emerged as a possible risk factor for esophageal cancer. As much as one-third of the high incidence in northwestern France was linked to the local excess in butter consumption (Launoy et al, 1998), even though, in South Africa, butter and margarine emerged as protective factors. Consumption of poly- or monounsaturated fatty acids has been repeatedly found to be inversely associated with the occurrence of squamous cell carcinoma in the esophagus (Franceschi et al, 2000).

Salt and nitrosamines. Salt intake, although difficult to assess in epidemiologic studies, has been implicated in a few studies (Castellsague et al, 2000). Nitrosamine exposure is even more difficult than salt to estimate on the basis of a recalled dietary pattern. Although ecological studies in Iran did not find remarkably high levels of nitrosamines in the food consumed by high-

risk groups (Hormozdiari et al, 1975), data chiefly from China provide some support for the hypothesis that nitrosamines and related compounds play a causal role in esophageal carcinogenesis.

An ecological study showed that high-risk areas were characterized by frequent pollution with nitrogen compounds in well water (Yokokawa et al, 1999). Other studies from high-risk areas have reported high exposure to nitrate and nitrite (Turkdogan et al, 2003) or volatile N-nitrosamines (Lin et al, 2002) in the population. In a cohort study, subjects who drank surface water were at increased risk (Yu et al, 1993). Moreover, an ecological study revealed that the rates of esophageal cancer mortality in 69 counties correlated positively with urinary levels of excreted N-nitrosoproline after proline loading, indicating exposure to N-nitroso compounds (Wu et al, 1993).

A high intake of pickled vegetables—known to contain high concentrations of N-nitroso compounds—was shown to be strongly and independently associated with the risk of esophageal cancer (Cheng, Day, Duffy et al, 1992). Intake of moldy food and pickled vegetable juice was also positively linked to esophageal cancer. However, several other studies in China, among them a cohort study, were unable to verify this positive association (Yu et al, 1993). In a recent systematic review, Jakszyn and Gonzalez (2006) attempted to summarize the available literature with regard to the relationship between estimated nitrosamine exposure and risk of esophageal cancer. They estimated exposure to preformed nitrosamines from external sources by examining intake of processed meat, beer, pickled and dried vegetables, smoked fish or meat, as well as salted or dried fish or meat. The quantification of endogenous nitrosamine formation was based on the intake of haem-containing red meat. Although the authors concluded that there is insufficient evidence for a role of nitrosamines in esophageal carcinogenesis, they noted that a majority of the studies showed point estimates that supported the nitrosamine hypothesis. This was particularly true for processed meat, but less for preserved fish, preserved vegetables, assessed nitrite exposure, and measured nitrosamine exposure. Moreover, 11 of 18 case-control studies and 1 out of 2 cohort studies showed a positive association between meat intake and esophageal cancer risk.

Other dietary hypotheses. Evidence of a protective effect of green tea was obtained in one study from Shanghai (Gao, McLaughlin, Blot, Ji, Dai et al, 1994). This may seem biologically plausible in view of documented anticarcinogenic effects of green tea in animal models. However, one study from Japan (Inoue et al, 1998) found no association, while a third study reported a statistically significant positive dose-risk trend of increasing esophageal squamous cell carcinoma risk with increasing number of cups per day (Ishikawa et al, 2006). Interpretation of such data is, however, complicated by the difficulties in disentangling the independent effects of tea from the effects of the temperature at which it is drunk. The association between drinking scalding hot beverages or very hot food and the risk of esophageal squamous cell carcinoma (Castellsague et al, 2000) is almost as consistent among studies as is the inverse association between fruit/vegetables and cancer risk. The only reported exception comes from Sweden (Terry, Lagergren, Wolk et al, 2001), where the range of exposure may be narrower than in the high-risk countries.

Heterocyclic amines are carcinogenic substances formed through pyrolysis of amino acids and creatine or creatinine when meats are cooked at high temperature, particularly by pan-frying. Heterocyclic amine levels increase with cooking temperature, with the type and shape of the cooked piece of meat, with the degree of browning on the surface, and with the cooking method. Several investigators have tried to shed light on a possible relationship between heterocyclic amine levels and risk of esophageal cancer, with cooking method, doneness preferences, or pictures of surface browning as markers of exposure. Frequent frying of

food (Galeone et al, 2005) or broiling of meat (De Stefani et al, 1998) was associated with risk of esophageal cancer or upper-aerodigestive cancer (of which approximately half were esophageal) in two European studies, while cooking method was unrelated to esophageal cancer in a third study from the US (Ward et al, 1997). A Swedish case-control study with a more detailed quantification of heterocyclic amine levels showed a statistically significant 2.4-fold excess risk for esophageal squamous cell carcinoma, but not for esophageal adenocarcinoma, among individuals with the highest intake of all three major heterocyclic amines, relative to those with the lowest intake (Terry et al, 2003).

For the sake of completeness, a few other hypotheses about food-related reasons for the excess of esophageal cancer in the high-incidence areas should be mentioned. Contamination of mycotoxins in the crop is one possibility and has, indeed, been documented in South Africa. However, its etiologic relevance has not been addressed in any analytical epidemiologic study. Another possible mechanism is an action of silica fragments that come from the grinding of millet bran. Silica fragments have been observed in the mucosa surrounding esophageal tumors of patients in northern China (O'Neill et al, 1982). Finally, high hepatic iron concentrations in South African black patients with esophageal cancer have led to the hypothesis that iron overload is a potential causal factor for these cancers (Isaacson et al, 1985). The iron is thought to emanate from alcoholic drinks that are home-brewed in cast iron containers.

Adenocarcinoma

Epidemiologic studies addressing dietary factors in esophageal adenocarcinoma remain sparse. The overall risk factor pattern seems to be similar to that observed in squamous cell carcinoma, notably a clear inverse relationship between intake of fruits and vegetables—or the corresponding microconstituents—and adenocarcinoma risk (Tzonou et al, 1996; Terry et al, 2000; Mayne et al, 2001; Bollschweiler et al,

2002; Chen, Ward et al, 2002; Chen, Tucker et al, 2002). US data indicated that 15.3% of all esophageal adenocarcinoma cases in the studied population could be attributed to low fruit and vegetable consumption (Engel et al, 2003).

The only dietary risk factor that differed between the two histological types of esophageal cancer in a US case-control study that included both histological types was dietary fat, the intake of which was a significant risk factor for esophageal adenocarcinoma but not for esophageal squamous cell carcinoma (Mayne et al, 2001). Saturated fat was a risk factor for esophageal adenocarcinoma also in a second US case-control study of esophageal adenocarcinoma (Chen, Tucker et al, 2002), but as saturated fat was reportedly a risk factor for esophageal squamous cell carcinoma in several other studies (see previous), it appears that the difference in the first US study may have been a chance finding.

A first analysis of the relationship between fruit and vegetable intake and risk of esophageal adenocarcinoma in the large European EPIC cohort (Gonzalez, Pera et al, 2006) yielded a nonsignificant negative association for the highest level of vegetable intake (hazard ratio 0.72, 95% confidence interval 0.32–1.64) and citrus intake (hazard ratio 0.77, 95% confidence interval 0.46–1.28), relative to the lowest. Although the low number of observed esophageal adenocarcinoma cases (n = 67) prohibits definite conclusions, it appears that the risk reduction in the cohort study was less than is typically seen in case-control studies, suggesting some recall bias in the latter.

The relationship to meat intake was also addressed in the EPIC cohort (Gonzalez, Jakszyn et al, 2006). The risk for esophageal adenocarcinoma was positively, albeit statistically nonsignificantly, associated with total meat intake (calibrated hazard ratio for a 100-g/day increase in intake 1.84, 95% confidence interval 0.78–4.39) and processed meat (calibrated hazard ratio for a 50-g/day increase in intake 1.44, 95% confidence interval 0.64–3.22), and statistically significantly with poultry intake

(calibrated hazard ratio for a 10-g/day increase in intake 1.14, 95% confidence interval 1.00–1.30).

The possible role of carbonated soft drinks, the consumption of which has increased in parallel with the increasing incidence of esophageal adenocarcinoma, and with a possible link to gastroesophageal reflux—the dominating risk factor for this cancer (see following)—was investigated in a US case-control study (Mayne et al, 2001). Contrary to the proposed hypothesis, the consumtion of carbonated soft drinks was inversely associated with esophageal adenocarcinoma risk. However, data from a similar Swedish case-control study did not confirm any important association between soft drink consumption and risk of esophageal adenocarcinoma (Lagergren et al, 2006).

Reproductive Factors and Hormones

Neither esophageal sqamous cell carcinoma nor adenocarcinoma are perceived as hormone-dependent cancers. There are practically no data on hormones and squamous cell carcinoma. The strong and unexplained male predominance among esophageal adenocarcinoma patients has attracted some attention. It was hypothesized that high estrogen levels might be protective. However, a study among more than 100 000 men receiving estrogen treatment for prostate cancer found no evidence of any protective effect (Lagergren and Nyren, 1998). The hypothesis postulating protection by female sex hormones has been tested further among women receiving hormone replacement therapy (Lindblad, Garcia Rodriguez et al, 2006), women with breast cancer being treated with the selective estrogen-receptor modulator Tamoxifen (Chandanos et al, 2006), and among women with varying parity (Lagergren and Jansson, 2005) without yielding any evidence in support of this theory. Given the already very low baseline incidence of esophageal adenocarcinoma among women, protective effects by any intervention are difficult to confirm. Breast-feeding was associated with a 60% reduction in esophageal adenocarcinoma risk among women in a study from Scotland, though (Cheng et al, 2000).

Anthropometric Measures

There are some reports of an inverse relation between relative weight (body mass index, BMI) and the risk of esophageal squamous cell carcinoma (Fig. 9–5). Since weight loss is an early consequence of the disease, the possibility of reversed causation or confounding by socioeconomic status cannot be ruled out. Other studies found BMI well before disease onset to be unrelated to the risk of squamous cell carcinoma (Chow, Blot et al, 1998; Lagergren, Bergstrom and Nyren, 1999).

Esophageal adenocarcinomas, on the other hand, are positively, independently, and strongly associated with relative weight (Chow, Blot et al, 1998; Lagergren, Bergsttom and Nyren 1999). This relationship has been confirmed in numerous studies, including a prospective study with meticulous registration of anthropometric measures and long follow up (MacInnis et al, 2006). Although the number of observed cases was small in the latter study, and esophageal and gastric cardia adenocarcinoma were lumped together, statistically significant risk gradients were confirmed in relation to BMI, waist circumference, and fat-free mass. It appears that the risk gradient goes through the whole spectrum of relative weights, from the leanest to the most obese. In a Swedish study persons with a BMI above 30 had a risk 16 times greater than that of persons with a BMI below 22 (Lagergren, Bergstrom and Nyren, 1999). Tall stature, possibly reflecting better socioeconomic conditions during childhood and adolescence, appears to be associated with a low risk (Lagergren, Bergstrom and Nyren, 1999).

Infections

Human papillomavirus

Infection with human papillomavirus (HPV), especially HPV type 16, has been implicated as a risk factor for squamous cell carcinoma of the esophagus. There are reports of HPV DNA detected in squamous cell carcinoma, although other studies are negative. Among six seroepidemiologic studies, three of which were nested within prospective cohorts, three found positive associations but with wide confidence intervals (Dillner et al, 1995; Han et al, 1996; Bjorge et al, 1997), whereas two retrospective studies, including the largest published to date (Lagergren, Wang et al, 1999; Van Doornum et al, 2003) and a prospective study in a Chinese high-risk area with precise odds ratio estimates for HPV 16, HPV 18, and HPV 73 (Kamangar, Qiao et al, 2006), were negative. The reasons for the inconsistent results remain conjectural. Although some authors express skepticism (Galloway and Daling, 1996), the issue about the role of HPV in esophageal squamous cell carcinoma is not yet settled. It appears, though, that esophageal adenocarcinomas are unrelated to HPV (Lagergren, Wang et al, 1999).

H. pylori

Another still enigmatic phenomenon is the inverse relationship between *Helicobacter pylori* type I seropositivity and the risk of adenocarcinoma of the esophagus and gastric cardia, confirmed in several studies conducted in Western populations (Chow, Blaser et al, 1998; Hansen et al, 1999; Siman et al, 2001; Wu, Crabtree et al, 2003; Ye et al, 2004; De Martel et al, 2005; Kamangar, Dawsey et al, 2006). The mechanism has been assumed to involve gastric atrophy, hypoacidity, and reduced acidic reflux into the esophagus. However, gastric atrophy, measured through the pepsinogen 1 biomarker, was unrelated to the risk of esophageal adenocarcinoma (Ye et al, 2004). Therfore, gastric atrophy is a less likely intermediate step.

Although a moderately strong inverse relationship appears to exist between *H. pylori* infection and prevalence of gastroesophageal reflux (Raghunath et al, 2003), the true character of the mechanism behind the mysterious protection against esophageal adenocarcinoma remains to be unveiled. Clearly, as *H. pylori* does not colonize the esophagus, esophageal carcinogenesis is in some way dependent on events that take place in the the stomach.

A twofold increased risk of esophageal squamous cell carcinoma was noted among individuals with serological evidence of CagA-positive *H. pylori* infections in a population-based Swedish case-control study (Ye et al, 2004). A similarly strong positive association with esophageal squamous cell carcinoma risk was found also for gastric atrophy, determined with pepsinogen I. However, a subsequent prospectice study from China found no link between *H. pylori* serostatus and risk of esophageal squamous cell carcinoma (Kamangar et al, 2007). More studies are needed in both high- and low-risk populations to clarify the possible role of *H. pylori* infection in the etiology of esophageal squamous cell carcinoma.

Occupation

Some occupational groups seem to be at increased risk for squamous cell carcinoma of the esophagus. There is substantial evidence that persons who work with vulcanization in the rubber or automobile industry run an increased risk of this cancer (Norell et al, 1983). Other occupations associated with an increased risk include chimney sweeps (Evanoff et al, 1993), mine workers (Vizcaino et al, 1995), chemical products workers (Sathiakumar et al, 1992), butchers (Besson et al, 2006), and medical x-ray workers. Significant positive associations have also been identified among workers in the cement industry (Jakobsson et al, 1990; Jansson et al, 2006), the plastics and composites industry (Wong et al, 1994), the dye production industry (Bulbulyan et al, 1995), and bookbindery (Bulbulyan et al, 1999).

Specific exposures tentatively linked to esophageal cancer include metal dust (Yu et al, 1988), asbestosis (Kang et al, 1997), silica dust (Pan et al, 1999; Wernli et al, 2006), combustion products (Gustavsson et al, 1993), metals (Wernli et al, 2006), organic solvents (Lynge et al, 1997; Hansen et al, 2001)—particularly perchlorethylene in dry-cleaning industries (Vaughan et al, 1997)—and PAH (Gustavsson et al, 1998).

Cumulative exposure to endotoxin, a contaminant of cotton dust, was found to be inversely related to esophageal cancer risk among female textile workers in China (Wernli et al, 2006). A problem in most of these studies was the inability to adjust for possible confounders, particularly smoking and alcohol use.

The strong gender imbalance among adenocarcinoma cases indicates that occupational exposures also may be important for this cancer type, but hard data are scarce. One case-control study reported a fourfold increased risk among white women with administrative jobs, while a twofold increase was found among female health professionals. Another study implicated employments in administrative support, financial, insurance, and real estate and health services (Engel et al, 2002). A third study found pesticide exposure to be borderline significantly associated with risk of esophageal adenocarcinoma (Jansson et al, 2006). More studies will be needed, but the rarity of esophageal adenocarcinoma constitutes an essentially insurmountable hurdle in the assessment of occupation-specific risks.

In a Swedish population-based case-control study, self-reported job strain, work-pace satisfaction, and coping was investigated in relation to risk of esophageal cancer by histology (Jansson et al, 2004). Subjects reporting low work-pace satisfaction had an almost fourfold elevated risk of esophageal squamous cell carcinoma and a nearly threefold increased risk of esophageal adenocarcinoma. Athough work-related stress did not seem to be important, the interaction of a stressful work environment and the individual's responses to it may be conducive to the developoment of esophageal cancer.

Medical Conditions

Some medical conditions confer a higher risk of esophageal cancer. The classic example is Plummer-Vinson or Paterson-Kelly syndrome (Ahlbom, 1936), characterized by hypochromic anemia and changes in the hypopharynx. This syndrome was formerly common in northern Europe but is rarely seen nowadays. It is thought to be caused by nutritional deficiencies and was often accompanied by esophageal squamous cell carcinomas. Achalasia, with stagnation of food debris and fluid in the esophagus because the lower sphincter fails to relax on swallowing, is associated with substantially elevated risks of both squamous cell carcinoma and adenocarcinoma, at least in men (Zendehdel et al, 2007). As the risks for both tumor types are more than tenfold increased 10 years or more after the achalasia diagnosis, reversed causation cannot explain the association.

Celiac disease has also been associated with an increased risk of esophageal cancer, although properly designed epidemiologic studies are lacking. Hemochromatosis was followed by an almost 50-fold excess risk of esophageal cancer in one cohort study (Hsing et al, 1995) with only two observed cases. A threefold increased risk of esophageal squamous cell carcinoma, but no significant risk elevation for adenocarcinoma, was noted among patients who had been hospitalized with pernicious anemia (Ye and Nyren, 2003).

Gastroesophageal reflux

Gastroesophageal reflux disease is the strongest known risk factor for adenocarcinoma of the esophagus (Fig. 9–5). In a large study, the risk gradient between those without any symptoms of reflux and those with the most severe and long-standing symptoms was more than 40-fold (Lagergren, Bergstrom, Lindgren et al, 1999). The association seems to be independent of other known or suspected risk factors for esophageal adenocarcinoma, including BMI. The presence of a hiatal hernia may interact synergistically with the reflux condition to inflate the relative risks more than multiplicatively (Wu, Tseng et al, 2003). Although the strength of the association varies among studies, the results are consistent and biologically plausible. The origin of adenocarcinoma in the esophagus could conceivably be in the submucosal glands or in ectopic gastric epithelium.

More commonly, though, adenocarcinomas seem to arise in Barrett's esophagus, a columnar cell metaplasia that replaces the native squamous cell epithelium of the distal part of the esophagus (Barrett, 1950; Spechler and Goyal, 1986).

Barrett's esophagus

There is a broad consensus that Barrett's esophagus in most cases is a consequence of long-standing gastroesophageal reflux (Winters et al, 1987). This metaplasia is seen in approximately 10% of patients who are investigated for reflux disease. Three histologic subtypes of Barrett's esophagus have been described: the fundic type, the junctional type, and the specialized intestinal-like type. Current definitions of Barrett's esophagus tend to require the presence of specialized intestinal metaplasia in addition to a macroscopically visible lesion. Early clinical observations indicated that the risk of developing adenocarcinoma in Barrett's esophagus is substantial. This increased risk appears to be confined to patients with the specialized intestinal-like subtype. The magnitude of the excess risk is a matter of controversy although review articles often mention a 50- to 100-fold increase (Streitz, 1994). Methodologically, studies of Barrett's esophagus and adenocarcinoma risk are hampered by small numbers (Shaheen et al, 2000), and by possible selection and publication bias. Selection bias might inflate risk estimates in clinical case series coming from centers with a special interest in esophageal cancer. And a systematic review gave clear indications of publication bias (Shaheen et al, 2000). Since then, a population based study of reasonable size has been published (Murray et al, 2003); among 2969 patients from Northern Ireland with Barrett's esophagus, contributing 11 068 person-years of follow-up, the crude overall esophageal cancer incidence was 260 per 100 000 person-years (400 per 100 000 person-years among patients with documented specialized intestinal metaplasia).

Another controversy related to the link between Barrett's esophagus and esophageal adenocarcinoma concerns whether or not the metaplasia is an obligatory intermediate step in the carcinogenic pathway. Earlier studies were unable to demonstrate metaplastic epithelium in approximately 30% of the adenocarcinoma cases (Kim et al, 1997). One study showed that the association between gastroesophageal reflux and adenocarcinoma was equally strong, regardless of whether or not the tumor was accompanied by Barrett's metaplasia (Lagergren, Bergstrom, Lindgren et al, 1999). However, several investigators claim that short metaplastic segments (Nandurkar et al, 1997) might be missed, perhaps due to destruction by the tumor (Sabel et al, 2000). If Barrett's esophagus is a necessary intermediate step, it appears that the neoplastic transformation of the metaplastic epithelium occurs much more often in men than in women; the male:female ratio in esophageal adenocarcinoma is considerably higher than in Barrett's esophagus (Johansson et al, 2007).

Other Risk Factors

It is well known that esophageal squamous cell carcinoma primarily affects the socioeconomically disadvantaged. For instance, the incidence in the United States is considerably higher among African-Americans than among whites. There is abundant evidence for a relatively steep inverse socioeconomic gradient in risk, regardless of whether the population is at high or low risk (Vassallo et al, 1985; Pukkala and Teppo, 1986; Segal et al, 1988; Van Loon et al, 1995; Gammon et al, 1997). The descriptive epidemiology of esophageal adenocarcinoma seems to imply that the distribution across socioeconomic strata is different from that of squamous cell carcinoma. In the United States, adenocarcinomas are more common among whites than among African-Americans. This does not mean, however, that socioeconomic status is positively associated with risk. British investigators found no relationship at all, while in the United States and Sweden, the risk increased more than threefold with decreasing socioeconomic status and income (Brown, Silverman et al, 1994; Jansson et al, 2005).

CONCLUSION

Esophageal cancer remains a challenge to health care and public health authorities. In large parts of the world, it is a very common disease, and the prospect of cure is worse than for most other malignancies. The remarkably uneven geographic distribution, and the apparently small proportion that can be attributed to genetic factors, seem to imply that strong external risk factors—possibly reinforced by genetically determined susceptibility—are in operation. This should raise hope that preventive measures will become a realistic option in the foreseeable future. The dramatic rise in incidence of the adenocarcinomas poses a special challenge to epidemiologists. Such a rapid change is bound to depend on changes in the exposure to important causal factors. The well-documented increase in the prevalence of obesity in many populations might be one such factor. However, given some conflicting observations, for instance the much lower risk among women despite the equally high prevalence of obesity, an uncertain link between obesity and reflux, and a clear association between obesity and adenocarcinoma risk observable also in the very low range of body mass, there is clearly room for alternative hypotheses. It appears that a number of other promising leads need be followed up, requiring joint and decisive efforts by epidemiologists and basic scientists.

REFERENCES

Abbas A, Delvinquiere K, Lechevrel M, Lebailly P, Gauduchon P, Launoy G, et al. GSTM1, GSTT1, GSTP1 and CYP1A1 genetic polymorphisms and susceptibility to esophageal cancer in a French population: different pattern of squamous cell carcinoma and adenocarcinoma. World J Gastroenterol 2004; 10:3389–93.

Ahlbom H. Simple achlorhydric anaemia, Plummer-Vinson syndrome and carcinoma of the mouth, pharynx and oesophagus in women. Br Med J 1936;2:331–33.

Akbari MR, Malekzadeh R, Nasrollahzadeh D, Amanian D, Sun P, Islami F, et al. Familial risks of esophageal cancer among the

Turkmen population of the Caspian littoral of Iran. Int J Cancer 2006;119:1047–51.

Barch DH. Esophageal cancer and microelements. J Am Coll Nutr 1989;8:99–107.

Barrett MT, Galipeau PC, Sanchez CA, Emond MJ, Reid BJ. Determination of the frequency of loss of heterozygosity in esophageal adenocarcinoma by cell sorting, whole genome amplification and microsatellite polymorphisms. Oncogene 1996;12:1873–78.

Barrett NR. Chronic peptic ulcer of the oesophagus and "oesophagitis." Br J Surg 1950; 38:175–82.

Bartsch H, Nair U, Risch A, Rojas M, Wikman H, Alexandrov K. Genetic polymorphism of CYP genes, alone or in combination, as a risk modifier of tobacco-related cancers. Cancer Epidemiol Biomarkers Prev 2000;9:3–28.

Besson H, Banks RBoffetta P. Cancer mortality among butchers: a 24-state death certificate study. J Occup Environ Med 2006;48:289–93.

Bizari L, Borim AA, Leite KR, Goncalves Fde T, Cury PM, Tajara EH, et al. Alterations of the CCND1 and HER-2/neu (ERBB2) proteins in esophageal and gastric cancers. Cancer Genet Cytogenet 2006;165:41–50.

Bjorge T, Hakulinen T, Engeland A, Jellum E, Koskela P, Lehtinen M, et al. A prospective, seroepidemiological study of the role of human papillomavirus in esophageal cancer in Norway. Cancer Res 1997;57:3989–92.

Blaser MJ, Saito D. Trends in reported adenocarcinomas of the oesophagus and gastric cardia in Japan. Eur J Gastroenterol Hepatol 2002;14:107–13.

Blot WJ, Devesa SS, Kneller RW, Fraumeni JF, Jr. Rising incidence of adenocarcinoma of the esophagus and gastric cardia. JAMA 1991;265:1287–89.

Blot WJ, Li JY, Taylor PR, Guo W, Dawsey S, Wang GQ, et al. Nutrition intervention trials in Linxian, China: supplementation with specific vitamin/mineral combinations, cancer incidence, and disease- specific mortality in the general population. J Natl Cancer Inst 1993;85:1483–92.

Boeing H, Dietrich T, Hoffmann K, Pischon T, Ferrari P, Lahmann PH, et al. Intake of fruits and vegetables and risk of cancer of the upper aero-digestive tract: the prospective EPIC-study. Cancer Causes Control 2006;17: 957–69.

Bollschweiler E, Wolfgarten E, Nowroth T, Rosendahl U, Monig SP, Holscher AH. Vitamin intake and risk of subtypes of esophageal cancer in Germany. J Cancer Res Clin Oncol 2002;128:575–80.

Boonyaphiphat P, Thongsuksai P, Sriplung H, Puttawibul P. Lifestyle habits and genetic susceptibility and the risk of esophageal cancer in the Thai population. Cancer Lett 2002;186:193–99.

Bosetti C, La Vecchia C, Talamini R, Simonato L, Zambon P, Negri E, et al. Food groups and risk of squamous cell esophageal cancer in northern Italy. Int J Cancer 2000;87: 289–94.

Bosetti C, Gallus S, Garavello WLa Vecchia C. Smoking cessation and the risk of oesophageal cancer: An overview of published studies. Oral Oncol 2006;42:957–64.

Botterweck AA, Schouten LJ, Volovics A, Dorant E, van Den Brandt PA. Trends in incidence of adenocarcinoma of the oesophagus and gastric cardia in ten European countries. Int J Epidemiol 2000;29:645–54.

Boynton RF, Blount PL, Yin J, Brown VL, Huang Y, Tong Y, et al. Loss of heterozygosity involving the APC and MCC genetic loci occurs in the majority of human esophageal cancers. Proc Natl Acad Sci USA 1992;89:3385–88.

Brown LM, Blot WJ, Schuman SH, Smith VM, Ershow AG, Marks RD, et al. Environmental factors and high risk of esophageal cancer among men in coastal South Carolina. J Natl Cancer Inst 1988;80:1620–25.

Brown LM, Hoover RN, Greenberg RS, Schoenberg JB, Schwartz AG, Swanson GM, et al. Are racial differences in squamous cell esophageal cancer explained by alcohol and tobacco use? J Natl Cancer Inst 1994;86:1340–45.

Brown LM, Silverman DT, Pottern LM, Schoenberg JB, Greenberg RS, Swanson GM, et al. Adenocarcinoma of the esophagus and esophagogastric junction in white men in the United States: alcohol, tobacco, and socioeconomic factors. Cancer Causes Control 1994;5:333–40.

Brown LM, Hoover R, Silverman D, Baris D, Hayes R, Swanson GM, et al. Excess incidence of squamous cell esophageal cancer among US Black men: role of social class and other risk factors. Am J Epidemiol 2001; 153:114–22.

Brown LM, Devesa SS. Epidemiologic trends in esophageal and gastric cancer in the United States. Surg Oncol Clin N Am 2002;11:235–56.

Bulbulyan MA, Figgs LW, Zahm SH, Savitskaya T, Goldfarb A, Astashevsky S, et al. Cancer incidence and mortality among beta-naphthylamine and benzidine dye workers in Moscow. Int J Epidemiol 1995;24:266–75.

Bulbulyan MA, Ilychova SA, Zahm SH, Astashevsky SV, Zaridze DG. Cancer mortality among women in the Russian printing industry. Am J Ind Med 1999;36:166–71.

Cai L, You NC, Lu H, Mu LN, Lu QY, Yu SZ, et al. Dietary selenium intake, aldehyde dehydrogenase-2 and X-ray repair cross-complementing 1 genetic polymorphisms, and the risk of esophageal squamous cell carcinoma. Cancer 2006;106:2345–54.

Cameron AJ, Lagergren J, Henriksson C, Nyren O, Locke GR, 3rd, Pedersen NL. Gastroesophageal reflux disease in monozygotic and dizygotic twins. Gastroenterology 2002; 122:55–59.

Carter CL, Hu N, Wu M, Lin PZ, Murigande C, Bonney GE. Segregation analysis of esophageal cancer in 221 high-risk Chinese families. J Natl Cancer Inst 1992;84:771–76.

Casson AG, Zheng Z, Chiasson D, MacDonald K, Riddell DC, Guernsey JR, et al. Associations between genetic polymorphisms of Phase I and II metabolizing enzymes, p53 and susceptibility to esophageal adenocarcinoma. Cancer Detect Prev 2003;27:139–46.

Casson AG, Zheng Z, Evans SC, Geldenhuys L, van Zanten SV, Veugelers PJ, et al. Cyclin D1 polymorphism (G870A) and risk for esophageal adenocarcinoma. Cancer 2005; 104:730–39.

Casson AG, Zheng Z, Evans SC, Veugelers PJ, Porter GA, Guernsey DL. Polymorphisms in DNA repair genes in the molecular pathogenesis of esophageal (Barrett) adenocarcinoma. Carcinogenesis 2005;26:1536–41.

Casson AG, Zheng Z, Porter GA, Guernsey DL. Genetic polymorphisms of microsomal epoxide hydroxylase and glutathione S-transferases M1, T1 and P1, interactions with smoking, and risk for esophageal (Barrett) adenocarcinoma. Cancer Detect Prev 2006;30:423–31.

Castellsague X, Munoz N, De Stefani E, Victora CG, Castelletto R, Rolon PA, et al. Independent and joint effects of tobacco smoking and alcohol drinking on the risk of esophageal cancer in men and women. Int J Cancer 1999;82:657–64.

Castellsague X, Munoz N, De Stefani E, Victora CG, Castelletto R, Rolon PA. Influence of mate drinking, hot beverages and diet on esophageal cancer risk in South America. Int J Cancer 2000;88:658–64.

Chak A, Ochs-Balcom H, Falk G, Grady WM, Kinnard M, Willis JE, et al. Familiality in Barrett's esophagus, adenocarcinoma of the esophagus, and adenocarcinoma of the gastroesophageal junction. Cancer Epidemiol Biomarkers Prev 2006;15:1668–73.

Chandanos E, Lindblad M, Jia C, Rubio CA, Ye W, Lagergren J. Tamoxifen exposure and risk of oesophageal and gastric adenocarcinoma: a population-based cohort study of breast cancer patients in Sweden. Br J Cancer 2006;95:118–22.

Chen F, Cole P, Mi Z, Xing L. Dietary trace elements and esophageal cancer mortality in Shanxi, China. Epidemiology 1992;3:402–6.

Chen H, Tucker KL, Graubard BI, Heineman EF, Markin RS, Potischman NA, et al. Nutrient intakes and adenocarcinoma of the esophagus and distal stomach. Nutr Cancer 2002;42:33–40.

Chen H, Ward MH, Graubard BI, Heineman EF, Markin RM, Potischman NA, et al. Dietary patterns and adenocarcinoma of the esophagus and distal stomach. Am J Clin Nutr 2002;75:137–44.

Chen YJ, Chen C, Wu DC, Lee CH, Wu CI, Lee JM, et al. Interactive effects of lifetime alcohol consumption and alcohol and aldehyde dehydrogenase polymorphisms on esophageal cancer risks. Int J Cancer 2006; 119:2827–31.

Cheng KK, Day NE, Davies TW. Oesophageal cancer mortality in Europe: paradoxical time trend in relation to smoking and drinking. Br J Cancer 1992;65:613–17.

Cheng KK, Day NE, Duffy SW, Lam TH, Fok M, Wong J. Pickled vegetables in the aetiology of oesophageal cancer in Hong Kong Chinese. Lancet 1992;339:1314–18.

Cheng KK, Duffy SW, Day NE, Lam TH, Chung SF, Badrinath P. Stopping drinking and risk of oesophageal cancer. Br Med J 1995; 310:1094–97.

Cheng KK, Day NE. Nutrition and esophageal cancer. Cancer Causes Control 1996;7:33–40.

Cheng KK, Sharp L, McKinney PA, Logan RF, Chilvers CE, Cook-Mozaffari P, et al. A case-control study of oesophageal adenocarcinoma in women: a preventable disease. Br J Cancer 2000;83:127–32.

Chow WH, Blaser MJ, Blot WJ, Gammon MD, Vaughan TL, Risch HA, et al. An inverse relation between cagA+ strains of Helicobacter pylori infection and risk of esophageal and gastric cardia adenocarcinoma. Cancer Res 1998;58:588–90.

Chow WH, Blot WJ, Vaughan TL, Risch HA, Gammon MD, Stanford JL, et al. Body mass index and risk of adenocarcinomas of the esophagus and gastric cardia. J Natl Cancer Inst 1998;90:150–55.

Crespi M, Munoz N, Grassi A, Qiong S, Jing WK, Jien LJ. Precursor lesions of oesophageal cancer in a low-risk population in China: comparison with high-risk populations. Int J Cancer 1984;34:599–602.

Cui Y, Morgenstern H, Greenland S, Tashkin DP, Mao J, Cao W, et al. Polymorphism of Xeroderma Pigmentosum group G and the risk of lung cancer and squamous cell carcinomas of the oropharynx, larynx and esophagus. Int J Cancer 2006;118:714–20.

Dandara C, Ballo R, Parker MI. CYP3A5 genotypes and risk of oesophageal cancer in two South African populations. Cancer Lett 2005;225:275–82.

Dandara C, Li DP, Walther G, Parker MI. Gene-environment interaction: the role of SULT1A1 and CYP3A5 polymorphisms as risk modifiers for squamous cell carcinoma of the oesophagus. Carcinogenesis 2006;27:791–97.

Dawsey SM, Wang GQ, Taylor PR, Li JY, Blot WJ, Li B, et al. Effects of vitamin/mineral supplementation on the prevalence of histological dysplasia and early cancer of the esophagus and stomach: results from the Dysplasia Trial in Linxian, China. Cancer Epidemiol Biomarkers Prev 1994;3:167–72.

de Martel C, Llosa AE, Farr SM, Friedman GD, Vogelman JH, Orentreich N, et al. Helicobacter pylori infection and the risk of development of esophageal adenocarcinoma. J Infect Dis 2005;191:761–67.

De Stefani E, Ronco A, Mendilaharsu M, Deneo-Pellegrini H. Case-control study on the role of heterocyclic amines in the etiology of upper aerodigestive cancers in Uruguay. Nutr Cancer 1998;32:43–48.

De Stefani E, Deneo-Pellegrini H, Ronco AL, Boffetta P, Brennan P, Munoz N, et al. Food groups and risk of squamous cell carcinoma of the oesophagus: a case-control study in Uruguay. Br J Cancer 2003;89:1209–14.

De Stefani E, Boffetta P, Deneo-Pellegrini H, Ronco AL, Correa P, Mendilaharsu M. The role of vegetable and fruit consumption in the aetiology of squamous cell carcinoma of the oesophagus: a case-control study in Uruguay. Int J Cancer 2005;116:130–35.

Dhillon PK, Farrow DC, Vaughan TL, Chow WH, Risch HA, Gammon MD, et al. Family history of cancer and risk of esophageal and gastric cancers in the United States. Int J Cancer 2001;93:148–52.

Dillner J, Knekt P, Schiller JT, Hakulinen T. Prospective seroepidemiological evidence that human papillomavirus type 16 infection is a risk factor for oesophageal squamous cell carcinoma. Br Med J 1995;311;1346.

di Martino E, Hardie LJ, Wild CP, Gong YY, Olliver JR, Gough MD, et al. The NAD(P)H:quinone oxidoreductase I C609T polymorphism modifies the risk of Barrett esophagus and esophageal adenocarcinoma. Genet Med 2007;9:341–7.

Drovdlic CM, Goddard KA, Chak A, Brock W, Chessler L, King JF, et al. Demographic and phenotypic features of 70 families segregating Barrett's oesophagus and oesophageal adenocarcinoma. J Med Genet 2003;40:651–6.

Ekström A-M. Factors related to the occurrence of gastric adenocarcinoma subtypes (Thesis). Stockholm, Karolinska Institutet, 2000.

Ellis A, Field JK, Field EA, Friedmann PS, Fryer A, Howard P, et al. Tylosis associated with carcinoma of the oesophagus and oral leukoplakia in a large Liverpool family—a review of six generations. Eur J Cancer B Oral Oncol 1994;2:102–12.

El-Omar EM, Rabkin CS, Gammon MD, Vaughan TL, Risch HA, Schoenberg JB, et al. Increased risk of noncardia gastric cancer associated with proinflammatory cytokine gene polymorphisms. Gastroenterology 2003;124:1193–201.

Engel LS, Vaughan TL, Gammon MD, Chow WH, Risch HA, Dubrow R, et al. Occupation and risk of esophageal and gastric cardia adenocarcinoma. Am J Ind Med 2002;42:11–22.

Engel LS, Chow WH, Vaughan TL, Gammon MD, Risch HA, Stanford JL, et al. Population attributable risks of esophageal and gastric cancers. J Natl Cancer Inst 2003;95:1404–13.

Evanoff BA, Gustavsson P, Hogstedt C. Mortality and incidence of cancer in a cohort of Swedish chimney sweeps: an extended follow up study. Br J Ind Med 1993;50:450–59.

Franceschi S, Bidoli E, Negri E, Barbone F, La Vecchia C. Alcohol and cancers of the upper aerodigestive tract in men and women. Cancer Epidemiol Biomarkers Prev 1994;3:299–304.

Franceschi S, Bidoli E, Negri E, Zambon P, Talamini R, Ruol A, et al. Role of macronutrients, vitamins and minerals in the aetiology of squamous-cell carcinoma of the oesophagus. Int J Cancer 2000;86:626–31.

Galeone C, Pelucchi C, Talamini R, Levi F, Bosetti C, Negri E, et al. Role of fried foods and oral/pharyngeal and oesophageal cancers. Br J Cancer 2005;92:2065–69.

Galeone C, Pelucchi C, Levi F, Negri E, Talamini R, Franceschi S, et al. Folate intake and squamous-cell carcinoma of the oesophagus in Italian and Swiss men. Ann Oncol 2006;17:521–25.

Galipeau PC, Cowan DS, Sanchez CA, Barrett MT, Emond MJ, Levine DS, et al. 17p (p53) allelic losses, 4N (G2/tetraploid) populations, and progression to aneuploidy in Barrett's esophagus. Proc Natl Acad Sci USA 1996;93:7081–84.

Galipeau PC, Prevo LJ, Sanchez CA, Longton GM, Reid BJ. Clonal expansion and loss of heterozygosity at chromosomes 9p and 17p in premalignant esophageal (Barrett's) tissue. J Natl Cancer Inst 1999;91:2087–95.

Galloway DA, Daling JR. Is the evidence implicating human papillomavirus type 16 in esophageal cancer hard to swallow? J Natl Cancer Inst 1996;88:1421–23.

Gammon MD, Schoenberg JB, Ahsan H, Risch HA, Vaughan TL, Chow WH, et al. Tobacco, alcohol, and socioeconomic status and adenocarcinomas of the esophagus and gastric cardia. J Natl Cancer Inst 1997;89:1277–84.

Gao C, Takezaki T, Wu J, Li Z, Wang J, Ding J, et al. Interaction between cytochrome P-450 2E1 polymorphisms and environmental factors with risk of esophageal and stomach cancers in Chinese. Cancer Epidemiol Biomarkers Prev 2002;11:29–34.

Gao CM, Takezaki T, Wu JZ, Li ZY, Liu YT, Li SP, et al. Glutathione-S-transferases M1 (GSTM1) and GSTT1 genotype, smoking, consumption of alcohol and tea and risk of esophageal and stomach cancers: a case-control study of a high-incidence area in Jiangsu Province, China. Cancer Lett 2002; 188:95–102.

Gao CM, Takezaki T, Wu JZ, Liu YT, Ding JH, Li SP, et al. Polymorphisms in thymidylate synthase and methylenetetrahydrofolate reductase genes and the susceptibility to esophageal and stomach cancer with smoking. Asian Pac J Cancer Prev 2004;5:133–38.

Gao CM, Toshiro T, Wu JZ, Cao HX, Liu YT, Ding JH, et al. [A case-control study on the polymorphisms of methylenetetrahydrofolate reductase 1298A—>C and susceptibility of esophageal cancer]. Zhonghua Liu Xing Bing Xue Za Zhi 2004;25:341–45.

Gao YT, McLaughlin JK, Blot WJ, Ji BT, Benichou J, Dai Q, et al. Risk factors for esophageal cancer in Shanghai, China. I. Role of cigarette smoking and alcohol drinking. Int J Cancer 1994;58:192–96.

Gao YT, McLaughlin JK, Blot WJ, Ji BT, Dai Q, Fraumeni JF, Jr. Reduced risk of esophageal cancer associated with green tea consumption. J Natl Cancer Inst 1994;86:855–58.

Garidou A, Tzonou A, Lipworth L, Signorello LB, Kalapothaki V, Trichopoulos D. Lifestyle factors and medical conditions in relation to esophageal cancer by histologic type in a low-risk population. Int J Cancer 1996;68:295–99.

Geddert H, Kiel S, Zotz RB, Zhang J, Willers R, Gabbert HE, et al. Polymorphism of p16 INK4A and cyclin D1 in adenocarcinomas of the upper gastrointestinal tract. J Cancer Res Clin Oncol 2005;131:803–8.

Ghadirian P. Familial history of esophageal cancer. Cancer 1985;56:2112–16.

Gonzalez CA, Jakszyn P, Pera G, Agudo A, Bingham S, Palli D, et al. Meat intake and risk of stomach and esophageal adenocarcinoma within the European Prospective Investigation Into Cancer and Nutrition (EPIC). J Natl Cancer Inst 2006;98:345–54.

Gonzalez CA, Pera G, Agudo A, Bueno-de-Mesquita HB, Ceroti M, Boeing H, et al.

Fruit and vegetable intake and the risk of stomach and oesophagus adenocarcinoma in the European Prospective Investigation into Cancer and Nutrition (EPIC-EURGAST). Int J Cancer 2006;118:2559–66.

Gough MD, Ackroyd R, Majeed AW, Bird NC. Prediction of malignant potential in reflux disease: are cytokine polymorphisms important? Am J Gastroenterol 2005;100:1012–18.

Graham S, Marshall J, Haughey B, Brasure J, Freudenheim J, Zielezny M, et al. Nutritional epidemiology of cancer of the esophagus. Am J Epidemiol 1990;131:454–67.

Gronbaek M, Becker U, Johansen D, Tonnesen H, Jense G, Sorensen TIA. Population based cohort study of the association between alcohol intake and cancer of the upper digestive tract. Br Med J 1998;317:844–48.

Guo W, Blot WJ, Li JY, Taylor PR, Liu BQ, Wang W, et al. A nested case-control study of oesophageal and stomach cancers in the Linxian nutrition intervention trial. Int J Epidemiol 1994;23:444–50.

Guo W, Wang N, Li Y, Zhang JH. Polymorphisms in tumor necrosis factor genes and susceptibility to esophageal squamous cell carcinoma and gastric cardiac adenocarcinoma in a population of high incidence region of North China. Chin Med J (Engl) 2005;118: 1870–78.

Guo W, Wang N, Wang YM, Li Y, Wen DG, Chen ZF, et al. Interleukin-10–1082 promoter polymorphism is not associated with susceptibility to esophageal squamous cell carcinoma and gastric cardiac adenocarcinoma in a population of high-incidence region of north China. World J Gastroenterol 2005;11:858–62.

Guo Y, Zhang X, Tan W, Miao X, Sun T, Zhao D, et al. Platelet 12-lipoxygenase Arg261Gln polymorphism: functional characterization and association with risk of esophageal squamous cell carcinoma in combination with COX-2 polymorphisms. Pharmacogenet Genomics 2007;17:197–205.

Gustavsson P, Evanoff B, Hogstedt C. Increased risk of esophageal cancer among workers exposed to combustion products. Arch Environ Health 1993;48:243–45.

Gustavsson P, Jakobsson R, Johansson H, Lewin F, Norell S, Rutkvist LE. Occupational exposures and squamous cell carcinoma of the oral cavity, pharynx, larynx, and oesophagus: a case-control study in Sweden. Occup Environ Med 1998;55:393–400.

Hamajima N, Matsuo K, Suzuki T, Nakamura T, Matsuura A, Hatooka S, et al. No associations of p73 G4C14-to-A4T14 at exon 2 and p53 Arg72Pro polymorphisms with the risk of digestive tract cancers in Japanese. Cancer Lett 2002;181:81–85.

Han C, Qiao G, Hubbert NL, Li L, Sun C, Wang Y, et al. Serologic association between human papillomavirus type 16 infection and esophageal cancer in Shaanxi Province, China. J Natl Cancer Inst 1996;88:1467–71.

Hansen J, Raaschou-Nielsen O, Christensen JM, Johansen I, McLaughlin JK, Lipworth L, et al. Cancer incidence among Danish workers exposed to trichloroethylene. J Occup Environ Med 2001;43:133–39.

Hansen S, Wiig JN, Giercksky KE, Tretli S. Esophageal and gastric carcinoma in Norway 1958–1992: incidence time trend variability according to morphological subtypes and organ subsites. Int J Cancer 1997;71: 340–44.

Hansen S, Melby KK, Aase S, Jellum E, Vollset SE. Helicobacter pylori infection and risk of cardia cancer and non-cardia gastric cancer. A nested case-control study. Scand J Gastroenterol 1999;34:353–60.

Hao B, Wang H, Zhou K, Li Y, Chen X, Zhou G, et al. Identification of genetic variants in base excision repair pathway and their associations with risk of esophageal squamous cell carcinoma. Cancer Res 2004;64:4378–84.

Harty LC, Caporaso NE, Hayes RB, Winn DM, Bravo-Otero E, Blot WJ, et al. Alcohol dehydrogenase 3 genotype and risk of oral cavity and pharyngeal cancers. J Natl Cancer Inst 1997;89:1698–705.

He YT, Hou J, Chen ZF, Qiao CY, Song GH, Meng FS, et al. Decrease in the esophageal cancer incidence rate in mountainous but not level parts of Cixian County, China, over 29 years. Asian Pac J Cancer Prev 2005;6:510–14.

Hong Y, Miao X, Zhang X, Ding F, Luo A, Guo Y, et al. The role of P53 and MDM2 polymorphisms in the risk of esophageal squamous cell carcinoma. Cancer Res 2005;65: 9582–87.

Hongo M. Review article: Barrett's oesophagus and carcinoma in Japan. Aliment Pharmacol Ther 2004;20 Suppl 8:50–54.

Hori H, Kawano T, Endo M, Yuasa Y. Genetic polymorphisms of tobacco- and alcohol-related metabolizing enzymes and human esophageal squamous cell carcinoma susceptibility. J Clin Gastroenterol 1997;25: 568–75.

Hormozdiari H, Day NE, Aramesh B, Mahboubi E. Dietary factors and esophageal cancer in the Caspian Littoral of Iran. Cancer Res 1975;35:3493–98.

Hsing AW, McLaughlin JK, Olsen JH, Mellemkjar L, Wacholder S, Fraumeni JF, Jr. Cancer risk following primary hemochromatosis: a population-based cohort study in Denmark. Int J Cancer 1995;60:160–62.

Hu J, Nyren O, Wolk A, Bergstrom R, Yuen J, Adami HO, et al. Risk factors for oesophageal cancer in northeast China. Int J Cancer 1994;57:38–46.

IARC. Acetaldehyde. IARC Monogr Eval Carcinog Risk Chem Hum 1985;36:101–32.

IARC. Alcohol drinking. IARC Working Group, Lyon, 13–20 October 1987. IARC Monogr Eval Carcinog Risks Hum 1988;44:1–378.

Inoue M, Tajima K, Hirose K, Hamajima N, Takezaki T, Kuroishi T, et al. Tea and coffee consumption and the risk of digestive tract cancers: data from a comparative case-referent study in Japan. Cancer Causes Control 1998;9:209–16.

Isaacson C, Bothwell TH, MacPhail AP, Simon M. The iron status of urban black subjects with carcinoma of the oesophagus. S Afr Med J 1985;67:591–93.

Ishikawa A, Kuriyama S, Tsubono Y, Fukao A, Takahashi H, Tachiya H, et al. Smoking, alcohol drinking, green tea consumption and the risk of esophageal cancer in Japanese men. J Epidemiol 2006;16:185–92.

Islami F, Kamangar F, Aghcheli K, Fahimi S, Semnani S, Taghavi N, et al. Epidemiologic features of upper gastrointestinal tract cancers in Northeastern Iran. Br J Cancer 2004; 90:1402–6.

Itoga S, Nomura F, Makino Y, Tomonaga T, Shimada H, Ochiai T, et al. Tandem repeat polymorphism of the CYP2E1 gene: an association study with esophageal cancer and lung cancer. Alcohol Clin Exp Res 2002;26:15S-19S.

Iwaya T, Maesawa C, Ogasawara S, Tamura G. Tylosis esophageal cancer locus on chromosome 17q25.1 is commonly deleted in sporadic human esophageal cancer. Gastroenterology 1998;114:1206–10.

Jain M, Kumar S, Rastogi N, Lal P, Ghoshal UC, Tiwari A, et al. GSTT1, GSTM1 and GSTP1 genetic polymorphisms and interaction with tobacco, alcohol and occupational exposure in esophageal cancer patients from North India. Cancer Lett 2006;242:60–67.

Jakobsson K, Attewell R, Hultgren B, Sjoland K. Gastrointestinal cancer among cement workers. A case-referent study. Int Arch Occup Environ Health 1990;62:337–40.

Jakszyn P, Gonzalez CA. Nitrosamine and related food intake and gastric and oesophageal cancer risk: a systematic review of the epidemiological evidence. World J Gastroenterol 2006;12:4296–303.

Jansson C, Johansson AL, Jeding K, Dickman PW, Nyren O, Lagergren J. Psychosocial working conditions and the risk of esophageal and gastric cardia cancers. Eur J Epidemiol 2004;19:631–41.

Jansson C, Johansson AL, Nyren O, Lagergren J. Socioeconomic factors and risk of esophageal adenocarcinoma: a nationwide Swedish case-control study. Cancer Epidemiol Biomarkers Prev 2005;14:1754–61.

Jansson C, Plato N, Johansson AL, Nyren O, Lagergren J. Airborne occupational exposures and risk of oesophageal and cardia adenocarcinoma. Occup Environ Med 2006; 63:107–12.

Jaskiewicz K, Marasas WF, Lazarus C, Beyers AD, Van Helden PD. Association of esophageal cytological abnormalities with vitamin and lipotrope deficiencies in populations at risk for esophageal cancer. Anticancer Res 1988;8:711–15.

Ji J, Hemminki K. Familial risk for esophageal cancer: an updated epidemiologic study from Sweden. Clin Gastroenterol Hepatol 2006; 4:840–45.

Johansson J, Hakansson HO, Mellblom L, Kempas A, Johansson KE, Granath F, et al. Risk factors for Barrett's oesophagus: a population-based approach. Scand J Gastroenterol 2007;42:148–56.

Jussawalla DJ, Deshpande VA. Evaluation of cancer risk in tobacco chewers and smokers: an epidemiologic assessment. Cancer 1971; 28:244–52.

Kabat GC, Ng SK, Wynder EL. Tobacco, alcohol intake, and diet in relation to adenocarcinoma of the esophagus and gastric cardia. Cancer Causes Control 1993;4:123–32.

Kamangar F, Dawsey SM, Blaser MJ, Perez-Perez GI, Pietinen P, Newschaffer CJ, et al. Opposing risks of gastric cardia and noncardia gastric adenocarcinomas associated with Helicobacter pylori seropositivity. J Natl Cancer Inst 2006;98:1445–52.

Kamangar F, Qiao YL, Schiller JT, Dawsey SM, Fears T, Sun XD, et al. Human papillomavirus serology and the risk of esophageal and gastric cancers: results from a cohort in a high-risk region in China. Int J Cancer 2006;119:579–84.

Kamangar F, Qiao YL, Blaser MJ, Sun XD, Katki H, Fan JH, et al. Helicobacter pylori and oesophageal and gastric cancers in a prospective study in China. Br J Cancer 2007;96:172–76.

Kang SK, Burnett CA, Freund E, Walker J, Lalich N, Sestito J. Gastrointestinal cancer mortality of workers in occupations with high asbestos exposures. Am J Ind Med 1997;31:713–18.

Kim R, Weissfeld JL, Reynolds JC, Kuller LH. Etiology of Barrett's metaplasia and esophageal adenocarcinoma. Cancer Epidemiol Biomarkers Prev 1997;6:369–77.

Kjaerheim K, Gaard M, Andersen A. The role of alcohol, tobacco, and dietary factors in upper aerogastric tract cancers: a prospective study of 10,900 Norwegian men. Cancer Causes Control 1998;9:99–108.

Kubo A, Corley DA. Marked multi-ethnic variation of esophageal and gastric cardia carcinomas within the United States. Am J Gastroenterol 2004;99:582–88.

Kuroki T, Trapasso F, Yendamuri S, Matsuyama A, Alder H, Mori M, et al. Promoter hypermethylation of RASSF1A in esophageal squamous cell carcinoma. Clin Cancer Res 2003a;9:1441–45.

Kuroki T, Trapasso F, Yendamuri S, Matsuyama A, Alder H, Mori M, et al. Allele loss and promoter hypermethylation of VHL, RAR-beta, RASSF1A, and FHIT tumor suppressor genes on chromosome 3p in esophageal squamous cell carcinoma. Cancer Res 2003b;63: 3724–28.

Kuwano H, Kato H, Miyazaki T, Fukuchi M, Masuda N, Nakajima M, et al. Genetic alterations in esophageal cancer. Surg Today 2005;35:7–18.

Lagergren J, Nyren O. Do sex hormones play a role in the etiology of esophageal adenocarcinoma? A new hypothesis tested in a population-based cohort of prostate cancer patients. Cancer Epidemiol Biomarkers Prev 1998;7:913–15.

Lagergren J. Cancer of the Esophagus and Gastric Cardia. Etiological Aspects (Thesis). Stockholm, Karolinska Institutet, 1999.

Lagergren J, Bergstrom R, Lindgren A, Nyren O. Symptomatic gastroesophageal reflux as a risk factor for esophageal adenocarcinoma. N Engl J Med 1999;340:825–31.

Lagergren J, Bergstrom R, Nyren O. Association between body mass and adenocarcinoma of the esophagus and gastric cardia. Ann Intern Med 1999;130:883–90.

Lagergren J, Wang Z, Bergstrom R, Dillner J, Nyren O. Human papillomavirus infection and esophageal cancer: a nationwide seroepidemiologic case-control study in Sweden. J Natl Cancer Inst 1999;91: 156–62.

Lagergren J, Bergstrom R, Lindgren A, Nyren O. The role of tobacco, snuff and alcohol use in the aetiology of cancer of the oesophagus and gastric cardia. Int J Cancer 2000;85: 340–46.

Lagergren J, Ye W, Lindgren A, Nyren O. Heredity and risk of cancer of the esophagus and gastric cardia. Cancer Epidemiol Biomarkers Prev 2000;9:757–60.

Lagergren J, Jansson C. Sex hormones and oesophageal adenocarcinoma: influence of childbearing? Br J Cancer 2005;93:859–61.

Lagergren J, Viklund P, Jansson C. Carbonated soft drinks and risk of esophageal adenocarcinoma: a population-based case-control study. J Natl Cancer Inst 2006;98:1158–61.

Lam AK. Molecular biology of esophageal squamous cell carcinoma. Crit Rev Oncol Hematol 2000;33:71–90.

Launoy G, Milan CH, Faivre J, Pienkowski P, Milan CI, Gignoux M. Alcohol, tobacco and oesophageal cancer: effects of the duration of consumption, mean intake and current and former consumption. Br J Cancer 1997; 75:1389–96.

Launoy G, Milan C, Day NE, Pienkowski MP, Gignoux M, Faivre J. Diet and squamous-cell cancer of the oesophagus: a French multicentre case-control study. Int J Cancer 1998; 76:7–12.

Launoy G, Milan C, Faivre J, Pienkowski P, Gignoux M. Tobacco type and risk of squamous cell cancer of the oesophagus in males: a French multicentre case-control study. Int J Epidemiol 2000;29:36–42.

Lee JM, Lee YC, Yang SY, Shi WL, Lee CJ, Luh SP, et al. Genetic polymorphisms of p53 and GSTP1,but not NAT2,are associated with susceptibility to squamous-cell carcinoma of the esophagus. Int J Cancer 2000;89:458–64.

Levi F, Pasche C, Lucchini F, Chatenoud L, Jacobs DR, Jr., La Vecchia C. Refined and whole grain cereals and the risk of oral, oesophageal and laryngeal cancer. Eur J Clin Nutr 2000;54:487–89.

Li D, Dandara C, Parker MI. Association of cytochrome P450 2E1 genetic polymorphisms with squamous cell carcinoma of the oesophagus. Clin Chem Lab Med 2005;43:370–75.

Li JY, Ershow AG, Chen ZJ, Wacholder S, Li GY, Guo W, et al. A case-control study of cancer of the esophagus and gastric cardia in Linxian. Int J Cancer 1989;43:755–61.

Li JY, Taylor PR, Li B, Dawsey S, Wang GQ, Ershow AG, et al. Nutrition intervention trials in Linxian, China: multiple vitamin/mineral supplementation, cancer incidence, and disease-specific mortality among adults with esophageal dysplasia. J Natl Cancer Inst 1993;85:1492–98.

Li L, Rao K. A statistical analysis of registered cancer morbidity and mortality in 11 counties, China (1988–1992). Bull Chinese Cancer (in Chinese) 2000;9:435–47.

Li T, Lu ZM, Guo M, Wu QJ, Chen KN, Xing HP, et al. p53 codon 72 polymorphism (C/G) and the risk of human papillomavirus-associated carcinomas in China. Cancer 2002;95:2571–76.

Limburg PJ, Wei W, Ahnen DJ, Qiao Y, Hawk ET, Wang G, et al. Randomized, placebo-controlled, esophageal squamous cell cancer chemoprevention trial of selenomethionine and celecoxib. Gastroenterology 2005;129: 863–73.

Lin DX, Tang YM, Peng Q, Lu SX, Ambrosone CB, Kadlubar FF. Susceptibility to esophageal cancer and genetic polymorphisms in glutathione S-transferases T1, P1, and M1 and cytochrome P450 2E1. Cancer Epidemiol Biomarkers Prev 1998;7:1013–18.

Lin K, Shen ZY, Lu SH, Wu YN. Intake of volatile N-nitrosamines and their ability to exogenously synthesize in the diet of inhabitants from high-risk area of esophageal cancer in southern China. Biomed Environ Sci 2002;15:277–82.

Lindblad M, Rodriguez LA, Lagergren J. Body mass, tobacco and alcohol and risk of esophageal, gastric cardia, and gastric non-cardia adenocarcinoma among men and women in a nested case-control study. Cancer Causes Control 2005;16:285–94.

Lindblad M, Garcia Rodriguez LA, Chandanos E, Lagergren J. Hormone replacement therapy and risks of oesophageal and gastric adenocarcinomas. Br J Cancer 2006;94:136–41.

Lindblad M, Ye W, Lindgren A, Lagergren J. Disparities in the classification of esophageal and cardia adenocarcinomas and their influence on reported incidence rates. Ann Surg 2006;243:479–85.

Liu G, Zhou W, Yeap BY, Su L, Wain JC, Poneros JM, et al. XRCC1 and XPD polymorphisms and esophageal adenocarcinoma risk. Carcinogenesis 2007;28:1254–8.

Lucas D, Menez C, Floch F, Gourlaouen Y, Sparfel O, Joannet I, et al. Cytochromes P4502E1 and P4501A1 genotypes and susceptibility to cirrhosis or upper aerodigestive tract cancer in alcoholic caucasians. Alcohol Clin Exp Res 1996;20:1033–37.

Lynge E, Anttila A, Hemminki K. Organic solvents and cancer. Cancer Causes Control 1997;8:406–19.

MacInnis RJ, English DR, Hopper JL, Giles GG. Body size and composition and the risk of gastric and oesophageal adenocarcinoma. Int J Cancer 2006;118:2628–31.

Mandard AM, Hainaut P, Hollstein M. Genetic steps in the development of squamous cell carcinoma of the esophagus. Mutat Res 2000;462:335–42.

Mayne ST, Risch HA, Dubrow R, Chow WH, Gammon MD, Vaughan TL, et al. Nutrient intake and risk of subtypes of esophageal and gastric cancer. Cancer Epidemiol Biomarkers Prev 2001;10:1055–62.

Miyake S, Nagai K, Yoshino K, Oto M, Endo M, Yuasa Y. Point mutations and allelic deletion of tumor suppressor gene DCC in human esophageal squamous cell carcinomas and their relation to metastasis. Cancer Res 1994;54:3007–10.

Montesano R, Hollstein M, Hainaut P. Genetic alterations in esophageal cancer and their relevance to etiology and pathogenesis: a review. Int J Cancer 1996;69:225–35.

Moons LM, Siersema PD, Kuipers EJ, van Vliet AH, Kusters JG. IL-1 RN polymorphism is not associated with Barrett's esophagus and esophageal adenocarcinoma. Am J Gastroenterol 2005;100:2818.

Mori T, Aoki T, Matsubara T, Iida F, Du X, Nishihira T, et al. Frequent loss of heterozygosity in the region including BRCA1 on chromosome 17q in squamous cell carcinomas of the esophagus. Cancer Res 1994;54:1638–40.

Morita M, Kuwano H, Nakashima T, Taketomi A, Baba H, Saito T, et al. Family aggregation of carcinoma of the hypopharynx and cervical esophagus: special reference to multiplicity of cancer in upper aerodigestive tract. Int J Cancer 1998;76:468–71.

Morita S, Yano M, Shiozaki H, Tsujinaka T, Ebisui C, Morimoto T, et al. CYP1A1, CYP2E1 and GSTM1 polymorphisms are not associated with susceptibility to squamous-cell carcinoma of the esophagus. Int J Cancer 1997;71:192–95.

Morita S, Yano M, Tsujinaka T, Ogawa A, Taniguchi M, Kaneko K, et al. Association between genetic polymorphisms of glutathione S-transferase P1 and N-acetyltransferase 2 and susceptibility to squamous-cell carcinoma of the esophagus. Int J Cancer 1998; 79:517–20.

Munoz N, Crespi M, Grassi A, Qing WG, Qiong S, Cai LZ. Precursor lesions of oesophageal cancer in high-risk populations in Iran and China. Lancet 1982;1:876–79.

Munoz N, Wahrendorf J, Bang LJ, Crespi M, Thurnham DI, Day NE, et al. No effect of riboflavine, retinol, and zinc on prevalence of precancerous lesions of oesophagus. Randomised double-blind intervention study in high-risk population of China. Lancet 1985; 2:111–14.

Munoz N, Hayashi M, Bang LJ, Wahrendorf J, Crespi M, Bosch FX. Effect of riboflavin, retinol, and zinc on micronuclei of buccal mucosa and of esophagus: a randomized double-blind intervention study in China. J Natl Cancer Inst 1987;79:687–91.

Munoz N, Day NE. Esophageal cancer. In: Schottenfeld D and Fraumeni JF (Eds): Cancer Epidemiology and Prevention. New York, Oxford University Press, 1996. pp 681–706.

Murphy SJ, Anderson LA, Johnston BT, Fitzpatrick DA, Watson PR, Monaghan P, et al. Have patients with esophagitis got an increased risk of adenocarcinoma? Results from a population-based study. World J Gastroenterol 2005;11:7290–95.

Murphy SJ, Hughes AE, Patterson CC, Anderson LA, Watson RG, Johnston BT, et al. A population-based association study of SNPs of GSTP1, MnSOD, GPX2 and Barrett's esophagus and esophageal adenocarcinoma. Carcinogenesis 2007;28:1323–8.

Murray L, Watson P, Johnston B, Sloan J, Mainie IM, Gavin A. Risk of adenocarcinoma in Barrett's oesophagus: population based study. Br Med J 2003;327:534–35.

Muto M, Hitomi Y, Ohtsu A, Ebihara S, Yoshida S, Esumi H. Association of aldehyde dehydrogenase 2 gene polymorphism with multiple oesophageal dysplasia in head and neck cancer patients. Gut 2000;47:256–61.

Nandakumar A, Anantha N, Pattabhiraman V, Prabhakaran PS, Dhar M, Puttaswamy K, et al. Importance of anatomical subsite in correlating risk factors in cancer of the oesophagus—report of a case—control study. Br J Cancer 1996;73:1306–11.

Nandurkar S, Talley NJ, Martin CJ, Ng TH, Adams S. Short segment Barrett's oesophagus: prevalence, diagnosis and associations. Gut 1997;40:710–15.

Newnham A, Quinn MJ, Babb P, Kang JY, Majeed A. Trends in the subsite and morphology of oesophageal and gastric cancer in England and Wales 1971–1998. Aliment Pharmacol Ther 2003;17:665–76.

Nimura Y, Yokoyama S, Fujimori M, Aoki T, Adachi W, Nasu T, et al. Genotyping of the CYP1A1 and GSTM1 genes in esophageal carcinoma patients with special reference to smoking. Cancer 1997;80:852–57.

Norell S, Ahlbom A, Lipping H, Osterblom L. Oesophageal cancer and vulcanisation work. Lancet 1983;1:462–63.

Nowell PC. The clonal evolution of tumor cell populations. Science 1976;194:23–28.

Ochs-Balcom HM, Falk G, Grady WM, Kinnard M, Willis J, Elston R, et al. Consortium approach to identifying genes for Barrett's esophagus and esophageal adenocarcinoma. Transl Res 2007;150:3–17.

O'Neill C, Pan Q, Clarke G, Liu F, Hodges G, Ge M, et al. Silica fragments from millet bran in mucosa surrounding oesophageal tumours in patients in northern China. Lancet 1982; 1:1202–6.

Pan G, Takahashi K, Feng Y, Liu L, Liu T, Zhang S, et al. Nested case-control study of esophageal cancer in relation to occupational exposure to silica and other dusts. Am J Ind Med 1999;35:272–80.

Parkin DM, Vizcaino AP, Skinner ME, Ndhlovu A. Cancer patterns and risk factors in the African population of southwestern Zimbabwe, 1963–1977. Cancer Epidemiol Biomarkers Prev 1994;3:537–47.

Parkin DM, Whelan SL, Ferlay J, Raymond LYoung J. Cancer Incidence in Five Continents. Volume VII. Lyon, International Agency for Research on Cancer, 1997.

Parkin DM, Pisani P, Ferlay J. Estimates of the worldwide incidence of 25 major cancers in 1990. Int J Cancer 1999;80:827–41.

Parkin DM, Bray F, Ferlay J, Pisani P. Global cancer statistics, 2002. CA Cancer J Clin 2005;55:74–108.

Pera M, Manterola C, Vidal O, Grande L. Epidemiology of esophageal adenocarcinoma. J Surg Oncol 2005;92:151–59.

Pohl H, Welch HG. The role of overdiagnosis and reclassification in the marked increase of esophageal adenocarcinoma incidence. J Natl Cancer Inst 2005;97:142–46.

Pukkala E, Teppo L. Socioeconomic status and education as risk determinants of gastrointestinal cancer. Prev Med 1986;15: 127–38.

Raghunath A, Hungin AP, Wooff D, Childs S. Prevalence of Helicobacter pylori in patients with gastro-oesophageal reflux disease: systematic review. Br Med J 2003;326:737.

Ransford RA, Jankowski JA. Genetic versus environmental interactions in the oesophagitis- metaplasia-dysplasia-adenocarcinoma sequence (MCS) of Barrett's oesophagus. Acta Gastroenterol Belg 2000;63:18–21.

Rao M, Liu FS, Dawsey SM, Yang K, Lipkin M, Li JY, et al. Effects of vitamin/mineral supplementation on the proliferation of esophageal squamous epithelium in Linxian, China. Cancer Epidemiol Biomarkers Prev 1994;3:277–79.

Riboli E, Norat T. Epidemiologic evidence of the protective effect of fruit and vegetables on cancer risk. Am J Clin Nutr 2003;78:559S-569S.

Romero Y, Cameron AJ, Locke GR, 3rd, Schaid DJ, Slezak JM, Branch CD, et al. Familial aggregation of gastroesophageal reflux in patients with Barrett's esophagus and esophageal adenocarcinoma. Gastroenterology 1997;113:1449–56.

Ryan BM, McManus R, Daly JS, Carton E, Keeling PW, Reynolds JV, et al. A common p73 polymorphism is associated with a reduced incidence of oesophageal carcinoma. Br J Cancer 2001;85:1499–503.

Sabel MS, Pastore K, Toon H, Smith JL. Adenocarcinoma of the esophagus with and without Barrett mucosa. Arch Surg 2000;135:831–35; discussion 6.

Sarbia M, Bitzer M, Siegel D, Ross D, Schulz WA, Zotz RB, et al. Association between NAD(P)H: quinone oxidoreductase 1 (NQ01) inactivating C609T polymorphism and adenocarcinoma of the upper gastrointestinal tract. Int J Cancer 2003;107:381–86.

Sathiakumar N, Delzell E, Austin H, Cole P. A follow-up study of agricultural chemical production workers. Am J Ind Med 1992;21: 321–30.

Savage SA, Abnet CC, Haque K, Mark SD, Qiao YL, Dong ZW, et al. Polymorphisms in interleukin -2, -6, and -10 are not associated with gastric cardia or esophageal cancer in a high-risk chinese population. Cancer Epidemiol Biomarkers Prev 2004;13:1547–49.

Segal I, Reinach SG, de Beer M. Factors associated with oesophageal cancer in Soweto, South Africa. Br J Cancer 1988;58:681–86.

Semnani S, Sadjadi A, Fahimi S, Nouraie M, Naeimi M, Kabir J, et al. Declining incidence of esophageal cancer in the Turkmen Plain, eastern part of the Caspian Littoral of Iran: a retrospective cancer surveillance. Cancer Detect Prev 2006;30:14–19.

Shaheen NJ, Crosby MA, Bozymski EM, Sandler RS. Is there publication bias in the reporting of cancer risk in Barrett's esophagus? Gastroenterology 2000;119:333–38.

Shibagaki I, Shimada Y, Wagata T, Ikenaga M, Imamura M, Ishizaki K. Allelotype analysis of esophageal squamous cell carcinoma. Cancer Res 1994;54:2996–3000.

Shibuta J, Eto T, Kataoka A, Inoue H, Ueo H, Suzuki T, et al. Genetic polymorphism of N-acetyltransferase 2 in patients with esophageal cancer. Am J Gastroenterol 2001;96: 3419–24.

Siman HJ, Forsgren A, Berglund G, Floren CH. Helicobacter pylori infection is associated with a decreased risk of developing oesophageal neoplasms. Helicobacter 2001;6:310–16.

Song C, Xing D, Tan W, Wei Q, Lin D. Methylenetetrahydrofolate reductase polymorphisms increase risk of esophageal squamous cell carcinoma in a Chinese population. Cancer Res 2001;61:3272–75.

Souza RF, Spechler SJ. Concepts in the prevention of adenocarcinoma of the distal esophagus and proximal stomach. CA Cancer J Clin 2005;55:334–51.

Spechler SJ, Goyal RK. Barrett's esophagus. N Engl J Med 1986;315:362–71.

Steinmetz KA, Potter JD. Vegetables, fruit, and cancer prevention: a review. J Am Diet Assoc 1996;96:1027–39.

Stolzenberg-Solomon RZ, Qiao YL, Abnet CC, Ratnasinghe DL, Dawsey SM, Dong ZW, et al. Esophageal and gastric cardia cancer risk and folate- and vitamin B(12)-related polymorphisms in Linxian, China. Cancer Epidemiol Biomarkers Prev 2003;12:1222–26.

Streitz JM. Barrett's esophagus and esophageal cancer. Chest Surg Clin N Am 1994;4:227–40.

Strong MS, Incze J, Vaughan CW. Field cancerization in the aerodigestive tract—its etiology, manifestation, and significance. J Otolaryngol 1984;13:1–6.

Suzuki H, Zhou X, Yin J, Lei J, Jiang HY, Suzuki Y, et al. Intragenic mutations of CDKN2B and CDKN2A in primary human esophageal cancers. Hum Mol Genet 1995;4:1883–87.

Takezaki T, Shinoda M, Hatooka S, Hasegawa Y, Nakamura S, Hirose K, et al. Subsite-specific risk factors for hypopharyngeal and esophageal cancer (Japan). Cancer Causes Control 2000;11:597–608.

Takezaki T, Gao CM, Wu JZ, Ding JH, Liu YT, Zhang Y, et al. Dietary protective and risk factors for esophageal and stomach cancers in a low-epidemic area for stomach cancer in Jiangsu Province, China: comparison with those in a high-epidemic area. Jpn J Cancer Res 2001;92:1157–65.

Tan W, Song N, Wang GQ, Liu Q, Tang HJ, Kadlubar FF, et al. Impact of genetic polymorphisms in cytochrome P450 2E1 and glutathione S-transferases M1, T1, and P1 on susceptibility to esophageal cancer among high-risk individuals in China. Cancer Epidemiol Biomarkers Prev 2000;9:551–56.

Tan W, Miao X, Wang L, Yu C, Xiong P, Liang G, et al. Significant increase in risk of gastroesophageal cancer is associated with interaction between promoter polymorphisms in thymidylate synthase and serum folate status. Carcinogenesis 2005;26:1430–35.

Taniere P, Martel-Planche G, Maurici D, Lombard-Bohas C, Scoazec JY, Montesano R, et al. Molecular and clinical differences between adenocarcinomas of the esophagus and of the gastric cardia. Am J Pathol 2001;158:33–40.

Tavani A, Negri E, Franceschi S, La Vecchia C. Risk factors for esophageal cancer in lifelong nonsmokers. Cancer Epidemiol Biomarkers Prev 1994;3:387–92.

Tavani A, La Vecchia C, Gallus S, Lagiou P, Trichopoulos D, Levi F, et al. Red meat intake and cancer risk: a study in Italy. Int J Cancer 2000;86:425–28.

Terry P, Lagergren J, Ye W, Nyren O, Wolk A. Antioxidants and cancers of the esophagus and gastric cardia. Int J Cancer 2000;87:750–54.

Terry P, Lagergren J, Hansen H, Wolk A, Nyren O. Fruit and vegetable consumption in the prevention of oesophageal and cardia cancers. Eur J Cancer Prev 2001;10:365–69.

Terry P, Lagergren J, Wolk A, Nyren O. Drinking hot beverages is not associated with risk of oesophageal cancers in a Western population. Br J Cancer 2001;84:120–21.

Terry PD, Lagergren J, Wolk A, Steineck G, Nyren O. Dietary intake of heterocyclic amines and cancers of the esophagus and gastric cardia. Cancer Epidemiol Biomarkers Prev 2003;12:940–44.

Thomas DB, Karagas MR. Cancer in first and second generation Americans. Cancer Res 1987;47:5771–76.

Thurnham DI, Zheng SF, Munoz N, Crespi M, Grassi A, Hambidge KM, et al. Comparison of riboflavin, vitamin A, and zinc status of Chinese populations at high and low risk for esophageal cancer. Nutr Cancer 1985;7:131–43.

Tian D, Feng Z, Hanley NM, Setzer RW, Mumford JL, DeMarini DM. Multifocal accumulation of p53 protein in esophageal carcinoma: evidence for field cancerization. Int J Cancer 1998;78:568–75.

Turkdogan MK, Testereci H, Akman N, Kahraman T, Kara K, Tuncer I, et al. Dietary nitrate and nitrite levels in an endemic upper gastrointestinal (esophageal and gastric) cancer region of Turkey. Turk J Gastroenterol 2003;14:50–53.

Tuyns AJ, Pequignot G, Jensen OM. [Esophageal cancer in Ille-et-Vilaine in relation to levels of alcohol and tobacco consumption. Risks are multiplying]. Bull Cancer 1977;64:45–60.

Tuyns AJ, Pequignot G, Abbatucci JS. Oesophageal cancer and alcohol consumption; importance of type of beverage. Int J Cancer 1979;23:443–47.

Tuyns AJ. Oesophageal cancer in non-smoking drinkers and in non-drinking smokers. Int J Cancer 1983;32:443–44.

Tzonou A, Lipworth L, Garidou A, Signorello LB, Lagiou P, Hsieh C, et al. Diet and risk of esophageal cancer by histologic type in a low-risk population. Int J Cancer 1996;68:300–4.

Van Doornum GJ, Korse CM, Buning-Kager JC, Bonfrer JM, Horenblas S, Taal BG, et al. Reactivity to human papillomavirus type 16 L1 virus-like particles in sera from patients with genital cancer and patients with carcinomas at five different extragenital sites. Br J Cancer 2003;88:1095–1100.

van Lieshout EM, Roelofs HM, Dekker S, Mulder CJ, Wobbes T, Jansen JB, et al. Polymorphic expression of the glutathione S-transferase P1 gene and its susceptibility to Barrett's esophagus and esophageal carcinoma. Cancer Res 1999;59:586–89.

van Loon AJ, Brug J, Goldbohm RA, van den Brandt PA, Burg J. Differences in cancer incidence and mortality among socio-economic groups. Scand J Soc Med 1995;23:110–20.

van Rensburg SJ. Epidemiologic and dietary evidence for a specific nutritional predisposition to esophageal cancer. J Natl Cancer Inst 1981;67:243–51.

Wang AH, Sun CS, Li LS, Huang JY, Chen QS. Relationship of tobacco smoking CYP1A1 GSTM1 gene polymorphism and esophageal cancer in Xi'an. World J Gastroenterol 2002;8:49–53.

Wang GQ, Dawsey SM, Li JY, Taylor PR, Li B, Blot WJ, et al. Effects of vitamin/mineral supplementation on the prevalence of histological dysplasia and early cancer of the esophagus and stomach: results from the General Population Trial in Linxian, China. Cancer Epidemiol Biomarkers Prev 1994;3: 161–66.

Wang LD, Zheng S, Liu B, Zhou JX, Li YJ, Li JX. CYP1A1, GSTs and mEH polymorphisms and susceptibility to esophageal carcinoma: study of population from a high-incidence area in north China. World J Gastroenterol 2003;9:1394–97.

Wang LD, Guo RF, Fan ZM, He X, Gao SS, Guo HQ, et al. Association of methylenetetrahydrofolate reductase and thymidylate synthase promoter polymorphisms with genetic susceptibility to esophageal and cardia cancer in a Chinese high-risk population. Dis Esophagus 2005;18:177–84.

Wang YP, Han XY, Su W, Wang YL, Zhu YW, Sasaba T, et al. Esophageal cancer in Shanxi Province, People's Republic of China: a case-control study in high and moderate risk areas. Cancer Causes Control 1992;3:107–13.

Wang Y, Guo W, He Y, Chen Z, Wen D, Zhang X, et al. Association of MTHFR C677T and SHMT(1) C1420T with susceptibility to ESCC and GCA in a high incident region of Northern China. Cancer Causes Control 2007;18:143–52.

Ward MH, Sinha R, Heineman EF, Rothman N, Markin R, Weisenburger DD, et al. Risk of adenocarcinoma of the stomach and esophagus with meat cooking method and doneness preference. Int J Cancer 1997;71:14–19.

Vassallo A, Correa P, De Stefani E, Cendan M, Zavala D, Chen V, et al. Esophageal cancer in Uruguay: a case-control study. J Natl Cancer Inst 1985;75:1005–9.

Vaughan TL, Stewart PA, Davis S, Thomas DB. Work in dry cleaning and the incidence of cancer of the oral cavity, larynx, and oesophagus. Occup Environ Med 1997;54: 692–95.

WCRF. World Cancer Research Fund—American Institute of Cancer Research. Food, Nutrition and the Prevention of Cancer: A Global Perspective. Menasha, USA, BANTA Book Group, 1997.

Wernli KJ, Fitzgibbons ED, Ray RM, Gao DL, Li W, Seixas NS, et al. Occupational risk factors for esophageal and stomach cancers among female textile workers in Shanghai, China. Am J Epidemiol 2006;163:717–25.

Winters C, Spurling TJ, Chobanian SJ, Curtis DJ, Esposito RL, Hacker JF, et al. Barrett's esophagus. A prevalent, occult complication of gastroesophageal reflux disease. Gastroenterology 1987;92:118–24.

Vizcaino AP, Parkin DM, Skinner ME. Risk factors associated with oesophageal cancer in

Bulawayo, Zimbabwe. Br J Cancer 1995;72: 769–73.

Vizcaino AP, Moreno V, Lambert R, Parkin DM. Time trends incidence of both major histologic types of esophageal carcinomas in selected countries, 1973–1995. Int J Cancer 2002;99:860–68.

von Rahden BH, Stein HJ, Langer R, von Weyhern CW, Schenk E, Doring C, et al. C609T polymorphism of the NAD(P)H:quinone oxidoreductase I gene does not significantly affect susceptibility for esophageal adenocarcinoma. Int J Cancer 2005;113:506–8.

Wong ML, Tao Q, Fu L, Wong KY, Qiu GH, Law FB, et al. Aberrant promoter hypermethylation and silencing of the critical 3p21 tumour suppressor gene, RASSF1A, in Chinese oesophageal squamous cell carcinoma. Int J Oncol 2006;28:767–73.

Wong O, Trent LS, Whorton MD. An updated cohort mortality study of workers exposed to styrene in the reinforced plastics and composites industry. Occup Environ Med 1994; 51:386–96.

Wu AH, Wan P, Bernstein L. A multiethnic population-based study of smoking, alcohol and body size and risk of adenocarcinomas of the stomach and esophagus (United States). Cancer Causes Control 2001;12:721–32.

Wu AH, Crabtree JE, Bernstein L, Hawtin P, Cockburn M, Tseng CC, et al. Role of Helicobacter pylori CagA+ strains and risk of adenocarcinoma of the stomach and esophagus. Int J Cancer 2003;103:815–21.

Wu AH, Tseng CC, Bernstein L. Hiatal hernia, reflux symptoms, body size, and risk of esophageal and gastric adenocarcinoma. Cancer 2003;98:940–48.

Wu CF, Wu DC, Hsu HK, Kao EL, Lee JM, Lin CC, et al. Relationship between genetic polymorphisms of alcohol and aldehyde dehydrogenases and esophageal squamous cell carcinoma risk in males. World J Gastroenterol 2005;11:5103–8.

Wu M, Zhao JK, Hu XS, Wang PH, Qin Y, Lu YC, et al. Association of smoking, alcohol drinking and dietary factors with esophageal cancer in high- and low-risk areas of Jiangsu Province, China. World J Gastroenterol 2006;12:1686–93.

Wu MT, Lee JM, Wu DC, Ho CK, Wang YT, Lee YC, et al. Genetic polymorphisms of cytochrome P4501A1 and oesophageal squamous-cell carcinoma in Taiwan. Br J Cancer 2002;87:529–32.

Wu MT, Wang YT, Ho CK, Wu DC, Lee YC, Hsu HK, et al. SULT1A1 polymorphism and esophageal cancer in males. Int J Cancer 2003;103:101–4.

Wu TT, Watanabe T, Heitmiller R, Zahurak M, Forastiere AA, Hamilton SR. Genetic alterations in Barrett esophagus and adenocarcinomas of the esophagus and esophagogastric junction region. Am J Pathol 1998;153:287–94.

Wu X, Chen VW, Ruiz B, Andrews P, Su LJ, Correa P. Incidence of esophageal and gastric carcinomas among American Asians/Pacific Islanders, whites, and blacks: subsite and histology differences. Cancer 2006;106:683–92.

Wu Y, Chen J, Ohshima H, Pignatelli B, Boreham J, Li J, et al. Geographic association between urinary excretion of N-nitroso compounds and oesophageal cancer mortality in China. Int J Cancer 1993;54:713–19.

Wynder EL, Bross IJ. A study of etiological factors in cancer of the esophagus. Cancer 1961;14:389–413.

Xing D, Qi J, Miao X, Lu W, Tan W, Lin D. Polymorphisms of DNA repair genes XRCC1 and XPD and their associations with risk of esophageal squamous cell carcinoma in a Chinese population. Int J Cancer 2002; 100:600–5.

Xing DY, Qi J, Tan W, Miao XP, Liang G, Yu CY, et al. [Association of genetic polymorphisms in the DNA repair gene XPD with risk of lung and esophageal cancer in a Chinese population in Beijing]. Zhonghua Yi Xue Yi Chuan Xue Za Zhi 2003;20:35–38.

Xing EP, Nie Y, Wang LD, Yang GY, Yang CS. Aberrant methylation of p16INK4a and deletion of p15INK4b are frequent events in human esophageal cancer in Linxian, China. Carcinogenesis 1999;20:77–84.

Yang CS, Sun Y, Yang QU, Miller KW, Li GY, Zheng SF, et al. Vitamin A and other deficiencies in Linxian, a high esophageal cancer incidence area in northern China. J Natl Cancer Inst 1984;73:1449–53.

Yang CX, Matsuo K, Ito H, Shinoda M, Hatooka S, Hirose K, et al. Gene-environment interactions between alcohol drinking and the MTHFR C677T polymorphism impact on esophageal cancer risk: results of a case-control study in Japan. Carcinogenesis 2005; 26:1285–90.

Yang CX, Matsuo K, Wang ZM, Tajima K. Phase I/II enzyme gene polymorphisms and esophageal cancer risk: a meta-analysis of the literature. World J Gastroenterol 2005;11: 2531–38.

Ye W. Aspects of Gastroesophageal Reflux and Risk of Esophageal Cancer. An Epidemiological Approach (Thesis). Stockholm, Karolinska Institutet, 2003.

Ye W, Nyren O. Risk of cancers of the oesophagus and stomach by histology or subsite in patients hospitalised for pernicious anaemia. Gut 2003;52:938–41.

Ye W, Held M, Lagergren J, Engstrand L, Blot WJ, McLaughlin JK, et al. Helicobacter py-

lori infection and gastric atrophy: risk of adenocarcinoma and squamous-cell carcinoma of the esophagus and adenocarcinoma of the gastric cardia. J Natl Cancer Inst 2004;96:388–96.

Ye W, Kumar R, Bacova G, Lagergren J, Hemminki K, Nyren O. The XPD 751Gln allele is associated with an increased risk for esophageal adenocarcinoma: a population-based case-control study in Sweden. Carcinogenesis 2006;27:1835–41.

Yokokawa Y, Ohta S, Hou J, Zhang XL, Li SS, Ping YM, et al. Ecological study on the risks of esophageal cancer in Ci-Xian, China: the importance of nutritional status and the use of well water. Int J Cancer 1999;83:620–24.

Yokoyama A, Muramatsu T, Ohmori T, Higuchi S, Hayashida M, Ishii H. Esophageal cancer and aldehyde dehydrogenase-2 genotypes in Japanese males. Cancer Epidemiol Biomarkers Prev 1996;5:99–102.

Yokoyama A, Ohmori T, Muramatsu T, Yokoyama T, Okuyama K, Makuuchi H, et al. Short-term follow-up after endoscopic mucosectomy of early esophageal cancer and aldehyde dehydrogenase-2 genotype in Japanese alcoholics. Cancer Epidemiol Biomarkers Prev 1998;7:473–76.

Yokoyama A, Muramatsu T, Omori T, Matsushita S, Yoshimizu H, Higuchi S, et al. Alcohol and aldehyde dehydrogenase gene polymorphisms influence susceptibility to esophageal cancer in Japanese alcoholics. Alcohol Clin Exp Res 1999;23:1705–10.

Yokoyama A, Muramatsu T, Omori T, Yokoyama T, Matsushita S, Higuchi S, et al. Alcohol and aldehyde dehydrogenase gene polymorphisms and oropharyngolaryngeal, esophageal and stomach cancers in Japanese alcoholics. Carcinogenesis 2001;22:433–39.

Yokoyama A, Kato H, Yokoyama T, Tsujinaka T, Muto M, Omori T, et al. Genetic polymorphisms of alcohol and aldehyde dehydrogenases and glutathione S-transferase M1 and drinking, smoking, and diet in Japanese men with esophageal squamous cell carcinoma. Carcinogenesis 2002;23:1851–59.

Younes M, Lebovitz RM, Lechago LV, Lechago J. p53 protein accumulation in Barrett's metaplasia, dysplasia, and carcinoma: a follow-up study. Gastroenterology 1993;105:1637–42.

Yu C, Lu W, Tan W, Xing D, Liang G, Miao X, et al. Lack of association between CCND1 G870A polymorphism and risk of esophageal squamous cell carcinoma. Cancer Epidemiol Biomarkers Prev 2003;12:176.

Yu HP, Wang XL, Sun X, Su YH, Wang YJ, Lu B, et al. Polymorphisms in the DNA repair gene XPD and susceptibility to esophageal squamous cell carcinoma. Cancer Genet Cytogenet 2004;154:10–15.

Yu MC, Garabrant DH, Peters JM, Mack TM. Tobacco, alcohol, diet, occupation, and carcinoma of the esophagus. Cancer Res 1988;48:3843–48.

Yu Y, Taylor PR, Li JY, Dawsey SM, Wang GQ, Guo WD, et al. Retrospective cohort study of risk-factors for esophageal cancer in Linxian, People's Republic of China. Cancer Causes Control 1993;4:195–202.

Zambon P, Talamini R, La Vecchia C, Dal Maso L, Negri E, Tognazzo S, et al. Smoking, type of alcoholic beverage and squamous-cell oesophageal cancer in northern Italy. Int J Cancer 2000;86:144–49.

Zendehdel K, Nyren O, Edberg A, Ye W. Risk of Esophageal Adenocarcinoma in Achalasia Patients, a Retrospective Cohort Study in Sweden. Am J Gastroenterol 2007;Epub ahead of print.

Zhang J, Li Y, Wang R, Wen D, Sarbia M, Kuang G, et al. Association of cyclin D1 (G870A) polymorphism with susceptibility to esophageal and gastric cardiac carcinoma in a northern Chinese population. Int J Cancer 2003;105:281–84.

Zhang J, Schulz WA, Li Y, Wang R, Zotz R, Wen D, et al. Association of NAD(P)H: quinone oxidoreductase 1 (NQ01) C609T polymorphism with esophageal squamous cell carcinoma in a German Caucasian and a northern Chinese population. Carcinogenesis 2003;24:905–9.

Zhang J, Cui Y, Kuang G, Li Y, Wang N, Wang R, et al. Association of the thymidylate synthase polymorphisms with esophageal squamous cell carcinoma and gastric cardiac adenocarcinoma. Carcinogenesis 2004;25:2479–85.

Zhang J, Zotz RB, Li Y, Wang R, Kiel S, Schulz WA, et al. Methylenetetrahydrofolate reductase C677T polymorphism and predisposition towards esophageal squamous cell carcinoma in a German Caucasian and a northern Chinese population. J Cancer Res Clin Oncol 2004;130:574–80.

Zhang JH, Li Y, Wang R, Geddert H, Guo W, Wen DG, et al. NQ01 C609T polymorphism associated with esophageal cancer and gastric cardiac carcinoma in North China. World J Gastroenterol 2003;9:1390–93.

Zhang JH, Li Y, Wang R, Wen DG, Wu ML, He M. [p53 gene polymorphism with susceptibility to esophageal cancer and lung cancer in Chinese population]. Zhonghua Zhong Liu Za Zhi 2003;25:365–67.

Zhang W, Bailey-Wilson JE, Li W, Wang X, Zhang C, Mao X, et al. Segregation analysis of esophageal cancer in a moderately high-incidence area of northern China. Am J Hum Genet 2000;67:110–19.

Zhang X, Miao X, Tan W, Ning B, Liu Z, Hong Y, et al. Identification of functional genetic variants in cyclooxygenase-2 and their association with risk of esophageal cancer. Gastroenterology 2005;129:565–76.

10

Stomach Cancer

OLOF NYRÉN AND HANS-OLOV ADAMI

Whereas cancer researchers have often faced the challenge of explaining dramatic temporal increases, for stomach cancer the situation is the reverse. As an "unplanned triumph," its incidence declined dramatically in the twentieth century. Yet on a global scale stomach cancer remains one of the most common causes of cancer death. Stomach cancer is the latest, but perhaps not the last, malignancy for which a predominant infectious etiology has been revealed.

Since the epidemiology of proximal gastric tumors, or cardia cancer, differs from that of distal tumors, reference will be made to these specific features where relevant. As there is no firm consensus about the anatomic definition of cardia cancer, available data on the frequency of this cancer vary by 10% to 35% of all gastric tumors and a corresponding variation in risk factor patterns would be expected. It appears, though, that the measures of association with putative risk factors are relatively robust with regard to these variations, at least as long as the lower borderline of what is considered to be the cardia does not

exceed 3 cm below the gastroesophageal junction (Lagergren et al, 1999).

CLINICAL SYNOPSIS

Subgroups

Because adenocarcinoma constitutes more than 95% of all stomach neoplasms, we will focus solely on this cancer. Other rare types, such as gastric lymphomas, carcinoids, and leiomyosarcomas, will not be covered here. Adenocarcinomas arising in the columnar epithelium of the esophagogastric junction (cardia cancer) are histologically identical to adenocarcinomas in the middle and distal parts of the stomach and are classified as stomach cancers.

Symptoms

Abdominal pain—often indistinguishable from that caused by peptic ulcer—anorexia, and weight loss are symptoms characteristic of stomach cancer. Anemia due to bleeding and obstruction of the gastric outlet due to tumor growth in the distal stomach are also common.

239

Diagnosis

Endoscopic examination with biopsy and histopathologic confirmation has now largely replaced contrast x-ray as the primary diagnostic tool. Computed tomography, ultrasound, and other modern imaging techniques may further clarify the extent of local tumor growth and reveal metastases in lymph nodes, the liver, and elsewhere.

Treatment

Cure can be achieved only by radical surgical removal—typically a subtotal or total gastrectomy—of a localized cancer. There is no established adjuvant systemic treatment. In advanced stages, chemotherapy and radiotherapy may offer short-term palliation.

Prognosis

Because most deaths occur within the first couple of months to years following diagnosis, 5-year relative survival is a good approximation of the long-term cure rate. Five-year relative survival varied between 10% and 20% among patients diagnosed during the 1980s in the United States and Europe. Based on recent SEER data, the 5-year survival rate is now 21% in the United States (Parkin et al, 2005).

Progress

Despite developments in diagnostic methods, notably the widespread use of endoscopy, and constant efforts to improve surgical treatment, the prognosis has remained grim. Although the prognosis may, in fact, have changed somewhat for the better, it appears that prevention is the most realistic way to reduce the burden of this dreaded disease.

DESCRIPTIVE EPIDEMIOLOGY

Notwithstanding that a remarkable spontaneous global decline has halved the age-specific incidence of stomach (gastric) cancer in most western countries in the past 30 to 40 years, this cancer is still the fourth most frequent one worldwide, surpassed only by cancers of the lung, breast, and colorectum (Parkin et al, 2005). Due to its poor prognosis stomach cancer ranks number 2 among all causes of cancer death. In fact, it accounts for more than 10% of all cancer deaths. Almost two-thirds of the cases occur in developing countries. The worldwide estimates of age-adjusted incidence (22.0 per 100 000 person-years in men and 10.3 per 100 000 person-years in women in 2002) are about 15% lower than the values estimated in 1985. However, due to the aging of the world's population and the steep age gradient in incidence among the elderly, stomach cancer continues to claim an increasing number of victims: 800 000 to 900 000 per year, corresponding to a 6% increase between 1985 and 1990.

Geographic and Demographic Distribution

International comparisons need to be interpreted cautiously in view of possible differences in the availability of medical services, diagnostic methods, and registration practices. The national incidence rates of stomach cancer vary approximately tenfold, with the lowest reliable rates observed among North Americans (age-standardized incidence of 7.4 per 100 000 person-years in men and 3.4 per 100 000 person-years in women, 2002) and the highest in Japan, where screening is ongoing (Parkin et al, 2005). The age-standardized incidence in Japan was 62.1 per 100 000 person-years in men and 26.1 per 100 000 person-years in women. In the US, stomach cancer now ranks number 11 among men and number 14 among women as far as incidence is concerned (American Cancer Society, 2006), with a corresponding 13 400 male and 8 800 female incident cases in 2006. In terms of deaths, the ranking is number 13 and 12 among US men and women, respectively, with 6 690 and 4 740 deaths.

With few exceptions, the incidence among women is approximately half of that among men, regardless of geographic area, culture, religion (Figs. 10–1 and 10–2). Stomach cancer is a cancer of the elderly. Except in Japan, it is rarely seen before the age of 50. The age-distribution patterns are similar in

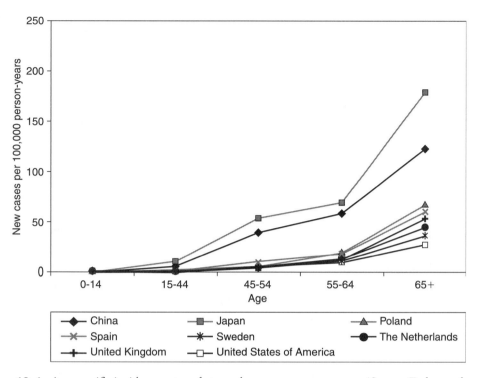

Figure 10–1. Age-specific incidence rates of stomach cancer among women. (*Source:* Ferlay et al, 2004)

most countries, and the 2:1 male/female ratio persists throughout all age groups in all countries (Figs. 10–3 and 10–4).

While the risk of stomach cancer seems to covary with socioeconomic conditions, there is no clear correlation between national level of economic development and national incidence rates, but suspected underreporting may distort comparisons. For instance, it has previously been suggested that gastric cancer is rare in Africa (Holcombe, 1992), but a closer look revealed that the incidence in Middle Africa is not very low (IARC, 2003). Although the highest rates are observed in eastern Asia (Japan, China, and Korea), low rates (< 10 per 100 000 person-years) are reported from South and Southeast Asia (eg, India, Thailand, and the Philippines). High incidence rates also are found in tropical Central and South America and in eastern Europe (Parkin et al, 2005).

Differences in incidence within nations further add to the variability. There is an increasing south-to-north gradient in incidence in the Northern Hemisphere. In Sweden, the difference between the lowest and highest incidence is approximately twofold (Swedish Oncological Centres, 1995). A similar 1.6-fold, south-north gradient also exists in China (Wong et al, 1998). Likewise, the incidence rates observed in 13 cancer registries in Italy varied threefold both in women and in men (Parkin et al, 1997). In the United States, the incidence is twice as high in blacks as in whites (Parkin et al, 1997), and the incidence among Japanese-Americans is three to six times higher than that of US-born whites (Kamineni et al, 1999). Immigrant Koreans have an incidence that is eightfold higher than that among whites (Cho et al, 1996), while the incidence among Filipino men, regardless of birthplace, is only 60% of that among US-born white men (Kamineni et al, 1999). Another example of marked differences within a limited geographic area comes from Singapore, where

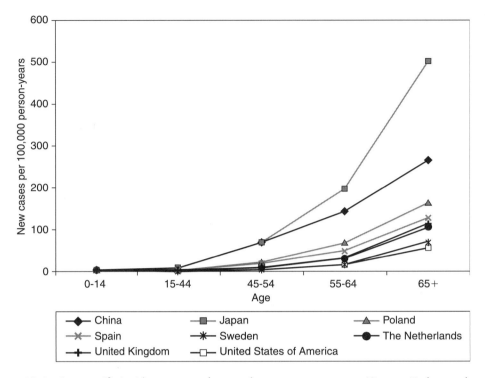

Figure 10–2. Age-specific incidence rates of stomach cancer among men. (*Source*: Ferlay et al, 2004)

the incidence rates among men of Malay and Chinese descent are 8.7 and 29.3 per 100 000 person-years, respectively (Parkin et al, 1997).

When people move between populations with different risks of stomach cancer, their

risk patterns are usually retained or only slightly modified, regardless of their country of origin and country of destination. In the succeeding generation, the rates adjust to that prevailing in the new environment, but this adaptation appears to be slower for

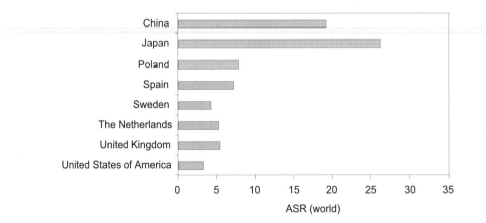

Figure 10–3. Age-standardized incidence rates of stomach cancer among women. (*Source*: Ferlay et al, 2004)

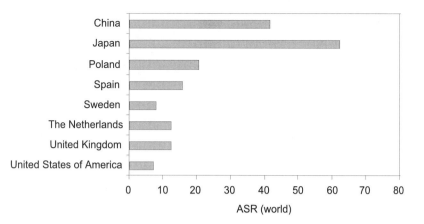

Figure 10–4. Age-standardized incidence rates of stomach cancer among men. (*Source*: Ferlay et al, 2004)

stomach cancer than for colorectal and some other cancers, particularly among Japanese emigrants to the United States (Kamineni et al, 1999). Though the patterns of risk in relation to migration are complex and defy simple dietary or other interpretation, it appears that early life exposures are important for the future risk of gastric cancer.

Secular Trends

The decline in the age-specific incidence of stomach cancer seems to have begun in the early 1930s in the Western Hemisphere and thereafter spread eastward. In the United States, stomach cancer was the leading cause of cancer death in 1930. The secular trend seems to fit well with a log-linear model—that is, the incidence decreases by a fixed percentage each year (Hansson et al, 1991). In multivariate modeling, with control for the effects of age, calendar period, and/or period of birth, this decline is best explained by a marked fall in incidence in successive birth cohorts (Hansson et al, 1991; Aragones et al, 1997).

Figure 10–5 depicts the age-adjusted relative risk of stomach cancer among Swedes between 1960 and 1984 by year of birth, with the risk among those born between 1876 and 1884 as a reference. With control for age, the relative risk among Swedish men and women born between 1906 and 1914 was 0.46 and 0.39, respectively, while

the corresponding figure for men born between 1956 and 1964 was no more than 0.07 (Hansson et al, 1991). In European countries engaged in World War II, there are transient rises in risk among the generations born around the 1940s (Aragones et al, 1997), consistent with the importance of exposures, possibly dietary, early in life.

Distribution of Histologic Types

There are several classifications of gastric adenocarcinoma. Most often used in epidemiologic research is the one proposed by Laurén (1965). It distinguishes between two main groups: *(1)* the intestinal type, with glandular epithelium composed of absorptive cells and globlet cells, and *(2)* the diffuse type, with poorly differentiated small cells in a dissociated, noncohesive growth pattern. In addition, mixed and unclassifiable tumors occur. Laurén noted that the intestinal type was more common among men than among women, and it was seen less often in young patients than in the elderly.

Some authors have attributed the overall decline in the incidence of stomach cancer to a selective decrease in the intestinal type (Munoz and Connelly, 1971; Nikulasson et al, 1992; Lauren and Nevalainen, 1993). This led to the hypothesis that the intestinal type, with its variation over time and across populations (Coleman et al, 1993), has a predominantly environmental

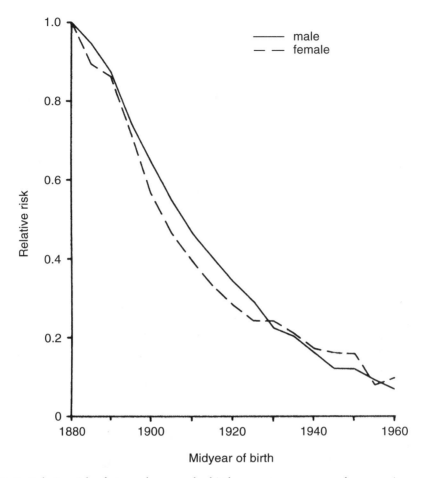

Figure 10–5. Relative risk of stomach cancer by birth year among men and women in Sweden, 1960–84. The birth year 1888 was set as the reference. The estimates were adjusted for attained age. (*Source*: Hansson et al, 1991)

etiology, while the diffuse type was postulated to be more genetically predetermined. Other investigators, however, have also noted falling incidence rates for the diffuse type (Sipponen et al, 1987; Nikulasson et al, 1992). There are reports from Sweden and Mexico of an unchanged ratio of intestinal to diffuse cancers in case series extending over decades (Lundegardh et al, 1991; Mohar et al, 1997). And a study in Sweden, with meticulous case ascertainment and histopathologic classification of all tumors, showed identical time trends for the two main histologic types when adjustments were made for age, gender, and local geographic differences in incidence (Ekstrom et al, 2000). Thus, the descriptive

epidemiology does not clearly support the notion that the occurrence of one histologic type of stomach cancer is more environmentally determined than the other.

Opposing Secular Trend for Cardia Cancer?

It appears that the decline in the incidence of gastric carcinoma overall has abated in the United States (Devesa et al, 1987; Devesa et al, 1998). For instance, the incidence among men (age-adjusted against the 1970 US standard) fell by no more than 0.2 per 100 000 person-years between 1974 to 1976 and 1992 to 1994 (Devesa et al, 1998). A closer look at the data, however, reveals that the steep downward trend persisted for distal stomach cancer in white men and women. Among the former, the incidence fell from 5.1 to 3.7 per 100 000 person-years. But this decline was balanced by an increase in the incidence of cardia cancer (from 2.1 to 3.3 per 100 000 person-years among white men).

Increasing incidence rates of cardia cancer have been noted in a number of cancer registers in Europe and the United States in the past 20 to 30 years (Blot et al, 1991; Hansson et al, 1993a). This deviating trend coincided with markedly increasing incidence rates of esophageal adenocarcinoma reported from several western countries (Blot et al, 1991; Hansson et al, 1993b). Given that a separate ICD code for cardia cancer was not introduced until after 1970 in most countries, and considering the potential for misclassification of esophageal adenocarcinoma as cardiac, there are reasons to be somewhat skeptical about the alleged rise in cardia cancer incidence.

Indeed, considerable misclassification of the site within the stomach has been demonstrated in the otherwise high-quality Swedish cancer registration (Ekstrom et al, 1999b); following careful classification of all tumors, no increasing trend could be confirmed for cardia cancer (Ekstrom et al, 2000). Some other studies have also failed to verify any upward trend, and even in the United States, the trend seems to have leveled off in the 1990s (Devesa et al, 1998). Regardless of whether the incidence curve for cardia cancer is flat or turning up, it is quite clear that it looks different from the descending one for distal gastric cancer.

GENETIC AND MOLECULAR EPIDEMIOLOGY

Familial Occurrence

Historically, stomach cancer is known for its unique, perhaps genetically determined, clustering in the family of Napoleon Bonaparte. More recently, familial aggregation of stomach cancer has been reported in the epidemiologic literature. Typically, a 50% to 130% excess risk was observed among subjects with a positive family history. Interestingly, a somewhat higher risk was noted when the mother was affected. Most epidemiologic studies have used an abbreviated family history approach and must, therefore, be cautiously interpreted. First, many laypeople refer to the whole abdomen as the stomach, so the specificity of positive reports of stomach cancer among relatives may be low. Second, recall bias may be substantial if the study is extended beyond first-degree relatives. Third, since having a large number of siblings is an established risk factor for gastric cancer (see following), and since the number of siblings is an important determinant of the likelihood of having a positive first-degree family history of any disease, there is a clear potential for confounding by family size.

Most studies have not adjusted for number of siblings. But even with more stringent study designs, familial aggregation is observed. In an analysis of 23 386 Swedish twin pairs, with case ascertainment in the virtually complete Swedish Cancer Register, the risk of stomach cancer among twins with a partner who developed the same cancer was five times as high as it was among twins whose partner did not have stomach cancer (Ahlbom et al, 1997). In a subsequent, bigger study including 44 788 Scandinavian twin pairs, the excess was 6.6-fold if the twin pair was dizygotic, and tenfold if the pair was monozygotic (Lichtenstein et al, 2000). In the latter study, it was estimated that inherited genes contribute 28% to the risk of gastric cancer, shared environmental effects contribute 10%, and nonshared environmental factors make up the remaining 62% of the risk. Therefore, studies on twins predict the involvement of major environmental factors plus minor genetic components.

Inherited Susceptibility

Germline mutations

An aggregation of two or more stomach cancers in the same family is noted in about 10% of all stomach cancer cases. Among them, a number of syndromes can be identified: *(1)* hereditary diffuse gastric cancer

(HDGC—requiring two or more documented cases of diffuse stomach cancer in first-/second-degree relatives, with at least one diagnosed before the age of 50; or three or more cases of documented diffuse stomach cancer in first-/second-degree relatives, independently of age)(Caldas et al, 1999); *(2)* familial diffuse gastric cancer (FDGC—families with aggregation of stomach cancer and an index case with diffuse stomach cancer, but not fulfilling the criteria for HDGC, for instance due to unknown histological type of the related cases); *(3)* familial intestinal gastric cancer (FIGC—families with a similar aggregation as in HDGC, but with intestinal type histology)(Shinmura et al, 1999); and *(4)* familial gastric cancer (FGC—familial aggregation of stomach cancer but with unknown histopathology).

Germline truncating mutations in the gene for the cell–cell adhesion protein E-cadherin (*CDH1*) were first discovered in three Maori families with autosomal dominant diffuse stomach cancer but have since been detected in an increasing proportion of families with aggregation of stomach cancer, notably HDGC (Gayther et al, 1998; Guilford et al, 1998). In a recent review of the accumulated literature (Oliveira et al, 2006), HDGC accounted for 26.9% of 439 screened families with any of the syndromes previously described. Another 23.7% had FDGC, 8.7% had FIGC, and 40.8% had FGC. Germline *CDH1* mutations were found in 36.4% of families with HDGC and in 12.5% of families with FDGC.

An additional small proportion has other familial cancer syndromes, for instance hereditary nonpolyposis colorectal cancer (HNPCC) (Aarnio et al, 1997) and Li-Fraumenis syndrome (Varley et al, 1995), which are both linked to an increased risk of stomach cancer. Recently, a *TP53*-truncating germline mutation was described in a family with characteristics of both HDGC and Li-Fraumeni syndrome (Kim et al, 2004). However, in about two-thirds of HDGC families, a large proportion of FDGC, and in the majority of FGC families,

cancer susceptibility is caused by presently unknown genetic defects.

Polymorphisms

The literature on genetic polymorphisms and stomach cancer risk is limited by a common lack of appropriate control of potential sources of bias; few studies are population-based, and the sample sizes are often insufficient even for the statistical verification of moderate main effects, let alone gene–environment interactions. Besides, information on exposure to relevant cofactors such as *Helicobacter pylori* infection, diet, and smoking is often lacking.

Interleukin-1

The role of functional polymorphisms in genes that code for various cytokines involved in the inflammatory response to *H. pylori* infection has attracted considerable attention in recent years. One of the key cytokines is interleukin-1 beta (IL-1β), which is an important driving force in the inflammatory responses and is also a potent inhibitor of gastric acid secretion. The *IL-1B* gene encoding IL-1β is highly polymorphic. Two of the polymorphisms are in the promoter region at positions -511 and -31, representing C–T and T–C transitions, respectively. The variant alleles of these loci are associated with more severe inflammation. Another cytokine that has an important influence on IL-1β levels is the endogenous interleukin-1 receptor antagonist (IL-1ra), whose gene (*IL-1RN*) is also known to be polymorphic. The *IL-1RN* gene has a penta allelic 86-bp tandem repeat polymorphism (variable number of tandem repeat, VNTR) in intron 2, of which the less common allele 2 (*IL-1RN*2*)—associated with enhanced IL-1β production in vitro—is linked to several chronic inflammatory conditions.

In a landmark case-control study from Poland, El-Omar and coworkers (2000) demonstrated that carriers of the C allele of *IL-1B*–31 (in positive linkage disequilibrium with *IL-1B*–511T) and homozygous carriers of the *2 allele of *IL-1RN* had 1.6- and

2.9-fold increased risks, respectively, of stomach cancer, compared to noncarriers of these variant alleles. Carriers of the *IL-1B–31T/ IL-1RN*2* haplotype had an odds ratio of 4.4. The estimated effects of these genotypes were similar in subgroups of gastric cancer defined by age, sex, histologic type, and anatomic site. These findings have been more or less replicated in several investigations.

A study from Portugal with genotyping of archived gastric biopsies suggested that the combination of proinflammatory genotypes in the host with infection with high-risk *H. pylori* strains (see section about *H. pylori* that follows) might involve major increases in risk, with relative risks as high as 87 (Figueiredo et al, 2002). However, others have failed to confirm any association of the *IL-1B–31/IL-1B–511* and/or *IL-1RN* polymorphisms with stomach cancer. To date, three meta-analyses, including between 25 and 39 reports, have been published. The most complete one, and the only one that has adequately handled multiple reports based on the same case series (Kamangar, Cheng et al, 2006), showed summary odds ratios (all gastric cancers) for, respectively, *IL-1B–511C/T* and T/T versus C/C, of 1.07 (95% confidence interval 0.91–1.25) and 1.16 (95% confidence interval 0.95–1.42). The summary odds ratios for *IL-1B–31C/T* and C/C versus T/T were 0.99 (95% confidence interval 0.83–1.19) and 0.98 (95% confidence interval 0.78–1.21), respectively. For *IL-1RN*2/L* versus L/L, the summary odds ratio was 1.15 (95% confidence interval 0.96–1.38) and for *IL-1RN*/2*2* versus L/L it was 1.23 (95% confidence interval 0.79–1.92). Thus, despite participation of a total of 5 503 cases and 7 865 controls, the summary estimates were still short of statistical significance. Interestingly, in cumulative meta-analysis, the associations were initially strong for each studied polymorphism, but they tended toward null associations with accumulation of more data over time. It has been claimed that the genotype-risk association might be confined to Caucasians

and not to Asians, but this impression has been partly driven by undue weight given to the Portuguese case series that has been included several times in each of the other meta-analyses. In the valid meta-analysis cited above (Kamangar et al, 2006), significant heterogeneity among studies was admittedly noted for all of the studied associations, but the investigators were unable to find a clear reason for the variation. However, point estimates for homozygous carriers of the variant alleles of *IL-1B–511* the *IL-1RN* VNTR in intron 2 tended to be slightly higher (but still non-significant) among Caucasians than among Asians. It appears that the relationship, if any, between polymorphisms in the *IL-1* gene cluster and stomach cancer risk may be more complex than first thought.

Other cytokines. Associations between functional polymorphisms of genes coding for other cytokines involved in the inflammatory response (*Tumor Necrosis Factor A* gene–308A/G, -857/C/T, -863C/T, -1031/C/T; *INFGR* (coding for the Interferon γ receptor 2) Ex7–128C/T; *Interleukin-4* gene diplotype 984 and 2983 AA/GA; *Interleukin-10* gene −592C/A, −819C/T, and −1082G/A; and *Interleukin-8* gene −251A/T) and risk of stomach cancer have been reported, but other investigators have found incompatible results or the reports have remained unconfirmed, casting doubt on the biological significance of the initial findings.

Toll-like receptor 4. The Toll-like receptor 4 (TLR4) is an important player in the defense against invading microorganisms. It is a transmembrane receptor that recognizes an array of conserved molecular patterns, including lipopolysaccharide (LPS), which is found in the cell wall of Gram-negative bacteria like *H. pylori*. A functional polymorphism (A>G transition) at position +896 in exon 4 of the *TLR4* gene was recently shown to be associated with a 2.3-fold increased risk of stomach cancer in a Polish case-control study (Hold et al, 2007), but studies from Mexico, Venezuela and China were unable to confirm this association, or associations with gastric precancerous lesions.

Human leukocyte antigen. Given the possible infectious etiology of stomach cancer, the human leukocyte antigen (HLA) class I and II molecules, encoding cell surface a-b heterodimers that bind and present peptides derived from foreign antigen to T cells, belong to the host factors that are of potential interest. Presence of the DQA1*0102 allele—inversely associated with the probability of *H. pylori* infection (Azuma et al, 1998; Magnusson et al, 2001)—was accompanied by a decreased risk of gastric cancer in a Japanese controlled-case series (Azuma et al, 1998), but not in a Swedish population-based case-control study (Magnusson et al, 2001). In the latter study, the *1601 allele at the DRB1 locus was associated with a tenfold increased gastric cancer risk, but it was unrelated to the risk of *H. pylori* infection. The excess risk was greater for Laurén's diffuse type (odds ratio 24) than for the intestinal type (odds ratio 5.6), and the association was particularly strong (odds ratio > 50) among *H. pylori*–negative subjects.

A similar, but weaker, association with the gastric cancer risk (odds ratio 3.2), without a positive link to *H. pylori* infection, has been noted for the *0301 allele at the DQB1 locus in an American study (Lee et al, 1996). This positive association was contradicted by data from Taiwan (Wu et al, 2002b), where the very same DQB1 allele was linked to a significantly reduced risk (odds ratio 0.33) for stomach cancer, possibly via a low prevalence of *H. pylori* infection. The Taiwanese investigators, instead, found a significantly increased risk (odds ratio 2.79) among carriers of the DQB1*0602 allele.

Mucins. Being part of the gastric mucosal protection, and constituting the medium in which *H. pylori* swims to its target cells, mucins are of potential interest in the search for susceptibility factors. Mucins exhibit a high degree of polymorphism because of the presence of a variable number of tandem repeats. Indeed, studies from Portugal indicate that smaller alleles at both MUC1 and MUC6 loci are significantly more common among gastric cancer patients than among blood donors (Carvalho et al, 1997; Garcia et al, 1997).

Metabolic enzymes. Metabolic phase I enzymes like the cytochrome P450 (CYP) superfamily catalyze oxidative reactions that introduce electrophilic groups in xenobiotic molecules and make them more reactive, typically leading to carcinogen activation. Phase II enzymes introduce a hydrophilic group into the activated intermediate molecules, usually leading to detoxification. Some of the polymorphic genes that code for phase I enzymes have been examined with regard to the association between presence of alleles of confirmed or suspected importance for the function of the gene product and risk of stomach cancer.

In a case-cohort analysis among Chinese high-risk individuals with cytologically proven esophageal dysplasia who participated in a cancer prevention trial, heterozygous or homozygous carriage of the variant *2A allele (3801T/C) of the CYP1A1 gene was associated with an almost halved risk of gastric cardia cancer (Roth et al, 2004). On the other hand, another Chinese study reported an almost fivefold increased risk of stomach cancer associated with homozygous presence of the variant CYP1AT*2C-allele (Li et al, 2005). Two other Chinese studies, one Japanese study, and a large European multinational cohort study failed to confirm any main effect of CYP1A1 polymorphisms, but suggestions of rather complex interactions with smoking, *H. pylori* infection, and GSTM1 genotypes make the interpretation of the CYP1A1 data difficult. In the European cohort study individuals carrying at least one variant allele CYP1AT*4 (KI nomenclature) had a twofold increased risk, but only if they were smokers (Agudo et al, 2006a).

The CYP2E1 gene, whose product is an important activator of nitrosamines, has also been investigated. A Taiwanese study found an almost threefold increased risk of stomach cancer among carriers of the c2/c2 genotype detected by *Rsa*I digestion, but no association with the *Dra*I polymorphism (Wu et al, 2002a). On the other hand, the *Rsa*I variant allele was shown to be protective against stomach cancer in non-Japanese Brazilians (Nishimoto et al, 2000). A recent meta-analysis (Boccia et al, 2007) including 13 case-control studies with 2066 stomach cancer cases and 2754 controls found no association overall (odds ratio among hetero- or homozygous carriers of the c2 allele, relative to homozygous carriers of the wild-type c1 allele, was 0.97 and it was non-significant 1.36 among c2 homozygotes). When only high-quality studies were considered, a statistically increased risk appeared among Asians for c2 carriers versus c1/c1 (odds ratio 1.50; 95% confidence interval 1.16–1.18) and for c2/c2 versus c1/c1 (odds ratio 2.62; 95% confidence interval 1.23–5.57).

Individuals who were homozygous with regard to the *CYP2A6* gene-deletion allele, causing a lack of enzyme activity, had a significant threefold increased risk of gastric cancer (Tsukino et al, 2002). Having either of the *2/*2, *3/*3, or *2/*3 variant genotypes of *CYP2C19*, associated with poor metabolizing ability, was associated with two- to threefold elevations in risk of stomach cancer, particularly of the diffuse histological type, in one Japanese (Sugimoto et al, 2005) and one Chinese study (Shi and Chen, 2004), but not in a Turkish study (Tamer et al, 2006).

MICROSOMAL EPOXIDE HYDROLASE. Microsomal epoxide hydrolase (mEH) is another Phase I enzyme that partly detoxifies CYP1A1-activated polycyclic aromatic hydrocarbons through hydrolysis, but also catalyzes additional oxidation of dihydrodiols to highly reactive diol epoxides. In the large-scale EPIC cohort study in Europe (Agudo et al, 2006a), homozygotes for the C (histidine) variant of the Ex3–28T>C polymorphism in the gene that codes for mEH (*EPHX1*) had an almost

doubled risk of stomach cancer (95% confidence interval 1.2–3.1). More studies are needed to confirm this result.

GLUTATHIONE S-TRANSFERASE (GST). GST enzymes belong to the metabolic phase II category and are involved in the detoxification of many potentially carcinogenic compounds. Due to rather common inherited deletions of the paternal and/or maternal alleles of the *GSTM1* and *GSTT1* genes (+/null or null/null genotypes), 10% to 60% of individuals, depending on the population, have reduced or no enzyme expression, with entailing reductions in the ability to detoxify certain xenobiotics. Therefore, these polymorphisms have attracted considerable interest. Although a number of studies have provided support for the hypothesis of an increased stomach cancer risk among carriers of the +/null or null/null genotypes, somewhat more consistently for *GSTM1* than for *GSTT1*, an approximately equal number of studies have been unable to confirm these findings, making the overall literature inconclusive (Gonzalez et al, 2002). The lack of association between *GSTT1* genotype and risk of gastric cancer was confirmed in a meta-analysis that included 16 case-control studies with a total of 6717 subjects (Saadat, 2006). It was noted, however, that a significant but moderate association emerged in Caucasians (odds ratio among carriers of the *GSTT1* null genotype was 1.27; 95% confidence interval 1.03–1.57), whereas no association (odds ratio 0.98) was seen in Asians. The bulk of the literature on *GSTP1* polymorphisms and stomach cancer risk weighs toward no association.

N-ACETYLTRANFERASES. The polymorphic phase II N-acetyltransferases *NAT1* and *NAT2* metabolize a number of aromatic and heterocyclic amine carcinogens and should also be of interest. According to a report from Japan, the variant *NAT1*10* allele was weakly associated with risk of gastric adenocarcinoma (Katoh et al, 2000). The association was found to be stronger and statistically significant among heavy smokers (odds ratio 3.0). A study from the UK could statistically confirm the positive association between carriage of the NAT1*10 allele and stomach cancer risk (Boissy et al, 2000). The latter study also reported a nonsignificant trend toward an increased stomach cancer risk among individuals who were homozygous for the wild type NAT2*4 allele (odds ratio 3.8). These individuals are rapid acetylators. Interestingly, the link with NAT2*4 carriage attained statistical significance in a study from Spain (odds ratio 1.95) (Ladero et al, 2002), thus adding to the consistency. However, subsequent studies from Poland (Lan et al, 2003), Japan (Suzuki et al, 2004), and within the EPIC cohort (Agudo et al, 2006b) did not find any relationship between NAT1 or NAT2 genotypes and stomach cancer risk.

Cyclooxygenase (COX). Given the possible role of COX, particularly COX-2, in human carcinogenicity, and its relation to H. pylori infection, effects of polymorphisms of the COX-2 gene are of interest. It has been proven that the −1195G/A polymorphism creates a C-MYB binding site, which may result in higher transcription activity of the COX-2 gene. Indeed, a study among Chinese stomach cancer patients and controls with superficial or chronic atrophic gastritis diagnosed in connection with a population-based screening effort in a high-risk Chinese population (Liu et al, 2006) confirmed a high expression of COX-2 in subjects with the −1195 AA genotype. More importantly, the investigators found a significantly increased risk of stomach cancer in subjects with the −1195 AA genotype (odds ratio 2.33). Stratified analysis indicated that the risk elevation was particularly marked in subjects infected with H. pylori (odds ratio 3.88) or subjects who were smokers (odds ratio 7.02). Confirmatory data are eagerly awaited.

Folate and MTMFR. Folate is a water-soluble B vitamin that plays an important role in the maintenance of DNA integrity.

Increasing evidence suggests that a low folate intake and/or an impaired folate metabolism may be implicated in the development of gastrointestinal cancers. The enzyme 5,10-methylenetetrahydrofolate reductase (MTHFR) irreversibly converts 5,10-methylenetetrahydrofolate to 5-methyltetrahydrofolate, the predominant form of folate in the circulation. Two common functional polymorphisms of the MTHFR gene, 677C/T and 1298A/C, have been identified, associated with up to 70% and 40% reductions, respectively, of MTHFR activity among individuals who are homozygous for the variant alleles.

A recent meta-analysis of 11 case-control and 2 cohort studies that examined the association between dietary folate intake and risk of stomach cancer arrived at statistically significant risk reductions for stomach cancer of both noncardia (summary relative risk 0.67, 95% confidence interval 0.51–0.88) and cardia (summary relative risk 0.73, 95% confidence interval 0.55–0.97) location among individuals with high intake relative to those with low intake (Larsson et al, 2006b). However, this inverse relationship was confined to studies conducted in the US and Europe, while studies done in other populations were essentially negative. The summary estimate of relative risk for stomach cancer among individuals with the variant TT genotype of MTHFR–677, relative to those with the CC genotype, was 1.68 (95% confidence interval 1.29–2.19) and the corresponding estimate for gastric cardia cancer was 1.90 (95% confidence interval 1.38–2.60). Available studies of the 1298A/C polymorphism did not provide any indications of a statistical relationship with stomach cancer risk. While another meta-analysis (Zintzaras, 2006) arrived at approximately the same overall conclusion, the author noted that the association between carriage of the MTHFR–677T allele and risk of stomach cancer was essentially confined to East Asians. The summary odds ratio for Caucasians was close to 1 and non-significant. Although there are single studies that have reported substantial associations also in Caucasians (Graziano et al, 2006), European studies published after the aforementioned meta-analyses add to the impression of no association (Gotze et al, 2007; Zhang et al, 2007).

DNA-repair. The normal functions of DNA repair proteins are critical for cells to remove damage and thus prevent carcinogenesis. The base excision repair (BER) pathway, among other DNA repair systems, is basically responsible for rectifying DNA base damage and single-strand breaks. Adenosine diphosphate ribosyl transferase (ADPRT) and x-ray repair cross-complementing 1 (XRCC1) play key roles. Genetic variants have been identified for both *ADPRT* and *XRCC1* genes. A T to C transition at codon 762 of the *ADPRT* gene causes Val-to-Ala amino acid substitution, and this polymorphism is associated with altered ADPRT function. In the *XRCC1* gene, the G to A polymorphism at codon 399 (*XRCC1* 28152G/A) results in Arg-to-Gln amino acid change, which is situated within the BRCT-1 region harboring the ADPRT-binding domain. An altered DNA repair activity has been suggested to be associated with the *XRCC1* 399Gln polymorphism.

A study from China examined the importance of this polymorphism, together with an *XRCC1* 26305C/T polymorphism in codon 194 (Shen et al, 2000). The risk elevation associated with carriage of the *XRCC1* 399Gln/Gln genotype alone was moderate and statistically nonsignificant, but combined with the *XRCC1* 194Arg/Arg genotype the odds ratio for total stomach cancer was 1.73 and statistically significant. A larger case-control study from China with 500 cardia cancer patients and 1000 controls found a moderately increased odds ratio (1.40) for cardia cancer among individuals with at least one *XRCC1* 399Gln allele, and a slightly higher odds ratio (1.61) among homozygous carriers (Miao et al, 2006). The odds ratio among homozygous carriers of the *ADPRT* 762Ala allele was 2.17. Gene–gene interaction of

ADPRT and *XRCC1* polymorphisms increased the relative risk for gastric cardia cancer in a multiplicative manner (odds ratio among individuals with both *ADPRT* Ala/Ala and *XRCC1* Gln/Gln genotypes was 6.43, 95% confidence interval 1.80–22.97, relative to individuals with *ADPRT* Val/Val and *XRCC1* Arg/Arg).

In contrast with this report, Ratnasinghe et al (2004) showed that subjects from Linxian, China, with at least one copy of the *XRCC1* 399Gln allele had a significantly reduced risk of gastric cardia cancer (odds ratio 0.60). A fourth study from Brazil found no evidence of a relationship between the polymorphisms *XRCC1* Arg194Trp, Arg399Gln, or *XRCC3* Thr241Met and the risk of chronic gastritis and gastric cancer (Duarte et al, 2005). Lastly, a population-based Swedish case-control study of gastric cardia cancer was also negative, although the odds ratio point estimate for the *XRCC1* Gln/Gln genotype in locus 399 was 1.7 (95% confidence interval 0.8–3.4) (Ye et al, 2006). The latter study also investigated the *XPD* Lys751Gln, *XPC* Lys939Gln, and *XRCC3* Thr241Met polymorphisms without any positive findings.

Growth factors. Epidermal growth factor (EGF), through interaction with its receptor (EGFR), induces growth signals and is important for tumor growth and progression. A G to A substitution at position 61 in the 5'-untranslated region (UTR) of the *EGF* gene is associated with reduced production of EGF. There are three Asian case-control studies (two from Japan and one from China) that have all demonstrated a reduced risk of stomach cancer among carriers of the variant *EGF*+61A allele (Goto et al, 2005; Hamai et al, 2005; Jin et al, 2007a). The odds ratios varied between 0.56 and 0.87 and were statistically significant in two of the three studies.

The transforming growth factor β (TGF-β) generally promotes tumor progression and metastasis, but it also suppresses early stage tumor growth. TGF-β exists in three isoforms (TGF-β1, TGF-β2, and TGF-β3).

Recently, investigators from China (Jin et al, 2007b) reported a decreased risk of stomach cancer in carriers of the variant alleles of one or both of two single nucleotide polymorphisms in the *TGFB1* (–509C/T) and *TGFB2* (–875G/A) genes, respectively. Odds ratio among carriers of *TGFB1*–509C/T or T/T, relative to those with C/C, was 0.65 (95% confidence interval 0.52–0.82), and among carriers of *TGFB2*–875G/A or A/A versus individuals with the G/G genotype it was 0.67 (95% confidence interval 0.53–0.85). Subjects with both variant genotypes had an odds ratio for stomach cancer of 0.44. Confirmatory studies are needed.

Somatic Events

Unlike in the adenoma-colorectal cancer sequence, no clear linear accumulation of genetic defects has been identified in gastric carcinogenesis (Vauhkonen et al, 2006). One important reason for the rather confusing overall picture is the fact that the histological subtypes of stomach cancer appear to arise through at least partly disparate molecular pathways. Moreover, Laurén's intestinal type may develop along three subpathways (Tahara, 2004): *(1)* an intestinal metaplasia (IM) → adenoma → carcinoma sequence; *(2)* an IM → carcinoma sequence; and *(3)* de novo. For the diffuse histological type, no premalignant lesion is known. However, most—if not all—stomach cancers, regardless of histological type, are preceded by *H. pylori* infection with entailing gastritis. The use of partly different morphological classifications further compounds the interpretation of existing data. But even among stomach cancers with apparently identical histopathological morphology there is a significant heterogeneity in expression of molecular markers.

In general, the number of genes in which mutations (ie, base substitutions, insertions, or deletions of a small number of base pairs) are regularly found is low in stomach cancer. As in several other cancers, however, mutation of the cellular gatekeeper and tumor suppressor gene *TP53*—largely missense point mutation—is common. The gene is usually inactivated through the classic two-hit mechanism, with loss of heterozygosity (LOH) and mutation of the remaining allele. The frequency of *TP53* mutations in intestinal-type stomach cancers is equally high (approximately 40%) regardless of whether the tumors are early or advanced. Therefore, the mutations are thought to be early events in the development of this histological subtype. *TP53* mutations are rare in early diffuse-type cancers but when the tumors are advanced the mutations occur with the same frequency as in the intestinal type (Tamura, 2006).

Similarly, mutation of the *CDH1/E-cadherin* gene, involved in calcium-dependent cell-to-cell adhesion and apparently important for morphogenesis, is rare in early but common (approximately 50%) in advanced diffuse-type stomach cancer. This mutation is always uncommon in the intestinal type, though, and when it occurs in tumors with mixed histology (both intestinal and diffuse), it is only seen in the diffuse component. These observations have fostered the hypothesis that the differentiated intestinal type may sometimes become "dedifferentiated" and turn into a diffuse-type tumor, and that acquisition of *CDH1/E-cadherin* mutations may be involved in this transition (Tamura, 2006).

Point mutations in the *KRAS* oncogene have been observed in up to one-fifth of stomach cancers (Vauhkonen et al, 2006), mainly in the intestinal type (Smith et al, 2006). Other oncogenes or proto-oncogenes may be amplified, *ERBB2/HER 2 (c-erbB2)* is amplified in approximately 20% of intestinal type cancers but not in cancers of the diffuse type, while *MET (c-met)* and *FGFR2* (K-sam) are each preferentially amplified in about one-third of diffuse-type cancers.

Deficient regulation of gene expression may also be caused by epigenetic changes. Tumor-suppressor genes may be silenced by hypermethylation of the promoter CpG islands. Accordingly, the promoter regions of *DCC* and *CDKN2A* (p16) exhibit frequent methylation. *DAP-kinase* promoter methylation is more frequent in the diffuse than in the intestinal type. *RASSF1A, RUNX3,* and *TCLC1* are other tumor-supressor genes that are frequently silenced through hypermethylation in stomach cancer (Tamura, 2006). In fact, increasing numbers of genes involved in cell-cycle control, DNA repair, cell-cell adhesion, apoptosis, and angiogenesis have been described as being silenced by hypermethylation; methylation of *CDH1/E-cadherin,* associated with decreased expression, is observed in more than 50% of early stage diffuse cancers and is also observable in surrounding noncancerous gastric epithelia. Thus, the epigenetic inactivation of *CDH1/E-cadherin* via promoter methylation may play a major role in the development of the diffuse type of stomach cancer. The present epigenetic data suggest that much, if not most, of the decrease (or loss) of gene expression may be explained by promoter hypermethylation.

In some cases promoter hypermethylation leads to activation of the gene. This is true for the human telomerase transcriptase gene (*hTERT*), an important determinant of telomerase activity. Reactivation of telomerase activity is necessary for cell immortality and is normally repressed in gastric cells. Such reactivation is seen in virtually all gastric cancers (Tahara et al, 1995). Over 50% of intestinal metaplasias express low levels of telomerase activity. While the association between *H. pylori* gastritis and CpG island methylation of genes is unclear, the microorganism may act as a trigger factor for hyperplasia in *hTERT* positive "stem cells" in intestinal metaplasia (Tahara, 2004).

Epigenetic methylation–associated inactivation of the mismatch repair gene *mutL homolog 1 colon cancer* (*hMLH1*) is of particular interest. It is a potent trigger of microsatellite instability (MSI), defined as the presence of replication errors in simple tandemly repeated stretches of DNA (microsatellites). MSI can be classified as either high frequency (MSI-H) or low frequency (MSI-L) and is found in 15% to 50% of stomach cancers, more often in the intestinal type than in the diffuse. Conversely,

among the microsatellite stable (MSS) tumors, ie, replication error negative, the diffuse histological type is dominating. In a study among early intestinal cancers, 20% of the tumors were classified as MSI-H (Ohmura et al, 2000), while another study among early diffuse cancers found no evidence of MSI at all (Tamura et al, 2001). Up to 90% of MSI-H tumors are associated with *hMLH1* promoter hypermethylation.

In MSI-H stomach cancers several genes undergo alterations in the repetitive segments of the coding regions leading to reading-frame mutations, for instance *transforming growth factor β receptor II* gene (*TGFβRII*—63%–92%), *insulin-like growth factor II receptor* gene (*IGFIIR*—5%–25%), proapoptotic *BAX* gene (15%–68%), DNA repair genes *hMSH6* (22%) and *hMSH3* (38%), and transcription factor gene *E2F-4* (37%–61%) (Vauhkonen et al, 2006). The MSI-L phenotype, also linked to the intestinal type of stomach cancer, is associated with the loss of heterozygosity (LOH) phenotype. Target gene mutations are infrequent in MSI-L tumors.

Frequent occurrence of LOH in a tumor has been suggested to indicate chromosomal instability (CIN). LOH is thought to represent the second inactivating hit in tumor-suppressor genes, characterizing the so-called suppressor pathway of carcinogenesis. In stomach cancer, LOH is mostly found on chromosomes 2q, 4p, 5q, 6p, 7q, 11q, 14q, 17p, 18q, and 21q. It can be detected in up to 80% of all tumors. It appears that the frequency is similar in intestinal and diffuse cancers, but few studies have addressed the occurrence of LOH in the diffuse histological type. The LOH rate in *TP53* is reportedly 26% to 83%, predominantly occurring in the intestinal histological type.

RISK FACTORS

Tobacco

A relationship between smoking and risk of gastric cancer is well established (Tredaniel et al, 1997; IARC 2004). The excess risk among current smokers is 1.5 to 2.5-fold. Although most earlier studies failed to confirm a dose-response relationship, more recent investigations have generally shown increasing risks with higher doses and/or longer duration of cigarette smoking (Gonzalez et al, 2003; Koizumi et al, 2004). It appears that the risk returns to baseline relatively soon after quitting smoking (Chow et al, 1999), but in a pooled analysis of two Japanese cohorts, a significant risk elevation remained for up to 14 years after cessation (Koizumi et al, 2004).

While some studies suggest that smoking is more strongly related to cardia cancer risk (Lagergren et al, 2000; Mao et al, 2002; Gonzalez et al, 2003), others indicate that the link with distal stomach cancer is not appreciably weaker, and in Japan it might even be stronger (Koizumi et al, 2004). In a Swedish study, the association between smoking and stomach cancer risk was largely confined to subjects with a low intake of fresh fruit and vegetables (Ye et al, 1999). There is also some evidence suggesting a multiplicative interaction between cigarette smoking and CagA-positive *H. pylori* infection, leading to 17-fold increased risks among people exposed to both risk factors, compared to those exposed to neither (Brenner et al, 2002).

Population-attributable risk percent (PAR) expresses the percent of the studied outcome disease that can be attributed to the exposure under study—or, in other words, the percent of all cases that might be prevented by eliminating this risk factor. PAR for smoking varies with the exposure prevalence, and thus between men and women, but within sexes the variation between American and European data is surprisingly small; thus, PAR among men varied between 21.5% and 28.6% and among women between 11% and 14% in three recent studies emanating from the US and Europe (Chao et al, 2002; Engel et al, 2003; Gonzalez et al, 2003).

Alcohol

Self-reports of alcohol consumption are notoriously unreliable. This leads to considerable nondifferential misclassification in epidemiological studies, and, in turn, to an attenuation of the estimates of association. The most authoritative review of the literature published up until the mid-1990s (World Cancer Research Fund, 1997) noted that the bulk of evidence weighed against the possibility of a substantial effect of alcohol consumption on the risk of stomach cancer, possibly with the exception for cardia cancer. However, more recent studies suggest that there are no important differences between cardia and noncardia stomach cancer. A meta-analysis in 2001 (Bagnardi et al, 2001) arrived at a summary relative risk estimate of 1.15 (95% confidence interval 1.09–1.22) and 1.32 (95% confidence interval 1.18–1.49) for an alcohol intake of 50g/day and 100 g/day, respectively, relative to no intake. A Swedish prospective study among women found no overall association of alcohol intake with stomach cancer risk but noted that frequent consumption of medium-strong/strong beer, which contains the animal carcinogen N-nitrosodimethylamine (NDMA), was associated with a statistically significant twofold risk elevation (Larsson et al, 2007). The link to beer intake, however, was not in accord with another Scandinavian cohort study (Barstad et al, 2005), which instead showed a significant 40% risk reduction per glass of wine drunk per day, a weak and nonsignificant trend toward positive association of stomach cancer with hard liquor consumption, no association with beer consumption, and no association with overall alcohol intake. The literature on specific relationships between different types of alcoholic beverages and stomach cancer risk was recently reviewed (Larsson et al, 2007) but no consistent pattern emerged.

Tea and Coffee

No causal association is established between tea or coffee and risk of stomach cancer; however, frequent intake of green tea, hypothesized to have a protective effect by virtue of its polyphenol content, was shown to be inversely associated, albeit sometimes without a clear dose-effect pattern, with risk of stomach cancer in the majority—but not all—of seven published case-control studies. Of seven prospective studies, however, only one (Sasazuki et al, 2004) found an inverse association and it was confined to distal stomach cancer among women. Coffee consumption has been unrelated to stomach cancer risk in most studies (World Cancer Research Fund, 1997), but three (Jacobsen et al, 1986; Galanis et al, 1998; Larsson et al, 2006c) out of five prospective studies showed an excess incidence (of borderline statistical significance) among highly exposed individuals, with relative risks in the highest-exposure versus lowest-exposure category ranging from 1.46 to 1.86.

Diet

Fruits, vegetables, and antioxidants

Until recently, the most consistent nutritional epidemiology finding in relation to stomach cancer has been inverse associations with fruit and vegetable intake. In 1997, an international expert panel at the World Cancer Research Fund–American Institute for Cancer Research concluded that there was convincing evidence that high intake of vegetables, particularly raw vegetables and allium vegetables, reduces the risk of stomach cancer (World Cancer Research Fund, 1997). A similar conclusion was also drawn with regard to high fruit intake. The apparently protective effects of these plant foods have been attributed to their high concentrations of antioxidant substances, notably carotenoids, vitamin C, and vitamin E compounds.

Additionally, there are many nonessential bioactive compounds with anticarcinogenic properties in fruits and vegetables, for example, phenolics (Steinmetz and Potter, 1996). These substances could conceivably act through several mechanisms, the most important ones being (1) scavenging of potentially mutagenic free radicals (vitamins C and E, β-carotene, and some phenolic compounds such as flavonoids); (2) inhibition of carcinogenic nitrosamine formation in the stomach (vitamins C and E); (3) regulation of cell differentiation and DNA synthesis (carot-

enoids and folate); and (4) inhibition of phase I metabolic enzymes (eg, P450 cytochromes), which may create reactive oxidative molecules, or induction of phase II enzymes (eg, glutathione transferase), which detoxify residual electrophilic metabolites generated by the phase I enzymes (flavonoids and allium compounds, isothiocyanates, glucosinolates, indoles, thiocyanates, and some carotenoids).

In a more recent meta-analysis (Riboli and Norat, 2003), however, the protective effect seemed to be weaker in cohort investigations than in case-control studies, suggesting that recall bias might have pushed the relative risk estimates away from the null value in the latter. The estimated overall relative risks that were based on all study types and an increment of 100 grams intake per day were 0.81 (95% confidence interval 0.75–0.87) for vegetables and 0.74 (95% confidence interval 0.69–0.81) for fruit. Although heterogeneity was observed in essentially all analyzed substrata, the estimates for both fruit and vegetables were always lower than 1 (Riboli and Norat, 2003). However, the most recent addition to the literature, a large European multinational cohort study with careful dietary assessments and a fairly wide range of exposure (Gonzalez et al, 2006b), failed to verify any overall association of stomach cancer risk with total or category-specific vegetable or fruit intake.

Even though the estimation of portion size and frequency of consumption of a wide range of vegetables is difficult and nondifferential misclassification may bias the relative risk estimates toward the null value, it is reasonable to assume that the more recent studies, particularly the cohort studies with increasingly sophisticated dietary assessments, are less affected by such bias compared to earlier studies. Therefore, previous research may have overestimated the protection conferred by these plant foods.

Vitamin C. Whereas there is almost total consensus among case-control studies that vitamin C intake is strongly protective, only one (Botterweck et al, 2000) out of four prospective studies (Zheng et al, 1995; Botterweck et al, 2000; Nouraie et al, 2005; Jenab et al, 2006b) reported a significant inverse association between estimated vitamin C intake and stomach cancer. The summary relative risk in a meta-analysis, however, was still statistically significant (relative risk among subjects with the highest intake, relative to those with the lowest, was 0.77 [95% confidence interval 0.61–0.97]) (Larsson, 2006). A similar meta-analysis of the three prospective studies concerned with predisease blood levels of vitamin C (Stahelin et al, 1991; Yuan et al, 2004; Jenab et al, 2006b) yielded a summary estimate that was also statistically significant (RR = 0.64, 95% confidence interval 0.41–0.98) (Larsson, 2006).

Vitamin E. Vitamin E (tocopherol), another important antioxidant in plant foods, has been investigated with regard to its relationship with stomach cancer risk in at least 18 case-control studies, close to half of which reported a statistically significant inverse association while the others were unable to statistically confirm any relationship at all. Among four prospective studies that related estimated dietary vitamin E intake to stomach cancer risk, only one— conducted among Finnish smokers (Nouraie et al, 2005)—showed a significantly reduced risk of noncardia stomach cancer among individuals with the highest intake. This study also noted an increased risk for cancer of the gastric cardia. The other three (Chyou et al, 1990; Zheng et al, 1995; Botterweck et al, 2000) found no association.

Six prospective studies that proceeded from predisease blood levels of tocopherols yielded mixed results; a recent large European study reported a strong and statistically significant inverse relationship with stomach cancer risk, albeit seemingly limited to the diffuse histologic type (Jenab et al, 2006a), while a Chinese study showed a positive association with noncardia cancer risk but no relationship with cardia cancer (Taylor et al, 2003). The other four could not confirm any association (Stahelin et al,

1991; Nomura et al, 1995; Yuan et al, 2004; Ito et al, 2005). Thus, the effect of vitamin E on risk of stomach cancer remains uncertain.

Vitamin A. At least 15 case-control studies have addressed the relationship between intake of total vitamin A (retinol and provitamin A carotenoids) and risk of stomach cancer and the overwhelming majority of them have shown a trend toward an inverse association, statistically significant in five of these. Of 12 case-controls studies that specifically examined retinol, mainly present in foods of animal origin, most reported either a null finding or a trend toward a positive association. Three prospective studies have related estimated dietary intake of retinol to stomach cancer risk; two found a nonsignificant trend toward an inverse association (Zheng et al, 1995; Nouraie et al, 2005) (in one study this trend was significant for cardia cancer [Nouraie et al, 2005]); while one suggested a positive association (Botterweck et al, 2000). The pooled estimate in a meta-analysis was nonsignificant (relative risk among subjects with the highest intake compared to those with the lowest was 0.77, 95% confidence interval 0.48–1.22) (Larsson, 2006).

Among seven prospective studies that investigated stomach cancer risk in relation to predisease blood levels of retinol, all but two found indications suggestive of an inverse relationship (Stahelin et al, 1991; Abnet et al, 2003; Yuan et al, 2004; Nouraie et al, 2005; Jenab et al, 2006a), but only two yielded statistically significant results (Stahelin et al, 1991; Jenab et al, 2006a). The summary estimate of relative risk (highest versus lowest category) in these seven studies was 0.80 (95% confidence interval 0.66–0.96) (Larsson, 2006).

With regard to β-carotene intake (provitamin A, mainly coming from plant foods and with additional antioxidative actions), case-control studies have generally shown statistically significant inverse associations with stomach cancer risk, or at least nonsignificant trends toward such inverse associations, but the prospective studies have been less persuasive. The summary estimate of relative risk related to dietary intake in prospective studies was 1.00 (95% confidence interval 0.64–1.56) and for predisease blood levels 0.77 (95% confidence interval 0.54–1.10) (Larsson, 2006).

Intervention trials. Unfortunately, not even randomized intervention trials have been able to provide an unambiguous answer regarding the protective effect of the antioxidative vitamins in plant foods. Two such studies argue in favor of a protective effect; a Chinese study, performed in subjects who were likely to be vitamin deficient, showed a reduced incidence of gastric cancer mortality after administration of a combination of β-carotene, vitamin E, and selenium (Blot et al, 1993). In the other study, carried out in South America (Correa et al, 2000), treatment with either β-carotene or ascorbic acid significantly increased the rates of regression of atrophic gastritis and intestinal metaplasia. A third randomized, double-blind, placebo-controlled trial from China was unable to statistically verify any beneficial effects of β-carotene on cancer incidence or progression of precancerous changes in the gastric mucosa but reported a significantly reduced incidence of all gastrointestinal cancers combined, and more reversions of gastric dysplasia, with folic acid in combination with vitamin B_{12} (Zhu et al, 2003).

Two other randomized intervention studies, conducted among Finnish male smokers (Malila et al, 2002; Virtamo et al, 2003) and American male physicians (Hennekens et al, 1996), respectively, showed no reduction in stomach cancer incidence during or after supplementation with either β-carotene or α-tocopherol, the most active form of vitamin E. Moreover, two additional randomized Chinese intervention studies did not observe any significant reductions in stomach cancer incidence or mortality after daily supplementation with 14 vitamins and 12 minerals for 6 years (Li et al, 1993; Dawsey et al, 1994) or in the prevalence of precancerous gastric lesions by a combination of vitamin C, vi-

tamin E, and selenium every second day for 7.3 years (You et al, 2006). A similar lack of effect on precancerous gastric lesions by treatment with a combination of vitamin C, vitamin E, and β-carotene was reported from a randomized, double-blind chemoprevention trial in a Venezuelan high-risk population (Plummer et al, 2007).

Other plant foods. Chili pepper, although generally rich in antioxidative vitamins, has been linked to a moderately increased stomach cancer risk, allegedly due to its capsaicin content (Lopez-Carrillo et al, 2003). Soyfoods, rich in presumably anticarcinogenic isoflavones, were found to confer protection according to several studies and a meta-analysis (Wu et al, 2000; Nagata et al, 2002), but appeared to act as a moderately strong risk factor (26% increased odds ratio according to the pooled analysis) when the product was fermented (Wu et al, 2000). Possible confounding from salt, fruit/vegetables, and other dietary factors precludes confident causal inference, though.

Dietary fibers

Several investigators have found a decreased risk of stomach cancer among people with a high consumption of fiber. A particularly strong inverse association has been demonstrated between cereal fiber intake and risk of cardia cancer (Terry et al, 2001), possibly attributable to the nitrite scavenging properties of wheat fiber. However, the only prospective study addressing the relationship between intake of whole-grain foods and stomach cancer mortality was negative (McCullough et al, 2001). High-starch/carbohydrate diets, on the other hand, were reportedly linked to an increased risk of stomach cancer in some studies, but others showed no association. It is conceivable that residual confounding by socioeconomic status explains the association noted in the positive studies.

Salt

Most textbooks list salt intake as an established risk factor for stomach cancer.

Ecological studies provide support for a relatively strong correlation between urinary salt excretion and stomach cancer mortality (Joossens et al, 1996; Kono and Hirohata, 1996; Tsugane, 2005). Further, there are abundant case-control and cohort data on intake of salt or salty foods and risk of stomach cancer. Although the results are somewhat divergent, the bulk of evidence weighs toward a positive association, albeit not particularly strong. However, confounding is a major concern; in some of the studied populations, consumption of salted foods may have correlated inversely with socioeconomic status, access to refrigeration, consumption of fruits and vegetables, and positively with the prevalence of *H. pylori* infection. Moreover, salted foods tend to contain significant amounts of N-nitroso compounds (NOCs), which may be the true culprits. The relative risk estimates in cohort and case-control studies are mostly in the range where undetected confounding might well explain the association. It should also be noted that there is no laboratory evidence that salt per se is a carcinogen for any site of the body (Cohen and Roe, 1997).

N-nitroso compounds

N-nitroso compounds (NOCs) have been found to be carcinogenic in multiple organs in at least 40 animal species. Humans are exposed to NOCs from diet (processed meats, smoked preserved foods, pickled and salty preserved foods, and foods dried at high temperatures such as the constituents of beer, whisky, and dried milk), tobacco smoke, and other environmental sources. But a large proportion of NOCs (typically more than 50%) comes from endogenous synthesis. Of 11 case-control studies addressing the possible association between estimated nitrite exposure and stomach cancer risk, 7 showed relative risks (highest versus lowest exposure category) above 1 (range 1.2 to 1.7), and the risk elevations were statistically significant in 5. The two available prospective studies showed effects in opposite directions, but none of the estimates were statistically significant (Van Loon et al, 1998a; Knekt et al, 1999).

All but one of six case-control studies that estimated NOC intake in relation to stomach cancer reported relative risks above 1 (range 1.1–7.0), and three of them yielded statistically significant results. Of three prospective studies that estimated NOC intake, two were negative (Knekt et al, 1999; Jakszyn et al, 2006), while a recent Swedish prospective study among women showed a positive association (relative risk among highest versus lowest exposure category 1.96, 95% confidence interval 1.08–3.58) (Larsson et al, 2006a).

Proceeding from the estimated intake of iron from meat, an index for endogenous NOC exposure was determined for each participant in the European prospective EPIC study (Jakszyn et al, 2006); when this measure was modeled with stomach cancer occurrence as the outcome, a statistically significant association emerged with noncardia stomach cancer (relative risk associated with a 40μg/day increase in endogenous NOC exposure was 1.42, 95% confidence interval 1.14–1.78) but not with cardia cancer. Thus, the epidemiological literature has been unable to unequivocally confirm a link between nitrite or NOC exposure and risk of gastric cancer, but the data are clearly suggestive of such a link.

Meat intake

Whilst meat consumption has been associated with increased risks of cancer of the colorectum, the epidemiologic evidence for a relationship with stomach cancer risk has so far been considered insufficient. However, recent cohort studies have reported up to twofold risk elevations among subjects in the highest intake categories, relative to those in the lowest (Ngoan et al, 2002; Van Den Brandt et al, 2003; Gonzalez et al, 2006a; Larsson et al, 2006a). These and other studies were included in a meta-analysis that encompassed six prospective cohort studies and nine case-control studies (Larsson et al, 2006d). The estimated summary relative risks of stomach cancer for an increase in processed meat consumption of 30 g/day, approximately half of an average serving, were 1.15 (95% confidence interval

1.04–1.27) for the cohort studies and 1.38 (95% confidence interval 1.19–1.60) for the case-control studies.

In three cohort and four case-control studies that examined the association between bacon consumption and stomach cancer, the summary relative risk was 1.37 (95% confidence interval 1.17–1.61) for highest versus lowest intake. Thus, it appears that high intake of processed meat should be added to the list of known—but moderately strong—risk factors for stomach cancer. In the European EPIC cohort, the association with processed meat was confined to noncardia stomach cancer; for every 50 grams per day increase in processed meat intake, the noncardia stomach cancer risk increased 2.45-fold (95% confidence interval 1.43–4.21) (Gonzalez et al, 2006a). Positive associations were also noted for nonprocessed meat, with significant 3.52- and 1.73-fold increases in noncardia stomach cancer risk per 50 grams/day increase in total meat and red-meat consumption, respectively. Since the results from previous epidemiological studies have been mixed, the relationships with red-meat and total-meat intake need to be further explored before they are accepted as causal.

Total energy and fat

There is no consistent data regarding the relationship between total energy intake and the risk of stomach cancer. A weak positive association has been noted for recent total intake, as well as an inverse association for total energy intake during adolescence.

Fat intake has been positively linked to risk. The excess risk was in some instances confined to persons consuming large amounts of animal fat or saturated lipids and cholesterol, whereas those on a diet rich in vegetable lipids or polyunsaturated lipids had an up to 70% reduced risk. One can only speculate about the extent to which residual confounding from fruit and vegetable intake might have contributed to these findings.

Trace elements

Selenium appears to have the potential for inhibiting the development of several tumors,

but its intake is impossible to assess through dietary questionnaires in epidemiologic studies since the selenium content of a specific food depends on the selenium content of the soil where it was produced. Toenail selenium levels were inversely associated with stomach cancer risk in a Dutch prospective study. Four prospective studies using determinations of serum levels of selenium reached different conclusions; one reported an inverse association (Knekt et al, 1990) while others found no relationship (e.g., [You et al, 2000]). The possible link to calcium intake has been addressed in a few studies. Their conflicting results are most likely an indication of no overall association.

Frying/grilling

Heterocyclic amines formed when fish or meat is fried are mutagenic in experimental studies (IARC, 1993). Polycyclic aromatic hydrocarbons (PAHs) are formed during incomplete combustion of organic material, for instance when food is smoked or fried over an open fire. Many PAHs are regarded as carcinogenic to humans. Some investigators, but not all, found a link between high consumption of hard-fried food and the risk of stomach cancer. In a case-control study from Uruguay, the subjects most exposed to 2-amino-1-methyl-6-phenylimidazo(4,5-b)pyridine had an almost fourfold increased risk of stomach cancer compared to those in the lowest exposure category (De Stefani et al, 1998). The effect of this heterocyclic amine interacted with the effect of nitrosodimethylamine in a multiplicative manner, yielding an almost 13-fold increased risk among persons highly exposed to both substances. However, studies addressing the relationship between exposure to PAH and gastric cancer risk have been negative, with one exception. Interpretation is complicated by the fact that grilling over an open fire seems to be closely linked to a high intake of fruits and vegetables in western settings.

Pickled food

Studies from China, Japan, Hawaii, and Spain reported an increased risk of gastric and/or cardia cancer among frequent consumers of pickled food. Extracts from pickled vegetables in China have been shown to be mutagenic and contain N-nitroso compounds and benzopyrenes.

Aspirin and Nonsteroidal Anti-Inflammatory Drugs (NSAIDs)

Several epidemiological studies have noted small reductions in risk of stomach cancer among users of aspirin and/or NSAIDs. A meta-analysis of eight case-control studies yielded a summary estimate of relative risk that indicated a statistically significant 22% risk reduction (Wang et al, 2003). Although some prospective studies have supported an inverse association (Thun et al, 1993; Lindblad et al, 2005), others did not (Friis et al, 2003). More importantly, a randomized trial among 40 000 US women suggests that low-dose aspirin use may not lower the risk of stomach cancer (Cook et al, 2005).

Infections

Helicobacter pylori

In the past 15 years, numerous observational studies of various designs have demonstrated a positive association between presence of anti-*H. pylori* antibodies and risk of stomach cancer. A recent review of published meta-analyses (Eslick, 2006) showed that serological evidence of *H. pylori* infection is associated with pooled odds ratios of stomach cancer ranging between 1.92 and 2.56, with little heterogeneity. In other words, carriers of antibodies to *H. pylori* allegedly run a risk for stomach cancer that is two to three times higher than among people without such antibodies. Already in 1994, the International Agency for Research on Cancer concluded that the evidence was sufficient that *H. pylori* causes stomach cancer and the microorganism was classified as a human carcinogen class I according to the established protocol (IARC, 1994).

However, because some infections disappear spontaneously due to changes in the gastric micro-environment during the precancerous stages, the strength of the association with stomach cancer risk may be underestimated (Maeda et al, 2000; Ekstrom et al, 2001). Moreover, it appears that the association is confined to noncardia gastric cancer, whereas the infection might even be inversely related to the risk of cardia cancer (Hansen et al, 1999; Kamangar, Dawsey et al, 2006). The lack of uniformity in the anatomic subsite definitions makes available data difficult to interpret, though, and the combined data suggest a small excess risk of 23% to 54% (Huang et al, 1998; Eslick et al, 1999).

In studies that restricted the outcome to noncardia stomach cancer and that took measures to overcome the misclassification of exposure due to spontaneous disappearance of the microorganism (Fig. 10–6), the relative risk linked to the infection was 20-fold or more (Ekstrom et al, 2001; Uemura et al, 2001; Brenner et al, 2004). According to such studies, the PAR may be 70% or higher even in Western populations (Ekstrom et al, 2001), while an American case-control study with conventional serotesting reported a PAR of only 10.4% (Engel et al, 2003).

The risk is similarly elevated for both the intestinal and diffuse histological types of stomach cancer, but it seems to be particularly high among carriers of CagA-positive strains (and among carriers of CagA-positive strains in those with strains having the 'A-B-D-type' CagA typically seen in Asian high-risk populations [Hatakeyama, 2004]), although CagA-negative strains are not without risk (Held et al, 2004). The *vacA* gene of *H. pylori*, encoding a vacuolating cytotoxin, comprises two variable regions: the s (signalling) and the m (mid) regions. *H. pylori* vacA type s1 and m1 strains appear to be more carcinogenic than strains with other vacA types (Figueiredo et al, 2002).

Although the ultimate proof of causality is still missing, a growing number of randomized trials have either shown trends toward reduced gastric cancer incidence or indications of slowing progression of precancerous lesions after *H. pylori* eradication (Correa et al, 2000; Sung et al, 2000; Leung et al, 2004; Wong et al, 2004; Mera et al,

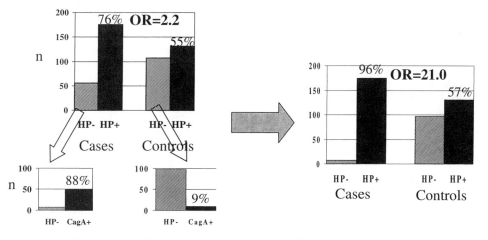

Figure 10–6. With conventional IgG ELISA serology, the odds ratio associated with *Helicobacter pylori (HP)* infection in a Swedish population-based case-control study was an unimpressive 2.2 (upper left panel). A large proportion of the seronegative cases, however, had antibodies to CagA as evidence of a previous infection (lower left panel). When the latter subjects were re-classified as *H. pylori* positive, the odds ratio rose to 21.0 (right hand panel). (Adapted from Ekström et al, 2001)

2005; You et al, 2006), thus gradually adding to our confidence in a causal inference.

The proposed mechanisms behind the putative carcinogenicity of *H. pylori* include *(1)* an intense inflammatory response with increased production of proinflammatory cytokines (tumor necrosis factor alpha [TNF-α], IL-1β, IL-6, IL-8, and IL-12) and secondary attraction and activation of macrophages and polymorphonuclear cells, with degranulation and production of mutagenic superoxide radicals; *(2)* induction of inducible nitric oxide synthase (iNOS) and proinflammatory cyclooxygenase (particularly COX-2) enzymes, resulting in release of reactive, mutagenic substances and possible alterations in epithelial cell growth; *(3)* increased cell proliferation, possibly due to the activation of the proto-oncogene *c-fos*, reduced expression of the cell-cycle regulatory protein p27, and CCK-β receptor activation; *(4)* decreased secretion of vitamin C into the gastric lumen, leading to a poorer inhibition of the mutagenicity of preformed N-nitroso compounds and deficient scavenging of reactive oxygen metabolites, nitrite ions, nitric oxide, and other free radicals; *(5)* development of atrophic gastritis, with decreased production of hydrochloric acid and entailing colonization of bacterial species that catalyze the nitrosation of dietary amines and amides to form carcinogenic N-nitroso compounds (unopposed by vitamin C); *(6)* altered mucus production and reduced mucosal blood flow, resulting in abnormal gastric surface permeability; *(7)* an upward expansion of the proliferative zone, paving the way for greater carcinogen penetration to the stem cells; *(8)* presence of larger pool of cells in S-phase, sensitive to mutation; *(9)* increased likelihood that mutations escape DNA repair and become fixed in progeny cells due to the increased cell turnover; *(10)* possible inhibition of the transcription of epithelial DNA repair genes; and *(11)* inhibition of apoptosis. Strains that are cagA-positive and harbor the *vacA* s1a m1 genotype stimulate mucosal cell proliferation in the host while simultaneously inhibiting apoptosis. The resulting hyperproliferation, not balanced by cell death, may contribute to malignant transformation.

It appears that mechanisms that potentially can be blocked by antioxidants play a quantitatively important role. The production of reactive oxygen metabolites in the gastric mucosa following *H. pylori* infection is well substantiated (Farinati et al, 1998). An inverse relation between the serum level of ascorbic acid and the risk of progression to mucosal dysplasia or gastric cancer was noted in a cohort study (You et al, 2000). In a population-based case-control study (Ekstrom et al, 2001), the association between *H. pylori* infection and the risk of non-cardia gastric cancer was significantly modified by ascorbic acid intake, so that the risk gradient was considerably steeper among subjects with a low intake of ascorbic acid compared to those with a high intake.

Experimental data in a mouse model demonstrated that treatment with the antioxidant astaxanthin reduces gastric inflammation and causes a shift of the T-lymphocyte response from a predominant Th1 response dominated by interferon-γ to a mixed Th1/Th2 response with interferon-γ and IL-4 (Bennedsen et al, 1999). Most persuasive is a report from a randomized chemoprevention trial in Colombia (Correa et al, 2000), in which treatment with β-carotene or ascorbic acid significantly increased the rates of regression of *H. pylori*–associated atrophy and intestinal metaplasia.

Helicobacter pylori infection appears to be the strongest and most important risk factor for noncardia gastric cancer now identified. Proceeding from the latest Swedish data, it was estimated that 71% of all noncardia adenocarcinomas occurring in the general Swedish population were attributable to *H. pylori* (Ekstrom et al, 2001). The sizeable risk associated with *H. pylori* infection was clearly demonstrated in a recent Japanese cohort study, in which 2.9% of 1 246 infected individuals developed gastric cancer during 7.8 years of follow-up, while no cancer was observed among 280 noninfected cohort members (Uemura et al, 2001).

Results from ongoing randomized intervention studies with cancer as the endpoint are critical both for causal inference and for future prevention strategies. Meanwhile, a number of intriguing questions need to be addressed: Why is the incidence of gastric cancer twice as high in men as in women when the prevalence of the infection is similar in both genders? This gender difference has not been explained by known risk factors. Further, why is the risk of gastric cancer in duodenal ulcer patients 40% lower than that in the general population (Hansson et al, 1996) despite an infection prevalence of almost 100% among the former? It appears that characteristics of the infecting strain or the host, or factors in the environment, or a combination thereof might radically modify the carcinogenicity of *H. pylori*.

Physical Activity

The relationship between physical activity and the risk of gastric cancer has been addressed in few studies. An analysis including 16 cohorts from seven countries revealed that adherence to the European Code Against Cancer recommendations regarding physical activity was associated with increased stomach cancer mortality (Ocke et al, 1998). Other studies, however, were negative (Dosemeci et al, 1993; Nomura et al, 1995). A recent US case-control study found no significant association between cardia or distal stomach cancer and an occupational activity index based on lifetime occupational histories and a simple job exposure matrix classifying jobs as sedentary, or moderately or highly physically active (Vigen et al, 2006). A nonsignificant trend toward risk reduction by 23% to 24% (highest activity level toward lowest) was, however, noted for both cardia and noncardia stomach cancer when the investigators used the average index before age 65 years as measure of exposure. With reservation for considerable misclassification due to imperfect instruments for exposure assessment, the combined data weigh against the possibility of an important association between physical activity and gastric cancer risk.

Ionizing Radiation

Among atomic bomb survivors in Hiroshima, Japan, the standardized mortality ratio for stomach cancer rose steadily with increasing radiation dose (Nakamura, 1977). The same pattern was seen in patients treated with x-rays for ankylosing spondylitis (Brown and Doll, 1965). Persons exposed to radiation at younger ages were reported to have a higher risk of stomach cancer, as were nonuranium miners exposed to α-emissions from radon daughters (Darby et al, 1995) and female radium dial workers (Stebbings et al, 1984). Although based on small numbers of observed cases, the consistency of the findings strongly suggests that the risk of gastric cancer increases with exposure to ionizing radiation.

Occupation

Small numbers and/or considerable heterogeneity with regard to factual exposure typically hamper the interpretation of data on site-specific cancer risks from occupational studies. Because the large literature on occupational exposures and gastric cancer risk is not strikingly consistent, the data need cautious interpretation. Occupations commonly associated with an increased risk of gastric cancer include work in dusty industries such as foundry, steel, and mining (Cocco et al, 1996; Ji and Hemminki, 2006). The reasoning is that when dust is inhaled, the particles are cleared from the lungs by the mucociliary system and swallowed. The majority of studies concerned with exposure to mineral and metal dusts have been positive (Cocco et al, 1996; Ekstrom et al, 1999a; Aragones et al, 2002; Ji and Hemminki, 2006). The evidence also weighs in favor of an increased gastric cancer risk among coal miners (Cocco et al, 1996), but several careful studies failed to observe any important association (Swaen et al, 1985; Weinberg et al, 1985; Coggon et al, 1990). If a true association exists, it is unclear which substance accounts for the observed excess.

The overall evidence of associations between exposure to asbestos or silica and stomach cancer risk is deemed to be uncertain (Cocco et al, 1996). A recent study among Swedish construction workers found exposure to quartz dust—but not asbestos—to be significantly and dose-dependently related to stomach cancer risk (Sjodahl et al, 2007), albeit with moderate strength (relative risk 1.3 in highest exposure tertile relative to lowest). An increased risk of stomach cancer among workers exposed to wood dust has often been noted (eg, Robinson et al, 1996; Jansson et al, 2005), but the findings across occupations are inconsistent, and support from exposure–response analyses is lacking. Textile dust has been implicated by some investigators (Simpson et al, 1999), while others found no association between textile work and stomach cancer risk (Aragones et al, 2002; Weiderpass et al, 2003; Ji and Hemminki, 2006; Wernli et al, 2006).

A small excess of stomach cancer was revealed in a large meta-analysis of studies concerned with cancer risks among farmers (Blair et al, 1992). The reasons for this excess remain to be clarified, but exposure to pesticides/herbicides and fertilizers has been specifically evaluated. Self-reported pesticide exposure was a moderately strong (odds ratio 2.1) risk factor for cardia cancer in a Swedish population-based case-control study (Jansson et al, 2006). Large studies among farmers and others with professional exposure to pesticides did not reveal any excess incidence or mortality of stomach cancer, though (Lee et al, 2004; Alavanja et al, 2005; Blair et al, 2005). Although a link to phenoxy acids has been suggested, the epidemiologic evidence for a causal association between chlorophenols and gastric cancer risk is weak (Cocco et al, 1996). A 70% excess risk among subjects exposed to phenoxyacetic acids was revealed in one study with detailed exposure assessment and control for potential confounding (Ekstrom et al, 1999a), but there was no clear trend with increasing duration of the exposure. Reports on fertilizers and gastric cancer risk were considered to be inconclusive (Cocco et al, 1996).

Exposure to preformed nitrosamines has been a concern in agriculture, the rubber industry, and foundries, as well as in the metal, leather, and chemical industries.

Excess cases of gastric cancer have been observed in several studies, notably among workers in the rubber industry, where the epidemiologic evidence is considered more consistent.

Exposure to diesel exhausts among construction workers (Sjodahl et al, 2007), motor vehicle operators, transport workers, or gas station workers (Aragones et al, 2002; Engel et al, 2002; Ji and Hemminki, 2006) has been shown with some consistency to be linked to an increased risk of stomach cancer. Although potentially carcinogenic polycyclic aromatic hydrocarbons and combustion particles might be involved, the causality remains uncertain.

An increased risk of gastric cancer was observed for workers in oil refineries, but work in the petroleum industry overall did not show an excess risk in a meta-analysis (Cocco et al, 1996). There is suggestive evidence that grinding operations, which can entail either mineral oil–based or ethanolamine-based oils, are associated with an excess risk of cancer of the esophagus, stomach, and pancreas (Tolbert, 1997). An excess gastric cancer risk also has been seen among workers exposed to sulfites and sulfates in the pulping process of the paper industry (Milham and Demers, 1984; Rix et al, 1997). A decreased risk, however, was reported among sulfite mill workers (Andersson et al, 1998).

Medical Conditions and Treatment

Peptic ulcer

Although gastric cancer and peptic ulcer share the same dominating risk factor, namely H. pylori infection, which could be considered to be close to a necessary cause of both diseases, all peptic ulcer patients do not have an increased risk of gastric cancer. A large retrospective cohort study among unoperated peptic ulcer patients hospitalized in Sweden from 1965 and onward revealed—as expected—an approximately twofold risk elevation among gastric ulcer patients, relative to the age, sex, and calendar period-matched Swedish general population (Hansson et al, 1996). Unoperated patients hospitalized for duodenal ulcer, on the other

hand, had a risk that was almost halved, despite a close to 100% H. pylori infection rate. A subsequent follow-up of the same cohort showed that this risk reduction pertained to noncardia gastric cancer only, while the risk of cardia cancer was close to, or slightly above, expectation (Bahmanyar et al, 2007). In contrast, the risk elevation linked to gastric ulcer was similar for both cardia and noncardia gastric cancer.

Gastric ulcer is associated with H. pylori colonization of both the lowermost part of the stomach (antrum) and the middle-upper part (corpus), where the hydrochloric acid is produced. This leads to corpus-predominant gastritis, and a tendency toward atrophy with decreased acid production, similar to the intragastric milieu in cases with stomach cancer. Conversely, duodenal ulcer is associated with H. pylori clonization exclusively in the antrum, where the gastric acidity is monitored and regulated. The antrum-predominant gastritis, therefore, is linked to a less efficient control of acid production and a tendency toward hyperacidity. It is hypothesized that the acididy in some way contributes to the apparent protection against noncardia stomach cancer, possibly through prevention of superinfection by other microorganisms.

Partial gastrectomy

Partial gastrectomy, but not vagotomy alone, is followed by an increased risk of gastric cancer. Probably due to the reduction in the amount of tissue at risk, the excess becomes apparent only after prolonged follow-up. But according to the largest cohort study published on the subject (Lundegardh et al, 1988), the risk increased by 28% for each successive 5-year interval after surgery. Moreover, Billroth II reconstructions, and operations performed for gastric rather than for duodenal ulcer, conferred a higher risk. The relative excess appears greater in women than in men. Meta-analyses of all published studies concerning partial gastrectomy and the risk of gastric cancer show significantly elevated risks following both Billroth I and Billroth II reconstructions, but only 15 years or more after the operation. The risk was even greater if a vagotomy had been added to the procedure (Tersmette et al, 1990).

A recent retrospective cohort study among all patients hospitalized for peptic ulcer in Sweden since 1965 (Bahmanyar et al, 2007) has added significant insights though; when compared to their unoperated peers, surgically resected duodenal ulcer patients had a significant 60% increased risk of noncardia gastric cancer in the long term following the operation. This meant that their advantage (as unoperated) relative to the general population (see previous) was reduced, albeit not entirely cancelled (SIR among unoperated duodenal ulcer patients = 0.5; SIR among resected ones = 0.8).

In contrast, patients who underwent gastric resection due to gastric ulcer, with an elevated baseline risk relative to the general population, experienced a risk reduction. In comparison with their unoperated gastric ulcer peers, the risk reduction was 40% (95% confidence interval 20%–50%). This changed the SIR, ie, the relative risk in relation to the general Swedish population, from 2.1 among the unoperated gastric ulcer patients to 1.2 among the operated. Thus it appears that following surgical intervention stomach cancer risks are shifted towrd normality, regardless of underlying ulcer type.

Acid inhibition

After the introduction of cimetidine—a potent H_2-receptor antagonist used for treatment of peptic ulcer—several gastroenterologists voiced the concern that the acid inhibition might lead to bacterial overgrowth, formation of N-nitroso compounds, growth stimulation by increased gastrin levels, and ultimately to the development of gastric cancer. Therefore, cancer risks among patients treated with H_2-receptor antagonists have been closely monitored. All studies, regardless of their design, have been reassuringly negative (eg, Johnson et al, 1996). A reverse causation arose because, in some patients, these drugs were prescribed for symptoms emanating from a yet-undiagnosed gastric cancer, and

an excessive incidence of gastric cancer was invariably observed during the first years after the start of treatment. But with longer follow-up, the relative risk estimates fell to unity (Moller et al, 1992). It is tempting to generalize these findings to the even more potent proton-pump inhibitors. However, indications of a more rapid development of atrophy when the drug was administered to *H. pylori*–infected subjects, and alterations in the gastric milieu favoring bacterial N-nitrosation (Kuipers et al, 1996; Mowat et al, 2000), are concerns.

Other Risk Factors

Although the biological correlates are yet to be determined, socioeconomic status has been a strong risk indicator for gastric cancer in epidemiologic studies. Generally, people who have low education and/or are economically underprivileged have at least a twofold higher risk than persons who are better off (Hansson et al, 1994; Brown et al, 1998; Van Loon et al, 1998b; Ji and Hemminki, 2006). The risk gradient across socioeconomic strata has never been fully explained. It is conceivable that occupational and dietary factors may play a role. Crowding during childhood due to poor living conditions and the presence of many siblings may increase the risk of transmission of *H. pylori*. Family size and birth order have also been positively associated with the risk of gastric cancer (Hansson et al, 1994; Blaser et al, 1995).

CONCLUSION

Efforts to improve the treatment of stomach cancer, the second most common cause of cancer death worldwide, have had limited success. In contrast, considerable knowledge about potentially causal factors has been gathered during the past few decades, and primary prevention no longer appears to be an unattainable goal. *Helicobacter pylori*, the strongest and most important risk factor, is likely to become the first target in future prevention strategies. A deeper understanding of effect-modifying factors or circumstances in the microorganism, in the host, and/or in the environment may help us to design precisely targeted interventions.

Dietary factors, particularly the intake of antioxidant-rich fruits and vegetables, are likely to be important, albeit perhaps somewhat overrated in older case-control data. Interesting interactions with *H. pylori* have been observed. New insights in bacterial and human genetics may enable us to focus even more precisely on the relevant high-risk groups. They may also allow selective prevention of infections predestined to trigger the carcinogenic process. To achieve these goals, epidemiologists, gastroenterologists, pathologists, tumor biologists, microbiologists, geneticists, and biochemists need to join forces in a coordinated effort.

REFERENCES

Aarnio M, Salovaara R, Aaltonen LA, Mecklin JP, Jarvinen HJ. Features of gastric cancer in hereditary non-polyposis colorectal cancer syndrome. Int J Cancer 1997;74:551–55.

Abnet CC, Qiao YL, Dawsey SM, Buckman DW, Yang CS, Blot WJ, et al. Prospective study of serum retinol, beta-carotene, beta-cryptoxanthin, and lutein/zeaxanthin and esophageal and gastric cancers in China. Cancer Causes Control 2003;14:645–55.

Agudo A, Sala N, Pera G, Capella G, Berenguer A, Garcia N, et al. Polymorphisms in metabolic genes related to tobacco smoke and the risk of gastric cancer in the European prospective investigation into cancer and nutrition. Cancer Epidemiol Biomarkers Prev 2006a;15:2427–34.

Agudo A, Sala N, Pera G, Capella G, Berenguer A, Garcia N, et al. No association between polymorphisms in CYP2E1, GSTM1, NAT1, NAT2 and the risk of gastric adenocarcinoma in the European prospective investigation into cancer and nutrition. Cancer Epidemiol Biomarkers Prev 2006b;15:1043–45.

Ahlbom A, Lichtenstein P, Malmstrom H, Feychting M, Hemminki K, Pedersen NL. Cancer in twins: genetic and nongenetic familial risk factors. J Natl Cancer Inst 1997; 89:287–93.

Alavanja MC, Sandler DP, Lynch CF, Knott C, Lubin JH, Tarone R, et al. Cancer incidence in the agricultural health study. Scand J Work Environ Health 2005;31 Suppl 1:39–45; discussion 5–7.

American Cancer Society. Cancer Facts and Figures 2006. Atlanta, American Cancer Society, 2006.

Andersson E, Nilsson T, Persson B, Wingren G, Toren K. Mortality from asthma and cancer among sulfite mill workers. Scand J Work Environ Health 1998;24:12–17.

Aragones N, Pollan M, Lopez-Abente G, Ruiz M, Vergara A, Moreno C, et al. Time trend and age-period-cohort effects on gastric cancer incidence in Zaragoza and Navarre, Spain. J Epidemiol Community Health 1997;51: 412–17.

Aragones N, Pollan M, Gustavsson P. Stomach cancer and occupation in Sweden: 1971–89. Occup Environ Med 2002;59:329–37.

Azuma T, Ito S, Sato F, Yamazaki Y, Miyaji H, Ito Y, et al. The role of the HLA-DQA1 gene in resistance to atrophic gastritis and gastric adenocarcinoma induced by Helicobacter pylori infection. Cancer 1998;82:1013–18.

Bagnardi V, Blangiardo M, La Vecchia C, Corrao G. A meta-analysis of alcohol drinking and cancer risk. Br J Cancer 2001;85:1700–5.

Bahmanyar S, Ye W, Dickman PW, Nyren O. Long-term risk of gastric cancer by subsite in operated and unoperated patients hospitalized for peptic ulcer. Am J Gastroenterol 2007;102:1185–91.

Barstad B, Sorensen TI, Tjonneland A, Johansen D, Becker U, Andersen IB, et al. Intake of wine, beer and spirits and risk of gastric cancer. Eur J Cancer Prev 2005;14:239–43.

Bennedsen M, Wang X, Willen R, Wadstrom T, Andersen LP. Treatment of H. pylori infected mice with antioxidant astaxanthin reduces gastric inflammation, bacterial load and modulates cytokine release by splenocytes. Immunol Lett 1999;70:185–89.

Blair A, Zahm SH, Pearce NE, Heineman EF, Fraumeni JF. Clues to cancer etiology from studies of farmers. Scand J Work Environ Health 1992;18:209–15.

Blair A, Sandler DP, Tarone R, Lubin J, Thomas K, Hoppin JA, et al. Mortality among participants in the agricultural health study. Ann Epidemiol 2005;15:279–85.

Blaser MJ, Chyou PH, Nomura A. Age at establishment of Helicobacter pylori infection and gastric carcinoma, gastric ulcer, and duodenal ulcer risk. Cancer Res 1995;55:562–65.

Blot WJ, Devesa S, Kneller R, Fraumeni JJ. Rising incidence of adenocarcinoma of the esophagus and gastric cardia. JAMA 1991; 265:1287–89.

Blot WJ, Li JY, Taylor PR, Guo W, Dawsey S, Wang GQ, et al. Nutrition intervention trials in Linxian, China: supplementation with specific vitamin/mineral combinations, cancer incidence, and disease-specific mortality in the general population. J Natl Cancer Inst 1993;85:1483–92.

Boccia S, De Lauretis A, Gianfagna F, van Duijn CM, Ricciardi G. CYP2E1PstI/RsaI polymorphism and interaction with tobacco, alcohol and GSTs in gastric cancer susceptibility: A meta-analysis of the literature. Carcinogenesis 2007;28:101–6.

Boissy RJ, Watson MA, Umbach DM, Deakin M, Elder J, Strange RC, et al. A pilot study investigating the role of NAT1 and NAT2 polymorphisms in gastric adenocarcinoma. Int J Cancer 2000;87:507–11.

Botterweck AA, van den Brandt PA, Goldbohm RA. Vitamins, carotenoids, dietary fiber, and the risk of gastric carcinoma: results from a prospective study after 6.3 years of follow-up. Cancer 2000;88:737–48.

Brenner H, Arndt V, Bode G, Stegmaier C, Ziegler H, Stumer T. Risk of gastric cancer among smokers infected with Helicobacter pylori. Int J Cancer 2002;98:446–49.

Brenner H, Arndt V, Stegmaier C, Ziegler H, Rothenbacher D. Is Helicobacter pylori infection a necessary condition for noncardia gastric cancer? Am J Epidemiol 2004;159: 252–58.

Brown J, Harding S, Bethune A, Rosato M. Longitudinal study of socio-economic differences in the incidence of stomach, colorectal and pancreatic cancers. Popul Trends 1998:35–41.

Brown WM, Doll R. Mortality from cancer and other causes after radiotherapy for ankylosing spondylitis. Br Med J 1965;5474:1327–32.

Caldas C, Carneiro F, Lynch HT, Yokota J, Wiesner GL, Powell SM, et al. Familial gastric cancer: overview and guidelines for management. J Med Genet 1999;36:873–80.

Carvalho F, Seruca R, David L, Amorim A, Seixas M, Bennett E, et al. MUC1 gene polymorphism and gastric cancer—an epidemiological study. Glycoconj J 1997;14:107–11.

Chao A, Thun MJ, Henley SJ, Jacobs EJ, McCullough ML, Calle EE. Cigarette smoking, use of other tobacco products and stomach cancer mortality in US adults: The Cancer Prevention Study II. Int J Cancer 2002;101:380–89.

Cho NH, Moy CS, Davis F, Haenszel W, Ahn YO, Kim H. Ethnic variation in the incidence of stomach cancer in Illinois, 1986–1988. Am J Epidemiol 1996;144:661–64.

Chow WH, Swanson CA, Lissowska J, Groves FD, Sobin LH, Nasierowska-Guttmejer A, et al. Risk of stomach cancer in relation to consumption of cigarettes, alcohol, tea and coffee in Warsaw, Poland. Int J Cancer 1999;81:871–76.

Chyou PH, Nomura AM, Hankin JH, Stemmermann GN. A case-cohort study of diet and stomach cancer. Cancer Res 1990;50: 7501–4.

Cocco P, Ward MH, Buiatti E. Occupational risk factors for gastric cancer: an overview. Epidemiol Rev 1996;18:218–34.

Coggon D, Barker DJ, Cole RB. Stomach cancer and work in dusty industries. Br J Ind Med 1990;47:298–301.

Cohen AJ, Roe FJ. Evaluation of the aetiological role of dietary salt exposure in gastric and other cancers in humans. Food Chem Toxicol 1997;35:271–93.

Coleman MP, Esteve J, Damiecki P, Arslan A, Renhard H. Trends in Cancer Incidence and Mortality. Lyon, International Agency for Research on Cancer, 1993.

Cook NR, Lee IM, Gaziano JM, Gordon D, Ridker PM, Manson JE, et al. Low-dose aspirin in the primary prevention of cancer: the Women's Health Study: a randomized controlled trial. Jama 2005;294:47–55.

Correa P, Fontham ET, Bravo JC, Bravo LE, Ruiz B, Zarama G, et al. Chemoprevention of gastric dysplasia: randomized trial of antioxidant supplements and anti-helicobacter pylori therapy. J Natl Cancer Inst 2000;92:1881–88.

Darby SC, Radford EP, Whitley E. Radon exposure and cancers other than lung cancer in Swedish iron miners. Environ Health Perspect 1995;103 Suppl 2:45–47.

Dawsey SM, Wang GQ, Taylor PR, Li JY, Blot WJ, Li B, et al. Effects of vitamin/mineral supplementation on the prevalence of histological dysplasia and early cancer of the esophagus and stomach: results from the Dysplasia Trial in Linxian, China. Cancer Epidemiol Biomarkers Prev 1994;3:167–72.

De Stefani E, Boffetta P, Mendilaharsu M, Carzoglio J, Deneo-Pellegrini H. Dietary nitrosamines, heterocyclic amines, and risk of gastric cancer: a case-control study in Uruguay. Nutr Cancer 1998;30:158–62.

Devesa SS, Silverman DT, Young JL, Jr., Pollack ES, Brown CC, Horm JW, et al. Cancer incidence and mortality trends among whites in the United States, 1947–84. J Natl Cancer Inst 1987;79:701–70.

Devesa SS, Blot WJ, Fraumeni JF, Jr. Changing patterns in the incidence of esophageal and gastric carcinoma in the United States. Cancer 1998;83:2049–53.

Dosemeci M, Hayes RB, Vetter R, Hoover RN, Tucker M, Engin K, et al. Occupational physical activity, socioeconomic status, and risks of 15 cancer sites in Turkey. Cancer Causes Control 1993;4:313–21.

Duarte MC, Colombo J, Rossit AR, Caetano A, Borim AA, Wornrath D, et al. Polymorphisms of DNA repair genes XRCC1 and

XRCC3, interaction with environmental exposure and risk of chronic gastritis and gastric cancer. World J Gastroenterol 2005; 11:6593–600.

Ekstrom AM, Eriksson M, Hansson LE, Lindgren A, Signorello LB, Nyren O, et al. Occupational exposures and risk of gastric cancer in a population-based case-control study. Cancer Res 1999a;59:5932–37.

Ekstrom AM, Signorello LB, Hansson LE, Bergstrom R, Lindgren A, Nyren O. Evaluating gastric cancer misclassification: a potential explanation for the rise in cardia cancer incidence. J Natl Cancer Inst 1999b;91:786–90.

Ekstrom AM, Hansson LE, Signorello LB, Lindgren A, Bergstrom R, Nyren O. Decreasing incidence of both major histologic subtypes of gastric adenocarcinoma—a population-based study in Sweden. Br J Cancer 2000;83:391–96.

Ekstrom AM, Held M, Hansson LE, Engstrand L, Nyren O. Helicobacter pylori in gastric cancer established by CagA immunoblot as a marker of past infection. Gastroenterology 2001;121:784–91.

El-Omar EM, Carrington M, Chow WH, McColl KE, Bream JH, Young HA, et al. Interleukin-1 polymorphisms associated with increased risk of gastric cancer. Nature 2000;404:398–402.

Engel LS, Vaughan TL, Gammon MD, Chow WH, Risch HA, Dubrow R, et al. Occupation and risk of esophageal and gastric cardia adenocarcinoma. Am J Ind Med 2002; 42:11–22.

Engel LS, Chow WH, Vaughan TL, Gammon MD, Risch HA, Stanford JL, et al. Population attributable risks of esophageal and gastric cancers. J Natl Cancer Inst 2003; 95:1404–13.

Eslick GD, Lim LL, Byles JE, Xia HH, Talley NJ. Association of Helicobacter pylori infection with gastric carcinoma: a meta-analysis. Am J Gastroenterol 1999;94:2373–79.

Eslick GD. Helicobacter pylori infection causes gastric cancer? A review of the epidemiological, meta-analytic, and experimental evidence. World J Gastroenterol 2006;12: 2991–99.

Farinati F, Cardin R, Degan P, Rugge M, Mario FD, Bonvicini P, et al. Oxidative DNA damage accumulation in gastric carcinogenesis. Gut 1998;42:351–56.

Figueiredo C, Machado JC, Pharoah P, Seruca R, Sousa S, Carvalho R, et al. Helicobacter pylori and interleukin 1 genotyping: an opportunity to identify high-risk individuals for gastric carcinoma. J Natl Cancer Inst 2002;94:1680–87.

Friis S, Sorensen HT, McLaughlin JK, Johnsen SP, Blot WJ, Olsen JH. A population-based cohort study of the risk of colorectal and other cancers among users of low-dose aspirin. Br J Cancer 2003;88:684–88.

Galanis DJ, Kolonel LN, Lee J, Nomura A. Intakes of selected foods and beverages and the incidence of gastric cancer among the Japanese residents of Hawaii: a prospective study. Int J Epidemiol 1998;27:173–80.

Garcia E, Carvalho F, Amorim A, David L. MUC6 gene polymorphism in healthy individuals and in gastric cancer patients from northern Portugal. Cancer Epidemiol Biomarkers Prev 1997;6:1071–74.

Gayther SA, Gorringe KL, Ramus SJ, Huntsman D, Roviello F, Grehan N, et al. Identification of germ-line E-cadherin mutations in gastric cancer families of European origin. Cancer Res 1998;58:4086–89.

Gonzalez CA, Sala N, Capella G. Genetic susceptibility and gastric cancer risk. Int J Cancer 2002;100:249–60.

Gonzalez CA, Pera G, Agudo A, Palli D, Krogh V, Vineis P, et al. Smoking and the risk of gastric cancer in the European Prospective Investigation Into Cancer and Nutrition (EPIC). Int J Cancer 2003;107:629–34.

Gonzalez CA, Jakszyn P, Pera G, Agudo A, Bingham S, Palli D, et al. Meat intake and risk of stomach and esophageal adenocarcinoma within the European Prospective Investigation Into Cancer and Nutrition (EPIC). J Natl Cancer Inst 2006a;98:345–54.

Gonzalez CA, Pera G, Agudo A, Bueno-de-Mesquita HB, Ceroti M, Boeing H, et al. Fruit and vegetable intake and the risk of stomach and oesophagus adenocarcinoma in the European Prospective Investigation into Cancer and Nutrition (EPIC-EURGAST). Int J Cancer 2006b;118:2559–66.

Goto Y, Ando T, Goto H, Hamajima N. No association between EGF gene polymorphism and gastric cancer. Cancer Epidemiol Biomarkers Prev 2005;14:2454–56.

Gotze T, Rocken C, Rohl FW, Wex T, Hoffmann J, Westphal S, et al. Gene polymorphisms of folate metabolizing enzymes and the risk of gastric cancer. Cancer Lett 2007;251:228–36.

Graziano F, Kawakami K, Ruzzo A, Watanabe G, Santini D, Pizzagalli F, et al. Methylenetetrahydrofolate reductase 677C/T gene polymorphism, gastric cancer susceptibility and genomic DNA hypomethylation in an at-risk Italian population. Int J Cancer 2006; 118:628–32.

Guilford P, Hopkins J, Harraway J, McLeod M, McLeod N, Harawira P, et al. E-cadherin germline mutations in familial gastric cancer. Nature 1998;392:402–5.

Hamai Y, Matsumura S, Matsusaki K, Kitadai Y, Yoshida K, Yamaguchi Y, et al. A single nucleotide polymorphism in the 5' untranslated region of the EGF gene is associated with occurrence and malignant progression of gastric cancer. Pathobiology 2005;72: 133–38.

Hansen S, Melby KK, Aase S, Jellum E, Vollset SE. Helicobacter pylori infection and risk of cardia cancer and non-cardia gastric cancer. A nested case-control study. Scand J Gastroenterol 1999;34:353–60.

Hansson LE, Bergstrom R, Sparen P, Adami HO. The decline in the incidence of stomach cancer in Sweden 1960–1984: a birth cohort phenomenon. Int J Cancer 1991;47:499–503.

Hansson LE, Sparen P, Nyren O. Increasing incidence of carcinoma of the gastric cardia in Sweden from 1970 to 1985. Br J Surg 1993a;80:374–77.

Hansson LE, Sparen P, Nyren O. Increasing incidence of both major histological types of esophageal carcinomas among men in Sweden. Int J Cancer 1993b;54:402–7.

Hansson LE, Baron J, Nyren O, Bergstrom R, Wolk A, Lindgren A, et al. Early-life risk indicators of gastric cancer. A population-based case-control study in Sweden. Int J Cancer 1994;57:32–37.

Hansson LE, Nyren O, Hsing AW, Bergstrom R, Josefsson S, Chow WH, et al. The risk of stomach cancer in patients with gastric or duodenal ulcer disease. N Engl J Med 1996;335:242–49.

Hatakeyama M. Oncogenic mechanisms of the Helicobacter pylori CagA protein. Nat Rev Cancer 2004;4:688–94.

Held M, Engstrand L, Hansson LE, Bergstrom R, Wadstrom T, Nyren O. Is the association between Helicobacter pylori and gastric cancer confined to CagA-positive strains? Helicobacter 2004;9:271–77.

Hennekens CH, Buring JE, Manson JE, Stampfer M, Rosner B, Cook NR, et al. Lack of effect of long-term supplementation with beta carotene on the incidence of malignant neoplasms and cardiovascular disease. N Engl J Med 1996;334:1145–49.

Holcombe C. Helicobacter pylori: the African enigma. Gut 1992;33:429–31.

Hold GL, Rabkin CS, Chow WH, Smith MG, Gammon MD, Risch HA, et al. A functional polymorphism of toll-like receptor 4 gene increases risk of gastric carcinoma and its precursors. Gastroenterology 2007;132: 905–12.

Huang JQ, Sridhar S, Chen Y, Hunt RH. Meta-analysis of the relationship between Helicobacter pylori seropositivity and gastric cancer. Gastroenterology 1998;114:1169–79.

IARC. Some Natural Occurring Substances: Food Items and Constituents, Heterocyclic Aromatic Amines and Mycotoxins. IARC Monogr Eval Carcinog Risk Chem Hum 1993;56.

IARC. Schistosomes, liver flukes and Helicobacter pylori. IARC Working Group on the Evaluation of Carcinogenic Risks to Humans. Lyon, 7–14 June 1994. IARC Monogr Eval Carcinog Risks Hum 1994;61:1–241.

IARC. Cancer in Africa: epidemiology and prevention. IARC Sci Publ 2003:1–414.

IARC. Tobacco smoke and involuntary smoking. IARC Monogr Eval Carcinog Risks Hum 2004;83:1–1438.

Ito Y, Kurata M, Hioki R, Suzuki K, Ochiai J, Aoki K. Cancer mortality and serum levels of carotenoids, retinol, and tocopherol: a population-based follow-up study of inhabitants of a rural area of Japan. Asian Pac J Cancer Prev 2005;6:10–15.

Jacobsen BK, Bjelke E, Kvale G, Heuch I. Coffee drinking, mortality, and cancer incidence: results from a Norwegian prospective study. J Natl Cancer Inst 1986;76:823–31.

Jakszyn P, Bingham S, Pera G, Agudo A, Luben R, Welch A, et al. Endogenous versus exogenous exposure to N-nitroso compounds and gastric cancer risk in the European Prospective Investigation into Cancer and Nutrition (EPIC-EURGAST) study. Carcinogenesis 2006;27:1497–1501.

Jansson C, Johansson AL, Bergdahl IA, Dickman PW, Plato N, Adami J, et al. Occupational exposures and risk of esophageal and gastric cardia cancers among male Swedish construction workers. Cancer Causes Control 2005;16:755–64.

Jansson C, Plato N, Johansson AL, Nyren O, Lagergren J. Airborne occupational exposures and risk of oesophageal and cardia adenocarcinoma. Occup Environ Med 2006; 63:107–12.

Jenab M, Riboli E, Ferrari P, Friesen M, Sabate J, Norat T, et al. Plasma and dietary carotenoid, retinol and tocopherol levels and the risk of gastric adenocarcinomas in the European prospective investigation into cancer and nutrition. Br J Cancer 2006a;95:406–15.

Jenab M, Riboli E, Ferrari P, Sabate J, Slimani N, Norat T, et al. Plasma and dietary vitamin C levels and risk of gastric cancer in the European Prospective Investigation into Cancer and Nutrition (EPIC-EURGAST). Carcinogenesis 2006b;27:2250–57.

Ji J, Hemminki K. Socio-economic and occupational risk factors for gastric cancer: a cohort study in Sweden. Eur J Cancer Prev 2006;15:391–97.

Jin G, Miao R, Deng Y, Hu Z, Zhou Y, Tan Y, et al. Variant genotypes and haplotypes of the epidermal growth factor gene promoter are associated with a decreased risk of gastric cancer in a high-risk Chinese population. Cancer Sci 2007a;98:864–68.

Jin G, Wang L, Chen W, Hu Z, Zhou Y, Tan Y, et al. Variant alleles of TGFB1 and TGFBR2 are associated with a decreased risk of gastric cancer in a Chinese population. Int J Cancer 2007b;120:1330–35.

Johnson AG, Jick SS, Perera DR, Jick H. Histamine-2 receptor antagonists and gastric cancer. Epidemiology 1996;7:434–36.

Joossens JV, Hill MJ, Elliott P, Stamler R, Lesaffre E, Dyer A, et al. Dietary salt, nitrate and stomach cancer mortality in 24 countries. European Cancer Prevention (ECP) and the INTERSALT Cooperative Research Group. Int J Epidemiol 1996;25:494–504.

Kamangar F, Dawsey SM, Blaser MJ, Perez-Perez GI, Pietinen P, Newschaffer CJ, et al. Opposing risks of gastric cardia and non-cardia gastric adenocarcinomas associated with Helicobacter pylori seropositivity. J Natl Cancer Inst 2006;98:1445–52.

Kamangar F, Cheng C, Abnet CC, Rabkin CS. Interleukin-1B polymorphisms and gastric cancer risk–a meta-analysis. Cancer Epidemiol Biomarkers Prev 2006;15:1920–28.

Kamineni A, Williams MA, Schwartz SM, Cook LS, Weiss NS. The incidence of gastric carcinoma in Asian migrants to the United States and their descendants. Cancer Causes Control 1999;10:77–83.

Katoh T, Boissy R, Nagata N, Kitagawa K, Kuroda Y, Itoh H, et al. Inherited polymorphism in the N-acetyltransferase 1 (NAT1) and 2 (NAT2) genes and susceptibility to gastric and colorectal adenocarcinoma. Int J Cancer 2000;85:46–49.

Kim IJ, Kang HC, Shin Y, Park HW, Jang SG, Han SY, et al. A TP53-truncating germline mutation (E287X) in a family with characteristics of both hereditary diffuse gastric cancer and Li-Fraumeni syndrome. J Hum Genet 2004;49:591–95.

Knekt P, Aromaa A, Maatela J, Alfthan G, Aaran RK, Hakama M, et al. Serum selenium and subsequent risk of cancer among Finnish men and women. J Natl Cancer Inst 1990; 82:864–68.

Knekt P, Jarvinen R, Dich J, Hakulinen T. Risk of colorectal and other gastro-intestinal cancers after exposure to nitrate, nitrite and N-nitroso compounds: a follow-up study. Int J Cancer 1999;80:852–56.

Koizumi Y, Tsubono Y, Nakaya N, Kuriyama S, Shibuya D, Matsuoka H, et al. Cigarette smoking and the risk of gastric cancer: a pooled analysis of two prospective studies in Japan. Int J Cancer 2004;112:1049–55.

Kono S, Hirohata T. Nutrition and stomach cancer. Cancer Causes Control 1996;7:41–55.

Kuipers EJ, Lundell L, Klinkenberg-Knol EC, Havu N, Festen HP, Liedman B, et al. Atrophic gastritis and Helicobacter pylori infection in patients with reflux esophagitis treated with omeprazole or fundoplication. N Engl J Med 1996;334:1018–22.

Ladero JM, Agundez JA, Olivera M, Lozano L, Rodriguez-Lescure A, Diaz-Rubio M, et al. N-acetyltransferase 2 single-nucleotide polymorphisms and risk of gastric carcinoma. Eur J Clin Pharmacol 2002;58:115–18.

Lagergren J, Bergstrom R, Lindgren A, Nyren O. Symptomatic gastroesophageal reflux as a risk factor for esophageal adenocarcinoma. N Engl J Med 1999;340:825–31.

Lagergren J, Bergstrom R, Lindgren A, Nyren O. The role of tobacco, snuff and alcohol use in the aetiology of cancer of the oesophagus and gastric cardia. Int J Cancer 2000;85:340–46.

Lan Q, Rothman N, Chow WH, Lissowska J, Doll MA, Xiao GH, et al. No apparent association between NAT1 and NAT2 genotypes and risk of stomach cancer. Cancer Epidemiol Biomarkers Prev 2003;12:384–86.

Larsson SC. Diet and Gastrointestinal Cancer. One Carbon Metabolism and Other Aspects (Thesis). Stockholm, Karolinska Institutet, 2006.

Larsson SC, Bergkvist L, Wolk A. Processed meat consumption, dietary nitrosamines and stomach cancer risk in a cohort of Swedish women. Int J Cancer 2006a;119:915–19.

Larsson SC, Giovannucci E, Wolk A. Folate intake, MTHFR polymorphisms, and risk of esophageal, gastric, and pancreatic cancer: a meta-analysis. Gastroenterology 2006b;131:1271–83.

Larsson SC, Giovannucci E, Wolk A. Coffee consumption and stomach cancer risk in a cohort of Swedish women. Int J Cancer 2006c;119:2186–89.

Larsson SC, Orsini N, Wolk A. Processed meat consumption and stomach cancer risk: a meta analysis. J Natl Cancer Inst 2006d;98:1078–87.

Larsson SC, Giovannucci E, Wolk A. Alcoholic beverage consumption and gastric cancer risk: A prospective population-based study in women. Int J Cancer 2007;120:373–77.

Lauren P. The two histological main types of gastric carcinoma:diffuse and so-called intestinal type carcinoma. An attempt at histoclinical classification. Acta Pathol Microbiol Scand 1965;64:31–49.

Lauren P, Nevalainen TJ. Epidemiology of intestinal and diffuse types of gastric carcinoma. A time-trend study in Finland with comparison between studies from high- and low-risk areas [see comments]. Cancer 1993;71:2926–33.

Lee JE, Lowy AM, Thompson WA, Lu M, Loflin PT, Skibber JM, et al. Association of gastric adenocarcinoma with the HLA class II gene DQB10301. Gastroenterology 1996; 111:426–32.

Lee WJ, Lijinsky W, Heineman EF, Markin RS, Weisenburger DD, Ward MH. Agricultural pesticide use and adenocarcinomas of the stomach and oesophagus. Occup Environ Med 2004;61:743–49.

Leung WK, Lin SR, Ching JY, To KF, Ng EK, Chan FK, et al. Factors predicting progression of gastric intestinal metaplasia: results of a randomised trial on Helicobacter pylori eradication. Gut 2004;53:1244–49.

Li H, Chen XL, Li HQ. Polymorphism of CYPIA1 and GSTM1 genes associated with susceptibility of gastric cancer in Shandong Province of China. World J Gastroenterol 2005;11:5757–62.

Li JY, Taylor PR, Li B, Dawsey S, Wang GQ, Ershow AG, et al. Nutrition intervention trials in Linxian, China: multiple vitamin/mineral supplementation, cancer incidence, and disease-specific mortality among adults with esophageal dysplasia. J Natl Cancer Inst 1993;85:1492–98.

Lichtenstein P, Holm NV, Verkasalo PK, Iliadou A, Kaprio J, Koskenvuo M, et al. Environmental and heritable factors in the causation of cancer—analyses of cohorts of twins from Sweden, Denmark, and Finland. N Engl J Med 2000;343:78–85.

Lindblad M, Lagergren J, Garcia Rodriguez LA. Nonsteroidal anti-inflammatory drugs and risk of esophageal and gastric cancer. Cancer Epidemiol Biomarkers Prev 2005;14:444–50.

Liu F, Pan K, Zhang X, Zhang Y, Zhang L, Ma J, et al. Genetic variants in cyclooxygenase-2: Expression and risk of gastric cancer and its precursors in a Chinese population. Gastroenterology 2006;130:1975–84.

Lopez-Carrillo L, Lopez-Cervantes M, Robles-Diaz G, Ramirez-Espitia A, Mohar-Betancourt A, Meneses-Garcia A, et al. Capsaicin consumption, Helicobacter pylori positivity and gastric cancer in Mexico. Int J Cancer 2003;106:277–82.

Lundegardh G, Adami HO, Helmick C, Zack M, Meirik O. Stomach cancer after partial gastrectomy for benign ulcer disease. N Engl J Med 1988;319:195–200.

Lundegardh G, Hansson LE, Nyren O, Adami HO, Krusemo UB. The risk of gastrointestinal and other primary malignant diseases following gastric cancer. Acta Oncol 1991; 30:1–6.

Maeda S, Yoshida H, Ogura K, Yamaji Y, Ikenoue T, Mitsushima T, et al. Assessment of gastric carcinoma risk associated with Helicobacter pylori may vary depending on the antigen used: CagA specific enzyme-linked immunoadsorbent assay (ELISA) versus commercially available H. pylori ELISAs. Cancer 2000;88:1530–35.

Magnusson PKE, Enroth H, Eriksson I, Held M, Nyren O, Engstrand L, et al. Gastric cancer and human leukocyte antigen: distinct DQ and DR alleles are associated with development of gastric cancer and infection by Helicobacter pylori. Cancer Res 2001;61:2684–89.

Malila N, Taylor PR, Virtanen MJ, Korhonen P, Huttunen JK, Albanes D, et al. Effects of alpha-tocopherol and beta-carotene supplementation on gastric cancer incidence in male smokers (ATBC Study, Finland). Cancer Causes Control 2002;13:617–23.

Mao Y, Hu J, Semenciw R, White K. Active and passive smoking and the risk of stomach cancer, by subsite, in Canada. Eur J Cancer Prev 2002;11:27–38.

McCullough ML, Robertson AS, Jacobs EJ, Chao A, Calle EE, Thun MJ. A prospective study of diet and stomach cancer mortality in United States men and women. Cancer Epidemiol Biomarkers Prev 2001;10: 1201–5.

Mera R, Fontham ET, Bravo LE, Bravo JC, Piazuelo MB, Camargo MC, et al. Long term follow up of patients treated for Helicobacter pylori infection. Gut 2005;54:1536–40.

Miao X, Zhang X, Zhang L, Guo Y, Hao B, Tan W, et al. Adenosine diphosphate ribosyl transferase and x-ray repair cross-complementing 1 polymorphisms in gastric cardia cancer. Gastroenterology 2006;131: 420–27.

Milham SJ, Demers RY. Mortality among pulp and paper workers. J Occup Med 1984;26: 844–46.

Mohar A, Suchil-Bernal L, Hernandez-Guerrero A, Podolsky-Rapoport I, Herrera-Goepfert R, Mora-Tiscareno A, et al. Intestinal type: diffuse type ratio of gastric carcinoma in a Mexican population. J Exp Clin Cancer Res 1997;16:189–94.

Moller H, Nissen A, Mosbech J. Use of cimetidine and other peptic ulcer drugs in Denmark 1977–1990 with analysis of the risk of gastric cancer among cimetidine users. Gut 1992;33:1166–69.

Mowat C, Williams C, Gillen D, Hossack M, Gilmour D, Carswell A, et al. Omeprazole, Helicobacter pylori status, and alterations in the intragastric milieu facilitating bacterial N-nitrosation. Gastroenterology 2000;119: 339–47.

Munoz N, Connelly R. Time trends of intestinal and diffuse types of gastric cancer in the United States. Int J Cancer 1971;8:158–64.

Nagata C, Takatsuka N, Kawakami N, Shimizu H. A prospective cohort study of soy product intake and stomach cancer death. Br J Cancer 2002;87:31–36.

Nakamura K. Stomach cancer in atomic-bomb survivors. Lancet 1977;2:866–67.

Ngoan LT, Mizoue T, Fujino Y, Tokui N, Yoshimura T. Dietary factors and stomach cancer mortality. Br J Cancer 2002;87:37–42.

Nikulasson S, Hallgrimsson J, Tulinius H, Sigvaldason H, Olafsdottir G. Tumours in Iceland. 16. Malignant tumours of the stomach. Histological classification and description of epidemiological changes in a high-risk population during 30 years. Apmis 1992;100:930–41.

Nishimoto IN, Hanaoka T, Sugimura H, Nagura K, Ihara M, Li XJ, et al. Cytochrome P450 2E1 polymorphism in gastric cancer in Brazil: case-control studies of Japanese Brazilians and non-Japanese Brazilians. Cancer Epidemiol Biomarkers Prev 2000;9:675–80.

Nomura AM, Stemmermann GN, Chyou PH. Gastric cancer among the Japanese in Hawaii. Jpn J Cancer Res 1995;86:916–23.

Nouraie M, Pietinen P, Kamangar F, Dawsey SM, Abnet CC, Albanes D, et al. Fruits, vegetables, and antioxidants and risk of gastric cancer among male smokers. Cancer Epidemiol Biomarkers Prev 2005;14:2087–92.

Ocke MC, Bueno-de-Mesquita HB, Feskens EJ, Kromhout D, Menotti A, Blackburn H. Adherence to the European Code Against Cancer in relation to long-term cancer mortality: intercohort comparisons from the Seven Countries Study. Nutr Cancer 1998;30:14–20.

Ohmura K, Tamura G, Endoh Y, Sakata K, Takahashi T, Motoyama T. Microsatellite alterations in differentiated-type adenocarcinomas and precancerous lesions of the stomach with special reference to cellular phenotype. Hum Pathol 2000;31:1031–35.

Oliveira C, Seruca R, Carneiro F. Genetics, pathology, and clinics of familial gastric cancer. Int J Surg Pathol 2006;14:21–33.

Parkin DM, Whelan SL, Ferlay J, Raymond L, Young J. Cancer Incidence in Five Continents. Volume VII. Lyon, International Agency for Research on Cancer, 1997.

Parkin DM, Bray F, Ferlay J, Pisani P. Global cancer statistics, 2002. CA Cancer J Clin 2005;55:74–108.

Plummer M, Vivas J, Lopez G, Bravo JC, Peraza S, Carillo E, et al. Chemoprevention of precancerous gastric lesions with antioxidant vitamin supplementation: a randomized trial in a high-risk population. J Natl Cancer Inst 2007;99:137–46.

Ratnasinghe LD, Abnet C, Qiao YL, Modali R, Stolzenberg-Solomon R, Dong ZW, et al.

Polymorphisms of XRCC1 and risk of esophageal and gastric cardia cancer. Cancer Lett 2004;216:157–64.

Riboli E, Norat T. Epidemiologic evidence of the protective effect of fruit and vegetables on cancer risk. Am J Clin Nutr 2003;78:559S–69S.

Rix BA, Villadsen E, Lynge E. Cancer incidence of sulfite pulp workers in Denmark. Scand J Work Environ Health 1997;23:458–61.

Robinson CF, Petersen M, Sieber WK, Palu S, Halperin WE. Mortality of Carpenters' Union members employed in the U.S. construction or wood products industries, 1987–1990. Am J Ind Med 1996;30:674–94.

Roth MJ, Abnet CC, Johnson LL, Mark SD, Dong ZW, Taylor PR, et al. Polymorphic variation of Cyp1A1 is associated with the risk of gastric cardia cancer: a prospective case-cohort study of cytochrome P-450 1A1 and GST enzymes. Cancer Causes Control 2004;15:1077–83.

Saadat M. Genetic polymorphisms of glutathione S-transferase T1 (GSTT1) and susceptibility to gastric cancer: a meta-analysis. Cancer Sci 2006;97:505–9.

Sasazuki S, Inoue M, Hanaoka T, Yamamoto S, Sobue T, Tsugane S. Green tea consumption and subsequent risk of gastric cancer by subsite: the JPHC Study. Cancer Causes Control 2004;15:483–91.

Shen H, Xu Y, Qian Y, Yu R, Qin Y, Zhou L, et al. Polymorphisms of the DNA repair gene XRCC1 and risk of gastric cancer in a Chinese population. Int J Cancer 2000;88:601–6.

Shi WX, Chen SQ. Frequencies of poor metabolizers of cytochrome P450 2C19 in esophagus cancer, stomach cancer, lung cancer and bladder cancer in Chinese population. World J Gastroenterol 2004;10:1961–63.

Shinmura K, Kohno T, Takahashi M, Sasaki A, Ochiai A, Guilford P, et al. Familial gastric cancer: clinicopathological characteristics, RER phenotype and germline p53 and E-cadherin mutations. Carcinogenesis 1999;20:1127–31.

Simpson J, Roman E, Law G, Pannett B. Women's occupation and cancer: preliminary analysis of cancer registrations in England and Wales, 1971–1990. Am J Ind Med 1999;36:172–85.

Sipponen P, Jarvi O, Kekki M, Siurala M. Decreased incidences of intestinal and diffuse types of gastric carcinoma in Finland during a 20-year period. Scand J Gastroenterol 1987;22:865–71.

Sjodahl K, Jansson C, Bergdahl IA, Adami J, Boffetta P, Lagergren J. Airborne exposures and risk of gastric cancer: A prospective cohort study. Int J Cancer 2007;120:2013–8.

Smith MG, Hold GL, Tahara E, El-Omar EM. Cellular and molecular aspects of gastric cancer. World J Gastroenterol 2006;12: 2979–90.

Stahelin HB, Gey KF, Eichholzer M, Ludin E, Bernasconi F, Thurneysen J, et al. Plasma antioxidant vitamins and subsequent cancer mortality in the 12-year follow-up of the prospective Basel Study. Am J Epidemiol 1991;133:766–75.

Stebbings JH, Lucas HF, Stehney AF. Mortality from cancers of major sites in female radium dial workers. Am J Ind Med 1984; 5:435–59.

Steinmetz KA, Potter JD. Vegetables, fruit, and cancer prevention: a review. J Am Diet Assoc 1996;96:1027–39.

Sugimoto M, Furuta T, Shirai N, Nakamura A, Kajimura M, Sugimura H, et al. Poor metabolizer genotype status of CYP2C19 is a risk factor for developing gastric cancer in Japanese patients with Helicobacter pylori infection. Aliment Pharmacol Ther 2005;22: 1033–40.

Sung JJ, Lin SR, Ching JY, Zhou LY, To KF, Wang RT, et al. Atrophy and intestinal metaplasia one year after cure of H. pylori infection: a prospective, randomized study. Gastroenterology 2000;119:7–14.

Suzuki S, Muroishi Y, Nakanishi I, Oda Y. Relationship between genetic polymorphisms of drug-metabolizing enzymes (CYP1A1, CYP2E1, GSTM1, and NAT2), drinking habits, histological subtypes, and p53 gene point mutations in Japanese patients with gastric cancer. J Gastroenterol 2004;39:220–30.

Swaen GM, Aerdts CW, Sturmans F, Slangen JJ, Knipschild P. Gastric cancer in coal miners: a case-control study in a coal mining area. Br J Ind Med 1985;42:627–30.

Swedish Oncological Centres 1995. Atlas of Cancer Incidence in Sweden. ISBN 91–86530-20-8.

Tahara E. Genetic pathways of two types of gastric cancer. IARC Sci Publ 2004;157:327–49.

Tahara H, Kuniyasu H, Yokozaki H, Yasui W, Shay JW, Ide T, et al. Telomerase activity in preneoplastic and neoplastic gastric and colorectal lesions. Clin Cancer Res 1995;1: 1245–51.

Tamer L, Ercan B, Ercan S, Ates N, Ates C, Ocal K, et al. CYP2C19 polymorphisms in patients with gastric and colorectal carcinoma. Int J Gastrointest Cancer 2006;37:1–5.

Tamura G, Sato K, Akiyama S, Tsuchiya T, Endoh Y, Usuba O, et al. Molecular characterization of undifferentiated-type gastric carcinoma. Lab Invest 2001;81:593–98.

Tamura G. Alterations of tumor suppressor and tumor-related genes in the development and progression of gastric cancer. World J Gastroenterol 2006;12:192–98.

Taylor PR, Qiao YL, Abnet CC, Dawsey SM, Yang CS, Gunter EW, et al. Prospective study of serum vitamin E levels and esophageal and gastric cancers. J Natl Cancer Inst 2003;95:1414–16.

Terry P, Lagergren J, Ye W, Wolk A, Nyren O. Inverse association between intake of cereal fiber and risk of gastric cardia cancer. Gastroenterology 2001;120:387–91.

Tersmette AC, Offerhaus GJ, Tersmette KW, Giardiello FM, Moore GW, Tytgat GN, et al. Meta-analysis of the risk of gastric stump cancer: detection of high risk patient subsets for stomach cancer after remote partial gastrectomy for benign conditions. Cancer Res 1990;50:6486–89.

Thun MJ, Namboodiri MM, Calle EE, Flanders WD, Heath CW, Jr. Aspirin use and risk of fatal cancer. Cancer Res 1993;53:1322–27.

Tolbert PE. Oils and cancer. Cancer Causes Control 1997;8:386–405.

Tredaniel J, Boffetta P, Buiatti E, Saracci R, Hirsch A. Tobacco smoking and gastric cancer: review and meta-analysis. Int J Cancer 1997;72:565–73.

Tsugane S. Salt, salted food intake, and risk of gastric cancer: epidemiologic evidence. Cancer Sci 2005;96:1–6.

Tsukino H, Kuroda Y, Qiu D, Nakao H, Imai H, Katoh T. Effects of cytochrome P450 (CYP) 2A6 gene deletion and CYP2E1 genotypes on gastric adenocarcinoma. Int J Cancer 2002;100:425–28.

Uemura N, Okamoto S, Yamamoto S, Matsumura N, Yamaguchi S, Yamakido M, et al. Helicobacter pylori infection and the development of gastric cancer. N Engl J Med 2001;345:784–89.

van den Brandt PA, Botterweck AA, Goldbohm RA. Salt intake, cured meat consumption, refrigerator use and stomach cancer incidence: a prospective cohort study (Netherlands). Cancer Causes Control 2003;14:427–38.

van Loon AJ, Botterweck AA, Goldbohm RA, Brants HA, van Klaveren JD, van den Brandt PA. Intake of nitrate and nitrite and the risk of gastric cancer: a prospective cohort study. Br J Cancer 1998a;78:129–35.

van Loon AJ, Goldbohm RA, van den Brandt PA. Socioeconomic status and stomach cancer incidence in men: results from The Netherlands Cohort Study. J Epidemiol Community Health 1998b;52:166–71.

Wang WH, Huang JQ, Zheng GF, Lam SK, Karlberg J, Wong BC. Non-steroidal anti-inflammatory drug use and the risk of gastric cancer: a systematic review and meta-analysis. J Natl Cancer Inst 2003;95:1784–91.

Varley JM, McGown G, Thorncroft M, Tricker KJ, Teare MD, Santibanez-Koref MF, et al. An extended Li-Fraumeni kindred with gastric carcinoma and a codon 175 mutation in TP53. J Med Genet 1995;32:942–45.

Vauhkonen M, Vauhkonen H, Sipponen P. Pathology and molecular biology of gastric cancer. Best Pract Res Clin Gastroenterol 2006;20:651–74.

Weiderpass E, Vainio H, Kauppinen T, Vasama-Neuvonen K, Partanen T, Pukkala E. Occupational exposures and gastrointestinal cancers among Finnish women. J Occup Environ Med 2003;45:305–15.

Weinberg GB, Kuller LH, Stehr PA. A case-control study of stomach cancer in a coal mining region of Pennsylvania. Cancer 1985;56:703–13.

Wernli KJ, Fitzgibbons ED, Ray RM, Gao DL, Li W, Seixas NS, et al. Occupational risk factors for esophageal and stomach cancers among female textile workers in Shanghai, China. Am J Epidemiol 2006;163:717–25.

Vigen C, Bernstein L, Wu AH. Occupational physical activity and risk of adenocarcinomas of the esophagus and stomach. Int J Cancer 2006;118:1004–9.

Virtamo J, Pietinen P, Huttunen JK, Korhonen P, Malila N, Virtanen MJ, et al. Incidence of cancer and mortality following alpha-tocopherol and beta-carotene supplementation: a postintervention follow-up. JAMA 2003;290:476–85.

Wong BC, Ching CK, Lam SK, Li ZL, Chen BW, Li YN, et al. Differential north to south gastric cancer-duodenal ulcer gradient in China. China Ulcer Study Group. J Gastroenterol Hepatol 1998;13:1050–57.

Wong BC, Lam SK, Wong WM, Chen JS, Zheng TT, Feng RE, et al. Helicobacter pylori eradication to prevent gastric cancer in a high-risk region of China: a randomized controlled trial. JAMA 2004;291:187–94.

World Cancer Research Fund—American Institute of Cancer Research. Food, Nutrition and the Prevention of Cancer: A Global Perspective. Menasha, USA, BANTA Book Group, 1997.

Wu AH, Yang D, Pike MC. A meta-analysis of soyfoods and risk of stomach cancer: the problem of potential confounders. Cancer Epidemiol Biomarkers Prev 2000;9:1051–58.

Wu MS, Chen CJ, Lin MT, Wang HP, Shun CT, Sheu JC, et al. Genetic polymorphisms of cytochrome p450 2E1, glutathione S-transferase M1 and T1, and susceptibility to gastric carcinoma in Taiwan. Int J Colorectal Dis 2002a;17:338–43.

Wu MS, Hsieh RP, Huang SP, Chang YT, Lin MT, Chang MC, et al. Association of HLA-DQB1*0301 and HLA-DQB1*0602 with different subtypes of gastric cancer in Taiwan. Jpn J Cancer Res 2002b;93:404–10.

Ye W, Ekstrom AM, Hansson LE, Bergstrom R, Nyren O. Tobacco, alcohol and the risk of gastric cancer by sub-site and histologic type. Int J Cancer 1999;83:223–29.

Ye W, Kumar R, Bacova G, Lagergren J, Hemminki K, Nyren O. The XPD 751Gln allele is associated with an increased risk for esophageal adenocarcinoma: a population-based case-control study in Sweden. Carcinogenesis 2006;27:1835–41.

You W, Zhang L, Gail MH, Chang Y, Liu W, Ma J, et al. Gastric dysplasia and gastric cancer: helicobacter pylori, serum vitamin C, and other risk factors. J Natl Cancer Inst 2000;92:1607–12.

You WC, Brown LM, Zhang L, Li JY, Jin ML, Chang YS, et al. Randomized double-blind factorial trial of three treatments to reduce the prevalence of precancerous gastric lesions. J Natl Cancer Inst 2006;98:974–83.

Yuan JM, Ross RK, Gao YT, Qu YH, Chu XD, Yu MC. Prediagnostic levels of serum micronutrients in relation to risk of gastric cancer in Shanghai, China. Cancer Epidemiol Biomarkers Prev 2004;13:1772–80.

Zhang FF, Terry MB, Hou L, Chen J, Lissowska J, Yeager M, et al. Genetic polymorphisms in folate metabolism and the risk of stomach cancer. Cancer Epidemiol Biomarkers Prev 2007;16:115–21.

Zheng W, Sellers TA, Doyle TJ, Kushi LH, Potter JD, Folsom AR. Retinol, antioxidant vitamins, and cancers of the upper digestive tract in a prospective cohort study of postmenopausal women. Am J Epidemiol 1995;142:955–60.

Zhu S, Mason J, Shi Y, Hu Y, Li R, Wahg M, et al. The effect of folic acid on the development of stomach and other gastrointestinal cancers. Chin Med J (Engl) 2003;116:15–19.

Zintzaras E. Association of methylenetetrahydrofolate reductase (MTHFR) polymorphisms with genetic susceptibility to gastric cancer: a meta-analysis. J Hum Genet 2006;51:618–24.

11

Colorectal Cancer

JOHN D. POTTER AND DAVID HUNTER

Colorectal cancer has at least two features that contribute to its preventability. First, tumors of the colon and rectum, being among the most common in western populations, have several established or suspected risk factors that are quantitatively important as well as potentially modifiable. Second, the existence of adenomatous polyps—a clearly preneoplastic lesion—and the accessibility of the colonic mucosa to endoscopy have enabled detailed molecular studies. A classic model describes how accumulating damage to key regulatory genes correlates with progression through the adenoma/carcinoma sequence, although it is now clear that several other pathways exist. Establishing the factors that determine progression to invasive cancer has become a central epidemiologic challenge.

The descriptive and analytic epidemiology of colon and rectal cancer have important characteristics in common as well as some notable differences. In most of this chapter, the colon and rectum will be considered together. Specific differences will be noted where relevant.

CLINICAL SYNOPSIS

Subtypes

Adenomatous polyps are established precursors of colorectal cancers, which are almost invariably adenocarcinomas. There is increasing evidence that hyperplastic polyps can give rise to serrated polyps and subsequently to cancer. Colorectal cancers have been distinguished mostly by their varying anatomic locations but molecular classification that is based on the presence of genomic instability versus chromosomal instability is increasingly applied. In the ICD classification, a small group of squamous cell anal cancers are included among rectal cancers, but they are not discussed in this chapter.

Symptoms

Colorectal cancers become symptomatic because they obstruct the bowel and often bleed—insidiously or overtly. Hence, changes in bowel habits, blood in the stool, and anemia are cardinal symptoms and signs. In later stages, fatigue, anorexia, weight loss, pain, jaundice, and other signs and symptoms of locally advanced and metastatic disease occur.

Diagnosis

Detection of blood in the stool is an early but nonspecific sign. The classic diagnostic tools—barium enema and rectoscopy—are now being increasingly replaced by sigmoidoscopy and colonoscopy with biopsy. Ultrasound, computed tomography, and other newer imaging techniques may provide complementary diagnostic information that is relevant for staging and treatment planning.

Treatment

Radical surgical removal of the primary lesion is the hallmark of curative treatment. Chemotherapy has an established role as an adjuvant to surgical treatment in stage III colon cancer; its role in stage II colon cancer and stage II and III rectal cancer is not established. In contrast, preoperative—and to a lesser extent postoperative—radiotherapy can markedly reduce the risk of local recurrence following removal of a rectal cancer and even improve long-term survival. The effects also are seen together with those of more optimized surgery such as total mesorectal excision. Chemotherapy is also used routinely for palliation in advanced disease. As with other tumors, it seems increasingly likely that the molecular characterizations of tumors will inform choice of therapeutic regimen.

Prognosis

For colorectal cancer, 5-year relative survival rates are now about 63% in the United States with substantial variation, not only by stage, but also among countries.

Progress

Although there have been only some minor therapeutic breakthroughs (eg, antiangiogenic agents), it has become obvious that chemotherapy can prevent some deaths. Optimal surgical resection and radiotherapy of rectal cancer are also important in reducing local recurrences, otherwise an incurable source of substantial suffering.

Survival rates have improved in many settings, possibly due in part to earlier diagnosis and state-of-the-art treatment.

DESCRIPTIVE EPIDEMIOLOGY

By the end of the twentieth century, approximately 950 000 cases of colorectal cancer occurred annually worldwide, accounting for about 9.5% of all new cases of cancer (Stewart and Kleihues, 2003). In the United States, colorectal cancer is the third most common incident cancer and the second most common cause of cancer death (ACS, 2006). Incidence rates vary more than 20-fold around the world, with the lowest rates in India and the highest in Japan. They increase sharply with age (Figs. 11–1 and 11–2), particularly in the more developed countries. The difference in age-standardized rates between the United States and China is more than threefold (Figs. 11–3 and 11–4). Colon cancer occurs with approximately equal frequency in men and women, whereas rectal cancer is up to twice as common in men.

The international differences and migrant data show that colorectal cancer is highly sensitive to changes in lifestyle. Among immigrants and their descendants, incidence rates may rapidly reach those of the host country (Haenszel, 1961; McMichael and Giles, 1988). Dietary and other environmental differences may explain most of the international variation in rates. Although incidence rates in Japan have long been low, the highest rates in the world are now seen among Japanese in Japan, where rates among men are now higher than those in the United States; among women, they are higher than in many European countries and approach those in the United States (Figs. 11–3 and 11–4).

Western countries have seen a shift in the distribution of cancers within the colon and rectum. In the mid-twentieth century, approximately 75% of all colorectal cancers occurred in the rectum, rectosigmoid, and sigmoid areas, compared to about 50% today; right-sided colon cancer, correspondingly, now accounts for a larger proportion.

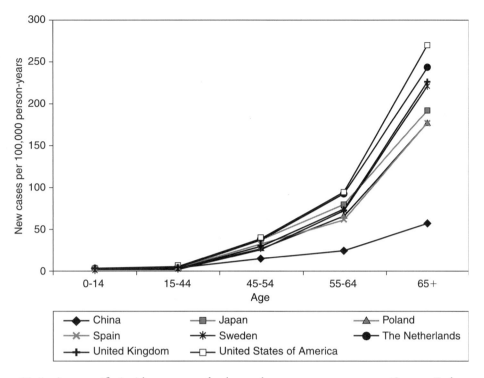

Figure 11–1. Age-specific incidence rates of colorectal cancer among women. (*Source*: Ferlay et al, 2004)

Increasing availability of sigmoidoscopy may account for a small part of the reduction in left-sided tumors because it leads to detection and removal of polyps—precursor lesions that would otherwise have progressed to invasive cancer.

GENETIC AND MOLECULAR EPIDEMIOLOGY

The underlying genetic events are better understood for cancer of the colon and rectum than for cancer at almost any other site. A small proportion of colorectal cancers occurs in the context of the familial syndromes discussed in the following. An emerging area is the study of the manner in which inherited variation in genes that are not directly associated with a high risk of colorectal cancer may nonetheless modify the effects of lifestyle factors, such as diet and smoking, as well as specific preventive agents, such as NSAIDs, on colorectal cancer risk.

The adenoma-carcinoma hypothesis developed in the 1970s (Hillet al, 1978) was stimulated by several observations including the following: *(1)* early cancers often arose in adenomatous polyps; *(2)* persons known to have polyps that were not removed were at higher risk of colorectal cancer; and *(3)* people with syndromes that present with multiple colorectal polyps (see following) are at very high risk of colorectal cancer. The current version of the sequence proposes that benign adenomatous polyps arise from proliferation of colonic crypt cells that lead to aberrant crypt foci and microadenomas. Macroscopic polyps undergo neoplastic transformation as they grow in size.

The fact that tissues at each stage of this process are accessible via colonoscopy or at surgery for cancer led Vogelstein and others to study molecular events at each stage of the transformation from normal epithelium to cancer (Fearon and Vogelstein, 1990). By studying somatic (acquired during life)

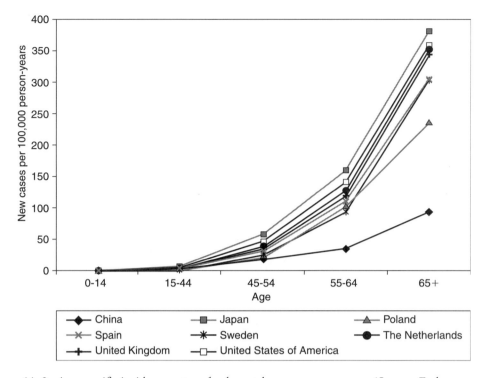

Figure 11–2. Age-specific incidence rates of colorectal cancer among men. (*Source*: Ferlay et al, 2004)

mutations in key genes controlling cellular proliferation and differention, they identified several genes that tend to mutate early in the adenoma-carcinoma sequence (especially mutation or loss of the *APC* gene), in the middle of the sequence (mutations in *KRAS*), and late in the sequence (the tumor-suppressor gene *p53*) (Fig. 11–5). This provided one of the first demonstrations in humans of the multihit theory, which implies that cancer arises in a cell that has sustained mutations or gene-activating or -

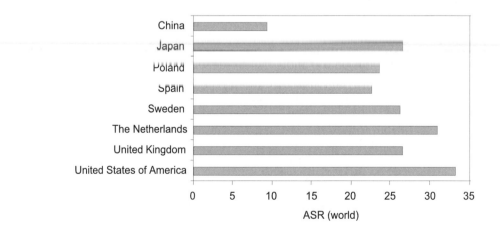

Figure 11–3. Age-standardized (to the world population) incidence rates of colorectal cancer among women. (*Source*: Ferlay et al., 2004)

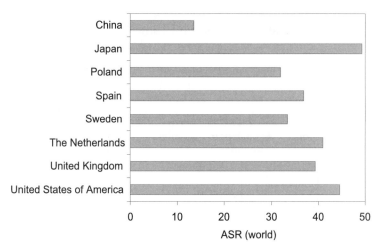

Figure 11–4. Age-standardized (to the world population) incidence rates of colorectal cancer among men. (*Source*: Ferlay et al, 2004)

inactivating events in multiple genes. This theory also accurately predicts that humans born with germline mutations (these are inherited and therefore in every cell in the body) in relevant genes would be at higher risk of colorectal cancer at an earlier age.

It is now clear that there are other pathways to colorectal cancer, the most important of these also having both an inherited and an acquired manifestation. Individuals with an inherited defect in DNA mismatch-repair genes are at elevated risk, particularly of colorectal cancer (see following). Silencing of these repair genes and other genes by hypermethylation is also a common event that gives rise to nonfamilial colorectal cancer, although the progression appears not to be via the canonical adenoma-carcinoma pathway but rather via hyperplastic polyp-serrated adenoma-carcinoma transitions and a process that produces the CpG island methylator phenotype (CIMP) (Issa, 2004). Other pathways and phenotypes have also been proposed (Jass et al, 2006).

Inherited Susceptibility

Individuals with a family history of colorectal cancer are themselves at increased risk of the disease. Having a first-degree relative with colorectal cancer approximately doubles the risk, and the risk increases with the proportion of relatives affected,

particularly if they are diagnosed at an early age (Woolf, 1958; Macklin, 1960). The major familial syndromes and key molecular mechanisms that underlie inherited susceptibility are the Mendelian dominant syndromes: familial adenomatous polyposis and hereditary nonpolyposis colorectal cancer, probably better called Lynch Syndrome. More recently, a recessive syndrome, associated with germline mutations in *MYH*, has been described.

Familial adenomatous polyposis

Familial adenomatous polyposis is a rare autosomal dominant syndrome (Veale, 1965) characterized by the development, sometimes from childhood, of multiple colorectal adenomas, numbering from a few polyps to several thousand. One or more of the polyps will almost always progress to cancer. Gardner syndrome is a closely related disorder in which adenomas also involve the small bowel, and extracolonic lesions such as osteomas and retinal changes may be present. These and some other rarer syndromes are caused by mutations in the *APC* gene, most of which introduce stop codons into the sequence and thus cause a truncated APC protein (Nishisho et al, 1991). The prevalence of these mutations is estimated to be about 1 in 10 000 individuals, and germline alterations in *APC*

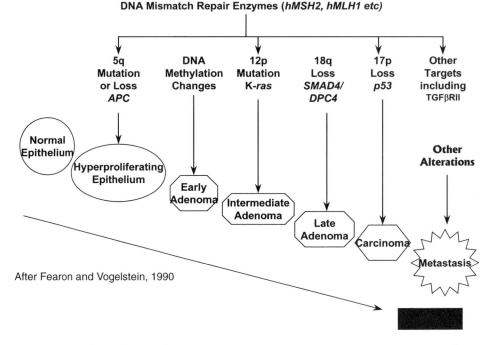

Figure 11–5. Hypothesized genes that are mutated in the pathway to colorectal cancers. (After Fearon and Vogelstein, 1990)

probably underlie less than 1% of all colorectal cancers.

This molecular model conforms to the classic two-hit model (Knudson, 1971), in which an inherited mutation in one allele combines with a somatic mutation in the other allele to produce a functionally homozygously deleted gene. Loss of both alleles is associated with the development of multiple initially benign adenomas, after which subsequent somatic mutations in other genes may cause malignant transformation of cells. Thus, as predicted by the multihit theory, multiple genetic events are needed to produce a cancer. A nontruncating intronic polymorphism of APC has been shown to occur among the Ashkenazim and to carry a modestly elevated risk of colorectal cancer (Laken et al, 1997). Similarly, a subset of APC mutations gives rise to an attenuated form of familial adenomatous polyposis, in

which only a few colon polyps appear (Spirio et al, 1998). Although the site and nature of the germline alterations in APC correlate somewhat with the different clinical entities, it is not possible to predict reliably the clinical consequences of a novel mutation. Nontruncating polymorphisms in APC may also be associated with modifications of risk (Slattery et al, 2001b).

Hereditary nonpolyposis colorectal cancer/Lynch Syndrome

Hereditary nonpolyposis colorectal cancer (HNPCC) is an inherited autosomal dominant syndrome (Lynch and Lynch, 1985) consisting of a tendency to early onset of colorectal cancer and a pattern of other cancers, particularly those involving the endometrium, urinary tract, stomach, and biliary system (Lynch et al, 1989). Initially, HNPCC was claimed to account for as many as 15%

of colorectal cancer cases. More recent studies suggest that this proportion may be around 2% or less (Aaltonen et al, 1998).

The DNA mismatch repair (MMR) system identifies and repairs errors that occur during DNA replication. A complex set of proteins recognize the mismatch, bind to it, excise the mismatched region, and resynthesize the correct sequence (Kolodner, 1995). Germline mutations in two genes in this system, *MSH2* and *MLH1*, account for a large majority of the HNPCC families identified to date (Peltomaki and de la Chapelle, 1997); germline mutations in *PMS1*, *PMS2*, and *MSH6* account for a small proportion.

The loss of MMR has several consequences, most crucially loss of proofreading and correction of small deletions and insertions in DNA (Umar and Kunkel, 1996). Runs of repetitive DNA sequences, such as (CA)n dinucleotide repeats, are particularly prone to expansion during replication in the presence of MMR deficiency, causing the microsatellite instability (MSI) characteristic of HNPCC tumors. The diagnosis of HNPCC can be suggested by examination of the tumor for microsatellite instability or by testing for germline mutations in the previously mentioned MMR genes. However, MSI, while common in HNPCC tumors, is neither sensitive nor specific, and screening for mutations in the relevant genes is expensive and less than 100% sensitive; current techniques may fail to detect some germline heterozygous mutations and deletions. Immunohistochemical techniques can be used to considerable advantage as a sensitive, highly specific, and cost-effective method of clinical diagnosis of specific MMR lesions, as well as in the research setting (Lindor et al, 2002). A proportion of MSI-positive tumors are due to somatic, not germline, mutation or hypermethylation occurring in the MMR genes.

Other hereditary syndromes
Biallelic inherited mutations in the base-excision repair gene, *MYH*, are associated with a specific pattern of polyposis and a considerably elevated risk of colorectal cancer (Al-Tassan et al, 2002; Jones et al,

2002; Sampson et al, 2003; Sieber et al, 2003; Croitoru et al, 2004).

Lindor et al (2005) and Mueller-Koch et al (2005) have recently described an inherited colorectal cancer syndrome, in which the families fit, broadly, Amsterdam-I criteria for a plausible diagnosis of Lynch Syndrome (HNPCC). However, two features clearly distinguish these families from Lynch Syndrome: *(1)* the absence of microsatellite instability; and *(2)* a family phenotype characterized largely by colorectal tumors rather than the multisite (especially endometrial and gastric cancers) phenotype characteristic of families with MMR defects. The genetic lesion in these Type X colorectal cancer families is not established.

Inherited polymorphisms that modify risk associated with exposures
A number of polymorphisms in a variety of pathways have now been established to modify risks associated with specific exposures. Others are suspected. Some are described in the following.

N-acetyltransferases (NAT1, NAT2) and CYP450 enzymes
Heterocyclic amines formed during the high-temperature cooking of animal protein are colorectal carcinogens in rodents. Thus, the question arises as to whether the metabolism of heterocyclic amines, which shows between-person genetic variability in at least three relevant enzymes—NAT1, NAT2, and CYP1A2—influences the risk of colorectal neoplasia associated with meat consumption (Kadlubar et al, 1992). Although CYP1A2 is phenotypically variable, the polymorphisms responsible for most of this variation have not been identified. The epidemiologic evidence for associations with genetic variants in *NAT1* and *NAT2* is mixed (Vineis and McMichael, 1996). The larger studies do not support an independent role for *NAT2* in cancer (Welfare et al, 1997; Chen et al, 1998; Slattery et al, 1998; Kampman et al, 1999) or in polyps (Probst-Hensch et al, 1995; Potter, 1999a). Although some investigators suggest an inter-

action with meat or tobacco smoke (Welfare et al, 1997; Chen et al, 1998; Chan et al. 2005b), the data are not consistent (Slattery et al, 1998; Potter et al, 1999; van der Hel et al, 2003; Tiemersma et al, 2004a; Tiemersma et al, 2004b). Results for NAT1 are also not consistent and suggest that there is no independent association with genotype (Bell et al, 1995; Probst-Hensch et al, 1996; Chen et al, 1998; Lin et al, 1998) Combinations of rapid NAT1, NAT2, and perhaps CYP1A2 genotypes may be associated with an elevated risk in the presence of tobacco smoking or high meat intake (Chen et al, 1998; Lilla et al, 2006).

Microsomal epoxide hydrolase

There have been at least 11 studies that have explored the role of polymorphisms in microsomal epoxide hydrolase (mEH) in relation to colrectal neoplasia—6 on cancer and 5 on adenomas. Most studies have examined polymorphisms in both Exon 3 (Tyr113His) and Exon 4 (His139Arg). None of the adenoma studies found any association with the genotypes themselves (Cortessis et al, 2001; Ulrich et al, 2001; Tiemersma et al, 2002); (Tranah et al, 2004) though Huang et al (2005) found a marginal association with advanced adenoma. Of the six studies of carcinoma, the smallest (101 cases/203controls) reported an elevated risk with the Exon 3 variant (Harrison et al, 1999). In contrast, Sachse et al (2002) reported an inverse association between Exon 3 variant alleles and cancer risk in a study of 433 case-control pairs, as did Tranah et al (Tranah et al, 2005) in the Harvard cohorts with the Exon 4 variant. The other three studies including the largest (1 593 cases/ 1 960 controls) found no association between the polymorphisms and CRC risk (Mitrou et al, 2002; Robien et al, 2005; van der Logt et al, 2006).

The data on interactions between mEH polymorphisms and smoking and meat consumption suggest that there may be an association between these interactions and adenoma risk but the specific exon involved and even the direction are not consistent, suggesting that, if there is an association, it is not simple (Cortessis et al, 2001; Ulrich et al, 2001; Tiemersma et al, 2002; Tranah et al, 2004; Huang et al, 2005). Of the six studies of CRC, three did not collect exposure data (Harrison et al, 1999; Sachse et al, 2002; van der Logt et al, 2006), one reported an elevated risk associated with Exon 4 variant alleles in smokers (Mitrou et al, 2002), and the other two found no evidence for interactions with either polymorphism (Robien et al, 2005; Tranah et al, 2005).

The folate pathway

Vegetables and multivitamin supplements have been suggested to be associated with a reduced risk of colorectal cancer. One of the postulated nutrients potentially responsible for these associations is folic acid. Folate is central to methyl-group metabolism and may influence both methylation of DNA and the available nucleotide pool for DNA replication and repair (Fig. 11–6). There is some evidence, albeit not entirely consistent, that folate and vitamin B12 (a cofactor in this pathway) are associated with a reduced risk of colorectal neoplasia (Freudenheim et al, 1991; Giovannucci et al, 1993b); (Giovannucci et al, 1995b; Slattery et al, 1997b). A growing body of evidence suggests that MTHFR, a polymorphic enzyme (C677T and A1298C), influences this association such that those at highest risk for both adenomas and cancer have the variant (677TT) genotype and low intakes of folate and vitamin B12 and high intakes of alcohol (Giovannucci et al, 1993b; Chen et al, 1996; Ma et al, 1997; Ulrich et al, 1999, Le Marchand et al, 2002; Marugame et al, 2003; Boyapati et al, 2004, Ulvik et al, 2004; Yin et al, 2004; Hirose et al, 2005; Le Marchand et al, 2005; Matsuo et al, 2005;).

Nonetheless, the complete story is more complex than was initially thought because those with the variant (TT) genotype in the presence of an adequate folate and vitamin B12 intake have, if anything, a somewhat reduced risk of colorectal neoplasia (Chen et al, 1996; Ulrich et al, 1999). The risk of carcinogenesis increases only when there is both a deficiency of folate and a variant

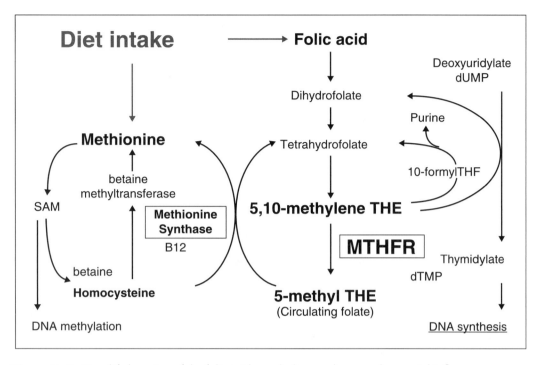

Figure 11–6. Simplifed version of the folic acid metabolism pathway and potential influences on DNA methylation and DNA synthesis. MTHFR:methylene-tetrahyrofolate reductase.

genotype (Ulrich et al, 1999), resulting in limited transfer of methyl groups as well as abnormalities of DNA synthesis, including misincorporation of uracil in place of thymidine. This misincorporation can cause increased chromosome breakage. Conversely, under conditions characterized by high folate/B12 intakes, among individuals with a variant genotype, 5,10-methylene-THF is increased, reducing uracil misincorporation during DNA synthesis and potentially reducing the risk of colonic neoplasia (Chen et al, 1996). These mechanisms are complex because both general hypomethylation of DNA and hypermethylation of specific gene-promoter regions are characteristic of colorectal cancer. Other possible interactions have been suggested (Curtin et al, 2004). Most recently, to identify low-penetrance alleles associated with colorectal cancer, Webb et al genotyped 1467 nonsynonymous SNPs in approximately 2500 cases and 2700 controls. They identified the *MTHFR* variant genotype as being associated with reduced risk

(OR = 0.82; 95% CI: 0.69–0.97) (Webb et al, 2006).

Other polymorphic genes in the folate pathway that have some suggested links to colorectal neoplasia, often with suggestions of specific environmental interactions, include thymidylate synthase (Ulrich et al, 2002; Chen et al, 2004a; Matsuo et al, 2005; Ulrich et al, 2005), methionine synthase (Ma et al, 1999; Le Marchand et al, 2002; Goode et al, 2004; Matsuo et al, 2005), methionine synthase reductase (Le Marchand et al, 2002), and reduced folate carrier (Chen et al, 2004b; Ulrich et al, 2005). Some folate-gene polymorphisms do not appear important (Chen et al, 2004b). For relevant reviews, also see Sharp and Little (2004) and Ulrich (2005).

NSAID metabolism and the prostaglandin pathway
There are extensive data now to show that aspirin and other nonsteroidal anti-inflammatory drugs (NSAIDs) reduce risk of colorectal neoplasia (see following).

Here we briefly consider the evidence that polymorphisms in both the metabolic pathway for NSAIDs and the downstream prostaglandin synthesis pathway are associated with altered risk.

There are data to show that variation in the metabolism of aspirin and NSAIDs, particularly a slow version of *UGT1A6* (with plausibly higher blood levels of aspirin and its metabolites), is associated with greater protection by aspirin (Bigler et al, 2001; Chan et al, 2005a), though there are null findings also (McGreavey et al, 2005). Other UGTs may also be important (Kuehl et al, 2005). Thus, genetic variability can modify the preventive potential of NSAIDs.

Polymorphisms also exist in key enzymes in the prostaglandin synthesis pathway, although a number of the enzymes (eg, PTGS 1 and 2, also known as COX 1 and 2) are not very polymorphic. Some of these are associated with alteration of risk of colorectal neoplasia, with some evidence of interactions with dietary sources of arachodanic acid and with NSAIDs; (see, for example: Lin et al, 2002; Cox et al, 2004; Goodman et al, 2004; Koh et al, 2004; Siezen et al, 2005; Ulrich et al, 2005; Poole et al, 2006). There is some suggestion that COX activity can be suppressed genetically or by NSAIDs, but that there is no synergy—an observation that has also been made for the *IL-10*–1082 G>A polymorphism (Sansbury et al, 2006). For a review, see Ulrich et al, (2006).

Other Genes

Other genes that have been implicated in the etiology or progression of human colorectal cancer, either as a result of biomarker studies or investigations of genetic polymorphisms, include: other DNA repair genes (Goode et al, 2002; Kim et al, 2004: Bigler et al, 2005; Jin et al, 2005; Slattery et al, 2005; Stern et al, 2005; Yu et al, 2006; Weiss et al, 2005); hormone receptors (Slattery et al, 2005); insulin, insulin-like growth factors and binding proteins, C-peptide, and glycosylated hemoglobin (Slattery et al, 2004; Le Marchand et al, 2005; Morimoto et al, 2005; Wong et al, 2005; Wei et al, 2006; Zecevic et al, 2006); and

possibly *PPARγ* and δ (Gong et al, 2005; Jiang et al, 2005; Murtaugh,et al, 2005; Siezen et al, 2005; Siezen et al, 2006).

In summary, a proportion of colorectal cancers, probably no more than 10%, are due to inherited mutations in single genes such as APC, hMSH2, and hMLH1. A higher but very uncertain proportion may be partially caused by inheritance of variants in metabolic or other genes that alter the way in which lifestyle factors, such as diet or specific agents such as NSAIDs, influence the risk. Much larger data sets will be needed to sort through the many variants in potential candidate genes before we can be certain of these interactions. Some of the relevant exposures are discussed in the following.

RISK FACTORS

Tobacco

Smoking cigarettes had originally not been associated with an elevated risk of colorectal cancer, although an association with cigar and pipe smoking has been described (Wynder and Shigematsu, 1967; Slattery et al, 1990). However, several more recent studies have noted an increased risk of colon cancer with early onset and a long history of cigarette smoking (Giovannucci et al, 1994a), although no association was seen in a large Italian case-control study (Tavani et al, 1998) or in a prospective study of male Swedish construction workers (Nyrén et al, 1996). More recent data suggest that smoking may be largely associated with microsatellite unstable (MSI+) colorectal cancer (Slattery et al, 2000) and, relatedly, in tumors that show loss of MLH1 expression rather than APC mutations (Lüchtenborg et al, 2005). The pathway is plausibly through hyperplastic polyps and serrated adenomas rather than the APC truncation-mutation pathway (Morimoto et al, 2002).

Tobacco smoke is a major source of a wide variety of carcinogens, including heterocyclic amines, polycyclic hydrocarbons, and nitrosamines. These are plausible bloodborne carcinogens. For instance, evidence from rat models shows that heterocyclic amines cause specific *APC* mutations (Kakiuchi et al, 1995); this pattern of deletion mutation does not occur in human tumors. However, if the association is essentially with MSI+ tumors, then smoking may act, in colon cancer, not just as a source of carcinogens but also as a stimulus to methylation of *MLH1*. Such a mechanism has not been identified. Although NSAIDs generally reduce the risk of colorectal neoplasia, they may not be effective in heavy smokers, especially against MSI+ tumors (Chia et al, 2006.

Diet

Ecologic studies correlating the international variation in per capita consumption of specific foods and nutrients with colorectal cancer incidence and mortality rates led to numerous hypotheses about an adverse influence of red meat and higher fat intake, and beneficial effects of fruit, vegetable, and fiber intakes. Evidence from case-control and cohort studies is less consistent (Potter et al, 1993; Steinmetz and Potter, 1996; WCRF Panel, 1997).

Vegetables, fruits, and constituent fiber and micronutrients

Several prospective studies examining vegetable and fruit consumption and colon cancer risk reported modest, but not entirely consistent, findings of lower risk associated with higher consumption (Potter et al, 1993; Steinmetz and Potter, 1996; WCRF Panel, 1997). One study reported on rectal cancer in Seventh-day Adventists, showing a small, statistically nonsignificant reduction in risk with higher consumption of green salad. In a cohort study of Adventists, a somewhat lower risk of colorectal cancer with higher intake of a variety of plant foods was observed, but this was statistically significant only for legumes (Singh and Fraser, 1998). In a follow-up study of 61 463 Swedish women in whom 460 cases of colorectal cancer occurred (Terry et al, 2001), low fruit and vegetable consumption (< 1.5 servings per day) was associated with a relative risk of 1.65; this association was due largely to low fruit intake. However, in a prospective study

among 88 776 women and 47 325 men, no relation of intake of either fruits or vegetables to the risk of colon or rectal cancer was apparent (Michels et al, 2000).

Almost all case-control studies of vegetable and fruit consumption and colon cancer have reported some degree of reduced risk with higher consumption of at least one category of vegetable or fruit (Potter et al, 1993; WCRF Panel, 1997). The results have been particularly consistent for raw, green, and cruciferous vegetables. In a meta-analysis of six case-control studies of vegetables and colon cancer (Trock et al, 1990), a combined relative risk of 0.48 for the highest versus the lowest quantiles of consumption was calculated. In about half of the case-control studies of rectal cancer, a statistically significant inverse association was observed for at least one vegetable or fruit category, most consistently for cruciferous vegetables. Each of five case-control studies of adenomas that examined vegetables as a broad category found an inverse association that was, however, not always statistically significant (Potter et al, 1993; WCRF Panel, 1997). Reported data on fruit consumption and colorectal cancer risk are less abundant and the findings less consistent than those for vegetables. A recent cohort study from the Netherlands suggested that any beneficial effects of fruits may be confined to those colon tumors that do not express MLH1 (Wark et al, 2005). Nurses' Health Study data suggest that fruit and legumes may be associated with a lower risk of adenomas (Michels et al, 2006). Neither of these studies found a statistically significant association with vegetable consumption.

Vegetables contain a large number of substances, both micronutrients with antioxidant activity, such as carotenoids and ascorbate, and other bioactive compounds with a variety of potent anticarcinogenic properties, such as phenols, flavonoids, isothiocyanates, and indoles (Wattenberg, 1978; Steinmetz and Potter, 1991). One comprehensive overview concluded that the "evidence that diets rich in vegetables protect against cancers of the colon and rectum is convincing" (WCRF Panel, 1997). The absent or much smaller inverse association seen in prospective studies published after this overview is disturbing, however. These results suggest that the association between fruit and vegetable intake may be limited to specific foods, may be nonlinear, may be part of a more complex dietary pattern rather than a simple function of fruit and vegetable intake, or may suggest that some aspects of vegetables themselves are changing (Potter, 2005).

Overall, the relationship of fiber to risk of colorectal cancer is inconsistent, perhaps because of the heterogeneous nature of fiber and differences in the way in which fiber intake is measured (WCRF Panel, 1997; Potter, 1999b). A role for dietary fiber—derived from vegetables as well as grains—in colon carcinogenesis was first proposed by Dennis Burkitt based on observations in Africa (Burkitt, 1969). Data from cohort studies are only weakly supportive of the fiber hypothesis, with two studies finding no association and two finding a weak inverse association. In a large cohort study of total dietary fiber, no association with either incident carcinoma or adenoma in women was reported (Fuchs et al, 1999). Only one prospective study has provided data on rectal cancer, and there was little evidence of an association. However, combined analysis of 13 case-control studies found a reduction in colorectal cancer risk with increasing intake of dietary fiber (Howe et al, 1992). Similar findings have been reported for a meta-analysis of 16 case-control studies (Trock et al, 1990).

In a prospective study, high intake of fiber from vegetables and cereals was associated with a halving of the risk for colorectal adenomas (Giovannucci et al, 1992). Case-control studies have found inverse associations with total fiber, fiber from cereals, and fiber from vegetables and fruits (WCRF Panel, 1997, p.196). The most recent cohort results on dietary fiber do not resolve the discrepancies. The PLCO cohort found that those in the highest quintile of dietary fiber intake had a 27% lower risk of distal colonic (but not rectal) adenoma than

those in the lowest quintile of intake (Peters et al, 2003). In the EPIC study of approximately two million person-years and more than 1000 cases of colorectal cancer in Europe, dietary fiber in foods was associated with a 25% reduction in risk from bottom to top quintile, with the strongest association in the left colon and the weakest in the rectum (echoing the PLCO findings) (Bingham et al, 2003).

However, in a comparable study (1.8 million person-years; approximately 1000 cases) in the US, a similar analysis to the EPIC study showed a hazard ratio of 0.91 (0.87–95), but adjusting for additional confounders (including folate, red meat, processed meat, and glycemic load) caused this association to disappear (Michels et al, 2005a). Two other differences in these studies involve dietary methods and the possibility that differences in the food supply on each side of the Atlantic matter. In a pooled analysis of 13 cohort studies with 8081 cases, findings were similar; a significant inverse age-adjusted association with dietary fiber intake was no longer significant after adjusting for other risk factors (Park et al, 2005). Fiber ferments in the large bowel to produce short-chain fatty acids and butyrate, an inducer of apoptosis in colonic cell lines (Hague and Paraskeva, 1995). Butyrate does modify carcinogenesis in animal models under some circumstances but not universally (for a review, see Sengupta et al, 2006). Other mechanisms have been proposed (Ishizuka et al, 2004).

Results of intervention studies have been much less supportive than observational studies of the hypotheses that vegetables and/or dietary fiber are inversely associated with risk. Data from an intervention trial in patients with familial adenomatous polyposis who were randomized to a diet that included higher fiber intake were not clearly supportive (DeCosse et al, 1989). Three randomized trials examined the risk of subsequent development of colorectal adenomas in patients diagnosed with a prior adenoma. In Australia, adenoma patients were randomized in a factorial design to an intervention including a low-fat diet, a

25-g wheat-bran supplement, and a 20-mg beta-carotene supplement daily. No overall significant reduction in metachronous adenoma incidence was detected after 4 years; however, the risk of large adenomas was reduced among patients in the low-fat-plus-wheat-bran arm (MacLennan et al, 1995).

In Arizona, 1429 men and women were randomized to either a high (13.5 g/day) or low (2 g/day) wheat-bran fiber supplement. After a median follow-up period of 3 years, the relative risk of metachronous adenoma in the high-fiber group was not significantly reduced (Alberts et al, 2000). In the largest such study, about 2000 American men and women were randomized either to a low-fat, high-fiber, increased fruit and vegetables diet, or to their usual diet. After 4 years, the relative risk of having at least one metachronous adenoma was 1.00 (Schatzkin et al, 2000).

These studies clearly demonstrate that short-term dietary interventions with increased fiber or fruit and vegetables do not reduce the risk of metachronous adenoma. Weaknesses in design include relatively short periods of intervention and study subjects who already have at least one adenoma and who thus may already be "primed" for the development of more adenomas. The multihit hypothesis of colorectal cancer (Fig. 11–5) implies the accumulation of damage in multiple genes over many years or decades. Thus, commencing an intervention among people who may already have many colonic epithelial cells well advanced on the pathway to colon adenoma may not be as good of a test of the intervention as one applied early in life for a longer period. These studies are also tests of new adenoma formation and thus do not test interventions that may modify the transition from adenoma to cancer.

Accordingly, interpretability of these randomized studies is somewhat limited. It is unlikely, however, that intervention studies large and long enough to test the influence of fruits, vegetables, and/or fiber on cancer risk will be designed and conducted. In the United States, the Womens' Health Initiative clinical trial had a major focus on assessing the effects of a low-fat diet on breast cancer risk among about 48 000 women. Women in the intervention arm were specifically counseled to increase fruit and vegetable intake; the results of this trial failed to provide evidence for benefits of this specific dietary pattern on the risk of colorectal cancer (Beresford et al, 2006).

Other nutrients have been invoked to explain the possibly reduced risk associated with vegetables (Steinmetz and Potter, 1991; Steinmetz and Potter, 1996). Freudenheim and colleagues, who first proposed the folate/colorectal cancer hypothesis, found lower risks of both colon and rectal cancer in association with high folate intakes in their case-control study (Freudenheim et al, 1991). Total folate intake and dietary folate were not associated, however, with differences in the risk of colon cancer in a cohort of men (Giovannucci et al, 1995b). Nonetheless, an increase in the risk of colon cancer was seen among men with a combination of low folate intake and methionine and high alcohol intake. Similar results were shown for adenomatous polyps in the same cohort study (Giovannucci et al, 1993b).

In a large multicenter case-control study, Slattery et al (1997b) found no association between micronutrients involved in methyl-group metabolism and the risk of colon cancer. In discussing a meta-analysis of seven cohort studies, Sanjoaquin et al (2005) cautiously concluded that folate from foods (but not supplements) may be associated with a reduced risk (RR = 0.75; 95% CI 0.64–0.89) of colorectal cancer. Some regard the evidence as insufficient to recommend folate to prevent colorectal cancer (Bollheimer et al, 2005).

In a large cohort of US women, long-term use of multivitamin supplements (that typically contain 400 mg of folate) was associated with a halving of the risk of colorectal cancer (Giovannucci et al, 1998). A similar halving of the risk associated with both vitamin E and multivitamin supplement use was observed by White et al (1997). In an observational study of adenoma recurrence, multivitamin use, vitamin E supplementation, and calcium supplementation (Whelan et al, 1999) were all associated with a 40% to 50% decreased risk of new adenoma development over a mean period of 37 months. Jacobs et al (2003) observed that, in the ACS Cancer Prevention Study II of almost 150 000 men and women, regular multivitamin use at baseline was not associated with reduced risk whereas reported use 10 years earlier showed a relative risk of 0.71 (95% CI: 0.57–0.89).

The Nurses' Health Study and Health Professionals Follow-up Study data show a lower risk for men who took vitamin E supplements, but not women (Wu et al, 2002). Satia-Abouta et al (2003) showed that a variety of micronutrients (including vitamins C and E) were higher in controls than colon cancer cases with most of the differences being explained by supplement use. Higher-serum selenum has been reported to be associated with a lower risk of adenoma (Connelly-Frost et al, 2006). In summary, colorectal adenoma and cancer development may be partly preventable through vitamin and mineral supplementation but the data are not entirely consistent.

Meat
The weight of the evidence points to an elevated risk of colorectal cancer with meat eating, even though the findings are neither strong nor entirely consistent. Several cohort studies have examined meat intake and the risk of colorectal neoplasia. In a study of nurses, women who consumed red meat frequently versus rarely had a 2.5-fold increase in the risk of colon cancer (Willett et al, 1990). Male health professionals who consumed five or more servings per week of beef, pork, or lamb also had a statistically significantly increased risk of colon cancer compared with men who consumed these meats less than once per month (Giovannucci et al, 1994b). In contrast, the large American Cancer Society mortality follow-up study (Cancer Prevention Study II) showed no difference in the risk of colo-

rectal cancer death between persons in the uppermost and lowest quintiles of meat consumption of either sex (Thun et al, 1992). Cohorts in the Netherlands, Finland, and Iowa (WCRF Panel, 1997) also showed no increase in risk with meat consumption.

The most recent cohort data from Europe (Norat et al, 2005), Australia (English et al, 2004), and the US (Chao et al, 2005) suggest that both fresh and processed meat are associated with elevated risks of colorectal cancer. However, reduction of meat intake in a randomized trial did not influence the incidence of metachronous adenomas (Mathew et al, 2004). Two of the four cohort studies that examined processed meat showed statistically significant higher risks of colorectal cancer with higher consumption, and one showed a weakly elevated risk (WCRF Panel, 1997). Processed meat has also been shown to be associated with adenoma risk (Robertson et al, 2005).

Most estimates of relative risk associated with meat consumption reported in these cohort studies are greater than 1.0, and none are less than 0.75 or statistically significantly less than 1.0 (WCRF Panel, 1997). Two cohort studies focused on meat consumption within low-consuming populations. One found no association with colorectal cancer mortality (Key et al, 1998), and the other found an elevated risk in Adventists with higher consumption of both red and white meat (Singh and Fraser, 1998).

As with the cohort studies, almost all estimates of risk from case-control studies of colorectal neoplasia are increased or null with higher meat intake. However, the largest case-control study observed no overall association with red or white meat consumption (Kampman et al, 1999). Some of these elevated risks were specific to or more marked in women; some findings were stronger for the rectum than for the colon. About half of the studies that reported on processed or cured meats found statistically significantly elevated risks, whereas the others showed no association. A study in Sweden reported a relative risk of 2.7 for colon cancer and 6.0 for rectal cancer among the most frequent consumers of fried meat with a heavily browned surface (Gerhardsson de Verdier et al, 1991). Schiffman and Felton (1990) also reported a 3.5-fold increase in risk for those preferring well-done meat.

Comparable findings have been seen in two case-control studies of adenomatous polyps (Probst-Hensch et al, 1997; Sinha et al, 1999) and in a large US case-control study (Kampman et al, 1999). However, a subsequent study in Sweden did not observe any positive association with method of meat preparation or with a calculated index of heterocyclic amine consumption with either site or colorectal cancer combined (Augustsson et al, 1999). As noted previously, heterocyclic amines and PAHs have been implicated earlier as the possible causal agents in meat. More recently, heme and nitrosation (Bingham et al, 2002; Cross et al, 2003) and 06 carboxymethyl guanine have been added to the list (Lewin et al, 2006).

Dietary fat
In the aggregate, modern epidemiologic studies have failed to find clear evidence for the association of colorectal cancer with dietary fat. Most cohort studies have found no association with total fat intake (WCRF Panel, 1997), although among female nurses, total fat intake in the highest versus the lowest quintile was associated with a twofold increased risk of colon cancer (Willett et al, 1990). In contrast, a decreased risk with higher intakes of total fat was found among Hawaiian-Japanese men. The large majority of the case-control studies of fat reported increased risks in association with higher intakes; relative risks ranged from 1.3 to 2.2. Following adjustment for energy intake, some investigators found no association, others a statistically significant increase in risk (WCRF Panel, 1997). In a combined analysis of 13 case-control studies from various populations with differing cancer risks and diets, no dietary fat variable was associated with colorectal cancer

after adjustment for total energy intake. Further, there were no convincing associations for any type of fat in subgroup analyses by sex, age, or anatomic location of the cancer (Howe et al, 1997).

Some cohort studies specifically analyzed saturated or animal fat. Among female nurses, the highest intakes of animal fat entailed an almost twofold greater risk than the lowest intakes (Willett et al, 1990). Smaller increases in risk were seen with high consumption of saturated fat. A small increase in the risk of colon cancer was reported for women but not men in the Netherlands cohort (Goldbohm et al, 1994). No substantial associations between saturated or animal fat were seen in another two cohort studies. Many case-control studies have examined associations between intake of saturated and/or animal fat and the risk of colon, rectal, or colorectal cancer; the results of these studies are inconsistent (WCRF Panel, 1997).

In summary, about half of the cohort and case-control studies show some evidence of elevated risk associated with higher intakes of saturated/animal fat, and no study shows the opposite. Thus, although the evidence of higher risk for saturated/animal fat is more consistent than that for total fat, the data are not entirely convincing. Giovannucci and Goldin (1997) concluded that the association with red meat does not appear to be mediated by its lipid content. Evidence for hypotheses related to the protein and iron content of red meat appears weaker still (WCRF Panel, 1997). Reduction of dietary fat in the randomized trial within the Womens Health Initiative did not reduce risk of colorectal cancer (Beresford et al, 2006).

Overall, the data suggest a stronger association with meat than with any of the associated nutrients. Moreover, although both processed meat and saturated/animal fat are possibly associated with an increased risk of colorectal cancer, neither total fat nor total protein seems to play a major role. Overall, the public health recommendation is clear, both for coronary heart disease and for cancer: "If eaten at all, limit intake of red meat to less than three ounces daily" (WCRF Panel, 1997, p199).

Calcium and Vitamin D

The association between higher intake of calcium, dairy foods, and colorectal neoplasia has been explored epidemiologically (for early studies, see references in Potter et al, 1993; WCRF Panel, 1997); initially, the results were tantalizing but inconsistent. Most of the early evidence, however, did suggest a reduced risk or no association. In one large case-control study, the adjusted relative risk for the highest quintile of dietary calcium consumption versus the lowest was 0.6 in both men and women (Kampman et al, 2000). Intervention data showed that calcium reduces proliferation in the upper part of the colonic crypt (Bostick et al, 1995), and observational data indicate that it reduces the likelihood of the growth of metachronous adenomas (Hyman et al, 1998). A double-blind, randomized trial comparing 1200 mg of elemental calcium per day with placebo showed a statistically significant 15% to 20% reduction in the incidence of metachronous colorectal adenomas (Baron et al, 1999).

Subsequent further analyses of these trial data showed that the reduction of metachronous adenoma risk with calcium was seen only among those with serum baseline 25-(OH) vitamin D levels above the median and, additionally, that those with high 25-(OH) vitamin D levels experienced a reduced risk only if they received calcium supplements (Grau et al, 2003). These data speak strongly to an interaction between vitamin D and calcium in determining risk. Other cohort and intervention studies have added to what is known. In relation to adenomas, two observational cohort studies within intervention studies showed that higher calcium and vitamin D (Hartman et al, 2005) or calcium alone (Peters et al, 2004) were associated with reduced risk of adenoma.

A pooled analysis of cohort studies (Cho et al, 2004a) and three other cohort studies (Terry et al, 2002; Flood et al, 2005; Lin et al, 2005) all showed a reduced risk of colorectal cancer with dietary calcium and sometimes with specific sources of calcium such as dairy products and supplements. The WHI Calcium plus Vitamin D Supplementation Trial showed no reduction in risk of colorectal cancer over 7 years, possibly due to the relatively low level of supplementation (Wactawski-Wende et al, 2006). A useful review summary of the majority of the calcium studies is Chia and Newcomb (2004).

There is thus evidence that both dairy foods and supplemental calcium may be inversely associated with risk, possibly especially in the presence of elevated vitamin D. Hence, either increased intake of dairy products, supplements, or both may be recommended in the future for colorectal cancer risk reduction.

Coffee

In a meta-analysis of 12 case-control studies and 5 cohort studies in the United States, Asia, and Europe, an overall inverse association of coffee consumption and colorectal cancer risk was observed (Giovannucci, 1998). Tavani and La Vecchia (2004) drew similar conclusions from many of the same data and commented on the lack of a similar association with decaffeinated coffee. Findings for both coffee preparations are exactly opposite to those reported specifically among the Harvard cohorts in which the association with caffeinated coffee was null but statistically significantly inverse for decaffeinated coffee (Michels et al, 2005b).

Other diet and food related variables

Certain other food and dietary-behavior variables have been, to varying degrees, associated with an increased risk of colorectal neoplasia—for example, egg consumption, sugar intake, and more frequent eating. Some others are associated with a possibly decreased risk—for example, complex carbohydrates (Potter et al, 1993; WCRF Panel, 1997). The evidence is sparse and insufficient to assess these associations adequately, although several of these are plausibly associated with a higher risk of obesity and an elevated glycemic load (Michaud et al, 2005).

Alcohol

Most studies have shown increased risk with higher alcohol consumption. Out of five general-population cohort studies, four showed statistically significant positive associations between alcohol consumption and the risk of colorectal cancer, as did each of the three studies that explored rectal cancer risk and two of the three studies that reported on colorectal cancer (WCRF Panel. 1997). A recent pooled cohort analysis showed an elevated risk for both colon and rectum, a dose-response relationship, no heterogeneity by study or sex, and no differences by specific alcoholic beverage (Cho et al, 2004b). Alcohol was also associated with an increased risk of colon and rectal cancer in about half of the case-control studies (WCRF Panel, 1997). Acetaldehyde (a metabolite of alcohol) is a potent DNA adduct former; alcohol may also inhibit DNA repair (Farinati et al, 1985) and may exert its effect through associated deficiencies in nutrients, particularly folate (Garro and Lieber, 1990; Giovannucci et al, 1995b).

The WCRF report concluded that "high alcohol consumption probably increases the risk of cancers of the colon and rectum" and that the association is likely to be "related to total ethanol intake, irrespective of the type of drink" (WCRF Panel, 1997, p.200).

Reproductive Factors

In 1969, an excess not only of some reproductive cancers but also of colon cancer was observed among nuns (Fraumeni et al, 1969). Several case-control studies in the 1970s and 1980s noted a higher risk of colon cancer among nulliparous women. It was initially hypothesized that this association might be due to changes in lipids and bile acids that occur with changes in the hormonal milieu (McMichael and Potter, 1980). Subsequent evidence that estrogen-receptor expression in the colonic epithelium declines with age is also compatible with a role of hormones in colon cancer (Issa et al, 1994; Potter et al, 1996).

More than 20 epidemiologic studies have reported on the relationships with reproductive history in women. Overall, age at first birth was not associated with colon cancer risk. The conservative interpretation of the parity data is similar, especially given that all the cohort studies show no association (Potter et al, 1993). Nevertheless, the differences between the findings of the cohort and population-based case-control studies remain to be explained (Slattery et al, 1994). Moreover, the hormone association may be with a particular molecular subset of colon tumors (see following). Also see the following for a discussion of the role of exogenous hormones in colon cancer, where the associations are more consistent.

Anthropometric Measures

Overall, the evidence suggests that obesity may increase the risk of colon cancer, particularly in men, but, as with physical activity (see following), this does not appear to apply to rectal cancer. Most epidemiologic studies have found that men who are in the highest quantile for body size, classifiable as obese, have as much as a twofold increased risk of colon cancer (Potter et al, 1993; WCRF Panel, 1997; Singh and Fraser, 1998). However, some studies have shown no association between body mass index (BMI) and colon cancer risk in men (Potter et al, 1993; WCRF Panel, 1997). Data on women are less consistent. Two cohort studies found no association between BMI and the risk of colorectal cancer (WCRF Panel, 1997). However, the Iowa Women's Health Study showed that subjects who were in the highest quintile of BMI had a statistically significant 40% higher risk than those in the lowest quintile (Bostick et al, 1994). Three case-control studies have also reported inconsistent findings for women (WCRF Panel, 1997). Recent data from a prospective study in Japan, in contrast, suggested that obesity and excessive weight gain were associated with risk of colon cancer in women but not men (Tamakoshi et al, 2004).

A large US multicenter case-control noted that while BMI was not associated with an elevated risk at high levels of long-term vigorous physical activity, at lower levels of such activity, risk appeared to be related both to total energy intake and to BMI. The relative risk for those who were least active, had the highest energy intake, and had the highest BMI was 3.4 compared with the opposite extreme. The association was explained solely by the findings for men, in whom the relative risk for a comparison of the extremes was 7.2; there was little association in women (Slattery et al, 1997a). A high waist/hip ratio is associated with increased risk in men (Giovannucci et al, 1995a) but not in women (Bostick et al, 1994). Data from the Framingham Study showed that waist circumference was a rather better predictor of lifetime colon cancer risk than BMI and that, unlike BMI, this association was similar in men and women (Moore et al, 2004).

The reduction of the risk of colon cancer in women associated with specific hormone exposures—whether oral contraceptives, postmenopausal hormones, parity, or postmenopausal obesity (obese women, as noted previously, are not at reduced risk but do not experience the same degree of risk elevation as seen in men (Slattery et al, 1997a; IARC, 2002))—may be confined to MSI-positive tumors (Slattery et al, 2001a). What remains to be established is the mechanistic link between hormones and DNA mismatch repair.

Physical Activity

The relation between physical activity and a reduced risk of colon cancer is among the most consistent findings in the epidemiologic literature, reported in studies of occupational activity, leisure activity, and total activity (Potter et al, 1993; WCRF Panel, 1997). Of nine cohort studies, only two reported no substantial association. Case-control studies are also consistent: Of 11 studies, only 1 noted an increased risk of colon cancer with higher total activity. The remainder showed inverse associations. Individuals with high levels of activity throughout their lives are at the lowest risk, whereas those who reported high levels of activity more recently show weaker inverse associations. There is little evidence that the rectal cancer risk is modified by physical activity. Two recent reviews (Lee, 2003; Slattery, 2004) and a meta-analysis (Samad et al, 2005) provide useful summaries of the state of play.

According to one hypothesis, physical activity stimulates colon peristalsis, thereby decreasing the time that colonic contents are in contact with the epithelium. However, transit time is not a well-established risk factor for colon neoplasia. Exercise has both acute and persistent hormonal effects, as well as favorable effects on the immune system (Potter et al, 1993). Furthermore, higher physical activity, especially in subjects with a low BMI, is associated with a general metabolic milieu (lower insulin, glucose, and triacylglycerol levels and possibly lower levels of other growth factors) that is less favorable to the growth of cancer in general and perhaps colon cancer in particular (McMichael and Potter, 1980; McMichael and Potter, 1985; McKeown-Eyssen, 1994; Giovannucci, 1995; WCRF Panel, 1997).

Infection

A number of infectious organisms have been suggested to increase risk of colorectal cancer. In a small study, a higher prevalence of IgG antibodies to *Helicobacter pylori* was observed in cases with colorectal adenoma than among controls. The authors speculate that increased gastrin levels in *H. pylori*-infected persons may exert a trophic effect on the colonic mucosa (Breuer-Katschinski et al, 1999). In one small study, a nonsignificant positive association between the presence of *H. pylori* antibodies and colorectal cancer was observed (Talley et al, 1991). A recent meta-analysis suggested a small elevation in risk (Zumkeller et al, 2006). Larger studies are needed to clarify this issue. Mucosa-associated lymphoid tissue (MALT) lymphoma in the colon has been reported to regress following antibiotic treatment (Raderer et al, 2000) and, as with gastric MALT lymphoma, presumably due to *H. pylori* eradication.

Limited ecologic and case-control data suggest an association of infection with Schistosoma japonicum in Japan and China and colorectal cancer risk. In one study, the association between a history of schistoso-miasis was statistically significant for pa-tients with rectal cancer but not colon cancer (Xu and Su, 1984).

JC Virus has been reported in colorectal cancers (Laghi et al, 1999; Enam et al, 2002), though not consistently (Newcomb et al, 2004). A mechanism of action has been proposed whereby the infection triggers the chromosomal instability pathway (Niv et al, 2005).

Ionizing Radiation

A significant excess of colon, but not rec-tum, cancer has been reported in follow-up of the Japanese atomic bomb survivors. However, the results of follow-up studies of medical exposures are inconsistent, and a precise dose–response relation has not been established (Thompson et al, 1994).

Occupation

Colon cancer risk is elevated in white-collar occupations, presumably due to the lower physical activity in these more sedentary jobs (Chow et al, 1994). An association with asbestos exposure has been observed intermittently; however, the excess risk, if any, is likely to be small (Kang et al, 1997). Recent data from the (female) Shanghai Textile Workers Cohort suggests that there may be an excess risk associated with dyes and metals and, intriguingly, a reduced risk associated with cotton and cotton dust (De Roos et al, 2005).

Medical Conditions and Treatment

Inflammatory bowel disease

Patients with the inflammatory bowel dis-eases (IBDs), ulcerative colitis and Crohn's disease, are at an increased risk of colorec-tal cancer (Ekbom et al, 1990a; Ekbom et al, 1990b). Up to 5% of all colorectal cancers in patients under the age of 50 occur in those with IBD. Among patients with ul-cerative colitis, younger age of onset, longer duration, and greater extent of disease, as well as primary sclerosing cholangitis, all increase the risk of colorectal cancer (Broome et al, 1992). Among patients with Crohn's disease, involvement of the colon and younger age at onset are established risk factors. The suggested decline in the risk of colorectal cancer among patients with IBD has been tentatively ascribed to greater use of anti-inflammatory drugs to control the disease (Moody et al, 1996).

The IBDs may increase the risk of colo-rectal cancer due to loss of the intestinal brush border, possibly bringing proliferat-ing stem cells into contact with the fecal stream without requiring prior adenoma formation (Potter, 1999a). Exposure to re-active oxygen and nitrogen species, as well as the processes associated with inflamma-tion, are plausible explanatory mechanisms (Itzkowitz and Yio, 2004) and some have noted that anti-IBD therapy (eg, 5-amino salicylic acid preparations) may explain why cancer risk in, eg, ulcerative colitis, is not higher (Munkholm, 2003).

Diabetes mellitus

Several studies support a positive relation between diabetes mellitus and subsequent risk of colorectal cancer (Hu et al, 1999). A recent meta-analysis suggests that diabetes mellitus carries an elevated risk of both colon and rectal cancer incidence in both sexes with summary relative risks around 1.3–1.4 and a comparable, if more hetero-geneous, association with colorectal cancer mortality (Larsson et al, 2005).

Cholecystectomy

Removal of the gallbladder alters the flow of bile into the small intestine, increasing exposure of the intestinal lumen to sec-ondary bile acids, and has been intensively studied as a possible risk factor for colo-rectal cancer. The results have been incon-sistent, with both strong positive associa-tions and null associations reported. Most of the positive associations have been re-ported from case-control studies in which selection bias in the choice of controls is of concern. In the largest case-control study of this issue, a 30% elevation in the risk of proximal colon cancer was balanced by a statistically nonsignificant inverse association with distal colon cancer, suggesting that only a very weak association, if any, exists overall (Todoroki et al, 1999).

Two large cohort studies from Scandinavia (Ekbom et al, 1993; Johansen et al, 1996) and two meta-analyses (Giovannucci et al, 1993a; Reid et al, 1996) suggest a 10% to 30% increased risk of right-sided colon cancer, 15 or more years after the operation. A study from Sweden (Lagergren et al, 2001) examined the risk of cancer in both the small and large bowel and observed a gradient of decreasing risk from the duodenum to the distal colon, consistent with the hypothesis that higher concentrations of bile acids more proximally are associated with a higher risk, and that the risk is reduced as the bile acids are diluted, thus also keeping viable the idea that bile acids may be important in the etiology of colorectal cancer.

Laxative use

It has been suggested that laxative use, independent of frequency of bowel movements, may be associated with an increased colorectal cancer risk. In the only published prospective analysis, however, no association with frequency of laxative consumption was seen (Dukas et al, 2000).

NSAIDs

Nonsteroidal anti-inflammatory drugs (NSAIDs), including aspirin, are consistently associated with a reduced risk of colorectal cancer. Most case-control studies of aspirin (Kune et al, 1988; Rosenberg et al, 1991; Suh et al, 1993; Muscat et al, 1994; Peleg et al, 1994; La Vecchia et al, 1997; Rosenberg et al, 1998; Bigler et al, 2001) have shown a lower risk of colorectal cancer and adenoma; most cohort studies have also reported a lower risk (Schreinemachers and Everson, 1994; Giovannucci et al, 1994c; Giovannucci et al, 1995b; Chan et al, 2005a) or lower mortality (Thun et al, 1991). An inverse association with adeno-

matous polyps is also seen with regular aspirin use (Greenberg et al, 1993; Logan et al, 1993; Suh et al, 1993; Giovannucci et al, 1994c). Sulindac induces regression of adenomas in patients with familial adenomatous polyposis (Giardiello et al, 1993).

In minor contrast, one cohort study (Paganini-Hill et al, 1989) and one low-dose aspirin-intervention study, analyzed both as an intervention trial (Gann et al, 1993) and at later follow-up (Stürmer et al, 1998), showed null results, perhaps due to the short duration (5 years) of the trial. In rodents, aspirin (Craven and DeRubertis, 1992), indomethacin (Pollard and Luckert, 1980; Narisawa et al, 1981), sulindac (Moorghen et al, 1988), piroxicam (Reddy et al, 1987), and celecoxib (a specific COX-2 inhibitor) (Kawamori et al, 1998) inhibit carcinogenesis.

Two randomized trials have shown that metachronous adenomas occur at lower frequency on aspirin versus placebo in those who have had a prior cancer (Sandler et al, 2003) or adenoma (Baron et al, 2003). The latter trial showed, paradoxically, that the low dose (81 mg/day) was more effective than the high (325 mg/day) both for all adenomas and for advanced lesions. In contrast, Sandler et al, who compared only the higher dose against placebo, saw a reduction in incidence. Specific COX-2 inhibitors are also effective in the clinical-trial setting (Arber et al, 2006; Bertagnolli et al, 2006), however, the increased heart disease risk associated with these drugs essentially precludes their use in cancer prevention in persons not at very high risk of colorectal cancer (Psaty and Potter, 2006).

NSAIDs suppress the enzyme COX-2 (Kalgutkar et al, 1998) and are capable of inhibiting polyp growth even in individuals with familial adenomatous polyposis. COX-2 inhibition reduces prostaglandin formation from arachidonic acid, decreases epithelial proliferation, increases apoptosis (Fig. 11–7) (Barnes et al, 1998), and reduces angiogenesis (Tsujii et al, 1998). That chronic inflammation may be relevant in colorectal cancer is evidenced by the risk associated with ulcerative colitis (see previous) and by the evidence that an elevated C-reactive protein is a biomarker of elevated risk of colorectal cancer (Gunter et al, 2006). There is evidence that NSAIDs (including aspirin) may directly suppress the HNPCC-associated mutator phenotype by genetic selection for a subset of cells that do not express MSI (Rüschoff et al, 1998). These agents show considerable promise for protecting even those at high genetically influenced risk. For a relevant review, see Ulrich et al, (2006).

Postmenopausal Hormone Use

The first investigation of postmenopausal hormones (PMH) and colorectal cancer risk found no association (Weiss et al, 1981). In 1983, a statistically significant lower risk of colon cancer was reported with use of the high-estrogen oral contraceptives (OCs) but not with non-OC hormone use (Potter and

McMichael, 1983). Since that time, there have been many other studies. Findings are not entirely consistent although, of the studies that provided separate data on colon cancer, about half showed a statistically significant lower risk with PMH or a less well-specified hormone variable (Chute et al, 1991; Gerhardsson de Verdier and London, 1992; Jacobs et al, 1994; Calle et al, 1995; Newcomb and Storer, 1995; Kampman et al, 1997; Fernandez et al, 1998), two showed a nonsignificantly lower risk (Potter and McMichael, 1983; Bostick et al, 1994), two were null (Peters et al, 1990; Risch and Howe, 1995), and one showed an elevated risk among users (Wu-Williams et al, 1991).

Consistent with other observations, several investigators report an approximate halving of risk with recent PMH use (Newcomb and Storer, 1995; Kampman

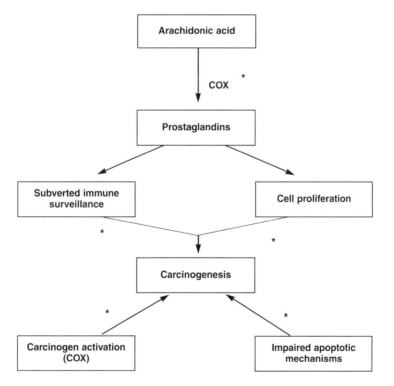

Figure 11–7. Proposed mechanisms of prevention of colon cancer by aspirin. *Indicates stages at which carcinogenesis can be blocked. Some of the effects could be due to metabolites of aspirin, including salicylate. (*Source*: International Agency for Research on Cancer, Handbooks of Cancer Prevention, Volume 1, 1997)

et al, 1997). This degree of risk reduction is maintained for about 10 years after cessation of use. Data on the duration of use suggest that longer use is associated with a lower risk. Most studies show that a similar pattern of association between PMH and risk exists for adenomatous polyps of both the colon and rectum (Jacobson et al, 1995; Potter et al, 1996).

In 2004, the WHI Estrogen plus Progestin Intervention Trial showed that those in the active arm had a considerably reduced risk of colorectal cancer although those who took estrogen plus progestin were diagnosed at a later stage than those on the placebo arm (Chlebowski et al, 2004). The estrogen-alone arm showed no reduction in risk (Anderson et al, 2004).

The evidence that estrogen-receptor hypermethylation increases with age and is a central feature of colon cancer initially suggested that declining levels of estrogen may be important (Issa,et al, 1994). The inverse relationship between PMH and both polyps and cancer may be a consequence of replacing the declining endogenous estrogen levels and thus reducing the likelihood that the estrogen-receptor gene will be silenced by methylation (Potter, 1995). MSI-positive tumors account for all of the reduced risk seen with PMH and with other hormonal exposures (Slattery et al, 2001a). As this is a small subset of colorectal tumors, it may explain the inconsistency of the findings. The WHI evidence that progestins may be crucial complicates the picture further. Identifying the hormone-responsive targets that are involved in colorectal carcinogenesis is an important research objective.

CONCLUSION

There is substantial evidence that colorectal cancer is, after lung cancer, one of the most preventable of the common cancers (see Table 11–1). Unlike the situation with many other cancer sites, there are several risk factors for which evidence of a causal association with colorectal cancer risk is strong. Increased BMI among men along with a sedentary lifestyle among both sexes is strongly implicated. The precise dietary patterns associated with increased risk are

Table 11–1. Colorectal cancer: some links between the epidemiologic risk factors and mechanisms

Epidemiology	Possible mechanisms	Direction of association
Family history	Familial adenomatous polyposis (APC mutation)	→Increased risk
	Hereditary nonpolyposis colorectal cancer (e.g. hMSH2, hMLH1 mutations)	→Increased risk
Meat and smoking	Nitrosamines and heterocylic amines	→Increased risk
Alcohol	Acetaldehyde	→Increased risk
	Effects via reduced folate	→Increased risk
Vegetables	Antioxidants	→Decreased risk
	Folate	→Decreased risk
	Fiber	→?Decreased risk
Calcium/dairy foods	Reduced cell proliferation	→?Decreased risk
Multivitamin supplements	?Folic acid	→?Decreased risk
Physical activity/low BMI	Reduced growth stimulus	→Decreased risk
	Reduced transit time	→Decreased risk
Nonsteroidal anti-inflammatory drugs	COX-2 inhibition	→Decreased risk
Hormone replacement therapy	?Prevention of estrogen receptor hypermethylation	→Decreased risk

less clear, but there is good evidence of an elevated risk with higher red-meat consumption and a reduced risk with higher intake of plant foods and calcium. In addition, good evidence links the over-the-counter drugs, aspirin and NSAIDs, as well as the prescription postmenopausal hormones, to a substantially reduced risk. Vitamin supplements, perhaps as simple as multivitamins containing 400 mg of folic acid, may also reduce colorectal cancer risk. Because there is a known precursor lesion (the adenomatous polyp), that is detectable at endoscopy, screening and early detection are feasible, effective, and reduce mortality. Thus, a variety of interventions are available for the primary prevention and early detection of colorectal cancer, suggesting that the incidence and mortality of this disease could be substantially reduced through a combination of lifestyle and social changes.

In a recently published randomized trial of folate in individuals with a history of adenoma, there was no overall effect of 1-mg/d supplementation on the development of metachronous adenomas, with risk ratios (RRs) of 1.04 (95% confidence interval [CI], 0.90-1.20) at 3 years and 1.13 (95% CI, 0.93-1.37) at the second follow-up. Moreover, at the second follow-up, there was a 67% increased risk of advanced lesions (RR, 1.67; 95% CI, 1.00-2.80), along with a more than 2-fold increased risk of having at least 3 adenomas (RR, 2.32; 95% CI, 1.23-4.35). Of concern, the risk of cancers other than colorectal cancer was statistically significantly increased in the intervention group ($P=.02$), an observation largely attributable to prostate cancer. Finally, the study showed no evidence that folate supplementation reduced cardiovascular outcomes, an expected benefit because of the homocysteine-lowering effects of folate.

REFERENCES

Aaltonen LA, Salovaara R, et al. Incidence of hereditary nonpolyposis colorectal cancer and the feasibility of molecular screening for the disease. N Engl J Med 1998;338:481–87.

ACS. Cancer Facts and Figures 2006. Atlanta, American Cancer Society.

Al-Tassan N, Chmiel NH, et al. Inherited variants of MYH associated with somatic G:C—>T:A mutations in colorectal tumors. Nat Genet 2002;30:227–32.

Alberts D., Martinez ME, et al. Lack of effect of a high-fiber cereal supplement on the recurrence of colorectal adenomas. Phoenix Colon Cancer Prevention Physicians' Network. N Engl J Med 2000;342:156–62.

Anderson GL, Limacher M, et al. Effects of conjugated equine estrogen in postmenopausal women with hysterectomy: the Women's Health Initiative randomized controlled trial. JAMA 2004;291:1701–12.

Arber N, Racz I, et al. Chemoprevention of colorectal adenomas with celecoxib in an international randomized, placebo-controlled, double-blind trial. 97th Annual Meeting of the American Association for Cancer Research. Washington DC, 2006.

Augustsson K, Skog K, et al. Dietary heterocyclic amines and cancer of the colon, rectum, bladder, and kidney: a population-based study [see comments].Lancet 1999; 353: 703–7.

Barnes C J, Cameron IL, et al. Non-steroidol anti-inflammatory drug effect on crypt cell proliferation and apoptosis during initiation of rat colon carcinogenesis. Br J Cancer 1998;77:573–80.

Baron JA., Beach M, et al. Calcium supplements for the prevention of colorectal adenomas. N Engl J Med 1999;340:101–7.

Baron JA, Cole BF, et al. A randomized trial of aspirin to prevent colorectal adenomas. N Engl J Med 2003;348:891–99.

Bell DA, Stephens EA, et al. Polyadenylation polymorphism in the acetyltransferase 1 gene (NAT1) increases risk of colorectal cancer. Cancer Research 1995;55:3537–42.

Beresford SA, Johnson KC, et al. Low-fat dietary pattern and risk of colorectal cancer: the Women's Health Initiative Randomized Controlled Dietary Modification Trial. JAMA 2006;295:643–54.

Bertagnolli MM, Eagle CJ, et al. Celecoxib reduces sporadic colorectal adenomas: Results from the Adenoma Prevention with Celecoxib (APC) trial. 97th Annual Meeting of the American Association for Cancer Research. Washington DC, 2006.

Bigler J, Whitton J, et al. CYP2C9 and UGT1A6 genotypes modulate the protective effect of aspirin on colon adenoma risk. Cancer Res 2001;61:3566–69.

Bigler J, Ulrich CM, et al. DNA repair polymorphisms and risk of colorectal adenomatous or hyperplastic polyps. Cancer Epidemiol Biomarkers Prev 2005; 14: 2501–8.

Bingham SA, Day NE, et al. Dietary fibre in food and protection against colorectal cancer in the European Prospective Investigation into Cancer and Nutrition (EPIC): an observational study. Lancet 2003; 361:1496–501.

Bingham S A, Hughes R, et al. Effect of white versus red meat on endogenous N-nitrosation in the human colon and further evidence of a dose response. J Nutr 2002;132(11 Suppl):3522S-3525S.

Bollheimer LC, Buettner R, et al. Folate and its preventive potential in colorectal carcinogenesis. How strong is the biological and epidemiological evidence? Crit Rev Oncol Hematol 2005;55:13–36.

Bostick R, Fosdick L, et al. Calcium and colorectoral epithelial cell proliferation in sporadic adenoma patients: a randomized, double-blinded, placebo-controlled clinical trial. J Natl Cancer Inst 1995;87:1307–15.

Bostick RM, Potter JD, et al. Sugar, meat, and fat intake, and non-dietary risk factors for colon cancer incidence in Iowa women (United States). Cancer Causes Control 1994; 5:38–52.

Boyapati SM, Bostick RM, et al. Folate intake, MTHFR C677T polymorphism, alcohol consumption, and risk for sporadic colorectal adenoma (United States). Cancer Causes Control 2004; 15: 493–501.

Breuer-Katschinski B, Nemes K, et al. Helicobacter pylori and the risk of colonic adenomas. Colorectal Adenoma Study Group. Digestion 1999;60:210–15.

Broome U, Lindberg G, et al. Primary sclerosing cholangitis in ulcerative colitis—a risk factor for the development of dysplasia and DNA aneuploidy? Gastroenterology 1992;102: 1877–80.

Burkitt DP. Related disease-related cause? Lancet 1969;1:1229–30.

Calle EE, Miracle-McMahill HL, et al. Estrogen replacement therapy and risk of fatal colon cancer in a prospective cohort of postmenopausal women. J Natl Cancer Inst 1995; 87:517–23.

Chan AT, Giovannucci EL, et al. Long-term use of aspirin and nonsteroidal anti-inflammatory drugs and risk of colorectal cancer. JAMA 2005;294:914–23.

Chan AT, Tranah GJ, et al. Prospective study of N-acetyltransferase-2 genotypes, meat intake, smoking and risk of colorectal cancer. Int J Cancer 2005a;115:648–52.

Chao A, Thun MJ, et al. Meat consumption and risk of colorectal cancer. JAMA 2005;293: 172–82.

Chen J, Giovannucci E, et al. A methylenetetrahydrofolate reductase polymorphism and the risk of colorectal cancer. Cancer Res 1996;56:4862–64.

Chen J, Kyte C, et al. Polymorphism in the thymidylate synthase promoter enhancer region and risk of colorectal adenomas. Cancer Epidemiol Biomarkers Prev 2004a;13:2247–50.

Chen J, Kyte C, et al. Polymorphisms in the one-carbon metabolic pathway, plasma folate levels and colorectal cancer in a prospective study. Int J Cancer 2004b;110:617–20.

Chen J, Stampfer MJ, et al. A prospective study of N-acetyltransferase genotype, red meat intake, and risk of colorectal cancer. Cancer Res 1998;58:3307–11.

Chia V, Newcomb P, et al. Risk of MSI colorectal cancer is associated jointly with smoking and NSAID use. Cancer Res 2007;66: 6877–83.

Chia V, Newcomb PA. Calcium and colorectal cancer: some questions remain. Nutr Rev 2004; 62:115–20.

Chlebowski RT, Wactawski-Wende J, et al. Estrogen plus progestin and colorectal cancer in postmenopausal women. N Engl J Med 2004;350:991–1004.

Cho E, Smith-Warner SA, et al. Alcohol intake and colorectal cancer: a pooled analysis of 8 cohort studies. Ann Intern Med 2004b; 140:603–13.

Cho E, Smith-Warner SA, et al. Dairy foods, calcium, and colorectal cancer: a pooled analysis of 10 cohort studies. J Natl Cancer Inst 2004a;96:1015–22.

Chow W, Malker H, et al. Occupational risks for colon cancer in Sweden. J Occup Med 1994;36:647–51.

Chute CG, Willett WC, et al. A prospective study of reproductive history and exogenous estrogens on the risk of colorectal cancer in women. Epidemiology 1991;2:201–7.

Cole et al, for the Polyp Prevention Study Group. Folic acid for the prevention of colorectal adenomas: a randomized clinical trial. JAMA. 2007;297:2351–2359.

Connelly-Frost A, Poole C, et al. Selenium, apoptosis, and colorectal adenomas. Cancer Epidemiol Biomarkers Prev 2006;15:486–93.

Cortessis V, Siegmund K, et al. A case-control study of microsomal epoxide hydrolase, smoking, meat consumption, glutathione S-transferase M3, and risk of colorectal adenomas. Cancer Res 2001;61:2381–85.

Cox DG, Pontes C, et al. Polymorphisms in prostaglandin synthase 2/cyclooxygenase 2 (PTGS2/COX2) and risk of colorectal cancer. Br J Cancer 2004; 91:339–43.

Craven PA, DeRubertis FR. Effects of aspirin on 1,2-dimethylhydrazine-induced colonic carcinogenesis. Carcinogenesis 1992;13:541–46.

Croitoru ME, Cleary SP, et al. Association between biallelic and monoallelic germline

MYH gene mutations and colorectal cancer risk. J Natl Cancer Inst 2004;96:1631–34.

Cross AJ, Pollock JR, et al. Haem, not protein or inorganic iron, is responsible for endogenous intestinal N-nitrosation arising from red meat. Cancer Res 2003;63:2358–60.

Curtin K, Bigler J, et al. MTHFR C677T and A1298C polymorphisms: diet, estrogen, and risk of colon cancer. Cancer Epidemiol Biomarkers 2004;Prev 13:285–92.

De Roos AJ, Ray RM, et al. Colorectal cancer incidence among female textile workers in Shanghai, China: a case-cohort analysis of occupational exposures. Cancer Causes Control 2005;16:1177–88.

DeCosse JJ, Miller HH, et al. Effect of wheat fiber and vitamins C and E on rectal polyps in patients with familial adenomatous polyposis. J Natl Cancer Inst 1989;81:1290–97.

Dukas L, Willett WC, et al. Prospective study of bowel movement, laxative use, and risk of colorectal cancer among women. Am J Epidemiol 2000;151:958–64.

Ekbom A, Helmick C et al. Ulcerative colitis and colorectal cancer. A population-based study. N Engl J Med 1990a;323:1228–33.

Ekbom A, Helmick C, et al. Increased risk of large-bowel cancer in Crohn's disease with colonic involvement. Lancet 1990b;336:357–59.

Ekbom A, Yuen J, et al. Cholecystectomy and colorectal cancer. Gastroenterology 1993;105:142–47.

Enam S, Del Valle L, et al. Association of human polyomavirus JCV with colon cancer: evidence for interaction of viral T-antigen and beta-catenin. Cancer Res 2002;62:7093–7101.

English DR, MacInnis RJ, et al. Red meat, chicken, and fish consumption and risk of colorectal cancer. Cancer Epidemiol Biomarkers Prev 2004;13:1509–14.

Farinati F, Espina N, et al. In vivo inhibition by chronic ethanol exposure of methylguanine transferase activity and DNA repair. Ital J Gastroenterol 1985;17:48–49.

Fearon ER, Vogelstein B. A genetic model for colorectal tumorigenesis. Cell 1990; 61:759–67.

Fernandez E, La Vecchia C, et al. Hormone replacement therapy and risk of colon and rectal cancer. Cancer Epidemiol Biomarkers Prev 1998;7:329–33.

Flood A, Peters U, et al. Calcium from diet and supplements is associated with reduced risk of colorectal cancer in a prospective cohort of women. Cancer Epidemiol Biomarkers Prev 2005;14:126–32.

Fraumeni JF Jr, Lloyd JW, et al. Cancer mortality among nuns: role of marital status in etiology of neoplastic disease in women. J Natl Cancer Inst 1969;42:455–68.

Freudenheim JL, Graham S, et al. Folate intake and carcinogenesis of the colon and rectum. Int J Epidemiol 1991;20:368–74.

Fuchs CS, Colditz GA, et al. Dietary fiber and the risk of colorectal cancer and adenoma in women. N Engl J Med 1999;340:169–76.

Gann PH, Manson JE, et al. Low-dose aspirin and incidence of colorectal tumors in a randomized trial. J Natl Cancer Inst 1993;85:1220–24.

Garro AJ, Lieber CS. Alcohol and cancer. Annu Rev Pharmacol Toxicol 1990;30:219–49.

Gerhardsson de Verdier M, Hagman U, et al. Meat, cooking methods and colorectal cancer: a case-referent study in Stockholm. Int J Cancer 1991;49:520–25.

Gerhardsson de Verdier M, London S. Reproductive factors, exogenous female hormones, and colorectal cancer by subsite. Cancer Causes Control 1992;3:355–60.

Giardiello FM, Hamilton SR, et al. Treatment of colonic and rectal adenomas with sulindac in familial adenomatous polyposis. N Engl J Med 1993;328:1313–16.

Giovannucci E. Insulin and colon cancer. Cancer Causes Control 1995;6:164–79.

Giovannucci E. Meta-analysis of coffee consumption and risk of colorectal cancer. Am J Epidemiol 1998;147:1043–52.

Giovannucci E, Ascherio A, et al. Physical activity, obesity, and risk for colon cancer and adenoma in men. Ann Intern Med 1995;122:327–34.

Giovannucci E, Colditz GA, et al. A meta-analysis of cholecystectomy and risk of colorectal cancer. Gastroenterology 1993;105:130–41.

Giovannucci E, Egan KM, et al. Aspirin and the risk of colorectal cancer in women. N Engl J Med 1995;333:609–14.

Giovannucci E, Goldin B. The role of fat, fatty acids, and total energy intake in the etiology of human colon cancer. Am J Clin Nutr 1997;66(6 Suppl):1564S-1571S.

Giovannucci E, Rimm EB, et al. Alcohol, low-methionine—low-folate diets, and risk of colon cancer in men. J Natl Cancer Inst 1995;87:265–73.

Giovannucci E, Rimm EB, et al. A prospective study of cigarette smoking and risk of colorectal adenoma and colorectal cancer in U.S. men. J Natl Cancer Inst 1994a;86:183–91.

Giovannucci E, Rimm EB, et al. Intake of fat, meat, and fiber in relation to risk of colon cancer in men. Cancer Res 1994b;54:2390–97.

Giovannucci E, Rimm EB, et al. Aspirin use and the risk for colorectal cancer and adenoma in male health professionals. Ann Intern Med 1994c;121:241–46.

Giovannucci E, Stampfer MJ, et al. Relationship of diet to risk of colorectal adenoma in men. J Natl Cancer Inst 1992;84:91–98.

Giovannucci E, Stampfer MJ, et al. Multivitamin use, folate, and colon cancer in women in the Nurses' Health Study. Ann Intern Med 1998;129:517–24.

Giovannucci E, Stampfer MJ, et al. Folate, methionine, and alcohol intake and risk of colorectal adenoma. J Natl Cancer Inst 1993;85:875–84.

Goldbohm RA, van den Brandt PA, et al. A prospective cohort study on the relation between meat consumption and the risk of colon cancer. Cancer Res 1994;54:718–23.

Gong Z., Xie D, et al. The PPAR{gamma} Pro12Ala polymorphism and risk for incident sporadic colorectal adenomas. Carcinogenesis 2005;26:579–85.

Goode EL, Potter JD, et al. Methionine synthase D919G polymorphism, folate metabolism, and colorectal adenoma risk. Cancer Epidemiol Biomarkers Prev 2004;13:157–62.

Goode EL, Ulrich CM, et al. Polymorphisms in DNA repair genes and associations with cancer risk. Cancer Epidemiol Biomarkers Prev 2002; 12:1513–30.

Goodman JE, Bowman ED, et al. Arachidonate lipoxygenase (ALOX) and cyclooxygenase (COX) polymorphisms and colon cancer risk. Carcinogenesis 2004; 25: 2467–72.

Grau MV, Baron JA, et al. Vitamin D, calcium supplementation, and colorectal adenomas: results of a randomized trial. J Natl Cancer Inst 2003;95:1765–71.

Greenberg ER, Baron JA, et al. Reduced risk of large-bowel adenomas among aspirin users. J Natl Cancer Inst 1993;85:912–16.

Gunter MJ, Stolzenberg-Solomon R, et al. A prospective study of serum C-reactive protein and colorectal cancer risk in men. Cancer Res 2006;66:2483–87.

Haenszel W. Cancer mortality among the foreign born in the United States. J Natl Cancer Inst 1961, 26.37–132.

Hague A, Paraskeva C. The short-chain fatty acid butyrate induces apoptosis in colorectal tumour cell lines. Eur J Cancer Prev 1995; 4:359–64.

Harrison D J, Hubbard AL, et al. Microsomal epoxide hydrolase gene polymorphism and susceptibility to colon cancer. Br J Cancer 1999;79:168–71.

Hartman TJ, Albert PS, et al. The association of calcium and vitamin D with risk of colorectal adenomas. J Nutr 2005;135:252–59.

Hill MJ, Morson BC, et al. Aetiology of adenoma-carcinoma sequence in large bowel. Lancet 1978;8058:245–47.

Hirose M, et al. Genetic polymorphisms of methylenetetrahydrofolate reductase and

aldehyde dehydrogenase 2, alcohol use and risk of colorectal adenomas: Self- Defense Forces Health Study. Cancer Sci 2005; 96: 513–8.

Howe G, Aronson K, et al. The relationship between dietary fat intake and risk of colorectal cancer: evidence from the combined analysis of 13 case-control studies. Cancer Causes Control 1997;8:215–28.

Howe GR, Benito E, et al. Dietary intake of fiber and decreased risk of cancers of the colon and rectum: evidence from the combined analysis of 13 case-control studies. J Natl Cancer Inst 1992;84:1887–96.

Hu FB, Manson JE, et al. Prospective study of adult onset diabetes mellitus (type 2) and risk of colorectal cancer in women. J Natl Cancer Inst 1999;91:542–47.

Huang WY, Chatterjee N, et al. Microsomal epoxide hydrolase polymorphisms and risk for advanced colorectal adenoma. Cancer Epidemiol Biomarkers Prev 2005;14:152–57.

Hyman J, Baron JA, et al. Dietary and supplemental calcium and the recurrence of colorectal adenomas. Cancer Epidemiol 1998; 7:291–95.

IARC. Weight Control and Physical Activity. Lyon, IARC Press, 2002.

Ishizuka S, Tanaka S, et al. Fermentable dietary fiber potentiates the localization of immune cells in the rat large intestinal crypts. Exp Biol Med (Maywood) 2004;229:876–84.

Issa JP. CpG island methylator phenotype in cancer. Nat Rev Cancer 2004;4:988–93.

Issa JP, Ottaviano YL, et al. Methylation of the oestrogen receptor CpG island links ageing and neoplasia in human colon. Nat Genet 1994;7:536–40.

Itzkowitz SH, Yio X. Inflammation and cancer IV. Colorectal cancer in inflammatory bowel disease: the role of inflammation. Am J Physiol Gastrointest Liver Physiol 2004; 287:G7–17.

Jacobs EJ, Connell CJ, et al. Multivitamin use and colorectal cancer incidence in a US cohort: does timing matter? Am J Epidemiol 2003;158:621–28.

Jacobs EJ, White E, et al. Exogenous hormones, reproductive history, and colon cancer (Seattle, Washington, USA). Cancer Causes Control 1994;5:359–66.

Jacobson JS, Neugut AI, et al. Reproductive risk factors for colorectal adenomatous polyps (New York City, NY, United States). Cancer Causes Control 1995;6:513–18.

Jass J, Baker K, et al. Advanced colorectal polyps with the molecular and morphological features of serrated polyps and adenomas: concept of a 'fusion' pathway to colorectal cancer. Histopathology 2006;49:121–31.

Jiang J, Gajalakshmi V, et al. Influence of the C161T but not Pr012Ala polymorphism in the peroxisome proliferator-activated receptor-gamma on colorectal cancer in an Indian population. Cancer Sci 2005;96:507–12.

Jin MJ, Chen K, et al. The association of the DNA repair gene XRCC3 Thr241Met polymorphism with susceptibility to colorectal cancer in a Chinese population. Cancer Genet Cytogenet 2005; 163: 38–43.

Johansen C, Chow WH, et al. Risk of colorectal cancer and other cancers in patients with gall stones. Gut 1996;39:439–43.

Jones S, Emmerson P, et al. Biallelic germline mutations in MYH predispose to multiple colorectal adenoma and somatic G:C→T:A mutations. Hum Mol Genet 2002;11: 2961–67.

Kadlubar FF, Butler MA, et al. Polymorphisms for aromatic amine metabolism in humans: relevance for human carcinogenesis. Environ Health Perspect 1992;98:69–74.

Kakiuchi H, Watanabe M, et al. Specific 5'-GGGA-3'—>5'-GGA-3' mutation of the Apc gene in rat colon tumors induced by 2-amino-1-methyl-6-phenylimidazo[4,5-b]pyridine. Proceedings of the National Academy of Sciences of the United States of America 1995;92:910–14.

Kalgutkar AS, Crews BC, et al. Aspirin-like molecules that covalently inactivate cyclooxygenase-2. Science 1998;280(5367):1268–70.

Kampman E, Potter JD, et al. Hormone replacement therapy, reproductive history, and colon cancer: a multicenter, case-control study in the United States. Cancer Causes Control 1997;8:146–58.

Kampman E, Slattery ML, et al. Meat consumption, genetic susceptibility, and colon cancer risk: a United States multicenter case-control study. Cancer Epidemiol Biomarkers Prev 1999;8:15–24.

Kampman E, Slattery ML, et al. Calcium, vitamin D, sunshine exposure, dairy products and colon cancer risk (United States). Cancer Causes & Control 2000;11:459–66.

Kang S, Burnett C, et al. Gastrointestinal cancer mortality of workers in occupations with high asbestos exposures. Am J Ind Med 1997;31:713–18.

Kawamori T, Rao CV, et al. Chemopreventive activity of celecoxib, a specific cyclooxygenase-2 inhibitor, against colon carcinogenesis. Cancer Res 1998;58:409–12.

Key TJ, Fraser GE, et al. Mortality in vegetarians and non-vegetarians: a collaborative analysis of 8300 deaths among 76,000 men and women in five prospective studies. Public Health Nutr 1998;1:33–41.

Kim JC, et al. Characterization of mutator phenotype in familial colorectal cancer patients not fulfilling amsterdam criteria. Clin Cancer Res 2004;10: 6159–68.

Knudson AG. Mutation and cancer: Statistical study of retinoblastoma. Proc Nat Acad Sci 1971;68:820–23.

Koh WP, Yuan JM, et al. Interaction between cyclooxygenase-2 gene polymorphism and dietary n-6 polyunsaturated fatty acids on colon cancer risk: the Singapore Chinese Health Study. 2004; 90:1760–4.

Kolodner RD. Mismatch repair: mechanisms and relationship to cancer susceptibility. Trends Biochem Sci 1995;20:397–401.

Kuehl GE, Lampe JW, et al. Glucuronidation of nonsteroidal anti-inflammatory drugs: identifying the enzymes responsible in human liver microsomes. Drug Metab Dispos 2005;33:1027–35.

Kune GA, Kune S, et al. Colorectal cancer risk, chronic illnesses, operations, and medications: case control results from the Melbourne Colorectal Cancer Study. Cancer Res 1988; 48:4399–4404.

La Vecchia C, Negri E, et al. Aspirin and colorectal cancer. Br J Cancer 1997;76:675–77.

Lagergren J, Ye W, et al. Intestinal cancer after cholecystectomy: is bile involved in carcinogenesis? Gastroenterology 2001;121:542–47.

Laghi L, Randolph AE, et al. JC virus DNA is present in the mucosa of the human colon and in colorectal cancers. Proc Natl Acad Sci U S A 1999;96:7484–89.

Laken S, Petersen G, et al. Familial colorectal cancer in Ashkenazim due to a hypermutable tract in APC. Nature Genetics 1997;17: 79–83.

Larsson SC, Orsini N, et al. Diabetes mellitus and risk of colorectal cancer: a meta-analysis. J Natl Cancer Inst 2005;97:1679–87.

Le Marchand L, Donlon T, et al. B-vitamin intake, metabolic genes, and colorectal cancer risk (United States). Cancer Causes Control 2002;13:239–48.

Le Marchand L, Kolonel LN, et al. Association of an exon 1 polymorphism in the IGFBP3 gene with circulating IGFBP-3 levels and colorectal cancer risk: the multiethnic cohort study. Cancer Epidemiol Biomarkers Prev 2005;14:1319–21.

Le Marchand L, Wilkens LR, et al. The MTHFR C677T polymorphism and colorectal cancer: the multiethnic cohort study. Cancer Epidemiol Biomarkers Prev 2005; 14 1198–203.

Lee IM. Physical activity and cancer prevention—data from epidemiologic studies. Med Sci Sports Exerc 2003;35:1823–27.

Lewin MH, Bailey N, et al. Red meat enhances the colonic formation of the DNA adduct 06-carboxymethyl guanine: implications for colorectal cancer risk. Cancer Res 2006; 66:1859–65.

Lilla C, Verla-Tebit E, et al. Effect of NAT1 and NAT2 genetic polymorphisms on colorectal cancer risk associated with exposure to tobacco smoke and meat consumption. Cancer Epidemiol Biomarkers Prev 2006;15:99–107.

Lin HJ, Probst-Hensch NM, et al. Variants of N-acetyltransferase NAT1 and a case-control study of colorectal adenomas. Pharmacogenetics 1998;8:269–81.

Lin HJ, et al. Prostaglandin H synthase 2 variant (Val511Ala) in African Americans may reduce the risk for colorectal neoplasia. Cancer Epidemiol Biomarkers Prev 2002; 11: 1305–15.

Lin J, Zhang SM, et al. Intakes of calcium and vitamin D and risk of colorectal cancer in women. Am J Epidemiol 2005;161:755–64.

Lindor NM, Burgart LJ, et al. Immunohistochemistry versus microsatellite instability testing in phenotyping colorectal tumors. J Clin Oncol 2002;20:1043–48.

Lindor NM, Rabe K, et al. Lower cancer incidence in Amsterdam-I criteria families without mismatch repair deficiency: familial colorectal cancer type X. JAMA 2005;293:1979–85.

Logan RF, Little J, et al. Effect of aspirin and non-steroidal anti-inflammatory drugs on colorectal adenomas: case-control study of subjects participating in the Nottingham faecal occult blood screening programme. BMJ 1993;307:285–89.

Lüchtenborg M, Weijenberg MP, et al. Cigarette smoking and colorectal cancer: APC mutations, hMLH1 expression, and GSTM1 and GSTT1 polymorphisms. Am J Epidemiol 2005;161:806–15.

Lynch HT, Cristofaro G, et al. Genetic Epidemiology of Colon Cancer. Genetic Epidemiology of Cancer. H. T. Lynch HT. Boca Raton, FL, CRC Press 1989, pp251–77.

Lynch PM, Lynch HT. Colon Cancer Genetics 1985. New York, Van Nostrand Rheinhold

Ma J Stampfer MJ, et al. Methylenetetrahydrofolate reductase polymorphism, dietary interactions, and risk of colorectal cancer. Cancer Res 1997;57L1098–102.

Ma J, Stampfer MJ, et al. A polymorphism of the methionine synthase gene: association with plasma folate, vitamin B12, homocyst(e)ine, and colorectal cancer risk. Cancer Epidemiol Biomarkers Prev 1999;8:825–29.

Macklin MT. Inheritance of cancer of the stomach and large intestine in man. J Natl Cancer Inst 1960;24:551–71.

MacLennan R, Macrae F, et al. Randomized trial of intake of fat, fiber, and beta carotene to prevent colorectal adenomas. J Natl Cancer Inst 1995;87:1760–66.

Marugame T, Tsuji E, et al. Relation of plasma folate and methylenetetrahydrofolate reductase C677T polymorphism to colorectal adenomas. Int J Epidemiol 2003;32:67–70.

Mathew A, Sinha R, et al. Meat intake and the recurrence of colorectal adenomas. Eur J Cancer Prev 2004;13:159–64.

Matsuo K, Ito H, et al. One-carbon metabolism related gene polymorphisms interact with alcohol drinking to influence the risk of colorectal cancer in Japan. Carcinogenesis 2005;26:2164–71.

McGreavey LE, Turner F, et al. No evidence that polymorphisms in CYP2C8, CYP2C9, UGT1A6, PPARdelta and PPARgamma act as modifiers of the protective effect of regular NSAID use on the risk of colorectal carcinoma. Pharmacogenet Genomics 2005;15:713–21.

McKeown-Eyssen GE. Epidemiology of colorectal cancer revisited: are serum triglycerides and/or plasma glucose associated with risk? Cancer Epidemiol Biomarkers Prev 1994;3:687–95.

McMichael AJ, Giles GG. Cancer in migrants to Australia: extending the descriptive epidemiological data. Cancer Res 1988;48:751–56.

McMichael AJ, Potter JD. Reproduction, endogenous and exogenous sex hormones, and colon cancer: a review and hypothesis. J Natl Cancer Inst 1980;65:1201–7.

McMichael AJ, Potter JD. Host factors in carcinogenesis: certain bile-acid metabolic profiles that selectively increase the risk of proximal colon cancer. J Natl Cancer Inst 1985;75:185–91.

Michaud DS, Fuchs CS, et al. Dietary glycemic load, carbohydrate, sugar, and colorectal cancer risk in men and women. Cancer Epidemiol Biomarkers Prev 2005;14:138–47.

Michels KB, Fuchs CS, et al. Fiber intake and incidence of colorectal cancer among 76,947 women and 47,279 men. Cancer Epidemiol Biomarkers Prev 2005;14:842–49.

Michels KB, Giovannucci E, et al. Fruit and vegetable consumption and colorectal adenomas in the Nurses' Health Study. Cancer Res 2006;66:3942–53.

Michels KB, Giovannucci E, et al. Prospective study of fruit and vegetable consumption and incidence of colon and rectal cancers. J Nat Cancer Inst 2000;92:1740–52.

Michels KB, Willett WC, et al. Coffee, tea, and caffeine consumption and incidence of colon and rectal cancer. J Natl Cancer Inst 2005; 97:282–92.

Mitrou P, Watson M, et al. NQ01 and mEH exon 4 (mEH4) gene polymorphisms, smoking and colorectal cancer risk. IARC Sci Publ 2002;156:495–97.

Moody GA, Jayanthi V, et al. Long-term therapy with sulphasalazine protects against colorectal cancer in ulcerative colitis: a retrospective study of colorectal cancer risk and compliance with treatment in Leicestershire. Eur J Gastroenterol Hepatol 1996;8:1179–83.

Moore LL, Bradlee ML, et al. BMI and waist circumference as predictors of lifetime colon cancer risk in Framingham Study adults. Int J Obes Relat Metab Disord 2004;28:559–67.

Moorghen M, Ince P, et al. A protective effect of sulindac against chemically-induced primary colonic tumours in mice. J Pathol 1988; 156:341–47.

Morimoto LM, Newcomb PA, et al. Risk factors for hyperplastic and adenomatous polyps: evidence for malignant potential? Cancer Epidemiol Biomarkers Prev 2002;11:1012–18.

Morimoto LM, Newcomb PA, et al. Insulin-like growth factor polymorphisms and colorectal cancer risk. Cancer Epidemiol Biomarkers Prev 2005;14:1204–11.

Mueller-Koch Y, Vogelsang H, et al. Hereditary non-polyposis colorectal cancer: clinical and molecular evidence for a new entity of hereditary colorectal cancer. Gut 2005;54:1733–40.

Munkholm P. The incidence and prevalence of colorectal cancer in inflammatory bowel disease. Aliment Pharmacol Ther 2003;18 Suppl 2:1–5.

Murtaugh MA, Ma KN, et al. Interactions of peroxisome proliferator-activated receptor {gamma} and diet in etiology of colorectal cancer. Cancer Epidemiol Biomarkers Prev 2005;14:1224–29.

Muscat JE, Stellman SD, et al. Nonsteroidal antiinflammatory drugs and colorectal cancer. Cancer 1994;74:1847–54.

Narisawa T, Sato M, et al. Inhibition of development of methylnitrosourea-induced rat colon tumors by indomethacin treatment. Cancer Res 1981;41:1954–57.

Newcomb PA, Bush AC, et al. No evidence of an association of JC virus and colon neoplasia. Cancer Epidemiol Biomarkers Prev 2004; 13:662–66.

Newcomb PA, Storer, BE. Postmenopausal hormone use and risk of large-bowel cancer. J Natl Cancer Inst 1995;87:1067–71.

Nishisho I, Nakamura Y, et al. Mutations of chromosome 5q21 genes in FAP and colorectal cancer patients. Science 1991;253:665–69.

Niv Y, Goel A, et al. JC virus and colorectal cancer: a possible trigger in the chromosomal instability pathways. Curr Opin Gastroenterol 2005;21:85–89.

Norat T, Bingham S, et al. Meat, fish, and colorectal cancer risk: the European Prospective Investigation into cancer and nutrition. J Natl Cancer Inst 2005;97:906–16.

Nyrén O, Bergström R, et al. Smoking and colorectal cancer: a 20-year follow-up study of Swedish construction workers. J Natl Cancer Inst 1996;88:1302–7.

Paganini-HillA, Chao A, et al. Aspirin use and chronic diseases: a cohort study of the elderly. Br Med J 1989;299:1247–50.

Park Y, Hunter DJ, et al. Dietary fiber intake and risk of colorectal cancer: a pooled analysis of prospective cohort studies. JAMA 2005; 294:2849–57.

Peleg II, Maibach HT, et al. Aspirin and nonsteroidal anti-inflammatory drug use and the risk of subsequent colorectal cancer. Arch Intern Med 1994;154:394–99.

Peltomaki P, de la Chapelle, A. Mutations predisposing to hereditary nonpolyposis colorectal cancer. Adv Cancer Res 1997;71:93–119.

Peters RK, Pike MC, et al. Reproductive factors and colon cancer. Br J Cancer 1990;61:741–48.

Peters U, Chatterjee N, et al. Calcium intake and colorectal adenoma in a US colorectal cancer early detection program. Am J Clin Nutr 2004;80:1358–65.

Peters U, Sinha R, et al. Dietary fibre and colorectal adenoma in a colorectal cancer early detection programme. Lancet 2003;361: 1491–95.

Pollard M, Luckert PH. Indomethacin treatment of rats with dimethylhydrazine-induced intestinal tumors. Cancer Treat Rep 1980; 64:1323–27.

Poole EM, Bigler J, et al. Prostacyclin synthase and arachidonate 5-lipoxygenase polymorphisms and risk of colorectal polyps. Cancer Epidemiol Biomarkers Prev 2006;15: 502–8.

Potter JD. Hormones and colon cancer. J Natl Cancer Inst 81995;7:1039–40.

Potter JD. Colorectal cancer: molecules and populations. J Natl Cancer Inst 1999a;91:916–32.

Potter JD. Fiber and colorectal cancer—where to now? N Engl J Med 1999b;340:223–24.

Potter JD. Vegetables, fruit, and cancer. Lancet 2005;366:527–30.

Potter JD, Bostick RM, et al. Hormone replacement therapy is associated with lower risk of adenomatous polyps of the large bowel: the Minnesota Cancer Prevention Research Unit Case-Control Study. Cancer Epidemiol Biomarkers Prev 1996;5:779–84.

Potter JD, Cerhan JR, et al. Colorectal adenomatous and hyperplastic polyps: smoking and N-acetyltransferase 2 polymorphisms. Cancer Epidemiology, Biomarkers & Prevention 1999;8:69–75.

Potter JD, McMichael AJ. Large bowel cancer in women in relation to reproductive and hormonal factors: a case-control study. J Natl Cancer Inst 1983;71:703–9.

Potter JD, Slattery ML, et al. Colon cancer: a review of the epidemiology. Epidemiol Rev 1993; 15:499–545.

Probst-Hensch NM, Haile RW, et al. Acetylation polymorphism and prevalence of colorectal adenomas. Cancer Res 1995;55:2017–20.

Probst-Hensch NM, Haile RW, et al. Lack of association between the polyadenylation polymorphism in the NAT1 (acetyltransferase 1) gene and colorectal adenomas. Carcinogenesis 1996;17:2125–29.

Probst-Hensch NM, Sinha R, et al. Meat preparation and colorectal adenomas in a large sigmoidoscopy-based case-control study in California (United States). Cancer Causes Control 1997;8:175–83.

Psaty BM, Potter JD. Risks and benefits of celecoxib to prevent recurrent adenomas. New Engl J Med 2006;355:950–52.

Raderer M, Pfeffel F, et al. Regression of colonic low greade B cell lymphoma of the mucosa associated lymphoid tissue type after eradication of Helicobacter pylori. Gut 2000;46: 133–35.

Reddy BS, Maruyama H, et al. Dose-related inhibition of colon carcinogenesis by dietary piroxicam, a nonsteroidal antiinflammatory drug, during different stages of rat colon tumor development. Cancer Res 1987;47: 5340–46.

Reid FD, Mercer PM, et al. Cholecystectomy as a risk factor for colorectal cancer: a meta-analysis. Scand J Gastroenterol 1996;31: 160–69.

Risch HA,Howe GR. Menopausal hormone use and colorectal cancer in Saskatchewan: a record linkage cohort study. Cancer Epidemiol Biomarkers Prev 1995;4:21–28.

Robertson DJ, Sandler RS, et al. Fat, fiber, meat and the risk of colorectal adenomas. Am J Gastroenterol 2005;100:2789–95.

Robien K, Curtin K, et al. Microsomal epoxide hydrolase polymorphisms are not associated with colon cancer risk. Cancer Epidemiol Biomarkers Prev 2005;14:1350–52.

Rosenberg L, Louik C, et al. Nonsteroidal antiinflammatory drug use and reduced risk of large bowel carcinoma. Cancer 1998;82: 2326–33.

Rosenberg L, Palmer J, et al. A hypothesis: nonsteroidal anti-inflammatory drugs reduce the incidence of large-bowel cancer. J Natl Cancer Inst 1991;83:355–58.

Rüschoff J, Wallinger S, et al. Aspirin suppresses the mutator phenotype associated with hereditary nonpolyposis colorectal cancer by genetic selection. Proc Natl Acad Sci U S A 1998;95:11301–6.

Sachse C, Smith G, et al. (2002). A pharmacogenetic study to investigate the role of dietary carcinogens in the etiology of colorectal cancer. Carcinogenesis 23(11):1839–49.

Samad AK, Taylor RS, et al. A meta-analysis of the association of physical activity with reduced risk of colorectal cancer. Colorectal Dis 2005;7:204–13.

Sampson JR, Dolwani S, et al. Autosomal recessive colorectal adenomatous polyposis due to inherited mutations of MYH. Lancet 2003;362:39–41.

Sandler RS, Halabi S, et al. A randomized trial of aspirin to prevent colorectal adenomas in patients with previous colorectal cancer. N Engl J Med 2003;348:883–90.

Sanjoaquin MA, Allen N, et al. Folate intake and colorectal cancer risk: a meta-analytical approach. Int J Cancer 2005;113:825–28.

Sansbury LB, Bergen AW, et al. Inflammatory cytokine gene polymorphisms, nonsteroidal anti-inflammatory drug use, and risk of adenoma polyp recurrence in the polyp prevention trial. Cancer Epidemiol Biomarkers Prev 2006;15:494–501.

Satia-Abouta J, Galanko JA, et al. Associations of micronutrients with colon cancer risk in African Americans and whites: results from the North Carolina Colon Cancer Study. Cancer Epidemiol Biomarkers Prev 2003; 12:747–54.

Schatzkin A, Lanza E, et al. Lack of effect of a low-fat, high-fiber diet on the recurrence of colorectal adenomas. Polyp Prevention Trial Study Group. N Engl J Med 2000;342:1149–55.

Schiffman MH, Felton, JS. Re: Fried foods and the risk of colon cancer. Am J Epidemiol 1990;131:376–78.

Schreinemachers D, Everson R. Aspirin use and lung, colon, and breast cancer incidence in a prospective study. Epidemiology 1994;5: 138–46.

Sengupta S, Muir JG, et al. Does butyrate protect from colorectal cancer? J Gastroenterol Hepatol 2006;21:209–18.

Sharp L, Little J. Polymorphisms in genes involved in folate metabolism and colorectal neoplasia: a HuGE review. Am J Epidemiol 2001;159:123–13.

Sieber OM, Lipton L, et al. Multiple colorectal adenomas, classic adenomatous polyposis, and germ-line mutations in MYH. N Engl J Med 2003;348:791–99.

Siezen C, Tijhuis M, et al. Protective effect of nonsteroidal anti-inflammatory drugs on colorectal adenomas is modified by a polymorphism in peroxisome proliferator-activated receptor delta. Pharmacogenet Genomics 2006;16:43–50.

Siezen CL, van Leeuwen AI, et al. Colorectal adenoma risk is modified by the interplay between polymorphisms in arachidonic acid pathway genes and fish consumption. Carcinogenesis 2005;26:449–57.

Singh PN, Fraser GE. Dietary risk factors for colon cancer in a low-risk population. Am J Epidemiol 1998;148:761–74.

Sinha R, Chow WH, et al. Well-done, grilled red meat increases the risk of colorectal adenomas. Cancer Res 1999;59:4320–24.

Slattery ML. Physical activity and colorectal cancer. Sports Med 2004;34:239–52.

Slattery ML., Curtin K, et al. Associations between cigarette smoking, lifestyle factors, and microsatellite instability in colon tumors. J Natl Cancer Inst 2000;92:1831–36.

Slattery ML, Potter J, et al. Energy balance and colon cancer—beyond physical activity. Cancer Res 1997;57:75–80.

Slattery ML, Potter JD, et al. Estrogens reduce and withdrawal of estrogens increases risk of microsatellite instability-positive colon cancer. Cancer Res 2001;61:126–30.

Slattery ML, Potter JD, et al. NAT2, GSTM-1, cigarette smoking, and risk of colon cancer. Cancer Epidemiol Biomarkers Prev 1998;7:1079–84.

Slattery ML, Potter JD, et al. Age and risk factors for colon cancer: Are there implications for understanding differences in case control and cohort studies? Cancer Causes Control 1994;5:557–63.

Slattery ML, Samowitz W, et al. A molecular variant of the APC gene at codon 1822: its association with diet, lifestyle, and risk of colon cancer. Cancer Res 2001;61:1000–4.

Slattery ML, Samowitz W, et al. Associations among IRS1, IRS2, IGF1, and IGFBP3 genetic polymorphisms and colorectal cancer. Cancer Epidemiol Biomarkers Prev 2004;13:1206–14.

Slattery ML, Schaffer D, et al. Are dietary factors involved in DNA methylation associated with colon cancer? Nutr Cancer 1997;28:52–62.

Slattery ML, Sweeney C, et al. Associations between ERalpha, ERbeta, and AR genotypes and colon and rectal cancer. Cancer Epidemiol Biomarkers Prev 2005;14:2936–42.

Slattery ML, West DW, et al. Tobacco, alcohol, coffee, and caffeine as risk factors for colon cancer in a low-risk population. Epidemiology 1990;1:141–45.

Spirio LN, Samowitz W, et al. Alleles of APC modulate the frequency and classes of mutations that lead to colon polyps. Nat Genet 1998;20:385–88.

Steinmetz KA, Potter JD. Vegetables, fruit, and cancer. II. Mechanisms. Cancer Causes Control 1991;2:427–42.

Steinmetz KA, Potter JD. Vegetables, fruit, and cancer prevention: a review. J Am Diet Assoc 1996;96:1027–39.

Stern MC, Siegmund KD, et al. XRCC1 and XRCC3 polymorphisms and their role as effect modifiers of unsaturated fatty acids and antioxidant intake on colorectal adenomas risk. Cancer Epidemiol Biomarkers Prev 2005; 14: 609–15.

Stewart BW, Kleihues PE. World Cancer Report. Lyon, IARC Press, 2003.

Stürmer T, Glynn RJ et al. Aspirin use and colorectal cancer: post-trial follow-up data from the Physicians' Health Study. Ann Intern Med 1998;128:713–20.

Suh O, Mettlin C, et al. Aspirin use, cancer, and polyps of the large bowel. Cancer 1993;72:1171–77.

Talley NJ, Zinsmeister AR, et al. Gastric adenocarcinoma and helicobacter pylori infection. J Nat Cancer Inst 1991;83:1734–39.

Tamakoshi K, Wakai K, et al. A prospective study of body size and colon cancer mortality in Japan: The JACC Study. Int J Obes Relat Metab Disord 2004;28:551–58.

Tavani A, Gallus S, et al. Cigarette smoking and risk of cancers of the colon and rectum: a case-control study from Italy. Eur J Epidemiol 11998;4:675–81.

Tavani A, La Vecchia C. Coffee, decaffeinated coffee, tea and cancer of the colon and rectum: a review of epidemiological studies, 1990–2003. Cancer Causes Control 2004; 15:743–57.

Terry P, Baron JA, et al. Dietary calcium and vitamin D intake and risk of colorectal cancer: a prospective cohort study in women. Nutr Cancer 2002;43:39–46.

Terry P, Giovannucci E, et al. Fruit, vegetables, dietary fiber, and risk of colorectal cancer. J Natl Cancer Inst 2001;93:525–33.

Thompson DE, Mabuchi K, et al. Cancer incidence in atomic bomb survivors. Part II: Solid tumors, 1958–1987. Radiat Res 1994;137(2 Suppl):S17–67.

Thun MJ, Calle EE, et al. Risk factors for fatal colon cancer in a large prospective study. J Natl Cancer Inst 1992;84:1491–1500.

Thun MJ, Namboodiri MM, et al. Aspirin use and reduced risk of fatal colon cancer. N Engl J Med 1991;325:1593–96.

Tiemersma EW, Bunschoten A, et al. Effect of SULT1A1 and NAT2 genetic polymorphism on the association between cigarette smoking and colorectal adenomas. Int J Cancer 2004;108:97–103.

Tiemersma EW, Kloosterman J, et al. Role of EPHX genotype in the associations of smoking and diet with colorectal adenomas. IARC Sci Publ 2002;156:491–93.

Tiemersma EW, Voskuil DW, et al. Risk of colorectal adenomas in relation to meat consumption, meat preparation, and genetic susceptibility in a Dutch population. Cancer Causes Control 2004; 15:225–36.

Todoroki I, Friedman GD, et al. Cholecystectomy and the risk of colon cancer. Am J Gastroenterol 1999;94:41–46.

Tranah GJ, Chan AT, et al. Epoxide hydrolase and CYP2C9 polymorphisms, cigarette smoking, and risk of colorectal carcinoma in the Nurses' Health Study and the Physicians' Health Study. Mol Carcinog 2005; 44:21–30.

Tranah GJ, Giovannucci E, et al. Epoxide hydrolase polymorphisms, cigarette smoking and risk of colorectal adenoma in the Nurses' Health Study and the Health Professionals Follow-up Study. Carcinogenesis 2004;25: 1211–18.

Trock B, Lanza E, et al. Dietary fiber, vegetables, and colon cancer: critical review and meta-analyses of the epidemiologic evidence. J Natl Cancer Inst 1990;82:650–61.

Tsujii M, Kawano S, et al. Cyclooxygenase regulates angiogenesis induced by colon cancer cells. Cell 1998;93:705–16.

Ulrich CM Kampman E, et al. Colorectal adenomas and the C677T MTHFR polymorphism: evidence for gene-environment interaction? Cancer Epidemiol Biomarkers Prev 1999;8:659–68.

Ulrich CM. Nutrigenetics in cancer research—folate metabolism and colorectal cancer. J Nutr 2005; 135:2698–702.

Ulrich CM, Bigler J, et al. Thymidylate synthase promoter polymorphism, interaction with folate intake, and risk of colorectal adenomas. Cancer Res 2002;62:3361–64.

Ulrich CM, Bigler J, et al. Non-steroidal anti-inflammatory drugs for cancer prevention: promise, perils and pharmacogenetics. Nat Rev Cancer 2006;6:130–40.

Ulrich CM, Bigler J, et al. Epoxide hydrolase Tyr113His polymorphism is associated with elevated risk of colorectal polyps in the presence of smoking and high meat intake. Cancer Epidemiol Biomarkers Prev 2001; 10;875–82.

Ulrich CM, Curtin K, et al. Polymorphisms in the reduced folate carrier, thymidylate synthase, or methionine synthase and risk of colon cancer. Cancer Epidemiol Biomarkers Prev 2005;14:2509–16.

Ulrich CM, Kampman E, et al. Colorectal adenomas and the C677T MTHFR polymorphism: evidence for gene-environment interaction? Cancer Epidemiol Biomarkers Prev 1999;8:659–68.

Ulrich and Potter. Folate and cancer—timing is everything. JAMA 2007; 297:2408–2409.

Ulrich CM, Whitton J, et al. PTGS2 (COX-2) -765G > C promoter variant reduces risk of colorectal adenoma among nonusers of nonsteroidal anti-inflammatory drugs. Cancer Epidemiol Biomarkers Prev 2005; 14: 616–19.

Ulvik A, et al. Colorectal cancer and the methylenetetrahydrofolate reductase 677C -> T and methionine synthase 2756A -> G polymorphisms: a study of 2,168 case- control pairs from the JANUS cohort. Cancer Epidemiol Biomarkers Prev 2004; 13: 2175–80.

Umar A, Kunkel TA. DNA-replication fidelity, mismatch repair and genome instability in cancer cells. Eur J Biochem 1996;238:297–307.

van der Hel OL, Bueno de Mesquita HB, et al. No modifying effect of NAT1, GSTM1, and GSTT1 on the relation between smoking and colorectal cancer risk. Cancer Epidemiol Biomarkers Prev 2003; 12:681–82.

van der Logt EM, Bergevoet SM, et al. Role of epoxide hydrolase, NAD(P)H:quinone oxidoreductase, cytochrome P450 2E1 or alcohol dehydrogenase genotypes in susceptibility to colorectal cancer. Mutat Res 2006; 593:39–49.

Veale AML. Intestinal Polyposis. Cambridge, Cambridge University Press, 1965.

Vineis P, McMichael A. Interplay between heterocyclic amines in cooked meat and metabolic phenotype in the etiology of colon cancer. Cancer Causes Control 1996;7:479–86.

Wactawski-Wende J, Kotchen JM, et al. Calcium plus vitamin D supplementation and the risk of colorectal cancer. N Engl J Med 2006;354:684–96.

Wark PA, Weijenberg MP, et al. Fruits, vegetables, and hMLH1 protein-deficient and -proficient colon cancer: The Netherlands cohort study. Cancer Epidemiol Biomarkers Prev 2005;14:1619–25.

Wattenberg LW. Inhibition of chemical carcinogenesis. J Natl Cancer Inst 1978;60:11–8.

WCRF Panel. Food, Nutrition and the Prevention of Cancer: a Global Perspective. Washington, DC, American Instituue for Cancer Research, 1997

Webb EL, Rudd MF, et al. Search for low penetrance alleles for colorectal cancer through a scan of 1467 non-synonymous SNPs in 2575 cases and 2707 controls with validation by kin-cohort analysis of 14704 first-degree relatives. Human Mol Genet 2006;15:3263–71.

Wei EK, Ma J, et al. C-peptide, insulin-like growth factor binding protein-1, glycosylated hemoglobin, and the risk of distal colorectal adenoma in women. Cancer Epidemiol Biomarkers Prev 2006; 15:750–55.

Weiss JM, Goode EL, et al. Polymorphic variation in hOGG1 and risk of cancer: a review of the functional and epidemiologic literature. Mol Carcinog 2005;14:127–41.

Weiss NS, Daling JR, et al. Incidence of cancer of the large bowel in women in relation to reproductive and hormonal factors. J Natl Cancer Inst 1981;67:57–60.

Welfare MR, Cooper J, et al. Relationship between acetylator status, smoking, and diet and colorectal cancer risk in the north-east of England. Carcinogenesis 1997;18:1351–54.

Whelan RL, Horvath KD, et al. Vitamin and calcium supplement use is associated with decreased adenoma recurrence in patients with a previous history of neoplasia. Dis Colon Rectum 1999;42:212–17.

White E, Shannon JS, et al. Relationship between vitamin and calcium supplement use and colon cancer. Cancer Epidemiol Biomarkers Prev 1997;6:769–74.

Willett WC, Stampfer MJ, et al. Relation of meat, fat, and fiber intake to the risk of colon cancer in a prospective study among women. N Engl J Med 1990;323:1664–72.

Wong HL, Delellis K, et al. A new single nucleotide polymorphism in the insulin-like growth factor I regulatory region associates with colorectal cancer risk in singapore chinese. Cancer Epidemiol Biomarkers Prev 2005;14:144–51.

Woolf CM. A genetic study of carcinoma of the large intestine. Am J Hum Genet 1958;10: 42–47.

Wu-Williams AH, Lee M, et al. Reproductive factors and colorectal cancer risk among Chinese females. Cancer Res 1991;51:2307–11.

Wu K, Willett WC, et al. A prospective study on supplemental vitamin E intake and risk of colon cancer in women and men. Cancer Epidemiol Biomarkers Prev 2002;11:1298–304.

Wynder EL, Shigematsu T. Environmental factors of cancer of the colon and rectum. Cancer 1967;20:1520–61.

Xu Z, Su DL. Schistosoma japonicum and colorectum cancer: an epidemiological study in the People's Republic of China. Int J Cancer 1984;34:315–18.

Yin G, et al. Methylenetetrahydrofolate reductase C677T and A1298C polymorphisms and colorectal cancer: the Fukuoka Colorectal Cancer Study. Cancer Sci 2004; 95: 908–13.

Yu JH, Bigler J, et al. Mismatch repair polymorphisms and colorectal polyps: hMLH1–93G>A variant modifies risk associated with smoking. Am J Gastroenterol 2006; 101: 1313–19.

Zecevic M, Amos CI, et al. IGF1 gene polymorphism and risk for hereditary nonpolyposis colorectal cancer. J Natl Cancer Inst 2006; 98:139–43.

Zumkeller N, Brenner H, et al. Helicobacter pylori infection and colorectal cancer risk: a meta-analysis. Helicobacter 2006;11:75–80.

12

Cancer of the Liver and Biliary Tract

SHERRI STUVER AND DIMITRIOS TRICHOPOULOS

Primary liver cancer is an uncommon disease in the western world, but the liver is an important cancer site for several reasons. Liver cancer is very frequent in sub-Saharan Africa and the Far East—that is, areas of the world with rapid population growth. It is a rapidly and almost uniformly fatal disease for which treatment is generally ineffective, but there is already sufficient knowledge and technology for effective primary prevention. Indeed, more important causal factors have been identified for three histologic forms of primary liver cancer (hepatocellular carcinoma [HCC], cholangiocarcinoma, and angiosarcoma) than for any of the common cancers except lung and cervix cancer. Liver cancer is also the first common human cancer that was found to have an infectious etiology. Following clinical observations first made in the 1940s, the causal role of hepatitis B virus (HBV) began to be documented in the 1970s, while the corresponding role of hepatitis C virus (HCV) started to emerge about a decade later. Hence, the discovery of the causes of liver cancer, and in particular HCC, is a success story of epidemiology with rich input from ecologic, case-control, and cohort studies.

CLINICAL SYNOPSIS

Subgroups

Hepatobiliary cancers encompass a variety of anatomic and histopathologic types. Predominant are HCC and cholangiocarcinoma of the liver and adenocarcinomas of the gallbladder and extrahepatic bile ducts.

Symptoms

Predominant symptoms are those of an advanced abdominal malignancy such as pain, anorexia, weight loss, weakness, fever, and abdominal swelling. Jaundice is particularly common in bile duct cancers.

Diagnosis

Clinical examination and analysis of α-phetoprotein in the serum, as well as ultrasound, computed tomography, and other imaging techniques, are used for diagnosis and staging. Histopathologic confirmation requires liver biopsy specimens obtained percutaneously, laparoscopically, or via open surgery. Percutaneous transhepatic or endoscopic retrograde cholangiography documents biliary anatomy in bile duct tumors.

Treatment

Hepatobiliary cancers are curable only through radical surgical resection or, occasionally, hepatectomy followed by liver transplantation. For intrahepatic bile duct cancer, the surgical approach is similar to that of HCC. More recently, progress has been made in the development of ablative localized treatments, which have demonstrated some effectiveness among patients with early stage, limited disease; these therapies include percutaneous ethanol injection, radiofrequency ablation, and transarterial embolization and chemoembolization. However, most cancers are diagnosed in advanced stages, when curative treatment is beyond reach.

Prognosis

The prognosis for patients with hepatobiliary cancer is extraordinarily gloomy. The median survival time following diagnosis is short, and 5-year relative survival rates in Europe are on average 6%, approaching zero in some countries. For biliary tract cancers, the corresponding survival rate is 12%. When liver and intrahepatic biliary tract cancers are analyzed together in the United States, 5-year relative survival is about 8%.

Progress

Notwithstanding the development of numerous, often advanced, techniques, there has been no substantial progress in the treatment of hepatobiliary cancer. The most promising development in the control of this dreaded disease is primary prevention of HCC through vaccination against HBV and interruption of HCV transmission and chronic infection.

CANCER OF THE LIVER DESCRIPTIVE EPIDEMIOLOGY

Liver cancer is one of the most frequently occurring malignancies in the world. Incidence estimates for the year 2002 rank liver cancer sixth with regard to the global cancer burden (Parkin et al, 2005). It has a very high fatality rate and thus is an even more important cause of cancer mortality worldwide. International liver cancer rates are extremely variable (Stuver and Trichopoulos, 1994; Bosch et al, 2004), but the overwhelming majority, over 80%, of all liver cancer cases occur in the developing world (Parkin et al, 2005). Rates are highest in eastern and southeastern Asia and sub-Saharan Africa and lowest in the Americas, Australia, and northern Europe (Figs. 12–1

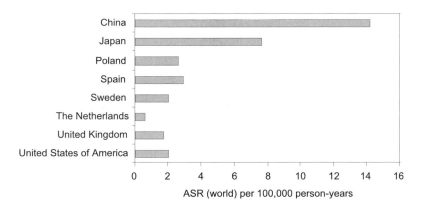

Figure 12–1. Age-standardized (to the world population) incidence rates of liver cancer among women. (*Source*: Ferlay et al, 2004)

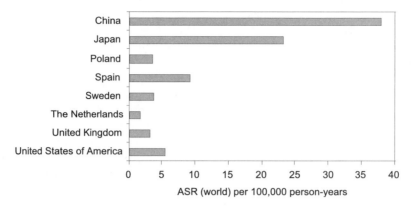

Figure 12–2. Age-standardized (to the world population) incidence rates of liver cancer among men. (*Source*: Ferlay et al, 2004)

and 12–2). Intracountry variation in liver cancer occurrence also can be quite pronounced (McGlynn et al, 2001). Men have a higher risk of liver cancer than women (Figs. 12–1 and 12–2), and this excess is more evident in populations with elevated liver cancer rates (Stuver and Trichopoulos, 1994; Parkin et al, 2005). In addition, the occurrence of liver cancer in persons less than 45 years of age is higher in high-risk countries for both genders (Figs. 12–3 and 12–4). Due to revisions in the classification and coding of liver cancer, as well as changes in diagnostic and certification practices, secular trends in liver cancer occurrence are difficult to describe (Stuver

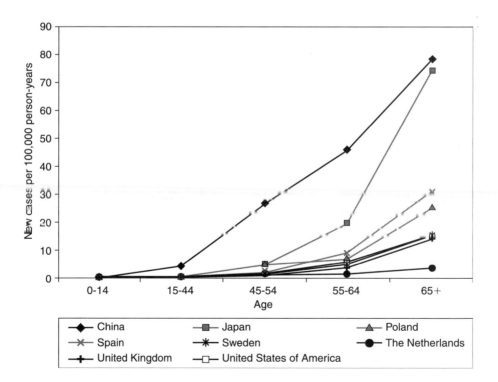

Figure 12–3. Age-specific incidence rates of liver cancer among women. (*Source*: Ferlay et al, 2004)

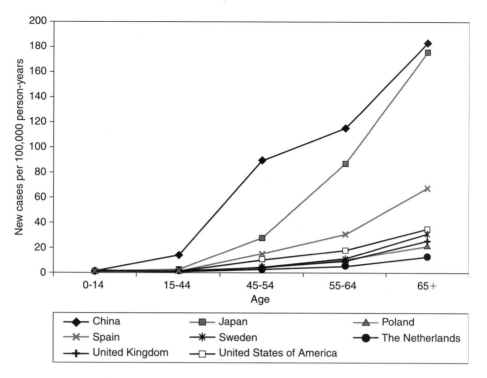

Figure 12–4. Age-specific incidence rates of liver cancer among men. (*Source*: Ferlay et al, 2004)

and Trichopoulos, 1994). Nonetheless, liver cancer rates seem to be increasing in Japan (Okuda, 1997) and a number of Western countries including the United States (El-Serag et al, 2003), the United Kingdom (Taylor-Robinson et al, 1997), and France (La Vecchia et al, 2000). Decreasing trends in liver cancer occurrence have been suggested for such countries as Spain, Singapore, and India (Stuver and Trichopoulos, 1994; McGlynn et al, 2001).

Although the global burden of liver cancer is substantial, this malignancy is largely preventable. We know as much about its etiology as about that of any other common form of human cancer; more than 10 distinct biological, chemical, and physical agents have been conclusively incriminated. Indeed, HCC, the most frequent histologic type, is the first common cancer for which a viral etiology has been conclusively established. It is also important that the research that revealed the etiology of liver cancer was overwhelmingly epidemiologic, although many of the leading researchers in this field were not mainstream epidemiologists.

GENETIC AND MOLECULAR EPIDEMIOLOGY

Inherited Susceptibility

Most clustering of HCC observed within families likely reflects shared risk factors, most notably chronic HBV infection. However, family history has remained associated even with adjustment for other known risk factors (Chen et al, 1997). Moreover, several inherited disorders, including α1-antitrypsin deficiency, hemochromatosis, and porphyria cutanea tarda, have been associated with HCC (Deugnier and Turlin, 1997; McGlynn and London, 2005). Most of the support for an effect of these diseases comes from case series studies, although some analytic epidemiologic investigations have provided important data (Sparos et al, 1984). A large cohort study of porphyria patients in Norway and Sweden found a more than 20-fold increased rate of primary liver cancer compared to that of the general population (Linet et al, 1999). The inherited metabolic disorders often result in inflammation, fibrosis, and/or cirrhosis of the liver, which likely is the mechanism by which they may be associated with the development of liver cancer (Deugnier and Turlin, 1997).

Specific genetic studies have yielded conflicting results. Directly opposite effects have been reported, occasionally by the same research group, for the association of specific genotypes of several enzymes, including cytochrome P450 2E1 (CYP2E1) (Yu et al, 1995a; Lee et al, 1997), the glutathione S-transferases (GSTM1 and GSTT1) (McGlynn et al, 1995, 2003; Yu et al, 1995a), and the epoxide hydrolases (EPHX) (McGlynn et al, 1995, 2003). The CYP2E1 enzyme is involved in the oxidation and metabolic activation of N-nitrosamines, including those in tobacco smoke. Alcohol consumption can induce CYP2E1, and the highest levels of the enzyme are found in the liver (Lee et al, 1997). The GSTs and EPHX are involved in the process of aflatoxin B1 detoxification in hepatocytes. Given the observed relationship of excessive alcohol consumption with the occurrence of HCC, polymorphisms in the genes encoding alcohol-metabolizing enzymes also have been examined, but with no apparent associations observed (Takeshita et al, 2000). At this point, it is difficult to draw any firm conclusions with regard to the role of inherited polymorphisms in the etiology of liver cancer.

Somatic Events

Liver cancer appears to be a disease with a long latency. Hepatocarcinogenesis likely involves a multistep process representing an accumulation of genetic changes. Cirrhosis, observed in the majority of HCC cases, appears to play an important role in those mutation events through the associated cycles of liver necrosis and regeneration (Tabor, 1998; Thorgeirsson and Grisham, 2002). Allelic loss has been reported in

conjunction with the occurrence of chronic hepatitis and cirrhosis and the development of HCC, and somatic changes in several cellular genes involved in DNA damage response, cell-cycle control, and apoptosis have been related to the development of HCC (Ozturk, 1999; Thorgeirsson and Grisham, 2002). The application of microarray technology to the study of the molecular pathogenesis of HCC will be useful in identifying new genes important in hepatocarcinogenesis (Shirota et al, 2001; Thorgeirsson and Grisham, 2002).

Mutations of tumor-suppressor genes, in particular *TP53*, and inactivation of their proteins are often observed in HCC. About 30% of HCC cases worldwide, and up to 60% of cases in high-risk areas, are reported to have *TP53* gene mutations (Tabor, 1998; Ozturk, 1999). Aflatoxin B1 exposure has been linked to specific mutations of codon 249 of the *TP53* gene (IARC, 1993; Montesano et al, 1997). It is hypothesized that these TP53-related events occur late in the progression of tumor development, resulting in the loss of cell-growth control through TP53-mediated apoptosis (Tabor, 1997; Thorgeirsson and Grisham, 2002). The retinoblastoma protein also plays an important role in cell-cycle regulation; loss of heterozygosity of the retinoblastoma gene (*RB1*) has been found in some HCC cases (Tabor, 1994; Ozturk, 1999). In addition, mutations to *RB1*, which result in suppression of transcription of the *C-MYC* and *C-FOS* promoters in vitro, may lead to uncontrolled expression of these oncogenes. Other genes important to cell-cycle regulation, including *P15INK4A* and cyclins *D* and *A*, have been found to be mutated in 10% to 20% of HCCs (Ozturk, 1999).

Several growth factors have been implicated in hepatocarcinogenesis (Tabor, 1994; Thorgeirsson and Grisham, 2002). The level of transforming growth factor alpha (TGF-α) frequently is increased in HCC tissue, as detected by immunohistochemistry. Overexpression of TGF-α in tumorous livers may result from liver regeneration and lead to enhanced tumor progression. Insulin-like growth factor II (IGF-II) also can be expressed at abnormally high levels in HCC, with changes in allelic expression possibly contributing to upregulation of the *IGF-II* gene (Aihara et al, 1998). Recent evidence suggests that cyclooxygenase 2 (COX-2), a proangiogenic and growth-promoting factor, may play a role in the development of HCC, particularly HBV-related disease (Tang et al, 2005).

RISK FACTORS

Like cancer of the lung and the cervix, liver cancer is one of the malignancies for which the major etiologic factors have been identified (see Table 12–1). A chronic process of liver damage and regeneration appears to play an important role, possibly through the accumulation of mutations in a stochastic manner over a long latent period (Tabor, 1998). Persistent infection with HBV or HCV, which accounts for over three-quarters of all liver cancer cases in the world, results in this type of injury to the liver. In the minority of cases in which viral infection is not involved in the occurrence of cancer, exposures that also damage the liver—for example, excessive alcohol consumption—or that may be directly genotoxic—for example, tobacco smoke or dietary aflatoxin—appear to be important. Such environmental exposures, as well as host-related factors such as male gender, may also act to modify the development of virus-associated liver malignancy.

Unlike the situation with most other cancers, a substantial fraction of liver cancer cases and deaths could actually be prevented given the existing knowledge and technology. However, because liver cancer remains a malignancy primarily of developing countries and disadvantaged groups, efforts to reduce its burden are advancing slowly. Eradication of HBV infection, reduction of HCV transmission, and improvement of socioeconomic conditions could dramatically diminish the occurrence of this cancer in the affected populations. In addition, moderation of alcohol consumption and avoidance of smoking may have an

Table 12–1. Risk factors for primary liver cancer

Established
  Chronic HBV infection
  Chronic HCV infection
  Alcoholic cirrhosis
  Dietary aflatoxins
  Opisthorchis viverrini infection (cholangiocarcinoma)
  Diagnostic thorium dioxide [α-particles] (mostly angiosarcoma)
  Vinyl chloride (angiosarcoma)
  Gallstones (gallbladder cancer)
  Tobacco smoking
Likely
  Diabetes mellitus
  Inherited metabolic disorders- α-antitrypsin deficiency, hemochromatosis,
    porphyria cutanea tarda
  Cirrhosis of any etiology
  Primary sclerosing cholangitis (cholangiocarcinoma)
  Inorganic arsenic (angiosarcoma)
  Obesity (gallbladder cancer)
Possible
  Decreased consumption of vegetables
  Oral contraceptives
  High parity
  Ionizing radiation [x- and γ-rays]
  Organic trichloroethylene solvent
  Clonorchis sinensis infection (cholangiocarcinoma)
  Androgenic-anabolic steroids (mostly angiosarcoma)

impact on the occurrence of liver cancer, particularly in more-developed areas of the world.

Tobacco

Tobacco smoke is a potent carcinogen, and it is possible that, in some industrialized countries where the prevalence of chronic hepatitis virus infection is low, tobacco smoking is important in the development of HCC (Trichopoulos et al, 1987). In 2004, the International Agency for Research on Cancer (IARC) indicated that there is sufficient evidence that the association between tobacco smoking and liver cancer is causal and, thus, tobacco smoking can be considered as an established liver carcinogen (IARC, 2004).

In the early 1980s, a more than twofold positive association was reported between tobacco smoking and HCC cases who were negative for the hepatitis B surface antigen (HBsAg), the marker for chronic infection with HBV (Trichopoulos et al, 1980; Lam et al, 1982). Although some subsequent studies that examined the association between tobacco smoking and HCC had no information on HBV status, a review (Austin, 1991) concluded that tobacco smoking likely increases the risk of HCC. Beginning in the 1990s, a number of studies have found a significant effect of smoking on HCC risk after controlling for the potentially confounding effect of chronic HBV and/or HCV infections (Yu and Chen, 1993; Chen et al, 1997; Yang et al, 2002; Wang et al, 2003; Yuan et al, 2004). While many studies have focused on smoking as a risk factor for HCC among men (Yu and Chen, 1993; Yang et al, 2002; Wang et al, 2003), a cohort study in China found an independent increased risk of HCC related to high levels of cigarette smoking among women (Evans et al, 2002). In a commentary by the epidemiologists of the IARC Working Group to update the monograph on the carcinogenecity of tobacco smoke, it was estimated that the relative risk estimates for HCC among smokers compared to nonsmokers range from 1.5 to 2.5 (IARC, 2004; Vineis et al, 2004).

A significant positive interaction between cigarette smoking and both HBV and/or HCV infection has been observed in some studies (Mori et al, 2000; Sun et al, 2003), although not in others (Wang et al, 2003; Yuan et al, 2004). A synergistic effect of tobacco smoking and heavy alcohol consumption also has been reported (Kuper et al, 2000b; Marrero et al, 2005).

Diet

A positive association of aflatoxins with the development of HCC has been supported by a number of studies, as has a protective effect of vegetables and, possibly, high levels of the antioxidants retinol and selenium. An inverse association with coffee intake has been reported in some studies, but the evidence is far from conclusive.

Aflatoxin contamination

Aflatoxins are produced primarily by two Aspergillus species of mold and can contaminate such dietary staples as corn, peanuts, and rice stored in hot, humid environments. Aflatoxins have been classified as established carcinogens (IARC, 1993) and are believed to be an important cause of HCC in some areas of the developing world (Montesano et al, 1997). The level and prevalence of aflatoxin exposure are highest in sub-Saharan Africa and southern China (Montesano et al, 1997). Correlation analyses conducted in those areas revealed significant associations between estimated aflatoxin intake and HCC incidence and mortality (IARC, 1993). Although limited in number, some analytic epidemiologic studies using food-frequency questionnaires in conjunction with data from aflatoxin-contamination food surveys supported an association between aflatoxin consumption and liver cancer risk (IARC, 1993), although some studies found no such relationship (Lam et al, 1982; Srivatanakul et al, 1991).

Aflatoxin and its oxidative metabolites can be measured in urine and serum and can be useful as markers of dietary intake and biologically effective dose. In Shanghai, the risk of HCC was increased fourfold among men with detectable urinary aflatoxin B1 and its metabolites (Ross et al, 1992), with an even stronger association with the detection of the N7-guanine adduct (Qian et al, 1994). Excretion of urinary aflatoxins and HBsAg interacted strongly positively with respect to risk of HCC (Ross et al, 1992; Qian et al, 1994). A similar strong interaction between aflatoxin B1 and HBV chronic infection also was observed in cohort studies in Taiwan (Wang et al, 1996; Lunn et al, 1997). Early exposure to aflatoxin and HBV may explain the younger age peak in HCC incidence observed in some parts of Africa and China.

Molecular evidence for a role of aflatoxin in the development of HCC has been convincingly presented (Montesano et al, 1997). Consumption of aflatoxin B1 appears to induce the frequent G:C to T:A transversion at codon 249 of the *TP53* gene observed in liver cancer cells from cases in southern China and sub-Saharan Africa. This *TP53* mutation is rarely observed in HCC cases in the United States or Europe, where aflatoxin exposure is low. In vitro experiments involving human cells show the same mutational effect of aflatoxin B1, with the N7-guanine adduct being primarily responsible. This one base-pair change results in a serine substitution of the arginine amino acid, which is important for the proper folding of the DNA-binding domain of the TP53 protein.

A higher frequency of this specific *TP53* mutation in HBsAg-positive HCC cases, as well as data from experimental studies in woodchucks and HBV-transgenic mice (which have an HBV gene inserted into their chromosomal DNA), support an interaction between chronic HBV infection and aflatoxin exposure in the development of liver cancer (Montesano et al, 1997). Although a meta-analysis of 48 studies revealed no significant modifying effect of HBV infection on the correlation between aflatoxin exposure level and frequency of the *TP53* 249ser mutation in HCC cases (Stern et al, 2001), aflatoxin B1 and HBV do appear to positively interact to cause HCC. The exact nature of this interaction, however, is not clear. It is possible that chronic HBV infection and the associated liver damage may lead to the selective proliferation of aflatoxin-mutated hepatocytes, via modulation of relevant metabolizing or detoxifying enzymes, increased hepatocyte turnover, increased oxidative stress, or interference with DNA repair pathways by the HBV X gene (Kew, 2003).

Food groups, macronutrients, micronutrients

An effect of diet on the risk of liver cancer development has been evaluated by the World Cancer Research Fund (1997). The evidence with regard to vitamins and food groups appears to be most consistent for a decreased risk with increased consumption of vegetables. Several case-control and cohort studies have reported a significant inverse trend with increasing level of vegetable intake (Lam et al, 1982; La Vecchia et al, 1988; Srivatanakul et al, 1991; Yu et al, 1995b). However, case-control studies in Greece (Kuper et al, 2000d) and Japan (Fukuda et al, 1993) did not find a protective effect. More recently, data from several studies suggest a possible, independent protective effect of coffee consumption on HCC development (Kuper et al, 2000b; Inoue et al, 2005).

With respect to micronutrient intake, an inverse relationship between dietary and serum retinol levels and HCC risk has been observed in studies of men in both Taiwan (Yu et al, 1995b) and China (Yuan et al, 2006), most apparent among those with chronic HBV infection. A study in Italy also found that low serum retinol strongly predicted the incidence of HCC in patients with cirrhosis (Clemente et al, 2002). In addition, evidence is now emerging to support a protective effect of high selenium intake on HCC development (McGlynn and London, 2005). Nested case-control studies in Taiwan (Yu et al, 1999b) and China (Sakoda et al, 2005) reported an inverse association between lower selenium levels and HCC incidence. However, the two studies differed with respect to the subgroups in which the protective effect was most apparent: cigarette smokers and those with low levels of serum retinol or carotenoids, in Taiwan; women and nondrinkers, in China.

Alcohol

Results of a number of studies strongly support the hypothesis that alcoholic cirrhosis as well as heavy drinking increase the risk of HCC (Austin, 1991; Adami et al, 1992; Kuper et al, 2000b, 2001a; Donato et al, 2002; Yuan et al, 2004; Morgan et al, 2004). In 1988, the IARC classified alcohol as a human carcinogen and specifically implicated alcohol consumption in the etiology of liver cancer (IARC, 1988). Although alcohol metabolism results in the generation of acetaldehyde and reactive oxygen species, which could directly damage hepatocytes (Morgan et al, 2004), alcohol intake might be a liver carcinogen mainly or only by being causally involved in the development of cirrhosis (Adami et al, 1992). A large historical cohort study based on hospital discharge diagnoses in Sweden found a relative risk of 22.4 for the incidence of HCC among patients hospitalized for alcoholism and cirrhosis but only a 2.4-fold increased risk among patients hospitalized for alcoholism alone (Kuper et al, 2001a). Thus, alcohol abuse leading to cirrhosis may be an important cause of HCC (Vall Mayans et al, 1990), whereas light and moderate drinking may have no major influence on HCC risk (Trichopoulos et al, 1987; La Vecchia et al, 1988). Based on epidemiologic studies that examined level of alcohol intake, chronic consumption greater than 80 grams per day appears to be associated with a roughly fivefold relative risk of HCC and likely represents an important cause of HCC in Western populations (Morgan et al, 2004). In addition, a more than additive effect of heavy alcohol consumption and hepatitis virus infection has been reported (Donato et al, 2002; Hassan et al, 2002; Yuan et al, 2004).

Reproductive Factors

Stanford and colleagues (1992) have postulated that endogenous hormones, primarily estrogens, may play a role in the development of HCC among women. In support of this hypothesis, increased parity appears to be positively associated with the risk of this cancer (Hsing et al, 1992; La Vecchia et al, 1992; Stanford et al, 1992; Tzonou et al, 1992); however, the association may be limited to HBsAg-negative women (Tzonou et al, 1992). A case-control study conducted in Greece found that the risk of HCC was higher for women with lower age at menarche or higher age at menopause (Mucci et al, 2001); the HCC cases also had somewhat higher levels of estradiol than did the controls. An increased risk of HCC with earlier age at menarche, but not with older age at menopause or increasing parity, was reported for women in Taiwan (Yu et al, 2003).

Hormones

Overall, the evidence is suggestive of a role for steroid hormones in the incidence of liver cancer, which may be further modified by HBV status in a complex manner that differs for men and women.

Three cohort studies of Asian men have investigated the relationship between serum testosterone level at recruitment and the development of HCC, with mixed results. In two studies by the same research group in Taiwan, having testosterone levels in the highest tertile was associated with an independent and significant fourfold increased risk of HCC in one (Yu and Chen, 1993) and with a significant twofold increased risk among HBV carriers in the other (Yu et al, 2000). A study in Shanghai reported only a nonsignificant 50% increased risk of HCC in the highest tertile among HBV carriers (Yuan et al, 1995). In a case-control study in Greece (Mucci et al, 2001), levels of testosterone and sex hormone-binding protein among women were found to be slightly higher for HCC cases than for controls; however, analysis of sex steroid levels among men suggested that the differences observed were more likely due to liver damage per se (Kuper et al, 2001b). Nonetheless, the consistently higher incidence of HCC in men than in women, particularly in developing countries where liver cancer rates are high and chronic HBV infection is endemic, suggests a role for testosterone in hepatocarcinogenesis, which is also supported by evidence from animal studies (Yu and Chen, 1993). Of interest, HBV-carrier Taiwanese men with 20 or fewer CAG repeats in the androgen receptor gene, indicating increased androgen receptor transactivation ability, had an increased risk of developing HCC, which was further elevated for those men with the highest levels of testosterone (Yu et al, 2000). In addition, limited case-report data point to an effect of androgenic-anabolic steroids on liver cancer risk (IARC, 1987; Trichopoulos, 1992).

Exogenous sex hormones also may have an effect on the occurrence of HCC. Case-control studies, primarily conducted in developed countries, investigated oral contraceptive use as a risk factor and found a two- to threefold increased risk of HCC among oral contraceptive users (Yu et al, 1991; The Collaborative MILTS Project Team, 1997). In contrast, among women from HBV-endemic areas, users showed a nonsignificant decrease in this risk (WHO Collaborative Study of Neoplasia and Steroid Contraceptives, 1989b; Yu et al, 2003). Other reports from developed countries also have not supported an effect of oral contraceptive use on liver cancer in general (Colditz, 1994; Bosch et al, 2004).

Anthropometric Measures

Recent epidemiologic data suggest that obesity (ie, body mass index $\geq$ 30) may be associated with an increased risk of liver cancer. Prospective cohort studies conducted in Sweden (Wolk et al, 2001), the United States (Calle et al, 2003; Samanic et al, 2004), and Korea (Oh et al, 2005) reported relative risks from about 1.5 to 4.5, for men and women; the results of two of the studies indicated that the effect might be stronger in men than in women (Wolk et al, 2001; Calle et al, 2003). In addition, a fourfold association was observed in a case-control study of HCC cases compared to cirrhotic controls (Marrero et al, 2005). The effect of obesity on liver cancer incidence may be mediated, at least in part, through the strong relationship of overweight with diabetes mellitus and nonalcoholic fatty liver disease/steatohepatitis, both of which are associated with the development of HCC (Calle and Kaaks, 2004).

Infections

Virus infection is involved in the majority of liver cancers. Convincing evidence has been provided for a causal role of chronic HBV and HCV infections in the development of HCC.

Hepatitis B virus

Hepatitis B virus, a DNA virus, requires a reverse-transcription step, similar to retroviruses, in order to replicate. When replicating, HBV does not directly copy its DNA genome, as all other DNA viruses do. Instead, a new DNA genome is made via reverse transcription of a full-length RNA copy of the viral DNA. The virus preferentially infects hepatocytes and can establish a chronic, persistent infection within the liver. The chronic carrier state of HBV infection is characterized by the serologic detection of HBsAg. The development of chronic infection is directly related to the age at first infection with HBV. Thus, 80% to more than 90% of babies born to infected mothers become chronic carriers of HBV compared to fewer than 10% of exposed adolescents and adults. With regard to the expression of acute, symptomatic disease upon initial infection, the reverse situation is true. Both phenomena are the result of the host's immune response to the virus, with neonates and children having a weaker immune response that leads to minimal symptoms and chronic infection and adults having a stronger response that leads to overt disease and viral clearance.

The global distribution of chronic HBV infection varies. Low levels of endemicity (ie, < 2% HBsAg prevalence) can be found in the Americas, western and northern Europe, and Australia. Areas with a more moderate prevalence of HBV carriers (2% to 7%) include eastern and southern Europe, the Middle East, Japan, and southern Asia. China, Southeast Asia, and sub-

Saharan Africa have the highest levels of chronic HBV infection ($\geq$ 8%) (IARC, 1994a). As would be expected, transmission around the time of birth and during childhood are important routes of infection with regard to HBV endemicity and are major sources of infection in areas where the prevalence of HBsAg is high. A strong geographic correlation has been demonstrated between the prevalence of chronic HBV infection and the incidence of HCC (Maupas and Melnick, 1981), with populations in the United States and Europe having low HCC rates as well as a low prevalence of HBV carriers.

The most convincing evidence for a causal role of chronic HBV infection in HCC development can be found in the overwhelmingly consistent results from the extensive number of analytic studies, representing over 2 decades of epidemiologic research in more than 25 countries throughout the world (IARC, 1994a). Most of the studies have been case-control in design and have yielded relative risk estimates ranging from 5 to 30 for the association of HCC with HBsAg positivity. The relative risk has been even higher in cohort studies (IARC, 1994a; Mori et al, 2000; Evans et al, 2002; Yang et al, 2002), exceeding 100-fold in a study from Taiwan (Beasley, 1988). In addition, early establishment of chronic HBV infection during childhood appears to increase the future risk of HCC (Muñoz et al, 1989; Kuper et al, 2000a). This hypothesis is also supported by the differential in risk observed for the younger age groups in high- and low-risk populations. In populations from low- and intermediate-risk areas, liver cancer is rarely observed in persons less than 40 years old, in contrast to populations with a high incidence of liver cancer, in which the disease is quite frequent in the younger age groups (Bosch et al, 2004). No association of HBV infection with cholangiocarcinoma has been reported in the few studies that have examined the relationship (IARC, 1994a).

On a molecular level, HBV DNA has been detected in the liver tissue specimens from over 90% of HBsAg-positive HCC cases as well as in some cases with no HBV serum markers (Tabor, 1998). These HBV sequences appear to be clonally integrated in the tumor cells. Although the woodchuck hepatitis virus causes liver cancer through insertional mutagenesis at the *myc* gene locus (Tennant et al, 2004), until recently no notable integration site for HBV-associated human HCC had been identified (Tabor, 1998). Newer polymerase chain reaction (PCR)–based methods, however, have shown that HBV integration may occur more frequently in or adjacent to host genes related to cell growth (Bréchot et al, 2000; Momosaki et al, 2003; Murakami et al, 2005). Moreover, insertion of multiple copies of the HBV genome can generate various random chromosomal abnormalities (Tabor, 1994).

The *X* and *PRE S2/S* regions of the HBV genome appear able to transactivate cellular oncogenes including *C-MYC* and *C-FOS* (Tabor, 1994; Bréchot et al, 2000). The HBV *X* gene encodes a viral protein whose function has not been established, but that can transactivate the transcription of viral and host genes in vitro. The *PRE S2/S* gene encodes for the middle protein of the HBV surface antigen. Sequences from both viral genes are systematically retained in HBV inserts in tumor cells (Bréchot et al, 2000). The deletions occurring in the integrated subviral DNA likely are important for transactivation, since the native PRE S2/S protein has no detectable transactivation potential and the truncated X protein is a stronger transactivator than the wild-type form. Furthermore, the X protein has been shown to inhibit the function of TP53 by binding this tumor suppressor in HCC tissue and in transgenic mice; of interest, there are reports of the development of HCC in 90% of male mice transgenic for the HBV *X* gene (Tabor, 1997). It is not clear whether HBV infection can lead directly to the mutations or allelic losses observed for the *TP53* and retinoblastoma genes in human HCC.

The potential etiologic relevance of so-called *occult* or *silent* HBV infection in the development of HCC has been the focus of several investigations (Bréchot et al, 2000; Tabor, 2002). Low levels of HBV DNA have been found in both HBsAg-negative HCC cases and noncases including blood donors, whose only marker of infection is antibody to the HBV core protein. Existing data support that such occult HBV infection does play a role in HCC (Bréchot et al, 2000; Tabor, 2002; Pollicino et al, 2004). The exact nature of this role is not clear and may be primarily in conjunction with other cofactors.

An effect of occult HBV on HCC has been most notable in hepatitis C virus (HCV)–associated disease (Bréchot et al, 2000; Tabor, 2002; Pollicino et al, 2004; Momosaki et al, 2005). The presence of HBsAg-negative HBV infection in HCC cases may be related to reduced virus replication associated with integration of the virus into the host genome or to mutations to the virus genome itself. Of interest, a specific double mutation in nucleotides 1762 (A→T) and 1764 (G→A) within the core promoter and X genes of the detected HBV DNA sequences has been reported in HBsAg-negative HCV-associated HCC cases (Momosaki et al, 2005). This same mutation has been found in HBsAg-positive tumors, and its detection in stored samples has been shown to predict the incidence of HCC, up to 5 years before diagnosis, in a prospective cohort study in China (Kuang et al, 2004).

Other markers of HBV infection also may prove to be useful in identifying carriers at high risk of progression to HCC. Two nested case-control studies within cohorts of HBsAg-positive men in Taiwan found a six- to sevenfold association of high prediagnostic serum levels of HBV DNA with the incidence of HCC, suggesting that increased virus replication might play a role in HBV-induced hepatocarcinogenesis (Yang et al, 2002; Yu et al, 2005). Moreover, some studies have shown that HBV carriers infected with genotype C may be at increased risk of HCC (Fujie et al, 2001; Yu et al, 2005); of interest, the 1762/1764 double mutation has been found more frequently in conjunction with HBV genotype C infection (Kuang et al, 2004).

Additionally, chronic HBV infection may also promote tumorogenesis through the continual turnover of hepatocytes resulting from constant inflammation and damage to the liver. In fact, most cases of HCC arise within cirrhotic livers (Tabor, 1998; Bréchot et al, 2000). Thus, due to its potential ability to both initiate and promote HCC development, HBV has been viewed as a complete carcinogen (Trichopoulos et al, 1987; Tabor, 1994).

In 1994, the IARC concluded that there was sufficient evidence to classify HBV as a human carcinogen (IARC, 1994a). Globally, an estimated 54% of all liver cancer—about 340 000 cases in 2002—can be attributed to HBV infection (Parkin, 2006). Most of the HBV-associated liver cancer occurs in the developing world (attributable fraction, 59%); those areas with the greatest burden include Melanesia (77%), western and central Africa (70%), and China (69.5%). In developed countries, only 23% of liver cancer is likely due to HBV infection, with as little as 9% in North America and western and northern Europe (Parkin, 2006).

The development of a safe, effective vaccine against HBV infection provides the opportunity to prevent a substantial proportion of HCC. Childhood vaccination programs initiated in HBV-endemic areas have led to a distinct reduction in the prevalence of carriers in those populations (Chen et al, 1996; Blumberg, 1997). Of singular importance is the report of a significant decline in HCC incidence among children in Taiwan between 1981 and 1994 following the introduction of a nationwide HBV immunization program (Chang et al, 1997). These data demonstrate the effectiveness of HBV vaccination in preventing the occurrence of HCC. Programs aimed at the universal immunization of infants have been established in over 100 countries (Bosch et al, 2004).

Hepatitis C virus

Hepatitis C virus, an RNA virus in the Flaviviridae family, was first identified in 1988 (Choo et al, 1989). With no reverse transcriptase, HCV does not integrate into the host's DNA (Tabor, 1998). The current multiantigen tests appear to have sufficient sensitivity and specificity to reliably detect antibody to HCV (anti-HCV). The presence of viremia also can be determined using reverse transcriptase-PCR for the detection of HCV RNA.

Characterization of the natural history of HCV has been challenging, primarily due to the largely asymptomatic nature of the infection. Based for the most part on studies of patients identified by the presence of clinical hepatitis or by transfusion exposure, as well as on population-based cross-sectional studies of HCV RNA prevalence, about 70% to 85% of those infected with HCV will develop a chronic, persistent infection (Alter et al, 1999; Bellentani et al, 1999; Hoofnagle, 2002; Okayama et al, 2002); persistence of infection may be less frequent in women and those who are younger or who experience symptomatic acute infection (Alter et al, 1999; Bellentani et al, 1999; Kenny-Walsh et al, 1999; Hoofnagle, 2002).

Among persons with chronic HCV infection, 50% to 80% progress to chronic hepatitis (Alter et al, 1992; Takahashi et al, 1993; Kenny-Walsh et al, 1999; Hoofnagle, 2002; Okayama et al, 2002). The rate of subsequent progression to cirrhosis appears to be quite variable and to be related to characteristics of the infected individual, including age at infection and underlying disease status (Poynard et al, 1997). In an analysis by Freeman et al (2001), the 20-year incidence of cirrhosis was estimated to range from 4% in blood donors and 7% in community-based populations to 22% in liver disease patients and 24% in persons with transfusion-related infection. After the development of cirrhosis, 4% or more progress to malignancy (Alter and Seeff, 2000).

In most populations throughout the world, the prevalence of anti-HCV is below 2.5%; however, the level of infection is very high (> 10%) in Egypt and appears to be linked to mass schistosomiasis treatment campaigns (IARC, 1994a; Lavanchy and McMahon, 2000). Pockets of relatively high HCV seroprevalence also have been reported in areas of Japan (Kiyosawa et al,

1994; Tanaka et al, 1997). Percutaneous transmission of the virus appears to be the major route of infection, with exposure to contaminated blood products (prior to screening), intravenous drug use (in the United States and other Western populations), and utilization of nondisposable needles/syringes (previously, in Japan, other Southeast Asia populations, some European countries, Egypt) representing important modes of transmission (Alter et al, 2000).

Epidemiologic studies have consistently supported a strong association between HCV and HCC, with relative risks greater than 10 in some cohort studies (IARC, 1994a; Yu and Chen, 1993; Boschi-Pinto et al, 2000; Mori et al, 2000; Sun et al, 2003). A similarly strong association has been observed in case-control studies conducted in a variety of populations (IARC, 1994a; Donato et al, 1998; Tagger et al, 1999; Kuper et al, 2000c). In Japan, anti-HCV seroprevalence has been correlated with HCC rates (Tanaka et al, 1994). Some studies have reported that HCV genotype 1b may contribute disproportionately to the virus' hepatocarcinogenic effect (Tanaka et al, 1996; Tagger et al, 1999). Patients with genotype 1 infection are also known to have a poorer response to interferon treatment (Hoofnagle, 2002). However, questions have been raised as to whether HCV genotype actually affects liver disease progression, based on a lack of association observed in other studies (Davis, 1999; Tagger et al, 1999). In addition, recent data suggest that HCV infection, in contrast to HBV infection (Kuper et al, 2001), may be associated with the risk of developing cholangiocarcinoma (Shaib et al, 2005).

The mechanisms by which HCV may cause liver cancer are not well understood. Since most HCV-associated HCC occurs in the presence of cirrhosis (Alter and Seeff, 2000), HCV infection may lead to cancer through the indirect mechanism of immune-mediated damage and subsequent liver cell turnover (Tabor, 1998). As a nonintegrating virus, HCV would be unlikely to have a direct role in HCC initiation. However, the HCV core protein has been shown to exhibit oncogenic properties in vitro. In particular, the core protein may affect cell-cycle control through repression of TP53 (Ray et al, 1997; Anzola, 2004) and interference with tumor necrosis factor alpha-inducted apoptosis (Block et al, 2003). Of note, HCC can develop in male mice that are transgenic for the HCV core gene (Moriya et al, 1998). The nonstructural virus proteins NS3 and NS5A also may play a role in HCV-inducted hepatocarcinogenesis via interaction with TP53 and intracellular signaling pathways (Block et al, 2003; Anzola, 2004). Last, HCV infection may be associated with increased levels of TGF-α and IGF-II, which could induce transformation of hepatocytes (Tanaka et al, 1996).

Hepatitis C virus–associated HCC appears to affect older patients and to follow more severe liver disease than does HBV-associated HCC (Shiratori et al, 1995). Thus, a prolonged period of hepatocellular damage progressing from chronic hepatitis to cirrhosis to HCC may be required for the development of HCV-related malignancy (Kiyosawa et al, 1990). There is considerable evidence for a strong interaction between heavy alcohol consumption and HCV infection, more so than for HBV infection, on the occurrence of liver damage and the progression of liver disease (Poynard et al, 1997; Tagger et al, 1999; Mori et al, 2000; Donato et al, 2002). Several studies have found that heavy alcohol consumption may markedly enhance the risk of HCC among those with HCV-associated cirrhosis (Chen et al, 1997; Okuda, 1997).

An interaction between HBV and HCV infections in the development of HCC has been suggested in some studies (Kaklamani et al, 1991; Kew et al, 1997; Tagger et al, 1999). In a meta-analysis, the synergism was superadditive, with summary relative risks of 165 for dual infection; 22.5 for infection with HBV alone; and 17.3 for infection with HCV alone (Donato et al, 1998). Several studies also have reported a negative association between prevalence of HBsAg and anti-HCV among control subjects, which would suggest some type of interference between the two infections (Tanaka et al, 1991; Donato et al, 1998; Tagger et al, 1999). Nonetheless, it would seem that when coinfection does occur, the effect is to further enhance virus-associated hepatocarcinogenesis. Coinfection with human immunodeficiency virus also appears to increase the risk of HCV-induced liver disease progression, most likely due to insufficient immune control of chronic HCV infection and increased hepatocellular damage (Graham et al, 2001; Thomas, 2002).

Hepatitis C virus has been designated as carcinogenic to humans by the IARC (1994a). Just under one-third of the liver cancers occurring in the world are estimated to be attributable to HCV infection; this figure represents 195 000 cases in 2002 (Parkin, 2006). The impact of HCV-associated HCC appears to be greatest in Asia, where the attributable fraction is 30% in Japan, 36% in China, and 41% in Southeast Asia, as well as in northern (61%) and central (55%) Africa (Parkin, 2006). Overall, the proportion of liver cancer due to HCV is higher in developing (33%) than in developed (20%) countries. A large part of the observed increase in HCC incidence in Japan (Okuda, 1997), and also in the United States (El-Serag et al, 2003), is considered to be the result of HCV infection.

Although at present there is no vaccine to prevent HCV infection, evidence exists to support significant reductions in new infections through the interruption of parenteral transmission of the virus. The testing of blood donations for anti-HCV has led to substantial decreases in the number of posttransfusion hepatitis C cases in Taiwan (Wang et al, 1995), Japan (Japanese Red Cross Non A, Non B-Hepatitis Research Group, 1991), and the United States (Tobler and Busch, 1997). The use of disposable needles and syringes and other changes in medical procedures also likely have helped to reduce HCV infection in Japan (Okuda, 1997) and Taiwan (Sung, 1997). Since parenteral exposure appears to be a major route of transmission, such interventions may be important for a future decline of HCV-associated liver cancer. In addition, some studies, albeit of mixed quality, have shown a possible protective effect of interferon treatment on the development of HCC among HCV carriers with and without cirrhosis, which is most evident among those patients who experienced a sustained response to treatment (Papatheodoridis et al, 2001; Heathcote, 2004).

Liver flukes

So far, we have discussed only the causal role of infections in the etiology of HCC. However, cholangiocarcinoma, occurring predominantly in Asia, has also been linked to infection, namely with the liver flukes *Opisthorchis viverrini*, *Opisthorchis felineus*, and *Clonorchis sinensis* (Parkin et al, 1991; IARC, 1994b). Chronic infection with these food-borne parasites usually occurs in the intrahepatic bile ducts. High endemic levels of infection can be found in Thailand and Laos (*O. viverrini*), in China, Taiwan, and the Republic of Korea (*C. sinensis*), and in the then Russian Federation (*O. felineus*) (IARC, 1994b).

The epidemiologic evidence linking liver fluke infection to cholangiocarcinoma is based on correlation studies primarily from Thailand, as well as on a limited number of case-control studies. One hospital-based study in Thailand found a fivefold association of elevated antibodies to *O. viverrini* with cholangiocarcinoma (Parkin et al, 1991), but no significant association with HCC (Srivatanakul et al, 1991); a more recent population-based case-control study in Thailand reported a more than 20-fold higher risk of cholangiocarcinoma with elevated levels of *O. viverrini* (Honjo et al, 2005). Based on the available data, an IARC Working Group concluded that infection with *O. viverrini* is carcinogenic to humans and infection with *C. sinensis* is probably carcinogenic (IARC, 1994b).

Ionizing Radiation

Exposure to diagnostic thorium dioxide, that is, Thorotrast, from the 1930s to the 1950s has been strongly associated with an increased risk of liver cancer (IARC, 1987).

Data on the relationship of Thorotrast exposure to cancer occurrence have originated from follow-up studies of patients injected with this radioactive contrast medium, in which relative risk estimates ranging from 13 to 126 were reported (Andersson and Storm, 1992; Mori et al, 1999; dos Santos Silva et al, 2003; Travis et al, 2003). Despite the potential limitations of these study cohorts, including selection of an appropriate unexposed group, differential loss to follow-up, quality of the cancer outcome information, and lack of data on important confounders, it is unlikely that bias could account for the strong associations observed. The malignancy appears to occur long after the exposure, with the majority of cases being of the cholangiocarcinoma and angiosarcoma subtypes.

Results from the Life Span Study of the atomic bomb survivors cohort in Hiroshima and Nagasaki, Japan, have shown a dose–response relationship between whole-body radiation exposure and the incidence of primary liver cancer (Thompson et al, 1994). In contrast to the findings of the studies of Thorotrast, the effect of the atomic bomb radiation exposure appears to be related to the development of HCC and not to the other histologic subtypes (Cologne et al, 1999). Additional analyses suggest that the radiation-related excess risk is higher in men and in persons who were exposed in their 20s; however, the investigators noted that confounding by known risk factors for HCC might account, in part, for these observations (Cologne et al, 1999).

Occupation

Vinyl chloride and inorganic arsenic exposure are considered to increase the risk of developing angiosarcoma in the liver (IARC, 1987; Chen et al, 1997; Ishak, 1997). The evidence for a causal association is strongest for vinyl chloride (IARC, 1987). A number of epidemiologic studies that examined the carcinogenic effect of occupational exposure to vinyl chloride have reported an increased risk of angiosarcoma (IARC, 1987; Lewis and Rempala, 2003;

Boffetta et al, 2003). In addition, specific *TP53* mutation patterns appear to occur in vinyl chloride–associated angiosarcomas (Ishak, 1997). Exposure to this chemical also has been linked to the occurrence of HCC (IARC, 1987; Boffetta et al, 2003; Mastrangelo et al, 2004).

The possible association of angiosarcoma with arsenic includes exposure not only in occupational settings but also via medical treatment (eg, Fowler's solution) and contaminated drinking water (IARC, 1987; Chen et al, 1997; Ishak, 1997). Intake of inorganic arsenic from well water also has been associated with HCC in epidemiologic studies conducted in Taiwan (Chen et al, 1997). In 1987, IARC judged both vinyl chloride and arsenic as being carcinogenic to humans (IARC, 1987).

In an extensive review and meta-analysis of the epidemiologic evidence for the carcinogenicity of the organic solvent trichloroethylene (TCE), Wartenberg et al (2000) concluded that the available data support an effect of TCE exposure on liver cancer occurrence. The investigators estimated an overall relative risk of 1.9 for the association of occupational exposure to this solvent and liver cancer incidence, based on data from occupational cohorts with the best-quality exposure assessment.

Medical Conditions

A fairly strong positive association of liver cancer with diabetes mellitus has been noted in a number of epidemiologic studies conducted in several different countries (Adami et al, 1996; Lagiou et al, 2000; El-Serag et al, 2004; Yuan et al, 2004; Davila et al, 2005). In a meta-analysis of published studies conducted between 1996 and 2005, a pooled odds ratio of 2.5 was found, for the association of diabetes with HCC, in both case-control and cohort studies (El-Serag et al, 2006). Although the nature of this association and its biological significance are not well understood, exposure of the liver to elevated levels of insulin, which may have important mitogenic properties, or the increased risk of liver disease among

diabetics could possibly contribute to hepatocarcinogenesis (Adami et al, 1996; Lagiou et al, 2000). Both hepatitis virus infection, particularly with HCV, and heavy alcohol consumption have been reported to act synergistically with diabetes to increase the occurrence of HCC (Donato et al, 2002; Hassan et al, 2002; Davila et al, 2005; Yuan et al, 2004).

Of related importance is the emerging evidence that nonalcoholic fatty liver disease (NAFLD), and its more serious manifestation—nonalcoholic steatohepatitis (NASH)—may play a role in hepatocarcinogenesis (Bugianesi et al, 2002). Several case series reports have suggested a possible association between NASH and HCC (Bugianesi et al, 2002; Shimada et al, 2002), and a fourfold increased risk of liver cancer was found for patients with NAFLD in Denmark (Sorensen et al, 2003). Both diabetes and obesity are known to be associated with NAFLD and NASH (Bugianesi et al, 2002; El-Serag et al, 2003) and, thus, may contribute to the development of HCC through a process of metabolic dysregulation and insulin resistance leading to NAFLD and NASH, with subsequent fibrosis and cirrhosis and progression to malignancy (Bugianesi et al, 2002).

Two medical conditions that directly affect the biliary ducts also appear to be associated with the development of liver cancer. Based on studies in Europe, patients with primary sclerosing cholangitis, a relatively rare disease, have a high incidence of cholangiocarcinoma (Bergquist et al, 1998; Chalasani et al, 2000). In one study, smoking seemed to enhance the risk of the malignancy among patients with this condition (Bergquist et al, 1998); in another, alcohol consumption did (Chalasani et al, 2000). An increased occurrence of HCC also has been observed in patients with primary biliary cirrhosis (Lööf et al, 1994) and it is likely that any type of cirrhosis, although to a variable degree, may act as a growth-enhancing factor in hepatocarcinogenesis (Kew and Popper 1984; Trichopoulos et al, 1987).

CANCER OF THE BILIARY TRACT DESCRIPTIVE EPIDEMIOLOGY

Cancers of the biliary tract primarily include malignancies occurring in the gallbladder and extrahepatic bile ducts. Gallbladder cancer occurs more frequently than bile duct cancer and is more common in women than in men. On a global level, the incidence of these cancers is relatively low. The highest incidence rates of gallbladder cancer are found in India, Japan, Korea, Latin America, and eastern Europe; low incidence rates occur in northern Europe, the United States, and Canada (Lazcano-Ponce et al, 2001; Randi et al, 2006). Differences in rates also are observed within countries, with respect to area of residence and racial group. Biliary tract cancer rates appear to be increasing in Japan, Chile, Italy, and Spain and decreasing in the United States, Canada, the United Kingdom, and Colombia (Lazcano-Ponce et al, 2001; Randi et al, 2006).

RISK FACTORS

Gallbladder Disease

Probably due to its infrequent occurrence and rapidly fatal outcome, little epidemiologic research has been done on the etiology of biliary tract cancer. The most consistently observed association is that between a history of gallstones or gallbladder disease and the occurrence of gallbladder cancer. On a global level, a strong geographic correlation exists between gallstone prevalence and gallbladder cancer incidence (Lazcano-Ponce et al, 2001; Randi et al, 2006). Variations in incidence within countries also correspond to differences in the frequency of gallstone disease; for example, a high prevalence of gallstones has been observed in Native Americans and Hispanics in the United States, populations in which gallbladder cancer rates are high (Lazcano-Ponce et al, 2001; Randi et al, 2006).

A number of case-control studies (Kato et al, 1989; WHO Collaborative Study of Neoplasia and Steroid Contraceptives, 1989a; Zatonski et al, 1997), as well as a

few cohort studies (Chow et al, 1999; Randi et al, 2006), have evaluated the association between history of gallstones or gallbladder disease and the risk of gallbladder cancer. In a review and meta-analysis of risk factors for gallbladder cancer by Randi et al (2006), summary relative risk estimates of 7.1 for the case-control studies and 2.2 for the cohort studies were obtained for history of gallbladder disease.

In addition, a family history of gallbladder disease or cancer appears to increase the risk of development of gallbladder cancer (Kato et al, 1989; Fernandez et al, 1994). The frequency of cholecystectomy operations would affect the incidence of biliary tract cancer and likely explains some of the observed variations among countries and over time (Lazcano-Ponce et al, 2001). Cholecystectomy also is associated with a reduced risk of bile duct cancer (Ekbom et al, 1993; Chow et al, 1999).

Obesity and Diet

Obesity may be another major risk factor for biliary tract cancer, probably through the strong relationship between overweight and the occurrence of gallstones (World Cancer Research Fund, 1997; Calle and Kaaks, 2004). An association of obesity with gallbladder cancer has been observed for both men and women (Calle et al, 2003; Samanic et al, 2004), although sometimes the effect is more evident for women (Zatonksi et al, 1997; Wolk et al, 2001; Randi et al, 2006). With respect to dietary intake and biliary tract cancer occurrence, frequent consumption of fruits and vegetables appears to be protective (Kato et al, 1989). A consistent association with an intake of high-fat foods has not been observed (Kato et al, 1989; Zatonksi et al, 1997). An increased level of total energy intake also may be related to an elevated occurrence of gallbladder cancer (Zatonksi et al, 1997).

Hormonal Factors

Reproductive factors appear to play a role in the development of biliary tract cancer. Increasing parity, which also is associated with gallstones, has been linked to an increased risk of gallbladder cancer (Lambe et al, 1993; Zatonski et al, 1997; Randi et al, 2006). Older age at first birth, however, may decrease this risk (Lambe et al, 1993; Zatonski et al, 1997). Reports of oral contraceptive use in relation to biliary tract cancer do not support a strong association (WHO Collaborative Study of Neoplasia and Steroid Contraceptives, 1989a; Zatonski et al, 1997). The limited studies conducted have not found a consistent association of hormone replacement therapy with biliary tract cancer risk (Zatonski et al, 1997; Gallus et al, 2002).

Mechanisms

Although all of the potential risk factors identified for biliary tract cancer also are associated with the development of gallstones (Lambe et al, 1993; Zatonski et al, 1997; Lazcano-Ponce et al, 2001), it is not established that common etiology is involved. Genetic susceptibility also has been postulated (Lazcano-Ponce et al, 2001). The mechanism by which cholelithiasis contributes to biliary tract carcinogenesis is not clear. Chronic inflammation probably plays a role (Lazcano-Ponce et al, 2001), a hypothesis that is supported by the strong long-term protective effective of removal of the gallbladder on the development of bile duct cancer (Ekbom et al, 1993). Alternatively, metabolic abnormalities or changes in bile composition are relevant to both gallstone formation and biliary tract cancer development (Lambe et al, 1993; Lazcano-Ponce et al, 2001). Nonetheless, avoidance of behaviors and exposures that may increase the risk of gallbladder disease would likely reduce the incidence of biliary tract cancer.

CONCLUSION

Primary liver cancer encompasses hepatocellular carcinoma ($> 90\%$), cholangiocarcinoma ($< 10\%$), and some other rare histologic types. Hepatocellular carcinoma is one of the most common cancers in Southeast Asia and in sub-Saharan Africa, and it is almost uniformly fatal. During the last 30 years, epidemiologic research has revealed the causes of most HCC cases. Chronic infection with HBV and HCV dominates the etiology of the disease in developing countries. Aflatoxin exposure also likely contributes to the causation of HCC in Africa. In developed countries, however, these factors are less prevalent, and alcoholic cirrhosis, cirrhosis of other etiology, and tobacco smoking assume a relatively more important role. Diet may also affect the development of liver cancer, but the relevant evidence is not conclusive. Rare chemical exposures, such as inorganic arsenic and vinyl chloride monomer, and, in the past, internal radiation from the contrast medium Thorotrast have been responsible for a small proportion of cases. Some inherited conditions, notably α1-antitrypsin deficiency, hemochromatosis, and porphyria cutanea tarda, also increase the risk of HCC. Cholangiocarcinoma has been linked to chronic infection with *O. viverrini* and perhaps other liver flukes, all food-borne parasites. Cancer of the extrahepatic bile ducts is closely associated with cholelithiasis and its attending risk factors, in particular female gender, obesity, and high parity.

REFERENCES

Adami HO, Chow WH, Nyrén O, Berne C, Linet MS, Ekbom A, et al. Excess risk of primary liver cancer in patients with diabetes mellitus [see comments]. J Natl Cancer Inst 1996;88:1472–77.

Adami HO, Hsing AW, McLaughlin JK, Trichopoulos D, Hacker D, Ekbom A, et al. Alcoholism and liver cirrhosis in the etiology of primary liver cancer. Int J Cancer 1992;51:898–902.

Aihara T, Noguchi S, Miyoshi Y, Nakano H, Sasaki Y, Nakamura Y, et al. Allelic imbalance of insulin-like growth factor II gene expression in cancerous and precancerous lesions of the liver. Hepatology 1998;28:86–89.

Alter HJ, Seeff LB. Recovery, persistence, and sequelae in hepatitis C virus infection: a perspective on long-term outcome. Semin Liver Dis 2000;20:17–35.

Alter MJ, Hutin YYF, Armstrong GL. Epidemiology of hepatitis C. In: Liang TJ, Hoofnagle JH (Eds): Biomedical Research

Reports, Hepatitis C. San Diego, Academic Press, 2000, pp 169–83.

Alter MJ, Kruszon-Moran D, Nainan OV, McQuillan GM, Gao F, Moyer LA, et al. The prevalence of hepatitis C virus infection in the United States, 1988 through 1994. N Engl J Med 1999;341:556–62.

Alter MJ, Margolis HS, Krawczynski K, Judson FN, Mares A, Alexander WJ, et al. The natural history of community-acquired hepatitis C in the United States. The Sentinel Counties Chronic non-A, non-B Hepatitis Study Team. N Engl J Med 1992;327:1899–1905.

Andersson M, Storm HH. Cancer incidence among Danish Thorotrast-exposed patients. J Natl Cancer Inst 1992;84:1318–25.

Anzola M. Hepatocellular carcinoma: role of hepatitis B and hepatitis C viruses proteins in hepatocarcinogenesis. J Viral Hepatitis 2004; 11:383–93.

Austin H. The role of tobacco use and alcohol consumption in the etiology of hepatocellular carcinoma. In: Tabor E, Di Bisceglie AM, Purcell RH (Eds): Etiology, Pathology, and Treatment of Hepatocellular Carcinoma in North America. Vol. 13. Houston, Advances in Applied Biotechnology Series, 1991, pp 57–75.

Beasley RP. Hepatitis B virus. The major etiology of hepatocellular carcinoma. Cancer 1988;61:1942–56.

Bellentani S, Pozzato G, Saccoccio G, Crovatto M, Croce LS, Mazzoran L, et al. Clinical course and risk factors of hepatitis C virus related liver disease in the general population: report from the Dionysos study. Gut 1999;44:874–80.

Bergquist A, Glaumann H, Persson B, Broome U. Risk factors and clinical presentation of hepatobiliary carcinoma patients with primary sclerosing cholangitis: a case-control study. Hepatology 1998;27:311–16.

Block TM, Mehta AS, Fimmel CJ, Jordan R. Molecular viral oncology of hepatocellular carcinoma. Oncogene 2003;44:5093–107.

Blumberg BS. The current state of the prevention of HBV infection, the carrier state and hepatocellular carcinoma. Res Virol 1997;148: 91–94.

Boffetta P, Matisane L, Mundt KA, Dell LD. Meta-analysis of studies of occupational exposure to vinyl chloride in relation to cancer mortality. Scand J Work Environ Health 2003;29:220–29.

Bosch FX, Ribes J, Diaz M, Cleries R. Primary liver cancer: worldwide incidence and trends. Gastroenterol 2004;127:S5–S16.

Boschi-Pinto C, Stuver S, Okayama A, Trichopoulos D, Orav EJ, Tsubouchi H, et al. A follow-up study of morbidity and mortality associated with hepatitis C virus infection and its interaction with human T lymphotropic virus type I in Miyazaki, Japan. J Infect Dis 2000;181:35–41.

Bréchot C, Gozuacik D, Murakami Y, Paterlini-Brechot P. Molecular bases for the development of hepatitis B virus (HBV)-related hepatocellular carcinoma (HCC). Sem Cancer Biology 2000;10:211–31.

Bugianesi E, Leone N, Vanni E, Marchesini G, Brunello F, Carucci P, et al. Expanding the natural history of nonalcoholic steatohepatitis: from cryptogenic cirrhosis to hepatocellular carcinoma. Gastroenterol 2002;123:134–40.

Calle EE, Kaaks R. Overweight, obesity and cancer: epidemiological evidence and proposed mechanisms. Nat Rev Cancer 2004;4:579–91.

Calle EE, Rodriguez C, Walker-Thurmond K, Thun MJ. Overweight, obesity, and mortality from cancer in a prospectively studied cohort of U.S. adults. N Engl J Med 2003;348:1625–38.

Chalasani N, Baluyut A, Ismail A, Zaman A, Sood G, Ghalib R, et al. Cholangiocarcinoma in patients with primary sclerosing cholangitis: a multicenter case-control study. Hepatology 2000;31:7–11.

Chang MH, Chen CJ, Lai MS, Hsu HM, Wu TC, Kong MS, et al. Universal hepatitis B vaccination in Taiwan and the incidence of hepatocellular carcinoma in children. Taiwan Childhood Hepatoma Study Group. N Engl J Med 1997;336:1855–59.

Chen C-J, Yu M-W, Liaw Y-F. Epidemiological characteristics and risk factors of hepatocellular carcinoma. J Gastroenterol Hepatol 1997;12(Suppl):S294–S308.

Chen HL, Chang MH, Ni YH, Hsu HY, Lee PI, Lee CY, et al. Seroepidemiology of hepatitis B virus infection in children: Ten years of mass vaccination in Taiwan. JAMA 1996; 276:906–8.

Choo QL, Kuo G, Weiner AJ, Overby LR, Bradley DW, Houghton M. Isolation of a cDNA clone derived from a blood-borne non-A, non-B viral hepatitis genome. Science 1989;244:359–62.

Chow WH, Johansen C, Gridley G, Mellemkjaer L, Fraumeni Jr JF. Gallstones, cholecystectomy and risk of cancers of the liver, biliary tract and pancreas. Br J Cancer 1999; 79: 640–44.

Clemente C, Elba S, Buongiorno G, Berloco P, Guerra V, Di Leo A. Serum retinol and risk of hepatocellular carcinoma in patients with child-Pugh class A cirrhosis. Cancer Letters 2002;178:123–29.

Colditz GA. Oral contraceptive use and mortality during 12 years of follow-up: the Nurses' Health Study. Ann Intern Med 1994; 120:821–26.

Cologne JB, Tokuoka S, Beebe GW, Fukuhara T, Mabuchi K. Effects of radiation on incidence of primary liver cancer among atomic bomb survivors. Radiation Res 1999;152:364–73.

Davila JA, Morgan RO, Shaib Y, McGlynn KA, El-Serag HB. Diabetes increases the risk of hepatocellular carcinoma in the United States: a population based case control study. Gut 2005;54:533–39.

Davis GL. Hepatitis C virus genotype and quasispecies. Am J Med 1999;107:S21–S26.

Deugnier Y, Turlin B. Other causes of hepatocellular carcinoma. In: Okuda K, Tabor E (Eds): Liver Cancer. New York, Churchill Livingstone, 1997, pp 97–110.

Donato F, Boffetta P, Puoti M. A meta-analysis of epidemiologic studies on the combined effect of hepatitis B and C virus infections in causing hepatocellular carcinoma. Int J Cancer 1998;75:347–54.

Donato F, Tagger A, Gelatti U, Parrinello G, Boffetta P, Albertini A, et al. Alcohol and hepatocellular carcinoma: the effect of lifetime intake and hepatitis virus infections in men and women. Am J Epidemiol 2002;255:323–31.

dos Santos Silva I, Malveiro F, Jones ME, Swerdlow AJ. Mortality after radiological investigation with radioactive Thorotrast: a follow-up study of up to fifty years in Portugal. Radiation Res 2003;159:521–34.

Ekbom A, Hsieh CC, Yuen J, Trichopoulos D, McLaughlin JK, Lan SJ, et al. Risk of extrahepatic bile duct cancer after cholecystectomy. Lancet 1993;342:1262–65.

El-Serag HB, Davila JA, Petersen NJ, McGlynn KA. The continuing increase in the incidence of hepatocellular carcinoma in the United States: an update. Ann Intern Med 2003;139:817–23.

El-Serag HB, Hampel H, Javadi F. The association between diabetes and hepatocellular carcinoma: a systematic review of epidemiologic evidence. Clin Gastroenterol Hepatol 2006;4:369–80.

El-Serag HB, Tran T, Everhart JE. Diabetes increases the risk of chronic liver disease and hepatocellular carcinoma. Gastroenterol 2004;126:460–68.

Evans AA, Chen G, Ross EA, Sheu F-M, Lin W-Y, London WT. Eight-year follow-up of the 90,000-person Haimen City Cohort: I. Hepatocellular carcinoma mortality, risk factors, and gender differencers. Cancer Epidemiol Biomarkers Prev 2002;11:369–76.

Fernandez E, La Vecchia C, D'Avanzo B, Negri E, Franceschi S. Family history and the risk of liver, gallbladder, and pancreatic cancer. Cancer Epidemiol Biomarkers Prev 1994;3:209–12.

Freeman AJ, Dore GJ, Law MG, Thorpe M, Von Overbeck J, Lloyd AR, et al. Estimating progression to cirrhosis in chronic hepatitis C virus infection. Hepatology 2001;34:809–16.

Fujie H, Moriya K, Shintani Y, Yotsuyanagi H, Iino S, Koike K. Hepatitis B virus genotypes and hepatocellular carcinoma in Japan. Gastroenterology 2001;120:1564–65.

Fukuda K, Shibata A, Hirohata I, tanikawa K, Yamaguchi G, Ishii M. A hospital-based case-control study on hepatocellular carcinoma in Fukuoka and Saga Prefectures, northern Kyushu, Japan. Jpn J Cancer Res 1993; 84:708–14.

Gallus S, Negri E, Chatenoud L, Rosetti C, Franceschi S, La Vecchia C. Post-menopausal hormonal therapy and gall bladder cancer risk. Int J Cancer 2002;99:762–63.

Graham CS, Baden LR, Yu E, Mrus JM, Carnie J, Heeren T, et al. Influence of human immunodeficiency virus infection on the course of hepatitis C virus infection: a meta-analysis. Clin Infect Dis 2001;33:562–69.

Hassan MM, Hwang L-Y, Hatten CJ, Swaim M, Li D, Abbruzzese JL, et al. Risk factors for hepatocellular carcinoma: synergism of alcohol with viral hepatitis and diabetes mellitus. Hepatology 2002;36:1206–13.

Heathcote EJ. Prevention of hepatitis C virus-related hepatocellular carcinoma. Gastroenterol 2004;127:S294–S302.

Honjo S, Srivatanakul P, Sriplung H, Kikukawa H, Hanai S, Uchida K, et al. Genetic and environmental determinants of risk for cholangiocarcinoma via Opisthorchis viverrini in a densely infested area in Nakhon Phanom, northeast Thailand. Int J Cancer 2005;117:854–60.

Hoofnagle JH. Course and outcome of hepatitis C. Hepatology 2002;36(Suppl 1):S21–S29.

Hsing AW, McLaughlin JK, Hoover RN, Co-Chien HT, Blot WJ, Fraumeni Jr JF. Parity and primary liver cancer among young women. J Natl Cancer Inst 1992;84:1118–19.

Inoue M, Yoshimi I, Sobue T, Tsugane S. For the JPHC Study Group. Influence of coffee drinking on subsequent risk of hepatocellular carcinoma: a prospective study in Japan. J Natl Cancer Inst 2005;97:293–300.

International Agency for Research on Cancer. Overall Evaluations of Carcinogenicity: An Updating of IARC Monographs 1–42. IARC Monogr Eval Carcinog Risk Humans. Suppl 7. Lyon, IARC, 1987.

International Agency for Research on Cancer. Alcohol Drinking. IARC Monogr Eval Carcinog Risk Humans. Vol. 44. Lyon, IARC, 1988.

International Agency for Research on Cancer. Some Naturally Occurring Substances: Food Items and Constituents, Heterocyclic Aromatic Amines and Mycotoxins. IARC

Monogr Eval Carcinog Risk Humans. Vol 56. Lyon, IARC, 1993.

International Agency for Research on Cancer. Hepatitis Viruses. IARC Monogr Eval Carcinog Risk Humans. Vol. 59. Lyon, IARC, 1994a.

International Agency for Research on Cancer. Schistosomes, Liver Flukes and Helicobacter pylori. IARC Monogr Eval Carcinog Risk Humans. Vol. 61. Lyon, IARC, 1994b.

International Agency for Research on Cancer. Tobacco Smoke and Involuntary Smoking. IARC Monogr Eval Carcinog Risk Humans. Vol. 83. Lyon, IARC 2004, pp 679 and 1182–83.

Ishak KG. Malignant mesenchymal tumors and some other nonhepatocellular tumors of the liver. In: Okuda K, Tabor E (Eds): Liver Cancer. New York, Churchill Livingstone, 1997, pp 291–314.

Japanese Red Cross Non A, Non B-Hepatitis Research Group. Effect of screening for hepatitis C virus antibody and hepatitis B virus core antibody on incidence of post-transfusion hepatitis. Lancet 1991;338:1040–41.

Kaklamani E, Trichopoulos D, Tzonou A, Zavitsanos X, Koumantaki Y, Hatzakis A, et al. Hepatitis B and C viruses and their interaction in the origin of hepatocellular carcinoma. JAMA 1991;265:1974–76.

Kato K, Akai S, Tominaga S, Kato I. A case-control study of biliary tract cancer in Niigata Prefecture, Japan. Jpn J Cancer Res 1989;80:932–38.

Kenny-Walsh E. For the Irish Hepatology Research Group. Clinical outcomes after hepatitis C infection from contaminated anti-D immune globulin. N Engl J Med 1999;340:1228–33.

Kew MC. Synergistic interaction between aflatoxin B1 and hepatitis B virus in hepatocarcinogenesis. Liver Intl 2003;23:405–9.

Kew MC, Popper H. Relationship between hepatocellular carcinoma and cirrhosis. Semin Liver Dis 1984;4:136–46.

Kew MC, Yu MC, Kedda M-A, Coppin A, Sarkin A, Hodkinson J. The relative roles of hepatitis-B and -C viruses in the etiology of hepatocellular carcinoma in southern African blacks. Gastroenterology 1997;112:184–87.

Kiyosawa K, Sodeyama T, Tanaka E, Gibo Y, Yoshizawa K, Nakano Y, et al. Interrelationship of blood transfusion, non-A, non-B hepatitis and hepatocellular carcinoma: analysis by detection of antibody to hepatitis C virus. Hepatology 1990;12:671–75.

Kiyosawa K, Tanaka E, Sodeyama T, Yoshizawa K, Yabu K, Furuta K, et al. Transmission of hepatitis C in an isolated area in Japan: community-acquired-infection. The South Kiso Hepatitis Study Group. Gastroenterology 1994;106:1596–1602.

Kuang SY, Jackson PE, Wang JB, Lu PX, Munoz A, Qian GS, et al. Specific mutations of hepatitis B virus in plasma predict liver cancer development. Proc Natl Acad Sci U.S.A. 2004;101:3575–80.

Kuper H, Hsieh CC, Stuver SO, Mucci LA, Tzonou A, Zavitsanos X, et al. Birth order, as a proxy for age at infection, in the etiology of hepatocellular carcinoma. Epidemiology 2000a;11:680–83.

Kuper H, Lagiou P, Mucci LA, Tamimi R, Benetou V, Trichopoulos D. Risk factors for cholangiocarcinoma in a low risk Caucasian population. Soz Praventivmed 2001;46:182–85.

Kuper H, Mantzoros C, Lagiou P, Tzonou A, Tamimi R, Mucci L, et al. Estrogens, testosterones and sex hormone binding globulin in relation to liver cancer in men. Oncology 2001b;60:355–60.

Kuper H, Tzonou A, Kaklamani E, Hadziyannis A, Tasopoulos N, Lagiou P, et al. Hepatitis B and C viruses in the etiology of hepatocellular carcinoma; a study in Greece using third-generation assays. Cancer Causes Control 2000c;11:171–75.

Kuper H, Tzonou A, Kaklamani E, Hsieh C-C, Lagiou P, Adami HO, et al. Tobacco smoking, alcohol consumption, and their interaction in the causation of hepatocellular carcinoma. Int J Cancer 2000b;85:498–502.

Kuper H, Tzonou A, Lagiou P, Mucci LA, Trichopoulos D, Stuver SO, et al. Diet and hepatocellular carcinoma: a case-control study in Greece. Nutrition and Cancer 2000d;38:6–12.

Kuper H, Ye W, Broomé U, Romelsjö A, Mucci LA, Ekbom A, et al. The risk of liver and bile duct cancer in patients with chronic viral hepatitis, alcoholism, or cirrhosis. Hepatology 2001a;34:714–18.

Lagiou P, Kuper H, Stuver SO, Tzonou A, Trichopoulos D, Adami H-O. Role of diabetes mellitus in the etiology of hepatocellular carcinoma. J Natl Cancer Inst 2000;92:1096–99.

Lam KC, Yu MC, Leung JWC, Henderson BE. Hepatitis B virus and cigarette smoking: risk factors for hepatocellular carcinoma in Hong Kong. Cancer Res 1982;42:5246–48.

Lambe M, Trichopoulos D, Hsieh C-C, Ekbom A, Adami H-O, Pavia M. Parity and cancer of the gall bladder and the extrahepatic bile ducts. Int J Cancer 1993;54:941–44.

Lavanchy D, McMahon B. Worldwide prevalence and prevention of hepatitis C. In: Liang TJ, Hoofnagle JH (Eds): Hepatitis C. San Diego, CA: Academic Press, 2000, pp 185–201.

La Vecchia C, Lucchini F, Franceschi S, Negri E, Levi F. Trends in mortality from primary liver cancer in Europe. Eur J Cancer 2000; 36:909–15.

La Vecchia C, Negri E, Decarli A, D'Aranzo B, Franceschi S. Risk factors for hepatocellular carcinoma in northern Italy. Int J Cancer 1988;42:872–76.

La Vecchia C, Negri E, Franceschi S, D'Avanzo B. Reproductive factors and the risk of hepatocellular carcinoma in women. Int J Cancer 1992;52:351–54.

Lazcano-Ponce EC, Miquel JF, Munoz N, Herrero R, Ferrecio C, Wistuba II, et al. Epidemiology and molecular pathology of gallbladder cancer. CA Cancer J Clin; 2001:51: 349–64.

Lee H-S, Yoon J-W, Kamimura S, Iwata K, Watanabe H, Kim CY. Lack of association of cytochrome P450 2E1 genetic polymorphisms with the risk of human hepatocellular carcinoma. Int J Cancer 1997;71:737–40.

Lewis R, Rempala G. A case-cohort study of angiosarcoma of the liver and brain cancer at a polymer production plant. J Occup Environ Med 2003;45:538–45.

Linet MS, Gridley G, Nyrén O, Mellemkjaer L, Olsen JH, Keehn S, et al. Primary liver cancer, other malignancies, and mortality risks following porphyria: a cohort study in Denmark and Sweden. Am J Epidemiol 1999; 149:1010–15.

Lööf L, Adami HO, Sparen P, Danielsson A, Eriksson LS, Hultcrantz R, et al. Cancer risk in primary biliary cirrhosis: a population-based study in Sweden. Hepatology 1994;20: 101–4.

Lunn Rm, Zhang YJ, Wang LY, Chen CJ, Lee PH, Lee CS, et al. p53 mutations, chronic hepatitis B virus infection, and aflatoxin exposure in hepatocellular carcinoma in Taiwan. Cancer Res 1997;57:3471–77.

Marrero JA, Fontana RJ, Fu S, Conjeevaram HS, Su GL, Lok AS. Alcohol, tobacco and obesity are synergistic risk factors for hepatocellular carcinoma. J Hepatology 2005;42:218–24.

Mastrangelo G, Fedell U, Fadda E, Valentini F, Agnesi R, Magarotto G, et al. Increased risk of hepatocellular carcinoma and liver cirrhosis in vinyl chloride workers: synergistic effect of occupational exposure with alcohol intake. Environ Health Perspec 2004;112: 1188–92.

Maupas P, Melnick JL. Hepatitis B infection and primary liver cancer. Prog Med Virol 1981; 27:1–5.

McGlynn KA, Hunter K, LeVoyer T, Roush J, Wise P, Michielli RA, et al. Susceptibility to aflatoxin B1-related primary hepatocellular carcinoma in mice and humans. Cancer Res 2003;63:4594–4601.

McGlynn KA, London WT. Epidemiology and natural history of hepatocellular carcinoma. Best Prac & Res Clin Gastroenterol 2005;19: 3–23.

McGlynn KA, Rosvold EA, Lustbader ED, Hu Y, Clapper ML, Zhou T, et al. Susceptibility to hepatocellular carcinoma is associated with genetic variation in the enzymatic detoxification of aflatoxin B1. Proc Natl Acad Sci USA 1995;92:2384–87.

McGlynn KA, Tsao L, Hsing AW, Devesa SS, Fraumeni Jr JF. International trends and patterns of primary liver cancer. Int J Cancer 2001;94:290–96.

Momosaki S, Hsia CC, Nakashima Y, Kojiro M, Tabor E. Integration of hepatitis B virus containing mutations in the core promoter/X gene in patients with hepatocellular carcinoma. Dig Liver Dis 2003;35:795–800.

Momosaki S, Nakashima Y, Kojiro M, Tabor E. HBsAg-negative hepatitis B virus infections in hepatitis C virus-associated hepatocellular carcinoma. J Viral Hepatitis 2005;12:325–29.

Montesano R, Hainaut P, Wild CP. Hepatocellular carcinoma: from gene to public health. J Natl Cancer Inst 1997;89:1844–51.

Morgan TR, Mandayam S, JAMAl MM. Alcohol and hepatocellular carcinoma. Gastroenterology 2004;127:S87–S96.

Mori M, Hara M, Wada I, Hara T, Yamamoto K, Honda M, et al. Prospective study of hepatitis B and C viral infections, cigarette smoking, alcohol consumption, and other factors associated with hepatocellular carcinoma risk in Japan. Am J Epidemiol 2000;151:131–39.

Mori T, Kido C, Fukutomi K, Kato Y, Hatakeyama S, Machinami R, et al. Summary of entire Japanese Thorotrast follow-up study: updated 1998. Radiation Res 1999;152: S84–S87.

Moriya K, Fujie H, Shintani Y, Yotsuyanagi H, Tsutsumi T, Ishibashi K, et al. The core protein of hepatitis C virus induces hepatocellular carcinoma in transgenic mice. Nat Med 1998;4:1065–67.

Mucci LA, Kuper HE, Tamimi R, Lagiou P, Spanos E, Trichopoulos D. Age at menarche and age at menopause in relation to hepatocellular carcinoma in women. Br J Obstet Gynaec 2001;108:291–94.

Muñoz N, Lingao A, Lao J, Esteve J, Viterbo G, Domingo EO, et al. Patterns of familial transmission of HBV and the risk of developing liver cancer: a case-control study in the Philippines. Int J Cancer 1989;44:981–84.

Murakami Y, Saigo K, Takashima H, Minami M, Okanoue T, Brechot C, et al. Large scaled analysis of hepatitis B virus (HBV) DNA integration in HBV related hepatocellular carcinomas. Gut 2005;54:1162–68.

Oh SW, Yoon YS, Shin S-A. Effects of excess weight on cancer incidences depending on cancer sites and histologic findings among men: Korea National Health Insurance Corporation Study. J Clin Oncol 2005;23:4742–54.

Okayama A, Stuver SO, Tabor E, Tachibana N, Kohara M, Mueller NE, et al. Incident hepatitis C virus infection in a community-based population in Japan. J Viral Hepatitis 2002; 9:43–51.

Okuda K. Hepatitis C virus and hepatocellular carcinoma. In: Okuda K, Tabor E (Eds): Liver Cancer. New York, Churchill Livingstone, 1997, pp 39–50.

Ozturk M. Genetic aspects of hepatocellular carcinogenesis. Sem Liver Dis 1999;19:235–42.

Papatheodoridis GV, Papadimitropoulos VC, Hadziyannis SJ. Effect of interferon therapy on the development of hepatocellular carcinoma in patients with hepatitis C virus-related cirrhosis: a meta-analysis. Aliment Pharmacol Ther 2001;15:689–98.

Parkin DM. The global health burden of infection-associated cancers in the year 2002. Int J Cancer 2006;118:3030–44.

Parkin DM, Bray F, Ferlay J, Pisani P. Global cancer statistics, 2002. CA Cancer J Clin 2005; 55:74–108.

Parkin DM, Srivatanakul P, Khlat M, Chenvidhya D, Chotiwan P, Insiripong S, et al. Liver cancer in Thailand. I. A case-control study of cholangiocarcinoma. Int J Cancer 1991;48: 323–28.

Pollicino T, Squadrito G, Cerenzia G, Cacciola I, Raffa G, Craxi A, et al. Hepatitis B virus maintains its pro-oncogenic properties in the case of occult HBV infection. Gastroenterology 2004;126:102–10.

Poynard T, Bedossa P, Opolon P. Natural history of liver fibrosis progression in patients with chronic hepatitis C. Lancet 1997;349: 825–32.

Qian GS, Ross RK, Yu MC, Yuan JM, Gao YT, Henderson BE, et al. A follow-up study of urinary markers of aflatoxin exposure and liver cancer risk in Shanghai, People's Republic of China. Cancer Epidemiol Biomarkers Prev 1994;3:3–10.

Randi G, Franceschi S, La Vecchia C. Gallbladder cancer worldwide: Geographical distribution and risk factors. Int J Cancer 2006; 118:1591–1602.

Ray RB, Steele R, Meyer K, Ray R. Transcriptional repression of p53 promoter by hepatitis C virus core protein. J Biol Chem 1997; 272:10983–86.

Ross RK, Yuan JM, Yu MC, Wogan GN, Qian GS, Tu JT, et al. Urinary aflatoxin biomarkers and risk of hepatocellular carcinoma. Lancet 1992;339:943–46.

Sakoda LC, Graubard BI, Evans AA, London WT, Lin W-Y, Shen F-M, et al. Toenail selenium and risk of hepatocellular carcinoma mortality in Haimen City, China. Int J Cancer 2005;115:618–24.

Samanic C, Gridley G, Chow W-H, Lubin J, Hoover RN, Fraumeni Jr JF. Obesity and cancer risk among white and black United Stataes veterans. Cancer Causes Control 2004;15:35–43.

Shaib YH, El-Serag HB, Davila JA, Morgan R, McGlynn KA. Risk factors of intrahepatic cholangiocarcinoma in the United States: a case-control study. Gastroenterology 2005;128:620–26.

Shimada M, Hashimoto E, Taniai M, Hasegawa K, Okuda H, Hayashi N, et al. Hepatocellular carcinoma in patients with non-alcoholic steatohepatitis. J Hepatol 2002;37:154–60.

Shiratori Y, Shiina S, Imamura M, Kato N, Kanai F, Okudaira T, et al. Characteristic difference of hepatocellular carcinoma between hepatitis B- and C-viral infection in Japan. Hepatology 1995;22:1027–33.

Shirota Y, Kaneko S, Honda M, Kawai HF, Kobayashi K. Identification of differentially expressed genes in hepatocellular carcinoma with cDNA microarrays. Hepatology 2001; 33:832–40.

Sorensen HT, Mellemkjaer L, Jepsen P, Thulstrup AM, Baron J, Olsen JH, et al. Risk of cancer in patients hospitalized with fatty liver: a Danish cohort study. J Clin Gastroenterol 2003;36:356–59.

Sparos L, Tountas Y, Chapuis-Cellier C, Theodoropoulos G, Trichopoulos D. Alpha1-antitrypsin levels and phenotypes and hepatitis B serology in liver cancer. Br J Cancer 1984;49:567–70.

Srivatanakul P, Parkin DM, Khlat M, Chenvidhya D, Chotiwan P, Insiripong S, et al. Liver cancer in Thailand. II. A case-control study of hepatocellular carcinoma. Int J Cancer 1991;48:329–32.

Stanford J, Thomas D, the WHO Collaborative Study of Neoplasia and Steroid Contraceptives. Reproductive factors in the etiology of hepatocellular carcinoma. Cancer Causes Control 1992;2:37–42.

Stern MC, Umbach DM, Yu MC, London SJ, Zhang Z-Q, Taylor JA. Hepatitis B, aflatoxin B1, and p53 codon 249 mutation in hepatocellular carcinomas from Guangxi, People's Republic of China, and a meta-analysis of existing studies. Cancer Epidemiol Biomarkers Prev 2001;10:617–25.

Stuver SO, Trichopoulos D. Liver cancer. In: Doll R, Fraumeni J, Muir C (Eds): Trends in Cancer Incidence and Mortality. Cancer Surveys, Vol. 19/20. London, Imperial Cancer Research Fund, 1994, pp 99–124.

Sun C-A, Wu D-M, Lin C-C, Lu S-N, You S-L, Wang L-Y, et al. Incidence and cofactors in hepatitis C virus-related hepatocellular carcinoma: a prospective study of 12,008 men in Taiwan. Am J Epidemiol 2003;157:674–82.

Sung J-L. Prevention of hepatitis B and C virus infection for prevention of cirrhosis and hepatocellular carcinoma. J Gastroenterol Hepatol 1997;12(Suppl):S370–S376.

Tabor E. Tumor suppressor genes, growth factor genes, and oncogenes in hepatitis B virus–associated hepatocellular carcinoma. J Med Virol 1994;42:357–65.

Tabor E. The role of tumor suppressor genes in the development of hepatocellular carcinoma. In: Okuda K, Tabor E (Eds): Liver Cancer. New York, Churchill Livingstone, 1997, pp 89–95.

Tabor E. Viral hepatitis and liver cancer. In: Goldin RD, Thomas HC, Gerber MA (Eds): Pathology of Viral Hepatitis. London, Arnold, 1998, pp 161–77.

Tabor E. Global epidemiology of hepatocellular carcinoma associated with hepatitis B and C virus infections. In: Margolis HS, Alter MJ, Liang TJ, Dienstag JL (Eds): Viral Hepatitis Liver Disease. Atlanta, International Medical Press, 2002, pp 400–3.

Tagger A, Donato F, Ribero ML, Chiesa R, Portera G, Gelatti U, et al. Case-control study on hepatitis C virus (HCV) as a risk factor for hepatocellular carcinoma: the role of HCV genotypes and the synergism with hepatitis B virus and alcohol. Brescia HCC Study. Int J Cancer 1999;81:695–99.

Takahashi M, Yamada G, Miyamoto R, Doi, T, Endo H, Tsuji T. Natural course of chronic hepatitis C. Am J Gastroenterol 1993;88: 240–43.

Takeshita T, Yang X, Inoue Y, Sato S, Morimoto K. Relationship between alcohol drinking, ADH2 and ALDH2 genotypes, and risk for hepatocellular carcinoma in Japanese. Cancer Letters 2000;149:69–76.

Tanaka H, Hiyama T, Okubo Y, Kitada A, Fujimoto I. Primary liver cancer incidence rates related to hepatitis-C virus infection: a correlational study in Osaka, Japan. Cancer Causes Control 1994;5:61–65.

Tanaka K, Hirohata T, Koga S, Sugimachi K, Kanematsu T, Ohryohji F, et al. Hepatitis C and hepatitis B in the etiology of hepatocellular carcinoma in the Japanese population. Cancer Res 1991;51:2842–47.

Tanaka K, Ikematsu H, Hirohata T, Kashiwagi S. Hepatitis C virus infection and risk of hepatocellular carcinoma among Japanese: possible role of type 1b (II) infection. J Natl Cancer Inst 1996;88:742–46.

Tanaka K, Stuver SO, Ikematsu H, Okayama A, Tachibana N, Hirohata T, et al. Hetero-

sexual transmission of hepatitis C virus among married couples in southwestern Japan. Int J Cancer 1997;72:50–55.

Tanaka S, Takenaka K, Matsumata T, Mori R, Sugimachi K. Hepatitis C virus replication is associated with expression of transforming growth factor-alpha and insulin-like growth factor-II in cirrhotic livers. Dig Dis Science 1996;41:208–15.

Tang TC-M, Poon RT-P, Fan S-T. The significance of cyclooxygenase-2 expression in human hepatocellular carcinoma. Biomed Pharmacothera 2005;59(Suppl 2):S311–S316.

Taylor-Robinson SD, Foster GR, Arora S, Hargreaves S, Thomas HC. Increase in primary liver cancer in the UK, 1979–94. Lancet 1997;350:1142–43.

Tennant BC, Toshkov IA, Peek SF, Jacob JR, Menne S, Hornbuckle WE, et al. Hepatocellular carcinoma in the woodchuck model of hepatitis B virus infection. Gastroenterol 2004;127:S283–S293.

The Collaborative MILTS Project Team. Oral contraceptives and liver cancer. Contraception 1997;56:275–84.

Thomas DL. Hepatitis C and human immunodeficiency virus infection. Hepatology 2002; 36(Suppl 1):S201–S209.

Thompson DE, Mabuchi K, Ron E, Soda M, Tokunaga M, Ochikubo S, et al. Cancer incidence in atomic bomb survivors. Part II: solid tumors, 1958–1987. Radiation Res 1994;137:S17–S67.

Thorgeirsson SS, Grisham JW. Molecular pathogenesis of human hepatocellular carcinoma. Nature Genetics 2002;31:339–46.

Tobler LH, Busch MP. History of posttransfusion hepatitis. Clin Chem 1997;43:1487–93.

Travis LB, Hauptmann M, Gaul LK, Storm HH, Goldman MB, Nyberg U, et al. Site-specific cancer incidence and mortality after cerebral anigography with radioactive Thorotrast. Radiation Res 2003;160:691–706.

Trichopoulos D. Etiology of primary liver cancer and the role of steroidal hormones. Cancer Causes Control 1992;3:3–5.

Trichopoulos D, Day NE, Kaklamani E, Tzonou A, Munoz N, Zavitsanos X, et al. Hepatitis B virus, tobacco smoking and ethanol consumption in the etiology of hepatocellular carcinoma. Int J Cancer 1987;39:45–49.

Trichopoulos D, MacMahon B, Sparros L, Merikas G. Smoking and hepatitis B–negative primary hepatocellular carcinoma. J Natl Cancer Inst 1980;65:111–14.

Tzonou A, Zavitsanos X, Hsieh CC, Trichopoulos D. Liveborn children and risk of hepatic-cellular carcinoma. Cancer Causes Control 1992;3:171–74.

Vall Mayans M, Calvet X, Bruix J, Bruguera M, Costa J, Esteve J, et al. Risk factors for hepatocellular carcinoma in Catalonia, Spain. Int J Cancer 1990;46:378–81.

Vineis P, Alavanja M, Buffler P, Fontham E, Franceschi S, Gao YT, et al. Tobacco and cancer: recent epidemiological evidence. J Natl Cancer Inst 2004;96:99–106.

Wang JT, Wang TH, Lin JT, Lee CZ, Sheu JC, Chen DS. Effect of hepatitis C antibody screening in blood donors on post-transfusion hepatitis in Taiwan. J Gastroenterol Hepatol 1995;10:454–58.

Wang L-Y, Hatch M, Chen C-J, Levin B, You SL, Lu SN, et al. Aflatoxin exposure and risk of hepatocellular carcinoma in Taiwan. Int J Cancer 1996;67:620–25.

Wang L-Y, You S-L, Lu S-N, Ho H-C, Wu M-H, Sun C-A, et al. Risk of hepatocellular carcinoma and habits of alcohol drinking, betel quid chewing and cigarette smoking; a cohort of 2416 HBsAg-seropositive and 9421 HBsAg-seronegative male residents in Taiwan. Cancer Causes and Control 2003;14:241–50.

Wartenberg D, Reyner D, Scott CS. Trichloroethylene and cancer: epidemiologic evidence. Environ Health Perspect 2000;108:161–76.

WHO Collaborative Study of Neoplasia and Steroid Contraceptives. Combined oral contraceptives and gall bladder cancer. Int J Epidemiol 1989a;18:309–14.

WHO Collaborative Study of Neoplasia and Steroid Contraceptives. Combined oral contraceptives and liver cancer. Int J Cancer 1989b;43:254–59.

Wolk A, Gridley G, Svensson M, Nyren O, McLaughlin JK, Fraumeni Jr, JF, et al. A prospective study of obesity and cancer risk (Sweden). Cancer Causes Control 2001;12:13–21.

World Cancer Research Fund. Food, Nutrition and the Prevention of Cancer: A Global Perspective. Washington, DC, American Institute for Cancer Research, 1997.

Yang H-I, Lu S-N, Liaw Y-F, You S-L, Sun C-A, Wang L-Y, et al. Hepatitis B e antigen and the risk of hepatocellular carcinoma. N Engl J Med 2002;347:168–74

Yu MC, Tong MJ, Govindarajan S, Henderson BE. Nonviral risk factors for hepatocellular carcinoma in a low-risk population, the non-Asians of Los Angeles County, California. J Natl Cancer Inst 1991;83:1820–26.

Yu M-W, Chang H-C, Chang S-C, Liaw Y-F, Lin S-M, Liu C-J, et al. Role of reproductive factors in hepatocellular carcinoma: impact on hepatitis B- and C-related risk. Hepatology 2003;38:1393–1400

Yu M-W, Chen C-J. Elevated serum testosterone levels and risk of hepatocellular carcinoma. Cancer Res 1993;53:790–94.

Yu M-W, Cheng S-W, Lin M-W, Yang S-Y, Liaw, Y-F, Chang H-C, et al. Androgen-receptor gene CAG repeats, plasma testosterone levels, and risk of hepatitis B-related hepatocellular carcinoma. J Natl Cancer Inst 2000;92:2023–28.

Yu M-W, Gladek-Yarborough A, Chiamprasert S, Santella RM, Liaw Y-F, Chen C-J. Cytochrome P450 2E1 and S-transferase M1 polymorphisms and susceptibility to hepatocellular carcinoma. Gastroenterology 1995a;109:1266–73.

Yu M-W, Homg I-S, Hsu K-H, Chiang Y-C, Liaw Y-F, Chen C-J. Plasma selenium levels and risk of hepatocellular carcinoma among men with chronic hepatitis virus infection. Am J Epidemiol 1999b;150:367–74.

Yu M-W, Hsieh HH, Pan WH, Yang CS, Chen CJ. Vegetable consumption, serum retinol level, and risk of hepatocellular carcinoma. Cancer Res 1995b;55:1301–5.

Yu M-W, Yeh S-H, Chen P-J, Liaw Y-F, Lin C-L, Liu C-J, et al. Hepatitis B virus genotype and DNA level and hepatocellular carcinoma: a prospective study in men. J Natl Cancer Inst 2005;97:265–72.

Yuan J-M, Gao Y-T, Ong C-N, Ross RK, Yu MC. Prediagnostic level of serum retinol in relation to reduced risk of hepatocellular carcinoma. J Natl Cancer Inst 2006;98:482–90.

Yuan J-M, Govindarajan S, Arakawa K, Yu MC. Synergism of alcohol, diabetes, and viral hepatitis on the risk of hepatocellular carcinoma in blacks and whites in the U.S. Cancer 2004;101:1009–17.

Yuan J-M, Ross RK, Stanczyk FZ, Govindarajan S, Gao Y-T, Henderson BE, et al. A cohort study of serum testosterone and hepatocellular carcinoma in Shanghai, China. Int J Cancer 1995;63:491–93.

Zatonski WA, Lowenfels AB, Boyle P, Maisonneuve P, Bueno de Mesquita HB, Ghadirian P, et al. Epidemiologic aspects of gallbladder cancer: a case-control study of the SEARCH Program of the International Agency for Research on Cancer. J Natl Cancer Inst 1997;89:1132–38.

13

Pancreatic Cancer

ANDERS EKBOM AND DIMITRIOS TRICHOPOULOS

Pancreatic cancer is probably one of the most dreaded diagnostic alternatives for a clinician facing a patient with wasting as the major symptom. Before the introduction of new imaging techniques such as ultrasound and computed tomography, explorative laparotomy was the only way to ensure—or rule out—the diagnosis. An alternative approach was to wait and see. If the patient was still alive 6 months later, the diagnosis of pancreatic cancer should probably be ruled out. If the diagnosis could not be ruled out, there would follow a demeaning process that ended with an anorectic and dehydrated patient, quite frequently in severe pain. The absence of survivors and the nature of the disease process are probably the major reasons for the anonymity surrounding pancreatic cancer. Count Basie (a famous jazz pianist), opera singer Luciano Pavarotti, Michael Landon (a popular actor), and the mother and siblings of former US President Jimmy Carter are among the exceptional few who have given faces to this malignancy. There is a similar anonymity in the world literature, although the novel *The Death of a Bee Keeper* by the Swedish author Lars Gustafsson is a notable exception.

CLINICAL SYNOPSIS

Subgroups

Ninety-five percent of all pancreatic cancers develop in the exocrine pancreas, about two-thirds in the head of the pancreas. Tumors located in the head of the pancreas are sometimes hard to distinguish from those of the papilla Vateri, duodenum, or distal common bile duct—that is, tumors with a different prognosis and possibly a different etiology.

Symptoms

Pancreatic cancer has an insidious onset. The presenting symptom is often jaundice caused by blockage of the common bile duct. Pain, anorexia, weight loss, onset of diabetes, or diffuse abdominal symptoms may preceed the diagnosis.

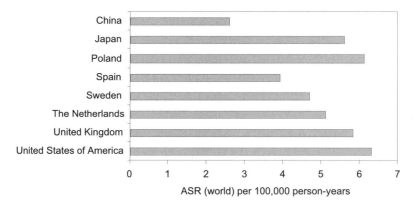

Figure 13–1. Age-standardized (to the world population) incidence rates of pancreatic cancer among women. (*Source*: Ferlay et al, 2004)

Diagnosis

Ultrasonography and computed tomography are the general methods; with either of them, tumors as small as 1 to 2 cm can be diagnosed. A histopathologic diagnosis can then be established by a guided percutaneous biopsy. Endoscopic retrograde cholangiopancreatography (ERCP) is also utilized, especially to find the cause for a silent jaundice and make it possible to relieve the jaundice by stenting.

Treatment

In essence, only palliative treatment is available, more precisely through resection of the tumor, stenting of the common bile duct, or other bypass procedures that give symptomatic relief.

Progress and Prognosis

The median survival following diagnosis is less than 6 months. Patients who survive for more than 5 years are frequently found to have been misdiagnosed. Notwithstanding many reports concerning various chemotherapeutic regimens, no randomized clinical trial has shown any survival benefit. The prognosis is as poor today as it was 50 years ago.

DESCRIPTIVE EPIDEMIOLOGY

As indicated, most pancreatic cancers derive from the exocrine part of the pancreas. The endocrine tumors (around 5%) that arise from the acinar cells will not be dealt with in this chapter.

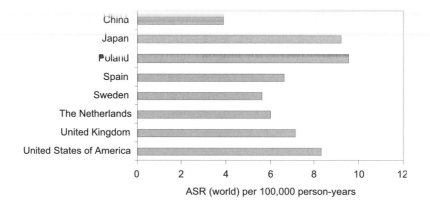

Figure 13–2. Age-standardized (to the world population) incidence rates of pancreatic cancer among men. (*Source*: Ferlay et al., 2004)

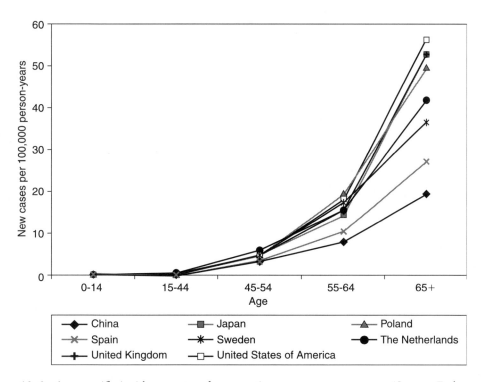

Figure 13–3. Age-specific incidence rates of pancreatic cancer among women. (*Source*: Ferlay et al, 2004)

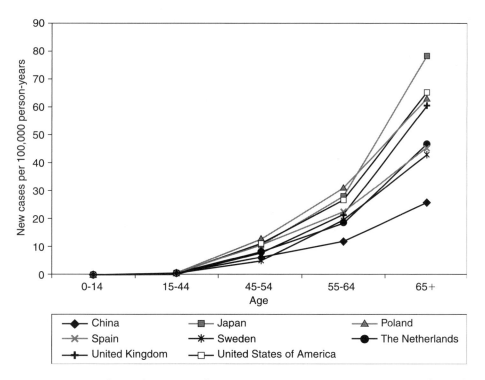

Figure 13– 4. Age-specific incidence rates of pancreatic cancer among men. (*Source*: Ferlay et al, 2004)

Close to 200 000 new cases of pancreatic cancer are registered annually worldwide with modest geographic differences (Figs. 13–1 and 13–2). The highest rates are from the SEER Registry for African Americans in the United States, with about 15 new cases per 100 000 person-years, compared to just under 6 in Spain. It is the malignancy with the worst prognosis, the only one for which the annual incidence is higher than the prevalence. In the United States, pancreatic cancer is the fifth most common cause of cancer death but only the twelfth most common cancer diagnosis. The male/female incidence ratio is around 1.5 in the industrialized world and 1.1 in the developing nations.

A decrease in incidence rates has been observed in the United States since 1994, especially among African American men (Parkin et al 1992). In Sweden, a declining trend is evident for both women and men during the last 20 years (National Board of Health and Welfare, 2005).

Pancreatic cancer is a disease of the elderly. The age-specific incidence rates are similar in different populations (Figs. 13–3 and 13–4), although in some the incidence is decreasing in the highest age groups. This decrease has been attributed to a lower prevalence of ever-smokers in the oldest age groups. Another, more likely explanation is lower diagnostic intensity among elderly persons who develop a silent jaundice sometimes preceded by or associated with weight loss (Warshaw and Fernandez del Castillo, 1992). As the median survival is less than 6 months—and even less in the age group over 80—autopsy frequency is an important determinant of the reported incidence among the elderly (Lindstrom et al, 1997).

GENETIC AND MOLECULAR EPIDEMIOLOGY

Several instances of family clusters have been reported, the best known being the family of former US President Jimmy Carter. A family history of pancreatic cancer has been associated with a substantially increased risk of the disease (Ghadirian et al, 1991; Fernandez et al, 1994), as have cancer susceptibility syndromes such as hereditary nonpolyposis colon cancer in association with microsatellite instability (Lynch et al, 1991), familial breast cancer with *BRCA2* gene alteration (Ozcelik et al, 1997), familial melanoma (Schenk et al, 1998), and ataxia-telangiectasia (Swift et al, 1991). A family history of pancreatic cancer is associated with an almost tenfold increased risk compared to the general population and is even more pronounced— a 30-fold excess risk—if there are three or more affected first-degree relatives (Klein at al, 2004). Moreover, those with family history are frequently diagnosed at younger ages, a finding that due to the natural history of the disease cannot be explained by surveillance bias (Petersen et al, 2006). Significant interactions have been reported between cigarette smoking and different genotypes, such as polymorphism of DNA repair gene *XRCC1*. This supports the hypothesis that individuals who have a deficient carcinogen detoxification and DNA repair capacities are at increased risk of pancreatic cancer (Duell et al, 2002). Finally, inflammatory gene polymorphism in combination with inflammatory conditions and possibly tobacco smoking also seem to increase the risk of pancreatic cancer (Duell et al, 2006).

RISK FACTORS

Tobacco

Smoking is the only exposure that has been consistently shown to increase the risk of pancreatic cancer, albeit rather modestly.

The increased risk is about twofold when current smokers are compared with non-smokers (Doll et al, 1994; Silverman et al, 1994; Boyle et al, 1996); some studies, however, give higher relative risk estimates (Cuzick and Babiker, 1989; Zheng et al, 1993). The fraction of pancreatic cancers attributable to smoking in an Italian study was 20% of the male cases (Fernandez et al,

1996). Most investigations reported an exposure–response relationship, whereas others failed to show such an association (Howe et al, 1991). The underlying biological mechanism remains elusive. Nitrosamines, shown to induce pancreatic cancer in animal models (Rivenson et al, 1988), and aromatic amines, known human bladder carcinogens (Cohen, 1998), have been proposed as causal agents (Hecht et al, 1993), since both are present in high levels in tobacco smoke.

Smoking cessation seems to lower the risk rather rapidly. A risk in former smokers similar to that in nonsmokers has been seen within 10 to 15 years after cessation (Howe et al, 1991; Zheng et al, 1993; Boyle et al, 1996; Lin et al, 2002), although in some reports the risk reduction was less pronounced (Cuzick and Babiker, 1989; Silverman et al, 1994). It is therefore tempting to attribute the decrease in incidence among men in the United States and Sweden to a preceding reduction in the prevalence of male smoking, although a decrease in the incidence of pancreatic cancer among females indicate that this cannot be the sole reason.

The rapid reduction in the risk of pancreatic cancer after smoking cessation suggests that tobacco smoke is a late-stage component in the carcinogenic process. According to a Finnish study, an interaction exists between smoking and levels of serum folate and/or pyridoxal-59phosphate, the coenzyme form of vitamin B6 in serum (Stolzenberg-Solomon et al, 1999), such that adequate folate and pyridoxine intake may reduce the risk of pancreatic cancer in smokers. The folic acid grain fortification implemented in the United States to reduce the risk of neural tube defects could therefore also have an impact on the incidence of pancreatic cancer, especially among smokers.

Smokeless tobacco has also been implicated as a risk factor for pancreatic cancer. Data from the US, however, indicate that smokeless tobacco use in Northern America is not associated with an increased risk of pancreatic cancer (Alguacil and Silverman, 2004; Accortt et al, 2005). In a Scandinavian setting "snus," the smokeless tobacco product widely used there, has been reported to be associated with a 70% significant excess risk (Boffetta et al, 2005). However, that study was criticized for methodological reasons and because there were very few cases (Rutqvist and Lewin, 2006). Thus, an association between smokeless tobacco and pancreatic cancer still remains to to established.

Diet

One of the few relatively consistent findings from the large number of case-control studies that have analyzed the possible association between various dietary compounds and pancreatic cancer is a decreased risk following high consumption of vegetables or fruits (Norell et al, 1986; Howe and Burch, 1996). The general lack of consistency of nutritional epidemiological studies can be explained, at least in part, by the methodologic difficulties that researchers face when using the case-control approach. As for cohort studies, data are hampered by low statistical power because of the relatively low incidence of pancreatic cancer. In a pooled analysis of 124 000 participants yielding 366 cases of pancreatic cancer, no association betweeen different dietary patterns and pancreatic cancer was evident (Michaud et al, 2005).

For high levels of vitamin C an apparently protective effect has been reported (Howe and Burch, 1996). For lycopene, a fairly consistent inverse association was reported when either tomato intake or lycopene serum level was examined (Giovannucci, 1999). Although the serum-based study involved only 22 cases, the results were statistically significant (Burney et al, 1989). For total carotenoids or beta-carotene, no association was found. Dietary fiber intake has also been associated with decreased risk (Howe and Burch, 1996). A reported positive association with high intake of carbohydrates may be related to high consumption of refined carbohydrates devoid of fiber components (Weiderpass et al, 1998).

Both ecologic studies (Yanai et al, 1979) and animal models (Longnecker et al, 1985) have implicated high fat intake as a risk factor for pancreatic cancer. High intake of total fat and cholesterol did appear to increase the risk in some studies (Norell et al, 1986; Mills et al, 1988) but not in others (Farrow and Davis, 1990; Howe and Burch, 1996; Skinner et al, 2004). Analyses of meat or protein intake showed similar inconsistencies (Farrow and Davis, 1990; Howe and Burch, 1996; Nothlings et al, 2005). High intake of folate was found in one study to be protective but was confined to folate from food sources but not from supplements (Larsson et al, 2006). Results from the United States have failed to reveal any such associations (Skinner et al, 2004). Comparing populations with variable and changing dietary habits present almost unsolvable problems and preclude interpretation of all but the most striking and consistent findings. The suggested interaction between smoking and folate or pyridoxal-59phosphate further highlights the problems in evaluating diet in relation to pancreatic cancer (Stolzenberg-Solomon et al, 1999). Thus, apart from a likely beneficial diet rich in vegetables and fruits, no dietary preventive measures can presently be recommended.

Coffee

Coffee is probably the dietary compound most widely assessed and discussed as a potential risk factor for pancreatic cancer. In spite of some residual concerns (Kuper et al, 2000), the consensus today is that there is no association (Gordis, 1990; Michaud et al, 2001a).

A positive association was suggested in the 1970s (MacMahon et al, 1981) and supported by several investigators. Subsequent studies, however, especially during the 1990s, came to a different conclusion (Michaud et al, 2001a). A Spanish study added a new twist to the convoluted story of coffee in relation to pancreatic cancer by suggesting an association only with

respect to K-ras positive cases (Porta et al, 1999).

These divergent results are a good illustration of the problems that investigators face when studying etiologic factors for pancreatic cancer. Because of the nonspecific abdominal symptoms in the early stages and the potential role of smoking as an important confounder, high-quality instruments to assess exposures and associated latencies are of special importance, as is careful selection of controls in case-control studies. The rapid clinical course after diagnosis also introduces problems with the representativeness of cases: Are the extreme short-term survivors similar to or different from the longer-term survivors?

Alcohol

Whether there is a causal link between alcohol use and pancreatic cancer remains to be established; the methodologic problems are considerable.

The use of alcohol has been associated with an increased risk of pancreatic cancer by several (Cuzick and Babiker, 1989; Zheng et al, 1993; Silverman et al, 1995) but not all (Zatonski et al, 1993; Ye et al, 2002) investigators. Alcohol abuse is more consistently found to increase the risk (Zheng et al, 1993; Silverman et al, 1995), the most pronounced association reported among African Americans (Silverman et al, 1995). It should be kept in mind, however, that smoking is frequent among alcohol abusers (Veenstra et al, 1993). Although most authors have tried to control for the confounding effect of smoking, the positive association of pancreatic cancer with alcohol might, at least to some extent, be a result of residual confounding. The fact that abusers' diets are frequently low in vegetables and fruits may further complicate the interpretation of results of studies focusing on alcohol.

Reproductive Factors

Although a link between reproductive factors and pancreatic cancer has been indicated repeatedly, and is biologically plausible, no direct evidence is available.

High parity might increase the risk of pancreatic cancer in women, according to studies from China (Ji et al, 1996), Norway (Kvale et al, 1994), and Sweden (Karlson et al, 1998), although opposite results have also been reported (; Fernandez et al, 1995; Teras et al, 2005). The link, if it exists, could lie on hormonal influences during pregnancy (Bueno de Mesquita et al, 1992). The presence of estrogen receptors in the exocrine pancreas (Andren-Sandberg, 1986) and high serum levels of estrogens in patients with pancreatic cancer compared to controls (Greenway et al, 1981) point in the same direction. Further, patients with endometriosis or hyperplasia of the ovaries may be at increased risk (Soloway and Sommers, 1966). Antiestrogen agents such as tamoxifen inhibited the growth of pancreatic cancer both in animal models and in human cell lines (Benz et al, 1986), but in clinical trials tamoxifen did not affect the clinical course of the disease (Keating et al, 1989).

Hormones

The global incidence of pancreatic cancer is consistently larger among men than among women, although the difference is more pronounced in developed countries. This excess might be explained by a higher prevalence of smokers among men and possibly by occupational exposures. It is tempting to also infer that sex hormones may be of importance. The presence of estrogen receptors in the normal pancreas as well as in pancreatic cancers indirectly supports an association (Andren-Sandberg, 1986). However, this association, if it exists, is unlikely to have a major impact and observational studies have so far failed to reveal any strong association (Duell and Holly, 2005).

Gastrointestinal hormones, which stimulate the growth of the gastrointestinal mucosa and the pancreas, have been suggested to promote the development of tumors in these locations. The role of cholecystokinin (CCK), in particular, has been discussed (Axelson et al, 1992). Cholecystokinin stimulates pancreatic enzyme secretion with a negative feedback mechanism involving intraluminal pancreatic proteases, especially trypsin. Lack of trypsin in the duodenum and upper jejunum results in release of CCK, whereas the presence of trypsin inhibits release. In animal models, exogenous CCK stimulated pancreatic growth (Gasslander et al, 1990), and the presence of CKK shortened the induction time and increased the incidence of pancreatic tumors (Howatson and Carter, 1985).

Human pancreatic cancer has receptors for CCK, and the growth of some human pancreatic cancer cell lines is stimulated by this hormone (Edwards et al, 1989). Although these results were not confirmed by other investigators (Liehr et al, 1990), they give some credence to a promoting role of CCK in pancreatic cancer development, either directly or indirectly by stimulating the release of local promoters. However, CCK is also substantially elevated in individuals with high fat intake (Axelson et al, 1992) and following cholecystectomy (Hyvarinen and Partanen, 1987). The absence of a consistent association between these two factors and pancreatic cancer argues against a causal role of CCK.

Gastrin, another gastrointestinal hormone with a trophic effect on the gastrointestinal mucosa, has also been proposed to play a role in pancreatic carcinogenesis (Petersen et al, 1978). The increased risk found in patients with pernicious anemia (Borch et al, 1988), which is associated with high gastrin levels, has been an argument for a causal relationship (Hsing et al, 1993). However, pernicious anemia is an autoimmune disorder linked to diabetes mellitus, itself a risk factor for pancreatic cancer. Moreover, considering that in a clinical setting pernicious anemia is difficult to distinguish from chronic gastritis (Karlson et al, 2000), which is associated with smoking, the evidence for gastrin as a causal factor in pancreatic cancer is equivocal.

Anthropometric Measures

A positive association between obesity and pancreatic cancer has been reported repeatedly and a meta-analysis in 2003 involving more than 6000 cases of pancreatic cancer documented an association between pancreatic cancer and obesity (Barrington de Gonzalez et al, 2003). The finding has been further substantiated in later studies in which the strongest association was evident among nonsmokers (Fryzek et al, 2005).

Infections

No reliable information is available.

Physical Activity

As for some other cancer types, physical activity seems to be protective albeit rather modestly (Michaud et al, 2001b; Barrington de Gonzalez et al, 2006). In one of the relevant studies, however, the inverse association was confined to those with a BMI higher than 25 kg/m2 (Michaud et al, 2001b).

Ionizing Radiation

Reports—notably from an early study on British radiologists (Matanoski et al, 1975)—have linked occupational exposure to ionizing radiation with an increased risk of pancreatic cancer. These reports, however, have not been confirmed after prolonged follow-up or in other settings (Smith and Doll, 1981; Tolley et al, 1983).

Occupation

With the possible exception of chlorinated hydrocarbon solvents, occupational exposures have not been convincingly linked to the risk of pancreatic cancer.

No socioeconomic gradient has been observed with respect to the incidence of pancreatic cancer (Stone et al, 1978) and this argues against a major role of occupational exposure in pancreatic cancer etiology. Many occupational studies of the malignancy have implicated various types of jobs and exposures to different chemical agents or processes. In general, associations with specific jobs or exposures were suggested in a single study and not confirmed in subsequent ones. Estimates of the population-attributable fraction have therefore been, in most instances, low (Weiderpass et al, 1998; Romundstad et al, 2000).

In a review, Ojajarvi and colleagues (2000) have linked occupational exposure to chlorinated hydrocarbon solvents with an up to 80% increased risk of pancreatic cancer; the higher the quality of the study, the higher the gradient of risk. The conclusion was, however, challenged by a well-conducted cohort study from Norway in which no such association was found (Romundstad et al, 2000). Occupational exposures to chromium and chromic compounds, as well as to nickel and nickel compounds, have also been considered as possible risk factors, but for these, as well as for asbestos, formaldehyde, gasoline, diesel exhaust, and wood dust, no firm conclusions have been drawn.

Medical Conditions and Treatment

Associated morbidity and changes in the incidence pattern following different medical or surgical interventions might help to explain the etiology of pancreatic cancer. However, few clues of this kind have been found.

Diabetes mellitus

Pancreatic cancer has, as already stated, an insidious onset, and clinical symptoms or signs frequently develop years before a manifest tumor. This may be one reason why diabetes mellitus is consistently reported as a strong risk factor (Everhart and Wright, 1995), although, in fact, diabetes is often the first clinical manifestation of an emerging pancreatic cancer (Warshaw and Fernandez del Castillo, 1992).

Most cohort studies found a substantially increased risk of pancreatic cancer in the first 5 years after the onset of diabetes mellitus (Adami et al, 1991; Calle et al, 1998). Results of case-control studies should be interpreted with caution, as some of them do not take into account the recency of the onset of diabetes and others exclude only "exposures" 1 year or less before the diagnosis of pancreatic cancer. However, even in studies that probe diabetes mellitus in the remote past, this condition has emerged as a consistent risk factor for pancreatic cancer (Adami et al,

1991; Everhart and Wright, 1995; Calle et al, 1998).

In analyses of diabetes mellitus, the disease has generally been treated as one entity, although juvenile or insulin-dependent diabetes and noninsulin-dependent diabetes have different etiologies and underlying pathophysiologies. In the few studies that analyzed the two types separately, the far more common noninsulin-dependent diabetes (NIDD) was associated with an increased risk (Everhart and Wright, 1995), whereas insulin-dependent diabetes (IDD) was in some instances even associated with a decreased risk (Green and Jensen, 1985). As IDD patients are exposed to low levels of insulin and NIDD patients to high levels of this hormone for many years, both before and after the onset of clinical diabetes mellitus, insulin has been proposed as important in pancreatic carcinogenesis.

Hyperinsulinemia increases local blood flow and cell divisions within the pancreas (Williams and Goldfine, 1985). Moreover, insulin may promote growth in human pancreatic cell lines (Takeda and Escribano, 1991). The exocrine pancreas is also exposed to higher concentrations of pancreatic islet cell hormones because it receives a large proportion of its blood supply through the islets. This is one possible pathway. Alternatively, pancreatic cancer and NIDD could have common etiologic characteristics, determined either genetically or environmentally. Smoking could be one of them, as smoking may be a risk factor for NIDD (Rimm et al, 1995) and is a known risk factor for pancreatic cancer. However, a positive association between diabetes and pancreatic cancer remains in most studies that have controlled for tobacco use, although residual confounding cannot be ruled out (Everhart and Wright, 1995).

Cholecystectomy and gallbladder disease

Gallstones, as well as cholecystectomy, have repeatedly been implicated as independent risk factors for pancreatic cancer (Wynder et al, 1973; Hyvarinen and Partanen, 1987), although the epidemiologic evidence is not strong. Three different biological mechanisms would be possible:

- Cholecystectomy leads to increased secretion of CCK. In animal models as well as in human cell lines, CCK has been shown to have a trophic effect on, and to stimulate the growth of, the exocrine pancreas.
- Cholecystectomy reduces the pools of primary bile salts and increases those of secondary bile salts. In animal models, secondary bile acids and salts have enhanced tumor formation in different gastrointestinal organs including the pancreas (Roda et al, 1978).
- Reflux of bile or duodenal juice into the pancreas might be an etiologic factor for pancreatic cancer (Wynder et al, 1973). Indirect evidence consists of the fact that pancreatic cancer is more frequent in the head of the gland than in the rest of the organ, size taken into account. The surgical procedure or the presence of choledocholitiasis frequently causes injury to the sphincter of Oddi, resulting in a continuous flow of bile and/or duodenal contents (Karlson et al, 1997a), which exposes the ductal epithelium of the pancreas to potentially carcinogenic products.

However, because early signs of pancreatic cancer include nonspecific abdominal symptoms that lead to higher diagnostic intensity and thereby perhaps to an increased frequency of cholecystectomies in patients with "silent" gallstones, a confounded association can emerge. In cohort studies of patients subjected to cholecystectomy, the incidence of pancreatic cancer compared to that of the background population was increased up to 5 years after the operation, but not thereafter (Ekbom et al, 1996; Chow et al, 1999). This illustrates well the problems encountered in epidemiologic studies of pancreatic cancer and the need to disregard "exposures" consequent to early symptoms from the tumor.

Pernicious anemia

Pernicious anemia is an autoimmune disorder characterized by vitamin B12 deficiency.

Antibodies to parietal cells in the stomach result in gastric atrophy and subsequent achlorhydria. Achlorhydria entails elevated levels of gastrin, which could explain the reported association with pancreatic cancer (Borch et al, 1988; Hsing et al, 1993). Smoking, a reported correlate of vitamin B12 deficiency, may act as a confounder.

Pancreatitis

Three different forms of pancreatitis have been investigated in relation to pancreatic cancer.

Hereditary pancreatitis. Hereditary pancreatitis is a rare autosomal dominant disorder with incomplete penetrance associated with a mutation in the trypsinogen gene on chromosome 7q35 (Lowenfels et al, 1997). Patients have recurrent episodes of pancreatitis often beginning during childhood. Their cumulative risk of developing pancreatic cancer has been estimated to be up to 40% (Lowenfels et al, 1997), although substantially lower risks have also been reported (Andren-Sandberg et al, 1997). The earlier belief that the increased risk was confined to those who inherited the disease from their fathers was contradicted in a study showing maternal inheritance as well (Lerch et al, 1999).

Chronic pancreatitis. Chronic pancreatitis has been implicated as a risk factor for pancreatic cancer (Lowenfels et al, 1993). Indeed, chronic inflammation appears to play a role in the malignant transformation of several organs, such as the liver in patients with hepatitis (Colombo, 1999; Kuper et al, 2001), the colon following inflammatory bowel disease (Ekbom et al, 1990), the bile duct among patients with sclerosing cholingitis (Broome et al, 1996), and the lung among patients with lung fibrosis (Askling et al, 1999).

The problems in distinguishing a noncausal from a causal relationship between chronic pancreatitis and pancreatic cancer are essentially the same as for diabetes mellitus and cholecystectomy. This is illustrated in a multicenter study in which the increased risk of pancreatic cancer was reported as 15-fold among patients with chronic pancreatitis compared to the general population (Lowenfels et al, 1993). Selection bias, however, is possible because the risk estimates are likely to be inflated during a short follow-up period (Ekbom et al, 1993). Furthermore, the most common causal factor in chronic pancreatitis, alcohol abuse, is strongly associated with smoking (Andren-Sandberg et al, 1997), as well as with a diet low in fruits and vegetables, which have both been asssociated with increased pancreatic cancer risk. In a study by Karlson et al (1997b), the excess risk of pancreatic cancer was only twofold 10 years or more after a discharge for chronic pancreatitis.

Thus, although patients with chronic pancreatitis are at increased risk of pancreatic cancer, the evidence of causality is not conclusive. In a review of 9 case-control studies including 2034 cases of pancreatic cancer and 4039 controls, there were 65 cases of pancreatitis among the cases and 37 among the controls (Fernandez et al, 1994). If there is a causal relationship, the population-attributable fraction of chronic pancreatitis for pancreatic cancer is low.

Other forms of pancreatitis. A single episode of acute pancreatitis (Ekbom et al, 1993), as well as one of tropical pancreatitis (Thomas et al, 1990), has been associated with an increased risk of pancreatic cancer. Because this association appears to be confined to the first few years of follow-up, the episodes of pancreatitis might be an early clinical manifestation of pancreatic cancer.

Partial gastrectomy

A history of peptic ulcer surgery, especially partial gastrectomy, has been reported to increase the risk of pancreatic cancer (Offerhaus et al, 1988). Nitrosamines, produced by nitrate reductase–producing bacteria that proliferate in the hypoacidic stomach, could be the intermediate link. However, for peptic ulcer disease, smoking is one of the main risk factors, and surgical patients have an increased risk over time of smoking-related cancers in general (Ekbom et al, 1998). It appears that taking up smoking again after surgery could generate a confounded association between partial gastrectomy and pancreatic cancer.

Cystic fibrosis
Patients with cystic fibrosis have, among other things, substantial pancreatic disturbance leading to insufficiency of the pancreas. Long-standing cystic fibrosis has been linked to an increased risk of pancreatic cancer (Sheldon et al, 1993; Neglia et al, 1995).

Allergies
A medical history of allergy has repeatedly been reported to be inversely associated with the risk of pancreatic cancer (Mack et al, 1986; Howe et al, 1991). Immunoglobulin E–mediated allergy might stimulate pancreatic secretions through histamine-mediated mechanisms operating via the gastric mucosa. However, the data are not consistent and there are reports of no such associations (Lindelof et al, 2005).

Primary Sclerosing Cholangitis
Patients with primary sclerosing cholangitis have a substantially excess risk for cancer in the bileducts but also have a more than tenfold excess risk of pancreatic cancer (Bergquist et al, 2002).

Other Risk Factors

Chlorinated municipal water (Ijsselmuiden et al, 1992), cadmium (Schwartz and Reis, 2000), and organochlorines (Hoppin et al, 2000) have occasionally been brought up as risk factors. However, the evidence is fragmentary and inconsistent.

CONCLUSION

Cancer of the pancreas is slightly more common among men than among women, and its incidence increases with increasing age. It has the worst prognosis among all forms of cancer, survival rarely exceeding 6 months. Trends in pancreatic cancer in- cidence in developed countries are slightly declining. The disease shows evidence of a familial occurrence, but neither major genes nor genetic polymorphisms that may play a crucial role have been identified. Tobacco smoking is the only established exogenous cause of the disease, and smoking cessation is quickly followed by a reduction in excess risk. Consumption of fruits and vegetables is inversely associated with the risk of pancreatic cancer, and there is evidence that vitamin C, folate, and lycopene may be the instrumental compounds. The current consensus is that alcohol, either consumed in moderate amounts or abused, does not substantially affect the risk of pancreatic cancer, although pancreatitis, frequently linked to excessive alcohol intake, has been found to slightly increase the risk of the disease. Occupational factors may play a role, but the evidence is relatively strong only for chlorinated hydrocarbon solvents frequently used in dry cleaning. Adult-onset diabetes mellitus and perhaps pernicious anemia may increase the risk of pancreatic cancer, possibly through the action of gastrointestinal hormones or insulin. Several reports indicate that allergies may be inversely related to the risk of pancreatic cancer.

REFERENCES

Accortt NA, Waterbor JW, Beall C, Howard G. Cancer incidence among cohort of smokeless tobacco users (United States). Cancer Cuses Control 2005;16:1107–15.

Adami HO, McLaughlin J, Ekbom A, Berne C, Silverman D, Hacker D, et al. Cancer risk in patients with diabetes mellitus. Cancer Causes Control 1991;2:307–14.

Alguacil J, Silverman DT. Smokeless and other noncigarette tobacco use and pancreatic cancer: a case-control study based on direct interviews. Cancer Epidemiol Biomarkers Prev 2004;13:55–58.

Andren-Sandberg A. Estrogens and pancreatic cancer: some recent aspects. Scand J Gastronterol 1986;21:129–33.

Andren-Sandberg A, Dervenis C, Lowenfels B. Etiologic links between chronic pancreatitis and pancreatic cancer. Scand J Gastroenterol 1997;32:97–103.

Askling J, Grunewald J, Eklund A, Hillerdal G, Ekbom A. Increased risk for cancer following sarcoidosis. Am J Respir Crit Care Med 1999;160:1668–72.

Axelson J, Ihse I, Hakanson R. Pancreatic cancer: the role of cholecystokinin? Scand J Gastroenterol 1992;27:993–98.

Barrington de Gonzalez A, Sepencer EA, Bueno-deMesquita HB, Roddam A, Stolzenberg-Solomon R, Halkjaer J, et al. Anthropometry, psysical activity, and the risk of pancreatic cancer in the European prospective investigation into cancer and nutrition. Cancer Epidemiol Biomarkers Prev 2006;15:879–85.

Barrington de Gonzalez A, Sweetland S, Spencer E. A meta-analysis of obesity and the risk of pancreatic cancer. Br J Cancer 2003;89:519–23.

Benz C, Hollander C, Miller B. Endocrine-responsive pancreatic carcinoma: steroid binding and cytotoxicity studies in human tumor cell lines. Cancer Res 1986;46:2276–81.

Bergquist A, Ekbom A, Olsson R, Kornfeldt D, Loof L, Danielsson A, et al. Hepatic and extrahepatic malignancies in primary sclerosing cholangitis. J Hepatol 2002;36:321–27.

Boffetta P, Aagnes B, Weiderpass E, Andersen A. Smokeless tobacco use and risk of cancer of the pancreas and other organs. Int J Cancer 2005;114:992–95.

Borch K, Kullman E, Hallhagen S, Ledin T, Ihse I. Increased incidence of pancreatic neoplasia in pernicious anemia. World J Surg 1988;12:866–70.

Boyle P, Maisonneuve P, Bueno de Mesquita B, Ghadirian P, Howe GR, Zatonski W, et al. Cigarette smoking and pancreas cancer: a case control study of the search programme of the IARC. Int J Cancer 1996;67:63–71.

Broome U, Olsson R, Lööf L, Bodemar G, Hultcrantz R, Danielsson A, et al. Natural history and prognostic factors in 305 Swedish patients with primary sclerosing cholangitis. Gut 1996;30.610 15.

Bueno de Mesquita HB, Maisonneuve P, Moerman CJ, Walker AM. Anthropometric and reproductive variables and exocrine carcinoma of the pancreas: a population-based case-control study in the Netherlands. Int J Cancer 1992;52:24–29.

Burney PG, Comstock GW, Morris JS. Serologic precursors of cancer: serum micronutrients and the subsequent risk of pancreatic cancer. Am J Clin Nutr 1989;49:895–900.

Calle EE, Murphy TK, Rodriguez C, Thun MJ, Heath CW Jr. Diabetes mellitus and pancreatic cancer mortality in a prospective cohort of United States adults. Cancer Causes Control 1998;9:403–10.

Chow WH, Johansen C, Gridley G, Mellemkjaer L, Olsen JH, Fraumeni JF Jr. Gallstones, cholecystectomy and risk of cancers of the liver, biliary tract and pancreas. Br J Cancer 1999;79:640–44.

Cohen SM. Urinary bladder carcinogenesis. Toxicol Pathol 1998;26:121–27.

Colombo M. Natural history and pathogenesis of hepatitis C virus related hepatocellular carcinoma. J Hepatol 1999;31(Suppl 1):25–30.

Cuzick J, Babiker AG. Pancreatic cancer, alcohol, diabetes mellitus and gall-bladder disease. Int J Cancer 1989;43:415–21.

Doll R, Peto R, Wheatley K, Gray R, Sutherland I. Mortality in relation to smoking: 40 years' observations on male British doctors. Br Med J 1994;309:901–11.

Duell EJ, Casella DP, Burk RD, Kelsey KT, Holly EA Inflammation, genetic polymorphisms in proinflammatory genes TNF-A, RANTES, and CCR5, and risk of pancreatic adenocarcinoma. Cancer Epidemiol Biomarkers Prev 2006;15:726–31.

Duell EJ, Holly EA. Reproductive and mentrual risk factors for pancreatic cancer: a population-based study of San Francisco Bay Area Women. Am J Epidemiol 2005;161:741–47.

Duell EJ, Holly EA, Bracci PM, Wiencke JK, Kelsey KT. A population-based study of the Arg399Gln polymorphism in X-ray repair cross-complementing group 1 (XRCC1) and risk of pancreatic adenocarcinoma. Cancer Res 2002;15:4630–36.

Edwards BF, Redding TW, Schally AV. The effect of gastrointestinal hormones on the incorporation of tritiated thymidine in the pancreatic adenocarcinoma cell line (WD PaCa). Int J Pancreatol 1989;5:191–201.

Ekbom A, Helmick C, Zack M, Adami HO. Ulcerative colitis and colorectal cancer. A population-based study. N Engl J Med 1990;323:1228–33.

Ekbom A, Lundegardh G, McLaughlin JK, Nyrén O. Relation of vagotomy to subsequent risk of lung cancer: population based cohort study. Br Med J 1998;316:518–19.

Ekbom A, McLaughlin JK, Nyrén O. Pancreatitis and the risk of pancreatic cancer. N Engl J Med 1993;329:1502–3.

Ekbom A, Yuen J, Karlsson BM, McLaughlin JK, Adami HO. Risk of pancreatic and periampullar cancer following cholecystectomy: a population-based cohort study. Dig Dis Sci 1996;41:387–91.

Everhart J, Wright D. Diabetes mellitus as a risk factor for pancreatic cancer. A meta-analysis. JAMA 1995;273:1605–9.

Farrow DC, Davis S. Diet and the risk of pancreatic cancer in men. Am J Epidemiol 1990;132:423–31.

Ferlay J, Bray F, Pisani P, Parkin DM. GLO-BOCAN 2000: Cancer Incidence, Mortality and Prevalence Worldwide. International Agency for Research on Cancer, Lyon, 2001.

Fernandez E, La Vecchia C, D'Avanzo B, Negri E. Menstrual and reproductive factors and pancreatic cancer risk in women. Int J Cancer 1995;62:11–14.

Fernandez E, La Vecchia C, D'Avanzo B, Negri E, Franceschi S. Family history and the risk of liver, gallbladder, and pancreatic cancer. Cancer Epidemiol Biomarkers Prev 1994;3:209–12.

Fernandez E, La Vecchia C, Decarli A. Attributable risks for pancreatic cancer in northern Italy. Cancer Epidemiol Biomarkers Prev 1996;5:23–27.

Fryzek JP, Schenk M, Kinnard M, Greenson JK, Garabrant DH. The association of body mass index and pancreatic cancer in residents of southeastern Michigan, Am J Epidemiol 2005;162:222–28.

Gasslander T, Axelson J, Hakanson R, Ihse I, Lilja I, Rehfeld JF. Cholecystokinin is responsible for growth of the pancreas after pancreaticobiliary diversion in rats. Scand J Gastroenterol 1990;25:1060–65.

Ghadirian P, Boyle P, Simard A, Baillargeon J, Maisonneuve P, Perret C. Reported family aggregation of pancreatic cancer within a population-based case-control study in the Francophone community in Montreal, Canada. Int J Pancreatol 1991;10:183–96.

Giovannucci E. Tomatoes, tomato-based products, lycopene, and cancer: review of the epidemiologic literature. J Natl Cancer Inst 1999;91:317–31.

Gordis L. Consumption of methylxanthine-containing beverages and risk of pancreatic cancer. Cancer Lett 1990;52:1–12.

Green A, Jensen OM. Frequency of cancer among insulin-treated diabetic patients in Denmark. Diabetologia 1985;28:128–30.

Greenway B, Iqbal MJ, Johnson PJ, Williams R. Oestrogen receptor proteins in malignant and fetal pancreas. Br Med J (Clin Res Ed) 1981;283:751–53.

Hecht SS, Carmella SG, Foiles PG, Murphy SE, Peterson LA. Tobacco-specific nitrosamine adducts: studies in laboratory animals and humans. Environ Health Perspect 1993;99:57–63.

Hoppin JA, Tolbert PE, Holly EA, Brock JW, Korrick SA, Altshul LM, et al. Pancreatic cancer and serum organochlorine levels. Cancer Epidemiol Biomarkers Prev 2000; 9:199–205.

Howatson AG, Carter DC. Pancreatic carcinogenesis—enhancement by cholecysto-kinin in the hamster-nitrosamine model. Br J Cancer 1985;51:107–14.

Howe GR, Burch JD. Nutrition and pancreatic cancer. Cancer Causes Control 1996;7:69–82.

Howe GR, Jain M, Burch JD, Miller AB. Cigarette smoking and cancer of the pancreas: evidence from a population-based case-control study in Toronto, Canada. Int J Cancer 1991;47:323–28.

Hsing AW, Hansson LE, McLaughlin JK, Nyrén O, Blot WJ, Ekbom A, et al. Pernicious anemia and subsequent cancer. A population-based cohort study. Cancer 1993;71:745–50.

Hyvarinen H, Partanen S. Association of cholecystectomy with abdominal cancers. Hepatogastroenterology 1987;34:280–84.

Ijsselmuiden CB, Gaydos C, Feighner B, Novakoski WL, Serwadda D, Caris LH, et al. Cancer of the pancreas and drinking water: a population-based case-control study in Washington County, Maryland. Am J Epidemiol 1992;136:836–42.

Ji BT, Hatch MC, Chow WH, McLaughlin JK, Dai Q, Howe GR, et al. Anthropometric and reproductive factors and the risk of pancreatic cancer: a case-control study in Shanghai, China. Int J Cancer 1996;66:432–37.

Karlson BM, Ekbom A, Arvidsson D, Yuen J, Krusemo UB. Population-based study of cancer risk and relative survival following sphincterotomy for stones in the common bile duct. Br J Surg 1997a;84:1235–38.

Karlson BM, Ekbom A, Josefsson S, McLaughlin JK, Fraumeni JF Jr, Nyrén O. The risk of pancreatic cancer following pancreatitis: an association due to confounding? Gastroenterology 1997b;113:587–92.

Karlson BM, Hsing AW, Ekbom A, Wacholder S, McLaughlin JK. Cancer of the upper gastrointestinal tract among patients with pernicious anemia. Scand J Gastroenterol 2000; 35:847–51.

Karlson BM, Wuu J, Hsieh CC, Lambe M, Ekbom A. Parity and the risk of pancreatic cancer: a nested case-control study. Int J Cancer 1998;77:224–27.

Keating JJ, Johnson PJ, Cochrane AM, Gazzard BG, Krasner N, Smith PM, et al. A prospective randomised controlled trial of tamoxifen and cyproterone acetate in pancreatic carcinoma. Br J Cancer 1989;60:789–92.

Klein AP, Brune KA, Peterse4n GM, Goggins M, Tersmette AC, Offerhaus GJ et al. Prospective risk of pancreatic cancer in familial pancreatic cancer kindreds. Cancer Res 2004;64:2634–38.

Kuper HE, Mucci LA, Trichopoulos D. Coffee, pancreatic cancer and the question of causation. J Epidemiol Community Health 2000; 54:650–51.

Kuper H, Ye W, Broome U, Romelsjö A, Mucci LA, Ekbom A, et al. The risk of liver and bile duct cancers in patients with chronic viral hepatitis, alcoholism, or cirrhosis. Hepatology 2001;34:714–18.

Kvale G, Heuch I, Nilssen S. Parity in relation to mortality and cancer incidence: a prospective study of Norwegian women. Int J Epidemiol 1994;23:691–99.

Larsson SC, Hakansson N, Giovannucci E, Wolk A. Folate intake and pancreatic cancer incidence: a prospective study of Swedish Women and men. J Natl Cancer Inst 2006; 98:407–13.

Lerch MM, Ellis I, Whitcomb DC, Keim V, Simon P, Howes N, et al. Maternal inheritance pattern of hereditary pancreatitis in patients with pancreatic carcinoma. J Natl Cancer Inst 1999;91:723–24.

Liehr RM, Melnykovych G, Solomon TE. Growth effects of regulatory peptides on human pancreatic cancer lines PANC-1 and MIA PaCa-2. Gastroenterology 1990;98: 1666–74.

Lindelof B, Granath F, Tengvall-Linder, Ekbom A. Allergy and cancer 2005;60:1116–20.

Lin Y, Tamakoshi A, Kawamura T, Inaba Y, Kikuchi S, Motohashi Y, et al. JACC Study Group. Japan Collaborative cohort. A prospective cohort study of cigarette smoking and pancreatic cancer in Japan. Cancer Cases Control 2002;13:249–54.

Lindstrom P, Janzon L, Sternby NH. Declining autopsy rate in Sweden: a study of causes and consequences in Malmo, Sweden. J Intern Med 1997;242:157–65.

Longnecker DS, Roebuck BD, Kuhlmann ET. Enhancement of pancreatic carcinogenesis by a dietary unsaturated fat in rats treated with saline or N-nitroso(2-hydroxypropyl) (2-oxopropyl)amine. J Natl Cancer Inst 1985;74:219–22.

Lowenfels AB, Maisonneuve P, Cavallini G, Ammann RW, Lankisch PG, Andersen JR, et al. Pancreatitis and the risk of pancreatic cancer. International Pancreatitis Study Group. N Engl J Med 1993;328:1433–37.

Lowenfels AB, Maisonneuve P, DiMagno EP, Elitsur Y, Gates LK Jr, Perrault J, et al. Hereditary pancreatitis and the risk of pancreatic cancer. International Hereditary Pancreatitis Study Group. J Natl Cancer Inst 1997;89:442–46.

Lynch HT, Richardson JD, Amin M, Lynch JF, Cavalieri RJ, Bronson E, et al. Variable gastrointestinal and urologic cancers in a Lynch syndrome II kindred. Dis Colon Rectum 1991;34:891–95.

Mack TM, Yu MC, Hanisch R, Henderson BE. Pancreas cancer and smoking, beverage consumption, and past medical history. J Natl Cancer Inst 1986;76:49–60.

MacMahon B, Yen S, Trichopoulos D, Warren K, Nardi G. Coffee and cancer of the pancreas. N Engl J Med 1981;304:630–33.

Matanoski GM, Seltser R, Sartwell PE, Diamond EL, Elliott EA. The current mortality rates of radiologists and other physician specialists: specific causes of death. Am J Epidemiol 1975;101:199–210.

Michaud DS, Giovannucci E, Willett WC, Colditz GA, Fuchs CS. Coffee and alcohol consumption and the risk of pancreatic cancer in two prospective United States cohorts. Cancer Epidemiol Biomarkers Prev 2001;10: 429–37.

Michaud DS, Giovannucci E, Willett WC, Colditz GA, Stampfer MJ, Fuchs CS. Physical activity, obesity, height, and the risk of pancreatic cancer. JAMA 2001;286:921–29.

Michaud DS, Skinner HG, Wu K, Hu F, Giovannucci E, Willett W, Colditz GA, Fuchs CS. Dietary patterns and pancreatic cancer risk in men and women. J Natl Cancer Inst 2005;97:518–24.

Mills PK, Beeson WL, Abbey DE, Fraser GE, Phillips RL. Dietary habits and past medical history as related to fatal pancreas cancer risk among Adventists. Cancer 1988;61: 2578–85.

National Board of Health and Welfare. Cancer Incidence in Sweden 2005. Stockholm, Centre of Epidemiology, 2005.

Neglia JP, FitzSimmons SC, Maisonneuve P, Schoni MH, Schoni-Affolter F, Corey M, et al. The risk of cancer among patients with cystic fibrosis. Cystic Fibrosis and Cancer Study Group. N Engl J Med 1995;332:494–99.

Norell SE, Ahlbom A, Erwald R, Jacobson G, Lindberg-Navier I, Olin R, et al. Diet and pancreatic cancer: a case-control study. Am J Epidemiol 1986;124:894–902.

Nothlings U, Wilkens LR, Murphy SP, Hankin JH, Henderson BE, Kolonel LN. Meat and fat intake as risk factors for pancreatic cancer: the multiethnic cohort study. J Natl Cancer Inst 2005;97:1458–65.

Offerhaus GJ, Tersmette AC, Tersmette KW, Tytgat GN, Hoedemaeker PJ, Vandenbroucke JP. Gastric, pancreatic, and colorectal carcinogenesis following remote peptic ulcer surgery. Review of the literature with the emphasis on risk assessment and underlying mechanism. Mod Pathol 1988;1:352–56.

Ojajarvi IA, Partanen TJ, Ahlbom A, Boffetta P, Hakulinen T, Jourenkova N, et al. Occupational exposures and pancreatic cancer: a meta-analysis. Occup Environ Med 2000; 57:316–24.

Ozcelik H, Schmocker B, Di Nicola N, Shi XH, Langer B, Moore M, et al. Germline BRCA2 6174delT mutations in Ashkenazi Jewish pancreatic cancer patients. Nat Genet 1997; 16:17–18.

Parkin DM, Muir CS, Whelan SL, Gao YT, Ferlay J, and Powell J (Eds): Cancer Incidence in Five Continents. Vol. VI. IARC Sci Pub. No. 120. Lyon, International Agency for Research on Cancer, 1992.

Petersen GM, de Andrade M, Goggins M, Hruban RH, Bondy M, Korczak JF, et al. Pancreatic cancer genetic epidemiology consortium. Cancer Epidemiol Biomarkers Prev 2006;15:704–10.

Petersen H, Solomon T, Grossman MI. Effect of chronic pentagastrin, cholecystokinin, and secretin on pancreas of rats. Am J Physiol 1978;234:E286–93.

Porta M, Malats N, Guarner L, Carrato A, Rifa J, Salas A, et al. Association between coffee drinking and K-ras mutations in exocrine pancreatic cancer. PANKRAS II Study Group. J Epidemiol Community Health 1999;53: 702–9.

Rimm EB, Chan J, Stampfer MJ, Colditz GA, Willett WC. Prospective study of cigarette smoking, alcohol use, and the risk of diabetes in men. Br Med J 1995;310:555–59.

Rivenson A, Hoffmann D, Prokopczyk B, Amin S, Hecht SS. Induction of lung and exocrine pancreas tumors in F344 rats by tobacco-specific and Areca-derived N-nitrosamines. Cancer Res 1988;48:6912–17.

Roda E, Aldini R, Mazzella G, Roda A, Sama C, Festi D, et al. Enterohepatic circulation of bile acids after cholecystectomy. Gut 1978; 19:640–49.

Romundstad P, Andersen A, Haldorsen T. Cancer incidence among workers in six Norwegian aluminum plants. Scand J work Environ Health 2000;26:461–69.

Rutqvist LE, Lewin F. Flawed methods. Int J Cancer 2006;118:1581.

Schenk M, Severson RK, Pawlish KS. The risk of subsequent primary carcinoma of the pancreas in patients with cutaneous malignant melanoma. Cancer 1998;82:1672–76.

Schwartz GG, Reis IM. Is cadmium a cause of human pancreatic cancer? Cancer Epidemiol Biomarkers Prev 2000;9:139–45.

Sheldon CD, Hodson ME, Carpenter LM, Swerdlow AJ. A cohort study of cystic fibrosis and malignancy. Br J Cancer 1993; 68:1025–28.

Silverman DT, Brown LM, Hoover RN, Schiffman M, Lillemoe KD, Schoenberg JB, et al. Alcohol and pancreatic cancer in blacks and whites in the United States. Cancer Res 1995; 55:4899–4905.

Silverman DT, Dunn JA, Hoover RN, Schiffman M, Lillemoe KD, Schoenberg JB, et al. Cigarette smoking and pancreas cancer: a case-control study based on direct interviews. J Natl Cancer Inst 1994;86:1510–16.

Skinner HG, Michaud DS, Giovannucci EL, Rimm EB, Stampfer MJ, Willett WC, et al. A prospective study of folate intake and the risk of pancreatic cancer in men and women. Am J epidemiol 2004;160:248–58.

Smith PG, Doll R. Mortality from cancer and all causes among British radiologists. Br J Radiol 1981;54:187–94.

Soloway HB, Sommers SC. Endocrinopathy associated with pancreatic carcinomas. Review of host factors including hyperplasia and gonadotropic activity. Ann Surg 1966;164:300–4.

Stolzenberg-Solomon RZ, Albanes D, Nieto FJ, Hartman TJ, Tangrea JA, Rautalahti M, et al. Pancreatic cancer risk and nutrition-related methyl-group availability indicators in male smokers. J Natl Cancer Inst 1999;91:535–41.

Stone BJ, Blot WJ, Fraumeni JF Jr. Geographic patterns of industry in the United States. An aid to the study of occupational disease. J Occup Med 1978;20:472–77.

Swift M, Morrell D, Massey RB, Chase CL. Incidence of cancer in 161 families affected by ataxia-telangiectasia. N Engl J Med 1991; 325:1831–36.

Teras LR, Patel AV, Rodriguez C, Thun MJ, Calle EE. Parity, other reproductive factors, and risk of pancreatic cancer mortality in a large cohort of U.S. women (United States). Cancer Causes control 2005;16:1035–40.

Takeda Y, Escribano MJ. Effects of insulin and somatostatin on the growth and the colony formation of two human pancreatic cancer cell lines. J Cancer Res Clin Oncol 1991; 117:416–20.

Thomas PG, Augustine P, Ramesh H, Rangabashyam N. Observations and surgical management of tropical pancreatitis in Kerala and southern India. World J Surg 1990;14:32–42.

Tolley HD, Marks S, Buchanan JA, Gilbert ES. A further update of the analysis of mortality of workers in a nuclear facility. Radiat Res 1983;95:211–13.

Veenstra J, Schenkel JA, van Erp-Baart AM, Brants HA, Hulshof KF, Kistemaker C, et al. Alcohol consumption in relation to food intake and smoking habits in the Dutch National Food Consumption Survey. Eur J Clin Nutr 1993;47:482–89.

Warshaw AL, Fernandez-del Castillo C. Pancreatic carcinoma. N Engl J Med 1992;326: 455–65.

Weiderpass E, Partanen T, Kaaks R, Vainio H, Porta M, Kauppinen T, et al. Occurrence, trends and environment etiology of pancreatic cancer. Scand J Work Environ Health 1998;24:165–74.

Williams JA, Goldfine ID. The insulin-pancreatic acinar axis. Diabetes 1985;34:980–86.

Wynder EL, Mabuchi K, Maruchi N, Fortner JG. A case control study of cancer of the pancreas. Cancer 1973;31:641–48.

Yanai H, Inaba Y, Takagi H, Yamamoto S. Multivariate analysis of cancer mortalities for selected sites in 24 countries. Environ Health Perspect 1979;32:83–101.

Ye W, Lagergren J, Weiderpass E, Nylen O, Adami HO, Ekbom A. Alcohol abuse and the risk of pancreatic cancer. Gut 2002;51:236–39.

Zatonski WA, Boyle P, Przewozniak K, Maisonneuve P, Drosik K, Walker AM. Cigarette smoking, alcohol, tea and coffee consumption and pancreas cancer risk: a case-control study from Opole, Poland. Int J Cancer 1993;53:601–7.

Zheng W, McLaughlin JK, Gridley G, Bjelke E, Schuman LM, Silverman DT, et al. A cohort study of smoking, alcohol consumption, and dietary factors for pancreatic cancer (United States). Cancer Causes Control 1993;4:477–82.

14

Cancer of the Lung, Larynx, and Pleura

PAOLO BOFFETTA AND DIMITRIOS TRICHOPOULOS

The history of lung cancer epidemiology parallels the history of modern chronic disease epidemiology. In the nineteenth century, an excess of lung cancer was observed among miners and some other occupational groups, but otherwise the disease was very rare. An epidemic increase in lung cancer began in the first half of the twentieth century, and there were much speculation and controversy about its possible environmental causes. Later, lung cancer became a milestone in epidemiology when its predominant cause, tobacco smoking, was established in a series of landmark studies beginning in 1950. Indeed, the challenge to demonstrate this causal association convincingly was a driving force in the remarkable development of epidemiologic methods during the second half of the century. Therefore, it is a tragedy that today, and in the foreseeable future, this highly preventable disease will remain among the most common and most lethal cancers globally. Although cancer of the larynx is much less common than lung cancer, it is also closely linked with tobacco smoking,

while mesothelioma, the typical malignancy of the pleura, arises mainly after exposure to asbestos, another avoidable cause.

Methodologically, epidemiologic studies of cancer of the lung and larynx have been straightforward because the site of origin is well defined, progressive symptoms prompt diagnostic activity, and the predominant causes are comparatively easy to ascertain. Novel approaches on the classification of lung cancer based on molecular techniques will likely bring new insights in its aetiology, in particular among nonsmokers.

CLINICAL SYNOPSIS

Subgroups

The main histologic types of lung cancer are squamous cell carcinoma (30% to 50%), small (10% to 30%) and large (5% to 15%) cell carcinoma, and the increasingly common adenocarcinoma (10% to 30%). Malignant neoplasms of the lung originate mainly from the bronchial, bronchiolar, and alveolar epithelium, more rarely from the tracheal epithelium or from interstitial tissue of the lung.

Symptoms

Cough, sometimes with bleeding (hemoptysis), and recurring pneumonia and bronchitis are the predominant symptoms. Locally advanced and metastatic disease may cause a multitude of symptoms besides those typical of an advanced malignancy, namely, breathlessness, obstruction of the airway and esophagus, enlarged lymph nodes, and loss of appetite or weight.

Diagnosis

Sputum cytology is a simple test that could be used when lung cancer is suspected. For staging, imaging by pulmonary x-ray, computed tomography, and magnetic resonance imaging are required. A majority of all lung cancers can be reached via the bronchoscope and confirmed histopathologically by means of a biopsy. Whenever surgical treatment is considered, a mediastinoscopy may clarify whether the tumor has metastasized into regional lymph nodes.

Treatment

Cure by means of radical surgical removal of a lobe or of one entire lung can be achieved only rarely. Five years after surgery with a curative intent, approximately one-third of all patients are still alive. Radiation therapy can produce cure in a minority and palliation in a majority of patients. In advanced tumors, chemotherapy produces a modest effect, with little influence on overall survival

Prognosis

Lung cancer remains a largely lethal disease, with 5-year relative survival rates of about 10% both in the United States and in Europe.

Progress

No remarkable improvement in treatment has been made over the last several decades, and no therapeutic breakthrough is within sight. Spiral computed tomography has been proposed as a screening tool. In selected series of high-risk individuals, this technique has resulted in the identification of a large number of *nodules* of uncertain biological behavior and clinical significance. The usefulness of this approach to reduce mortality from lung cancer is currently being studied in randomized controlled trials. Because no effective screening strategies are currently available, primary prevention through a reduction in tobacco smoking remains the only realistic strategy to control this globally dominant malignancy.

TUMORS OF THE LUNG
DESCRIPTIVE EPIDEMIOLOGY

Lung cancer, a rare disease until the beginning of the twentieth century, has become the most frequent malignant neoplasm among men in most countries, and a parallel increase in incidence is now seen among women, notably in western countries. In 2002, lung cancer accounted for an estimated 965 000 new cases among men, which is 17% of all cancers excluding skin cancer, and 387 000, that is, 8%, of new cancer cases among women. After nonmelonocytic skin cancer, it is the most frequent malignant neoplasm in humans and the most important cause of death from neoplasia. Approximately 50% of all cases occur in developing countries (Ferlay et al, 2004).

Among both women and men, the incidence of lung cancer is low in persons under age 40 and increases up to age 70 or 75 (Figs 14–1 and 14–2). The decline in incidence in the older age groups can be explained, at least in part, by incomplete diagnosis or by a generation (birth-cohort) effect.

The geographic and temporal patterns of lung cancer incidence are determined chiefly by consumption of tobacco (Figs. 14–3 and 14–4). An increase in tobacco consumption is paralleled a few decades later by an increase in the incidence of lung cancer, and a decrease in consumption is followed by a decrease in incidence. Other

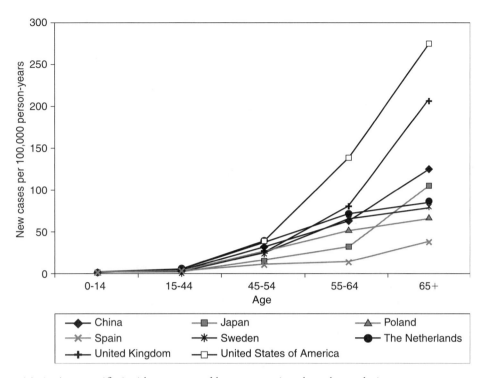

Figure 14–1. Age-specific incidence rates of lung cancer in selected populations—women.

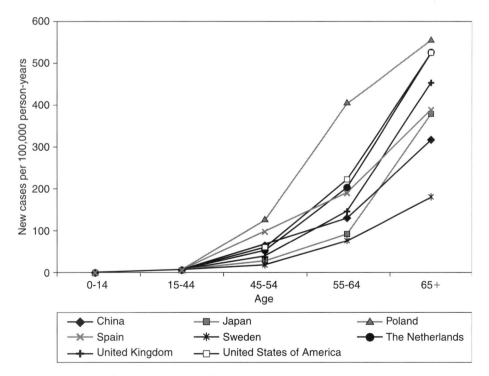

Figure 14–2. Age-specific incidence rates of lung cancer in selected populations—men.

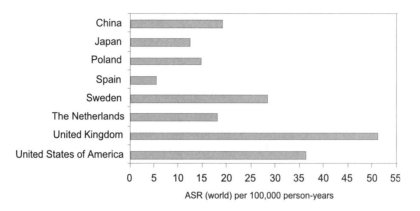

Figure 14–3. Age-standardized incidence rates of lung cancer in selected populations—women.

factors, such as genetic susceptibility, poor diet, and indoor air pollution, may act in concert with tobacco smoking in shaping the descriptive epidemiology of lung cancer.

The pattern we observe today in men (Fig. 14–3) is composed of populations at high risk, in which consumption of tobacco has been persistently high for decades, and populations at low risk, either because tobacco consumption has not been increasing for long (eg, China, Africa) or because a decrease in consumption has been relatively low for several decades (eg, Sweden).

In most countries, the risk of lung cancer among men is consistently two- to threefold higher in lower than in higher socioeconomic classes (Singh et al, 2002) (Fig. 14–5). The pattern among women is less consistent. In countries with populations con-

sisting of different ethnic groups, differences in lung cancer rates are frequently observed: For example, in the United States, the rates are high among male and female African Americans (Table 14–1).

Over the last 20 years, the distribution of histologic types has been changing. In the United States, squamous cell carcinoma, which was formerly the predominant type, is decreasing, while adenocarcinoma has increased in both genders (Travis et al, 1996). In Europe, similar changes are occurring in men, while in women, both squamous cell carcinoma and adenocarcinoma are increasing (Tyczynski et al, 2003). Although the increase in the incidence of adenocarcinoma may be due, at least in part, to improved diagnostic techniques, changes in composition and patterns of tobacco consumption

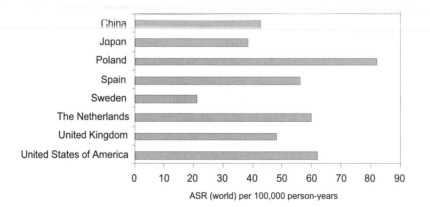

Figure 14–4. Age-standardized incidence rates of lung cancer in selected populations—men.

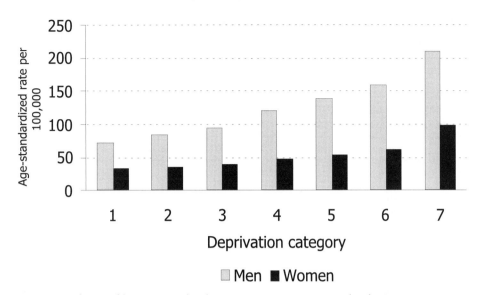

Figure 14–5. Incidence of lung cancer by deprivation category in Scotland. (*Source*: McLaren and Bain, 1998)

(deeper inhalation of low-nicotine and tar tobacco smoke) are an additional explanation (Surgeon General, 2004).

GENETIC AND MOLECULAR EPIDEMIOLOGY

Family History

A positive family history of lung cancer has been found to be a risk factor in several studies (reviewed by Sellers and Bailey-Wilson, 1998). In several registry-based studies, a high familial risk for early onset cases was found. Athough shared smoking patterns within families may explain a large part of the associaton with family history, increased related risks were found even after adjustment for smoking (Bermejo and Hemminki, 2005).

High-penetrance genes

Segregation analyses suggest inheritance of a major gene that, in conjunction with tobacco smoking, might account for more than 50% of cases diagnosed below age 60 (Gauderman et al, 1997). A pooled analysis of high-risk pedigrees identified a major susceptibility locus to chromosome 6q23–25 (Bailey-Wilson et al, 2004). Lung cancer risk is also increased within the framework of the Li-Fraumeni syndrome, characterized by germline mutation in the tumor-suppressor gene *p53* (Malkin et al, 1990).

Genetic polymorphisms

In addition to the possible effect of relatively rare genes with high penetrance, there is growing evidence of a role for genetic polymorphisms in lung carcinogenesis. Variants in several genes have been investigated in association studies. Table 14–2 summarizes the evidence of an association between genetic variants and lung cancer

Table 14–1. Age-standardized rates (per 100,000 person-years) of lung cancer in different ethnic groups. Los Angeles County, USA, 1993–1997 (Parkin et al, 2002).

Ethnic group	Men	Women
Non-Hispanic White	50.2	37.6
Hispanic White	34.6	15.5
Black	80.2	35.6
Chinese	25.8	15.5
Filipino	50.0	12.4
Japanese	27.3	16.3
Korean	35.8	10.6

(Spitz et al, 2006). Most genes whose polymorphisms have been analyzed with respect to lung cancer risk are involved either in the metabolism of exogenous compounds or in DNA repair. For a few genes, the accumulated evidence points toward an increased risk of lung cancer among carriers of the rare variants (eg, *GSTM1* deletion,

Table 14–2. Summary of the evidence from genetic association studies of polymorphisms and lung cancer (from Spitz et al, 2006).

Gene	Polymorphism	N studies	Main populations	Summary of the evidence
Metabolism				
CYP1A1	Ile462Val	10–20	Asia, Europe, USA, South America	increased risk suggested
	Msp 1	10–20	Asia, Europe, USA	weakly increased risk suggested
	African-Americans	<5	USA	increased risk suggested
CYP2D6	*3–10	10–20	Asia, Europe, USA	no association
CYP2C9	*2	<5	USA	inconsistent results
CYP2E1	RsaI	5–10	Asia, Europe, USA	inconsistent results
	DraI	5–10	Asia, Europe, USA	inconsistent results
	PstI	5–10	Asia, Europe, USA	inconsistent results
MPO	463G>A	5–10	Europe, USA	null to reduced risk suggested
EPHX	Tyr113His	10–20	Europe, North America	inconsistent results
	Arg139His	10–20	Europe, North America	inconsistent results
NQO1	Pro187Ser	10–20	various	inconsistent results
GSTM1	deletion	>20	various	weakly increased risk likely
GSTT1	deletion	>20	various	no association likely
GSTP 1	Ile105 Val	10–20	Europe, USA	inconsistent results
	Ala114Val	10–20	Europe, USA	inconsistent results
NAT2	'slow' phenotype	10–20	Europe, USA, Aisa	inconsistent results
NAT1	'fast' phenotype (*10)	<5	Europe, USA	inconsistent results
MTHFR	Ala222Val	<5	Asia, USA	null to increased risk suggested
DNMT3B	Promoter (C149T)	<5	Asia	increased risk suggested
DNA repair				
XPA	23A>G	<5	Asia, USA, Europe	inconsistent results
XPD	Asp312Asn	5–10	Asia, Europe, USA	inconsistent results
ERCC1	8092 A>C	<5	Europe, USA	inconsistent results
XRCC1	Arg399Gln	5–10	Asia, Europe, USA	inconsistent results
	Arg194Trp	5–10	Asia, Europe, USA	decreased risk suggested
XRCC3	Thr241Met	5–10	Europe, USA	inconsistent results
hOGG1/MMH	Ser326Cys	5–10	Asia, USA, Europe	increased risk suggested
Cell cycle control				
p53	Arg72Pro	15–20	Asia, Europe, USA	weakly increased risk suggested
	intron 3 16bp duplications	<5	Europe, USA	increased risk suggested
	intron 6	<5	Europe, USA	inconsistent results

with a relative risk among carriers in the order of 1.15—Houlston et al, 1999, or toward the lack of an effect (eg, *GSTT1* deletion—Stucker et al, 2001). For most genes, however, the available results do not allow conclusions on the presence or absence of an effect. This is due to methodological limitations in the available studies (eg, choice of convenience control groups) and low statistical power.

Polymorphisms are likely to act by modifying the effect of other risk factors, such as tobacco smoking and diet. One particularly interesting example of a gene–environment interaction in lung carcinogenesis is that of the protective effect of dietary intake of cruciferous vegetables, which is likely due to isothiocyanates (see following).

DNA Repair Capacity

There is abundant evidence that reduced capacity to repair DNA damage represents an important component of the individual susceptibility to lung cancer. Different assays have been developed to measure DNA repair capacity: The mutagen sensitivity assay involves challenging lymphocytes with mutagens such as benzo[a]pyrene diol epoxide and bleomycin, and measuring chromatid breaks after recovery. Several studies have shown increased number of breaks in lung cancer cases than in matched controls, and the difference is greater for light smokers and young patients (Zheng et al, 2003). In the host-cell reactivation assay a nonreplicating recombinant plasmid harboring a reporter gene is transfected to lymphocytes: The activity of the reporter gene is then measured as marker of the excision repair activity of the host cell–Lower activity has been reported among more cases than controls (Wei et al, 1996; Spitz et al, 2003). Persistence of DNA adducts in lymphocytes treated with a standard dose of benzo[a]pyrene diol epoxide, the active metabolite of benzo[a]pyrene, is measured by 32P-postlabeling and indicates the individual ability to repair DNA damage: Cases of lung cancer have been shown to have higher adduct level than controls (Li et al, 2001). Cases also had lower expression of

several genes involved in nucleotide excision repair as measured by mRNA level (Cheng et al, 2000).

Somatic Cells and Genetic Events

There is strong evidence for stepwise accumulation in lung carcinogenesis of genetic alterations, including allelic losses, chromosomal instability, mutations in proto-oncogenes and tumor-suppressor genes, epigenetic changes, and expression alterations (Gazdar et al, 2004). There are quite distinct patterns of alterations in small-cell lung cancer and nonsmall-cell lung cancer, likely reflecting the different origin of these two categories of tumors (epithelial cell with neuro-endocrine characteristics versus bronchial and alveolar cell). In the latter group, squamous cell carcinoma, originating from bronchial cells undergoing squamous metaplasia and dysplasia, shows distinct genetic alterations from adenocarcinoma, deriving from alveolar or bronchiolar cells. The data on the other, more rare, types of lung cancer are sparse (Fig. 14–6). Table 14–3 shows the most important genetic alterations observed in lung cancer and their possible association with etiologic agents.

Mutations in the tumor-suppressor gene *TP53* are the most frequent events in lung cancer. Adenocarcinoma cases present a lower prevalence of *p53* mutations than other histologic types (Pfeifer et al, 2002). Among lung cancer cases, the proportion of *p53* mutations increases with the duration and amount of tobacco smoking (Le Calvez et al, 2005). Also, a higher proportion of *p53* alterations has been reported from studies in lung cancer patients with exposure to polycyclic aromatic hydrocarbons (PAHs), asbestos, or radon than in patients without these exposures. The wide distribution and variety of types of *p53* mutations following environmental exposures might ultimately elucidate mechanisms in lung carcinogenesis (Pfeifer et al, 2002).

Inactivation of the pathway controlling the retinoblastoma gene, *RB1*, that acts as a gatekeeper for the G1 to S transition of the cell cyle is another common alteration in all types of lung cancer. Alterations are

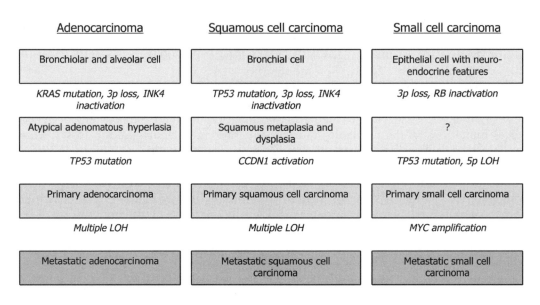

Genetic alterations are marked in bold.

Figure 14–6. Model of lung carcinogenesis. (*Source*: Yokota and Kohno, 2004)

particularly frequent in three genes involved in the pathway: loss of *RB1* expression, detectable in almost all small-cell lung cancers, inactivation of p16, and overexpression of *CCND1*, encoding cyclin D1 (Brambilla et al, 1999).

Activating point mutations at codon 12 in the *KRAS* oncogene occurs in 30% to

Table 14–3. Main acquired somatic genetic alternations in human lung cancer and their suspected associations with etiological agents

Gene	Locus	Main alterations	Percentage of tumours with alteration			Exposures	Comments
			SCC	AC	SqCC		
p53	17p13	M(G:C>T:A)	70–90	30	50	Tobacco, asbestos, radon	Early event
RB1	13q14	LE	80–100	15		?	Inverse
p16^{INK4}	9p21	LOH, M, HM	rare	50–70		Tobacco	correlation of
CCND1	11q13	OE	rare	rare	10	?	Rb loss, p16 inactivation, CCD1 OE
KRAS	12p21	M (GGT>TGT)	rare	30–40	<5	Tobacco, asbestos	Early event
FHIT, RASSF1, SEMA3B	3p1–2	LOH, HM?	80	50–80		Tobacco	Role of specific genes unclear
APC		M	5	rare	5	?	
MYC	8q21–23	LOH	30	<10		?	
?	5q	LOH	10–40	<5			

SCC: small cell carcinoma; AC: adenocarcinoma, SqCC: squamous cell carcinoma; LE: loss of expression; HM: hypermetilation; LOH: loss of heterozygosity; M: mutation; TD: transcriptional dysregulation; OE: overexpression; PAH: polycyclic aromatic hydrocarbons

40% of adenocarcinoma of the lung (Sekido et al, 2001). This alteration may be a relatively early event in lung carcinogenesis.

Data showing a high frequency of allelic losses and loss of expression in the short arm of chromosome 3 (3p) in human lung tumors firmly suggest the presence of one or several important tumor-suppressor genes in this region: Candidates include *FHIT, RASSF1*, and *SEMA3B*. The role of these genes in lung carcinogenesis, however, is poorly understood. Other oncogenes have also been implicated in lung carcinogenesis, in particular *eMYC, APC, ErbB2*, and *Bc12*. They have been associated with clinical parameters such as stage, differentiation, and survival. In addition, comparative genomic hybridization studies have detected amplifications in 1p, 3q, 5p, 17q, and Xq26 regions, suggesting the involvement of other unknown genes (Sekido et al, 2001; Gazdar et al, 2004).

RISK FACTORS

Tobacco

There is overwhelming evidence that tobacco smoking causes all major histologic types of lung cancer.

A carcinogenic effect of tobacco smoke on the lung has been demonstrated in epidemiologic studies conducted since the early 1950s and has been recognized by public health and regulatory authorities since the mid-1960s. Tobacco smoking is the main cause of lung cancer in most human populations, and the geographic and temporal patterns of the disease largely reflect tobacco consumption accumulated during the previous decades. Because of the strong carcinogenic potency of tobacco smoke, a major reduction in tobacco consumption would result in the prevention of a large fraction of human cancers (Peto et al, 1992; IARC, 2004a).

The excess risk among continuous smokers relative to that among never-smokers is on the order of 10- to 20-fold. The overall relative risk reflects the contribution of the different aspects of tobacco smoking: average consumption, duration of smoking, time since quitting, age at start, type of tobacco product, and inhalation pattern, as well as the absolute risk in never-smokers.

Time variables

Several large cohort and case-control studies have provided detailed information on the relative contributions of duration and amount of cigarette smoking in excess lung cancer risk. Doll and Peto (1978) analyzed data from a large cohort of British doctors. They concluded that the excess lung cancer risk rises in proportion to the square of the number of cigarettes smoked per day but to the fourth power of the duration of smoking. Therefore, duration of smoking should be considered the strongest determinant of lung cancer risk in smokers. These results have been confirmed by the analysis of the same cohort after 50 years of follow-up (Doll et al, 2004).

An important aspect of tobacco-related lung carcinogenesis is the effect of cessation of smoking. The excess risk sharply decreases in ex-smokers starting approximately 5 years after quitting, and an effect is apparent even for cessation late in life. However an excess risk throughout life likely persists even in long-term quitters (IARC, 2004a).

Tar content

The risk of lung cancer is lower among smokers of low-tar cigarettes than among smokers of high-tar cigarettes and among smokers of filtered cigarettes than smokers of unfiltered cigarettes. Smokers of black (air-cured) tobacco cigarettes are at two- to threefold higher risk of lung cancer than smokers of blond (flue-cured) tobacco cigarettes (IARC, 2004a). Tar content, the presence of a filter, and the type of tobacco are not independent, however: High-tar cigarettes tend to be unfiltered and, in the countries where both black and blond tobacco are used, they are more frequently made of black tobacco.

Although cigarettes are the main tobacco product smoked in western countries, an exposure–response relationship with lung cancer risk has also been shown for cigars, cigarillos, and pipes, indicating a carcinogenic effect of these products, as well (IARC, 2004a). An increased risk of lung cancer has also been shown following consumption of bidi and hookah in India, khii yoo in Thailand, and water pipe in China (IARC, 2004a). Limited data suggest an increased lung cancer risk following consumption of other tobacco products, such as narghile in western Asia and northern Africa, and toombak in Sudan.

Differences in effect according to histology, sex, and race

Although the evidence is abundant that tobacco smoking causes all major histologic types of lung cancer, the associations are strongest for squamous cell and small-cell carcinoma and lower for adenocarcinoma. The incidence of the latter histologic type has greatly increased during the last decades. Some of the increase might be attributable to improved diagnostic techniques, but it is possible that aspects of tobacco smoking have also played a role; it is unclear, however, which aspects of smoking might explain these changes.

A few studies have suggested a difference in the risk of lung cancer between men and women who have smoked a comparable amount of tobacco (Zang and Wynder, 1996), but most of the available evidence does not support this gender difference (IARC, 2004a).

The higher rate of lung cancer among African Americans as compared to other ethnic groups in the United States is probably explained by their higher tobacco consumption (Devesa et al, 1999). The lower risk of lung cancer among smokers in China and Japan as compared to Europe and North America might be due to relatively recent introduction of regular heavy smoking in Asia, although differences in susceptibility might also play a role (IARC, 2004a).

Involuntary smoking

The collective epidemiologic evidence and biological plausibility support a causal association between involuntary (or passive) exposure to cigarette smoke and lung cancer risk in nonsmokers (IARC, 2004b). The evidence of a high relative risk in the original studies (Trichopoulos et al, 1981; Hirayama, 1981) has been challenged on the basis of possible confounding by active smoking, diet, or other factors, and of possible reporting bias. When these factors were taken into account the association was confirmed, although the excess risk was in the order of 20% to 25% (Hackshaw et al, 1997; IARC, 2004b).

The effect of involuntary smoking appears to be present for both household exposure, mainly from the spouse, and workplace exposure (IARC, 2004b). On the other hand, there is little evidence of an effect of childhood involuntary smoking exposure (Boffetta et al, 2000).

Confounding effects of tobacco smoking

The importance of tobacco smoking in the causation of lung cancer complicates the investigation of the other causes of this disease because tobacco smoking may act as a powerful confounder. For example, a population of industrial workers exposed to a suspected carcinogen may smoke more than the unexposed comparison population. An excessive lung cancer risk in the exposed group, especially if small, might be due to the difference in smoking rather than to the effect of the occupational agent. One solution is to restrict the investigation of other risk factors to lifetime nonsmokers. However, they represent a selected group, with low prevalence of exposure to many agents of interest. An alternative is to collect detailed information on smoking habits and to compare the effect of the suspected carcinogens across different groups of smokers. This approach has shown that tobacco smoking as a confounder rarely explains completely excess risks larger than about 50% (Siemiatycki et al, 1988).

Interactive effects of tobacco smoke

Other carcinogens might interact with tobacco smoke in the determination of their carcinogenic action on the lung. In other words, the risk from exposure to another agent might be greater (or smaller) among heavy smokers compared to the corresponding risk among light smokers and nonsmokers. The interaction might take place at the stage of external exposure; that is, the other agent has to be absorbed on the tobacco particles to penetrate the lung or at some stage of the carcinogenic process, for example, induction of common activating or detoxifying enzymes. The empirical evidence on interaction between tobacco smoking and other agents is scanty, mainly because of lack of data among light smokers and nonsmokers (Boffetta and Saracci, 1993). A synergism has been suggested between asbestos exposure and tobacco smoking in causing lung cancer, but its degree remains uncertain (IARC, 2004a). The interaction between radon exposure and tobacco smoking best fits a submultiplicative model; data for other agents are too sparse to allow conclusions.

Use of smokeless tobacco products

Few studies have investigated the risk of lung cancer among users of smokeless tobacco products. In two large cohorts of US volunteers, the relative risk (RR) for spit tobacco use among nonsmokers was 1.08 (95% CI 0.64–1.83) and 2.00 (95% CI 1.23–3.24) (Henley et al, 2005). In a Norwegian cohort, the RR for ever use of snus was 0.80 (95% CI 0.61–1.05) (Boffetta et al, 2005). In a large case-control study from India the RR of lung cancer for ever use of tobacco-containing chewing products was 0.74 (95% CI 0.57-.96) (Gajalakshmi et al, 2003). Overall, the evidence of an increased risk of lung cancer from use of smokeless tobacco products is weak; the apparent protective effect detected in studies including smokers might be due to uncontrolled negative confounding.

Diet

Vegetables and fruits

A diet rich in vegetables and fruits probably exerts a protective effect against lung cancer (IARC, 2003). Although most case-control studies reported a protective effect

of high vegetable and fruit intake (WCRF, 1997), most prospective studies with detailed information on dietary intake did not provide consistent evidence of a protective effect. Possible reasons for the inconsistent results include bias from retrospective dietary assessment, misclassification of exposure in cohort studies, and variability in food composition. Although a weak protection from high intake of vegetables, and in particular cruciferous vegetables, is compatible with the data, it is unlikely that these foods represent a strong protective factor against lung cancer.

Meat and other foods

It has been suggested that high intake of meat, in particular fried or well-done red meat, increases the risk of lung cancer (Sinha et al, 1998). If real, the association might be explained by formation of nitrosamines during cooking of the meat (Sinha et al, 2000), as well as by saturated fat content of meat (see below). Although some studies reported risk estimates for intake of other foods, such as cereals, pulses, eggs, milk, and dairy products, these results are inadequate for a judgment of the evidence of an effect (WCRF, 1997).

Coffee and tea

In a few studies, high consumption of coffee has been associated with an increased risk of lung cancer. Residual confounding by tobacco smoking, however, remains a distinct possibility, and no conclusion can be drawn at present (WCRF, 1997). There is some evidence of a chemopreventive effect of tea, notably green tea, in smokers (Clark and You, 2006). The overall evidence, however, is not consistent.

Lipids

Several ecologic studies show a positive association between total lipid intake and lung cancer risk that appears to be independent of that of tobacco consumption (WCRF, 1997). The analytic studies that have addressed this association, however, have produced mixed results. Although no study provided evidence of a protective effect of total lipid intake, an increased risk was shown only in case-controls studies, while a pooled analysis of eight cohort studies provided no evidence of an increased risk of lung cancer for high intake of either total fat or saturated fat (Smith-Warner et al, 2002).

Carotenoids

Many studies have addressed the risk of lung cancer according to estimated intake of either β-carotene or total carotenoids (which in most cases correspond to the sum of α- and β-carotene) (reviewed by Albanes, 1999; IARC, 1998a). Five cohort and 18 case-control studies published up to 1994 (WCRF, 1997) provided 28 risk estimates in different populations; with some notable exceptions (Kalandidi et al, 1990), 25 of them indicated a protective effect of high β-carotene intake. The protective effect provided a 30% to 80% reduction in the risk of lung cancer between the highest and lowest intake categories (WCRF, 1997). The risk decreased for all major histologic types of lung cancer in many countries, in both genders, and in both smokers and non-smokers. Similar results have been obtained in studies based on measurement of β-carotene in prospectively collected sera (Holick et al, 2002).

The evidence of a protective effect from most observational studies has been refuted by the results of randomized intervention trials based on β-carotene supplementation

(Table 14–4). In two of them, which included smokers or workers exposed to asbestos, a significant increase in the incidence of lung cancer was observed in the treated groups; in the remaining studies, no effect was ascertained. An evaluation by the International Agency for Research on Cancer (IARC) concluded that available evidence suggests lack of preventive activity of β-carotene used as a supplement in high doses and inadequate evidence with regard to its activity at usual dietary levels (IARC, 1998a).

A difference in results between observational studies and preventive trials would arise if fruits and vegetables are protective due to constituents other than β-carotene (confounding). Alternatively, at very high nonphysiological doses, β-carotene might cause oxidative damage, in particular among smokers (Greenwald, 2003).

Other vitamins

For none of the antioxidant vitamins is there conclusive evidence of a protective effect against lung cancer. In the case of vitamin A, lutein, lycopene, and α-carotene, in particular, the data are inconclusive (Ruano-Ravina et al, 2006). The results of studies of serum level of these micronutreints are insufficient for an evaluation: Given the high correlation with β-carotene, however, it is not surprising that results of many epidemiologic studies indicate a protective effect (WCRF, 1997; IARC, 1998a).

Table 14–4. Preventive trials on supplementation of β-carotene and lung cancer risk.

Reference	Setting, population, age	Follow-up	Daily dose	RR	95% CI
Kamangar et al. 2006	Linxian, China; 29,584, 40–69	1986–2001	15 mg*	0.98	0.71–1.35
ATBCCP Study Group 1994	Finland; 29,133 male smokers, 50–69	1985–93**	20 mg	1.18	1.03–1.36
Hennekens et al. 1996	USA; 22,071 male physicians, 40–84	1982–95	25 mg***	0.93	NA
Omenn et al. 1994	USA; 18,314 smokers or asbestos workers, 45–74	1985–95	30 mg	1.28	1.04–1.57

* combined with selenium (50 μg) and α-tocopherol (30 mg)

** follow-up for cancer incidence

*** 50 mg on alternate days

RR: relative risk; CI: confidence interval; NA: not available

Selenium

A meta-analysis of 16 observational studies has indicated a reduced risk of lung cancer for high intake of selenium (RR 0.74, 95% CI 0.57–0.97) (Zhuo et al, 2004). The effect was stronger in studies conducted in areas with low selenium intake (RR 0.72, 95% CI 0.45–1.16) than in other areas (RR 0.86, 95% CI 0.61–1.22). The results of one intervention study are consistent with a protective effect (RR 0.70, 95% CI 0.40–1.21) (Duffield-Lillico et al, 2002).

Isothiocyanates

Isothiocyanates are a group of chemicals with cancer-preventive activity in experimental systems, and may be responsible for the possibly reduced risk of lung cancer in relation to high intake of cruciferous vegetables. The enzymes, glutathione-S-transferases M1 and T1 are involved in their metabolism: As indicated, these enzymes are polymorphic, with 5% to 10% of Europeans and 30% to 40% of Asians being carriers of a deletion in both. In four studies it has been shown that the protective effect of high intake of isothiocyanates is stronger in carriers of both deletions than in other subjects (Fig. 14–7). No final conclusions

can be drawn at present, but this is an example of possible gene–environment interaction in lung carcinogenesis.

Alcohol

Given the strong correlation between alcohol drinking and tobacco smoking in many populations, it is difficult to disentangle the contribution of alcohol to lung carcinogenesis while properly controlling for the potential confounding effect of tobacco. Meta-analyses have indicated that the increased risk of lung cancer observed among alcoholics is mainly attributable to such residual confounding, but a smoking-adjusted association was suggested for high alcohol consumption (Bandera et al, 2001; Korte et al, 2002). This conclusion was confirmed by a pooled analysis of seven cohort studies (Freudenheim et al, 2005).

Overall, it might be premature to conclude that an association between alcohol drinking and lung cancer has been refuted by the available data. If the association is causal, alcohol might act as a solvent for carcinogens such as those in tobacco smoke. In addition, it can induce metabolic enzymes or act through direct DNA damage via the active metabolite acetaldehyde (Fang and Vaca, 1997).

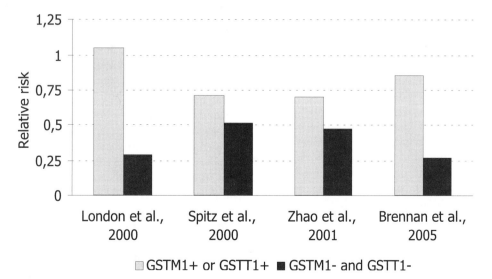

Figure 14–7. Relative risk of lung cancer for high intake of isothiocyanates, by GST polymorphism.

Reproductive Factors

Only few studies have reported estimates of lung cancer risk according to reproductive factors such as parity, age at first pregnancy, or history of abortion, and no conclusions can be drawn at present.

Hormones

Estrogen and progesterone receptors are expressed in the normal lung and in lung cancer cell lines, and estradiol has a proliferative effect on the latter type of cells. Although an effect of estrogens on lung carcinogenesis has not been demonstrated, they might act via formation of DNA adducts and activation of growth factors (Thomas et al, 2005). Data on risk of lung cancer following use of hormone replacement therapy have been reported from five case-control studies, two cohort studies, and one randomized trial (Wu et al, 1988; Adami et al, 1989; Taioli and Wynder, 1994; Blackman et al, 2002; WGWHII, 2002; Kreuzer et al, 2003; Olsson et al, 2003; Schabath et al, 2004). A small increased risk of lung cancer has been reported in the early studies, while a decreased risk was detected in the more recent studies. No effect was observed in the only randomized trial (WGWHII, 2002). While the different results might be explained by changes in the formulations used for replacement therapy, the lack of an effect in the only study with an experimental design argues against an effect of this type of exposure on lung cancer.

Three cohorts and one case-control study were included in a meta-analysis of serum IGF-I level and lung cancer. The overall RR was 1.01 (95% CI 0.49–2.11) (Renehan et al, 2004). The results on IGFBP-3 level were also negative (summary RR 0.83, 95% CI 0.38–1.84), although exclusion of a deviant study resulted in a decreased risk of lung cancer for high level of IGFBP-3 (RR 0.53, 95% CI 0.34–0.83).

Anthropometric Measures

There is some evidence that a reduced body mass index (BMI) is associated with an increased risk of lung cancer. However, this inverse association can be explained, at least in part, by negative confounding by smoking (Henley et al, 2002), and no clear association has been demonstrated among never-smokers. The relevant studies have been reviewed by an IARC Working Group, which concluded that there is inadequate evidence for an association between BMI and lung cancer risk (IARC, 2001). Subsequent studies supported this conclusion (eg, Calle et al, 2003).

There is evidence suggesting a direct association between height and lung cancer risk (reviewed in Gunnell et al, 2001). Subsequent studies supported this finding (Gunnell et al, 2003; Batty et al, 2006), although the evidence is not fully consistent (Rodriguez et al, 2001; Song et al, 2003).

Infections

Patients with pulmonary tuberculosis have been found to be at increased risk of lung cancer (Aoki, 1993). A similar association was reported from community-based studies among smoking and nonsmoking women (Gao et al, 1987; Wu et al, 1988; Alavanja et al, 1992; Ko et al, 1997). In the most informative study, involving a large cohort of tuberculosis patients from Shanghai, China (Zheng et al, 1987), the relative risk of lung cancer in the whole cohort was 1.5, and it was 2.0 20 years after the diagnosis of tuberculosis; a correlation was also seen with the location of the tuberculosis lesions. Whether the excess risk is caused by the chronic inflammatory status of the lung parenchyma or by the specific action of the Mycobacterium is not clear. A role of isoniazid, a widely used tuberculosis drug that causes lung tumors in experimental animals, was excluded in one large study (Boice and Fraumeni, 1980).

Chlamydia pneumoniae is a cause of acute respiratory infection. Six studies have been published on risk of lung cancer among individuals with markers of *C. pneumoniae* infection: They consistently detected a positive association (Littman et al, 2005). However, studies based on prediagnostic samples had lower risk estimates than studies based on postdiagnostic samples.

An association between infection with human papilloma virus and lung cancer, in particular the adenocarcinoma type, has been suggested by the results of analysis of series of cases (Chen et al, 2004) and the growing evidence of an increased risk among workers potentially exposed to this agent, such as butchers (Durusoy et al, 2006). The results are currently insufficient to conclude on the presence or absence of a causal association. Other biological agents that have been suggested to play a role in lung carcinogenesis include simian virus 40 (Galateau-Salle et al, 1998) and the fungus *Microsporum canis* (Nakachi et al, 1999).

Physical Activity

Available evidence suggests that high physical activity might reduce lung cancer risk (WCRF, 1997), but confounding by other lifestyle activities of health-conscious people cannot be confidently excluded. The risk of lung cancer relative to occupational or leisure-time physical activity has been assessed in several studies that were reviewed by an IARC Working Group (IARC, 2001). The conclusion was that there is inadequate evidence for a protective effect of physical activity on lung cancer. The results of recent studies do not alter this conclusion (Steindorf et al, 2006).

Ionizing Radiation

There is conclusive evidence that high exposure to ionizing radiation increases the risk of lung cancer (IARC, 2000). Atomic bomb survivors and patients treated with radiotherapy for ankylosing spondylitis or breast cancer are at moderately increased risk of lung cancer (RR 1.5–2 for cumulative exposure in excess of 100 rads) (for review see Boice et al, 1996). The association with high doses of ionizing radiation was stronger for small-cell carcinoma than for other histologic types of lung cancer. Studies of nuclear industry workers exposed to relatively low levels, however, provided no evidence of an increased risk of lung cancer (IARC, 2000).

Underground miners exposed to radioactive radon and its decay products, which emit α-particles, have been consistently found to be at increased risk of lung cancer (IARC, 2001). The risk increased with estimated cumulative exposure and decreased with attained age and time since cessation of exposure (Lubin et al, 1994). A pooled analysis of 11 cohorts estimated an apparently linear, approximately 6% risk increase per working-level year of exposure (Lubin et al, 1994). There was also evidence that, for comparable cumulative exposure, the risk is greater for lower rates over a longer period (Lubin et al, 1995a) and that smoking modifies the carcinogenic effect of radon (Lubin et al, 1994).

Today the main concern about lung cancer risk from radon and its decay products comes from residential rather than occupational exposure. A pooled analysis of 13 European case-control studies resulted in a RR of 1.084 (95% CI 1.030–1.158) per 100 Bq/m3 increase in measured indoor radon (Darby et al, 2005). After correction for the dilution caused by measurement error, the RR was 1.16 (95% CI 1.05–1.31). The exposure-response relationship was linear with no evidence of a threshold. A similar analysis of North American studies came to the same conclusion (Krewski et al, 2006). These results suggest that indoor radon exposure might be an important cause of lung cancer, in particular among nonsmokers unexposed to occupational carcinogens.

Occupation

The important role of specific occupational exposures in lung cancer etiology is well established in reports dating back to the 1950s. The risk of lung cancer is increased among workers employed in a number of industries and occupations. The responsible agent(s) have been identified for several, but not all, of these high-risk workplaces. Evidence for the carcinogenicity of many occupational agents has been reviewed in the IARC Monographs Program since 1972, and several agents have been classified as lung carcinogens (Table 14–5) (Siemiatycki et al, 2006; IARC, 1972–2006).

Table 14–5. Occupational agents, groups of agents, mixtures and exposure circumstances classified by the IARC Monographs Programme, Volumes 1–94 (IARC, 1972–2006) into groups 1 or 2A, which have the lung as target organ

Agents, mixture, circumstance	Main industry, use	Evidence of carcinogenicity in humans	Other target organs
Group 1—Carcinogenic to humans			
Agents, groups of agents			
Arsenic and arsenic compounds	Glass, metals, pesticides	S	Skin
Asbestos	Insulation, filters, textiles	S	Pleura
Benzo[a]pyrene	Many	L	Skin, bladder
Beryllium and beryllium compounds	Aerospace	S	
Bis(chloromethyl)ether and chloromethyl methyl ether	Chemical intermediate	S	
Cadmium and cadmium compounds	Dye/pigment	S	
Chromium[VI] compounds	Metal plating, dye/pigment	S	Nose
Dioxin (TCDD)	Chemical industry	L	Several
Involuntary tobacco smoking	Hospitality	S	
Nickel compounds	Metallurgy, alloy, catalyst	S	Nose
χ- and γ-radiation	Medical	S	Many
Radon and its decay products	Mining	S	
Silica, crystalline	Stone cutting, mining, glass, paper	S	
Mixtures			
Coal-tar pitches	Construction, electrodes	S	Skin, bladder
Coal-tars	Fuel	S	Skin, bladder
Mineral oils, untreated & mildly treated	Metallurgy	S	Skin, bladder
Soots	Pigments	S	Skin
Exposure circumstances			
Aluminum production		S	Skin
Coal gasification		S	
Coke production		S	
Haematite mining (underground) with exposure to radon		S	
Iron and steel founding		S	
Painter (occupational exposure as a)		S	
Group 2A—Probably carcinogenic to humans			
Agents and groups of agents			
χ-Chlorinated toluenes and benzoyl chloride (combined exposure)	Chemical intermediate	l	
Diesel engine exhaust	Transport	L	
Non-arsenical insecticides (occupational exposures in spraying and application of)	Farming	L	
Exposure circumstances			
Art glass, glass containers and pressed ware (manufacture of)		L	

S: sufficient; L: limited

Metals

Exposure to inorganic arsenic, known as a lung carcinogen since the late 1960s, occurs mainly among workers employed in hot smelting; other groups at increased risk are fur handlers, manufacturers of sheep-dip compounds and pesticides, and vineyard workers (IARC, 1987; Hayes, 1997). Chromium [VI] compounds increase the risk of lung cancer among chromate-production workers, chromate-pigment manufacturers, chromium platers, and ferrochromium producers (IARC, 1990a; Hayes, 1997). No such risk has been detected among workers exposed only to chromium [III] compounds (IARC, 1990a).

Studies of nickel miners, smelters, electrolysis workers, and high-nickel alloy manufacturers showed an increased risk of lung cancer (IARC, 1990b; Hayes, 1997). There is debate on whether all nickel compounds are carcinogenic for humans; the available evidence does not allow a clear separation between different nickel salts to which workers are exposed. An increased risk of lung cancer has been demonstrated among workers in cadmium-based battery manufacture, copper-cadmium alloy workers, and cadmium smelters (IARC, 1993a; Hayes, 1997). The increased risk does not seem to be attributable to concomitant exposure to nickel or arsenic.

Studies of beryllium-exposed workers from the United States showed an excess risk of lung cancer (IARC, 1993b), although the causal nature of the association has been challenged (BISAC, 1997).

Asbestos

The first evidence of increased risk of lung cancer following inhalation of asbestos fibers dates from the 1950s (Hughes and Weil, 1994). All different forms of asbestos—chrysotile and amphiboles, including crocidolite, amosite, and tremolite—are carcinogenic to the human lung, although the potency of chrysotile might be lower than that of other types (WHO, 2006). Although asbestos has been banned in many countries, a substantial number of workers is still exposed, mainly in the construction industry. In many low- and medium-resource countries, occupational exposure is widespread. In many countries, asbestos is the agent responsible for a large number of occupationally related lung cancers.

Silica and other mineral dusts

An increased risk of lung cancer has been consistently reported in cohorts of silicotic patients (IARC, 1997a; Steenland and Stayner, 1997). Many authors investigated crystalline silica–exposed workers in foundries, pottery making, ceramics, diatomaceous earth mining, brick making, and stone cutting, some of whom might have developed silicosis. An increased risk of lung cancer was reported by some, but not all, studies, and in the positive studies the increase was small (IARC, 1997a; Steenland and Stayner, 1997), with evidence of an exposure–response relationship (Steenland et al, 2001).

Polycyclic aromatic hydrocarbons

Polycyclic aromatic hydrocarbons (PAHs) are a complex and important group of chemicals formed during combustion of organic material. They are widespread in the human environment; for most people, diet and tobacco smoke are the main sources of exposure of PAHs. A number of occupational settings entail exposure to high levels of PAHs. These chemicals, however, occur inevitably as complex mixtures of variable composition; an assessment of the risk from individual PAHs is therefore difficult. An increased risk of lung cancer has been demonstrated in several industries and occupations entailing exposure to PAHs such as aluminium production, coal gasification, coke production, iron and steel founding, tar distillation, roofing, and chimney sweeping (IARC, 2006a). An increase has also been suggested in a few other industries, including shale oil extraction, wood impregnation, road paving, carbon black production, and carbon electrode manufacture, with an exposure–response relationship in the studies with detailed exposure information.

Motor vehicle and other engine exhausts represent an important group of mixtures of PAHs, since they contribute significantly to air pollution. The available epidemiologic evidence suggests a 40% to 50% excess risk among those occupationally exposed to diesel engine exhaust (Boffetta et al, 1997).

Medical Conditions and Treatment

As discussed under "Infections," an increased risk of lung cancer has been described after tuberculosis. In addition, lung fibrosis from chronic exposure to high levels of fibers and dusts may result in a condition that increases the risk of lung cancer, such as silicosis and asbestosis (see "Occupation"). Chronic respiratory diseases have been associated with lung cancer risk. Patients with chronic bronchitis and emphysema are at moderately increased risk, which is greater for squamous cell carcinoma, after adjustment for tobacco smoking (Gao et al, 1987; Wu et al, 1995; Mayne et al, 1999). The roles of shared exposures, namely tobacco smoking and chronic inflammation,, have not been disentangled. A meta-analysis of studies of lung cancer and asthma resulted in a summary RR of 1.8 (95% CI 1.3–2.3) (Santillan et al, 2003); the results were similar when the analysis was restricted to studies that controlled for smoking. Since the evidence is mainly based on case-control studies, recall bias cannot be fully excluded.

The risk of lung cancer is increased in patients surviving other tobacco- and lifestyle-related cancers (Li and Hemminki, 2003). Commonality of risk factors, long-term effects of radiotherapy, and increased susceptibility probably interact in the causation of second primary cancers. The effect of chemotherapy and radiotherapy on the risk of a second primary lung cancer has been extensively investigated among long-term survivors of breast cancer, 2% to 9% of whom develop lung cancer (Daly and Costalas, 1999). The increased risk is restricted to patients receiving radiotherapy. Among them, a clear exposure–response relationship has been shown, together with an interactive effect of tobacco smoking.

Several studies have assessed lung cancer risk among regular users of aspirin and other nonsteroidal anti-inflammatory drugs. A meta-analysis of 11 studies included in a recent review (Harris et al, 2005) resulted in a pooled RR of 0.75 (95% CI 0.59–0.94). There was however heterogeneity among the different studies, likely due in part to differences in the definition of the exposure. The protective effect was stronger for case-control studies (RR 0.60, 95% CI 0.41–0.89) than cohort studies (RR 0.90, 95% CI 0.74–1.09), suggesting a role for recall bias. In particular, a large cohort study of one million US volunteers did not report a reduction in risk (Thun et al, 1991).

Other Risk Factors

Indoor air pollution

Indoor air pollution is thought to be responsible for the elevated risk of lung cancer experienced by nonsmoking women living in several regions of China and other Asian countries. The evidence is stronger for coal burning in poorly ventilated houses, but also burning of wood and other solid fuels, as well as fumes from high-temperature cooking using unrefined vegetable oils such as rapeseed oil (IARC, 2006b). A positive association between various indicators of indoor air pollution and lung cancer risk has also been reported in populations exposed to less extreme conditions than those encountered by some Chinese women, for example populations in Central and Eastern Europe (Lissowska et al, 2005).

Outdoor air pollution

There is abundant evidence that lung cancer rates are higher in cities than in rural settings (Katsouyanni and Pershagen, 1997). This pattern, however, might result from confounding by other factors, notably tobacco smoking, and occupational exposures, rather than from air pollution. Cohort and case-control studies are limited by difficulties in assessing past exposure to the relevant air pollutants. The exposure to air pollution has been assessed either on the basis of proxy indicators—for example, the number of inhabitants in the community of residence, residence near a major pollution source—or on the basis of actual data on pollutant levels. These data, however, reflect mainly present levels or levels in the recent past and refer to total suspended particulates, sulfur oxides, and nitrogen oxides, which are not likely to be the agents responsible for the carcinogenic effect, if any, of air pollution. Furthermore, the sources of data might cover quite a wide area, masking small-scale differences in exposure levels.

The combined evidence suggests that urban air pollution might entail a small excess risk of lung cancer on the order of 50%, but residual confounding cannot be excluded. In four cohort studies, assessment of exposure to fine particles was based on environmental measurements (Table 14–6). The results of these studies are suggestive of a small increase in risk among people classified as most highly exposed to air pollution.

For asbestos, a distinct air pollutant, there is debate on whether environmental, as opposed to occupational, exposure, mainly from indoor air in contaminated buildings, represents a lung cancer hazard (Bourdes et al, 2000). Studies on domestic

exposure are fairly consistent in showing a small increase in lung cancer risk that is not due to confounding by tobacco smoking. In contrast, studies on outdoor air contamination are in most cases negative.

Drinking water contamination
An increased risk of lung cancer has been consistently reported among people exposed to arsenic in drinking water. Investigations include ecologic studies from Argentina, Chile, and Taiwan, and case-control and cohort studies from Taiwan—in particular, in areas endemic for blackfoot disease, caused by chronic arsenic poisoning—Japan, USA, and Chile (IARC, 2004c). An exposure-response relationship was observed in most of these studies. In particular, in a cohort study from a contaminated area in Taiwan, the relative risk of lung cancer according to cumulative estimated exposure to arsenic from drinking water was 4.0 for 20 or more milligrams per liter of average drinking water contamination compared to uncontaminated water (Chiou et al, 1995).

Table 14–6. Results of selected cohort studies on fine particle exposure and risk of lung cancer.

Study; population; reference	No and Sex	RR	95% CI	Exposure contrast*	Basis for exposure assessment	Range, mean
Seventh-day Adventists; USA, 1977–1992 (McDonnell et al., 2000)	6 338, M	2.23	0.56–8.94	per 24.3 $\mu g/m^3$ $PM_{2.5}$	Residential history 1966–1992 and local monthly pollutant estimates based on airport visibility data 1966–1992	Mean (SD) $PM_{2.5}$: 59.2 (16.8) $\mu g/m^3$
ASC/CPS-II; USA, 1982–1998 (Pope et al., 2002)	500 000, M+F	1.08	1.01–1.16	per 10 $\mu g/m^3$ $PM_{2.5}$	City of residence in 1982. Pollutant averages of 1979–1983	Mean (SD) $PM_{2.5}$: 21.1 (4.6); range roughly 5–30 $\mu g/m^3$
Six Cities; USA, 1975–1998 (Laden et al., 2006)	8 111, M+F	1.27	0.96–1.69	per 10 $\mu g/m^3$ $PM_{2.5}$	City of residence in 1975. Pollutant average 1979–1985	Range $PM_{2.5}$: 34.1–89.9 $\mu g/m^3$
GENAIR; Europe; 1990–1999 (Vineis et al., 2006)	NA M+F	0.91	0.70–1.18	per 10 $\mu g/m^3$ PM_{10}	Place of residence. Traffic-related air pollution 1990–1999	Range PM_{10}: 19.9–73.4 $\mu g/m^3$

NA, not available

CANCER OF THE LARYNX

More than 90% of cancers of the larynx are squamous cell carcinomas, and the majority originate from the supraglottic and glottic regions of the organ. The incidence in women is below 1/100 000 in most populations (Figs. 14–8 and 14–9). The incidence in men is high (10/100 000 or more) in southern and central Europe, Brazil, Uruguay, and Argentina, as well as among African Americans in the United States (Figs. 14–10 and14–11), while the lowest rates (1/100 000) are recorded in Southeast Asia and central Africa (Parkin et al, 1997). Rates have not changed markedly during the last 2 decades. An estimated 160 000 new cases occurred worldwide in 2002, of which 140 000 were among men (Ferlay et al, 2004). The estimated number of deaths in the same year is 80 000.

Most cases of laryngeal cancer in western countries are attributable to tobacco smoking, alcohol drinking, and the interaction between these two factors (Olshan,

2006). The effect of tobacco, with risks in smokers on the order of 10 relative to non-smokers, seems to be stronger for glottic than for supraglottic neoplasms (IARC, 2004a; De Stefani et al, 2004). Studies in several populations have shown an exposure–response relationship and a beneficial effect of quitting smoking. Smoking black tobacco cigarettes entails a stronger risk than smoking blond tobacco cigarettes. Studies from India have also reported an effect of chewing tobacco-containing products. The effect of alcohol is stronger for supraglottic tumors than for tumors in other sites. It is not clear, however, whether different alcoholic beverages exert a different carcinogenic effect (Boffetta and Hashibe, 2006).

A protective effect is possibly exerted by high intake of fruits and vegetables, although the evidence regarding specific micronutrients such as carotenoids and vitamin C is inadequate for drawing a conclusion (IARC, 2003; Olshan, 2006). Hot maté drinking has been suggested to be a risk factor in studies from Brazil and Ur-

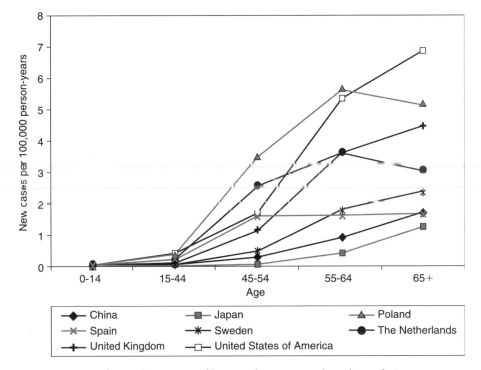

Figure 14–8. Age-specific incidence rates of laryngeal cancer in selected populations—women.

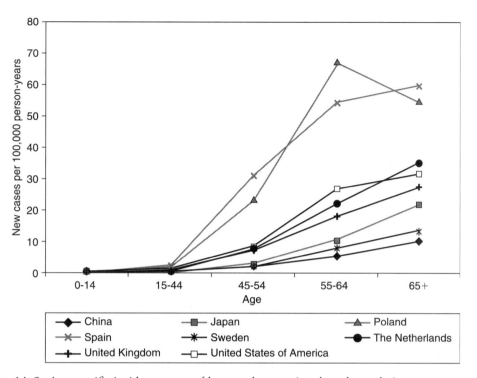

Figure 14–9. Age-specific incidence rates of laryngeal cancer in selected populations—men.

uguay (Goldenberg et al, 2003). Data concerning a possible effect of other food items are not consistent.

Occupational exposure to mists of strong inorganic acids, sulfuric acid in particular, is an established risk factor for laryngeal cancer (IARC, 1992). A possible effect has been suggested for other occupational ex-

posures, including nickel, asbestos, and ionizing radiation, but the evidence is not conclusive (Siemiatycki et al, 2006).

Laryngeal papillomatosis, a condition characterized by multiple benign tumors called papillomas, is caused by infection with human papillomavirus (HPV) types 6 and 11, the same types that cause genital

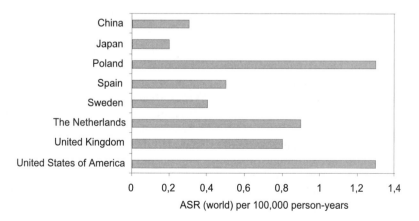

Figure 14–10. Age-standardized incidence rates of laryngeal cancer in selected populations—women.

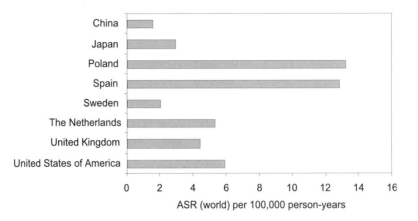

Figure 14–11. Age-standardized incidence rates of laryngeal cancer in selected populations—men.

condylomata acuminata. Infection in children occurs in both genders during delivery; in adults, infection is common among men and may occur via orogenital sexual contact. Papillomatosis patients have an increased risk of laryngeal cancer; however, studies aimed at assessing the presence of HPV DNA have not provided conclusive evidence for a higher prevalence of infection in cases of laryngeal cancer than in controls (Lindeberg and Krogdahl, 1999).

There is no evidence of strong genetic factors in laryngeal carcinogenesis; however, polymorphisms of enzymes implicated in the metabolism of alcohol and tobacco, such as alcohol and aldehyde dehydrogenases, may act as susceptibility factors (Olshan, 2006).

CANCER OF THE PLEURA

The most important malignant neoplasm arising from the pleura is the mesothelioma. Occurrence of mesothelioma has been linked conclusively to asbestos exposure, in particular amphiboles such as crocidolite and amosite. Past occupational exposure to asbestos is the main determinant of the descriptive epidemiology of pleural mesothelioma. High-exposure industries include mining, shipyard working, and asbestos cement manufacture (Boffetta and Stayner, 2006).

Despite a reduction or ban of asbestos use in many countries, the incidence of mesothelioma is increasing, which reflects the long latency of the disease (Peto et al, 1995). In the absence of occupational exposure to asbestos, incidence rates on the order of 0.1–0.2/100 000 are estimated in both genders. In heavily exposed workers, relative risks on the order of 1000 have been reported. There is evidence of an increased risk of pleural mesothelioma following environmental exposure to asbestos: Rates in polluted areas have been reported to be two- to tenfold higher than those in nonpolluted areas (Bourdes et al, 2000). Epidemics of mesothelioma have been reported from areas with environmental contamination by other natural mineral fibers, such as some districts of central Turkey, where erionite, a fibrous substance similar to amphibole asbestos, contaminated the materials used for building construction (Artvinli and Baris, 1979).

In several populations, DNA of simian virus 40 has been reported in a high proportion of mesothelioma cases; however, a causal role of this virus, which contaminated polio vaccines used in the 1950s in many countries, has not been confirmed (Shah et al, 2004). Exposure to ionizing radiation entails an increased risk of pleural mesothelioma, as it has been shown in cohorts of patients treated with thorotrast, a radiological contrast medium (Boffetta and

Stayner, 2006). Tobacco smoking, alcohol drinking, and diet do not appear to be risk factors for pleural mesothelioma.

CONCLUSION

Given the poor prognosis of lung cancer and the lack of effective screening procedures, primary prevention remains the main weapon against this neoplasm, and control of tobacco smoking is by far the most important preventive measure. In some populations, reduced tobacco consumption decreased the incidence of the disease. Much, however, remains to be done, in particular among women and the young, as well as in low-income countries. Control of exposure to other lung carcinogens, in both the general and the occupational environment, is another measure that has been taken and, at least in some instances, has had substantial effects. Priorities for the prevention of lung cancer, in addition to tobacco control, include understanding the carcinogenic and preventive effects of dietary and other lifestyle factors, avoidance of high exposure to known carcinogens, such as indoor pollution in some regions of China, and elucidation of conditions entailing increased genetic predisposition.

Lung cancer among nonsmokers is not rare. Occupational factors, passive smoking, and indoor exposure to radon do not explain more than a minor proportion of these cases, and dietary, infectious, and genetic factors are currently receiving attention.

Lung cancer was the most important epidemic of the twentieth century, and it will likely remain a major public health problem in the twenty-first century also. It is ironic that this cancer causes more deaths than any other malignancy in the world, even though epidemiology has led to the identification of more than 10 causes of the disease, including the quantitatively dominant tobacco smoking. Lung cancer is also a paradigm of the superiority of prevention over treatment and a sad reminder that scientific knowledge is not sufficient to ensure human health.

Cancer of the larynx is mostly caused by tobacco, alcohol, and their interaction, but dietary factors are also likely to be important. Pleural mesothelioma is almost specifically linked to occupational exposure to asbestos.

REFERENCES

Adami HO, Persson I, Hoover R, Schairer C, Bergkvist L. Risk of cancer in women receiving hormone replacement therapy. Int J Cancer 1989;44:833–39.

Albanes, D. Beta-carotene and lung cancer: a case study. Am J Clin Nutr 1999;69:1345s–1350s.

Alavanja MCR, Brownson RC, Boice JD Jr, Hock E. Preexisting lung disease and lung cancer among nonsmoking women. Am J Epidemiol 1992;136:623–32.

Aoki K. Excess incidence of lung cancer among pulmonary tuberculosis patients. Jpn J Clin Oncol 1993;23:205–20.

Artvinli M, Baris YI. Malignant mesotheliomas in a small village in the Anatolian region of Turkey: an epidemiologic study. J Natl Cancer Inst 1979;63:17–22.

ATBCCP Study Group (Alpha-Tocopherol, Beta-Carotene Cancer Prevention Study Group). The effect of vitamin E and beta-carotene on the incidence of lung cancer and other cancers in male smokers. N Engl J Med 1994;330:1029–35.

Bailey-Wilson JE, Amos CI*, Pinney SM, Petersen GM, de Andrade M, Wiest JS, et al. A major lung cancer susceptibility locus maps to chromosome 6q23–25. Am J Hum Genet 2004;75:460–74.

Bandera EV, Freudenheim J, Vena JE. Alcohol consumption and lung cancer. Cancer Epidemiol Biomarkers Prev 2001;10:813–21.

Batty GD, Shipley MJ, Langenberg C, Marmot MG, and Davey Smith G. Adult height in relation to mortality from 14 cancer sites in men in London (UK): evidence from the original Whitehall study. Ann Oncol 2006; 17:157–66.

Bermejo JL, Hemminki K. Familial lung cancer and aggregation of smoking habits: a simulation of the effect of shared environmental factors on the familial risk of cancer. Cancer Epidemiol Biomarkers Prev 2005;14:1738–40.

BISAC (Beryllium Industry Scientific Advisory Committee). Is beryllium carcinogenic in humans? J Occup Environ Med 1997; 39:205–8.

Blackman JA, Coogan PF, Rosenberg L, Strom BL, Zauber AG, Palmer JR. Estrogen replacement therapy and risk of lung cancer. Pharmacoepidemiol Drug Saf 2002;11:561–67.

Boffetta P, Aagnes B, Weiderpass E, Andersen A. Smokeless tobacco use and risk of cancer of the pancreas and other organs. Int J Cancer 2005;114: 992–95.

Boffetta P, Hashibe M. Alcohol and cancer. Lancet Oncol 2006;7:149–56.

Boffetta P, Jourenkova N, Gustavsson P. Cancer risk from occupational and environmental exposure to polynuclear aromatic hydrocarbons. Cancer Causes Control 1997;8:444–72.

Boffetta P, Saracci R. Occupational factors of lung cancer. In: Hirsch A, Goldberg M, Martin JP, Masse R (Eds): Prevention of Respiratory Diseases. New York, Marcel Dekker, 1993, pp 37–63.

Boffetta P, Stayner LT. Pleural and Peritoneal Neoplasms. In: Schottenfeld D, Fraumeni JF Jr (Eds): Cancer Epidemiology and Prevention, 3rd ed. New York, Oxford University Press, 2006, pp 659–73.

Boffetta P, Tredaniel J, Grecco A. Risk of childhood cancer and adult lung cancer after childhood exposure to passive smoke: A meta-analysis. Environ Health Perspect 2000;108:73–82.

Boice JD Jr, Fraumeni JF Jr. Late effects following isoniazid therapy. Am J Public Health 1980;70:987–89.

Boice JD Jr, Land CE, Preston DL. Ionizing radiation. In: Schottenfeld D, Fraumeni JF Jr (Eds): Cancer Epidemiology and Prevention, 2nd ed. New York, Oxford University Press, 1996, pp 319–54.

Bourdes V, Boffetta P, Pisani P. Environmental exposure to asbestos and risk of pleural mesothelioma: review and meta-analysis. Eur J Epidemiol 2000;16:411–17.

Brambilla E, Moro D, Gazzeri S, Brambilla C. Alterations of expression of Rb, p16(INK4A) and cyclin D1 in non-small cell lung carcinoma and their clinical significance. J Pathol 1999;188:351–60.

Brennan P, Hsu CC, Moullan N, Szeszenia-Dabrowska N, Lissowska J, Zaridze D, et al. Effect of cruciferous vegetables on lung cancer in patients stratified by genetic status: a mendelian randomisation approach. The Lancet 2005;366:1558–60.

Calle EE, Rodriguez C, Walker-Thurmond K, Thun MJ. Overweight, obesity, and mortality from cancer in a prospectively studied cohort of U.S. adults. New Engl J Med 2003;348;1625–38.

Chen YC, Chen JH, Richard K, Chen PY, Christiani DC. Lung adenocarcinoma and Human Papillomavirus infection. Cancer 2004;101:1428–36.

Cheng L, Spitz MR, Hong WK, Wei Q. Reduced expression levels of nucleotide excision repair genes in lung cancer: A case-control analysis. Carcinogen 2000;21:1527–30.

Chiou HY, Hsueh YM, Liaw KF, Horng SF, Chiang MH, Pu YS, et al. Incidence of internal cancers and ingested inorganic arsenic: a seven-year follow-up study in Taiwan. Cancer Res 1995;55:1296–1300.

Clark J, You M. Chemoprevention of lung cancer by tea. Mol Nutr Food Res 2006;50;144–51.

Daly MB, Costalas J. Breast cancer. In: Neugut AI, Meadows AT, Robinson E (Eds): Multiple Primary Cancers. Philadephia, Lippincott Williams & Wilkins, 1999, pp 303–17.

Darby S, Hill D, Auvinen A, Barros-Dios JM, Baysson H, Bochicchio F, et al. Radon in homes and risk of lung cancer: collaborative analysis of individual data from 13 European case-control studies. BMJ 2005;330:223.

De Stefani E, Boffetta P, Deneo-Pellegrini H, Brennan P, Correa P, Oreggia F, et al. Supraglottic and glottic carcinomas: epidemiologically distinct entities? Int J Cancer 2004; 112(6):1065–71.

Devesa SS, Grauman DJ, Blot WJ, Fraumeni JF Jr. Cancer surveillance series: changing geographic patterns of lung cancer mortality in the United States, 1950 through 1994. J Natl Cancer Inst 1999;91:1040–50.

Doll R, Peto R. Cigarette smoking and bronchial carcinoma: dose and time relationships among regular smokers and lifelong non-smokers. J Epidemiol Commun Health 1978;32: 303–13.

Doll R, Peto R, Boreham J, Sutherland I. Mortality in relation to smoking: 50 years' observations on male British doctors. BMJ 2004;328(7455):1519–28.

Duffield-Lillico AJ, Reid ME, Turnbull BW, Combs GF Jr, Slate EH, Fischbach LA, et al. Baseline characteristics and the effect of selenium supplementation on cancer incidence in a randomized clinical trial: A summary report of the Nutritional Prevention of Cancer Trial. Cancer Epidemiol Biom Prev 2002;11:630–39.

Durusoy R, Boffetta P, 't Mannetje A, Zaridze D, Szeszenia-Dabrowska N, Rudnai P, et al. Lung cancer risk and occupational exposure to meat and live animals. Int J Cancer 2006;118:2543–47.

Fang JL, Vaca CE. Detection of DNA adducts of acetaldehyde in peripheral white blood cells of alcohol abusers. Carcinogenesis 1997; 18:627–32.

Ferlay J, Bray F, Pisani P, et al. 2004. Globocan 2002: Cancer Incidence, Mortality and Prevalence Worldwide, Version 2.0. IARC Cancer Base No. 5. Lyon, IARC Press, 2004: WHO IARC.

Freudenheim JL, Ritz J, Smith-Warner SA, Albanes D, Bandera EV, van den Brandt PA, et al. Alcohol consumption and risk of lung cancer: a pooled analysis of cohort studies. Am J Clin Nutr 2005;82:657–67.

Gao YT, Blot WJ, Zheng W, Ershow AG, Hsu CW, Levin LI, et al. Lung cancer among Chinese women. Int J Cancer 1987;40:604–9.

Gajalakshmi V, Hung RJ, Mathew A, Varghese C, Brennan P, Boffetta P. Tobacco smoking and chewing, alcohol drinking and lung cancer risk among men in southern India. Int J Cancer 2003;107:441–47.

Galateau-Salle F, Bidet P, Iwatsubo Y, Gennetay E, Renier A, Letourneux M, et al. Detection of SV40-like DNA sequences in pleural mesothelioma, bronchopulmonary carcinoma and other pulmonary diseases. Dev Biol Stand 1998;94:147–52.

Gauderman WJ, Morrison JL, Carpenter CL, Thomas DC. Analysis of gene–smoking interaction in lung cancer. Genet Epidemiol 1997;14:199–214.

Gazdar A, Franklin WA, Brambilla E, Hainaut P, Yokota J, Harris CC. Genetic and molecular alterations. In Pathology & Genetics. Tumors of the Lung, Pleura, Thymus and Heart. William D. Travis, Elizabeth Brambilla, H. Konrad Müller-Hermelink and Curtis C. Harris (Eds). Lyon, IARC Press 2004, pp 21–23.

Goldenberg D, Golz A, Joachims HZ. The beverage mate: a risk factor for cancer of the head and neck. Head Neck 2003;25:595–601.

Greenwald P. B-carotene and lung cancer: A lesson for future chemoprevention investigations? J Natl Cancer Inst 2003;95.

Gunnell D, May M, Ben-Shlomo Y, Yarnell J, Davey Smith G. Height, leg length, and cancer: The Caerphilly Study. Nutr Cancer 2003;47:34–39.

Gunnell D, Okasha M, Smith GD, Oliver SE, Sandhu J, Holly JM. Height, leg length, and cancer risk: a systematic review. Epidemiol Rev 2001;23:313–42.

Hackshaw AK, Law MR, Wald NJ. The accumulated evidence on lung cancer and environmental tobacco smoke. Br Med J 1997; 315:980–88.

Harris RE, Beebe-Donk J, Doss H, Burr Doss D. Aspirin, ibuprofen, and other non-steroidal anti-inflammatory drugs in cancer prevention: A critical review of non-selective COX-2 blockade. Oncol Rep 2005;13:559–83.

Hayes RB. The carcinogenicity of metals in humans. Cancer Causes Control 1997;8:371–85.

Henley SJ, Flanders WD, Manatunga A, Thun MJ. Leanness and lung cancer risk: fact or artifact? Epidemiol 2002;13:268–76.

Henley SJ, Thun MJ, Connell C, Calle EE. Two large prospective studies of mortality among men who use snuff or chewing tobacco (United States). Cancer Causes Control 2005;16(4):347–58.

Hennekens CH, Buring JE, Manson JE, Stampfer M, Rosner B, Cook NR, et al. Lack of effect of long-term supplementation with beta carotene on the incidence of malignant neoplasms and cardiovascular disease. N Engl J Med 1996;334:1145–49.

Hirayama T. Non-smoking wives of heavy smokers have a higher risk of lung cancer: a study from Japan. Br Med J (Clin Res Ed) 1981;282:183–85.

Holick CN, Michaud DS, Stolzenberg-Solomon R, Mayne ST, Pietinen P, Taylor PR, et al. Dietary carotenoids, serum beta-carotene, and retinol and risk of lung cancer in the alpha-tocopherol, beta-carotene cohort study. Am J Epidemiol 2002;156:536–47.

Houlston RS. Glutathione S-transferase M1 status and lung cancer risk: a meta-analysis.Cancer Epidemiol Biomarkers Prev 1999;8:675–82.

Hughes JM, Weill H. Asbestos and man-made fibers. In: Samet JM (Ed): Epidemiology of Lung Cancer. Lung Biology in Health and Disease, Vol. 74. New York, Marcel Dekker, 1994, pp 185–205.

International Agency for Research on Cancer. Overall evaluations of carcinogenicity: an updating of IARC monographs Vols. 1 to 42. IARC Monographs on the Evaluation of the Carcinogenic Risk of Chemicals to Humans. Suppl 7. Lyon, IARC, 1987.

International Agency for Research on Cancer. Chromium and chromium compounds. In: Chromium, Nickel and Welding. IARC Monographs on the Evaluation of Carcinogenic Risks to Humans. Vol. 49. Lyon, IARC, 1990a, pp 49–256.

International Agency for Research on Cancer. Nickel and nickel compounds. In: Chromium, Nickel and Welding. IARC Monographs on the Evaluation of Carcinogenic Risks to Humans. Vol. 49. Lyon, IARC, 1990b, pp 257–445.

International Agency for Research on Cancer. Occupational exposures to mists and vapours from sulfuric acid and other strong inorganic acids. In: Occupational Exposures to Mists and Vapours from Strong Inorganic Acids and Other Industrial Chemicals. IARC Monographs on the Evaluation of Carcinogenic Risks to Humans. Vol. 54. Lyon, IARC, 1992, pp 41–119.

International Agency for Research on Cancer. Cadmium and cadmium compounds. In: Beryllium, Cadmium, Mercury and Exposures in the Glass Manufacturing Industry.

IARC Monographs on the Evaluation of Carcinogenic Risks to Humans. Vol. 58. Lyon, IARC, 1993a, pp 119–237.

International Agency for Research on Cancer. Beryllium and beryllium compounds. In: Beryllium, Cadmium, Mercury and Exposures in the Glass Manufacturing Industry. IARC Monographs on the Evaluation of Carcinogenic Risks to Humans. Vol. 58. Lyon, IARC, 1993b, pp 41–117.

International Agency for Research on Cancer. Silica. In: Silica, Some Silicates, Coal Dust and Para-Aramid Fibrils. IARC Monographs on the Evaluation of Carcinogenic Risks to Humans. Vol. 68. Lyon, IARC, 1997a, pp 41–242.

International Agency for Research on Cancer. Carotenoids. IARC Handbooks of Cancer Prevention. Vol. 2. Lyon, IARC, 1998a.

International Agency for Research on Cancer. Lung Cancer. In: Ionizing Radiation, Part 1: X- And Gamma (y)-Radiation, and Neutrons. IARC Monographs on the Evaluation of Carcinogenic Risks to Humans. Vol. 75. Lyon, IARC, 2000, pp 253–54.

International Agency for Research on Cancer. Weight Control and Physical Activity. IARC Handbooks of Cancer Prevention, Vol. 6. Lyon, IARC, 2001.

International Agency for Research on Cancer. Fruit and Vegetables. IARC Handbooks of Cancer Prevention, Vol. 8. Lyon, IARC, 2003.

International Agency for Research on Cancer. Tobacco smoke. In: Tobacco Smoke and Involuntary Smoking. IARC Monographs on the Evaluation of Carcinogenic Risks to Humans. Vol. 83. Lyon, IARC, 2004a, pp 51–1187.

International Agency for Research on Cancer. Tobacco smoke. In: Tobacco Smoke and Involuntary Smoking. IARC Monographs on the Evaluation of Carcinogenic Risks to Humans. Vol. 83. Lyon, IARC, 2004b, pp 1191–1413.

International Agency for Research on Cancer. Arsenic in drinking-water. In: Some Drinking-water Disinfectants and Contaminants, including Arsenic. IARC Monographs on the Evaluation of Carcinogenic Risks to Humans. Vol. 84. Lyon, IARC, 2004c, pp 39–267.

International Agency for Research on Cancer. Air Pollution, Part I. In: Some non-heterocyclic polycyclic aromatic hydrocarbons and some related exposures. IARC Monographs on the Evaluation of Carcinogenic Risks to Humans. Vol. 92. Lyon, IARC, 2006a, (in press).

International Agency for Research on Cancer. Household use of solid fuels and high-temperature frying. Vol. 95. Lyon, IARC, 2006b, (in press).

International Agency for Research on Cancer. IARC Monographs on the Evaluation of Carcinogenic Risks to Humans. Volumes 1–94. Lyon, IARC, 1972–2006.

Kalandidi A, Katsouyanni K, Voropoulou N, Bastas G, Saracci R, Trichopoulos D. Passive smoking and diet in the etiology of lung cancer among non-smokers. Cancer Causes Control 1990; 1:15–21.

Kamangar F, Qiao YL, Yu B, Sun XD, Abnet CC, Fan JH, et al. Lung cancer chemoprevention: a randomized, double-blind trial in Linxian, China. Cancer Epidemiol Biom Prev 2006;15:1562–64.

Katsouyanni K, Pershagen G. Ambient air pollution exposure and cancer. Cancer Causes Control 1997;8:284–91.

Ko YC, Lee CH, Chen MJ, Huang CC, Chang WY, Lin HJ, et al. Risk factors for primary lung cancer among non-smoking women in Taiwan. Int J Epidemiol 1997:26:24–31.

Korte JE, Brennan P, Henley SJ, Boffetta P. Dose-specific meta-analysis and sensitivity of the relation between alcohol consumption and lung cancer risk. Am J Epidemiol 2002;155:496–506.

Krewski D, Lubin JH, Zielinski JM, Alavanja M, Catalan VS, Field RW, et al. A combined analysis of North American case-control studies of residential radon and lung cancer. J Toxicol Environ Health A 2006;69:533–97.

Kreuzer M, Gerken M, Heinrich J, Kreienbrock L, Wichmann HE. Hormonal factors and risk of lung cancer among women? Int J Epidemiol 2003:32:263–71.

Laden F, Schwartz J, Speizer FE, Dockery DW. Reduction in fine particulate air pollution and mortality: Extended follow-up of the Harvard Six Cities study. Am J Respir Crit Care Med 2006;173(6):667–72.

Le Calvez F, Mukeria A, Hunt JD, Kelm O, Hung RJ, Taniere P, et al. TP53 and KRAS mutation load and types in lung cancers in relation to tobacco smoke: distinct patterns in never, former, and current smokers. Cancer Res 2005;65:5076–83.

Li D, Firosi PF, Wang LE, Bosken CH, Spitz MR, Hong WK, et al. Sensitivity to DNA damage induced by benzo(a)pyrene diol epoxide and risk of lung cancer: a case-control analysis. Cancer Res 2001;61:1445–50.

Li X, Hemminki K. Familial and second lung cancers: a nation-wide epidemiologic study from Sweden. Lung Cancer 2003;39(3):255–63.

Lindeberg H, Krogdahl A. Laryngeal cancer and human papillomavirus: HPV is absent in the majority of laryngeal carcinomas. Cancer Lett 1999;146:9–13.

Lissowska J, Bardin-Mikolajczak A, Fletcher T, Zaridze D, Szeszenia-Dabrowska N, Rudnai P, et al. Lung cancer and indoor pollution from heating and cooking with solid fuels: the IARC international multicentre case-control study in Eastern/Central Europe and the United Kingdom. Am J Epidemiol 2005;162:326–33.

Littman AJ, Jackson LA, and Vaughan TL. Chlamydia pneumoniae and lung cancer: Epidemiologic evidence. Cancer Epidemiol Biom Prev 2005;14:773–78.

London SJ, Yuan JM, Chung FL, Gao YT, Coetze GA, Ross RK, et al. Isothiocyanates, glutathione S-transferase M1 and T1 polymorphisms, and lung-cancer risk: a prospective study of men in Shanghai, China. Lancet 2000;356:724–29.

Lubin JH, Boice JD, Edling C, Hornung RW, Howe G, Kunz E. Radon and lung cancer risk: a joint analysis of 11 underground miners studies. In: Public Health Service and National Institute of Health (Eds). NIH Pub. No. 94–3644. Washington, DC U.S. Department of Health and Human Services, 1994.

Lubin JH, Boice JD, Edling C, Hornung RW, Howe G, Kunz E, et al. Radon-exposed underground miners and inverse dose-rate (protraction enhancement) effects. Health Phys 1995a;69:494–500.

Malkin D, Li FP, Strong LC, Fraumeni JF Jr, Nelson CE, Kim DH, et al. Germ line p53 mutations in a familial syndrome of breast cancer, sarcomas, and other neoplasms. Science 1990;250:1233–38.

Mayne ST, Buenconsejo J, Janerich DT. Previous lung cancer disease and risk of lung cancer among men and women nonsmokers. Am J Epidemiol 1999;149:13–20.

McDonnell WF, Nishino-Ishikawa N, Petersen FF, Chen LH, Abbey DE. Relationships of mortality with the fine and coarse fractions of long-term ambient PM10 concentrations in nonsmokers. J Expo Anal Environ Epidemiol 2000;10:427–36.

Nakachi K, Limtrakul P, Sonklin P, Sonklin O, Jarern CT, Lipigorngoson S, et al. Risk factors for lung cancer among Northern Thai women: epidemiological, nutritional, serological, and bacteriological surveys of residents in high- and low-incidence areas. Jpn J Cancer Res 1999;90:1187–95.

Olshan AF. Cancer of the Larynx. In: Schottenfeld D, Fraumeni JF Jr. (Eds): Cancer Epidemiology and Prevention (3rd ed). Oxford University Press, 2006, pp 627–37.

Olsson H, Bladström A, Ingvar C. Are smoking-associated cancers prevented or postponed in women using hormone replacement therapy? Obst Gynecol 2003;102:565–70.

Omenn GS, Goodman GE, Thornquist M, Brunzell JD. Long-term vitamin A does not produce clinically significant hypertriglyceridemia: results from CARET, the beta-carotene and retinol efficacy trial. Cancer Epidemiol Biomarkers Prev 1994;3:711–13.

Parkin DM, Whelan SL, Ferlay J, Raymond L, Young J (Eds): Cancer Incidence in Five Continents, Vol. VII. IARC Sci. Pub. No. 143. Lyon, International Agency for Research on Cancer, 1997.

Parkin DM, Whelan SL, Ferlay J, Teppo L, Thomas DB (Eds): Cancer Incidence in Five Continents, Vol. VIII. IARC Scientific Publ. No. 155. Lyon: IARC, 2002.

Peto J, Hodgson JT, Matthews FE, Jones JR. Continuing increase in mesothelioma mortality in Britain. Lancet 1995;345:535–39

Peto R, Lopez AD, Boreham J, Thun M, Heath C Jr. Mortality from tobacco in developed countries: indirect estimation from national vital statistics. Lancet 1992;339:1268–78.

Pfeifer GP, Denissenko MF, Olivier M, Tretyakova N, Hecht SS, Hainaut P. Tobacco smoke carcinogens, DNA damage and p53 mutations in smoking-associated cancers. Oncogene 2002;21:7435–51.

Pope CA III, Burnett RT, Thun MJ, Calle EE, Krewski D, Ito K, et al. Lung cancer, cardiopulmonary mortality, and long-term exposure to fine particulate air pollution. JAMA 2002;287:1132–41.

Renehan AG, Zwahlen M, Minder C, O'Dwyer ST, Shalet SM, Egger M. Insulin-like growth factor (IGf)-I, IGF binding protein-3, and cancer risk: systematic review and meta-regression analysis. Lancet 2004;363:1346–53.

Rodriguez C, Patel AV, Calle EE, et al. Body mass index, height, and prostate cancer mortality in two large cohorts of adult men in the United States. Cancer Epidemiol Biomarkers Prev 2001;10:345–53.

Ruano-Ravina A, Figueiras A, Freire-Garabal M, Barros-Dios JM. Antioxidant vitamins and risk of lung cancer. Curr Pharm Des 2006;12:599–613.

Santillan AA, Camargo CA Jr, Colditz GA. A meta-analysis of asthma and risk of lung cancer. Cancer Causes Control 2003;14:327–34.

Schabath MB, Wu X, Vassilopoulou-Sellin R, Vaporciyan AA, Spitz MR. Hormone replacement therapy and lung cancer risk: A case-control analysis. Clin Cancer Res 2004;10:113–23.

Sekido Y, Fong KM, Minna JD. Molecular biology of lung cancer. In: DeVita VT, Hellman S, Rosenberg SA (Eds): Cancer Principles and Practice of Oncology, 6th ed. Philadelphia: Lippincott and Williams and Wilkins, 2001, pp 917–25.

Sellers TA, Bailey-Wilson JE. Familial predisposition to lung cancer. In: Roth JA, Cox JD, Hong WK (Eds): Lung Cancer. Malden, MA: Blackwell, 1998, pp 57–71.

Shah KV, Galloway DA, Knowles WA, Viscidi RP. Simian virus 40 (SV40) and human cancer: a review of the serological data. Rev Med Virol 2004;14:231–39.

Siemiatycki J, Wacholder S, Dewar R, Cardis E, Greenwood C, Richardson L. Degree of confounding bias related to smoking, ethnic group, and socioeconomic status in estimates of the associations between occupation and cancer. J Occup Med 1988;30:617–25.

Siemiatycki J, Richardson L, Boffetta P. Occupation. In: Schottenfeld D, Fraumeni JF Jr. (Eds): Cancer Epidemiology and Prevention (3rd ed). Oxford University Press, 2006, pp 322–54.

Singh GK, Miller BA, Hankey BF. Changing area socioeconomic patterns in US cancer mortality, 1950–1998: Part II—lung and colorectal cancers. J Natl Cancer Inst 2002;94:916–25.

Sinha R, Kulldorff M, Curtin J, Brown CC, Alavanja MC, Swanson CA. Fried, well-done red meat and risk of lung cancer in women (United States). Cancer Causes Control 1998;9:621–30.

Sinha R, Kulldorff M, Swanson CA, Curtin J, Brownson RC, Alavanja MC. Dietary heterocyclic amines and the risk of lung cancer among Missouri women. Cancer Res 2000; 60:3753–56.

Smith-Warner SA, Ritz J, Hunter DJ, Albanes D, Beeson WL, van den Brandt PA, et al. Dietary fat and risk of lung cancer in a pooled analysis of prospective studies. Cancer Epidemiol Biomarkers Prev 2002;11:987–92.

Song YM, Davey Smith G, Sung J. Adult height and cause-specific mortality: a large prospective study of South Korean men. Am J Epidemiol 2003;158:479–85.

Spitz MR, Duphorne CM, Detry MA, Pillow PC, Amos CI, Lei L, et al. Dietary intake of isothiocyanates: evidence of a joint effect with glutathione S transferase polymorphisms in lung cancer risk. Cancer Epidemiol Biomarkers Prev 2000;9:1017–20.

Spitz MR, Wei Q, Dong Q, Amos CI, Wu X. Genetic susceptibility to lung cancer: the role of DNA damage and repair. Cancer Epidemiol Biomarkers Prev 2003;12:689–98.

Spitz MR, Wu X, Wilkinson A, Wei Q. Cancer of the Lung. In: Schottenfeld D, Fraumeni JF Jr. (Eds): Cancer Epidemiology and Prevention (3rd ed). Oxford University Press, 2006, pp 638–58.

Steenland K, t' Mannetje A, Boffetta P, Stayner L, Attfield M, Chen J, et al. Pooled exposure-response analyses and risk assessment for lung cancer in 10 cohorts of silica-exposed workers: an IARC multicentre study. Cancer Causes Control 2001;12:773–84.

Steenland K, Stayner L. Silica, asbestos, man-made mineral fibers, and cancer. Cancer Causes Control 1997;8:491–503.

Steindorf K, Friedenreich C, Linseisen J, Rohrmann S, Rundle A, Veglia F, et al. Physical activity and lung cancer risk in the European Prospective Investigation into Cancer and Nutrition cohort. Int J Cancer 2006;119: 2389–97.

Stucker I, Boffetta P, Antilla S, Benhamou S, Hirvonen A, London S, et al. Lack of interaction between asbestos exposure and glutathione S-transferase M1 and T1 genotypes in lung carcinogenesis. Cancer Epidemiol Biomarkers Prev 2001;10:1253–58.

Surgeon General's 2004 Report: The Health Consequences of Smoking. US Department of Health and Human Services, Rockville, MD

Taioli E, Wynder EL. Endocrine factors and adenocarcinoma of the lung in women. J Natl Cancer Inst 1994;86:869–70

Thomas L, Austin Doyle L, Edelman MJ. Lung cancer in women: Emerging differences in epidemiology, biology, and therapy. Chest 2005;128:370–81.

Thun MJ, Namboodiri MM, Heath CW Jr. Aspirin use and reduced risk of fatal colon cancer. N Engl J Med 1991;325:1593–96.

Travis WD, Lubin J, Ries L, Devesa S. United States lung carcinoma incidence trends: declining for most histologic types among males, increasing among females. Cancer 1996;77:2464–70.

Trichopoulos D, Kalandidi A, Sparros L, MacMahon B. Lung cancer and passive smoking. Int J Cancer 1981;27:1–4.

Tyczynski JE, Bray F, Parkin DM. Lung cancer in Europe in 2000: epidemiology, prevention, and early detection. The Lancet Oncology 2003;4:45–55.

Vineis P, Hoek G, Krzyzanowski M, Vigna-Taglianti F, Veglia F, Airoldi L, et al. Air pollution and risk of lung cancer in a prospective study in Europe. Int J Cancer 2006;119:169–74.

Wei Q, Cheng L, Hong WK, Spitz MR. Reduced DNA repair capacity in lung cancer patients. Cancer Res 1996:56:4103–7.

World Cancer Research Fund. Lung. In: Food, Nutrition and the Prevention of Cancer: A Global Perspective (Part II, Cancers, Nutrition and Food). Washington, DC, American Institute for Cancer Research, 1997, pp 130–47.

World Health Organization. WHO Workshop on Mechanisms of Fibre Carcinogenesis and

Assessment of Chrysotile Asbestos Substitutes 8–12 November 2005, Lyon, France. Summary Consensus Report. WHO, Geneva, 2006 (http://www.who.int/ipcs/publications/new_issues/summary_report.pdf)

Writing Group for the Women's Health Initiative Investigators. Risks and benefits of estrogen plus progestin in healthy postmenopausal women. Principal results from the Women's Health Initiative randomized controlled trial. JAMA 2002;288:321–33.

Wu AH, Fontham ETH, Reynolds P, Greenberg RS, Buffler P, Liff J, et al. Previous lung disease and risk of lung cancer among lifetime nonsmoking women in the United States. Am J Epidemiol 1995;141:1023–32.

Wu AH, Yu MC, Thomas DC, Pike MC, Henderson BE. Personal and family history of lung cancer and disease as risk factors for adenocarcinoma of the lung. Cancer Res 1988;48: 7279–84.

Zang EA, Wynder EL. Differences in lung cancer risk between men and women: examination of the evidence. J Natl Cancer Inst 1996;88: 183–92.

Zheng YL, Loffredo CA, Yu Z, Jones RT, Krasna MJ, Alberg AJ, et al. Bleomycin-induced chromosome breaks as a risk marker for lung cancer: a case-control study with population and hospital controls. Carcinogen 2003;24: 269–74.

Zheng W, Blot WJ, Liao ML, Wang ZX, Levin LI, Zhao JJ, et al. Lung cancer and prior tuberculosis infection in Shanghai. Br J Cancer 1987;56:501–4.

Zhao B, Seow A, Lee EJD, Poh WT, Teh M, Eng P, et al. Dietary Isothiocyanates, Glutathione S-transferase -M1, -T1 Polymorphisms and Lung Cancer Risk among Chinese Women in Singapore. Cancer Epidemiology Biomarkers & Prev 2001;10:1063–67.

Zhuo H, Smith AH, Steinmaus C. Selenium and lung cancer: A quantitative analysis of heterogeneity in the current epidemiologicall Literature. Cancer Epidemiol Biom Prev 2004; 13:771–78.

15

Skin Cancer

ADÈLE GREEN, JOLIEKE VAN DER POLS
AND DAVID HUNTER

Skin cancer presents unusual opportunities for, and challenges to, the use of epidemiologic methods. It is one of the few types of cancer for which the major carcinogenic exposure, sunlight, is strongly implicated on the basis of descriptive epidemiologic data alone. But there are three major forms of skin cancer—melanoma, basal cell carcinoma (BCC), and squamous cell carcinoma (SCC)—and each appears to have a different relation to pattern and total amount of sunlight exposure. Although conceptually we think we understand the exposure we would like to measure, past sunlight exposure is a complex variable, and questionnaire or interview-based methods have limited ability to precisely capture exposure patterns that may vary with age and region of residence. This leaves us uncertain about the relative importance of factors such as intermittent high-intensity exposure compared with lower-level chronic exposure in the etiology of these three major forms. The development of molecular methods of dosimetry may be helpful in dealing with this uncertainty, and skin tissues can be sampled

with relative ease to permit these measurements. Because we know the key carcinogen, and because exposure of skin to sunlight is modifiable, skin cancers are in theory substantially preventable.

CLINICAL SYNOPSIS

Subgroups

Three distinct forms of cancer are considered together in this chapter: BCC, SCC, and melanoma. For BCC and melanoma, subgroups can be readily identified, but the descriptive and analytic epidemiology has mostly considered each of them as a single entity.

Symptoms

A nonhealing skin lesion is the predominant symptom of BCC and SCC, while melanoma usually appears as a new and changing pigmented lesion on the skin. Occasionally, melanomas are first detected due to symptoms of metastases to lymph nodes or other organs.

Diagnosis

Often, visual inspection allows a preliminary diagnosis, which is confirmed histopathologically by biopsy or, in the case of melanoma, by excision. A dermatoscope—a magnifying device—may be used to improve diagnostic accuracy.

Treatment

Adequate surgical excision is the method of treatment of BCC, SCC, and primary melanoma. There is no established curative treatment for melanoma that has spread beyond the regional lymph nodes.

Prognosis

Although fatality from BCC and SCC is low, patients with BCC and SCC require follow-up to detect recurrence or spread. For melanoma, overall 5-year relative survival rates approach—or even exceed—80% in most western countries, with higher relative survival in women than in men. Prognosis is strongly dependent on the level of invasion and for melanoma, the thickness of the tumor.

Progress

There has been substantial improvement in the prognostic outlook among melanoma patients. Because this progress was not preceded by any therapeutic breakthrough—but rather by more limited surgical excisions—it is attributable largely to increased general awareness and treatment in early, curable stages. New approaches, including treatment with cell-based therapies, are under evaluation.

DESCRIPTIVE EPIDEMIOLOGY

A major problem in the descriptive epidemiology of keratinocyte cancers (ie, BCC and SCC) is that they are not registered by most cancer surveillance systems. Registration is not attempted for three main reasons: (1) there is a very high cure rate when medical attention is available, and thus these cancers are perceived as somewhat less important than cancers with higher fatality rates; (2) the sheer numbers of these cancers would place a major burden on most systems; and (3) since multiple lesions may be diagnosed simultaneously, and since many people have multiple lesions in their lifetimes, there are substantial methodologic difficulties in distinguishing these cancers. In the United States, over one million diagnosed cases of BCC and SCC were expected in 2007 (Jemal et al, 2007).

Keratinocyte skin cancer rates are much higher in white-skinned populations than in darker-skinned populations in Africa and Asia. Between 1985 and 1996, rates of BCC in the United States were almost 14 times higher in whites than in Hispanics, whereas rates of SCC were 11-fold higher in whites than in Hispanics (Harris et al, 2001). The highest rates in the world are recorded in Australia, in which survey data in 2002 suggested a cumulative risk to age 70 years of having at least one keratinocyte skin cancer of 70% for men and 58% for women, a BCC:SCC ratio of 2.3:1, and a threefold gradient in incidence between the northern latitudes closest to the equator compared with the southern latitudes (Staples et al, 2006). In this survey it was estimated that rates of keratinocyte skin cancer had increased between 1985 and 2002 in particular for persons aged 60 years and older, but rates in younger age groups had stabilized.

In the US, incidence rates of BCC in persons younger than 40 years were modestly higher for women than for men, but after 50 years of age men were around two times more likely to develop BCC than women. The incidence of SCC in men was approximately two times higher than for women in all age groups (Harris et al, 2001; Christenson et al, 2005). Rates were higher in the southern latitudes than in the northern ones, the gradient being more pronounced for SCC than BCC. In Germany, between 1998 and 2001, 80% of all skin cancers were BCC and 17% were SCC (Katalinic et al, 2003). In the Netherlands, between 1973 and 2000, age-adjusted incidence rates of BCC increased in both sexes, most markedly among young females (de Vries et al, 2004). The data on increasing risk

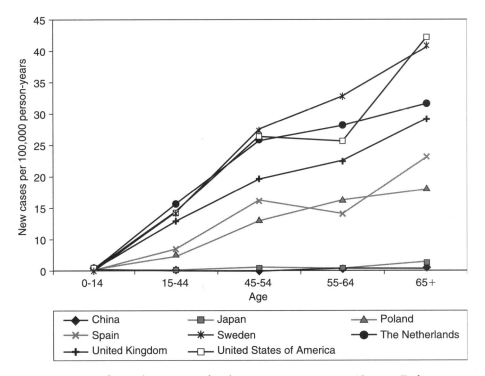

Figure 15–1. Age-specific incidence rates of melanoma among women. (*Source*: Ferlay et al, 2004)

associated with proximity to the equator, combined with the predominance of keratinocyte cancers on sun-exposed skin, strongly point to exposure to sunlight as the main causal factor in white populations.

Melanoma

Melanoma rates are also much higher in the predominantly white-skinned populations of Europe and the United States than in Africa or Asia (Figs. 15–1 and 15–2). Again the highest rates are recorded in the north of Australia, and increasing rates with proximity to the equator have been reported from northern Europe, the United States, and New Zealand (Whiteman and Green, 1999). Incidence rates increased between the 1950s and the 1990s as high as up to tenfold in Northern Europe, although mortality rates increased less rapidly and appeared to have reached a plateau, presumably because of improved early detection and treatment (de Vries et al, 2003). In the US in particular, incidence of lentigo maligna melanoma has

been increasing at a higher rate compared to other subtypes in persons aged 45 years or older (Swetter et al, 2005). In many populations, rates among women are comparable to, or even higher than, rates among men (Figs. 15–3 and 15–4).

Migrant studies suggest that exposure to latitudes close to the equator early in life is more strongly associated with melanoma risk than is exposure later in life, though adult exposure is also important (Whiteman et al, 2001).

GENETIC AND MOLECULAR EPIDEMIOLOGY

Inherited Susceptibility

Basal cell carcinoma

Much insight into the pathogenesis of BCC has been obtained from the study of patients with Gorlin's syndrome (nevoid basal cell carcinoma syndrome), an autosomal dominant disorder characterized by the development of multiple BCCs at an early

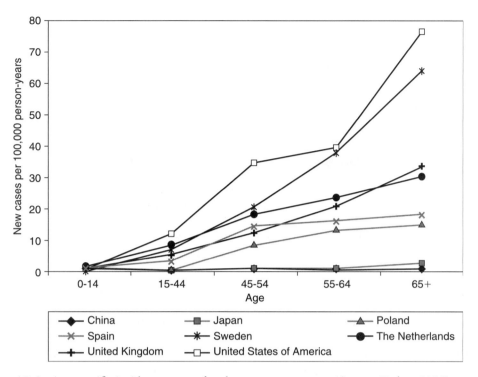

Figure 15–2. Age-specific incidence rates of melanoma among men. (*Source*: Ferlay, 2004)

age, as well as diverse internal tumors and other phenotypic abnormalities including pitting of the palms and soles, and dental and brain malformations (Gorlin, 2004). Gorlin's syndrome patients develop BCCs as early as two years of age, with a clear increase in tumor numbers between puberty and 35 years of age. The most common site of their initial appearance is the nape of the neck—they are rarely found below the waist. Ninety percent of white-skinned Gorlin's syndrome patients develop BCC, but only 40% of black patients do (Goldstein et al, 1994); thus sun exposure is likely

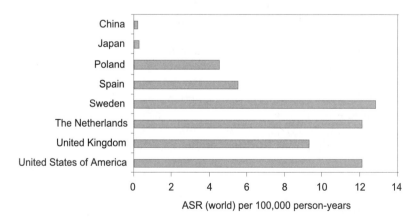

Figure 15–3. Age-standardized (to the world population) incidence rates of melanoma among women. (*Source*: Ferlay et al, 2004)

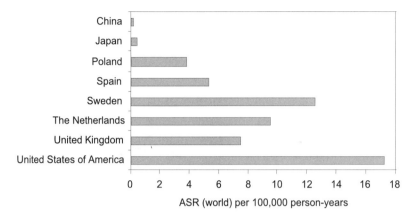

Figure 15–4. Age-standardized (to the world population) incidence rates of melanoma among men. (*Source*: Ferlay et al, 2004)

to play a role in addition to the genetic component in BCCs associated with this syndrome.

Gorlin's patients carry mutations in the *patched* gene, which acts as a tumor-suppressor gene. As predicted by the classic two-hit model, one defective copy of this gene is inherited but tumors arise after in-activation of the remaining allele (Tilli et al, 2005). The *patched* gene product is part of a receptor for the sonic hedgehog protein involved in embryonic development. When sonic hedgehog binds to patched it releases smoothened, a transmembrane signaling protein. Mutations of the *patched* and *smoothened* genes result in upregulation of the hedgehog signaling pathway and acti-vation of downstream target genes that are associated with cell growth and differenti-ation (Bale and Yu, 2001), including the Gli family of transcription factors (High and Zedan, 2005). Only around 0.5% of BCC cases arise in persons with Gorlin's syn-drome, but up to 95% of sporadic BCCs show somatic mutations or allelic loss in the *patched* gene (Teh et al, 2005) and 10% carry *smoothened* gene mutations (Reifen-berger et al, 2005).

DNA repair defects
Xeroderma pigmentosum is a rare autoso-mal recessive disorder that is part of an expanding family of nucleotide excision re-pair defect diseases (Cleaver, 2005). Mani-fested as an extreme photosensitivity to ul-traviolet radiation resulting from a defect in any one of the seven genes that regulate ex-cisional repair of ultraviolet (UV)-damaged DNA, Xeroderma pigmentosum occurs in approximately 1 in 250 000 people in the United States and Europe and 1 in 40 000 in Japan (Horenstein and Diwan, 2005). Al-though common in these patients, skin can-cer is not common in some other diseases with nucleotide excision repair defects such as Cockayne syndrome, despite the sun sen-sitivity in both disorders. Hence the in-creased mutation rates in both xeroderma pigmentosum and Cockayne syndrome pa-tients may be necessary but not sufficient for carcinogenesis. Additional chromosome instability as seen in xeroderma pigmento-sum may therefore be required for cancer development (Cleaver, 2005).

Skin tumors in xeroderma pigmentosum patients show high levels of *ras* oncogene activation, *Ink4a-Arf* and *p53* tumor-suppressor gene modifications, and aberra-tions of the sonic hedgehog pathway (Daya-Grosjean and Sarasin, 2005). UV-specific mutations of the *smoothened* gene are three times higher in xeroderma pigmentosum patients than in those with sporadic BCCs, confirming the high rate of UV-induced mutations in these DNA-repair deficient persons (Couve-Privat et al, 2002). Although mutations in the *sonic hedgehog* gene are relatively rare in sporadic BCCs, they are found in 15% of BCCs from xeroderma pigmentosum patients (Couve-Privat et al, 2004).

Detoxifying proteins

The enzyme family glutathione-S-transferase is part of the skin's defense mechanism against UV-induced oxidative stress. Polymorphisms in *GSTM1, GSTM3, GSTT1,* and *GSTP1* in particular appear to be associated with increased occurrence of BCC (Lear et al, 1996; Ramachandran et al, 2000).

Squamous cell carcinoma

In addition to xeroderma pigmentosum, the rare Ferguson-Smith syndrome may predispose to the development of lesions that are indistinguishable from SCCs, although they tend to resolve spontaneously. Recent gene mapping has excluded *patched* as a causative gene but has shown loss of heterozygosity in the 9q22-q31 region, suggesting that the gene for this syndrome is likely to be a tumor-suppressor gene (Bose et al, 2006).

Melanoma

Approximately 5% to 10% of melanomas occur among people with a strong family history of the disease. In the early 1990s, linkage analyses of melanoma kindreds identified a familial melanoma susceptibility locus on the short arm of chromosome 9 (Cannon-Albright et al, 1992; Nancarrow et al, 1993). The same region of chromosome 9 was also shown to suffer high frequencies of deletion, indicating the existence of a tumor-suppressor gene (Fountain et al, 1992). This led to the identification, from the 9p21 region, of the *CDKN2A* gene (Kamb et al, 1994), now known as the most common cause of inherited susceptibility to melanoma (Bishop et al, 2002).

CDKN2A encodes two proteins, p16INK4A (commonly referred to as p16) and p14ARF (Alternative Reading Frame) both of which are tumor suppressors involved in regulation of the cell cycle. Some

melanoma families have *p14ARF* gene defects only, and thus the ARF locus can also be considered a melanoma susceptibility gene in its own right (de Snoo and Hayward, 2005). Germline *CDKN2A* mutations have been identified in patients with familial melanoma in Australia, Europe, and North America; however, the penetrance varies markedly, being higher among families sampled from high-incidence populations. The analysis of 80 families across eight international populations showed that by age 80 years *CDKN2A* mutation penetrance reached 0.58 in Europe, 0.76 in the United States, and 0.91 in Australia (Bishop et al, 2002).

Additional candidate genes for familial melanoma have been sought among other regulators of the G1 checkpoint for cell-cycle regulation: Some seven melanoma families around the world have been identified with mutations in the *CDK4* gene, the protein product of which forms a complex with p16. It has also been speculated that the *BRAF* proto-oncogene may be mutated in the germline of some melanoma cases, though this remains to be confirmed (de Snoo and Hayward, 2005). There is no evidence that people with Li-Fraumeni syndrome, characterized by germline mutations in the *p53* gene, have an increased risk of melanoma; conversely, melanoma kindreds do not carry germline *p53* mutations (Platz et al, 1998).

Several other inherited cancer syndromes are associated with an increased risk of melanoma. Patients with xeroderma pigmentosum (described previously) develop cutaneous melanoma at more than 1000 times the rate of the normal population (Kraemer et al, 1994). However, there is a difference in melanoma types and their anatomic distribution compared with the general population. A large proportion of melanomas occurring in xeroderma pigmentosum patients appear to be lentigo maligna melanoma occurring on chronically sun-exposed body sites (Kraemer et al, 1994; Spatz et al, 2001).

Several other germline defects underlie syndromes whose sufferers have secondarily been reported to be at increased risk for melanoma. These include mutations in the Werner syndrome (WRN) gene that also encodes a DNA helicase involved in DNA repair; in the NF1 gene that causes neurofibromatosis type I and affects cells originating from the neural crest, as melanoma is a tumor of cells of neural crest origin; and in the *BRCA2* gene (de Snoo and Hayward, 2005). A common link between *BRCA2, WRN,* and the *xeroderma pigmentosum* gene family is that they encode proteins involved in DNA repair, suggesting that aberrations of this cellular process is important in melanoma development (de Snoo and Hayward, 2005).

Somatic Events

Basal cell carcinoma

Aberrant upregulation of the sonic hedgehog signaling pathway is commonly found in sporadic BCCs, and either inactivating mutations in the *patched* gene or activating mutations in *smoothened* genes (or both) appear to be the cause. Mutations and allelic loss in the *patched* gene are found in up to 95% of sporadic BCCs and may at least partly arise from uniparental disomy (loss of one allele and its replacement with the allele inherited from the other parent) due to somatic recombination (Teh et al, 2005). The most recent estimates of *patched* mutation rates in somatic BCC, derived from genome-wide single nucleotide polymorphism microarray mapping, are higher than previous estimates, probably due to the limitations of previous techniques. Under normal circumstances, patched represses hedgehog target gene expression through its interaction with smoothened. In around 10% of sporadic BCCs (Reifenberger et al, 2005), activating mutations in the *smoothened* gene cause constitutive sonic hedgehog pathway activation (Xie et al, 1998). Inhibition of smoothened can prevent UV-induced BCCs in mice (Athar et al, 2004).

Increased expression levels of Gli1 and Gli2, members of the Gli family of zinc-finger transcription factors and downstream targets of sonic hedgehog, are also known to play a role in BCC carcinogenesis (Kasper et al, 2006; Regl et al, 2002). Further evidence for the importance of sonic hedgehog pathway activation in BCC carcinogenesis comes from transgenic human-skin models in which sonic hedgehog expressing human keratinocytes formed BCC-like lesions when grafted onto the skin of immune-deficient mice (Fan et al, 1997). Also, *patched* heterozygous knockout mice develop BCC-like lesions when exposed to UV or ionizing radiation (Aszterbaum et al, 1999).

Mutations in the *p53* tumor-suppressor gene are detected in around half of all BCC tumors. However, people suffering from the Li-Fraumeni syndrome, characterized by germline mutations in the *p53* gene, do not show increased incidence of BCC and thus *p53* mutations are presumed to be secondary events in BCC pathogenesis (Tilli et al, 2005).

Squamous cell carcinoma

Mutations of the *p53* tumor-suppressor gene are found in the majority of SCCs (Ahmadian et al, 1998). These mutations are often "UV-signature mutations," indicating that they are caused by exposure to UV radiation. Mutations in the *p53* gene can lead to uncontrolled cell proliferation and loss of apoptosis, thus promoting cancerous growth. Immunohistochemically detectable clusters of epidermal cells with accumulated nuclear p53 protein ("p53 patches") are found in normal skin before tumors arise. These patches are thought to be an early step in the development of actinic keratoses and subsequent SCCs, though the progression rate is low (Rebel et al, 2005).

Melanoma

Mutations and deletions affecting the *CDKN2A/ARF* locus are found in melanoma cell lines but rarely in primary sporadic melanomas (Pollock et al, 1995). This is believed to occur due to p16INK4A's central role in senescence: Cells in vitro lacking p16 escape senescence and can readily become immortalized (Bennett, 2003). The same appears to be true for mutations in the tumor-suppressor gene *PTEN* in cell lines and tumors (de Snoo and Hayward, 2005). In primary melanoma, the *CDKN2A/ARF* locus shows loss of heterozygosity (LOH) in around 50% of melanomas, but mutations in the *CDKN2A* or *ARF* genes are found only in a small proportion of tumors (Pollock et al, 2001). When deletions are accounted for, however, the overall proportion of tumors showing inactivation of either *CDKN2A* or *ARF* increases (de Snoo and Hayward, 2005). LOH of this region occurs frequently in dysplastic nevi, less so in banal nevi (Birindelli et al, 2000; Hussein et al, 2003), consistent with a melanoma precursor role of some nevi; but the importance of such events in melanomagenesis including that from benign nevi is unknown. Although loss of either *CDKN2A* or the retinoblastoma (*RB1*) tumor-suppressor genes results in the same cell-cycle dysregulation, few studies to date have assessed the possible role of pRB pathway in melanoma formation (de Snoo and Hayward, 2005).

Prevalence of overexpression of the *p53* gene in melanoma appears to vary according to the anatomic site of melanomas (Whiteman et al, 1998), which may explain the widely varying estimates (0%–24%) (de Snoo and Hayward, 2005) between series of tumor samples that have not accounted for tumor site. Mutations of the UV-signature type are seen in *p53* but frequency is similarly variable. In a case-control study in Queensland men, p53-immunopositive melanomas were twice as likely as p53-immunonegative melanomas to have occurred on the head and neck and legs as on the back or arms. Compared with men who had no melanoma (or had a p53-negative melanoma), men with p53-positive melanomas were more likely to have had a past BCC or SCC or to have sun-sensitive skin (Whiteman et al, 1998). In contrast, p53-negative melanomas were strongly associated with having a large number of nevi on the skin of the arm, back, and shoulders and with having many freckles in childhood.

Prevalence of mutations in the *BRAF* proto-oncogene in melanoma also varies according to the histological subtype and site of melanomas. Mutations in mucosal melanomas are rare but present in some 50% of cutaneous melanomas (Maldonado et al, 2003; Thomas et al, 2004). A lower incidence of *BRAF* mutations in tumors on chronically sun-exposed skin has been reported (Maldonado et al, 2003), though the majority of lesions on sun-exposed body sites were of the lentigo maligna melanoma subtype, which has a reduced mutation rate compared with other subtypes. The frequency of *BRAF* mutations in benign melanocytic nevi appears even higher than in melanomas but, like melanoma, varies markedly by histological subtype of tumor (0%–90%) (de Snoo and Hayward, 2005).

In summary, tumor-suppressor genes and proto-oncogenes appear to be involved in development of sporadic melanoma and confer moderate to high risk of melanoma. So far most of the genes implicated encode products that assist in either cell-cycle regulation, DNA repair, or receptor-mediated signal transduction (de Snoo and Hayward, 2005). Beyond these moderate- to high-risk genes, there are many possible candidates for lower risk or modifier predisposition genes (Hayward, 2003), perhaps the most prominent being the melanocortin-1 receptor gene that partly determines hair color, skin color, and freckling (Sturm et al, 2003) and is strongly associated with melanoma (Palmer et al, 2000). A number of nonsynonymous polymorphisms in *MC1R* are strong predictors of red hair color, and may convey modest additional information in melanoma risk prediction over and above self-reported hair color (Han et al, 2006a).

RISK FACTORS

Tobacco

Basal cell carcinoma

Smoking has not been linked to BCC in the majority of large studies that have investigated the association (Hunter et al, 1990; Green et al, 1996; Lear et al, 1997; van

Dam et al, 1999; Corona et al, 2001; De Hertog et al, 2001; Freedman et al, 2003a).

Squamous cell carcinoma

Squamous cell carcinoma specifically of the lip is associated with tobacco use (Moore et al, 1999), as well as with other tobacco-associated cancers (Soderholm et al, 1994).

Most but not all (Green et al, 1996; Odenbro et al, 2005) studies of cutaneous SCC and cigarette smoking support a positive association (Karagas et al, 1992; Grodstein et al, 1995). Smokers in the Nurses Health Study had a 50% increased risk of SCC compared to nonsmokers (Grodstein et al, 1995). Furthermore, studies of second primary cancers in patients with squamous cell carcinoma show that tobacco-associated primary cancers—including cancers of the lung, lip, salivary gland, oesophagus, larynx, and pharynx—as well as melanoma are increased in people previously diagnosed with SCC of the skin (Maitra et al, 2005).

Melanoma

There is no evidence that cutaneous melanoma is positively associated with tobacco use (Gallagher et al, 1986; Green et al, 1986), but melanoma on the soles and palms has been found to be inversely associated with smoking (Green et al, 1999a).

Diet

Although melanoma and basal and squamous cell carcinomas of the skin are cancers with distinct clinical, etiological, and genetic profiles, dietary factors have been hypothesized to modify risk of these cancers through a number of common pathways. These include the role of antioxidant nutrients in the skin's defense against UV-induced genetic and cellular damage, and the effect of dietary fats on the UV-induced inflammatory response, through modification of prostaglandin production.

Basal cell carcinoma

A large cohort study showed a small (13%) but significant increase in risk of BCC for men with a high intake of long chain n-3

fatty acids and an inverse association with intake of total and monounsaturated fat (van Dam et al, 2000). In an intervention study, a low-fat (20%) diet was shown to reduce the risk of keratinocytic cancers (Black et al, 1995), but since BCC and SCC were combined it is not clear how this intervention affected each specific type of skin cancer. Other studies have not found clear evidence for an association between dietary fat and BCC risk (McNaughton et al, 2005).

Studies of BCC risk and intake of antioxidant nutrients have shown weak and inconsistent results for retinol, beta-carotene, vitamin E, vitamin C, and selenium, while evidence regarding other carotenoids is lacking (McNaughton et al, 2005).

Squamous cell carcinoma

Results from a case-control study of North American SCC patients suggested 30% decreased risk of SCC associated with a diet high in n-3 fatty acids and for diets with a high n-3/n-6 fatty acid ratio (Hakim et al, 2000). A possible protective effect on SCC of n-3 fatty acids is in agreement with a blinded experimental study in which persons who took n-3 fatty acid supplements for 3 months showed reduced sensitivity to sunburn and reduced UV-induced p53 expression in comparison to persons who took an oleic acid supplement (Rhodes et al, 2003).

A prospective study of food intake and SCC risk showed a 55% reduced SCC risk for high intake of green leafy vegetables and a doubling of SCC risk associated with high intake of unmodified dairy products (eg, full cream dairy milk and cheese) in Australian adults with a history of skin cancer (Hughes et al, 2006).

Further study of this population extended this finding to show that a "meat and fat" dietary pattern, characterized by other components such as processed meat, discretionary fat, and white bread, had an additional association over and above the association with the high-fat dairy food group alone in the development of subsequent SCC tumors (Ibiebele et al, 2007).

Although animal studies have suggested a protective effect of antioxidant intake (which may underlie a protective effect of green leafy vegetable consumption), human studies have been few and have shown inconsistent results (McNaughton et al, 2005). Intervention studies of beta-carotene supplementation in relation to the incidence of SCC showed no effect of supplementation (Greenberg et al, 1990; Green et al, 1999b; Frieling et al, 2000). Risk of SCC was actually increased after 13 years of selenium supplementation compared to a placebo (Duffield-Lillico et al, 2003).

Melanoma

A large North-American case-control study showed a lower risk for melanoma in persons with high versus low consumption levels of alpha-carotene, beta-carotene, cryptoxanthin, lutein, and lycopene (Millen et al, 2004). In the same study there were inverse dose-response relationships with consumption of fruits and vegetables, including dark green and yellow fruit and vegetables. It has been suggested that redox-cycling of melanin and its precursors is an etiologically important component in melanoma pathogenesis (Meyskens et al, 2005). A number of other case-control studies, however, have shown weak or no associations with antioxidant-rich foods (Le Marchand et al, 2006; Naldi et al, 2004; Vinceti et al, 2005). An inverse association of high intake of vitamin D–rich foods has been seen in two North-American studies (Millen et al, 2004; Weinstock et al, 1992). The role of vitamin D in skin cancer risk warrants further investigation.

Alcohol

Basal cell carcinoma

The results of recent cohort studies suggest that the association between alcohol intake and BCC may vary between different types of alcoholic beverages (Freedman et al, 2003b; Fung et al, 2002; Soleas et al, 2002). These studies showed a positive association between BCC risk and total alcohol intake, white wine consumption, and liquor consumption, and an inverse association with red wine consumption. Others have found no overall association between BCC risk and total alcohol consumption (Kune et al, 1992; Sahl et al, 1995).

Squamous cell carcinoma

The relationship between alcohol and SCC risk has not been specifically reported.

Melanoma

Melanoma patients were more likely to be moderate or high alcohol consumers in case-control studies from Hawaii (Le Marchand et al, 2006) and North America (Freedman et al, 2003b; Millen et al, 2004), but two case-control studies from Italy did not show this association (Naldi et al, 2004; Vinceti et al, 2005). It has been hypothesized that melanoma pathogenesis is partly driven by a changed redox state and that alcohol affects this by enhancement of a pro-oxidant state (Meyskens et al, 2005).

Reproductive factors

Basal cell and squamous cell carcinoma

No human studies have addressed the association between reproductive factors and these keratinocyte cancers.

Melanoma

Some studies (Lambe et al, 1996; Naldi et al, 2005; Neale et al, 2005), including a pooled analysis (Karagas et al, 2006a), have reported an association between age at first birth and melanoma risk, although most individual studies have not found such an association (Holman et al, 1984; Green and Bain, 1985; Osterlind et al, 1988; Holly et al, 1995; Westerdahl et al, 1996). One of the possible explanations for the inconsistent findings may be residual confounding—adjustment for sun-exposure history mitigated associations between reproductive history and melanoma risk in some studies (Neale et al, 2005).

Hormones

Basal cell and squamous cell carcinoma

There is no evidence that sex hormones are associated with BCC or SCC risk.

Melanoma

Although a case-control study in 1977 suggested a positive association between long-term oral contraceptive use and melanoma, further studies, including meta-analyses (Gefeller et al, 1998; Pfahlberg et al, 1997) and a pooled analysis (Karagas et al, 2002) of case-control studies, have not confirmed this finding. One of the few cohort studies reported an increased risk of melanoma in current but not past users of oral contraceptives (Feskanich et al, 1999), although lack of correction for use of sunscreen or sunbathing habits may partly explain the findings (Leslie and Espey, 2005).

There is no evidence that use of hormone replacement therapy is associated with an increased risk of melanoma (Westerdahl et al, 1996; Smith et al, 1998; Freedman et al, 2003b; Naldi et al, 2005).

Anthropometric Measures

Anthropometric indicators such as height, weight, and body surface are thought to affect skin cancer risk through modification of metabolism and/or immune function, physiological programming in early life, or simply through the association of body size with number of target cells.

Basal cell carcinoma

One small case-control study (Sahl et al, 1995) showed a positive association between BCC and body weight, but neither a large case-control study (Milan et al, 2003) nor a cohort study (Olsen et al, 2006) found any association between anthropometric measures and BCC risk.

Squamous cell carcinoma

Anthropometric measures in relation to SCC have not been specifically investigated.

Melanoma

A number of cohort (Gallus et al, 2006; Oh et al, 2005; Samanic et al, 2004; Thune et al, 1993; Veierod et al, 1997; Veierod et al, 2003) and case-control studies (Bain et al, 1993; Cutler et al, 1996; Gallus et al, 2006; Green et al, 1999a; Holly et al, 1995;

Kirkpatrick et al, 1994) have shown associations between anthropometric measures and melanoma risk. Although the pattern of associations with height, weight, BMI, and body surface area has been inconsistent, most of these studies suggest a small increased melanoma risk associated with either increased weight, BMI, or body surface area. A pooled analysis showed that greater height and weight gain may be risk factors for melanoma in women (Olsen et al, *In Press*). However, other studies have not shown these associations (Calle et al, 2003; Freedman et al, 2003b; Gallagher et al, 1985; Holman et al, 1984; Moller et al, 1994; Wolk et al, 2001). Variable levels of correction for confounders such as sun-exposure history may partly explain some of these discrepancies.

Infections

Basal cell carcinoma

To date there is no evidence that infectious agents are associated with BCC in the general population.

Squamous cell carcinoma

The main evidence of the involvement of infectious agents in skin cancer concerns specific cutaneous human papilloma virus (HPV) types and SCC. Originally identified in studies of patients with epidermodysplasia verruciformis (Orth et al, 1980), these cutaneous HPV types are classified in the beta genus of papilloma viruses (de Villiers et al, 2004) and infection is common not only in immunosuppressed organ transplant recipients but among the general population as well (Pfister, 2003). A number of studies that have measured beta-HPV antibodies, as well as those that have assessed the presence of beta-HPV DNA, have shown beta-HPVs to be associated with solar keratoses and SCC (Boxman et al, 2000; Feltkamp et al, 2003; Struijk et al, 2006; Karagas et al, 2006b). It is likely that beta-HPV, if etiologically involved, acts to potentiate the effect of UV radiation possibly via viral inhibition of DNA repair and apoptosis following UV radiation (Hall et al, 2006; McBride et al, 2007).

Melanoma

A small hospital-based case-control study found a significant reduction in the risk of melanoma associated with self-reported febrile infections during adulthood but not childhood (Kolmel et al, 1992), but the finding has not been confirmed.

Physical Activity

The possible relationship between skin cancer and physical activity has not been studied adequately. The scant available evidence of an association of outdoor leisure activity and melanoma is likely to be explained by sun exposure (Schnohr et al, 2005).

Ionizing Radiation

Elevated risks of BCC have been reported among atomic bomb survivors after long latent periods (Ron et al, 1998) and among people exposed to occupational (Wang et al, 1988; Yoshinaga et al, 2005) and therapeutic ionizing radiation (Karagas et al, 1996; Levi et al, 2006), usually before the age of 40 years. Squamous cell carcinomas have been described in patients decades after they received ionizing radiation therapy for a variety of benign skin conditions (Johnson et al, 1992). However, increased SCC risk has not been found in other epidemiologic studies (Karagas et al, 1996; Ron et al, 1998). Results of studies of nuclear workers and of participants in nuclear tests have been inconsistent with regard to melanoma mortality in relation to radiation exposure. Taken together, epidemiologic data offer little support to the hypothesis linking melanoma to ionizing radiation (Wilkinson, 1997).

Occupation

Historically various occupations have been described as associated with skin cancer: most famously, Potts' link of SCCs of the scrotum with soot among chimney sweeps in the late eighteenth century, and industrial exposures to chemical exposures, which now are limited in most Western countries (Gawkrodger, 2004). Many present occupations linked to skin cancer are associated with, and therefore partly explained by, high levels of UV exposure.

Although increased risks of melanoma have been observed in workers in a range of occupations, these have not been clearly related to specific exposures, with the possible exception of polychlorinated biphenyls and some other organic chemicals (Wilkinson, 1997). Similarly, the link between indoor occupation and melanoma observed in a number of studies is most likely explained by a higher level of recreational sun exposure (sunbathing, vacations spent in sunny countries, and sunburns) seen among indoor workers compared with outdoor workers (Nelemans et al, 1993). Overall, specific occupational associations have not been consistent and, in many studies, host characteristics and sun exposure have not been adequately taken into account.

Medical Conditions and Treatment

Basal cell carcinoma

Exposure to various medicines containing inorganic arsenic, including Chinese proprietary medicines (Wong et al, 1998) and drugs used in the past to treat various dermatologic conditions (Reymann et al, 1978), as well as some asthma medications (Boonchai et al, 2000), have been associated with the development of BCC after long latent periods. Use of glucocorticoids—a group of drugs with immunosuppressive properties and widely used to treat acute and chronic inflammatory disease—has been associated with increased risk of BCC (Sorenson et al, 2004).

Squamous cell carcinoma

It is well established that renal transplant recipients and other immunosuppressed patients are at increased risk of skin cancer, especially SCC (London et al, 1995). Time of onset after transplantation is inversely related to intensity of ambient sun exposure. In Queensland, Australia, cumulative incidence of SCCs is approximately 30% at 10 years and 60% at 20 years, whereas comparable rates in European transplant recipients are delayed in onset by some 10 years relative to those in Queensland (London et al, 1995; Bouwes Bavinck et al, 1996). There is also an increase in the incidence of cutaneous SCC in patients with skin disorders such as psoriasis who are treated with psoralen and ultraviolet A (PUVA) (Lindelof et al, 1999) and in patients treated with glucocorticoids (Sorenson et al, 2004).

Melanoma

Studies conducted among various populations have pointed out that patients with SCC of the skin have about a threefold increased risk of cutaneous melanoma (Green and O'Rourke, 1985; Levi et al, 1997a, 1997b). In contrast, there is no association between SCC and ocular melanoma (Swerdlow et al, 1995a). There has been concern that patients with various skin disorders treated with PUVA may be at increased risk of melanoma; however, a Swedish study found no evidence of an association (Lindelof et al, 1999). No other therapeutic associations with melanoma have been reported.

Ultraviolet Radiation

Solar ultraviolet radiation

Sunlight is the principal environmental cause of the three major types of skin cancer: BCC, SCC, and melanoma (IARC, 1992). The UV radiation spectral regions of sunlight—wavelengths of 280–320 nm (UVB) and to a lesser extent, 320–400 nm (UVA)—are those specifically implicated in skin carcinogenesis. There is a diversity of evidence for this causal link, ranging from migrant to clinical studies. Among white populations, permanent residents of high-latitude regions with low daily hours of sunlight are largely protected from skin cancers, while those who migrate from high to low latitudes early in life and materially increase their lifetime level of sun exposure take on a higher risk of all types of skin cancer (Kricker et al, 1991; Swerdlow et al, 1995b; Whiteman and Green, 1999). All skin cancer types are most common on the most highly sun-exposed body site, the face (Franceschi et al, 1996).

Analytic epidemiologic studies show that skin cancer patients have skin that tans poorly and sunburns easily (IARC, 1992) because it is unprotected by melanin. Moreover, different skin cancer types tend to occur in the same patients, confirming common etiologic processes. People with a history of BCC or SCC have a significantly increased risk of melanoma and vice versa (Green and O'Rourke, 1985; Karagas et al, 1992; Swerdlow et al, 1995a). More evidence of the causal role of solar UV radiation in the development of skin cancer is the extremely high rate at which xeroderma pigmentosum patients suffer all types of skin cancers (Kraemer et al, 1994).

Despite their overall association with high levels of sun exposure, BCC, SCC, and melanoma all appear to show different patterns of dependence on solar UV radiation, which is perhaps not unexpected given their different cells of origin within the dermo-epidermis. Heterogeneity among histological subtypes of both BCC and melanoma adds to the complexity. While detailed descriptive data about anatomic site distributions provide the first clues that these differences exist, the one common feature remains: Continually exposed sites on the head are those most affected per unit area of skin for all skin cancers.

Thereafter only the anatomic distribution of SCC reflects sites of maximal UV exposure, as illustrated by data from the Vaud Cancer Registry in Switzerland, which has paid specific attention to skin neoplasms. These registry data show that incidence rates on the face are 120–130 times higher for SCC, some 40–50 times higher for BCC, and only 3–6 times higher for melanoma than the corresponding incidence rates per unit surface area on the relatively unexposed trunk in both men and women (Franceschi et al, 1996). It is of note that the body-site distributions of BCC and SCC, as well as of melanoma (lentigo maligna type), in patients with xeroderma pigmentosum are the same as those seen in the corresponding general population (Kraemer et al, 1994).

In analytic epidemiologic studies, accurate measurement of an individual's overall sun exposure prior to the development of skin cancer, in order to investigate details of the sunlight–skin cancer association, is extremely difficult and assessment of exposure at specific anatomic sites even more so. Traditionally, subjective measures have been used, namely, individuals' recall of the amount of time spent outdoors or the number of sunburns experienced during various age periods from childhood on, as proxies for their exposure to solar UV in these age periods. This information has been gathered using variable definitions of what constitutes *outdoors*—for example, whether "in the sun," "not in shade," or unqualified. Variable definitions have also been used with respect to *sunburn*—whether associated with peeling or pain for a certain period of time, unqualified, or given in quantitative or qualitative form.

Further details such as geographic location, season, and time of day when exposure occurred, whether protective clothing or sunscreen was used, and which skin sites were protected each have a bearing on the level of UV exposure received at the skin surface. Furthermore, skin color influences the final UV dose at the target cells beneath the superficial layers of the epidermis (Green et al, 1986). No epidemiologic studies have been able to gather details of this scope and complexity, and investigators have differed in the degree to which they attempted to take such details into account. Assessments of UV exposure necessarily have been based on memories of average behavior and assumptions about constancy of habits during various life periods. Thus the possibility of misclassification of cumulated hours of self-reported sun exposure or cumulated sunburns is substantial and needs to be borne in mind when assessing any lack of association between sun exposure and skin cancers.

Results may be distorted in other ways as well. Significant self-selection can be seen among those with the highest sun-exposure levels, namely, outdoor workers, whereby people with fair complexions and a tendency to sunburn are systematically underrepresented among those in long-term outdoor occupations, thus partly explaining the frequently observed lack of association between occupational sun exposure and skin cancers (Green et al, 1996).

Notwithstanding these severe limitations operating in studies of sun exposure and skin cancer, several differences between BCC, SCC, and melanoma have been revealed.

Squamous cell carcinoma

Overall it appears that increasing hours of sun exposure are consistently associated with an increasing risk of SCC (Rosso et al, 1996; English et al, 1998). In contrast, neither BCC (Kricker et al, 1995; Rosso et al, 1996) nor melanoma (Elwood and Jopson, 1997; Whiteman et al, 2003) have shown consistent evidence of such a monotonic increase in risk.

Basal cell carcinoma

Various explanations have been proposed to explain the overall lack of a monotonic association between BCC and chronic sun exposure. The intermittent UV exposure theory proposes that the pattern of sun exposure rather than the total amount of exposure determines the risk of BCC. In particular, it is suggested that a certain dose of solar UV delivered in infrequent, intense increments will increase the risk of BCC more than the same total dose delivered continuously over the same period (Kricker et al, 1995; Zanetti et al, 2006). The intermittent pattern theory does not explain all the epidemiologic evidence of BCC's UV dose dependence (Kricker et al, 1991; Green et al, 1996), and the same empirical evidence could perhaps be interpreted otherwise. Strong positive dose-response relationships with childhood sun exposure suggest that the ultraviolet radiation dose received early in life is an important predictor of BCC risk (Corona et al, 2001).

Because the epithelial cells from which BCCs arise are believed to be stem cells, the threshold of total solar radiation for malignant transformation may be low. Current evidence increasingly points to the hair follicle stem cell as the likely cell of origin of BCC (Kruger et al, 1999; Tilli et al, 2005). In comparison, a higher dose appears to be needed to transform the more differentiated epithelial keratinocytes of the epidermis from which SCCs arise. The occurrence of BCC at earlier ages than SCC and on less sun-exposed sites like the trunk is consistent with a lower dose of solar UV being required for basal cell compared with squamous cell carcinogenesis (Rosso et al, 1996).

Ultraviolet dose dependence may also vary among BCC subtypes, as suggested by their clinical and histologic differences. In particular, superficial BCCs (approximately 15% of the total) appear to differ from other subtypes, as demonstrated in two large series from Australia (McCormack et al, 1997) and the Netherlands (Bastiaens et al, 1998). Superficial BCCs, diagnosed in younger patients (Bastiaens et al, 1998), also differ markedly in their site distribution. In the Australian series, for example, 23% of superficial BCCs occurred on the head and neck and 49% on the trunk, compared with 65% of other types on the head and neck and 20% on the trunk (McCormack et al, 1997).

In a recent cohort study, BCCs of the trunk had a relatively strong association with sunburns and truncal lentigines, but were not associated with sun sensitivity, compared with BCCs of the head and neck (Neale et al, 2007). These findings were thought to suggest that superficial (truncal) BCCs result from acute, intense sun exposure sufficient to cause sunburn among people whose ability to tan makes the skin of their face less susceptible to UV carcinogenesis.

Melanoma

A causal link specifically between sun exposure and melanoma was first suggested because the disease was more common on sun-exposed skin (McGovern, 1952). The sunlight hypothesis was supported by the first published evidence that as latitude decreased (and by inference exposure to ambient solar radiation rose), melanoma mortality rates rose among white-skinned populations (Lancaster, 1956). Latitude gradients in both incidence and mortality rates were described subsequently in white populations in northern Europe, the United States, and New Zealand (Whiteman and Green, 1999); it is estimated that the incidence of melanoma increases at a rate of about 5% per degree of latitude toward the equator (Bulliard et al, 1994).

Fair skin signifies that skin (epidermal) transmission of solar radiation to the target cell (here, the melanocyte) is high (Green et al, 1986). Its importance is illustrated in Australia, where melanoma is exceedingly rare in indigenous Australians, while Australians of predominantly European ancestry have the world's highest incidence rates (IARC, 1992). In migrants, the risk of melanoma depends on age at arrival in or departure from sunny countries. Thus it is thought that UV induction of melanoma probably occurs early in life (Whiteman et al, 2001).

Numerous case-control studies have confirmed that exposure to the UV component of sunlight is the major environmental determinant of melanoma, but the results are complicated (Whiteman et al, 2003). Indeed, the intermittent UV exposure theory—whereby a short, intense UV exposure is more important than chronic exposure—was first suggested to explain the lack of association between melanoma and chronic sun exposure when subjective assessment (recall) of outdoor exposure is used to assess the level of sun exposure (Elwood et al, 1985; Armstrong, 1988). As for BCC, however, this suggestion that the pattern rather than the total amount of UV exposure to the target cell causes melanoma appears somewhat inconsistent with other evidence.

From a systematic review of 21 case-control studies, it has been inferred that a past history of multiple sunburns throughout life is a strong predictor of melanoma (Elwood and Jopson, 1997). Multiple sunburns, a key marker of intermittent sun exposure, represent repeated episodes of acute UV-induced burn injuries to the dermo-epidermis. Their effects appear cumulative because a history of multiple sunburns strongly predicts the risk of solar keratoses (Frost et al, 1998) and SCCs (English et al, 1998), diseases that are UV dose-dependent. Melanoma's predilection for the face and the male ear (Green et al, 1993; Franceschi et al, 1996), and its strong association with a history of other skin cancers or the presence of solar keratoses (Holman and Armstrong, 1984; Green and O'Rourke, 1985), also point to a role for chronic sun exposure.

When cutaneous melanomas are analyzed by histologic subtype, lentigo maligna melanoma is found to have the strongest relationship with cumulative sun exposure, but nodular (Chamberlain et al, 2002) and superficial spreading melanoma have also been strongly associated with signs of chronic solar damage to the skin (Holman and Armstrong, 1984). Moreover, most case-control studies of cutaneous melanoma have excluded lentigo maligna melanoma from analyses because of its distinctive UV dose dependence. Thus, the apparently paradoxical findings of case-control studies are not fully explained by the histologic heterogeneity of melanomas.

A *divergent pathway* model has been proposed to explain the associations of melanoma with both chronic and intermittent patterns of sun exposure (Whiteman et al, 1998, 2003, 2006). This model predicts that people with many nevi who have an inherently high propensity for nevus development require a lower threshold dose of solar UV for malignant transformation to occur probably early in life (Whiteman et al, 2001). This is because their melanocytes are manifestly prone to proliferation—hence they develop melanoma on relatively sun-protected anatomic sites at young or middle ages. In contrast, melanomas in people with few nevi will tend to be associated with cumulative sun exposure and will thus arise on the head and neck at older ages.

Supporting the existence of multiple causal pathways to melanoma, head and neck melanomas as a whole are more likely to overexpress the p53 protein than those on the trunk (Whiteman et al, 1998), whereas trunk melanomas are more likely to arise from a preexisting nevus (Skender-Kalnenas et al, 1995; Carli et al, 1999). People with head and neck melanomas are less likely to have many nevi than people with trunk melanomas but are more likely to have many solar keratoses and a past history of excised skin cancers (Whiteman et al, 2003). Patients with head and neck melanoma are more likely than those with trunk melanoma to report high levels of sun exposure in adulthood and, specifically, higher levels of occupational (cumulative) exposure, but lower levels of recreational (intermittent) sun exposure (Whiteman et al, 2006). These findings together with somatic mutational differences in melanomas arising on sun-exposed and nonexposed skin (Maldonado et al, 2003; Curtin et al, 2005; Liu et al, 2007) and data showing that melanomas with and without neval remnants differ in their risk factor profiles (Lee et al, 2006) are consistent with melanomas arising through different causal pathways.

The subgroup of melanomas on the unexposed skin of the soles, palms, and digits (including subungually) traditionally have also been excluded from case-control studies of cutaneous melanoma because of their location and their relatively low incidence. Three case-control studies have been conducted to date, one of plantar melanoma in Paraguayans (Rolon et al, 1997) and two of plantar, palmar, and digit melanoma—one in Caucasians (Green et al, 1999a) and the other in Japanese (Rokuhara et al, 2004). The first two found approximate doubling of the risk of these melanomas among people with outdoor occupational exposure compared to others. This finding suggests a role for systemic mediators of the effects of UV exposure in the evolution of melanomas on sites that are not directly sun exposed. Plantar, palmar, and digital nevi were risk factors for melanomas on these sites in the Caucasian (Green et al, 1999a) but not the Japanese (Rokuhara et al, 2004) study populations.

Artificial Ultraviolet Radiation

Sources of artificial UV radiation include various lamps used in medicine and industry and for domestic and cosmetic purposes (IARC Working Group on artificial UV light and skin cancer, 2007). Sun beds and sunlamps used for tanning purposes are becoming a major source of deliberate exposure to UV radiation. In a meta-analysis of summary results from relevant studies, there was no consistent evidence that use of indoor tanning facilities in general was associated with the development of melanoma or skin cancer. However, there was a consistent increase in risk of melanoma in people who first used indoor tanning facilities in their twenties or teen years (IARC Working Group on artificial UV light and skin cancer, 2007). In a prospective study, ever use of sunlamps for tanning was associated with a twofold increase in risk of melanoma, after control for sun exposure and constitutional susceptibility (Han et al, 2006b). Limited data suggested that SCC may also be increased with first use of artificial tanning facilities as a teenager (IARC Working Group on artificial UV light and skin cancer, 2007)

Trauma

Mostly SCCs, but also BCCs and melanoma, can arise from sites of chronic injury or scar tissue especially thermal burn scars; the historical evidence includes the nineteenth century reports of *Kangri* cancers—SCCs of the abdomen in Kashmiris who used a Kangri or cooking pot filled with coals under their clothes for warmth in winter (Kowal-Vern and Criswell, 2005). Although there is little evidence that acute trauma is a risk factor for BCC, SCC, or the majority of cutaneous melanomas, two case-control studies of melanomas on the extremities have both implicated local trauma, specifically penetrating injuries, as a risk factor (Rolon et al, 1997; Green et al, 1999a). In a cross-sectional survey however it was observed that 9% of patients with melanoma of any histologic type reported a prior history of trauma at the site of their lesion. Many of the injuries in that series (Kaskel et al, 2000), however, occurred in the 12 months before diagnosis, constituting weak evidence of a causal association.

CONCLUSION

Although the predominant carcinogen for all three forms of skin cancer is known, substantial research questions remain that pose a formidable challenge to epidemiologic methods. The relationship of age at first high-level sun exposure, pattern, and total amount of sun exposure, and the ways these interact with the host phenotype require elucidation for the three major types of skin cancer. Molecular techniques of UV dosimetry may be useful in helping to answer these questions, given the limitations of conventional epidemiologic methods in measuring the key exposure. In theory, skin cancers in fair-skinned people are substantially preventable by avoiding UV-radiation exposure. Behavior modification programs have been remarkably successful in some countries, for instance the "Slip (on a shirt), Slap (on a hat), and Slop (on sunscreen)" campaign in Australia. In the coming decades, the extent to which these programs translate into a lower incidence of skin cancer will become apparent.

REFERENCES

Ahmadian A, Ren ZP, Williams C, Ponten F, Odeberg J, Ponten J, et al. Genetic instability in the 9q22.3 region is a late event in the development of squamous cell carcinoma. Oncogene 1998;17:1837–43.

Armstrong BK. Epidemiology of malignant melanoma: intermittent or total accumulated exposure to the sun. J Dermatol Surg Oncol 1988;14:835–49.

Aszterbaum M, Epstein J, Oro A, Douglas V, LeBoit PE, Scott MP, et al. Ultraviolet and ionizing radiation enhance the growth of BCCs and trichoblastomas in patched heterozygous knockout mice. Nat Med 1999; 5:1285–91.

Athar M, Li CX, Tang XW, Chi SM, Zhang XL, Kim AL, et al. Inhibition of Smoothened signaling prevents ultraviolet B-induced basal cell carcinomas through regulation of Fas expression and apoptosis. Cancer Research 2004;64:7545–52.

Bain C, Green A, Siskind V, Alexander J, Harvey P. Diet and melanoma. An exploratory case-control study. Ann Epidemiol 1993;3:235–38.

Bale AE, Yu KP. The hedgehog pathway and basal cell carcinomas. Hum Mol Genet 2001; 10:757–62.

Bastiaens MT, Hoefnagel JJ, Bruijn JA, Westendorp RGJ, Vermeer BJ, Bouwes Bavinck JN. Differences in age, site distribution, and sex between nodular and superficial basal cell carcinomas indicate different types of tumors. J Invest Dermatol 1998;110:880–84.

Bennett DC. Human melanocyte senescence and melanoma susceptibility genes. Oncogene 2003; 22: 3063–69.

Birindelli S, Tragni G, Bartoli C, Ranzani GN, Rilke F, Pierotti MA, et al. Detection of microsatellite alterations in the spectrum of melanocytic nevi in patients with or without individual or family history of melanoma. Int J Cancer 2000; 86: 255–261.

Bishop DT, Demenais F, Goldstein AM, Bergman W, Newton Bishop J, Bressac-de Paillerets B, et al. Geographical variation in the penetrance of CDKN2A mutations for melanoma J Natl Cancer Inst 2002; 94: 894–903.

Black HS, Thornby JI, Wolf JE, Jr., Goldberg LH, Herd JA, Rosen T, et al. Evidence that a low-fat diet reduces the occurrence of non-melanoma skin cancer. Int J Cancer 1995;62:165–69.

Boonchai W, Green A, Ng J, Dicker A, Chenevix-Trench G. Basal cell carcinoma in chronic arsenicism in Queensland after ingestion of an asthma medication. J Am Acad Dermatol 2000;43:664–69.

Bose S, Morgan LJ, Booth DR, Goudie DR, Ferguson-Smith MA, Richards FM. The elusive multiple self-healing squamous epithelioma (MSSE) gene: further mapping, analysis of candidates, and loss of heterozygosity. Oncogene 2006:25:806–12.

Bouwes Bavinck JN, Hardie DR, Green A, Cutmore S, MacNaught A, O'Sullivan B, et al. The risk of skin cancer in renal transplant recipients in Queensland, Australia. A follow-up study. Transplantation 1996;61: 715–21.

Boxman ILA, Russell A, Mulder LHC, Bouwes Bavinck JN, ter Schegget J, Green A. Case-control study in a subtropical Australian population to assess the relation between nonmelanoma skin cancer and EV-HPV DNA in plucked eyebrow hairs. Int J Cancer 2000;86:18–121.

Bulliard JL, Cox B, Elwood JM. Latitude gradients in melanoma incidence and mortality in the non-Maori population of New Zealand. Cancer Causes Control 1994;5:234–40.

Calle EE, Rodriguez C, Walker-Thurmond K, Thun MJ. Overweight, obesity, and mortality from cancer in a prospectively studied cohort of US adults. N Engl J Med 2003;348:1625–38.

Cannon-Albright LA, Goldgar DE, Meyer LJ, Lewis CM, Fountain JW, Hegi ME, et al. Assignment of a locus for familial melanoma, MLM, to chromosome 9p13-p22. Science 1992;258:1148–52.

Carli P, Massi D, Santucci M, Biggeri A, Giannotti B. Cutaneous melanoma histologically associated with a nevus and melanoma de novo have a different profile of risk: Results from a case-control study. J Am Acad Dermatol 1999;40:549–557.

Cleaver JE. Cancer in xeroderma pigmentosum and related disorders of DNA repair. Nat Rev Cancer 2005;5:564–73.

Chamberlain AJ, Fritschi L, Giles GG, Dowling JP, Kelly JW. Nodular type and older age as the most significant associations of thick melanoma in Victoria, Australia. Arch Dermatol 2002;138:609–14.

Christenson, L. J., T. A. Borrowman, et al. (2005). "Incidence of basal cell and squamous cell carcinomas in a population younger than 40 years." JAMA 294(6):681–90.

Corona R, Dogliotti E, D'Errico M, Sera F, Iavarone I, Baliva G, et al. Risk factors for basal cell carcinoma in a Mediterranean population: role of recreational sun exposure early in life. Arch Dermatol 2001;137:1162–68.

Couve-Privat S, Bouadjar B, Avril MF, Sarasin A, Daya-Grosjean L. Significantly high levels of ultraviolet-specific mutations in the smoothened gene in basal cell carcinomas from DNA repair-deficient xeroderma pigmentosum patients. Cancer Res 2002;62: 7186–89.

Couve-Privat S, Le Bret M, Traiffort E, Queille S, Coulombe J, Bouadjar B, et al. Functional analysis of novel sonic hedgehog gene mutations identified in basal cell carcinomas from xeroderma pigmentosum patients. Cancer Res 2004;64:3559–65.

Curtin JA, Fridlyand J, Kageshita T, Patel HN, Busam KJ, Kutzner H, et al. Distinct sets of genetic alterations in melanoma. N Engl J Med 2005;353:2135–47.

Cutler C, Foulkes WD, Brunet JS, Flanders TY, Shibata H, Narod SA. Cutaneous malignant melanoma in women is uncommonly associated with a family history of melanoma in first-degree relatives: a case-control study. Melanoma Res 1996;6:435–40.

Daya-Grosjean L, Sarasin A. The role of UV induced lesions in skin carcinogenesis: an overview of oncogene and tumor suppressor gene modifications in xeroderma pigmentosum skin tumors. Mutat Res 2005;571:43–56.

De Hertog SAE, Wensveen CAH, Bastiaens MT, Kielich CJ, Berkhout MJP, Westendorp RGJ, et al. Relation between smoking and skin cancer. Journal of Clinical Oncology 2001; 19:231–38.

De Snoo FA, Hayward NK. Cutaneous melanoma susceptibility and progression genes. Cancer Letters 2005;230:153–86.

De Villiers E-M, Fauquet C, Broker TR, zur Hausen H. Classification of papillomaviruses. Virology 2004;324:17–27.

de Vries E, Bray FI, et al. Changing epidemiology of malignant cutaneous melanoma in Europe 1953–1997: rising trends in incidence and mortality but recent stabilizations in western Europe and decreases in Scandinavia. Int J Cancer 2003;107(1):119–26.

de Vries E. Louwman M, et al. Rapid and continuous increases in incidence rates of basal cell carcinoma in the southeast Netherlands since 1973. J Invest Dermatol 2004;123(4): 634–38.

Duffield-Lillico AJ, Slate EH, Reid ME, Turnbull BW, Wilkins PA, Combs GF, Jr. et al. Selenium supplementation and secondary prevention of nonmelanoma skin cancer in a randomized trial. J Natl Cancer Inst 2003:95(19),1477–81.

Elwood JM, Gallagher RP, Hill GB, Pearson JC. Cutaneous melanoma in relation to intermittent and constant sun exposure—the Western Canada Melanoma Study. Int J Cancer 1985;35:427–33.

Elwood JM, Jopson J. Melanoma and sun exposure: an overview of published studies. Int J Cancer 1997;73:198–203.

English DR, Armstrong BK, Kricker A, Winter MG, Heenan PJ, Randell PL. Case-control study of sun exposure and SCC of the skin. Int J Cancer 1998;77:347–53.

Fan H, Oro AE, Scott MP, Khavari PA. Induction of basal cell carcinoma features in transgenic human skin expressing Sonic Hedgehog. Nat Med 1997;3:788–92.

Feltkamp MC, Broer R, di Summa FM et al. Seroreactivity to epidermodysplasia verruciformis-related human papillomavirus types is associated with nonmelanoma skin cancer. Cancer Res 2003;63:2695–2700.

Feskanich D, Hunter DJ, Willett WC, Spiegelman D, Stampfer MJ, Speizer FE, et al. Oral contraceptive use and risk of melanoma in premenopausal women. Br J Cancer 1999; 81:918–23.

Fountain JW, Karayiorgou M, Ernstoff MS, Kirkwood JM, Vlock DR, Titus-Ernstoff L,

et al. Homozygous deletions within human chromosome band 9p21 in melanoma, Proc Natl Acad Sci USA 1992;89:10557–61.

Franceschi S, Levi F, Randimbison L, La Vecchia C. Site distribution of different types of skin cancer: new etiological clues. Int J Cancer 1996;67:24–28.

Freedman DM, Sigurdson A, Doody MM, Mabuchi K, Linet MS. Risk of Basal Cell Carcinoma in Relation to Alcohol Intake and Smoking. Cancer Epidemiol Biomarkers Prev 2003a;12:1540—43.

Freedman DM, Sigurdson A, Doody MM, Rao RS, Linet MS. Risk of melanoma in relation to smoking, alcohol intake, and other factors in a large occupational cohort. Cancer Causes Control 2003b;14:847–57.

Frieling U, Schaumberg D, Kupper T, Muntwyler J, Hennekens C. A randomized, 12-year primary-prevention trial of beta carotene supplementation for nonmelanoma skin cancer in the Physician's Health Study. Arch Dermatol 2000;136:179–84.

Frost C, Green A, Williams G. The prevalence and determinants of solar keratoses at a subtropical latitude. Br J Dermatol 1998; 139:1033–39.

Fung TT, Hunter DJ, Spiegelman D, G.A Colditz, Rimm EB, Willet WC. Intake of alcohol and alcoholic beverages and the risk of basal cell carcinoma of the skin. Cancer Epidemiol Biomarkers Prev 2002;11:1119–22.

Gallagher RP, Elwood JM, Hill GB, Coldman AJ, Threlfall WJ, Spinelli JJ. Reproductive factors, oral contraceptives and risk of malignant melanoma: Western Canada Melanoma Study. Br J Cancer 1985;52:901–7.

Gallagher RP, Elwood JM, Hill GB. Risk factors for cutaneous malignant melanoma: the Western Canada Melanoma Study. Recent Results Cancer Res 1986;102:38–55.

Gallus S, Naldi L, Martin L, Martinelli M, La Vecchia C. Anthropometric measures and risk of cutaneous malignant melanoma: a case-control study from Italy. Melanoma Res 2006;16:83–87.

Gawkrodger DJ. Occupational skin cancers. Occ Med 2004; 54:458–63.

Gefeller O, Hassan K, Wille L. Cutaneous malignant melanoma in women and the role of oral contraceptives. Br J Dermatol 1998;138: 122–24.

Goldstein AM, Pastakia B, DiGiovanna JJ, Poliak S, Santucci S, Kase R, et al. Clinical findings in two African-American families with the nevoid basal cell carcinoma syndrome (NBCC). Am J Med Genet 1994;50: 272–81.

Gorlin RJ. Nevoid basal cell carcinoma (Gorlin) syndrome. Genet Med 2004;6:530–39.

Green A, Bain C, McLennan R, Siskind V. Risk factors for cutaneous melanoma in Queensland. Recent Results Cancer Res 1986;102: 76–97.

Green A, Bain C. Hormonal factors and melanoma in women. Med J Aust 1985;142: 446–48.

Green A, Battistutta D, Hart V, Leslie D, Weedon D, Nambour Study Group. Skin cancer in a subtropical Australian population: incidence and lack of association with occupation. Am J Epidemiol 1996;144: 1034–40.

Green A, MacLennan R, Youl P, Martin N. Site distribution of cutaneous melanoma in Queensland. Int J Cancer 1993;53:232–36.

Green A, McCredie M, MacKie R, Giles G, Young P, Morton C, et al. A case-control study of melanomas of the soles and palms (Australia and Scotland). Cancer Causes Control 1999a;10:21–25.

Green A, Williams G, Neale R, Hart V, Leslie D, Parsons P, et al. Daily sunscreen application and beta-carotene supplementation in prevention of BCC and SCC of the skin: a randomised controlled trial. Lancet 1999b;354: 723–29.

Green AC, O'Rourke MGE. Cutaneous malignant melanoma in association with other skin cancers. J Natl Cancer Inst 1985;74: 977–80.

Greenberg E, Baron J, Stukel T, Stevens M, Mandel J, Spencer S, et al. A clinical trial of beta carotene to prevent basal-cell and squamous-cell cancers of the skin. N Engl J Med 1990;323:789–95.

Grodstein F, Speizer FE, Hunter DJ. A prospective study of incident squamous cell carcinoma of the skin in the nurses' health study. J Natl Cancer Inst 1995;87:1061–66.

Hakim IA, Harris RB, Ritenbaugh C. Fat intake and risk of squamous cell carcinoma of the skin. Nutrition and Cancer 2000;36:155–62.

Hall L, Struijk L, Neale R, Feltkamp MC. Human papillomavirus infection and incidence of squamous cell and basal cell carcinomas of the skin. JNCI 2006; 15: 529–35.

Han J, Kraft P, Colditz GA, Wong J, Hunter DJ. Melanocortin 1 receptor variants and skin cancer risk. Int J Cancer 2006a;119(8): 1976–84.

Han J, Colditz GA, Hunter DJ. Risk factors for skin cancers: a nested case-control study in the Nurses' Health Study. Int J Epidemiol 2006b:35:1514–21.

Harris RB, Griffith K, et al. Trends in the incidence of nonmelanoma skin cancers in southeastern Arizona, 1985–1996. J Am Acad Dermatol 2001;45:528–36.

Hayward NK. Genetics of melanoma predisposition. Oncogene 2003; 22: 3053–62.

High A, Zedan W. Basal cell nevus syndrome. Curr Opin Oncol 2005;17:160–66

Holly EA, Aston DA, Cress RD, Ahn DK, Kristiansen JJ. Cutaneous melanoma in women. II. Phenotypic characteristics and other host-related factors. Am J Epidemiol 1995;141: 934–42.

Holman CD, Armstrong BK, Heenan PJ. Cutaneous malignant melanoma in women: exogenous sex hormones and reproductive factors. Br J Cancer 1984;50:673–80.

Holman CD, Armstrong BK. Cutaneous malignant melanoma and indicators of total accumulated exposure to the sun: an analysis separating histogenetic types. J Natl Cancer Inst 1984;73:75–82.

Horenstein M, Diwan A. 2005. Xeroderma pigmentosum. E-medicine http://www .emedicine.com/DERM/topic462.htm.

Hughes MC, van der Pols JC, Marks GC, Green AC. 2006. Food intake and risk of squamous cell carcinoma of the skin in a community: the Nambour skin cancer cohort study. Int J Cancer 2006;119:1953–60.

Hunter DH, Colditz GA, Stampfer MJ, Rosner B, Willett WC, Speizer FE. Risk factors for basal cell carcinoma in a prospective cohort of women. Ann Epidemiol 1990;1:13–23.

Hussein MR, Roggero E, Tuthill RJ, Wood GS, Sudilovsky O. Identification of novel deletion loci at 1p36 and 9p22–21 in melanocytic dysplastic nevi and cutaneous malignant melanomas. Arch. Dermatol 2003;139:816– 17.

Ibiebele TI, van der Pols JC, Hughes MC, Marks GC, Williams GM, Green AC. Dietary pattern in association with squamous cell carcinoma of the skin: a prospective study. Am J Clin Nutr 2007;85:1401–8.

International Agency for Research on Cancer (IARC) Working Group on artificial ultraviolet (UV) light and skin cancer. The association of use of sunbeds with cutaneous malignant melanoma and other skin cancers: A systematic review. Int J Cancer 2007;120: 1116–22. Erratum in: Int J Cancer. 2007; 120:2526.

International Agency for Research on Cancer. IARC Monographs on the Evaluation of Carcinogenic Risks to Humans. Vol. 55, Solar and Ultraviolet Radiation. Lyon, IARC, 1992.

Jemal A, Siegel R, Ward E, Murray T, Xu J, Thun MJ. Cancer statistics, 2007. CA Cancer J Clin 2007;57(1):43–66.

Johnson TM, Rowe DE, Nelson BR, Swanson NA. Squamous cell carcinoma of the skin (excluding lip and oral mucosa). J Am Acad Dermatol 1992;26:467–84.

Kamb A, Shattuck-Eidens D, Eeles R, Liu Q, Gruis A, Ding W, et al. Analysis of the p16 gene CDKN2 as a candidate for the chromosome 9p melanoma susceptibility locus. Nature Genetics 1994;8:22–26.

Karagas MR, McDonald JA, Greenberg ER, Stukel TA, Weiss JE, Baron JA, et al. Role of basal cell and squamous cell skin cancers after ionizing radiation therapy. For The Skin Cancer Group. J Natl Cancer Inst 1996;88:1848–53.

Karagas MR, Nelson HH, Waterboer T, Stukel T, Andrew A, Green AC et al. Serologic evidence of human papillomaviruses and the incidence of squamous cell and basal cell carcinomas. J Nat Cancer Instit 2006b;98: 389–95.

Karagas MR, Stukel TA, Dykes J, Miglionico J, Greene MA, Carey M, et al. A pooled analysis of 10 case-control studies of melanoma and oral contraceptive use. Br J Cancer 2002;86:1085–92.

Karagas MR, Stukel TA, Greenberg ER, Baron JA, Mott LA, Stern RS. Risk of subsequent basal cell carcinoma and squamous cell carcinoma of the skin among patients with prior skin cancer. Skin Cancer Prevention Study Group. JAMA 1992;267:3305–10.

Karagas MR, Zens MS, Stukel TA, Swerdlow AJ, Rosso S, Osterlind A, et al. Pregnancy history and incidence of melanoma in women: a pooled analysis. Cancer Causes Control 2006a;17:11–19.

Kaskel P, Kind P, Sander S, Peter RU, Krähn G. Trauma and melanoma formation: a true association? Br J Dermatol 2000;143:749–53.

Kasper M, Regl G, Frischauf AM, Aberger F. GLI transcription factors: mediators of oncogenic Hedgehog signalling. Eur J Cancer 2006;42:437–45.

Katalinic A, Kunze U, et al. Epidemiology of cutaneous melanoma and non-melanoma skin cancer in Schleswig-Holstein, Germany: incidence, clinical subtypes, tumour stages and localization (epidemiology of skin cancer). Br J Dermatol 2003;149(6):1200–6.

Kirkpatrick CS, White E, Lee JA. Case-control study of malignant melanoma in Washington State. II. Diet, alcohol, and obesity. Am J Epidemiol 1994;139;869–80.

Kolmel KF, Gefeller O, Haferkamp B. Febrile infections and malignant melanoma: results of a case-control study. Melanoma Res 1992;2:207–11.

Kowal-Vern A, Criswell BK. Burn scar neoplasms: a literature review and statistical analysis. Burns 2005;31:403–13.

Kraemer KH, Lee MM, Andrews AD, Lambert WC. The role of sunlight and DNA repair in melanoma and nonmelanoma skin cancer. The xeroderma pigmentosum paradigm. Arch Dermatol 1994;130:1018–21.

Kricker A, Armstrong BK, English DR, Heenan PJ. Does intermittent sun exposure cause BCC? A case-control study in western Australia. Int J Cancer 1995;60:489–94.

Kricker A, Armstrong BK, English DR, Heenan PJ. Pigmentary and cutaneous risk factors for non-melanocytic skin cancer—a case-control study. Int J Cancer 1991;48:650–62.

Kruger K, Blume-Peytavi U, Orfanos CE. Basal cell carcinoma possibly originates from the outer root sheath and/or the bulge region of the vellus hair follicle. Arch Dermatol Res 1999; 291: 253–59.

Kune GA, Bannerman S, Field B, Watson LF, Cleland H, Merenstein D, et al. Diet, alcohol, smoking, serum beta-carotene, and vitamin A in male nonmelanocytic skin cancer patients and controls. Nutr Cancer. 1992;18: 237–44.

Lambe M, Thorn M, Sparen P, Bergstrom R, Adami HO. Malignant melanoma: reduced risk associated with early childbearing and multiparity. Melanoma Res 1996;6:147–53.

Lancaster HO. Some geographical aspects of the mortality from melanoma in Europeans. Med J Aust 1956;i:1082–87.

Le Marchand L, Saltzman BS, Hankin JH, Wilkens LR, Franke AA, Morris SJ, et al. Sun exposure, diet and melanoma in Hawaii Caucasians. Am J Epidemiol 2006 164(3): 232–45.

Lear JT, Heagerty AH, Smith A, Bowers B, Payne CR, Smith CA, et al. Multiple cutaneous basal cell carcinomas: glutathione S-transferase (GSTM1, GSTT1) and cytochrome P450 (CYP2D6, CYP1A1) polymorphisms influence tumour numbers and accrual. Carcinogenesis 1996;17:1891–96.

Lear JT, Tan BB, Smith AG, Bowers W, Jones PW, Heagerty AH, et al. Risk factors for basal cell carcinoma in the UK: case-control study in 806 patients. J R Soc Med 1997;90:371–74.

Lee EY, Williamson R, Watt P, Hughes MC, Green AC, Whiteman DC. Sun exposure and host phenotype as predictors of cutaneous melanoma associated with neval remnants or dermal elastosis. Int J Cancer 2006,119, 636–42.

Leslie KK, Espey E. Oral contraceptives and skin cancer: is there a link? Am J Clin Dermatol 2005;6:349–55.

Levi F, Moeckli R, Randimbison L, Te VC, Maspoli M, La Vecchia C. Skin cancer in survivors of childhood and adolescent cancer. Eur J Cancer 2006; 42:656–59.

Levi F, La-Vecchia C, Randimbison L, Te VC, Erler G. Incidence of invasive cancers following cutaneous malignant melanoma. Int J Cancer 1997a;72:776–79.

Levi F, Randimbison L, La-Vecchia C, Erler G, Te VC. Incidence of invasive cancers following squamous cell skin cancer. Am J Epidemiol 1997b;146:734–39.

Lindelof B, Sigurgeirsson B, Tegner E, Larko O, Johannesson A, Berne B, et al. PUVA and cancer risk: the Swedish follow-up study. Br J Dermatol 1999;141:108–12.

Liu W, Kelly JW, Trivett M, Murray WK, Dowling JP, Wolfe R, Mason G, Magee J, Angel C, Dobrovic A, McArthur GA. Distinct clinical and pathological features are associated with the BRAF(T1799A(V600E)) mutation in primary melanoma. J Invest Dermatol 2007;127:900–905

London NJ, Farmery SM, Will EJ, Davison AM, Lodge JPA. Risk of neoplasia in renal transplant patients. Lancet 1995;346:403–6.

Maitra SK, Gallo H, Rowland-Payne C, Robinson D, Moller H. Second primary cancers in patients with squamous cell carcinoma of the skin. Br J Cancer 2005;92:570–71.

Maldonado JL, Fridlyand J, Patel H, Jain AN, Busam K, Kageshita T, et al. Determinants of BRAF mutations in primary melanomas. J Natl Cancer Inst 2003;95:1878–90.

McBride P, Neale R, Pandeya N, Green A. Sun-related factors, beta papillomavirus and actinic keratoses: a prospective study. Arch Dermatol 2007;143:862–68.

McCormack CJ, Kelly JW, Dorevitch AP. Differences in age and body site distribution of the histological subtypes of basal cell carcinoma. A possible indicator of differing causes. Arch Dermatol 1997;133:593–96.

McGovern VJ. Melanoblastoma. Med J Aust 1952;i:139–42.

McNaughton SA, Marks GC, Green AC. Role of dietary factors in the development of basal cell cancer and squamous cell cancer of the skin. Cancer Epidemiol Biomarkers Prev 2005;14:1596–1607.

Meyskens FL, Jr., Farmer PJ, Anton-Culver H. Diet and melanoma in a case-control study. Cancer Epidemiol Biomarkers Prev 2005;14:293.

Milan T, Verkasalo PK, Kaprio J, Koskenvuo M. Lifestyle differences in twin pairs discordant for basal cell carcinoma of the skin. Br J Dermatol 2003;149:115–23.

Millen AE, Tucker MA, Hartge P, Halpern A, Elder DE, Guerry Dt, et al. Diet and melanoma in a case-control study. Cancer Epidemiol Biomarkers Prev 2004;13:1042–51.

Moller H, Mellemgaard A, Lindvig K, Olsen JH. Obesity and cancer risk: a Danish record-linkage study. Eur J Cancer 1994;30A:344–50.

Moore S, Johnson N, Pierce A, Wilson D. The epidemiology of lip cancer: a review of global incidence and etiology. Oral Dis 1999; 5:185–95.

Naldi L, Altieri A, Imberti GL, Giordano L, Gallus S, La Vecchia C. Cutaneous malignant melanoma in women. Phenotypic characteristics, sun exposure, and hormonal factors: a case-control study from Italy. Ann Epidemiol 2005;15:545–50.

Naldi L, Gallus S, Tavani A, Imberti GL, La Vecchia C. Risk of melanoma and vitamin A, coffee and alcohol: a case-control study from Italy. Eur J Cancer Prev 2004;13:503–8.

Nancarrow DJ, Mann GJ, Holland EA, Walker GJ, Beaton SC, Walters MK, et al. Confirmation of chromosome 9p linkage in familial melanoma. Am J Hum Genet 1993; 53:936–42.

Neale RE, Darlington S, Murphy MF, Silcocks PB, Purdie DM, Talback M. The effects of twins, parity and age at first birth on cancer risk in Swedish women. Twin Res Hum Genet 2005;8:156–62.

Neale RE, Batista M, Pandeya N, Whiteman DC, Green AC. Basal cell carcinoma on the trunk is associated with excessive sun exposure. J Am Acad Dermatol 2007; 56: 380–86.

Nelemans PJ, Groenendal H, Kiemeney LA, Rampen FH, Ruiter DJ, Verbeek AL. Effect of intermittent exposure to sunlight on melanoma risk among indoor workers and sun-sensitive individuals. Environ Health Perspect 1993;101:252–55.

Odenbro A, Bellocco R, Boffetta P, Lindelof B, Adami J. Tobacco smoking, snuff dipping and the risk of cutaneous squamous cell carcinoma: a nationwide cohort study in Sweden. Br J Cancer 2005;92:1326–28.

Oh SW, Yoon YS, Shin SA. Effects of excess weight on cancer incidences depending on cancer sites and histologic findings among men: Korea National Health Insurance Corporation Study. J Clin Oncol 2005;23:4742–54.

Olsen CM, Hughes MC, Pandeya N, Green AC. Anthropometric measures in relation to Basal Cell Carcinoma: a longitudinal study. BMC Cancer 2006;6:82.

Olsen CM, Green AC, Zens MS, Stukel TA, Bataille V, Berwick M, Elwood JM, Gallagher R, Holly EA, Kirkpatrick C, Mack T, Osterlind A, Rosso S, Swerdlow AJ, Karagas MR. Anthropometric factors and risk of melanoma in women: a pooled analysis. Int J Cancer, *In Press*

Orth G, Favre M, Breitburd F. Epidermodysplasia verruciformis: a model for the role of papillomaviruses in human cancer. In: Essex M, Todaro G, zur Hausen H (Eds): Viruses in Naturally Occurring Cancers. Vol. 7. Cold Spring Harbor, NY, Cold Spring Harbor Laboratory, 1980, pp 259–82.

Osterlind A, Tucker MA, Stone BJ, Jensen OM. The Danish case-control study of cutaneous malignant melanoma. III. Hormonal and reproductive factors in women. Int J Cancer 1988;42:821–24.

Palmer JS, Duffy DL, Box NF, Aitken JF, O'Gorman LE, Green AC, et al. MC1R polymorphisms and risk of melanoma: is the association explained solely by pigmentation phenotype? Am J Hum Genet 2000;66: 176–86.

Pfahlberg A, Hassan K, Wille L, Lausen B, Gefeller O. Systematic review of case-control studies: oral contraceptives show no effect on melanoma risk. Public Health Rev 1997; 25:309–15.

Pfister H. Chapter 8: Human papillomavirus and skin cancer. J Nat Cancer Inst Mongraphs 2003;31:52–56.

Platz A, Hansson J, Ringborg U. Screening of germline mutations in the CDK4, CDKN2C and TP53 genes in familial melanoma: a clinic-based population study. Int J Cancer 1998;78:13–15.

Pollock PM, Welch J, Hayward NK. Evidence for three tumor suppressor loci on chromosome 9p involved in melanoma development. Cancer Res 2001;61:1154–61.

Pollock PM, Yu F, Qiu L, Parsons PG, Hayward NK. Evidence for UV induction of CDKN2 mutations in melanoma cell lines. Oncogene 1995;11:663–68.

Ramachandran S, Hoban PR, Ichii-Jones F, Pleasants L, Ali-Osman F, Lear JT, et al. Glutathione S-transferase GSTP1 and cyclin D1 genotypes: association with numbers of basal cell carcinomas in a patient subgroup at high-risk of multiple tumours. Pharmacogenetics 2000;10:545–56.

Rebel H, Kram N, Westerman A, Banus S, van Kranen HJ, de Gruijl FR. Relationship between UV-induced mutant p53 patches and skin tumours, analysed by mutation spectra and by induction kinetics in various DNA-repair-deficient mice. Carcinogenesis 2005; 26:2123–30.

Regl G, Neill GW, Eichberger T, Kasper M, Ikram MS, Koller J, et al. Human GLI2 and GLI1 are part of a positive feedback mechanism in Basal Cell Carcinoma. Oncogene 2002;21:5529–39.

Reifenberger J, Wolter M, Knobbe CB, Kohler B, Schonicke A, Scharwachter C, et al. Somatic mutations in the PTCH, SMOH, SUFUH and TP53 genes in sporadic basal cell carcinomas. Br J Dermatol 2005;152:43–51.

Reymann F, Moller R, Nielsen A. Relationship between arsenic intake and internal malignant neoplasms. Arch Dermatol 1978;114: 378–81.

Rhodes LE, Shahbakhti H, Azurdia RM, Moison RMW, Steenwinkel M, Homburg MI, et al. Effect of eicosapentaenoic acid, an omega-3 polyunsaturated fatty acid, on UVR-related cancer risk in humans. An assessment of early genotoxic markers. Carcinogenesis 2003;24:919–25.

Rokuhara S, Saida T, Oguchi M, Matsumoto K, Murase S, Oguchi S. Number of acquired melanocytic nevi in patients with melanoma and control subjects in Japan: Nevus count is a significant risk factor for nonacral melanoma but not for acral melanoma. J Am Acad Dermatol 2004;50:695–700.

Rolon PA, Kramarova E, Rolon HI, Khlat M, Parkin DM. Plantar melanoma: a case-control study in Paraguay. Cancer Causes Control 1997;8:850–56.

Ron E, Preston DL, Kishikawa M, Kobuke T, Iseki M, Tokuoka S, et al. Skin tumor risk among atomic-bomb survivors in Japan. Cancer Causes Control 1998;9:393–401.

Rosso S, Zanetti R, Martinez C, Tormo MJ, Schraub S, Sancho-Garnier H, et al. The multicentre south Euoropean study 'Helios' II: different sun exposure patterns in the etiology of basal cell and squamous cell carcinomas of the skin. Br J Cancer 1996;73: 1447–54.

Sahl WJ, Glore S, Garrison P, Oakleaf K, Johnson SD. Basal cell carcinoma and lifestyle characteristics. Int J Dermatol 1995;34:398–402.

Samanic C, Gridley G, Chow WH, Lubin J, Hoover RN, Fraumeni JF, Jr. Obesity and cancer risk among white and black United States veterans. Cancer Causes Control 2004;15:35–43.

Schnohr P. Gronbaek M. Petersen L. Hein HO. Sorensen TI. Physical activity in leisure-time and risk of cancer: 14-year follow-up of 28,000 Danish men and women. Scandinavian Journal of Public Health 2005;33: 244–49.

Skender-Kalnenas TM, English DR, Heenan PJ. Benign melanocytic lesions: risk markers or precursors of cutaneous melanoma? J Am Acad Dermatol 1995, 33.1000–1007.

Smith MA, Fine JA, Barnhill RL, Berwick M. Hormonal and reproductive influences and risk of melanoma in women. Int J Epidemiol 1998;27:751–57.

Soderholm AL, Pukkala E, Lindqvist C, Teppo L. Risk of new primary cancer in patients with oropharyngeal cancer. Br J Cancer 1994;69:784–87.

Soleas GJ, Grass L, Josephy PD, Goldberg DM, Diamandis EP. A comparison of the anticarcinogenic properties of four red wine polyphenols. Clin. Biochem 2002;35:119–24.

Sorensen HT, Mellemkjaer L, Nielsen GL, Baron JA, Olsen JH, Karagas MR. Skin cancers and non-hodgkin lymphoma among users of systemic glucocorticoids: a population-based cohort study. J Natl Cancer Inst 2004;96:709–11.

Spatz A, Giglia-Mari G, Benhamou S, Sarasin A. Association between DNA repair-deficiency and high level of p53 mutations in melanoma of Xeroderma pigmentosum. Cancer Res 2001;61:2480–86.

Staples, M. P., M. Elwood, et al. Non-melanoma skin cancer in Australia: the 2002 national survey and trends since 1985. Med J Aust 2006;184(1): 6–10.

Struijk L, Hall L, van der Meijden E, Wanningen P, Bouwes Bavinck J-Nico, Neale R et al. Prevalence of cutaneous human papillomavirus infections in people with tumor-free skin, actinic keratoses and squamous cell carcinoma. Cancer Epidem Biomark Prev 2006;15:529–35.

Sturm RA, Duffy DL, Box NF, Chen W, Smit DJ, Brown DL et al. The role of melanocortin-1 receptor polymorphism in skin cancer risk phenotypes. Pigment Cell Res 2003;16:266–72.

Swerdlow A, Cooke KR, Skegg DCG, Wilkinson J. Cancer incidence in England and Wales and New Zealand and in migrants between the two countries. Br J Cancer 1995b;72:236–43.

Swerdlow AJ, Storm HH, Sasieni PD. Risks of second primary malignancy in patients with cutaneous and ocular melanoma in Denmark, 1943–1989. Int J Cancer 1995a;61:773–79.

Swetter SM, Boldrick JC, et al. Increasing incidence of lentigo maligna melanoma subtypes: northern California and national trends 1990–2000. J Invest Dermatol 2005;125(4):685–91.

Teh MT, Blaydon D, Chaplin T, Foot NJ, Skoulakis S, Raghavan M, et al. 2005. Genomewide single nucleotide polymorphism microarray mapping in basal cell carcinomas unvcils uniparental disomy as a key somatic event. Cancer Res 65:8597–603.

Thomas NE, Alexander A, Edmiston SN, Parrish E, Millikan RC, Berwick M, et al. Tandem BRAF mutations in primary invasive melanomas. J Invest Dermatol 2004;122:1245–50.

Thune I, Olsen A, Albrektsen G, Tretli S. Cutaneous malignant melanoma: association with height, weight and body-surface area. a prospective study in Norway. Int J Cancer 1993;55:555–61.

Tilli CM, Van Steensel MA, Krekels GA, Neumann HA, Ramaekers FC. Molecular aetiology and pathogenesis of basal cell carcinoma. Br J Dermatol 2005;152:1108–24.

van Dam RM, Huang Z, Giovannucci E, Rimm EB, Hunter DJ, Colditz GA, et al. Diet and basal cell carcinoma of the skin in a prospective cohort of men. Am J Clin Nutr 2000;71:135–41.

van Dam RM, Huang Z, Rimm EB, Weinstock MA, Spiegelman D, Colditz GA, et al. Risk factors for basal cell carcinoma of the skin in men: results from the health professionals follow-up study. Am J Epidemiol 1999;50:459–68.

Wang JX, Boice JD Jr, Li BX, Fraumeni JF Jr. Cancer among medical diagnostic X-ray workers in China. J Natl Cancer Inst 1988;80:344–50.

Veierod MB, Thelle DS, Laake P. Diet and risk of cutaneous malignant melanoma: a prospective study of 50,757 Norwegian men and women. Int J Cancer 1997;71:600–4.

Veierod MB, Weiderpass E, Thorn M, Hansson J, Lund E, Armstrong B, et al. A prospective study of pigmentation, sun exposure, and risk of cutaneous malignant melanoma in women. J Natl Cancer Inst 2003;95:1530–38.

Weinstock MA, Stampfer MJ, Lew RA, Willett WC, Sober AJ. Case-Control Study of Melanoma and Dietary Vitamin-D—Implications for Advocacy of Sun Protection and Sunscreen Use. Journal of Investigative Dermatology 1992;98:809–11.

Westerdahl J, Olsson H, Masback A, Ingvar C, Jonsson N. Risk of malignant melanoma in relation to drug intake, alcohol, smoking and hormonal factors. Br J Cancer 1996;73:1126–31.

Whiteman DC, Green A, Parson PG. p53 expression and risk factors for cutaneous melanoma: a case-control study. Int J Cancer 1998;77:843–48.

Whiteman DC, Green AC. Melanoma and sun exposure: where are we now? Int J Dermatol 1999;38:481–89.

Whiteman DC, Stickley M, Watt P, Hughes MC, Green AC. Melanomas of the head and trunk have different associations with chronic and intermittent patterns of sun exposure. J Clin Oncol 2006;24:3172–77.

Whiteman DC, Watt P, Purdie DM, Balajadia-Hughes M-C, Green AC. Melanocytic nevi, actinic keratoses and the origins of cutaneous melanoma. J Nat Cancer Instit 2003;95:806–12.

Whiteman DC, Whiteman CA, Green AC. Childhood sun exposure as a risk factor for melanoma: a systematic review of epidemiologic studies. Cancer Causes Control 2001;12:69–82.

Wilkinson GS. Invited commentary: are low radiation doses or occupational exposures really risk factors for malignant melanoma. Am J Epidemiol 1997;145:532–35.

Vinceti M, Pellacani G, Malagoli C, Bassissi S, Sieri S, Bonvicini F, et al. A population-based case-control study of diet and melanoma risk in northern Italy. Public Health Nutr 2005;8:1307–14.

Wolk A, Gridley G, Svensson M, Nyren O, McLaughlin JK, Fraumeni JF, et al. A prospective study of obesity and cancer risk (Sweden). Cancer Causes Control 2001; 12:13–21.

Wong SS, Tan KC, Goh CL. Cutaneous manifestations of chronic arsenicism: review of seventeen cases. J Am Acad Dermatol 1998; 38:179–85.

Xie J, Murone M, Luoh SM, Ryan A, Gu Q, Zhang C, et al. Activating Smoothened mutations in sporadic basal-cell carcinoma. Nature 1998;391:90–92.

Yoshinaga S, Hauptmann M, Sigurdson AJ, Doody MM, Freedman DM. Alexander BH, et al. Nonmelanoma skin cancer in relation to ionizing radiation exposure among US radiologic technologists. Int J Cancer 2005; 115:828–34.

Zanetti R, Rosso S, Martinez C, Nieto A, Miranda A, Mercier M, et al. Comparison of risk patterns in carcinoma and melanoma of the skin in men: a multi-centre case-case-control study. British Journal of Cancer 2006;94:743–51.

16

Breast Cancer

SUSAN HANKINSON, RULLA TAMIMI,
AND DAVID HUNTER

Breast cancer has probably attracted more scientific interest among epidemiologists than any other malignancy. The profound importance of reproductive factors was first revealed in the eighteenth century, when the Italian researcher Ramazzini noted that breast cancer was more common among nuns than among other women. During the last decades of the twentieth century, thousands of research papers described in increasing detail the associations between a woman's reproductive life and her risk of developing breast cancer. In addition, large natural experiments on breast cancer risk began when oral contraceptives came into wide use in the 1960s, and later on when an increasing proportion of women began using postmenopausal hormone replacement therapy. During the 1990s, accumulating evidence that a woman's risk may be influenced even in utero further complicated our view of the breast cancer mechanism. Yet the wealth of available epidemiologic information can be synthesized into a consistent and testable, albeit still hypothetical, causal model.

CLINICAL SYNOPSIS

Subgroups

Virtually all breast cancers are adenocarcinomas. In general clinical practice, the distinction between different histopathologic types has limited implications for either diagnosis or treatment. Cancer in situ of the breast, notably the ductal (but not the lobular) type, is now detected more often due to widespread use of mammography. The etiology and natural history of in situ lesions and their relation to invasive cancer are largely unknown. Therefore, this chapter focuses on invasive cancer only.

Symptoms

Formerly, a palpable tumor was the most common initial symptom. Occasionally, however, changes in the nipple or spread to axillary lymph nodes or distant metastases, often in the lung or bone, prompted a consultation. Today many breast cancers are diagnosed before symptoms occur by means of mammography.

Diagnostic Methods

When breast cancer is suspected on the basis of clinical examination or mammography, pathologic confirmation is a necessary prelude to definitive primary treatment. Fine needle aspiration, core biopsy, or surgical excision can be used to establish the diagnosis. Sometimes a frozen section examination of a surgical biopsy specimen allows definite local treatment during the same period of anesthesia.

Treatment

Until the early 1980s, extensive surgical removal of the breast and regional lymph nodes was believed to improve both local tumor control and long-term cure. Accumulating scientific data, mostly from clinical trials, has forced a radical rethinking. Today, breast-conserving surgery is used increasingly in combination with postoperative radiation therapy, which limits local recurrences. Moreover, adjuvant treatment with chemotherapy or tamoxifen, an anti-estrogen, has become part of routine treatment. The most recent clinical guidelines are now recommending the inclusion of aromatase inihibtors as an initial therapy, or after tamoxifen therapy, for postmenopausal women with estrogen receptor positive (ER+) breast cancer.

Prognosis

In the United States, overall 5-year relative survival among women diagnosed between 1986 and 1993 was 84.2%, although it was substantially higher among white (85.3%) than among black (70.0%) breast cancer patients. In Europe, corresponding rates were consistently lower, on average about 70%.

Progress

Randomized, controlled trials have documented that breast cancer mortality can be reduced by early detection through mammography screening and by adjuvant systemic treatment following primary surgery. Increasing public awareness may also have contributed to earlier clinical diagnosis. Thanks to an improved prognosis, breast cancer mortality has remained fairly stable in many settings despite increasing incidence. Starting in the 1990s, breast cancer mortality began to decline both in the United States and in some European countries.

DESCRIPTIVE EPIDEMIOLOGY

Breast cancer is the most commonly occurring cancer in women, with an estimated 1.05 million cases newly diagnosed worldwide in 2000 (Parkin et al, 2001). Overall, breast cancer accounts for 21% of all cancer diagnoses in women.

The shape of the age-incidence curves is generally similar across countries, but with big differences in the absolute rates at every age (Fig. 16–1). Overall, rates increase substantially with increasing age. The diagnosis is rare in women under 40 years of age. In the United States, incidence rates per 100 000 women are 25 in the 30 to 34 age group, 200 in the 40 to 45 age group, and 463 in the 70 to 74 age group (National Center for Health Statistics, 1998). Of note, the rapid rise in rates with increasing age slows somewhat around age 50, near the time of menopause, which strongly suggests a role for reproductive hormones in the etiology of the disease.

There is a four- to fivefold variation in rates worldwide, with the highest rates observed in Europe and North America and the lowest rates in Asia (Fig. 16–2). Migrant studies, in which changes in breast cancer rates are evaluated in women who move from low- to high-risk countries—or vice versa—have shown that the rates of the host country are assumed over time, frequently one or two generations later (Tominaga, 1985; Ziegler et al, 1993). These data indicate that international differences in breast cancer rates are due, at least in part, to environmental and lifestyle differences.

Data from an ongoing cancer registry in the state of Connecticut begun in 1930 show that breast cancer rates have been steadily increasing, approximately 1.2% per year, since the 1930s, with a more marked increase in the 1980s (White et al, 1990; Devesa et al, 1995). The reasons for this

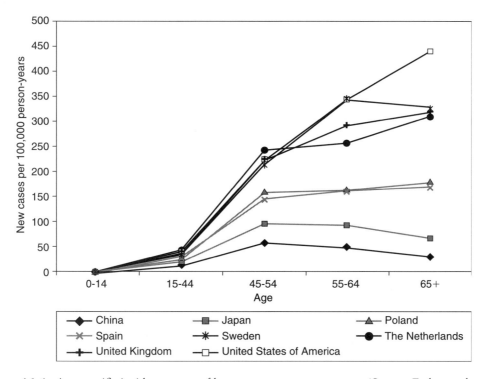

Figure 16–1. Age-specific incidence rates of breast cancer among women. (*Source*: Ferlay et al, 2004)

increase are unclear, although changes in reproductive patterns and other lifestyle factors—for example, increasing obesity in postmenopausal women and use of post-menopausal hormones—almost certainly have played an important role. Much of the increase in rates in the 1980s was attributable to increased diagnosis of small (≤ 2 cm), localized breast tumors. This finding, along with a subsequent decrease in cancer mortality in white women in the United States, indicates that the growing use of screening mammography—leading to earlier detection of preexisting cancer—most certainly played a major role. Since the 1950s, breast cancer rates have been increasing in a number of other countries as well, including low-risk countries such as China (Jin et al, 1993), Japan (Nagata et al, 1997), and Singapore (Chia et al, 2005). Changes in reproductive patterns, along with dramatic changes in other aspects of lifestyle such as diet and physical activity, likely account for much of this increase.

GENETIC AND MOLECULAR EPIDEMIOLOGY

Inherited Susceptibility

High-penetrance gene mutations

A family history of breast cancer in a first-degree relative is an established risk factor. A relative risk of 1.5–3.0 has generally been found when women whose mother or sister had breast cancer are compared to those whose first-degree female relatives did not have breast cancer (Greene, 1997). Among women whose mother and sister had breast cancer, particularly with an early age at onset, the risk is substantially higher.

It is estimated that 5% to 10% of all breast cancers can be attributed to highly penetrant germline mutations (Bennett et al, 1999). This proportion varies by age, with about one-third of breast cancer cases in women younger than 30 years of age attributed to inherited factors (Ellisen and Haber, 1998). Breast cancer gene 1 (*BRCA1*), located on chromosome 17q21, was identified

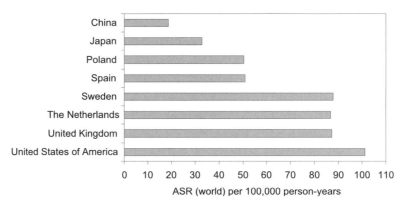

Figure 16–2. Age-standardized (to the world population) incidence rates of breast cancer among women. (*Source*: Ferlay et al, 2004)

in 1994 (Ellisen and Haber, 1998). Two years later *BRCA2*, located on chromosome 13q12–13, was identified. Accumulating evidence suggests that BRCA1 functions in cell-cycle control, genetic stability, and repair of DNA damage (Deng, 2006). A mutation in at least one of these genes is estimated to cause 2% to 5% of all breast cancers, with the highest frequency in those with multiply affected first-degree relatives and early onset of disease. Up to age 40, women with *BRCA1* are estimated to have a 20-fold greater risk of breast cancer compared to the general population and to have a lifetime risk of breast cancer of 60% to 85% (Ellisen and Haber, 1998). Factors that modify penetrance most strongly appear to be reproductive factors and exogenous hormones (Narod, 2006). Estimates of the prevalence of *BRCA1* or *BRCA2* mutations in the general population range from 1/200 to 1/1000 (Ellisen and Haber, 1998). *BRCA1* and *BRCA2* founder populations have been identified among the Ashkenazi Jews and Icelanders, respectively (Greene, 1997). Among Ashkenazi Jews, the prevalence of either mutation is estimated to be as high as 1 in 44.

The tumor-suppressor gene *P53* is associated with hereditary breast cancer. Breast cancer is one of several cancers that can occur in women with the rare Li-Fraumeni familial cancer syndrome, which is linked to mutations in *P53* (Ellisen and Haber, 1998).

Germline mutations in *P53* have low prevalence in the general population (< 1%) and are thus responsible for few breast cancers (Greene, 1997; Bennett et al, 1999). However, *P53* mutations may also play a role in tumor progression, independent of predisposition, since somatic mutations have been found in 50% of sporadic breast cancers (Ellisen and Haber, 1998).

By age 50, 30% to 50% of women with Cowden's disease—also called multiple hamartoma syndrome—develop breast cancer, including bilateral cancer (Bennett et al, 1999). The *PTEN* gene (phosphatase and tensin homologue deleted on chromosome 10), which is responsible for this disease, is located on chromosome 10q23 (Greene, 1997) and has an autosomal dominant inheritance pattern. PTEN functions as a tumor-suppressor gene, and it participates in intracellular signalling and control of cell division.

Ataxia-telangiectasia (AT) is inherited in an autosomal recessive pattern; homozygotes experience a range of severe, progressive neurologic and immunologic effects. An estimated 1.4% of the general population are heterozygotes (Greene, 1997; Warmuth et al, 1997; Bennett et al, 1999), with a markedly increased susceptibility to DNA damage through ionizing radiation, chemotherapy, or hydroxy radicals. Female relatives of children with homozygous *AT* mutations have a four- to sevenfold higher risk of breast cancer than controls who are not genetically related to the children (Ellisen and Haber, 1998; Bennett et al, 1999). In a meta-analysis of four studies, the relative risk of breast cancer was 3.9 (95% CI, 2.1–7.2) among heterozygotes (Greene, 1997; Sellers, 1997).

Low-penetrance polymorphisms
Hundreds of papers have now been published on associations between common (>5% allele frequency) polymorphisms and breast cancer risk. Most of these have focused on polymorphic variation in carcinogen-metabolizing genes or genes in the steroid metabolism pathways or receptor families. Other candidate genes include those in the growth factor, cell-cycle, apoptosis, and inflammation pathways. Due to the small to modest predicted relative risks, and the comparatively small sample sizes of most studies, most initial reports have not been replicated (Dunning et al, 1999). Publication bias also mitigates against the rapid publication of null reports following up on positive studies. It seems likely that formation of Consortia such as the Breast Cancer Association Consortium (Breast Cancer Association Consortium, 2006), the Genetic Susceptibility to Environmental Carcinogens Database (Paracchini et al, 2006), and the Breast & Prostate Cancer Cohort Consortium (Hunter et al, 2005), will help in the large-scale replication of candidate gene variants, and exploration of gene–environment interactions. The development of genome-wide association studies will provide an unbiased test of association at multiple (>500 000 on the current generation of "SNP chips") loci, and introduce some order into the search for low-penetrance alleles, although the challenges of replication are formidable due to the unprecedented multiple comparisons problem inherent in this approach (Hirschhorn and Daly, 2005).

HRAS1 and CHEK2 are two polymorphic genes that are exceptions in that data are quite consistent in showing an association with breast cancer. The *HRAS1* proto-oncogene, located on chromosome 11p15.5, is highly polymorphic, with a varying number of tandem nucleotide repeats (Greene, 1997; Ellisen and Haber, 1998). Mutant alleles are present in approximately 6% of the general population (Ellisen and Haber, 1998). The functional significance of the rare alleles has not been determined. In a meta-analysis of 23 studies, the rare *HRAS* alleles were associated with a significant 70% increase in breast cancer incidence (Krontiris et al, 1993). However, a large nested case-control study in which cases (n = 717) and controls (n = 798) arose from the same population found no overall association between rare alleles of the HRAS gene and breast cancer (Tamimi et al, 2003).

A rare variant (~1.1%) identified in the *CHEK2* gene has been reported to confer a 1.5-fold to 2.0-fold increase in breast cancer risk in individuals that carry this allele (Meijers-Heijboer et al, 2002; CHEK2 Breast Cancer Case-Control Consortium, 2004). CHEK2 is a tumor-suppressor gene. The 1100delC polymorphism leads to a truncated protein, in which kinase activity of the protein is abolished. To date, this is the first polymorphism to be successfully confirmed with strong statistical power. Additional confirmation of these results and identification of additional genes conferring modest risk will lend further support to a polygenic model of breast cancer risk, in which it is hypothesized that as many as 100 genes may confer a small amount of risk individually—yet in combination, this would result in modest susceptibility to breast cancer.

Recently, two genome-wide association studies identified a breast cancer susceptibility locus in *FGFR2* (Easton et al, 2007; Hunter et al, 2007). *FGFR2*, fibroblast growth factor receptor 2, encodes a receptor tyrosine kinase that is amplified and over-expressed in breast cancers. Additional work will be necessary to identify the causal variant at this locus. Relative to homozygotes with the wild type allele, the SNPs in *FGFR2* most strongly associated with breast cancer conferred a 20% increased risk of breast cancer among heterozygotes and a 60% increased risk among homozygotes with the variant allele (Easton et al, 2007; Hunter et al, 2007). Although this susceptibility locus confers a modest risk, the variant allele is common in the population and the population attributable risk is estimated to be 16% (Hunter et al, 2007).

RISK FACTORS

Tobacco

The relationship between cigarette smoking and breast cancer risk has been evaluated in many studies; overall, the data do not support any important association (Palmer and Rosenberg, 1993; Laden and Hunter, 1998). In the few studies that demonstrated an association, the increase in risk was generally modest (RR = 1.2–1.4), frequently with no dose–response relationship found. Although it is possible that any deleterious effects are more pronounced in persons exposed at a young age, study results have been inconsistent (Snedeker and Diaugustine, 1992; Laden and Hunter, 1998; Welp et al, 1998). However, among large, prospective studies, there is suggestive evidence of a positive association with long-term smoking prior to the first birth (Al-Delaimy et al, 2004; Reynolds et al, 2004; Gram et al, 2005). The Norwegian-Swedish Women's Lifestyle and Health Cohort Study of over 100 000 women found that women who initiated smoking during their teenage years and continued to smoke for 20 or more years were at an increased risk of breast cancer (comparing women who intitiated smoking before age 15 to never smokers RR = 1.48, 95% CI 1.03–2.13) (Gram et al, 2005). This association was not observed among women who smoked for 20+ years, but started smoking after their first birth. These results are consistent with the hypothesis that breast tissue is particularly susceptible to carcinogens between early puberty and the first full-term pregnancy (Russo et al, 1982).

Because secondhand smoke may contain more carcinogens than direct exposure due to the lack of filtration (Laden and Hunter, 1998), there has been some interest in evaluating passive-smoking exposure as a cause of breast cancer. In several case-control studies and one large cohort study of cancer mortality, either statistically significant yet modest or nonsignificant increases in risk have been observed; again, no dose–response relationship was seen. Although additional study is needed to resolve this issue, it is of limited public health importance because of the overwhelming evidence of the deleterious effects of cigarette smoking overall.

Diet

Fat intake

Overall, observational studies do not support any important relationship between total dietary fat intake in adulthood and the risk of breast cancer. However, the potential role of dietary fat intake in breast carcinogenesis has been of considerable interest over the last several decades, and hundreds of epidemiologic and laboratory studies have been conducted to evaluate the relationship. The interpretation of the results of these studies has been notably controversial, and these data will therefore be reviewed in some detail.

Animal studies and biological mechanisms. The interpretation of animal studies of high-fat diets in relation to mammary tumors has been controversial, in large part due to the difficulty of separating the effect of energy from that of fat intake per se. It is well established that high-calorie diets result in higher mammary tumor rates in animals (Hunter and Willett, 1993). Whether an independent effect of fat intake exists, after holding energy intake constant, is less clear (Stephen and Wald, 1990; Willett, 1998). In terms of biological mechanisms for an effect of fat intake on breast cancer risk, a number of studies have evaluated the influence of fat intake on circulating hormone levels. However, importantly, the majority did not have a concurrent control group, did not adequately account for changes in weight associated with the change in diet—important because lower weight is known to be associated with lower hormone levels—and were generally short-term. Thus, any effect of fat intake on hormone levels remains uncertain.

Descriptive data. The hypothesis that fat intake increases the risk of breast cancer was initially motivated by the strong international correlation between per capita fat intake and breast cancer mortality (Willett, 1998). Although this type of analysis is important as a first approach to evaluate differences in disease occurrence among countries, it is limited both by the quality of the data and by the inability to control for other possible risk factors. For example, the countries characterized by the lowest and highest breast cancer rates also tend to be the least and most economically developed, respectively. Hence, many factors that vary among those countries, such as age at first birth or body weight, could bias the observed association. In a second correlation study of fat intake and breast cancer incidence conducted in a number of counties within China—to make confounding less of a problem—the correlation was low (Chen et al, 1990).

Secular trends in fat intake and breast cancer risk within a country also have been assessed. Based on "food disappearance data"—which represent the amount of food available in a country and not the actual amount eaten—fat intake has increased in the United States over the last several decades, a period when breast cancer rates have increased by 1% to 2% per year. However, food disappearance data cannot account for food wastage, for example, if the amount of fat that individuals discard from their food, such as meat, varies over time. Better measures of total fat intake, based on estimates of individual intake from a number of epidemiologic studies, show that fat intake has actually decreased over the last several decades in the United States (Stephen and Wald, 1990).

Analytic epidemiologic studies. In a meta-analysis of 12 case-control studies including a total of 4312 cases and 5978 controls, the relative risk of breast cancer

for a 100-g increase in total fat intake was 1.35 overall and 1.48 among postmenopausal women (Howe et al, 1990). However, most women with a typical daily intake of 1600 to 1800 calories consume 50 to 80 g of fat daily, and a reduction of 100 g/day would not be possible. Based on a more realistic change in intake of 25 g of fat per day, the relative risk from the meta-analysis would be 1.08 overall and 1.10 for postmenopausal women. Relative risks of this magnitude could easily be due to bias, either related to differences between cases and controls in recalling past diet, or selection bias, or both. In another large case-control study, not included in the meta-analysis, no association with fat intake was seen (Graham et al, 1982).

In a pooled analysis of six prospective studies including 4980 cases among 337 819 women (Hunter et al, 1996), no association was noted for total fat intake; the relative risk associated with a 25 g/day increment in intake was 1.02 (Fig. 16–3). Long-standing concerns related to observational studies of this association were that fat intake could not be adequately assessed by means of a questionnaire—substantial measurement error would result in missing a true-positive association—and that the range of fat intake in the populations studied was too narrow and did not overlap the low intakes found in countries with the lowest breast cancer mortality rates. In each of the studies in the pooled analysis, a validation study was conducted among a subset of participants to allow an assessment of the validity of the reported diet. After using statistical methods to correct for the measurement error (using the validation data), the comparable relative risk for total fat was 1.07, suggesting, again, little if any association between fat intake and risk. In addition, the investigators were able to assess low fat intakes: Women obtaining less than 20% of their energy from fat were not observed to have a lower risk of breast cancer.

In a large-scale US randomized controlled trial—the Women's Health Initiative (WHI)—the effect of a low-fat dietary pattern on risk of breast cancer was evaluated. The

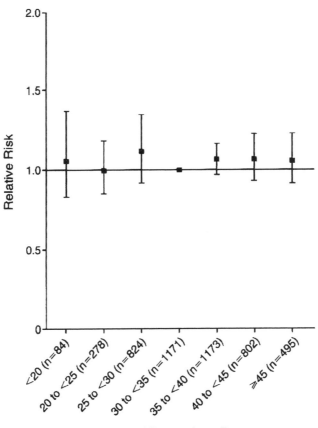

Figure 16–3. Pooled analyses: A level of 30% to less than 35% of total energy from fat was designated as the reference category, n denotes the number of cases in each category. Relative risks are adjusted for age at menarche, menopausal status, parity, age at birth of first child, body mass index, height, education, history of benign breast disease, maternal history of breast cancer in a sister, oral contraceptive use, fiber intake, alcohol intake, and energy intake. (*Source*: Hunter et al, 1996)

dietary intervention consisted of a low-fat (20% of calories), high-fruit and -vegetable (≥ 5 servings/day), and high-grain (≥ 6 servings/day) diet. After 8 years of follow-up, the dietary intervention group experienced a nonsignificant 9% lower incidence of breast cancer compared to the comparison group (RR = 0.91, 95% CI 0.83–1.01) (Prentice et al, 2006). These results suggest that short-term reductions in fat intake during the postmenopausal years do not reduce the risk of breast cancer. However, this does not preclude an association between fat intake earlier in life and subsequent breast cancer risk.

Fat subtypes have also been examined in a number of studies. In several case-control studies, intake of olive oil specifically was inversely related to breast cancer risk (Trichopoulou, 1995; Willett, 1998). Similarly, in one large prospective analysis, monounsaturated fats were inversely related to risk (Wolk et al, 1998), although this was not observed in the pooled analysis described previously (Hunter et al, 1996). In an updated pooled analysis of 7329 incident invasive breast cancer cases occurring among 351 821 women, the pooled relative risks (95% CI) for an increment of 5% of energy were 1.09 (1.00–1.19) for saturated fat,

0.93 (0.84–1.03) for monounsaturated fat, and 1.05 (0.96–1.16) for polyunsaturated fat compared with equivalent energy intake from carbohydrates (Smith-Warner et al, 2001a). Intake of olive oil specifically could not be addressed in the pooled analysis.

The relationship between total and specific subtypes of fat and fatty acids was evaluated in the Nurses' Health Study cohort (Holmes et al, 1999), a large study of 2956 cases that benefited from having dietary data collected four times over the 14 years of follow-up. Compared to women who obtained 30% to 35% of their energy from total fat, those obtaining less than 20% had a relative risk of 1.15 and those obtaining more than 50% of their energy from fat had a relative risk of 0.96. No substantial differences were found according to menopausal status or specific subtypes of fat (eg, saturated, polyunsaturated, transunsaturated fats).

In a similar cohort among largely premenopausal women, a weak positive association was observed for total fat that was due to a positive association with animal fat, but not vegetable fat (Cho et al, 2003). Women in the highest quintile of intake of animal fat intake were at 33% increased risk of breast cancer (RR = 1.33; 95% CI = 1.02 to 1.73; P-trend = 0.002). Intakes of both saturated and monounsaturated fat were related to modestly elevated breast cancer risk. Among food groups contributing to animal fat, red meat and high-fat dairy foods were each associated with an increased risk of breast cancer. Further assessment of fat subtypes, including monounsaturated fat and olive oil in particular, is needed.

Fiber intake

Fiber intake has been hypothesized to decrease the risk of breast cancer by inhibiting the intestinal reabsorption of estrogens secreted via the biliary tract, resulting in lower circulating estrogen levels. Epidemiologic studies have, however, not consistently supported such a relationship. In a meta-analysis of 10 case-control studies, dietary fiber intake was inversely associated with risk; the relative risk for a 20-g increment in fiber intake was 0.85 (Howe et al, 1990). However, in a number of large prospective studies (Willett, 2001), inverse associations have generally not been noted. It is important to recognize that *fiber* can be further divided into a number of subtypes—for example, soluble and insoluble. Data on the specific fiber content of individual foods have been limited, and the laboratory methods used to assess the fiber subtypes have been controversial. Until recently, these methodologic issues have limited our ability to evaluate fiber intake and breast cancer risk in detail, and further evaluations are therefore warranted.

Micronutrient intake

Of the micronutrients, the epidemiologic data most strongly support a protective role for vitamin A and the carotenoids, although the relationship appears modest in magnitude. Overall, the protective effect, if any, has been observed somewhat more consistently among premenopausal women.

Carotenoids and vitamin A. Vitamin A consists of both preformed vitamin A—that is, retinol, primarily from animal products—and several carotenoids, such as beta-carotene, which are found primarily in fruits and vegetables and can be converted to retinol. The carotenoids are well-established antioxidants and, as such, may protect against cellular and DNA damage caused by reactive oxygen species. Vitamin A is important in maintaining cellular differentiation and thus may help prevent the emergence of cells with a malignant phenotype.

In one of the first large case-control studies (Graham et al, 1982), a modest but significant 20% reduction in risk was noted between persons in the bottom and top quartiles of total vitamin A intake. In the pooled analysis of case-control studies (Howe et al, 1990), a similar association was noted that appeared to be somewhat stronger for carotenoids than for preformed vitamin A intake. Results of several prospective studies also support a modest protective association with vitamin A (Hunter and Willett, 1993; Zhang et al, 1999a).

In a population-based case-control study among premenopausal women (Freudenheim et al, 1996), an inverse association was noted with higher intakes of both beta-carotene and lutein/zeaxanthin. In the first large prospective study of specific dietary carotenoids (Zhang et al, 1999a), an inverse association of beta-carotene and lutein/zeaxanthin with the risk of breast cancer was noted in premenopausal but not in postmenopausal women. Premenopausal women in the top quintile of lutein/zeaxanthin intake (median intake = 8796 mg/day) had a 21% lower risk than women in the bottom quintile (median intake =1376 mg/day).

Micronutrients, specifically carotenoids, exhibit a great deal of interindividual variation in their absorption, metabolism, and excretion (Mathews-Roth, 1990; Stahl and Sies, 1992), therefore, plasma levels may give a more accurate measurement of the bioavailable amount of these nutrients than dietary intake estimates. Early studies, which focused on plasma beta-carotene and retinol and breast cancer were small and largely inconclusive (Wald et al, 1984; Willett et al, 1984; Coates et al, 1988; Knekt, 1988; Russell et al, 1988). More recently, four studies have prospectively evaluated other carotenoids including beta-carotene, alpha-carotene, lycopene, beta-cryptoxanthin, and lutein/zeaxanthin and tocopherols in relation to breast cancer risk (Dorgan et al, 1998; Toniolo et al, 2001; Sato et al, 2002). Although these studies were not consistent in terms of which carotenoid was inversely associated with breast cancer, in general, each of the studies reported an inverse association with at least one carotenoid. Because there is a high degree of collinearity between the different plasma carotenoids, it is difficult to conclude that any specific carotenoid is responsible for the observed inverse associations, but these findings do suggest that carotenoids in general are associated with a reduced risk of breast cancer.

Vitamin C. Vitamin C is an effective water-soluble antioxidant. This nutrient was noted to be inversely related to breast cancer risk in the pooled analysis of nine case-control studies (Howe et al, 1990); a significant 39% reduction in risk was noted for each 300 mg/day increase in vitamin C intake. This relationship has not been confirmed in a number of prospective studies (Hunter and Willett, 1993), even though a wide range of intake of vitamin C and extended durations of vitamin C supplement use were examined.

Vitamin E. Relatively few studies have evaluated the relationship between vitamin E intake and breast cancer, and in those that have, generally little if any association has been noted (Hunter and Willett, 1993). In a large prospective analysis (Zhang et al, 1999a), the relative risk for using specific vitamin E supplements for 10 or more years, compared to never-use, was 1.11. Similarly, no association was noted for vitamin E intake from food.

Selenium. Several studies have evaluated the relationship between selenium status (as measured in blood or toenails; Willett, 1998) and breast cancer risk because of selenium's important role in the function of the antioxidant enzyme glutathione peroxidase. In the largest study, one of about six prospective studies of this relationship, Hunter et al (1990) found no association between selenium and risk (RR = 0.9 for top versus bottom quintile comparison in toenail selenium levels). Most other case-control and cohort studies similarly found little evidence for an important protective effect of selenium.

Folate. Inadequate folate levels may result in abnormal DNA synthesis and disrupted DNA repair and hence may influence breast cancer risk. Several epidemiologic studies including three large prospective cohorts, the Nurses' Health Study (Zhang et al, 1999b; Zhang et al, 2003), the Canadian National Breast Screening Study (Rohan et al, 2000), and the Iowa Women's Health Study (Sellers et al, 2001), suggest that adequate folate levels may be important in the prevention of breast cancer, particularly among women who regularly consume alcohol.

Alcohol is a known folate antagonist and thus could plausibly increase the requirement for folate intake. Among women consuming about one or more alcoholic drinks per day, intake of at least 600 mg/day was associated with a 39% reduction in risk compared to those who consumed 190–299 mg/day (Zhang et al, 1999b). Most recently, higher total folate intake has been significantly associated with lower risk of developing ER-, but not ER+ breast cancer. The inverse association between total folate intake and ER- breast cancer was mainly present among women consuming at least 15 g/d of alcohol (RR = 0.46; 95% CI, = 0.25–0.86; top versus bottom quintile) (Zhang et al, 2005).

Vitamin D. Biologic, ecologic, and epidemiologic studies suggest that vitamin D may be involved in reducing the risk of breast cancer. Sunlight and dietary intake of fortified dairy products, cereals, and supplements are the major contributors to circulating levels of vitamin D (Webb et al, 1988; Webb et al, 1990; Salamone et al, 1994). In vitro and in vivo data suggest that vitamin D and its receptor function in inhibiting proliferation and inducing differentiation (Zinser et al, 2002). The NHANES I study found that measures of sunlight were associated with a significant 20%–33% reduction in breast cancer (John et al, 1999).

In the Nurses' Health Study, total intake of vitamin D was associated with a reduced risk of premenopausal breast cancer, but not postmenopausal breast cancer (Shin et al, 2002). Similarly, the Cancer Prevention Study II Nutrition cohort also observed no association with vitamin D intake and postmenopausal breast cancer risk (McCullough et al, 2005). Given that dietary intake of vitamin D is not a complete measure of vitamin D status, circulating levels of plasma vitamin D metabolites may provide a better measure. However, there have been conflicting results from studies examining plasma vitamin D metabolites and breast cancer (Cui and Rohan, 2006). More than 12 epidemiologic studies have examined genetic variation in the VDR and risk of breast cancer with inconsistent findings (Cui and Rohan, 2006).

Phytoestrogens

There is considerable interest in the relationship between breast cancer and phytoestrogens, compounds with estrogenic activity found in plants. Soy intake has been of particular interest because it is consumed in high quantities in Asian countries, where breast cancer rates are low. Both genistein and daidzein, the primary isoflavones in soy, can bind to estrogen receptors but are much less potent than estradiol—and thus could potentially serve as estrogen antagonists (Fournier et al, 1998). In addition, several, but not all, small studies have reported lower estrogen levels or lengthening of the follicular phase in the menstrual cycle in women consuming soy supplements. These mechanisms are not well established, however, and more work is needed.

Of four case-control studies conducted since 1990 among Asian or Asian-American women, one showed a significant inverse relationship, one a nonsignificant inverse association, and two no relationship with breast cancer risk (Wu et al, 1998). This association has not yet been evaluated in prospective studies and, because of the often low intake of soy products in these populations, most US and European studies have been unable to evaluate this association.

Food intake

Intake of specific food items has also been evaluated in a number of studies. The most consistent finding has been a modest inverse association between fruit and vegetable intake and breast cancer risk (Hunter and Willett, 1993; Trichopoulou et al, 1995; Zhang et al, 1999a). For example, in the prospective analysis by Zhang et al (1999a), premenopausal women who consumed five or more servings of fruits and vegetables per day had a relative risk of 0.77, compared to women consuming fewer than two servings per day on average. In an analysis of eight prospective studies with 7377 cases occurring among 351 825 women, in comparisons of the highest versus lowest quintiles of intake, only weak associations were seen for intake of total fruits (RR = 0.93), total vegetables (RR = 0.96), and total fruits and vegetables (RR = 0.93). No additional benefit was seen in the highest decile of intake, and results did not vary according to menopausal status (Smith-Warner et al, 2001b).

In addition to the micronutrients described previously, fruits and vegetables contain many other phytochemicals, including indoles, flavonoids, and protease inhibitors, and one or more of these substances could play a role in risk reduction.

Alcohol

Alcohol intake is the dietary factor most consistently associated with breast cancer risk, although the relationship observed has generally been modest. In a meta-analysis of 38 case-control and cohort studies, a positive association was noted in 31 studies (Longnecker, 1994). Substantial heterogeneity in relative risk estimates was observed among studies, perhaps due to the different ways alcohol consumption was measured—for example, past versus current use, updated versus nonupdated exposure. Overall, women who consumed two drinks per day experienced a 20% increase in risk compared to nondrinkers, and those consuming more than two drinks per day had a 40% increase in risk. These studies were conducted in diverse populations, and in most of them, other well-established breast cancer risk factors were accounted for in the analysis. Additionally, in the studies in which various types of alcohol were evaluated, beer, wine, and spirits were each positively associated with breast cancer risk, suggesting that the association is due to ethanol per se.

In a pooled analysis of six prospective studies (Smith-Warner et al, 1998) comprising 322 647 women, 4335 of whom developed breast cancer during follow-up, alcohol intake was again consistently related to an increased risk of breast cancer. The relative risk for each 10-g increase in alcohol intake (compared to nonuse) was 1.09; women who consumed 30–60 g of alcohol per day had a 41% higher risk of invasive breast cancer. The association was not observed to vary substantially within subgroups of women defined by other breast cancer risk factors—for example, women with and women without a family history of breast cancer.

A number of important details regarding this relation remained unresolved, however. Whether timing of the exposure in a woman's life is important is not known. In an initial assessment of the independent influence of alcohol intake before versus after age 30 on the subsequent breast cancer risk, drinking in young adulthood was most consistently associated with an increase in risk (Harvey et al, 1987). In contrast, in a large case-control study, recent and lifetime intake rather than early adult intake of alcohol were found to be the strongest predictors of risk (Longnecker et al, 1995). Few other studies have evaluated this aspect of the alcohol–breast cancer association. Other important details, such as the possible influence of drinking patterns, such as drinking 14 drinks each weekend versus 2 drinks per day, also still need to be resolved. Paradoxically, however, no appreciably increased risk has been demonstrated in women who are alcoholics (Kuper et al, 2000).

Several biological mechanisms have been proposed for this association, including an increase in circulating hormone levels, a direct carcinogenic effect of alcohol metabolites (eg, acetaldehyde, a known mutagen), and an antagonistic effect on folate absorption and metabolism (Willett, 2001; Zhang et al, 1999b). The best-supported mechanism to date is that related to circulating hormone levels—which has been observed in both premenopausal and postmenopausal women. In a controlled feeding study, two alcoholic drinks per day increased total and bioavailable estrogen levels in premenopausal women (Reichman et al, 1993). A positive relationship between alcohol intake and circulating estrogen levels in postmenopausal women has been observed in several, although not all, cross-sectional studies and in an intervention study of alcohol intake and postmenopausal hormone use (Willett et al, 1999). Alcohol intake was also found to be associated with estrogen-receptor positive breast tumors, but not estrogen-negative tumors (Suzuki et al, 2005). In a prospective analysis, high intake of folic acid appeared to negate the increased risk of breast cancer in women who consumed one or more drinks per day (Zhang et al, 1999b). Alcohol is known to interfere with folate absorption and metabolism, and low folate levels can result in misincorporation of uracil into DNA; hence, this may be another mechanism for the observed alcohol–breast cancer association.

Reproductive Factors

Age at menarche

Age at menarche has been consistently associated with the risk of both premenopausal and postmenopausal breast cancer; risk is reduced by 5% to 20% for each year that the onset of menarche is delayed (Hsieh et al, 1990; Kelsey et al, 1993). Several mechanisms have been proposed. Menarche marks the onset of the mature hormonal milieu—that is, cyclic hormonal changes that result in ovulation, menstruation, and cellular proliferation in the breast (Willett et al, 1999). The earlier the age at menarche, the earlier a young woman starts experiencing increased steroid hormone levels. An earlier age at menarche also has been related to an earlier onset of regular ovulatory cycles. In addition, although data are limited, women with earlier menarche may have higher circulating estrogen levels for a number of years afterward (MacMahon et al, 1982; Henderson et al, 1996). Although age at menarche is a relatively weak risk factor overall, substantial international variation—for example, mean age in China

of 16 to 17 years versus 12 to 13 years in the United States—makes it a contributor to the observed international variation in breast cancer rates.

Age at first birth and parity

Overall, parous women have a lower risk of breast cancer than nulliparous women, although the relationship is complex and varies with both time since childbirth and the total number of births (Kelsey et al, 1993; Adami et al, 1998). For 10 to 20 years after delivery, a woman's risk of breast cancer is higher than that of a comparable nulliparous woman (Lambe et al, 1994). This is thought to be due to the promotional effects of high pregnancy hormone levels on a preexisting malignancy. After this time, however, a parous woman experiences a long-lasting reduction in risk compared to that of a nulliparous woman. This risk is further reduced, although more modestly, with each subsequent birth (Trichopoulos et al, 1983; Rosner et al, 1994). Because the lower risk occurs when a woman is older and her baseline risk of breast cancer is relatively high, the long-term reduction in risk substantially outweighs the short-term postpregnancy increase in risk.

The biological mechanism behind this long-term reduction in risk associated with pregnancy has been studied extensively (Russo et al, 1990). The ductal system of the breast undergoes profound changes from birth through adulthood. After menarche but prior to a first pregnancy, the breast contains relatively undifferentiated ducts and associated alveolar buds (termed lobule types 1 and 2). Differentiation of the glandular epithelial cells takes place gradually, culminating in terminally differentiated tissue (termed lobule types 3 and 4). These changes take place largely after a first full-term pregnancy and, to a lesser extent, after subsequent pregnancies. The terminally differentiated epithelial cells have longer cell cycles (lower proliferation rates) and spend more time in G1, the resting phase that allows for DNA repair (Russo et al, 1990), both factors that decrease the risk of malignant transformation. Another possible explanation for the long-term reduction in breast cancer risk is a prolonged post-pregnancy reduction in levels of circulating hormones such as prolactin (Bernstein and Ross, 1993).

A woman's age at the time of a first full-term pregnancy is also important to her risk of breast cancer (MacMahon et al, 1970). Independent of parity, the younger a woman is at her first full-term birth, the lower her subsequent risk. Although the magnitude of the effect has varied among studies, the reduction in risk from having had a first birth by age 20 compared to age 35 or older is about 30% (Kelsey et al, 1993). Mechanistically, when the first pregnancy occurs at an early age, fewer cells are likely to have been initiated and the period of protection, afforded by the terminal differentiation of the breast glandular epithelium, covers a larger fraction of the woman's remaining lifetime.

Breast-feeding
The data relating breast-feeding practices to subsequent breast cancer risk have not been as consistent as those for other reproductive factors. A reduction has been seen most consistently among premenopausal women who breast-fed for an extended period, but even here the magnitude of the observed effect has varied substantially (Lipworth et al, 2000). In one large case-control study, a significant 22% reduction in risk was observed in premenopausal women who lactated. The risk decreased with increasing duration of lactation (Newcomb et al, 1994). In a pooled analysis of 47 epidemiologic studies in 30 countries, lifetime duration of breast feeding was associated with a significant reduction in breast cancer risk among parous women, which did not vary by menopausal status. The relative risk of breast cancer decreased by 4.3% (95% CI 2.9–5.8; p < 0.0001) for every 12 months of breast-feeding (Collaborative Group on Hormonal Factors in Breast Cancer, 2002). In a review of 32 published studies (Willett et al, 1999), 16 of the studies showed a statistically significant reduction in risk

with longer duration of breast-feeding. A number of factors may be responsible for these inconsistent results. Most studies conducted in western populations have had limited statistical power to detect an effect of long durations of lactation; for example, in the large Nurses' Health Study, less than 10% of the population breast-fed for at least 1 year. Additionally, the pattern of breast-feeding has generally not been taken into account in these studies; for example, whether the breast-feeding was exclusive or supplemental may influence the ultimate reduction in risk.

Several mechanisms may be responsible for any protective effect of lactation (Kelsey et al, 1993). Breast-feeding may result in further terminal differentiation of the breast epithelium, thus making it more resistant to carcinogenic change. Additionally, breast-feeding delays the postpregnancy reestablishment of the ovulatory menstrual cycle and hence may reduce the risk.

Spontaneous and induced abortions
Based on data from animal studies, it has been hypothesized that the incomplete differentiation of breast cells during the first trimester of a pregnancy could result in increased susceptibility of the tissue to malignant transformation (Kelsey et al, 1993). In a meta-analysis that included data from 28 studies, a positive association was indeed noted between induced abortion and breast cancer (Brind et al, 1996). However, most of these investigations were case-control studies and thus were potentially biased by differential recall of past induced abortions. A large population-based cohort study, composed of 1,5 million Danish women of whom 18% had had one or more abortions, provides the best available evaluation of this hypothesis (Melbye et al, 1997). After adjusting for age, age at first birth, parity, and calendar period, the risk of breast cancer for women with a history of one or more abortions was remarkably similar (RR = 1.0) to that of women with no history of abortion. No trend in risk was noted with an increasing number of abortions.

Age at menopause

The positive relationship between age at menopause and subsequent breast cancer risk is also well established. On average, the risk of breast cancer increases by about 3% per year that menopause is delayed (Kelsey et al, 1993). The reduction in risk associated with an earlier menopause is likely due to the cessation of ovarian function and the resultant dramatic reduction in circulating steroid hormone levels. An artificial menopause through bilateral oophorectomy confers more protection than a natural menopause at the same age because of the abrupt elimination of both ovarian estrogens and androgens. Although estrogen levels decline within 1 to 2 years of menopause, androgens ordinarily continue to be produced for a number of years. Women with a bilateral oophorectomy before age 45 have about half the risk of breast cancer of those with a natural menopause at age 55 or older (Trichopoulos et al, 1972). Most studies have observed that having a simple hysterectomy, with the ovaries left intact, does not influence the subsequent risk of breast cancer (Kelsey et al, 1993).

Hormones and Hormone Receptors

Endogenous hormones

Several lines of evidence have long suggested that sex hormones play a central role in the etiology of breast cancer. As just reviewed, several reproductive factors are consistently associated with breast cancer risk. In addition, after menopause, adipose tissue is the major source of estrogen, and obese postmenopausal women have both higher levels of endogenous estrogen and a higher risk of breast cancer (Harris et al, 1992; Huang et al, 1997). Further, estrogens and progesterone promote mammary tumors in animals (Briand, 1983). Also, tamoxifen, which acts as an antiestrogen in the breast (by blocking binding of estrogen to the estrogen receptor), decreases the incidence of breast cancer in high-risk women (Fisher et al, 1998).

Despite this strong body of evidence suggesting a central role of endogenous hormones, studies directly relating blood or urinary hormone levels to the risk of breast cancer have, until recently, been largely inconsistent. The complexity and expense of hormone assays, coupled with the need to collect urine or blood samples from study subjects—and timed samples in premenopausal subjects—have resulted in both a limited number of epidemiologic studies of these issues and small sample sizes. These factors, in conjunction with error in the laboratory assays (Hankinson et al, 1994), have likely contributed to the lack of consistent findings. A summary, which relies predominantly on the larger prospective studies where possible, is provided in the following section.

Estrogens. Estradiol, considered the most biologically active endogenous estrogen, circulates in blood either unbound ("free") or bound to sex hormone-binding globulin or albumin. Free or bioavailable (free plus albumin-bound) estradiol is thought to be readily available to breast tissue and thus may be more strongly related to risk than total estradiol. Postmenopausally, estrone is the source of most circulating estradiol, and estrone sulfate is the most abundant circulating estrogen (Roberts et al, 1980). Both normal and malignant breast cells have sulfatase and 17-beta-dehydrogenase activity (Pasqualini et al, 1996). Thus, estrone and estrone sulfate could serve as ready sources of intracellular estradiol.

In 2002, a pooled analysis was published consisting of all prospective studies of endogenous estrogens and androgens in postmenopausal women that had been available at that time (Key et al, 2002). Data were from nine prospective studies with a total of 663 breast cancer cases and 1765 healthy controls; none of the women were using exogenous hormones at blood collection. The risk of breast cancer increased with increasing estrogen levels. For example, the relative risks (95% CI) for increasing quintiles of estradiol level, all relative to the lowest quintile, were 1.4 (1.0–2.0), 1.2 (0.9–1.7), 1.8 (1.3–2.4), and 2.0 (1.5–2.7).

Estrone, estrone sulfate, and free estradiol were similarly related to risk. Subsequent to the pooled analysis, several additional prospective studies have been published and all have supported these findings (Manjer et al, 2003; Missmer et al, 2004; Kaaks et al, 2005a) (See Table 16-1).

Recently, these associations were reported to be stronger for estrogen and progesterone receptor–positive tumors, with little association for hormone receptor–negative tumors (Missmer et al, 2004). For example, for estradiol, the top versus bottom category RR (95% CI) was 3.3 (2.0–5.4) for ER+/PR+ tumors (p-trend < 0.001), 1.0 (0.4–2.6; p-trend = 0.82) for ER+/PR– tumors, and 1.0 (0.4–2.4; p-trend = 0.46) for ER-/PR- tumors. These data are in line with findings from the tamoxifen and raloxifene trials, where risk of only ER+ tumors was reduced (Cuzick et al, 2003; Martino et al, 2004), and also from epidemiologic studies of obesity and breast cancer where stronger associations have been noted for ER+ tumors.

Data on premenopausal estrogen levels and breast cancer risk are more limited, in large part because of the complexities related to sampling during the menstrual cycle. Data from several case-control studies, but not all, suggest that high levels of estradiol in premenopausal women increase the risk of breast cancer (Bernstein and Ross, 1993). In two recent cohort studies, a positive association was noted for follicular phase estradiol (Eliassen et al, 2006) in one, but no association was noted in a second (Kaaks et al, 2005b).

Estrogen metabolites. A woman's pattern of estrogen metabolism also has been hypothesized to influence her breast cancer risk. Estradiol and estrone can be metabolized through several pathways, including the 16-a and 2 (and 4-)-hydroxy pathways (Fig. 16–4) (Yager and Liehr, 1996). Products of these pathways have markedly different biological properties, and opposing hypotheses have been proposed concerning their influence on risk (Yager and Liehr, 1996). However, the epidemiologic studies evaluating associations between estrogen metabolites and breast cancer risk have been small, the largest having just 60 cases, and the results have been inconsistent (Meilahn et al, 1998; Willett et al, 1999).

Estrogen receptors. Given the role of estrogen receptors in estrogen response, and the consistently observed associations between plasma estrogen levels and breast cancer risk, the expression of estrogen receptors in normal breast tissue is of interest. The proportion of estrogen receptor–positive breast tumors has been reported to be higher among Caucasian than Asian patients (Adami et al, 1998). In addition, the likelihood of breast cancer has been reported to be higher when there is overexpression of estrogen receptor in the surrounding normal epithelium (Khan et al, 1998). Caucasians were found to have greater expression of estrogen receptor alpha in normal breast epithelial tissue than Japanese women of similar age (Lawson et al, 1999).

Androgens. Androgens have been hypothesized to increase the breast cancer risk either directly, by increasing the growth and proliferation of breast cancer cells, or indirectly, by their conversion to estrogen (Bernstein and Ross, 1993). Dehydroepiandrosterone (DHEA) administered to rodents can decrease tumor formation. In humans, DHEA may act like an antiestrogen premenopausally but an estrogen postmenopausally in stimulating cell growth (Ebeling and Koivisto, 1994); in part because of the estrogenic effect of its metabolite, 5-androstene-3b,17b-diol also can bind to the estrogen receptor (Seymour-Munn and Adams, 1983).

In postmenopausal women, the best summary of evidence on circulating androgens and breast cancer risk is from the pooled analysis of nine prospective studies described previously (Key et al, 2002), along with the recently published report from the EPIC study (see Table 16-1) (Kaaks et al, 2005a). In the pooled analysis, testosterone

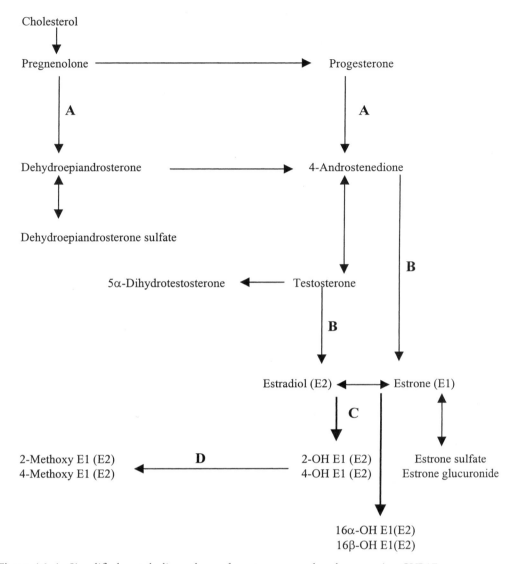

Figure 16–4. Simplified metabolic pathway for estrogens and androgens. A = CYP17, B = CYP19, C = CYP1A1, D = COMT.

was positively associated with breast cancer risk: The relative risks (95% CI) for increasing quintile category (all relative to the lowest quintile of levels) were 1.3 (1.0–1.9), 1.6 (1.2–2.2), 1.6 (1.1–2.2), and 2.2 (1.6–3.1). Findings were generally similar for several other androgens measured. In EPIC, similar positive associations were observed for each of the androgens measured. In each of these analyses, when estradiol was added to the statistical models, relative risks for the androgens were only modestly attenuated

suggesting some independent effect of circulating androgens on breast cancer risk. However, interpretation of these data is complicated because of possible differences between estradiol and the androgens in terms of assay precision, hormone stability within woman over time, and intracellular conversion of androgens to estrogens, which cannot be accounted for in epidemiologic analyses.

Among premenopausal women, although data are much more limited, prospective nested case-control studies are relatively consistent in showing a positive association, of similar magnitude to that reported among postmenopausal women, between circulating androgen levels and risk of breast cancer (Thomas et al, 1997b; Micheli et al, 2004; Kaaks et al, 2005b; Eliassen et al, 2006).

Progesterone. Progesterone exerts powerful influences on breast physiology and can influence tumor development in rodents (Kelsey, 1979). Based largely on indirect evidence, progesterone has been hypothesized both to decrease the breast cancer risk by opposing estrogenic stimulation of the breast (Kelsey, 1979) and to increase the risk because breast mitotic rates are highest in the luteal (high-progesterone) phase of the menstrual cycle (Bernstein and Ross, 1993). In three large prospective studies, results have not been consistent with inverse (Micheli et al, 2004; Kaaks et al, 2005a) and no association (Eliassen et al, 2006) reported. However, progesterone levels vary substantially throughout the menstrual cycle and are difficult to measure in the context of large epidemiologic studies, hence further assessments with better measures are warranted. In postmenopausal women, only a single prospective study has been conducted and no association found (Missmer et al, 2004).

Prolactin. Prolactin receptors have been found on more than 50% of breast tumors (Partridge and Hahnel, 1979), and prolactin can increase the growth of both normal and malignant breast cells in vitro (Malarkey et al, 1983). Prolactin administration also is well documented to increase mammary tumor development rates in mice. Because prolactin is influenced by both physical and emotional stress (Herman et al, 1981; Yen and Jaffe, 1991), levels in women with breast cancer may not reflect their predisease levels. Thus, evaluation of this association in prospective studies is particularly important.

In the only large prospective study among postmenopausal women (Hankinson et al, 1999; Tworoger et al, 2004), 851 cases and 1275 controls were evaluated over 10 years of follow-up. Prolactin levels were associated with a modestly increased risk of breast cancer overall, which was confined to invasive breast cancer cases (top versus bottom quartile categories for invasive: RR = 1.4, 95% CI = 1.1–1.9, p-trend = 0.003). In addition, the association significantly differed by estrogen (ER) and progesterone (PR) receptor status of the tumor with a RR, comparing the top to bottom 25% of levels, of 1.8 (95% CI = 1.3–2.5, p-trend < 0.001) for ER+/PR+, 0.8 (95% CI = 0.4–1.3, p-trend = 0.28) for ER-/PR-, and 1.9 (95% CI = 1.0–3.8, p-trend = 0.12) for ER+/PR- breast cancers. Even fewer data are available in premenopausal women, although in the one large study to date (316 cases and 633 controls) similar positive associations were observed (Tworoger et al, 2006). Cumulatively, the data support a role for prolactin in the etiology of breast cancer.

Insulin-like growth factors. Insulin-like growth factor I (IGF-I) is a protein hormone with a structural homology to insulin. The growth hormone–IGF-I axis can stimulate proliferation of both breast cancer and normal breast epithelial cells (Pollak, 1998). Rhesus monkeys treated with growth hormone or IGF-I show histologic evidence of mammary gland hyperplasia. In addition, positive associations have been observed between breast cancer and birth weight as well as height, which are both positively correlated with IGF-I levels (Pollak, 1998). In a recent meta-analysis of six prospective epidemiologic studies, a positive relationship was reported between circulating IGF-1 and premenopausal breast cancer (comparing the 75th with the 25th percentile OR = 1.65, 95% CI 1.26–2.08), but not with postmenopausal breast cancer (Renehan et al, 2004). In this same meta-analysis, high levels of IGF binding protein-3 (IGFBP-3) were also associated with increased premenopausal breast cancer (comparing the 75th with the 25th percentile OR = 1.51, 95% CI 1.01–2.27) (Renehan et al, 2004).

Subsequent to this meta-analysis, three large prospective studies have reported results challenging the earlier findings. Rinaldi et al reported no association between IGF1 and breast cancer in women under the age of 50, but a positive modest association among older women in the European Prospective Investigation into Cancer and Nutrition (EPIC) (Rinaldi et al, 2006). In the Nurses' Health Study II, Schernhammer et al also reported no association between IGF-1 and IGFBP3 with premenopausal breast cancer (Schernhammer et al, 2006). An updated analysis of the Nurses' Health Study found that circulating IGF-I levels were only modestly associated with breast cancer risk among premenopausal women, but not among postmenopausal women (Schernhammer et al, 2005). An updated analysis of the New York University Women's Health Study reported a significant positive association with circulating IGF in premenopausal women (top versus bottom quartile OR = 1.93, 95% CI 1.00–3.72), consistent with their initial findings (Rinaldi et al, 2005).

Although the earlier findings relating plasma IGF-I levels to breast cancer were promising, the most recent data highlight the need for larger studies, particularly among premenopausal women. In addition, there are a number of differences across these studies that may contribute to some of the inconsistency in results including differences in assays, age and menopausal cutoffs, adjustment for IGFBP-3 levels, and time since blood collection.

Oral contraceptives

Since oral contraceptives were first introduced in the 1960s, they have been used by millions of women (Committee on the Relationship Between Oral Contraceptives and Breast Cancer Institute of Medicine, 1991). Most combined oral contraceptives contain ethinyl estradiol (or mestranol, which is metabolized to ethinyl estradiol) and a progestin. The estrogen dose in oral contraceptives has ranged from at least 100 mg in 1960 to 20 to 30 mg, the doses most commonly used today; during this same time period, at least nine different progestins have been used (Annegers, 1989). Patterns of use also have changed considerably over time, with both increasing durations of use and a trend toward earlier age at first use. Over 50 epidemiologic studies have evaluated the relationship between oral contraceptive use and breast cancer risk.

Most studies have observed no significant increase in breast cancer risk even with long durations of use. Individual data from 54 epidemiologic studies were collected and analyzed centrally (Collaborative Group on Hormonal Factors in Breast Cancer, 1996). In this large pooled analysis, in which data from 53 297 women with and 100 239 women without breast cancer were evaluated, no overall relationship was observed between duration of use and risk of breast cancer. Similar findings were generally observed when long-term use was evaluated among either postmenopausal women or women over the age of 45 years. However, prior to the pooled analysis, findings for long-term use among young women were not quite as consistent or reassuring. In two meta-analyses, summary relative risks for long duration of use in young women were 1.5 (Romieu et al, 1990) and 1.4 (Thomas, 1991). The greatest increase tended to be observed in the youngest women, generally those less than 35 years of age; this observation also was noted in several more case-control studies.

In the pooled analysis (Collaborative Group on Hormonal Factors in Breast Cancer, 1996), current and recent users of oral contraceptives had an increased risk of breast cancer (for current versus never-users, RR = 1.24). This increased risk disappeared within 10 years of stopping oral contraceptive use (relative risk by years since stopping use versus never use: 1–4 years, 1.16; 5–9 years, 1.07; 10–14 years, 0.98; more than 15 years, 1.03). When the investigators evaluated both time since last use and duration of use, they observed a modestly increased risk only among current and recent users, and no independent effect of long duration of use on the risk of breast cancer even among very young women.

Thus, the increased risk of breast cancer observed among young, long-term users of oral contraceptives in past individual studies (and meta-analyses) appears due primarily to recency of use rather than to duration. These data suggest that oral contraceptives may act as late-stage promoters. Importantly, current and recent users, the women who appear to have a modest increase in risk, are generally young (under 45 years of age) and thus have a low absolute risk of breast cancer. Hence, a modest increase in their risk will result in few additional cases of breast cancer. Nevertheless, this apparently increased risk among current and recent users should be considered in deciding whether to use oral contraceptives.

Because any influence of oral contraceptives on the breast has been hypothesized to be greatest prior to the cellular differentiation that occurs with a full-term pregnancy (Russo et al, 1990), a number of investigators have evaluated the effect of oral contraceptive use prior to a first full-term pregnancy. In both meta-analyses, the summary relative risk indicated a modest increase in risk with long-term use (Romieu et al, 1990; Thomas, 1991). In the pooled analysis (Collaborative Group on Hormonal Factors in Breast Cancer, 1996), a significant trend of increasing risk with first use before age 20 years was observed. Among women ages 30 to 34 years, the relative risk associated with recent oral contraceptive use was 1.54 if use began before age 20 years and 1.13 if use began at age 20 years or older.

Overall, there is no consistent evidence of a differential effect according to type or dose of either estrogen or progestin, but few studies have examined this issue (Bernstein and Ross, 1993). Limited data exist regarding the influence of the newer oral contraceptive formulations on breast cancer risk (Collaborative Group on Hormonal Factors in Breast Cancer, 1996). Possible interactions with other breast cancer risk factors were evaluated in detail for the first time in the collaborative pooling project (Collaborative Group on Hormonal Factors in Breast Cancer, 1996). In this study, the investigators defined oral contraceptive use in terms of recency and age at first use, rather than "ever use," as done in most previous individual studies. Overall, the relationship between oral contraceptive use and breast cancer did not vary appreciably by family history of breast cancer, weight, alcohol intake, or other breast cancer risk factors.

The Women's CARE Study, a large population-based case-control study with 4575 breast cancer cases and 4682 controls, also examined the risk of breast cancer associated with oral contraceptives among different subgroups of women (Marchbanks et al, 2002). In this study, there was no increased risk of breast cancer among current users (RR = 1.0, 95% CI 0.8–1.0) or former users (RR = 0.9, 95% CI 0.8–1.0). This study found no increased risk among women with a family history or those who initiated use at an early age. In addition, the risk of breast cancer did not appear to vary by duration, dose, or type of progestin (Marchbanks et al, 2002).

Progestin-only contraceptives include progestin-only pills ("mini-pill"), depot-medroxyprogesterone (DMPA, an injectable contraceptive), and implantable levonorgestrel (Norplant); few epidemiologic studies have evaluated their association with breast cancer risk. To date, longer-term users of the progestin-only pill have been observed to have either a similar or lower risk of breast cancer than never users (Stanford and Thomas, 1993). In the most comprehensive study of DMPA (Waaler and Lund, 1983; WHO Collaborative Study of Neoplasia and Steroid Contraceptives, 1991), no significant increase in risk was observed with increasing duration of use (for more than 3 years of use versus never use, RR = 0.9). No data are available on the long-term use of Norplant, a long-acting contraceptive that is implanted subdermally, as it was introduced in the United States only in 1990. Further epidemiologic research is needed for each of these drugs.

Postmenopausal hormone use

Postmenopausal estrogens have been used for over half a century. By the mid-1970s, almost 30 million prescriptions were being filled annually in the United States (Kennedy and Baum, 1985). A challenge in studying the relationship between postmenopausal hormones and breast cancer is the substantial variation in formulations and patterns of use that has occurred over time. By the time sufficient use of one type of hormone has occurred to allow a detailed epidemiologic evaluation, new formulations are already being introduced.

Following publication of at least six meta-analyses during the 1990s, relationships betwen postmenopausal hormone use and breast cancer risk were evaluated in considerable detail in the pooled analysis that combined the results of 51 epidemiologic studies (Collaborative Group on Hormonal Factors in Breast Cancer, 1997). Importantly, in these analyses, women with an uncertain age at menopause were excluded (eg, women with simple hysterectomies), as inadequate accounting for age at menopause in the analysis can lead to substantial attenuation of the observed relationships between postmenopausal hormone use and breast cancer risk.

The investigators observed a statistically significant association between current or recent use of postmenopausal hormones and the risk of breast cancer; the positive association was strongest among those with the longest duration of use. For example, among women who had used postmenopausal hormones within the previous 5 years compared to never-users, the relative risks for duration of use were 1.08 for 1 to 4 years of use, 1.31 for 5 to 9 years, 1.24 for 10 to 14 years, and 1.56 for 15 years or more of use. No significant increase in breast cancer risk was noted for women who had stopped using postmenopausal hormones 5 or more years in the past, regardless of their duration of use.

Subsequent to this meta-analysis, findings from the Nurses' Health Study and the Million Women Study support the findings that short-term use of unopposed estrogen is not associated with an increased risk of breast cancer, while longer term use is (Beral et al, 2003; Chen et al, 2006). In addition, Chen et al reported that 15 years or more of use was significantly associated specifically with ER+/PR+ breast cancers (Chen et al, 2006).

One concern has been whether the increased risk observed is an artifact of increased surveillance for breast cancer among women taking hormones. Consistent with that possibility, a higher relative risk has been associated with in situ disease than with invasive disease (Schairer et al, 1994; Colditz et al, 1995). However, in both of these studies, a significant positive, although weaker, association was noted when only invasive breast cancer cases were considered. Also, in the Nurses' Health Study, mammography rates were uniformly high, exceeding 90% even among women who never used hormones. Moreover, past users, and current users of short duration, were not observed to have an elevated risk, despite higher mammography rates than the never-users. Finally, an elevated death rate from breast cancer was observed among current users of 10 or more years' duration at the time of diagnosis. These analyses indicate that the association cannot be explained simply as an artifact of screening.

Limited data are available regarding the effects of the dose or type of estrogen on breast cancer risk. Again, the best data come from the pooled analysis (Collaborative Group on Hormonal Factors in Breast Cancer, 1997). No significant differences in relative risk were observed according to either the type of estrogen used (conjugated estrogen versus other) or the estrogen dose (< 0.625 mg versus ≥ 1.25 mg), although some modest differences in estimates suggested that further evaluation is warranted. Although the effect of estrogen use on breast cancer risk could be reasonably hypothesized to vary by mode of estrogen delivery, for example, by avoiding the first-pass effect in the liver (patch estrogen does not increase

Table 16–1. Epidemiology of breast cancer: risk factor summary

Risk factor	Direction of effect*
Well-Confirmed Risk Factors	
Family history in first-degree relative	↑ ↑
Height	↑ ↑
Benign breast disease	↑ ↑
Mammographically dense breasts	↑ ↑
Age at first birth >30 years versus, <20	↑ ↑
Menopause at >54 years versus, <45	↑ ↑
High endogenous estrogen levels	↑ ↑
Postmenopausal hormone use	↑
Ionizing radiation exposure	↑ ↑
Menarche at <12 years versus >14	↑
Alcohol use (≥1 drink/day)	↑
High body mass index (postmenopausal)	↑
High body mass index (premenopausal)	↓
Tamoxifen	↓
Probable Relationship Exists, Based on Substantial Data	
High endogenous androgen levels	↑ ↑
Current oral contraceptive use	↑
Physical activity	↓
Lactation (longer durations)	↓
Folate	↓
Carotenoids	↓
Weak, if Any, Relationship Exists, Based on Substantial Data	
Total dietary fat intake during adulthood	—
Induced or spontaneous abortion	—
Cigarette smoking	—
Past oral contraceptive use	—
Exposure to electromagnetic fields	—
Inconsistent Findings or Limited Study to Date	
High endogenous insulin-like growth factor levels	↓ ↓
High plasma insulin-like growth factor levels	↑ ↑
High endogenous progesterone levels	↑
High endogenous vitamin D levels	↓
Childood bodyfatness	↓
In utero exposures	↑
Nonsteroidal anti-inflammatory drug use	↓
Organochlorine exposure	—
Adult-onset diabetes	↑
Thyroid disease	↑

*Arrows indicate the approximate magnitude of the relationship: ↑, slight to moderate increase in risk; ↑ ↑, moderate to large increase in risk; ↓, slight to moderate decrease in risk; ↓, moderate to large decrease in risk; —, no association

Note: The magnitude of the risk can vary substantially, depending on the exact comparison being made. For example, having a family history of breast cancer in a first-degree relative is a consistent breast cancer risk factor. However, the magnitude of the association increases substantially the earlier the age at diagnosis in the relative(s) and with the number of relatives affected.

sex hormone-binding globulin to the extent that oral preparations do), insufficient data are available to evaluate these potential differences.

The risk associated with postmenopausal hormone use was assessed in a number of specific subgroups in the pooled analysis (Collaborative Group on Hormonal Factors in Breast Cancer, 1997). Risk did not appear to vary according to reproductive history, alcohol or smoking history, or by family history of breast cancer. However, the relative risks associated with 5 or more years of postmenopausal hormone use were highest among the leanest women; this interaction has been consistently observed (Huang et al, 1997) and is biologically plausible since lean women tend to have the lowest estrogen levels. Hence, taking postmenopausal hormones will result in a greater proportional increase in estrogen levels compared to that in heavier women, who tend to have higher estrogen levels.

The Women's Health Initiative (WHI) randomized controlled trial in which 10 739 women with hysterectomy were randomized to estrogen-only therapy reported a nonsignificant inverse association between therapy and breast cancer after an average of 7 years of follow-up (RR = 0.77, 95% CI 0.59–1.01) (Anderson et al, 2004). At enrollment, the average age of WHI participants was 64 years and approximately 45% of the population had a body mass index $\geq 30 \text{ kg/m}^2$. Given that these women were randomized to hormone use many years after menopause and that a large proportion are considered obese, the difference between results from WHI and observational studies may reflect differences in study populations.

Estrogen plus progestin use. The addition of a progestin to estrogen regimens has become increasingly common, as it minimizes or eliminates the increased risk of endometrial hyperplasia and cancer associated with using unopposed estrogens. In the United States, by the mid-1980s, almost 30% of postmenopausal hormone prescriptions included a prescription for progestin (Hemminki et al, 1988). There are data suggesting that the addition of a progestin may increase the risk beyond that associated with estrogen alone (Bergkvist et al, 1989; Colditz and Rosner, 2000). In the PEPI double-blind, randomized trial of placebo, estrogens, and three estrogen-progestin regimens, the estrogen-progestin combinations were associated with a much larger increase in mammographic density than the estrogen-only formulation (Greendale et al, 1999). In the pooled analysis (Collaborative Group on Hormonal Factors in Breast Cancer, 1997), data on postmenopausal hormone formulation were available from only 39% of the women, and only 12% of these reported use of estrogen plus a progestin. The relative risk associated with 5 or more years of recent use, relative to never use, was 1.53. The comparable relative risk for estrogen use alone was 1.34.

Since the time of the pooled analysis, at least five large observational studies—three cohort studies (Schairer et al, 2000; Colditz and Rosner, 2000; Beral et al, 2003) and two case-control studies (Magnusson et al, 1999; Ross et al, 2000)—investigated the influence of combined estrogen-progestin treatment on breast cancer risk. Schairer et al reported a relative risk of 2.0 after at least 4 years of current or recent use of combined estrogen-progestin compared to never use in lean women. The corresponding relative risk for use of estrogen only was 1.0. In the most recent report from the Nurses' Health Study (Colditz and Rosner, 2000) of relative to never users, 10 years of unopposed estrogen use was associated with a 23% increase in the risk of breast cancer, while 10 years of estrogen plus progestin use increased the risk by 67%. In the United States, combined treatment contains mainly conjugated estrogens with cyclic addition of one specific progestin (methylprogesterone acetate). Lack of power, however, precluded detailed analyses of the impact of different types of estrogen-progestin treatments on risk. The Million Women Study, a prospective cohort of over one million UK women, was designed to specifically examine the effects of different postmenopausal hormone regimens. Current users of estrogen plus progestin preparations (RR = 2.00, 95% CI 1.88–2.12) were at increased risk of breast cancer compared to never users and risk increased with increasing duration (Beral et al, 2003).

In a Swedish case-control study, long-term use of any type of combined treatment was associated with a threefold increase in breast cancer risk (RR = 3.0) compared to never use (Magnusson et al, 1999). The excess risk was higher following use of continuously as compared to cyclically combined estrogen-progestin replacement (after more than 10 years of use, RR = 5.4 versus 2.4) (Magnusson et al, 1999). These data pertain mainly to the use of estradiol and testosterone-like progestin. In contrast, a more pronounced effect of the use of cyclically combined estrogen-progestin than of continuously combined treatment on breast cancer risk was noted (after more than 10 years of use, RR = 1.8 versus 1.5 compared to never use) in an American case-control study (Ross et al, 2000). The difference, however, was not statistically significant.

In 2002, the Women's Health Inititiave trial in which 16 608 postmenopausal women were randomized to either a combined estrogen plus progestin therapy or placebo demonstrated that this combination therapy increased the risk of invasive breast cancer and was stopped early. Over 7 years of follow-up there was a 24% increased risk of breast cancer (HR = 1.24, 95% CI 1.01–1.54) (Chlebowski et al, 2003). Since the publication of the WHI results, the prescription patterns for estrogen plus progesterone therapies have declined (Majumdar et al, 2004). In contrast, there is evidence that use of estrogen plus testosterone therapies are increasing (Davis, 1999; Tamimi et al, 2006). Consistent with the elevation in risk for endogenous testosterone levels, one prospective study reported that women currently using estrogen plus testosterone therapies were at a significant increased risk of invasive breast cancer (RR = 2.48; 95% CI, 1.53–4.04) (Tamimi et al, 2006).

It has now become well-accepted that current use of combined estrogen plus pro-gestin therapies increases the risk of breast cancer and that this increase in risk is greater than that observed for estrogen-only therapies. The difference between the breast and the endometrium in this regard is striking. Given the substantial evidence implicating combined estrogen plus pro-gestin therapy in breast cancer and other postmenopausal hormone therapies, it has been recommended that women and their physicians should reconsider use and, more specifically, long-term use of these therapies (Willett et al, 2000b).

Hormonal chemoprevention

A number of agents are being developed or undergoing testing as breast cancer chemo-preventives. One of the most widely studied, tamoxifen, is a member of an increasing family of agents called selective estrogen receptor modulators (SERMs), which have tissue-specific estrogen agonist/antagonist effects (MacGregor and Jordan, 1998). Tamoxifen widely used in the treatment of breast cancer may reduce breast cancer incidence by about 50% in high-risk women (Fisher et al, 1998). The International Breast Cancer Intervention Study (IBIS-I) is a placebo-controlled randomized trial of tamoxifen for the prevention of breast cancer in women at high risk. After a median of 50 months of follow-up, there was a 32% (RR = 0.68, 95% CI 0.50–0.92) reduction of breast cancer risk among women on the tamoxifen arm (Cuzick et al, 2002). However, there was also an increase in the number of thromboembolic events in the tamoxifen arm. After 7 years of follow-up, the National Surgical Adjuvant Breast and Bowel Project (NSABP) P-1 trial, reported a 43% (RR = 0.57, 95% CI 0.46–070) reduction in breast cancer incidence, very much in line with their initial findings prior to unblinding (Fisher et al, 2005). The risks of thromboembolic events including stroke and deep-vein thrombosis were also elevated in this study.

The breast cancer prevention trials of tamoxifen have demonstrated that tamoxifen is effective in reducing the incidence of breast cancer, and specifically ER+ breast cancer; however, concerns over side effects remain (Cuzick et al, 2003). Another SERM, raloxifene, has been evaluated for the prevention of breast cancer relative to tamoxifen in the NSABP Study of Tamoxifen and Raloxifene (STAR) P-2 trial. In the STAR raloxifene was as effective as tamoxifen in reducing risk of breast cancer with fewer thromboembolic events (Vogel et al, 2006). The Raloxifene Use for the Heart (RUTH) trial, a randomized double-blind trial of over 10 000 women, also found that women randomized to raloxifene had a reduced risk of breast cancer (RR = 0.56, 95% CI 0.38–0.83), and experienced greater thromoembolic events compared to women on placebo (Barrett-Connor et al, 2006).

Aromatase inhibitors, such as anastrazole, letrozole, and exemestane, suppress estrogen production by blocking the aromatase enzyme, which converts androgens to estrogens (Gradishar, 2006). Several trials have demonstrated that aromatase inhibitors have better efficacy than tamoxifen in treating ER+ breast cancer. These studies found that aromatase inhibitors reduced the risk of contralateral breast cancer by 39% to 56% among postmenopausal women (Gradishar, 2006). The International Breast Cancer Intervention Study (IBIS) II and MAP3 (National Cancer Institute, Canada) are two recently initiated randomized control trials comparing aromatase inhibitors to placebo among women at high risk for breast cancer (O'Regan, 2006). Other drugs, such as somatostatin analogues, which decrease levels of IGF-I, may be evaluated in the future (Pollak, 1998). Thus, chemoprevention for breast cancer is now becoming an option; however, the risk/benefit and cost/benefit ratios, including optimal criteria for use of these agents, have yet to be established.

Anthropometric Measures

Height

Height has been consistently associated with an increase in breast cancer risk, although the magnitude of the effect is modest. In a large prospective study from Nor-

way (Tretli, 1989) with over 8000 cases of breast cancer, a 40% increase in risk was observed with a 15-cm increment in height; comparable relative risks were noted for both premenopausal and postmenopausal women. Similarly, a positive linear trend between height and risk was noted in the birth cohort of women (1929–1932) who lived through their peripubertal period during the Second World War, a time when food was scarce and average attained height was reduced (Vatten and Kvinnsland, 1992). Height may indirectly reflect early energy intake, such that (for a given genetic makeup) short women may have been energy-restricted in childhood. It is well established that energy restriction in rodents substantially reduces mammary tumor rates. Adult height and mammary gland mass are likely to be positively associated, albeit weakly, since both reflect, to a certain extent, overall growth. Of note, IGF-1 levels in childhood are strongly correlated with height (Juul et al, 1994, 1995).

Body mass index

The relationship between body mass index (BMI) and breast cancer risk is complex and varies according to the menopausal status. In premenopausal women, an inverse association between BMI and risk has been reported in most case-control and cohort studies (Ursin et al, 1995). The summary relative risk for a BMI difference of 8 kg/m^2 was 0.70 for the 4 cohort studies and 0.88 for the 19 case-control studies. Several mechanisms likely explain this consistently observed association. First, obesity is inversely associated with mammographic density, and mammographic density is strongly and positively related to breast cancer risk (see "Mammographic Density and Parenchymal Patterns") (Adami et al, 1998). Second, obese women are less likely to ovulate, which reduces their lifetime number of ovulations and alters their circulating hormone levels.

Body mass index is positively related to postmenopausal breast cancer, although the magnitude of the relationship has frequently been modest and has varied substantially among studies (Hunter and Willett, 1993). The mechanism behind this increase in risk is likely related to the increase in circulating hormone levels. After menopause, plasma estrogens are derived primarily from adipose tissue, such that a linear relationship exists between BMI and estrogen levels. In addition, overweight women have low levels of sex hormone-binding globulin and thus a higher biologically available estrogen level; again, this may increase their risk of breast cancer.

Although the weak relationship observed in many studies between BMI and risk in postmenopausal women was unexpected (because of the strong relation between BMI and estrogen levels), it likely occurred for several reasons. First, the reduction in breast cancer risk due to overweight in early adulthood appears to continue into the postmenopausal years. In a prospective analysis, BMI at age 18 was inversely associated with breast cancer risk in both premenopausal and postmenopausal women after controlling for weight change from age 18 (Huang et al, 1997). Thus, women who are obese from early adulthood on would have some of their postmenopausal risk negated by the early protective effect of being overweight. For this reason, weight gain from adolescence to adulthood appears to be most strongly associated with the risk of postmenopausal breast cancer (Willett et al, 1999).

Second, because of the large elevation in estrogen levels they cause, past or current use of postmenopausal hormones appears to obscure much of the positive association that exists between BMI and breast cancer risk (Huang et al, 1997). In the same prospective analysis, although no association was observed between BMI and risk in postmenopausal women who used postmenopausal hormones, a strong positive relationship was observed among women who never used hormones. In this group, those with a BMI of more than 31 kg/m^2 had a relative risk of 1.6 compared to those with a BMI of 20 kg/m^2 or less. Similarly, those who gained 20 kg or more from age 18 to later adulthood had a relative risk of 2.0 compared to women who maintained stable weights, 62 kg, throughout adulthood.

Body fat distribution

As just described, both height and overall adiposity are consistent breast cancer risk factors. Whether body fat distribution contributes further to risk has also been of interest. Greater central or upper body fat distribution is associated with multiple hormonal and metabolic changes, including insulin resistance, decreases in sex hormone-binding globulin, and increases in androgen levels and the conversion of androgens to estrogens in peripheral tissues, and thus could increase the breast cancer risk. Several different measures of fat distribution have been used: waist circumference, waist/hip ratio, and various skinfold measurements. A positive association has been noted in most studies of postmenopausal women. For example, in one large prospective study (Huang et al, 1999) among postmenopausal women who never used postmenopausal hormone therapy, and controlling for BMI, women in the highest versus lowest quintile of waist circumference had an 83% increased risk of breast cancer. Associations among premenopausal women have been weaker and less consistent.

A variety of evidence suggests that early life factors and exposures between the time of menarche and first birth may play a critical role in the etiology of breast cancer. Given the importance of adult adiposity and breast cancer risk, it is plausible that earlier adiposity may also influence adult breast cancer risk. The majority of studies examining childhood fatness and breast cancer have been case-control studies, in which body size was recalled after breast cancer diagnosis, with inconsistent results. In studies with body size data collected prior to breast cancer diagnosis, a strong inverse association between body fatness during adolescence and subsequent risk of both premenopausal (Berkey et al, 1999; Weiderpass et al, 2004; Baer et al, 2005) and postmenopausal (Ahlgren et al, 2004; Berkey et al, 1999) breast cancer has been observed. The Women's Lifestyle and Health cohort study in Norway and Sweden observed a 30% reduction in premenopausal breast cancer risk among women reporting fatter body shapes at age 7 compared with an average body shape (RR = 0.69, 95% CI 0.50–0.93), which was only marginally significant after adjustment for adult BMI (RR = 0.73, 95% CI 0.53–1.01) (Weiderpass et al, 2004). In the Nurses' Health Study II body fatness during childhood and adolescence was also associated with a reduced risk of premenopausal breast cancer, with an approximate 50% lower risk of breast cancer comparing the most overweight to the most lean in childhood (Baer et al, 2005). This strong inverse relation was only slightly attenuated when additionaly adjusted for adult BMI.

Infections

In 1936, a virus that became known as the mouse mammary tumor virus (MMTV) was first reported to substantially increase breast cancer rates in certain strains of mice (Bittner, 1936). Since that time, speculation regarding the relationship between viral infection and human breast cancer has persisted. DNA sequences from several viruses have been found in human breast cancer cells, breast milk, sera, and cyst fluid (Wang et al, 1995). However, the relationship between the presence of these particles and breast cancer development and prognosis remains unknown.

In 1998, French researchers discovered the human mammary tumor virus (HMTV), which is genetically similar to MMTV, in 37% of 387 breast cancer tissue samples (Wang et al, 1995). Previously, most (albeit limited) attention had focused on several common viruses in humans. For example, the prevalence of Epstein-Barr virus (EBV) in breast cancer tissue was found to range from 20% to 46%, depending on the geographic subgroup. Studies of the association between the risk of breast cancer and viral transmission via breast milk have consistently been null (Egan et al, 1999). However, it has been hypothesized that later age at seroconversion, rather than in infancy, may be more important to the subsequent breast cancer risk (Richardson, 1997). To date, viruses appear to play little, if any, role in breast cancer etiology; however, research in this area is continuing.

Physical Activity

Physical activity has been hypothesized to reduce the risk of breast cancer but the epidemiologic data have been generally inconsistent. Strenuous activity in girls can delay both menarche and the onset of regular menstrual cycles. In women, strenuous activity, such as competitive running, can alter circulating hormone levels and increase the frequency of anovulation (Willett et al, 1999). The influence of more moderate activity on hormone levels and menstrual patterns is less well defined. An indirect result of increased physical activity in postmenopausal women is weight reduction, which would likely result in a decrease in breast cancer risk (see previous).

Epidemiologic studies of this association have varied in their approaches to defining physical activity, and this has likely contributed to the observed inconsistency in results (Gammon et al, 1998a; Willett et al, 1999). Studies have focused on activity in different periods of life (eg, earlylife only versus recent activity) or on different types of activity (eg, recreational versus occupational). The frequency and intensity of activity have been assessed in some, but not all, studies.

In a case-control study of premenopausal women using a detailed physical activity assessment (Bernstein et al, 1994), a significant 58% reduction in risk was observed among women with a lifetime average activity level of at least 3.8 hours per week compared to women with an average of 0 hours of activity per week. In a cohort study in Norway (Thune et al, 1997), where a simple survey of leisure-time activity was administered, a similar substantial reduction in risk was noted (RR = 0.63 for consistently active versus consistently inactive women). In contrast, in another large prospective study among premenopausal women in which a simple questionnaire querying leisure-time activity was used (Rockhill et al, 1998), neither adolescent nor adult activity was related to breast cancer risk (eg, for ≥ 7 hours of activity per week versus < 1 hour per week, RR = 1.1). In a second cohort of older women (Rockhill et al, 1999), a modest but significant inverse association was found. In only a few studies has a detailed lifetime assessment of both occupational and nonoccupational activity been collected, with attention paid to both the frequency and intensity of the reported activities. While this is due in large part to the difficulty of designing—and validating—such a questionnaire and to the burden inflicted on the participants, this type of information may need to be collected to fully resolve the relationship between physical activity and breast cancer risk (Gammon et al, 1998a). The International Agency for Research on Cancer of the World Health Organization concluded that there was sufficient evidence for the role of physical activity in preventing breast cancer (Vainio et al, 2002).

Ionizing Radiation

Exposure to ionizing radiation is a well-established cause of somatic DNA mutations. The relationship with breast cancer specifically has been evaluated in a number of cohorts exposed to moderate to high levels of ionizing radiation, including women exposed to the atomic bomb in Nagasaki and Hiroshima, Japan, and women who received repeated fluoroscopic exams for tuberculosis (John and Kelsey, 1993). Follow-up of these cohorts consistently supports a significantly increased risk of breast cancer. The magnitude of the effect increases as the radiation dose increases and as the age at exposure decreases, with the highest risk found in women exposed prepubertally (Miller et al, 1989; Wolff et al, 1996; Davis et al, 1998). As much as a ninefold increase in risk has been reported within this exposed subgroup.

Occupation

Goldberg and Labreche (1996) reviewed 115 studies that addressed the relationship between occupation and breast cancer risk. They found that, in most studies, exposure was categorized according to job title rather than by quantifying the known or hypothesized carcinogens to which women in those occupations may be exposed. In addition, few analyses controlled for potential confounders, such as reproductive factors or socioeconomic status, nor did they evaluate past occupation and current occupation independently. Therefore, conclusions regarding the relationship between specific occupations and breast cancer cannot be made.

Limited evidence suggests that there could be an increased risk for women working in the pharmaceutical industry, and as cosmetologists, and as beauticians. There was no evidence of an increased risk among textile workers, dry cleaners, shoe manufacturers, or nuclear industry workers (Goldberg and Labreche, 1996). In three studies, an increased risk was observed among teachers, bookbinders, nurses, social workers, and cashiers (Welp et al, 1998). An increased risk of breast cancer was reported among flight attendants, although no association has been found among radiologists or x-ray technicians who are also exposed to ionizing radiation (Goldberg and Labreche, 1996; Welp et al, 1998). Again, many of these studies had substantial methodologic problems, particularly no measure of actual exposure and limited, if any, data on potential confounders.

There has been accumulating evidence that occupations involving night-shift work may increase the risk of breast cancer. A meta-analysis of 13 observational studies found a 48% (RR = 1.48, 95% CI 1.36–1.61) increased risk of breast cancer among shift workers (Megdal et al, 2005). One underlying mechanism for an association is proposed to be the suppression of melatonin levels. Accumulating epidemiologic and laboratory data suggest that melatonin may influence breast cancer risk. In vitro studies indicate that melatonin reduces the growth of breast tumor cells and removal of the pineal gland, the source of melatonin, boosts tumor growth in rodent models (Tamarkin et al, 1981). To date, in the two studies to examine melatonin levels and breast cancer risk, an inverse association was observed in one (Schernhammer and Hankinson, 2005), but not in the other (Travis et al, 2004).

Medical Conditions and Treatment

Women with certain medical conditions may possibly be at higher risk of breast cancer. Talamini et al (1997) conducted a large hospital-based case-control study to evaluate the relationship between breast cancer risk and 23 medical conditions. The risk of breast cancer was increased in postmenopausal women with a history of diabetes mellitus. Women who had thyroid nodules had a lower breast cancer risk.

Adult-onset (type II) diabetes may increase the risk of breast cancer because of the associated hyperinsulinemia that can increase the growth of breast cancer cells and may increase levels of other growth factors, such as IGF-I (Willett et al, 1999). Compared to the general population, diabetic women were noted to have a higher incidence of breast cancer (RR = 1.3) (Weiderpass et al, 1997). In studies by Talamini et al (1997) and Weiderpass et al (1997), positive associations between diabetes and breast cancer risk in older women also were observed. Because insulin resistance is modifiable (eg, through maintenance of lean body weight), the relationship between diabetes and breast cancer risk should be further evaluated.

The relationship between thyroid disease and breast cancer has been evaluated in several studies, with inconsistent results. Reports of a modest positive association could reflect increased medical surveillance and thus provide an opportunity for diagnosis in those receiving medical attention for thyroid disorders. It has been reported that nontoxic goiter and high thyroid volumes are more common among women with breast cancer; however, to date, no detailed epidemiologic analyses have been carried out (Shering et al, 1996).

Given that nulliparity and later age at first birth are established breast cancer risk factors, the effect of infertility on risk has also been evaluated in several studies. Results of a population-based case-control study of women aged 20 to 54 (Weiss et al, 1998) suggested that first birth after age 35 was associated with an increased risk of breast cancer among women who reported having difficulty becoming pregnant or maintaining a pregnancy (OR=2.96), but not among those who did not report fertility problems (OR=1.1). In the Nurses' Health Study II cohort, a 60% decrease in risk was found among women reporting ovulatory infertility compared to fertile women (OR=0.4) (Garland et al, 1998).

While there is substantial evidence that the use of nonsteroidal anti-inflammatory drugs (NSAIDs) decreases the risk of colon cancer, the association between NSAID use and breast cancer is unclear. In a large case-control study (Harris et al, 1996), women who had used an NSAID three or more times per week for at least 1 year were at decreased risk of breast cancer compared to nonusers (OR=0.66). In contrast, in a large prospective study (Egan et al, 1996), no relationship was found with the use of two or more aspirin tablets per week with the heavy use of more than two aspirin tablets per day compared to nonusers. The California Teachers Study also observed no overall association between regular NSAID use and incidence of cancer (Marshall et al, 2005). In contrast, the observational study of the Women's Health Initiative (WHI), found that regular users of NSAIDs (2+ tablets/week) were at a 21% decreased risk of breast cancer (RR, 0.79; 95% CI, 0.60–1.04) (Harris et al, 2003). More detailed information on indications for and patterns of NSAID use, as well as specific categorization of types of both over-the-counter and prescription preparations, need to be evaluated before any conclusions can be drawn.

A growing body of literature suggests that statins have antitumor activity by interrupting cell-cycle progression and inducing apoptosis. Statins are a class of lipid-lowering drugs prescribed for the prevention of cardiovasuclar disease. A meta-analysis of randomized trials (Bonovas et al, 2005) and two large prospective studies (Eliassen et al, 2005; Cauley et al, 2006) suggest that statins as a group are not associated with breast cancer incidence. However, one study reported that the hydrophobic class of statins (eg, simvastatin and lovastatin) were associated with a 18% (HR = 0.82, 95% CI 0.70–0.97) reduction in breast cancer incidence (Cauley et al, 2006). Further evaluation of specific classes of statins and long-term use are necessary.

Other Risk Factors

In utero and perinatal exposures

There is evidence that intrauterine exposures play an important role in the etiology of adult-onset diseases. This, and the role of hormones in breast cancer etiology, leads to the hypothesis that the intrauterine hormonal environment might influence the risk of breast cancer in adulthood (Trichopoulos, 1990). Direct evidence of a role of in utero hormonal exposures influencing breast cancer risk comes from diethylstilbestrol (DES) exposed cohorts. DES is a synthetic estrogen that was prescribed to pregnant women in the 1940s to 1960s with the hope of preventing miscarriage, although was later found to provide no benefit against spontaneous abortion. Daughters who were exposed in utero to DES have a 40% increased risk of developing breast cancer (Palmer et al, 2006). This association may be stronger at older ages, with women 50+ experiencing the greatest risk (RR = 3.85, 95% CI 1.06–14.0). Animal evidence that supports the potential importance of early life exposures for subsequent breast cancer risk includes studies in which the female offspring of pregnant rodents fed a high-fat diet had a higher incidence of induced mammary tumors (Hilakivi-Clarke et al, 1997) and more aggressive mammary tumors (Walker and Kurth, 1997) than did the female offspring of pregnant rodents fed a low-fat diet. To address this hypothesis, factors likely to be associated with hormone levels during pregnancy have been evaluated in relation to breast cancer risk in the offspring.

Some, but not all, data suggest that women who are first-born are at increased risk of breast cancer in adulthood. Compared to subsequent pregnancies, first pregnancies have been associated with higher circulating estrogen levels (Lipworth, 1995). Maternal preeclampsia has been associated with a substantially decreased risk of breast cancer in the offspring in one large population-based study in Sweden (Ekbom et al, 1997), perhaps on account of the lower circulating estrogen levels in such pregnancies. Dizygotic twins also have been observed to have a higher risk of breast cancer (Weiss et al, 1997; Cerhan et al, 2000), once again because these pregnancies are associated with higher estrogen levels. Data on gestational age are inconsistent. One study, however, suggests an increased risk of breast cancer for women born before the 33rd week of gestation (Ekbom et al, 2000).

In a large study in Sweden (Ekbom et al, 1992), a positive association between birth weight and breast cancer risk was found, although in a subsequent study (Ekbom et al, 1997) the association was not observed. A recent study found a positive association between birth weight and breast cancer risk in a cohort of opposite-sex twins (Kaijser et al, 2001). In twins, the variation in levels of estrogen exposure is greater than in singletons. Lastly, in a case-control study nested in the Nurses' Health Study cohorts, a strong and statistically significant positive association was found between birth weight and breast cancer risk (Michels et al, 1996). Overall, the accumulated evidence suggests an influence of in utero exposures on the subsequent risk of breast cancer.

Benign breast disease

A number of benign breast conditions have been evaluated in terms of their influence on subsequent breast cancer risk (Bodian, 1993). A classification scheme for these lesions was proposed by Dupont and Page (1985); these criteria were subsequently adopted for use by the American College of Pathologists. The benign diseases were divided into three primary categories: nonproliferative breast disease (eg, cysts, apocrine metaplasia), proliferative breast disease without atypia (eg, intraductal papilloma, sclerosing adenosis), and proliferative disease with atypia (atypical hyperplasia). Compared to women with nonproliferative breast disease, those with proliferative disease without atypia have approximately a 1.3- to 1.9-fold higher risk of breast cancer (Bodian, 1993; Marshall et al, 1997). Women with atypical hyperplasia generally are observed to have a four- to sixfold higher risk of breast cancer; this appears to be somewhat more marked for women with atypical lobular (versus ductal) hyperplasia (Marshall et al, 1997). The subsequent breast cancer is as likely to be diagnosed in the contralateral breast as in the ipsilateral breast, which suggests that these benign conditions serve as general markers of increased risk rather than being precursor lesions. Further support for this concept is the observation that the increased risk of breast cancer following benign breast biopsy can last for several decades.

Mammographic Density and Parenchymal Patterns

The breast is made up of fat, stroma, and epithelial tissue. On a mammogram, fat tissue appears translucent, whereas stromal and epithelial tissue are radiographically dense. Mammographic parenchymal patterns were first described by Wolfe as consisting of predominantly fat (N1 pattern), having gradually increasing ductal prominence (P1 and P2 patterns), or having diffuse or nodular density (DY pattern) (Wolfe, 1976). Several additional classification schemes have been used subsequently, including a description of the overall percentage of dense tissue seen on the mammogram (ie, mammographic density).

The vast majority of case-control and cohort studies have observed a significant positive relationship between dense mammographic patterns and subsequent risk of breast cancer (Oza and Boyd, 1993); the association has been particularly strong when the exposure is defined as percent breast density. In a large prospective study, Byrne et al (1995) found a relative risk of 4.4 for women with more than 75% density versus 0% density on their mammogram. The relative risk was independent of other well-established breast cancer risk factors. Importantly, percent breast density predicted the breast cancer risk for 10 or more years, suggesting that the result was not due to a masking effect of the dense tissue on a preexisting lesion.

Percent breast density is an expression of the mammary gland mass as a fraction of the total breast area, and thus presumably the total number of breast cells at risk of malignant transformation (Trichopoulos and Lipman, 1992; Adami et al, 1998). Additional evidence supports the importance of breast size, that is, the total number of cells at risk, for breast cancer. Small-breasted women who were motivated to have augmentation mammoplasty, and whose mammary gland mass had to be small, were found to have a substantially reduced breast cancer risk, as were women who had undergone surgical reduction of their breasts (Adami et al, 1998). Breast size, as measured by bra size, was positively associated with breast cancer risk in postmenopausal women in some studies (Hsieh and Trichopoulos, 1991; Egan et al, 1999).

Epidemiologic studies examining the effects of hormone replacement therapy and tamoxifen on mammographic density have driven the hypothesis that estrogens are associated with breast density. Cross-sectional studies examining postmenopausal endogenous estrogen levels and mammographic density have been conflicting, reporting no association (Boyd et al, 2002; Tamimi et al, 2005) or only a slight positive association (Greendale et al, 2005). Future studies among premenopausal women will help to elucidate the relation between endogenous hormone levels and mammographic density.

Environmental Pollution

It has been hypothesized that environmental carcinogens, whether through occupational, dietary, or home exposure, act to increase the risk of breast cancer through interaction with hormone receptors, frequently termed *endocrine disruptors* (Adami et al, 1995). Geographic variation, cluster identification, and the increasing incidence of breast cancer over time have played a role in promoting the belief that environmental toxins are significant contributors to breast cancer development. Compounds under investigation include organochlorines such as dichlorodiphenyltrichloroethane (DDT) and polychlorinated biphenyls (PCBs), as well as polynuclear aromatic compounds such as benzópyrene and triazine herbicides (Snedeker and Diaugustine, 1992; Laden and Hunter, 1998; Welp et al, 1998). In animal studies, only DDT exposure has been found to increase the risk of breast neoplasms (Wolff et al, 1996). To date, several prospective epidemiologic investigations have been relatively consistent in showing no substantial increase in risk among those with higher DDT and PCB blood levels (Davis et al, 1998; Laden and Hunter, 1998). Although a modest positive association is difficult to exclude, it is unlikely that exposures to these compounds are important causes of breast cancer. Other environmental pollutants have received more limited evaluation in epidemiologic studies, and additional research is ongoing.

Electromagnetic Fields

A link between low-frequency electromagnetic field (EMF) exposure and breast cancer incidence has been suggested based on the hypothesis that the exposure upregulates estrogen and prolactin secretion by suppressing melatonin (Snedeker and Diaugustine, 1992; Laden and Hunter, 1998; Welp et al, 1998). A number of animal studies have supported a possible relationship, but the epidemiologic evidence has been inconsistent. One of the greatest difficulties in these studies is obtaining an accurate measure of EMF exposure; many studies have used indirect measures that may vary in the resultant degree of misclassification. In a study of 2619 Norwegian women who worked as radio and telegraph operators between 1920 and 1980 (Tynes et al, 1996), the incidence of breast cancer compared to the incidence in the general population was 1.5. In addition, four studies have found an increased risk of breast cancer in men who are electrical workers (Goldberg and Labreche, 1996). However, an association with the use of an electric blanket (a strong household source of EMFs) has not been found (Gammon et al, 1998b). Although additional studies are ongoing, it is unlikely that exposure to EMF contributes significantly to the breast cancer incidence.

Breast Cancer in Men

Admittedly, the incidence of female breast cancer far exceeds that of male breast cancer (1992–1996 age-adjusted US rates per 100 000 were 110.6 in women versus 0.9 in men), with fewer than 1% of all breast cancers occurring in men (SEER). However, both the histologic type of the tumor and the age distribution of the cancer are similar in men and women. And the geographic variation in incidence may mimic that of female breast cancer (Ewertz et al, 1989).

Known risk factors for male breast cancer include BRCA2 gene mutation, Klinefelter syndrome (XXY), and exogenous estrogen exposure (Hsing et al, 1998; Ravandi-Kashani and Hayes, 1998). Using next-of-kin interview data from the National Mortality Followback Survey (NMFS), Hsing et al (1998) compared 178 male fatal breast cancer cases with 512 controls who died from other causes. They found no association with cigarette or alcohol use and a significant positive association with BMI. As would be expected due to the rarity of the disease, few studies of breast cancer in men have been conducted.

CONCLUSION

We have learned a great deal about the lifestyle and genetic factors that influence breast cancer risk. As shown in Table 16–1, at least 14 risk factors are now well established. In addition to the confirmed risk factors, there are many that either have been reported only inconsistently in the literature or have received only limited study to date; these factors also are listed in Table 16–1. When interpreting this table, it is important to note that many factors are continuous variables; thus, the magnitude of the association is highly dependent upon what two groups are being compared. For example, the relative risk associated with a first birth at age 35 (versus less than age 20) is much higher than that associated with a first birth at age 25 (versus age 20).

The mechanisms underlying these confirmed or possible risk factors are known with varying levels of certainty. The epide-

miologic literature related to breast cancer risk has been summarized and integrated into a proposed etiologic model consisting of several components (Adami et al, 1998). Breast cancer appears to increase with the number of susceptible cells in the breast; this number is, in turn, influenced by early life, and perhaps even prenatal, exposures. Both mammographic density and mammary gland mass are likely to reflect, at least in part, the total number of at-risk cells. Several lines of evidence, such as the associations with height and early exposure to radiation, support an important influence of early life events on subsequent breast cancer risk.

Risk is further influenced by pregnancy, which can stimulate the growth of already initiated cells, but conveys long-term pro-

Table 16–2. Association (Relative risks and 95% confidence intervals) between circulating levels of estradiol and testosterone with subsequent risk of breast cancer in postmenopausal women*

Study	Cases/ controls	Categories of circulating hormones[†]				
		1 (low)	2	3	4	5 (high)
Estradiol						
EHBCCG (2002)[‡]	663/1765	1.0 (Ref)	1.4(1.0–2.0)	1.2(0.9–1.7)	1.8(1.3–2.4)	2.0(1.5–2.7)
Manjer et al. (2003)	173/438	1.0 (Ref)	1.7(1.0–2.9)			
Missmer et al. (2004)[∥]	322/643	1.0 (Ref)	1.3(0.9–1.9)	1.1(0.7–1.7)	2.1(1.5–3.2)	
Zeleniuch-Jacquotte et al. (2004)[§]	297/563	1.0 (Ref)	1.6(1.0–2.7)	1.2(0.7–1.9)	1.7(1.0–2.8)	2.5(1.5–4.2)
Kaaks et al. (2005)	677/1309	1.0 (Ref)	1.1(0.8–1.5)	1.4(1.0–2.0)	1.7(1.2–2.4)	2.3(1.6–3.2)
Testosterone						
EHBCCG (2002)[‡]	585/1574	1.0 (Ref)	1.3(1.0–1.9)	1.6(1.2–2.2)	1.6(1.1–2.2)	2.2(1.6–3.1)
Manjer et al. (2003)	154/417	1.0 (Ref)	1.2(0.7–2.2)	1.3(0.7–2.3)	1.9(1.1–3.3)	
Missmer et al. (2004)[∥]	312/628	1.0 (Ref)	0.9(0.6–1.4)	1.5(1.0–2.2)	1.6(1.0–2.4)	
Zeleniuch-Jacquotte et al. (2004)[§]	297/562	1.0 (Ref)	1.7(1.0–2.8)	1.6(0.9–2.6)	1.9(1.2–3.2)	2.4(1.4–4.0)
Kaaks et al. (2005)	668/1280	1.0 (Ref)	1.1(0.8–1.6)	1.3(1.0–1.8)	1.6(1.1–2.2)	1.9(1.3–2.6)

[*] All studies are prospective

[†] Hormone date are presented as quartiles or quintiles according to the original publication, except for Manjer et al, where the analysis compares women with the highest 20% of circulating level to the remaining women.

[‡] Endogenous hormone and breast cancer collaborative group

[∥] Extension to study included as part of EHBCCG. An additional 167 new breast cancer cases and 333 new controls are included in the updated analysis.

[§] Extension of study included as part of EHBCCG. An additional 168 new breast cancer cases and 316 new controls are included in the updated analysis.

tection, perhaps through permanent structural changes to the tissue or other still-unknown mechanisms. In adult life, levels of hormones (whether resulting from obesity or use of exogenous estrogens, for example) and their receptors may influence the number of target cells, the likelihood of retaining spontaneous somatic mutations, and the rate of growth of malignant cells. The role of circulating high estrogen levels is now well established to increase the risk; the role of other hormones such as prolactin or insulin-like growth factor is less clear but likely to be important.

Although a number of exposures are now well established to influence breast cancer risk, this knowledge, unfortunately, does not readily translate into a means for cancer prevention. Most of the established reproductive risk factors, such as age at menarche, age at first birth, and parity, are not readily altered or not appropriate for public health intervention. The established modifiable risk factors include postmenopausal hormone use, moderate alcohol intake, and adult weight gain. Individual decision making is complex, however, as several of these factors, such as hormone use, are probably beneficial in decreasing the risk of other chronic diseases such as osteoporosis. Other factors that may decrease the risk of breast cancer include breast-feeding, physical activity, and increased dietary intake of fruits and vegetables, although the evidence here is neither as strong nor as consistent as for other factors. With our increasing knowledge of the relation between endogenous hormones and breast cancer risk, and the development of selective estrogen receptor modulators, such as tamoxifen and raloxifene as well as aromatase inhibitors, chemoprevention also may be possible in the future. Substantial additional research, including risk/benefit and cost/benefit assessments, are needed, however.

REFERENCES

Adami HO, Lipworth L, Titus-Ernstoff L, Hsieh CC, Hanberg A, Ahlborg U, et al. Organochlorine compounds and estrogen-related cancers in women. Cancer Causes Control 1995;6:551–66.

Adami HO, Signorello LB, Trichopoulos D. Towards an understanding of breast cancer etiology. Semin Cancer Biol 1998;8:255–62.

Ahlgren M, Melbye M, Wohlfahrt J, Sorensen TI. Growth patterns and the risk of breast cancer in women. N Engl J Med 2004; 351(16):1619–26.

Al-Delaimy WK, Cho E, Chen WY, Colditz G, Willet WC. A prospective study of smoking and risk of breast cancer in young adult women. Cancer Epidemiol Biomarkers Prev 2004;13:398–404.

Anderson GL, Limacher M, Assaf AR, Bassford T, Beresford SA, Black H, et al. Effects of conjugated equine estrogen in postmenopausal women with hysterectomy: the Women's Health Initiative randomized controlled trial. JAMA 2004;291:1701–12.

Annegers JF. Patterns of oral contraceptive use in the United States. Br J Rheumatol 1989; 28:48–50.

Baer HJ, Colditz GA, Rosner B, Michels KB, Rich-Edwards JW, Hunter DJ, et al. Body fatness during childhood and adolescence and incidence of breast cancer in premenopausal women: a prospective cohort study. Breast Cancer Res 2005;7(3):R314–25.

Barrett-Connor E, Mosca L, Collins P, Geiger MJ, Grady D, Kornitzer M, et al. Effects of raloxifene on cardiovascular events and breast cancer in postmenopausal women. N Engl J Med 2006;355:125–37.

Bennett I, Gattas M, Teh B. The genetic basis of breast cancer and its clinical implications. Aust N Z J Surg 1999;69:95–105.

Beral V and Million Women Study Coordinators. Breast cancer and hormone-replacement therapy in the Million Women Study. Lancet 2003;362(9382):419–27.

Bergkvist L, Adami HO, Persson I, Hoover R, Schairer C. The risk of breast cancer after estrogen and estrogen-progestin replacement. N Engl J Med 1989;321:293–97.

Berkey CS, Frazier AL, Gardner JD, Colditz GA. Adolescence and breast carcinoma risk. Cancer 1999;85(11):2400–9.

Bernstein L, Henderson BE, Hanisch R, Sullivan-Halley J, Ross RK. Physical exercise and reduced risk of breast cancer in young women. J Natl Cancer Inst 1994;86:1403–8.

Bernstein L, Ross RK. Endogenous hormones and breast cancer risk. Epidemiol Rev 1993; 15:48–65.

Bittner, JJ. Some possible effects of nursing on the mammary gland tumor incidence in mice. Science 1936;84:162–63.

Bodian CA. Benign breast diseases, carcinoma in situ, and breast cancer risk. Epidemiol Rev 1993;15:177–87.

Bonovas S, Filioussi K, Tsavaris N, Sitaras NM. Use of statins and breast cancer: a meta-analysis of seven randomized clinical trials and nine observational studies. J Clin Oncol 2005;23:8606–12.

Boyd NF, Stone J, Martin LJ, Jong R, Fishell E, Yaffe M, et al. The association of breast mitogens with mammographic densities. Br J Cancer 2002;87:876–82.

Breast Cancer Association Consortium. Commonly studied single-nucleotide polymorphisms and breast cancer: results from the Breast Cancer Association Consortium. J Natl Cancer Inst 2006;98:1382–96

Briand P. Hormone-dependent mammary tumors in mice and rats as a model for human breast cancer [review]. Anticancer Res 1983;3:273–81.

Brind J, Chinchilli VM, Severs WB, Summy-Long J. Induced abortion as an independent risk factor for breast cancer: a comprehensive review and meta-analysis. J Epidemiol Commun Health 1996;50:481–96.

Byrne C, Schairer C, Wolfe J, Parekh N, Salane M, Brinton LA, et al. Mammographic features and breast cancer risk: effects with time, age, and menopause status. J Natl Cancer Inst 1995;87:1622–29.

Cauley JA, McTiernan A, Rodabough RJ, La-Croix A, Bauer DC, Margolis KL, et al. Statin use and breast cancer: prospective results from the Women's Health Initiative. J Natl Cancer Inst 2006;98:700–7.

Cerhan JR, Kushi LH, Olson JE, Rich SS, Zheng W, Folsom AR, et al. Twinship and risk of postmenopausal breast cancer. J Natl Cancer Inst 2000;92:261–65.

CHEK2 Breast Cancer Case-Control Consortium: CHEK2*1100delC and susceptibility to breast cancer: a collaborative analysis involving 10,860 breast cancer cases and 9,065 controls from 10 studies. Am J Hum Genet 2004;74:1175–82.

Chen WY, Manson JE, Hankinson SE, Rosner B, Holmes MD, Willett WC, et al. Unopposed estrogen therapy and the risk of invasive breast cancer. Arch Intern Med 2006; 166(9):1027–32.

Chen J, Campbell TC, Junyao L, Peto R. Diet, Lifestyle, and Mortality in China: A Study of the Characteristics of 65 Chinese Counties. Oxford, Oxford University Press, 1990.

Chia KS, Reilly M, Tan CS, Lee J, Pawitan Y, Adami HO, Hall P, Mow B. Profound changes in breast cancer incidence may reflect changes into a Westernized lifestyle: a comparative population-based study in Singapore and Sweden. Int J Cancer. 2005;10; 113:302–6.

Chlebowski RT, Hendrix SL, Langer RD, Stefanick ML, Gass M, Lane D, et al. Influence of estrogen plus progestin on breast cancer and mammography in healthy postmenopausal women: the Women's Health Initiative Randomized Trial. JAMA 2003; 289(24):3243–53.

Cho E, Spiegelman D, Hunter DJ, Chen WY, Stampfer MJ, Colditz GA, et al. Premenopausal fat intake and risk of breast cancer. J Natl Cancer Inst 2003; 95(14):1079–85.

Coates RJ, Weiss NS, Daling JR, Morris JS, Labbe RF. Serum levels of selenium and retinol and the subsequent risk of cancer. Am J Epidemiol 1988;128:515–23.

Colditz GA, Hankinson SE, Hunter DJ, Willett WC, Manson JE, Stampfer MJ, et al. The use of estrogens and progestins and the risk of breast cancer in postmenopausal women. N Engl J Med 1995;332:1589–93.

Colditz GA, Rosner B. Cumulative risk of breast cancer to age 70 years according to risk factor status: data from the Nurses' Health Study. Am J Epidemiol 2000;152: 950–64.

Collaborative Group on Hormonal Factors in Breast Cancer. Breast cancer and hormonal contraceptives: collaborative reanalysis of individual data on 53,297 women with breast cancer and 100,239 women without breast cancer from 54 epidemiological studies. Collaborative Group on Hormonal Factors in Breast Cancer. Lancet 1996;347: 1713–27.

Collaborative Group on Hormonal Factors in Breast Cancer. Breast cancer and hormone replacement therapy: collaborative reanalysis of data from 51 epidemiological studies of 52,705 women with breast cancer and 108,411 women without breast cancer. Collaborative Group on Hormonal Factors in Breast Cancer. Lancet 1997;350:1047–59.

Collaborative Group on Hormonal Factors in Breast Cancer. Breast cancer and breastfeeding: collaborative reanalysis of individual data from 47 epidemiological studies in 30 countries, including 50302 women with breast cancer and 96973 women without the disease. Lancet 2002;360:187–95.

Committee on the Relationship Between Oral Contraceptives and Breast Cancer Institute of Medicine. Oral contraceptives and Breast Cancer. Washington, DC, National Academy Press, 1991.

Cui Y, Rohan TE. Vitamin D, calcium, and breast cancer risk: a review. Cancer Epidemiol Biomarkers Prev 2006;15:1427–37.

Cuzick J, Forbes J, Edwards R, Baum M, Cawthorn S, Coates A, et al. First results from the International Breast Cancer Intervention Study (IBIS-I): a randomised prevention trial. Lancet 2002;360(9336):817–24.

Cuzick J, Powles T, Veronesi U, Forbes J, Edwards R, Ashley S, et al. Overview of the main outcomes in breast-cancer prevention trials. Lancet 2003;361(9354):296–300.

Davis DL, Axelrod D, Bailey L, Gaynor M, Sasco AJ. Rethinking breast cancer risk and the environment: the case for the precautionary principle. Environ Health Perspect 1998;106:523–29.

Davis S. Androgen replacement in women: a commentary. J Clin Endocrinol Metab 1999;84:1886–91.

Deng CX. BRCA1: cell cycle checkpoint, genetic instability, DNA damage response and cancer evolution. Nucleic Acids Res 2006;34:1416–26.

Devesa SS, Blot WJ, Stone BJ, Miller BA, Tarone RE, Fraumeni JF Jr. Recent cancer trends in the United States. J Natl Cancer Inst 1995;87:175–82.

Dorgan JF, Sowell A, Swanson CA, Potischman N, Miller R, Schussler N, et al. Relationships of serum carotenoids, retinol, alpha-tocopherol, and selenium with breast cancer risk: results from a prospective study in Columbia, Missouri (United States). Cancer Causes Control 1998;9:89–97.

Dunning AM HC, Pharoah PD, Teare MD, Ponder BA, Easton DF: A systematic review of genetic polymorphisms and breast cancer risk. Cancer Epidemiol Biomarkers Prev 1999; 8: 843–54.

Dupont WD, Page DL. Risk factors for breast cancer in women with proliferative breast disease. N Engl J Med 1985;312:146–51.

Easton DF, Pooley KA, Dunning AM, Pharoah PD, Thompson D, Ballinger DG, et al. Genome-wide association study identifies novel breast cancer susceptibility loci. Nature 2007;447:1087–93.

Ebeling P, Koivisto VA. Physiological importance of dehydroepiandrosterone. Lancet 1994;343:1479–81.

Egan KM, Newcomb PA, Titus-Ernstoff L, Trentham-Dietz A, Baron JA, Willett WC, et al. The relation of breast size to breast cancer risk in postmenopausal women (United States). Cancer Causes Control 1999;10:115–18.

Egan KM, Stampfer MJ, Giovannucci E, Rosner BA, Colditz GA. Prospective study of regular aspirin use and the risk of breast cancer. J Natl Cancer Inst 1996;88:988–93.

Ekbom A, Erlandsson G, Hsieh C, Trichopoulos D, Adami HO, Cnattingius S. Risk of breast cancer in prematurely born women. J Natl Cancer Inst 2000;92:840–41.

Ekbom A, Hsieh CC, Lipworth L, Adami HO, Trichopoulos D. Intrauterine environment and breast cancer risk in women: a population-based study. J Natl Cancer Inst 1997;89:71–76.

Ekbom A, Trichopoulos D, Adami HO, Hsieh CC, Lan SJ. Evidence of prenatal influences on breast cancer risk. Lancet 1992;340:1015–18.

Eliassen AH, Colditz GA, Rosner B, Willett WC, Hankinson SE. Serum lipids, lipid-lowering drugs, and the risk of breast cancer. Arch Intern Med 2005;165:2264–71.

Eliassen AH, Missmer SA, Tworoger SS, Spiegelman DS, Barbieri RL, Dowsett M, Hankinson SE. Endogenous steroid hormone concentrations and risk of breast cancer among premenopuasal women. J Natl Cancer Inst 2006; 98: 1406–15.

Ellisen LW, Haber DA. Hereditary breast cancer. Annu Rev Med 1998;49:425–36.

Ewertz M, Holmberg L, Karjalainen S, Tretli S, Adami HO. Incidence of male breast cancer in Scandinavia, 1943–1982. Int J Cancer 1989;43:27–31.

Ferlay J, Bray F, Pisani P, Parkin DM. GLOBOCAN 2000: Cancer Incidence, Mortality and Prevalence Worldwide. International Agency for Research on Cancer, Lyon, 2001.

Fisher B, Costantino JP, Wickerham DL, Redmond CK, Kavanah M, Cronin WM, et al. Tamoxifen for prevention of breast cancer: report of the National Surgical Adjuvant Breast and Bowel Project P-1 Study. J Natl Cancer Inst 1998;90:1371–88.

Fisher B, Costantino JP, Wickerham DL, Cecchini RS, Cronin WM, Robidoux A, et al. Tamoxifen for the prevention of breast cancer: current status of the National Surgical Adjuvant Breast and Bowel Project P-1 study. J Natl Cancer Inst 2005;97(22):1652–62.

Fournier DB, Erdman JW Jr, Gordon GB. Soy, its components, and cancer prevention: a review of the in vitro, animal, and human data. Cancer Epidemiol Biomarkers Prev 1998;7:1055–65.

Freudenheim JL, Marshall JR, Vena JE, Laughlin R, Brasure JR, Swanson MK, et al. Premenopausal breast cancer risk and intake of vegetables, fruits, and related nutrients. J Natl Cancer Inst 1996;88:340–48.

Gammon MD, John EM, Britton JA. Recreational and occupational physical activities and risk of breast cancer. J Natl Cancer Inst 1998a;90:100–17.

Gammon MD, Schoenberg JB, Britton JA, Kelsey JL, Stanford JL, Malone KE, et al. Electric blanket use and breast cancer risk among younger women. Am J Epidemiol 1998b;148:556–63.

Garland M, Hunter DJ, Colditz GA, Manson JE, Stampfer MJ, Spiegelman D, et al. Menstrual cycle characteristics and history of ovulatory infertility in relation to breast cancer risk in a large cohort of U.S. women. Am J Epidemiol 1998;147:636–43.

Goldberg MS, Labreche F. Occupational risk factors for female breast cancer: a review. Occup Environ Med 1996;53:145–56.

Gradishar W. Landmark trials in endocrine adjuvant therapy for breast carcinoma. Cancer 2006;106:975–81.

Graham S, Marshall J, Mettlin C, Rzepka T, Nemoto T, Byers T. Diet in the epidemiology of breast cancer. Am J Epidemiol 1982; 116:68–75.

Gram IT, Braaten T, Terry PD, et al. Breast cancer risk among women who start smoking as teenagers. Cancer Epidemiol Biomarkers Prev 2005;14:61–66.

Greendale GA, Reboussin BA, Sie A, Singh HR, Olson LK, Gatewood O, et al. Effects of estrogen and estrogen-progestin on mammographic parenchymal density. Postmenopausal Estrogen/Progestin Interventions (PEPI) Investigators. Ann Intern Med 1999;130:262–69.

Greendale GA, Palla SL, Ursin G, Laughlin GA, Crandall C, Pike MC, et al. The association of endogenous sex steroids and sex steroid binding proteins with mammographic density: results from the postmenopausal estrogen/progestin interventions mammographic density study. Am J Epidemiol 2005;162: 826–34.

Greene MH. Genetics of breast cancer. Mayo Clin Proc 1997;72:54–65.

Hankinson SE, Manson JE, London SJ, Willett WC, Speizer FE. Laboratory reproducibility of endogenous hormone levels in postmenopausal women. Cancer Epidemiol Biomarkers Prev 1994;3:51–56.

Hankinson SE, Willett WC, Michaud DS, Manson JE, Colditz GA, Longcope C, et al. Plasma prolactin levels and subsequent risk of breast cancer in postmenopausal women. J Natl Cancer Inst 1999;91:629–34.

Harris RE, Chlebowski RT, Jackson RD, Frid DJ, Ascenseo JL, Anderson G, et al. Breast cancer and nonsteroidal anti-inflammatory drugs: prospective results from the Women's Health Initiative. Cancer Res 2003;63:6096–6101.

Harris JR, Lippman ME, Veronesi U, Willett W. Breast cancer (1). N Engl J Med 1992;327: 319–28.

Harris RE, Namboodiri KK, Farrar WB. Nonsteroidal antiinflammatory drugs and breast cancer. Epidemiology 1996;7:203–5.

Harvey EB, Schairer C, Brinton LA, Hoover RN, Fraumeni JF Jr. Alcohol consumption and breast cancer. J Natl Cancer Inst 1987; 78:657–61.

Hemminki E, Kennedy DL, Baum C, McKinlay SM. Prescribing of noncontraceptive estrogens and progestins in the United States, 1974–1986. Am J Public Health 1988; 78:1479–81.

Henderson B, Pike M, Bernstein L, Ross R. Breast cancer. In: Schottenfeld D, Fraumeni J Jr (Eds): Cancer Epidemiology and Prevention. New York, Oxford University Press, 1996, pp 1022–39.

Herman V, Kalk WJ, de Moor NG, Levin J. Serum prolactin after chest wall surgery: elevated levels after mastectomy. J Clin Endocrinol Metab 1981;52:148–51.

Hilakivi-Clarke L, Clarke R, Onojafe I, Raygada M, Cho E, Lippman M. A maternal diet high in n-6 polyunsaturated fats alters mammary gland development, puberty onset, and breast cancer risk among female rat offspring. Proc Natl Acad Sci USA 1997; 94:9372–77.

Hirschhorn JN, Daly MJ: Genome-wide association studies for common diseases and complex traits. Nat Rev Genet 2005;6:95–108.

Holmes MD, Hunter DJ, Colditz GA, Stampfer MJ, Hankinson SE, Speizer FE, et al. Association of dietary intake of fat and fatty acids with risk of breast cancer. JAMA 1999; 281:914–20.

Howe GR, Hirohata T, Hislop TG, Iscovich JM, Yuan JM, Katsouyanni K, et al. Dietary factors and risk of breast cancer: combined analysis of 12 case-control studies. J Natl Cancer Inst 1990;82:561–69.

Hsieh CC, Trichopoulos D. Breast size, handedness and breast cancer risk. Eur J Cancer 1991;27:131–35.

Hsieh CC, Trichopoulos D, Katsouyanni K, Yuasa S. Age at menarche, age at menopause, height and obesity as risk factors for breast cancer: associations and interactions in an international case-control study. Int J Cancer 1990;46:796–800.

Hsing AW, McLaughlin JK, Cocco P, Co-Chien HT, Fraumeni JF Jr. Risk factors for male breast cancer (United States). Cancer Causes Control 1998;9:269–75.

Huang Z, Hankinson SE, Colditz GA, Stampfer MJ, Hunter DJ, Manson JE, et al. Dual effects of weight and weight gain on breast cancer risk. JAMA 1997;278:1407–11.

Huang Z, Willett WC, Colditz GA, Hunter DJ, Manson JE, Rosner B, et al. Waist circumference, waist:hip ratio, and risk of breast cancer in the Nurses' Health Study. Am J Epidemiol 1999;150:1316–24.

Hunter DJ, Morris JS, Stampfer MJ, Colditz GA, Speizer FE, Willett WC. A prospective study of selenium status and breast cancer risk. JAMA 1990;264:1128–31.

Hunter DJ, Spiegelman D, Adami HO, Beeson L, van den Brandt PA, Folsom AR, et al. Cohort studies of fat intake and the risk of breast cancer—a pooled analysis. N Engl J Med 1996;334:356–61.

Hunter DJ, Willett WC. Diet, body size, and breast cancer. Epidemiol Rev 1993;15:110–32.

Hunter DJ, Riboli E, Haiman CA, Albanes D, Altshuler D, Chanock SJ, Haynes RB, Henderson BE, Kaaks R, Stram DO, et al.: A candidate gene approach to searching for low-penetrance breast and prostate cancer genes. Nat Rev Cancer 2005;12:977–85.

Hunter DJ, Kraft P, Jacobs KB, Cox DG, Yeager M, Hankinson SE, et al. A genome-wide association study identifies alleles in FGFR2 associated with risk of sporadic postmenopausal breast cancer. Nat Genet 2007;39:870–74

Jin F, Shu XO, Devesa SS, Zheng W, Blot WJ, Gao YT. Incidence trends for cancers of the breast, ovary, and corpus uteri in urban Shanghai, 1972–1989. Cancer Causes Control 1993;4:355–60.

John EM, Kelsey JL. Radiation and other environmental exposures and breast cancer. Epidemiol Rev 1993;15:157–62.

John EM, Schwartz GG, Dreon DM, Koo J. Vitamin D and breast cancer risk: the NHANES I Epidemiologic follow-up study, 1971–1975 to 1992. National Health and Nutrition Examination Survey. Cancer Epidemiol Biomarkers Prev 1999;8:399–406.

Juul A, Bang P, Hertel NT, Main K, Dalgaard P, Jorgensen K, et al. Serum insulin-like growth factor-I in 1030 healthy children, adolescents, and adults: relation to age, sex, stage of puberty, testicular size, and body mass index. J Clin Endocrinol Metab 1994;78:744–52.

Juul A, Dalgaard P, Blum WF, Bang P, Hall K, Michaelsen KF, et al. Serum levels of insulin-like growth factor (IGF)-binding protein-3 (IGFBP-3) in healthy infants, children, and adolescents: the relation to IGF-I, IGF-II, IGFBP-1, IGFBP-2, age, sex, body mass index, and pubertal maturation. J Clin Endocrinol Metab 1995;80:2534–42.

Kaaks R, Rinaldi S, Key TJ, Berrino F, Peeters PH, Biessy C, et al. Postmenopausal serum androgens, oestrogens and breast cancer risk: the European prospective investigation into cancer and nutrition. Endocr Relat Cancer 2005a;12:1071–82.

Kaaks R, Berrino F, Key T, Rinaldi S, Dossus L, Biessy C, et al. Serum sex steroids in premenopausal women and breast cancer risk within the European Prospective Investigation into Cancer and Nutrition (EPIC). J Natl Cancer Inst 2005b;97:755–65.

Kaijser M, Lichtenstein P, Granath F, Erlandsson G, Cnattingius S, Ekbom A. In utero exposures and breast cancer: a study of opposite-sexed twins. J Natl Cancer Inst 2001; 93:60–62.

Kelsey JL. A review of the epidemiology of human breast cancer. Epidemiol Rev 1979;1: 74–109.

Kelsey JL, Gammon MD, John EM. Reproductive factors and breast cancer. Epidemiol Rev 1993;15:36–47.

Kennedy DL, Baum C, Forbes MB. Noncontraceptive estrogens and progestins: use patterns over time. Obstet Gynecol 1985;65: 441–46.

Key T, Appleby P, Barnes I, Reeves G, Group EHaBCC. Endogenous sex hormones and breast cancer in postmenopausal women: reanalysis of nine prospective studies. J Natl Cancer Inst 2002;94:606–16.

Khan SA, Rogers MA, Khurana KK, Meguid MM, Numann PJ. Estrogen receptor expression in benign breast epithelium and breast cancer risk. J Natl Cancer Inst 1998; 90:37–42.

Knekt P. Serum vitamin E level and risk of female cancers. Int J Cancer 1988;17:281–86.

Krontiris TG, Devlin B, Karp DD, Robert NJ, Risch N. An association between the risk of cancer and mutations in the HRAS1 minisatellite locus. N Engl J Med 1993;329: 517–23.

Kuper H, Ye W, Weiderpass E, Ekbom A, Trichopoulos D, Nyrén O, et al. Alcohol and breast cancer risk: the alcoholism paradox. Br J Cancer 2000;83:949–51.

Laden F, Hunter DJ. Environmental risk factors and female breast cancer. Annu Rev Public Health 1998;19:101–23.

Lambe M, Hsieh C, Trichopoulos D, Ekbom A, Pavia M, Adami HO. Transient increase in the risk of breast cancer after giving birth. N Engl J Med 1994;331:5–9.

Lawson JS, Field AS, Champion S, Tran D, Ishikura H, Trichopoulos D. Low oestrogen receptor alpha expression in normal breast tissue underlies low breast cancer incidence in Japan. Lancet 1999;354:1787–88.

Lipworth L. Epidemiology of breast cancer. Eur J Cancer Prev 1995;4:7–30.

Lipworth L, Bailey LR, Trichopoulos D. History of breast-feeding in relation to breast cancer risk: a review of the epidemiologic literature. J Natl Cancer Inst 2000;92:302–12.

Longnecker MP. Alcoholic beverage consumption in relation to risk of breast cancer: meta-analysis and review. Cancer Causes Control 1994;5:73–82.

Longnecker MP, Newcomb PA, Mittendorf R, Greenberg ER, Clapp RW, Bogdan GF, et al. Risk of breast cancer in relation to lifetime alcohol consumption. J Natl Cancer Inst 1995;87:923–29.

MacGregor JI, Jordan VC. Basic guide to the mechanisms of antiestrogen action. Pharmacol Rev 1998;50:151–96.

MacMahon B, Cole P, Lin TM, Lowe CR, Mirra AP, Ravnihar B, et al. Age at first birth and breast cancer risk. Bull World Health Organ 1970;43:209–21.

MacMahon B, Trichopoulos D, Brown J, Andersen AP, Cole P, deWaard F, et al. Age at menarche, urine estrogens and breast cancer risk. Int J Cancer 1982;30:427–31.

Magnusson C, Baron JA, Correia N, Bergström R, Adami HO, Persson I. Breast-cancer risk following long-term oestrogen- and oestrogen-progestin-replacement therapy. Int J Cancer 1999;81:339–44.

Majumdar SR, Almasi EA, Stafford RS. Promotion and prescribing of hormone therapy after report of harm by the Women's Health Initiative. Jama 2004;292(16):1983–88.

Manjer J, Johansson R, Berglund G, Janzon L, Kaaks R, Agren A, et al. Postmenopausal breast cancer risk in relation to sex steroid hormones, prolactin and SHBG (Sweden). Cancer Causes Control 2003;14:599–607.

Malarkey WB, Kennedy M, Allred LE, Milo G. Physiological concentrations of prolactin can promote the growth of human breast tumor cells in culture. J Clin Endocrinol Metab 1983;56:673–77.

Marchbanks PA, McDonald JA, Wilson HG, Folger SG, Mandel MG, Daling JR, et al. Oral contraceptives and the risk of breast cancer. N Engl J Med 2002;346:2025–32.

Marshall LM, Hunter DJ, Connolly JL, Schnitt SJ, Byrne C, London SJ, et al. Risk of breast cancer associated with atypical hyperplasia of lobular and ductal types. Cancer Epidemiol Biomarkers Prev 1997;6:297–301.

Marshall SF, Bernstein L, Anton-Culver H, Deapen D, Horn-Ross PL, Mohrenweiser H, et al. Nonsteroidal anti-inflammatory drug use and breast cancer risk by stage and hormone receptor status. J Natl Cancer Inst 2005;97:805–12.

Martino S, Cauley JA, Barrett-Connor E, Powles TJ, Mershon J, Disch D, et al. Continuing outcomes relevant to Evista: breast cancer incidence in postmenopausal osteoporotic women in a randomized trial of raloxifene. J Natl Cancer Inst 2004;96(23):1751–61.

Mathews-Roth M. Plasma concentrations of carotenoids after large doses of beta-carotene. Am J Clin Nutr 1990;52:500–1.

McCullough ML, Rodriguez C, Diver WR, Feigelson HS, Stevens VL, Thun MJ, et al. Dairy, calcium, and vitamin D intake and postmenopausal breast cancer risk in the Cancer Prevention Study II Nutrition Cohort. Cancer Epidemiol Biomarkers Prev 2005;14:2898–2904.

Megdal SP, Kroenke CH, Laden F, Pukkala E, Schernhammer ES. Night work and breast cancer risk: a systematic review and meta-analysis. Eur J Cancer 2005;41:2023–32.

Meijers-Heijboer H, van den Ouweland A, Klijn J, Wasielewski M, de Snoo A, Oldenburg R, Hollestelle A, Houben M, Crepin E, van Veghel-Plandsoen M, et al.: Low-penetrance susceptibility to breast cancer due to CHEK2(*) 1100delC in noncarriers of BRCA1 or BRCA2 mutations. Nat Genet 2002;31:55–59.

Meilahn EN, De Stavola B, Allen DS, Fentiman I, Bradlow HL, Sepkovic DW, et al. Do urinary oestrogen metabolites predict breast cancer? Guernsey III cohort follow-up. Br J Cancer 1998;78:1250–55.

Melbye M, Wohlfahrt J, Olsen JH, Frisch M, Westergaard T, Helweg-Larsen K, et al. Induced abortion and the risk of breast cancer. N Engl J Med 1997;336:81–85.

Micheli A, Muti P, Secreto G, Krogh V, Meneghini E, Venturelli E, et al. Endogenous sex hormones and subsequent breast cancer in premenopausal women. Int J Cancer 2004; 112:312–18.

Michels KB, Trichopoulos D, Robins JM, Rosner BA, Manson JE, Hunter DJ, et al. Birthweight as a risk factor for breast cancer. Lancet 1996;348:1542–46.

Miller AB, Howe GR, Sherman GJ, Lindsay JP, Yaffe MJ, Dinner PJ, et al. Mortality from breast cancer after irradiation during fluoroscopic examinations in patients being treated for tuberculosis. N Engl J Med 1989;321(19):1285–89

Missmer SA, Eliassen AH, Barbieri RL, Hankinson SE. Endogenous estrogen, androgen, and progesterone concentrations and breast cancer risk among postmenopausal women. J Natl Cancer Inst 2004;96:1856–65.

Nagata C, Kawakami N, Shimizu H. Trends in the incidence rate and risk factors for breast cancer in Japan. Breast Cancer Res Treat 1997;44:75–82.

Narod SA. Modifiers of risk of hereditary breast cancer. Oncogene 2006;25:5832–36.

National Center for Health Statistics. SEER Cancer Statistics Review, 1973–1995. Bethesda, MD, National Cancer Institute, 1998.

Newcomb PA, Storer BE, Longnecker MP, Mittendorf R, Greenberg ER, Clapp RW, et al. Lactation and a reduced risk of pre-menopausal breast cancer. N Engl J Med 1994;330:81–87.

O'Regan RM. Chemoprevention of breast cancer. Lancet 2006;367:1382–83.

Oza AM, Boyd NF. Mammographic parenchymal patterns: a marker of breast cancer risk. Epidemiol Rev 1993;15:196–208.

Palmer J, Rosenberg L. Cigarette smoking and risk of breast cancer. In: Kelsey J (Ed): Epidemiologic Reviews. Baltimore: John Hopkins University School of Hygiene and Public Health, 1993, pp 145–56.

Palmer JR, Wise LA, Hatch EE, Troisi R, Titus-Ernstoff L, Strohsnitter W, et al. Prenatal diethylstilbestrol exposure and risk of breast cancer. Cancer Epidemiol Biomarkers Prev 2006;15(8):1509–14.

Paracchini V, Raimondi S, Gram IT, et al. Meta- and Pooled Analyses of the Cytochrome P-450 1B1 Va1432Leu Polymorphism and Breast Cancer: A HuGE-GSEC Review. Am J Epidemiol 2007; 165: 115–25.

Parkin DM, Bray F, Ferlay J, Pisani P. Estimating the world cancer burden: Globocan 2000. Int J Cancer 2001;94:153–56.

Partridge RK, Hahnel R. Prolactin receptors in human breast carcinoma. Cancer 1979;43:643–46.

Pasqualini JR, Chetrite G, Blacker C, Feinstein MC, Delalonde L, Talbi M, et al. Concentrations of estrone, estradiol, and estrone sulfate and evaluation of sulfatase and aromatase activities in pre- and postmenopausal breast cancer patients. J Clin Endocrinol Metab 1996;81:1460–64.

Pollak M. IGF-I physiology and breast cancer. Recent Results Cancer Res 1998;152:63–70.

Prentice RL, Caan B, Chlebowski RT, Patterson R, Kuller LH, Ockene JK, et al. Low-fat dietary pattern and risk of invasive breast cancer: the Women's Health Initiative Randomized Controlled Dietary Modification Trial. JAMA 2006;295:629–42.

Ravandi-Kashani F, Hayes TG. Male breast cancer: a review of the literature. Eur J Cancer 1998;34:1341–47.

Reichman ME, Judd JT, Longcope C, Schatzkin A, Clevidence BA, Nair PP, et al. Effects of alcohol consumption on plasma and urinary hormone concentrations in premenopausal women. J Natl Cancer Inst 1993;85:722–27.

Renehan AG, Zwahlen M, Minder C, O'Dwyer ST, Shalet SM, Egger M. Insulin-like growth factor (IGF)-I, IGF binding protein-3, and cancer risk: systematic review and meta-regression analysis. Lancet 2004;363:1346–53.

Reynolds P, Hurley S, Goldberg DE, et al. Active smoking, household passive smoking, and breast cancer: evidence from the California Teachers Study. J Natl Cancer Inst 2004; 96:29–37

Richardson A. Is breast cancer caused by late exposure to a common virus? Med Hypotheses 1997;48:491–97.

Rinaldi S, Kaaks R, Zeleniuch-Jacquotte A, Arslan AA, Shore RE, Koenig KL, et al. Insulin-like growth factor-I, IGF binding protein-3, and breast cancer in young women: a comparison of risk estimates using different peptide assays. Cancer Epidemiol Biomarkers Prev 2005;14:48–52.

Rinaldi S, Peeters PH, Berrino F, Dossus L, Biessy C, Olsen A, et al. IGF-I, IGFBP-3 and breast cancer risk in women: The European Prospective Investigation into Cancer and Nutrition (EPIC). Endocr Relat Cancer 2006;13(2):593–605.

Roberts KD, Rochefort JG, Bleau G, Chapdelaine A. Plasma estrone sulfate levels in postmenopausal women. Steroids 1980;35: 179–87.

Rockhill B, Willett WC, Hunter DJ, Manson JE, Hankinson SE, Colditz GA. A prospective study of recreational physical activity and breast cancer risk. Arch Intern Med 1999; 159:2290–96.

Rockhill B, Willett WC, Hunter DJ, Manson JE, Hankinson SE, Spiegelman D, et al. Physical activity and breast cancer risk in a cohort of young women. J Natl Cancer Inst 1998; 90:1155–60.

Rohan TE, Jain MG, Howe GR, Miller AB. Dietary folate consumption and breast cancer risk. J Natl Cancer Inst 2000;92:266–69.

Romieu I, Berlin JA, Colditz G. Oral contraceptives and breast cancer. Review and meta-analysis. Cancer 1990;66:2253–63.

Rosner B, Colditz GA, Willett WC. Reproductive risk factors in a prospective study of breast cancer: the Nurses' Health Study. Am J Epidemiol 1994;139:819–35.

Ross RK, Paganini-Hill A, Wan PC, Pike MC. Effect of hormone replacement therapy on breast cancer risk: estrogen versus estrogen plus progestin. J Natl Cancer Inst 2000;92: 328–32.

Russell MJ, Thomas BS, Bulbrook RD. A prospective study of the relationship between serum vitamins A and E and risk of breast cancer. Br J Cancer 1988;57:213–15.

Russo J, Tay LK, Russo IH. Differentiation of the mammary gland and susceptibility to carcinogenesis. Breast Cancer Res Treat 1982;2:5–73.

Russo J, Gusterson BA, Rogers AE, Russo IH, Wellings SR, van Zwieten MJ. Comparative study of human and rat mammary tumorigenesis. Lab Invest 1990;62:244–78.

Salamone LM, Dallal GE, Zantos D, Makrauer F, Dawson-Hughes B. Contributions of vitamin D intake and seasonal sunlight exposure to plasma 25-hydroxyvitamin D concentration in elderly women. Am J Clin Nutr 1994;59:80–86.

Sato R, Helzlsouer KJ, Alberg AJ, Hoffman SC, Norkus EP, Comstock GW. Prospective study of carotenoids, tocopherols, and retinoid concentrations and the risk of breast cancer. Cancer Epidemiol Biomarkers Prev 2002;11:451–57.

Schairer C, Byrne C, Keyl PM, Brinton LA, Sturgeon SR, Hoover RN. Menopausal estrogen and estrogen-progestin replacement therapy and risk of breast cancer (United States). Cancer Causes Control 1994;5:491–500.

Schairer C, Lubin J, Troisi R, Sturgeon S, Brinton L, Hoover R. Menopausal estrogen and estrogen-progestin replacement therapy and breast cancer risk. JAMA 2000;283: 485–91.

Schernhammer ES, Holly JM, Pollak MN, Hankinson SE. Circulating levels of insulin-like growth factors, their binding proteins, and breast cancer risk. Cancer Epidemiol Biomarkers Prev 2005;14(3):699–704.

Schernhammer ES, Holly JM, Hunter DJ, Pollak MN, Hankinson SE. Insulin-like growth factor-I, its binding proteins (IGFBP-1 and IGFBP-3), and growth hormone and breast cancer risk in The Nurses Health Study II. Endocr Relat Cancer 2006;13(2):583–92.

Schernhammer ES, Hankinson SE. Urinary melatonin levels and breast cancer risk. J Natl Cancer Inst 2005;97(14):1084–87.

Sellers TA. Genetic factors in the pathogenesis of breast cancer: their role and relative importance. J Nutr 1997;127:929S–932S.

Sellers TA, Kushi LH, Cerhan JR, Vierkant RA, Gapstur SM, Vachon CM, et al. Dietary folate intake, alcohol, and risk of breast cancer in a prospective study of postmenopausal woman. Epidemiol 2001;12: 420–28.

Seymour-Munn K, Adams J. Estrogenic effects of 5-androstene-3 beta, 17 beta-diol at physiological concentrations and its possible implication in the etiology of breast cancer. Endocrinology 1983;112:486–91.

Shering SG, Zbar AP, Moriarty M, McDermott EW, O'Higgins NJ, Smyth PP. Thyroid disorders and breast cancer. Eur J Cancer Prev 1996;5:504–6.

Shin MH, Holmes MD, Hankinson SE, Wu K, Colditz GA, Willett WC. Intake of dairy products, calcium, and vitamin D and risk of breast cancer. J Natl Cancer Inst 2002; 94:1301–11.

Smith-Warner SA, Spiegelman D, Adami HO, Beeson WL, van Den Brandt PA, Folsom AR, et al. Types of dietary fat and breast cancer: a pooled analysis of cohort studies. Int J Cancer 2001a;92:767–74.

Smith-Warner SA, Spiegelman D, Yaun SS, Adami HO, Beeson WL, van den Brandt PA, et al. Intake of fruits and vegetables and risk of breast cancer: a pooled analysis of cohort studies. JAMA 2001b;285:769–76.

Smith-Warner SA, Spiegelman D, Yaun SS, van den Brandt PA, Folsom AR, Goldbohm RA, et al. Alcohol and breast cancer in women: a pooled analysis of cohort studies. JAMA 1998;279:535–40.

Snedeker S, Diaugustine R. Hormonal and environmental factors affecting cell proliferation and neoplasia in the mammary gland. In: Huff J, Boyd J, Barrett J (Eds): Cellular and Molecular Mechanisms of Hormonal Carcinogenesis: Environmental Influences. New York, Wiley-Liss, 1992: 211–53.

Stahl W, Sies H. Uptake of lycopene and its geometrical isomers is greater from heat-processed than from unprocessed tomato juice in humans. J Nutr 1992;122:2161–66.

Stanford JL, Thomas DB. Exogenous progestins and breast cancer. Epidemiol Rev 1993; 15(1):98–107.

Stephen AM, Wald NJ. Trends in individual consumption of dietary fat in the United States, 1920–1984. Am J Clin Nutr 1990;52:457–69.

Suzuki R, Ye W, Rylander-Rudqvist T, Saji S, Colditz GA, Wolk A. Alcohol and postmenopausal breast cancer risk defined by estrogen and progesterone receptor status: a prospective cohort study. J Natl Cancer Inst 2005;97:1601–9.

Talamini R, Franceschi S, Favero A, Negri E, Parazzini F, La Vecchia C. Selected medical conditions and risk of breast cancer. Br J Cancer 1997;75:1699–1703.

Tamarkin L, Cohen M, Roselle D, Reichert C, Lippman M, Chabner B. Melatonin inhibition and pinealectomy enhancement of 7,12-dimethylbenz(a)anthracene-induced mammary tumors in the rat. Cancer Res 1981;41:4432–36.

Tamimi RM, Hankinson SE, Ding S, Gagalang V, Larson GP, Spiegelman D, et al. The HRAS1 variable number of tandem repeats and risk of breast cancer. Cancer Epidemiol Biomarkers Prev 2003;12(12):1528–30.

Tamimi RM, Hankinson SE, Colditz GA, Byrne C. Endogenous sex hormone levels and mammographic density among postmenopausal women. Cancer Epidemiol Biomarkers Prev 2005;14:2641–47.

Tamimi RM, Hankinson SE, Chen WY, Rosner B, Colditz GA. Combined estrogen and testosterone use and risk of breast cancer in postmenopausal women. Arch Intern Med 2006;166(14):1483–89.

Thomas DB. Oral contraceptives and breast cancer: review of the epidemiologic literature. Contraception 1991;43:597–642.

Thomas HV, Key TJ, Allen DS, Moore JW, Dowsett M, Fentiman IS, et al. A prospective study of endogenous serum hormone concentrations and breast cancer risk in premenopausal women on the island of Guernsey. Br J Cancer 1997b;75:1075–79.

Thune I, Brenn T, Lund E, Gaard M. Physical activity and the risk of breast cancer. N Engl J Med 1997;336:1269–75.

Tominaga S. Cancer incidence in Japanese in Japan, Hawaii, and western United States. Natl Cancer Inst Monogr 1985;69:83–92.

Toniolo P, Van Kappel AL, Akhmedkhanov A, Ferrari P, Kato I, Shore RE, et al. Serum carotenoids and breast cancer. Am J Epidemiol 2001;153:1142–47.

Travis RC, Allen DS, Fentiman IS, Key TJ. Melatonin and breast cancer: a prospective study. J Natl Cancer Inst 2004;96(6):475–82.

Tretli S. Height and weight in relation to breast cancer morbidity and mortality. A prospective study of 570,000 women in Norway. Int J Cancer 1989;44:23–30.

Trichopoulou A. Olive oil and breast cancer. Cancer Causes Control 1995;6:475–76.

Trichopoulou A, Katsouyanni K, Stuver S, Tzala L, Gnardellis C, Rimm E, et al. Consumption of olive oil and specific food groups in relation to breast cancer risk in Greece. J Natl Cancer Inst 1995;87:110–16.

Trichopoulos D. Hypothesis: does breast cancer originate in utero? Lancet 1990;335:939–40.

Trichopoulos D, Hsieh CC, MacMahon B, Lin TM, Lowe CR, Mirra AP, et al. Age at any birth and breast cancer risk. Int J Cancer 1983;31:701–4.

Trichopoulos D, Lipman RD. Mammary gland mass and breast cancer risk. Epidemiology 1992;3:523–26.

Trichopoulos D, MacMahon B, Cole P. Menopause and breast cancer risk. J Natl Cancer Inst 1972;48:605–13.

Tworoger SS, Eliassen AH, Rosner B, Sluss P, Hankinson SE. Plasma prolactin concentrations and risk of postmenopausal breast cancer. Cancer Res 2004;64:6814–19.

Tworoger SS, Sluss P, Hankinson S. Association between plasma prolactin concentrations and risk of breast cancer among predominantly premenopausal women. Cancer Res 2006;66:2476–82.

Tynes T, Hannevik M, Andersen A, Vistnes AI, Haldorsen T. Incidence of breast cancer in Norwegian female radio and telegraph operators. Cancer Causes Control 1996;7:197–204.

Ursin G, Longnecker MP, Haile RW, Greenland S. A meta-analysis of body mass index and risk of premenopausal breast cancer. Epidemiology 1995;6:137–41.

Vatten LJ, Kvinnsland S. Prospective study of height, body mass index and risk of breast cancer. Acta Oncol 1992;31:195–200.

Vainio H, Kaaks R, Bianchini F. Weight control and physical activity in cancer prevention: international evaluation of the evidence. Eur J Cancer Prev 2002;11 Suppl 2:S94–S100.

Vogel VG, Costantino JP, Wickerham DL, Cronin WM, Cecchini RS, Atkins JN, et al. Effects of tamoxifen vs raloxifene on the risk of developing invasive breast cancer and other disease outcomes: the NSABP Study of Tamoxifen and Raloxifene (STAR) P-2 trial. JAMA 2006;295(23):2727–41.

Waaler HT, Lund E. Association between body height and death from breast cancer. Br J Cancer 1983;48:149–50.

Wald NJ, Boreham J, Hayward JL, Bulbrook RD. Plasma retinol, beta-carotene and vitamin E levels in relation to the future risk of breast cancer. Br J Cancer 1984;49:321–24.

Walker BE, Kurth LA. Multigenerational effects of dietary fat carcinogenesis in mice. Cancer Res 1997;57:4162–63.

Wang Y, Holland JF, Bleiweiss IJ, Melana S, Liu X, Pelisson I, et al. Detection of mammary tumor virus env gene-like sequences in human breast cancer. Cancer Res 1995;55:5173–79.

Warmuth MA, Sutton LM, Winer EP. A review of hereditary breast cancer: from screening to risk factor modification. Am J Med 1997;102:407–15.

Webb AR, Kline L, Holick MF. Influence of season and latitude on the cutaneous synthesis of vitamin D3: exposure to winter sunlight in Boston and Edmonton will not promote vitamin D3 synthesis in human skin. J Clin Endocrinol Metab 1988;67:373–78.

Webb AR, Pilbeam C, Hanafin N, Holick MF. An evaluation of the relative contributions of exposure to sunlight and of diet to the circulating concentrations of 25-hydroxyvitamin D in an elderly nursing home population in Boston. Am J Clin Nutr 1990;51:1075–81.

Weiderpass E, Braaten T, Magnusson C, Kumle M, Vainio H, Lund E, Adami HO. A prospective of body size in different periods of life and risk of premenopausal breast cancer. Cancer Epidemiol Biom Prev 2004;13:1121–27.

Weiderpass E, Gridley G, Persson I, Nyrén O, Ekbom A, Adami HO. Risk of endometrial and breast cancer in patients with diabetes mellitus. Int J Cancer 1997;71:360–63.

Weiss HA, Potischman NA, Brinton LA, Brogan D, Coates RJ, Gammon MD, et al. Prenatal and perinatal risk factors for breast cancer in young women. Epidemiology 1997;8:181–87.

Weiss HA, Troisi R, Rossing MA, Brogan D, Coates RJ, Gammon MD, et al. Fertility problems and breast cancer risk in young women: a case-control study in the United States. Cancer Causes Control 1998;9:331–39.

Welp EA, Weiderpass E, Boffetta P, Vainio H, Vasama-Neuvonen K, Petralia S, et al. Environmental risk factors of breast cancer. Scand J Work Environ Health 1998;24:3–7.

White E, Lee CY, Kristal AR. Evaluation of the increase in breast cancer incidence in relation to mammography use. J Natl Cancer Inst 1990;82:1546–52.

WHO Collaborative Study of Neoplasia and Steroid Contraceptives. Breast cancer and depot-medroxyprogesterone acetate: a multinational study. Lancet 1991;338:833–38.

Willett WC, Polk BF, Underwood BA, Stampfer MJ, Pressel S, Rosner B, et al. Relation of serum vitamins A and E and carotenoids to the risk of cancer. N Engl J Med 1984; 310:430–34.

Willett WC. Nutritional Epidemiology. New York, Oxford University Press, 1998.

Willett WC, Colditz G, Stampfer M. Postmenopausal estrogens—opposed, unopposed, or none of the above. JAMA 2000b;283(4):534–35.

Wolfe JN. Risk for breast cancer development determined by mammographic parenchymal pattern. Cancer 1976;37:2486–92.

Wolff MS, Collman GW, Barrett JC, Huff J. Breast cancer and environmental risk factors: epidemiological and experimental findings. Annu Rev Pharmacol Toxicol 1996;36:573–96.

Wolk A, Bergström R, Hunter D, Willett W, Ljung H, Holmberg L, et al. A prospective study of association of monounsaturated fat and other types of fat with risk of breast cancer. Arch Intern Med 1998;158:41–45.

Wu AH, Ziegler RG, Nomura AM, West DW, Kolonel LN, Horn-Ross PL, et al. Soy intake and risk of breast cancer in Asians and Asian Americans. Am J Clin Nutr 1998;68:1437S–1443S.

Yager JD, Liehr JG. Molecular mechanisms of estrogen carcinogenesis. Annu Rev Pharmacol Toxicol 1996;36:203–32.

Yen SSC, Jaffe RB. Reproductive Endocrinology. Philadelphia, WB Saunders, 1991.

Zeleniuch-Jacquotte A, Shore RE, Koenig KL, et al. Postmenopausal levels of oestrogen, androgen, and SHBG and breast cancer: long-term results of a prospective study. Br J Cancer 2004;90:153–59.

Zhang S, Hunter DJ, Forman MR, Rosner BA, Speizer FE, Colditz GA, et al. Dietary carotenoids and vitamins A, C, and E and risk of breast cancer. J Natl Cancer Inst 1999a; 91:547–56.

Zhang S, Hunter DJ, Hankinson SE, Giovannucci EL, Rosner BA, Colditz GA, et al. A prospective study of folate intake and the risk of breast cancer. JAMA 1999b; 281:1632–37.

Zhang SM, Willett WC, Selhub J, Hunter DJ, Giovannucci EL, Holmes MD, et al. Plasma folate, vitamin B6, vitamin B12, homocysteine, and risk of breast cancer. J Natl Cancer Inst 2003;95:373–80

Zhang SM, Hankinson SE, Hunter DJ, Giovannucci EL, Colditz GA, Willett WC. Folate intake and risk of breast cancer characterized by hormone receptor status. Cancer Epidemiol Biomarkers Prev 2005;14:2004–8.

Ziegler RG, Hoover RN, Pike MC, Hildesheim A, Nomura AM, West DW, et al. Migration patterns and breast cancer risk in Asian-American women. J Natl Cancer Inst 1993; 85:1819–27.

Zinser G, Packman K, Welsh J. Vitamin D(3) receptor ablation alters mammary gland morphogenesis. Development 2002;129:3067–76.

17

Cervical Cancer

NATHALIE YLITALO, SHERRI STUVER,
AND HANS-OLOV ADAMI

With cancer of the cervix as a striking example, there has been a long prelude to the current realization that infection has an important role in human cancer. Observations made as far back as the eighteenth and nineteenth centuries indicated that sexual behavior was associated with cancer of the cervix, because the disease was rare in nuns but common in prostitutes. However, it was not until the late 1970s that a sexually transmitted agent, namely human papillomavirus (HPV), was postulated to explain the association between sexual activity and cervical cancer (zur Hausen, 1977). Since then, numerous studies have confirmed the association and today persistent infection with certain oncogenic types of HPV are considered necessary, though not sufficient, causes of squamous cell cancer of the cervix (Bosch et al, 2002; IARC, 1995a). Needless to say, this understanding opens fascinating prospects for primary prevention through vaccination, hopefully soon to become a clinical reality at least in some parts of the world.

Methodologically, studies of the viral etiology of cervical cancer have offered and continue to offer numerous challenges both in designing epidemiologic studies and in measuring exposure to oncogenic viruses. Molecular biology allowed research to go beyond crude surrogate measures of sexually transmitted infection, such as age at first intercourse and number of sexual partners. Much work was necessary, however, before HPV infection could be ascertained with adequate specificity and sensitivity. Further progress will require even more advanced molecular tools to study viral load, viral microheterogeneity, cellular immunity, and their interactions in the initiation and progression of cervical cancer.

CLINICAL SYNOPSIS

Subgroups

Although squamous cell cancer accounts for 80% to 90% of all malignancies of the cervix in most settings, adenocarcinoma, the other main histopathologic type, is becoming increasingly common. Squamous cell cancer has a distinct, probably obligatory precursor detectable by cytologic screening, namely, carcinoma in situ (CIS). Likewise, the immediate precursor to adenocarcinoma is named adenocarcinoma in situ (AIS), but is generally more difficult to detect by cytological screening.

Dysplastic, noninvasive precursor lesions with varying grades of severity also can be detected in the cervix. It is thought that these intraepithelial lesions may represent precancerous neoplasias. The principal systems used to classify cervical abnormalities include one proposed by the World Health Organization (WHO), one advanced by Richart, and the Bethesda System developed in conjunction with the US National Cancer Institute (Kiviat et al, 1992; IARC, 1995a; Mitchell et al, 1996). The WHO system involves histologic classification of cervical dysplasia as mild, moderate, or severe, as well as a separate category for carcinoma in situ (CIS). Richart introduced the term *cervical intraepithelial neoplasia* (CIN) to classify cervical lesions into three stages: CIN I represents mild dysplasia; CIN II, moderate dysplasia; and CIN III, severe dysplasia or CIS. In the Bethesda System, which is based on cytology from Papanicolaou test readings, a low-grade squamous intraepithelial lesion (LSIL) corresponds to CIN I and includes condyloma, and a high-grade SIL (HSIL) encompasses both CIN II and CIN III.

Symptoms

Carcinoma in situ is typically symptomless, whereas invasive cancer of the cervix causes postcoital and spontaneous bleeding, discharge, and discomfort during intercourse. In advanced disease, which is predominant in large parts of the developing world, a wide variety of symptoms arise due to extensive local tumor growth and/or metastasis.

Diagnosis

A combination of visual inspection, aided by colposcopy, acetic acid application, and palpation are highly informative. Cytologic examination of a Papanicolaou test often reveals malignant cells. Nevertheless, biopsy with histopathologic confirmation is necessary for definite diagnosis.

Treatment

As with most other malignancies, treatment planning depends profoundly on the clinical stage. In localized disease, cure can be achieved by surgical removal, irradiation (internal or external), or a combination of these modalities. Although cobalt is now the preferable isotope for external radiation, local radium treatment is an attractive approach to cure early disease in settings with limited resources. Today, cisplatinum-based chemotherapy—most often administered weekly—is recommended to be given concurrently with radiotherapy to improve survival.

Prognosis

Cure rates depend strongly on the stage at diagnosis. In the United States and most European Countries, the 5-year relative survival rate is approximately 65% but ranges between 15% to 80%, depending on the extent of the disease.

Progress

During the twentieth century, earlier clinical diagnosis greatly reduced mortality from cervical cancer in many developed countries. However, since the 1970s, there has been little, if any, improvement in overall or stage-specific survival.

DESCRIPTIVE EPIDEMIOLOGY

Almost half a million women develop cervical cancer every year, which makes this cancer the second most frequently occurring malignancy among women worldwide (Parkin et al, 2005). More than half of the women developing cervical carcinoma will die as a result of their disease, with women in developing countries accounting for 80% of these deaths. There is only limited variation in age-standardized incidence between the countries shown in Figure 17–1, except for Poland. In several western

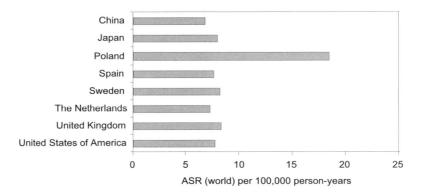

Figure 17–1. Age-standardized incidence rates of cervical carcinoma in different countries. *Source*: Ferlay et al, 2004)

countries there have been substantial declines in incidence rates following cytologic screening during the latter twentieth century (Gustafsson et al, 1997). On a global scale, however, incidence rates of invasive cervical cancer vary substantially between different regions, from less than 7 per 100 000 in China to more than 40 per 100 000 in parts of Eastern Africa (Parkin et al, 2005). In general, the highest incidence

rates are found in sub-Saharan Africa, Melanesia, and South-central and Southeast Asia, Latin America, and the Caribbean; whereas the lowest rates are observed in North America, Australia/New Zealand, China, and Western Asia (Parkin et al, 2005).

Unlike most other solid tumors, the incidence of cervical cancer becomes high during middle age, with limited further in-

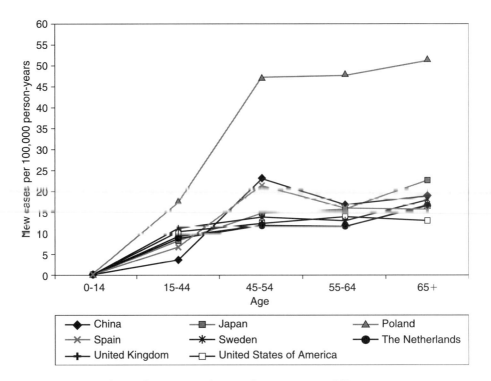

Figure 17–2. Age-specific incidence rates of cervical carcinoma in different countries. (*Source*: Ferlay et al, 2004)

crease at older ages in many settings (Fig. 17–2). Indeed, these age-specific incidence figures have been distorted markedly by screening for cervical cancer, which provides proportionally greater protection in younger than in older women (Gustafsson et al, 1997).

Mortality rates are much lower than incidence rates; average 5-year survival is about 50% worldwide but tends to be higher in low-risk areas (Parkié et al, 2005), due chiefly to earlier clinical diagnosis followed by adequate treatment (Pontén et al, 1995). However, because women are diagnosed with cervical cancer and die from the disease, on average, at younger ages than women with other types of cancer, the total years of life lost due to this malignancy are substantial (Herrero, 1996).

In countries where organized cytological screening has been implemented over the last 3 or 4 decades, the incidence of and mortality from cervical carcinoma have declined steadily (Gustafsson et al, 1997; Pontén et al, 1995). However, the decline is mainly attributed to the predominant squamous cell type of cervical carcinoma. For cervical adenocarcinomas, which constitute about 10% to 25% of all cervical cancers (Smith et al, 2000; Vizcaino et al, 1998), increases in the age-adjusted incidence rates, primarily among young women, have been reported in several populations, even where cytological screening programs are present and functioning (Bergström et al, 1999; Kjaer and Brinton, 1993; Sasieni and Adams, 2001; Vizcaino et al, 1998). These upward trends raise the concern that routine cytological screening might not be an efficient way to prevent against adenocarcinoma.

GENETIC AND MOLECULAR EPIDEMIOLOGY

Inherited Susceptibility

Not much research has been conducted on an inherited component of cervical cancer occurrence. Some family clustering has been observed (Brinton et al, 1987; Hemminki and Vaittinen, 1998). In addition, several polymorphisms of the human leukocyte antigen (HLA) complex are reported to be associated with the risk of both invasive cervical cancer and its precursor lesions (Odunsi and Ganesan, 1997). Although the findings are not necessarily consistent, different DRB1 and DQB1 haplotypes appear to be involved in susceptibility to as well as protection from cervical carcinogenesis (Apple et al, 1994; Lema et al, 2006; Odunsi and Ganesan, 1997; Wank and Thomssen, 1991). Two population-based studies in Scandinavia both identified HLA-DQ6 and HLA-DR15 as susceptibility markers for high-grade CIN (Helland et al, 1998; Sanjeevi et al, 1996). These associations were further confirmed in a meta-analysis on the relation between different HLA class II haplotypes and cervical cancer (Konya and Dillner, 2001) Of interest, some HLA associations were only evident among carriers of HPV type 16—the oncogenic HPV type that is most important for cervical cancer development. Thus, it is proposed that the role of HLA type in cervical cancer occurrence involves the host's immune response to HPV infection and the ability of the virus to persist and induce carcinogenesis.

In 1998, a polymorphism in codon 72 of the tumor-suppressor gene P53 was suggested to affect the risk of developing HPV-associated cervical cancer (Storey et al, 1998). However, subsequent reports revealed no such association (Hildesheim et al, 1998; Josefsson et al, 1998; Rosenthal et al, 1998; Sonoda et al, 1999). Considering the conflicting results, it remains to be seen whether heritable factors play a small, if any, role for cervical cancer development as suggested from a large study on twins (Lichtenstein et al, 2000), or if there is a significant genetic susceptibility and the major important gene loci still need to be identified (Magnusson et al, 2000).

Somatic Events

Unlike many other cancers, somatic mutations of tumor-suppressor genes or cellular oncogenes are not commonly observed for malignancies of the cervix (Southern and Herrington, 1998). Allelic loss does seem to occur, with loss of heterozygosity most frequently observed for chromosomes 3p, 11q, and 17p. The nature and relevance of these genetic changes remain unknown. Although *P53* mutations are infrequently found in cervical cancer cell lines and tissue, they do appear more often in cell lines and tumors without detectable HPV DNA (Southern and Herrington, 1998). Some limited evidence exists for overexpression of the *C-MYC* oncogene as well as, possibly, of the epidermal growth factor receptor and the *HER2/NEU* regulatory genes (Berchuk and Rodabaugh, 1996).

RISK FACTORS

Tobacco

In the late 1970s, Winkelstein hypothesized a possible role for tobacco smoking in the risk of cervical cancer (Winkelstein, 1977). A review of the relevant research during the ensuing decade by the same investigator found the epidemiologic and biologic evidence to be supportive of this hypothesis, even after control for the potentially strong confounding effects of sexual behavior (Winkelstein, 1990). However, with improved detection of HPV—the primary causal agent of cervical cancer—an independent effect of smoking was not consistently observed for invasive cervical cancer and CIN in well-conducted studies (Eluf-Neto et al, 1994; Kjaer et al, 1996; Koutsky et al, 1992). Nonetheless, an association of smoking with CIN, CIS, and cervical cancer has been reported in other studies after adjustment for HPV infection (Dillner et al, 1997; Chichareon et al, 1998; Ngelangel et al, 1998; Ylitalo et al, 1999). Of late, two large collaborative studies lent further support for the association between smoking and cervical carcinoma. One study used pooled data restricted to HPV-positive women only within IARC's multicentered case-control studies; the other pooled and reanalyzed data from 23 different epidemiological studies (International Collaborative Study of Cervical Cancer, 2006; Plummer et al, 2003). Both studies reported

an approximate doubling in risk among current smokers compared to never smokers. In the latter study, risk was further increased with number of cigarettes smoked per day and younger age at starting smoking. In both studies the effect of smoking appeared to be limited to squamous cell carcinoma of the cervix, a finding supported by previous work (International Collaborative Study of Cervical Cancer, 2006; Plummer et al, 2003; Schiffman and Brinton, 1995; Winkelstein, 1990). In addition, an increased risk of cervical cancer among women exposed passively to tobacco smoke has been reported (Winkelstein, 1990).

Cigarette smoking may promote carcinogenicity through various mechanisms, both by affecting local cell-mediated immune response and by inducing genetic damage (Barton et al, 1988; Palefsky and Holly, 1995). Both nicotine and cotinine have been found in the cervical secretions of smokers and passive smokers (Winkelstein, 1990; McCann et al, 1992; Palefsky and Holly, 1995). Moreover, polycyclic aromatic hydrocarbons from cigarette smoke can inhibit cell proliferation of normal cervical cell lines in vitro (Southern and Herrington, 1998).

In addition to its known mutagenic effects, tobacco smoking may produce local immune suppression that enhances HPV persistence (Brinton, 1992; Burger et al, 1993; zur Hausen 1982). This immunologic effect may be mediated through a reduction in the number of Langerhans cells, which are important antigen-presenting cells (Barton et al, 1988).

Diet

There are plausible biological mechanisms for a role of diet and nutrients in protecting against cervical cancer development (Potischman and Brinton, 1996). Yet, a review of epidemiological studies performed through 2004 concluded that the epidemiological evidence for an association between diet and nutritional status and cervical cancer is not convincing (Garcia-Closas, 2005). Research in this area has mainly focused on carotenoids, retinol, vitamins C and E, and folate (Potischman and Brinton, 1996; World Cancer Research Fund, 1997). However, earlier studies are limited by inadequate measurement of and adjustment for HPV status. A possible protective effect of serum carotenoids and dietary vitamin C against cervical cancer is a fairly consistent finding (Potischman and Brinton, 1996). Although not as uniform an observation, an inverse association between high dietary vitamin E intake and cervical cancer also is suggested (World Cancer Research Fund, 1997). Folate levels appear to be inversely related to the risk of CIN but not to that of invasive disease (Potischman and Brinton, 1996). Lastly, potential reductions in CIN and cervical cancer risk are suggested for women consuming large amounts of fruits and vegetables (World Cancer Research Fund, 1997), possibly through a protective effect on HPV persistence (Giuliano et al, 2003; Sedjo et al, 2002).

Reproductive Factors

The current epidemiologic data support an association between multiparity and invasive cervical cancer, independent of HPV infection or other potential reproductive and sexual behavior variables (Brinton, 1992; Schiffman and Brinton, 1995). An association with higher parity also has been observed for CIN and CIS, controlling for HPV status (Schiffman et al, 1993; Kjaer et al, 1996). Most studies performed in populations where multiparity is common have reported an increased risk for cervical cancer among both HPV-negative (Bosch et al, 1992) and HPV-positive women (Eluf-Neto et al, 1994; Muñoz et al, 1993, 2002; Ngelangel et al, 1998). A few case-control studies on CIS and invasive cervical cancer, however, failed to show an association between multiparity and invasive cervical cancer, (Chichareon et al, 1998) or CIS (Ylitalo et al, 1999).

Several hypotheses have been suggested to explain the risk associated with multiparity, including hormonal influence during pregnancy, changed nutrition, immunological mechanisms triggered at pregnancy, or trauma to the cervix during parturition.

Clearly, cervical dysplasia is more common during pregnancy (Schneider and Koutsky, 1992). Yet, these lesions often regress postpartum, which may be explained by a transient immune suppression during pregnancy. Thus, multiple pregnancies could modulate the immune response to HPV, enabling the virus to periodically evade immune control and thereby influence the risk of viral persistence. Alternatively, hormonal factors related to pregnancy may play a direct role in cervical carcinogenesis or may modify the effect of HPV (Muñoz et al, 2002; Muñoz and Bosch, 1996; Schiffman and Brinton, 1995).

Hormones

Because the use of oral contraceptives (OCs) is so closely associated with sexual behavior and, consequently, with the potential for HPV infection, it has been difficult to establish whether these exogenous hormones have an independent effect on the development of cervical cancer. Nonetheless, a moderate association of long-term OC use with cervical cancer has been reported in studies that have controlled for potential confounding factors (Brinton, 1992; Schiffman and Brinton, 1995; Madeleine et al, 2001). In studies restricted to HPV-positive women, a synergistic effect between duration of OC use and HPV has been observed for the risk of invasive cervical cancer (Bosch et al, 1992; Eluf-Neto et al, 1994; Hildesheim et al, 1990; Moreno et al, 2002). With regard to CIN and CIS, results are conflicting; investigators have found no effect (Koutsky et al, 1992), an independent effect (Ylitalo et al, 1999), a possible effect among HPV-negative women only (Schiffman et al, 1993), and an inconsistent effect of duration of OC use (Muñoz et al, 1993). From a public health perspective it is important to know whether an increased risk for cervical cancer among long-term OC users persists long after cessation of OC use. Currently, there are limited data in the literature to assess this risk (Smith et al, 2003).

The effect of OCs on cancer risk appears to be somewhat stronger for adenocarcinoma than for squamous cell carcinoma, suggesting that at least part of the increase in the rate of the adenocarcinoma subtype may be due to a higher prevalence of exposure to OCs (Kjaer and Brinton, 1993; Ursin et al, 1994; Schiffman and Brinton, 1995). There is experimental evidence for an influence of exogenous hormones on HPV genes (Schiffman and Brinton, 1995; von Knebel Doeberitz et al, 1997; Southern and Herrington, 1998). Oral contraceptives' hormones have been shown to enhance HPV-associated transformation in vitro through the upregulation of viral oncogene transcription.

In addition, steroid hormones may alter immune function by downregulating the expression of HLA class I antigens, which may be important in the cellular immune response to HPV infection (von Knebel Doeberitz et al, 1997; Southern and Herrington, 1998).

Anthropometric Measures

Obesity may be a risk factor for cervical carcinoma (Lacey et al, 2003) and particularly so for adenocarcinoma of the cervix (Kjaer and Brinton, 1993; Lacey et al, 2003). In one relatively large case-control study of cervical adenocarcinoma, weight gain since age 18 also was associated with increased risk (Ursin et al, 1996). Again, adequate control of the potential confounding effect of HPV, sexual behavior, and hormonal factors is of paramount importance for assessing the association with obesity and cervical cancer.

Sexual Behavior

Early in the study of cervical cancer, it was recognized that sexual behavior played an important role (Beral, 1974); low rates of disease were observed in nuns and virgins and high rates in women who married at young ages (Boyd and Doll, 1964; Brinton, 1992; Palefsky and Holly, 1995; Schiffman and Brinton, 1995). Risk factors related to a woman's sexual behavior and later shown to be associated with increased risk for cervical cancer and its precursor lesions include an increased number of life-time sex-

ual partners and an early age at first intercourse (Brinton, 1992; Schiffman and Brinton, 1995). Some investigations found that rates of cervical cancer and neoplasia were higher in women whose husbands had cancer of the penis or who were married to men whose former wives were diagnosed with cervical cancer. The male partner's number of previous and extramarital partners also has been associated with the risk of cervical cancer (Bosch et al, 1996). This so-called "male factor" was among the first clues that cervical cancer likely had an infectious etiology (Brinton, 1992).

Infections

Ever since the connection between sexual activity and cervical carcinoma became evident, researchers have speculated an involvement of various sexually transmitted agents (Beral, 1974). Before the strong association between HPV and cervical cancer was revealed, herpes simplex virus type 2 (HSV-2) was considered the likely etiologic infectious agent involved in cervical cancer; this hypothesis has since been dismissed due to insufficient supporting data (Brinton, 1992). However, HSV-2 may act as a cofactor with HPV in the causation of cervical cancer (zur Hausen, 1982). Some studies have found an increased risk of cervical cancer associated with the presence of antibodies to HSV-2 among HPV-positive women (Hildesheim et al, 1991), while others have not (de Sanjosé et al, 1994; Muñoz et al, 1995).

Chlamydia trachomatis infection also has been linked to increased risk for cervical carcinoma in several studies (Anttila et al, 2001; Dillner et al, 1997; Koutsky et al, 1992; Wallin et al, 2002). The association between infection with *C. trachomatis* and invasive cervical cancer was recently confirmed in a pooled analysis of the IARC multicentered case-control studies; among HPV DNA-positive women who were also *C. trachomatis* seropositive, risk was increased almost twofold compared to seronegativ women (Smith et al, 2004). It is, however, not clear whether *C. trachomatis* has an independent effect on cervical cancer risk or if its effect is mediated through an interaction with HPV. It has been hypothesized that concomitant genital infections may induce chronic cervicitis, which could promote HPV-associated oncogenesis (Schiffman and Brinton, 1995). Last, in addition to its known deleterious effects on host immune function and, thus, control of chronic virus infections, human immunodeficiency virus (HIV) may directly interact with HPV in coinfected individuals (Palefsky and Holly, 1995). The transactivating tat gene of HIV has been shown to upregulate the expression of certain HPV genes in vitro (Vernon et al, 1993).

Human Papillomavirus Infection

Almost 30 years have passed since zur Hausen first suggested a possible role for HPV in the development of squamous cell carcinomas (zur Hausen, 1977). Today, infection with certain oncogenic types of HPV is generally accepted as a necessary cause for the development of cervical carcinoma and its immediate precursor lesions (Bosch et al, 2002). This strong epidemiologic evidence has gradually emerged through a successful multidisiplinary approach using molecular epidemiological methods to study HPV and its association with other potential risk factors during cervical carcinogenesis. A prerequisite to this understanding has been the advent of more sensitive and reliable assays to detect HPV DNA in the late 1980s.

Virology. Papillomaviruses are nonenveloped DNA viruses about 55 nm in diameter (von Knebel Doeberitz, 1992; IARC, 1995a; Howley, 1996). Their circular, double-stranded genome of close to 8000 base pairs contains eight known viral genes; the "early" genes (E1, E2, E4, E6, and E7) encode regulatory proteins, and the "late" genes (L1 and L2) code for the structural capsid proteins. Currently, there are over 120 different HPV types described, of which more than 40 infect the genital mucosa (de Villiers et al, 2004). Specification of the HPV genotype is based on DNA homology, with less than 90% sequence similarity constituting a separate HPV type.

Squamous epithelial cells are the targets for HPV infection, which occurs at the basal cell layer and is facilitated by injury or abrasion of the affected tissue (Koutsky et al, 1988; von Knebel Doeberitz, 1992; IARC, 1995a). The virus itself replicates productively only in the terminally differentiated keratinocytes at the surface layer of the epithelium. The genital HPVs are further classified into high-risk and low-risk types, depending on their oncogenic potential (Muñoz et al, 2003). The low-risk HPV types (mainly types 6 and 11) are generally associated with low-grade dysplastic lesions and particularly so with genital warts (ie, condyloma); whereas, the high-grade lesions, the true precursor of invasive cervical cancer, are related to infection with high-risk HPV types (types 16, 18, 31, 33, 35 39, 45, 51, 52, 56, 58, 59, 68, 73, and 82).

Extensive experimental work has been done on the function of the HPV proteins, especially with regard to the oncogenic potential of this virus (IARC, 1995a; Palefsky and Holly, 1995; Howley, 1996; Southern and Herrington, 1998). Of most interest are the E6 and E7 proteins, both of which have transforming properties. Although the HPV genome exists in episomal form in benign cervical lesions, HPV DNA detected in cervical cancer cells most often is found to be integrated into the host chromosome. When the virus genome becomes integrated, the E6 and E7 regions appear to be retained as functional genes. In contrast, the E2 region, which exerts transcriptional control over these two genes, usually is disrupted or lost. Thus, as with hepatitis B virus and hepatocellular carcinoma, integration of HPV into the host genome is an event representing an important step in the progression to invasive disease. What induces this integration step is unknown, but it may involve factors affecting host immune control and is believed to be a property exclusive for high-risk HPV types.

The ability of E6 and E7 to transform cells appears to involve their interaction with host tumor-suppressor proteins (IARC, 1995a; Palefsky and Holly, 1995; Howley,

1996; Southern and Herrington, 1998). In vitro, E6 has been shown to abrogate the function of the p53 tumor-suppressor protein, by binding p53 and inducing its degradation through the ubiquitin pathway. p53 plays an important role in cell-cycle control; it prevents the transition from the checkpoint G1 phase to the replication S phase, thus allowing for the repair of damaged DNA or the induction of apoptosis (Fig. 17–3). The E7 protein of HPV is able to bind and inactivate the RB tumor-suppressor protein, which also participates in the dynamics of cell-cycle regulation. Of note, the E6 and E7 proteins of high-risk HPV types can bind and degrade their respective tumor suppressors more effectively than the same proteins of the low-risk HPVs. The evidence suggests that cells infected with high-risk HPV types do not have a functional G1 checkpoint, which leads to the suppression of cell-cycle arrest and apoptosis and the accumulation of genetic damage

(Fig. 17–3). The E6 protein also has been shown to induce telomerase activity (Southern and Herrington, 1998); the telomerase enzyme elongates chromosomal telomeres, a process that appears to be necessary for cell immortalization. Moreover, E7 may further induce transformation by binding the AP1 transcription factors and thus inhibiting differentiation of keratinocytes, as well as by interfering with other cell-cycle regulators such as cyclin A and cyclin-dependent kinase 2 (Palefsky and Holly, 1995; Southern and Herrington, 1998).

Detection. Cervical HPV infection can be characterized as: clinical, that is, symptomatic or visually detectable (eg, as condyloma or genital warts); subclinical, that is, asymptomatic but detectable by colposcopy or cytologic examination; or latent, that is, having normal cytology and detectable only by viral testing (Schneider and Koutsky, 1992).

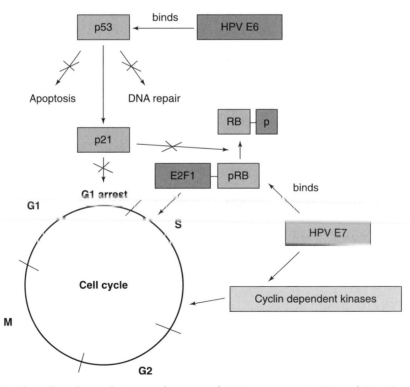

Figure 17–3. The cell cycle regulating mechanisms of HPV oncoproteins E6 and E7. (*Source:* Burd EM, 2003)

A number of methods have been used to detect HPV DNA in cervical specimens (Koutsky et al, 1988; Schiffman, 1992b; Schneider and Koutsky, 1992; IARC, 1995a). With in situ hybridization, DNA or RNA probes are hybridized to HPV DNA in tissue, which allows the histology of the biopsy to be preserved. It is a labor-intensive method, and the need for a tissue specimen makes it impractical for epidemiology studies. Filter in situ hybridization of exfoliated cells was the first test designed for use in epidemiologic research, but due to its low sensitivity and specificity as well as to its poor reproducibility, this assay is no longer used (Schiffman, 1992b). Southern blot hybridization of cervical specimens, usually of exfoliated cells, is a highly specific method of detection and was considered the gold standard until the advent of polymerase chain reaction (PCR) technology. Southern blot testing requires an adequate sample of DNA, and problems with interlaboratory reproducibility have occurred. The development of commercially available dot blot hybridization kits was an important breakthrough, since these assays are easier to use in large studies. With this assay, radiolabeled RNA probes are hybridized to DNA on filter paper in a dot blot format. The first such kit, ViraPap, could detect seven HPV types (Schiffman, 1992b; IARC, 1995a); the ViraPap and ViraType assays can be used in conjunction to type an HPV infection as being in one of three groups (6/11, 16/18, or 31/33/35).

The Hybrid Capture test represents a more recent version of the hybridization assays, using a liquid-based system with nonradioactive RNA probes to detect the DNA of 14 HPV types that can be identified as high-risk (16/18/31/33/35/45/51/52/56) or low-risk (6/11/42/43/44) (IARC, 1995a). The Hybrid Capture system is the only assay currently approved by the Food and Drug Adminstration for use in the United States.

The PCR detection of HPV DNA provided researchers with a highly sensitive assay that could identify as few as 10 to 100 copies of HPV in a very small amount of specimen (IARC, 1995a). The initial problems with specificity were resolved as the use of PCR became more standardized. Now PCR is the most commonly used assay. As would be expected, the higher validity and reliability of PCR in detecting HPV DNA greatly increased the strength of the association of HPV infection with cervical neoplasia as well as with sexual behavior variables (Guerrero et al, 1992; Schiffman and Schatzkin, 1994; IARC, 1995a). Sampling methods, including how the specimen is collected (eg, biopsy of the lesion versus cytologic sampling), also can affect the determination of HPV status (Muñoz et al, 1988; Bosch et al, 1994).

Epidemiology. Sexual transmission is the major route of genital HPV infection. In fact, HPV infection is considered the most common sexually transmitted disease in the world, with the lifetime risk of being infected with one or more HPV infections estimated to be at least 75% in some western countries (Cox, 2006). In concordance, a recent study on condom use and risk of HPV infection confirmed a protective effect of condom use; the incidence rates of both genital HPV infection and cervical intraepithelial lesions were reduced in condom users compared to nonusers (Winer et al, 2006). Most HPV infections appear to resolve without leading to detectable lesions, with the average duration of new infections believed to be only a few years (IARC, 1995a; Schiffman and Brinton, 1995; Ho et al, 1998). The prevalence of detectable cervical HPV infection ranges from about 4% to 40% in sexually active women with normal cervical cytology and appears to decrease with age (Schiffman, 1992a; IARC, 1995a).The decreasing prevalence may be explained by decreased transmission during later years of sexual activity. Or possibly, by the acquisition of a protective immune response as a result of previous exposure to the virus. Alternatively, women in adolescence may be more susceptible to infection for biological reasons (Cox, 2006; Schiffman, 1992a). It is further hypothesized that a small proportion of women becomes persistently infected with an oncogenic HPV type, which, in some, will progress to high-grade CIN in their late 20s to early 30s and then to invasive disease 10 or more years later.

Most of the epidemiologic evidence for an association between high-risk HPV types and cervical cancer has come from case-control studies (IARC, 1995a). Despite the methodologic difficulties inherent in the study of this relationship (Muñoz et al, 1988), including the potential for selection bias and for misclassification of both exposure and disease status, very strong relative risk estimates on the order of 10-fold to over 100-fold were observed. Improvements in the methods used to detect HPV and the utilization of PCR assays yielded even more striking results (Schiffman and Schatzkin, 1994; IARC, 1995a). Due to the long latency involved in cervical carcinogenesis as well as to the ethical imperative to treat early lesions, cohort studies have been few. A handful of studies have investigated the progression from normal cervical cytology to CIN, and somewhat more studies have focused on the progression from CIN I to CIN II/III (IARC, 1995a; Schiffman and Brinton, 1995; Muñoz and Bosch, 1996; Liaw et al, 1999). In all these studies, strong associations were reported between infection with high-risk HPV types and progression of neoplasia. It has been thought that the natural history of HPV infection leading to cervical cancer proceeds with an orderly increase in the degree of neoplasia (ie, from CIN I to CIN III and further to invasive cervical cancer) (Kiviat and Koutsky, 1993; Schiffman and Brinton, 1995; Mitchell et al, 1996). However, some women who develop CIN II/III appear never to have had CIN I (Koutsky et al, 1992; Liaw et al, 1999). Thus, although CIN I may precede the development of higher-grade lesions, such low-grade neoplasias may not always be involved in disease progression (Kiviat and Koutsky, 1993; Mitchell et al, 1996).

In 1995, the International Agency for Research on Cancer (IARC) classified HPV types 16 and 18 as being "carcinogenic to

humans" and types 31 and 33 as being "probably carcinogenic to humans" (IARC, 1995a); it was further determined that the evidence suggested a "lack of carcinogenicity" to the cervix for types 6 and 11. After revisiting all gathered data in 2005, however, HPV 6 and 11 were also classified as possibly carcinogenic (Trottier and Franco, 2006). A comprehensive study of nearly 900 squamous cell carcinoma cases from 22 different countries revealed an overall HPV DNA prevalence of 93% (Bosch et al, 1995). About 50% of the cases were positive for HPV 16, 12% for HPV 18, 8% for HPV 45, and 5% for HPV 31; the low-risk types HPV 6 and 11 were found in only one case each. The distribution of HPVs was fairly similar across different geographic regions, with some variation between countries with respect to the less common types. For adenocarcinoma of the cervix, a somewhat lower prevalence of HPV DNA is detected by PCR, although some estimates are similar to those for squamous cell cancer (Kjaer and Brinton, 1993; Bosch et al, 1995; IARC, 1995a). Human papillomavirus type 18 appears to be the predominant type occurring in adenocarcinomas (Madeleine et al, 2001), the prevalence being 56% in the large international study by Bosch and colleagues (1995).

Given the ubiquity of infection with HPV, the determination of what constitutes an etiologically relevant infection would be useful for research purposes, as well as for possible public health interventions. Although not much is known about the regression, recurrence, or persistence of HPV lesions, some studies have provided important details concerning the natural history of the infection and the progression to cancer. Risk factors for the development of persistent HPV infection (compared to transient infection) include older age and infection with a high-risk HPV, particularly HPV 16 and 18 (Franco et al, 1999; Hildesheim et al, 1994; Ho et al, 1998). An association between high viral load and persistence of HPV infection has also been postulated (Franco et al, 1997; Ho et al, 1995). In support of this hypothesis, a population-based cohort study in Sweden also found a strong association of persistent high viral load of HPV 16 and the development of CIS (Josefsson et al, 2000; Ylitalo et al, 2000a,b); the estimated cumulative risk of developing CIS within 15 years was 22.7% among women with a high viral load and only 6.6% in women with a medium viral load of HPV 16. In contrast, the risk among women with low viral load was similar to that among women who were HPV 16 negative (Fig. 17–4).

Cell-mediated immunity plays an important role in the clearance of HPV infection (Schneider and Koutsky, 1992; IARC, 1995a). Thus, the host's immune response, as well as the oncogenic potential of the infecting HPV, likely contributes to the persistence and progression of infection. Immune suppression frequently leads to the emergence of HPV-related lesions. Indeed, a high prevalence of HPV and SIL has been observed among women infected with HIV. Although an HIV-induced inability to clear and control HPV infection would reasonably be hypothesized to play a role in the risk of this malignancy, the literature is far

from conclusive. Some investigators report no increased risk of invasive cervical cancer among HIV-infected women (IARC, 1996a; Beral and Newton, 1998), while others suggest a higher incidence of invasive cervical cancer in women with HIV (Frisch et al, 2000). An important question is whether HIV-positive women have a higher likelihood of HPV infection due to shared transmission routes and/or whether the immunosuppressive effects of HIV enhance the progression of HPV infection to cervical cancer. The evidence does support the belief that HIV infection in women is related to persistent infection with HPV (Ahdieh et al, 2000).

An interesting area of research in the natural history of HPV involves the study of the humoral immune response to this infection. Within the last 10 years, serologic assays have been developed that enable the detection of type-specific antibodies to different HPV structural and regulatory proteins (Galloway, 1992; IARC, 1995a). The most studied antibodies are those to the HPV 16 E6 and E7 proteins, which are important in HPV transformation and

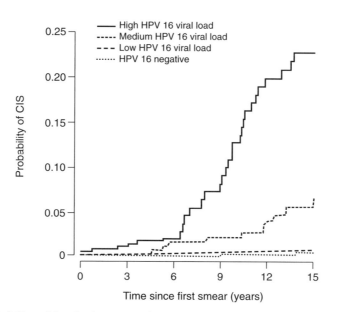

Figure 17–4. Probability of developing cervical carcinoma in situ in relation to HPV 16 viral load of first smear among women younger than 25 years at time of first smear. CIS = cervical carcinoma in situ. (*Source:* Ylitalo et al, 2000b.)

oncogenesis. In more than 10 case-control studies that have examined these antibodies, consistent positive associations were seen for cervical cancer, with a 2- to 40-fold relative risk (Viscidi et al, 1993; Dillner et al, 1995; IARC, 1995a). Assays have become available to detect antibodies to HPV 16 virus-like particles (VLPs) (Kirnbauer et al, 1994). The presence of these antibodies is predictive of progression to CIN II/III and invasive cervical cancer (Dillner et al, 1995, 1997; Wideroff et al, 1995; Lehtinen et al, 1996; Olsen et al, 1996; de Gruijl et al, 1997). In a nested case-control study of cervical cancer, HPV 16 seropositivity was associated with squamous cell carcinoma, whereas HPV 18 seropositivity was associated with adenocarcinoma (Dillner et al, 1997).

The weaker association of HPV antibodies with CIN and cervical cancer compared to that observed for HPV DNA in cervical cells likely reflects the fact that the presence of HPV antibodies represents past infection as well as current infection. Among subjects with normal cervical cytology, the prevalence of HPV VLP antibodies is higher than the prevalence of HPV DNA (Nonnenmacher et al, 1995). Antibody seroconversion appears to occur some months after infection (Carter et al, 1996), which could explain the reports of HPV DNA–positive women without HPV antibodies (Kirnbauer et al, 1994; Nonnenmacher et al, 1995). The prevalence of anti-VLPs has been reported to be higher in HPV 16–positive women with CIN III (~75%) than in HPV 18–positive women with cervical cancer (~50%) (Nonnenmacher et al, 1995). This finding contrasts with that for antibodies to HPV 16 E6 and E7 proteins, which are high in cancer but low in CIN III (Viscidi et al, 1993). It has been hypothesized that in the course of cancer development productive HPV infection may cease, including the synthesis of capsid proteins and thus their associated antibodies; however, levels of E6 and E7 likely increase with malignant progression, leading to higher titers of antibodies to these virus proteins (Dillner et al, 1995; Nonnenmacher et al, 1995).

Cervical cancer is a rare consequence of a genital HPV infection. Hence, presence of additional cofactors is needed for cervical carcinogenesis to occur (zur Hausen, 1982). With regard to the interaction between other cofactors and HPV, the findings have been mixed. Part of the difficulty relates to the possibility that the cofactors postulated may have roles both in the acquisition and persistence of HPV infection as well as in the progression of HPV-associated cervical cancer (Schneider and Koutsky, 1992; Palefsky and Holly, 1995). Moreover, different cofactors may act at different points in the natural history of HPV and the progression to invasive malignancy (Muñoz et al, 1993) (Fig. 17–5).

Many of the nonviral risk factors for cervical cancer were established before good methods were available to detect HPV DNA (Schiffman and Brinton, 1995). Subsequent studies suggested that HPV infection likely explains most of the associations reported for sexual risk factors in particular and also for other behavioral and demographic determinants. Nonetheless, residual effects of these factors are observed, even after adjusting for the presence of HPV.

As discussed previously, both epidemiological and biological evidence exist for a possible modifying effect of tobacco smoking, multiparity, and OC use on HPV-associated cervical carcinogenesis (Palefsky and Holly, 1995; Schiffman and Brinton, 1995; Muñoz and Bosch, 1996) (Fig. 17–5). Even some of the sexual behavior factors could be modifying the effect of HPV infection on cervical cancer risk. A weak effect of early age at first intercourse remains after adjustment for HPV status in some studies and may reflect an increased susceptibility of the cervix in younger women to persistent HPV infection as well as to HPV's oncogenic potential. Whether the nonviral risk factors for cervical cancer have independent or modifying effects needs further research. Since these variables tend to be highly correlated with HPV infection, the fact that their association with cervical cancer often is stronger among HPV-negative women than among HPV-positive

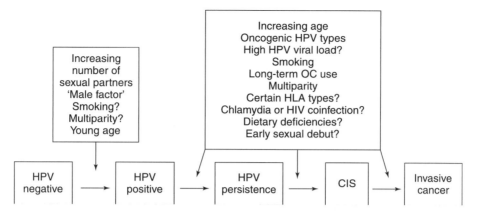

Figure 17–5. Established or possible(?) cofactors during different stages of the natural history of HPV infection and subsequent development of cervical cancer.

women may result from a misclassification of HPV status rather than a carcinogenic effect (Ylitalo et al, 1999).

Prevention. Papanicolaou test screening is recognized as an effective means of reducing cervical cancer morbidity and mortality through the detection of preclinical lesions. However, it is estimated that only about 20% or less of low-grade lesions will progress to invasive disease if left untreated (Schiffman and Brinton, 1995; Mitchell et al, 1996; Holowaty et al, 1999). There is currently no way to distinguish precursor lesions with a potential to progress from those that are prone to regress spontaneously. Consequently, test taking is of little help in predicting disease outcome in individual women, and the overtreatment of women with cervical dysplastic lesions, which would have been self-limited if left untreated, is substantial. Given the significant extra cost for this overtreatment, as well as the potential adverse effect on fertility and pregnancy outcome, the magnitude of the problem is not trivial (Kyrgiou et al, 2006).

HPV DNA testing of samples collected at Papanicolaou screening has been evaluated in some countries as a way to improve the clinical management of women with dysplastic or atypical lesions. Indeed, HPV DNA testing has proven to increase early detection of cervical cancer and its precursor lesions when used alone or in combination with cytological screening (Schiffman et al, 2005). Whether the implementation of HPV testing as part of a cervical screening program would have an effect on the current overtreatment by disentangling transient from persistent HPV infections remains to be seen. It has been proposed that HPV testing in conjunction with Papanicolaou screening could be implemented among women over 30 years old as a way to identify those women with a persistent high-risk HPV infection and to lengthen the interval between screening for women at low risk of developing cervical cancer (Cuzick, 1998). In the US such an approach has already been approved, whereas in Europe conventional cytological screening still remains the standard procedure (Arbyn et al, 2006). In younger women (less than 35) HPV testing alone together with cytological triage has been suggested as an alternative to traditional cytology screening (Ronco et al, 2006). Also, for many developing countries, cytological screening programs with Papanicolaou tests at regular visits every 1 to 3 years may not be realistic. Incorporating visual inspection of the cervix using acetoacid or HPV DNA testing on one or two occasions may be a cost-effective alternative in these settings (Goldie et al, 2005).

Much interest and research have been directed to the development of HPV vaccines, which hopefully should become important preventive tools for reducing the spread of the most prevalent high-risk HPV types. Lately, vaccines consisting of VLPs (which are empty shells of viral structural proteins) have been the most promising candidates. Animal studies of VLP-based vaccines of species-appropriate papillomaviruses have demonstrated protection from infection and development of neutralizing antibodies in the animals immunized (Lowy and Schiller, 1998; Sherman et al, 1998). Hope was raised in 2002 after the report of a double-blind clinical trial performed among 2392 young women, comparing three doses of HPV-16 VLP vaccine to placebo (Koutsky et al, 2002). All nine cases of HPV-16 CIN occurred within the placebo group during follow-up, indicating that the vaccine provided 100% protection. This clinical trial has been followed by several phase II and III trials testing either a bivalent VLP vaccine (against HPV types 16/18) or a quadrivalent VLP vaccine (against HPV types 6/11/16/18) (Villa et al, 2006). A sustained efficacy of 100% after 4.5 years follow-up was recently reported after 3 doses of a bivalent VLP vaccine (Harper et al, 2006).

By including the two most common HPV types, HPV 16 and 18, a vaccine could potentially prevent the over 70% of cervical cancers attributed to these two HPVs. Since these vaccines are preventive and thus not intended for treating infections already present, the ideal group targeted for vaccination would be young girls (around 12 years old) just before they become sexually active. Controversy remains however with regard to who should be vaccinated. A number of important questions have been raised, including the acceptability of a vaccine against an STD to be administered to adolescents not yet sexually active, the benefit of vaccination for adults already infected with HPV, as well as the length of time that protection will last. The issue of targeting men for vaccination against HPV also is under debate.

Vaccine programs by no means can replace traditional cytological screening, primarily because many women will have already been exposed to HPV and also because the current vaccines do not cover all potentially oncogenic HPV types. Therefore, despite the recent success of ongoing vaccination trials, there is no doubt that Papanicolaou test screening in combination with HPV DNA testing will remain as a key tool for the prevention of cervical cancer (Franco et al, 2006). Finally, since the incubation period from HPV infection to the development of cervical carcinoma in situ is long, the cancer-preventive potential of vaccination programs will not be evident within the next 10 years.

Physical Activity

A relationship between physical activity and cervical cancer occurrence has not been evaluated in a study specifically designed to test that hypothesis. A significant fivefold increased risk of cancer of the cervix was observed for self-reported inactivity in the first National Health and Nutrition Examination Study (Albanes et al, 1989); neither HPV status nor sexual behavior, however, was controlled for in that study. In contrast, a small hospital-based case-control study reported a nonsignificant inverse association between decreased occupational physical activity and cervical cancer occurrence, after controlling for smoking and socioeconomic status (Dosemeci et al, 1993).

Ionizing Radiation

Little evidence exists for an association between exposure to radiation and cervical cancer (Ron, 1998; IARC, 2000). Rates of cervical cancer do not appear to be increased in the Japanese atomic bomb survivors cohort or in patients receiving radiotherapy.

Occupation

Several studies have shown associations of particular occupations with cervical cancer in women. An excess occurrence has been observed primarily in service occupations (eg, maids, cleaners, waitresses, cooks) and in the manufacturing and textile industries (eg, machine operators, textile workers, printers, dry cleaners) (IARC, 1995b, 1996b; Savitz et al, 1995; Sala et al, 1998; Carpenter and Roman, 1999). Increased cervical cancer occurrence also has been associated with agricultural work (Savitz et al, 1995; Sala et al, 1998). Most of these studies were based on proportional risk estimates; none controlled for HPV status, and many did not adjust for socioeconomic status. Only the case-control study by Savitz et al (1995) was specifically designed to evaluate the relationship between occupation and cervical cancer; that study also controlled for the confounding effects of sexual behavior, Papanicolaou test screening, and tobacco smoking.

Several of the occupations that have been reported to be associated with cervical cancer involve potential exposure to hazardous chemicals such as organic solvents. In 1995, the IARC found limited evidence for a carcinogenic effect of tetrachloroethylene and trichloroethylene, solvents used in dry cleaning and textile processing and as degreasing agents, on the cervix (IARC, 1995b). An increased risk of cervical cancer was reported for a cohort of solvent-exposed workers (Berlin et al, 1995); however, a meta-analysis of mortality studies of workers exposed to organic solvents did not find a significantly elevated risk of death due to cervical cancer (Chen and Seaton, 1996).

Medical Conditions

There appears to be no evidence for an effect of a particular medical condition on the occurrence of cervical cancer.

CONCLUSION

A persistent infection with an oncogenic HPV type is today considered a causal factor for the occurrences of cervical cancer. The oncogenic potential of the virus appears to be mediated through the action of particular viral proteins that interact with host tumor-suppressor proteins, thereby suppressing cell-cycle control and apoptosis. Although the evidence is compelling that HPV is necessary for cervical carcinogenesis, infection alone likely is not sufficient for malignancy to occur. A number of cofactors have been identified as possible modifiers of HPV during the development of cervical cancer, including tobacco smoking, multiparity, OC use, and *Chlamydia trachomatis* infection. Because many of these factors are strongly correlated with HPV infection, it has been difficult to characterize their role in the development and progression of cervical neoplasia, as well as in the acquisition and persistence of HPV infection. Host immune control of the infection, including factors that would affect it, also may be important in HPV-induced carcinogenesis.

As one of the leading causes of cancer among women worldwide, cervical cancer remains an important public health problem, particularly in developing countries. Although Papanicolaou test screening has been highly effective in decreasing cancer incidence and mortality, the recent advancement in the development of a vaccine against HPV infection probably offers the best means of reducing the burden of this malignancy. Despite the advent of HPV vaccination, early detection of cytological changes within the screening programs will nonetheless continue to be a key element in the prevention of cervical cancer. The use of HPV testing to characterize virus status (ie, HPV genotype, persistence of infection) also may enhance the identification of those women most at risk for progression to cervical cancer. Thus, through a combination of public education about transmission of HPV, early detection of precursor lesions to cervical carcinoma by regular cytological screening with the incorporation of HPV testing and vaccination against certain high-risk types of HPV, carcinoma of the cervix may become one of the major forms of cancer that is most preventable on a global scale.

REFERENCES

Ahdieh L, Muñoz A, Vlahov D, Trimble CL, Timpson LA, Shah K. Cervical neoplasia and repeated positivity of human papillomavirus infection in human immunodeficiency virus–seropositive and–seronegative women. Am J Epidemiol 2000;151:1148–57.

Albanes D, Blair A, Taylor PR. Physical activity and risk of cancer in the NHANES I population. Am J Public Health 1989;79:744–50.

Anttila T, Saikku P, Koskela P, Bloigu A, Dillner J, Ikäheimo I, et al. Serotypes of Chlamydia trachomatis and risk for development of cervical squamous cell carcinoma. JAMA 2001; 285:47–51.

Apple RJ, Erlich HA, Klitz W, Manos MM, Becker TM, Wheeler CM. HLA DR-DQ associations with cervical carcinoma show papillomavirus-type specificity. Nat Genet 1994;6:157–62.

Arbyn M, Sasieni P, Meijer CJLM, Clavel C, Koliopoulos G, Dillner J. Clinical applications of HPV testing: a summary of a meta-analyses. Vaccine 2006;24:78–89.

Barton SE, Maddox PH, Jenkins D, Edwards R, Cuzick J, Singer A. Effect of smoking on cervical epithelial immunity: a mechanism for neoplastic change? Lancet 1988;2:652–54.

Beral V. Cancer of the cervix: a sexually transmitted infection? Lancet 1974;1:1037–40.

Beral V, Newton R. Overview of the epidemiology of immunodeficiency-associated cancers. J Natl Cancer Inst Monogr 1998;23:1–6.

Berchuk A, Rodabaugh KJ. Role of oncogene and tumor suppressor gene alterations in cervical carcinogenesis. In: Rubin SC, Hoskins W (Eds): Cervical Cancer and Preinvasive Neoplasia. Philadelphia, Lippincott-Raven, 1996, pp 49–57.

Bergström R, Sparen P, Adami HO. Trends in cancer of the cervix uteri in Sweden following cytological screening. Br J Cancer 1999: 81:159–66.

Berlin K, Edling C, Persson B, Ahlborg G, Hillert L, Hogstedt B, et al. Cancer incidence and mortality of patients with suspected solvent-related disorders. Scand J Work Environ Health 1995;21:362–67.

Bosch FX, Castellsague X, Muñoz N, de Sanjosé S, Ghaffari AM, Gonzalez LC, et al. Male sexual behavior and human papillomavirus DNA: key risk factors for cervical cancer in Spain. J Natl Cancer Inst 1996;88:1060–67.

Bosch FX, de Sanjosé S, Muñoz N. Correspondence re: M Schiffman and A Schatzkin, Test reliability is critically important to molecular epidemiology: an example from studies of human papillomavirus infection and cervical neoplasia. Cancer Res 1994;54:6288–89.

Bosch FX, Lorincz A, Munoz N, Meijer CJ, Shah KV. The causal relation between human papillomavirus and cervical cancer. J Clin Pathol 2002;55:244–65.

Bosch FX, Manos MM, Muñoz N, Sherman M, Jansen AM, Peto J, et al. Prevalence of human papillomavirus in cervical cancer: a worldwide perspective. International biological study on cervical cancer (IBSCC) Study Group. J Natl Cancer Inst 1995;87:796–802.

Bosch FX, Muñoz N, de Sanjosé S, Izarzugaza I, Gili M, Viladiu P, et al. Risk factors for cervical cancer in Colombia and Spain. Int J Cancer 1992;52:750–58.

Boyd JT, Doll R. A study of the aetiology of carcinoma of the cervix uteri. Br J Cancer 1964;18:419–34.

Brinton LA. Epidemiology of cervical cancer—overview. In: Muñoz N, Bosch FX, Shah KV, Meheus A (Eds): The Epidemiology of Cervical Cancer and Human Papillomavirus. Lyon, International Agency for Research on Cancer, 1992, pp 3–23.

Brinton LA, Tashima KT, Lehman HF, Levine RS, Mallin K, Savitz DA, et al. Epidemiology of cervical cancer by cell type. Cancer Res 1987;47:1706–11.

Burger MPM, Hollema H, Gouw ASH, Pieters WJ, Quint WG. Cigarette smoking and human papillomavirus in patients with reported cervical cytological abnormality. Br Med J 1993;306:749–52.

Carpenter L, Roman E. Cancer and occupation in women: identifying associations using routinely collected national data. Environ Health Perspect 1999;107(Suppl 2):299–303.

Carter JJ, Koutsky LA, Wipf GC, Christensen ND, Lee SK, Kuypers J, et al. The natural history of human papillomavirus type 16 capsid antibodies among a cohort of university women. J Infect Dis 1996;174:927–36.

Chen R, Seaton A. A meta-analysis of mortality among workers exposed to organic solvents. Occup Med 1996;46:337–44.

Chichareon S, Herrero R, Muñoz N, Bosch FX, Jacobs MV, Deacon J, et al. Risk factors for cervical cancer in Thailand: a case-control study. J Natl Cancer Inst 1998;90:50–57.

Cox JT. The development of cervical cancer and its precursors: what is the role of human papillomavirus infection? Curr Opin Obstet Gynecol 2006;18:S5-S13.

Cuzick J. HPV testing in cervical screening. Sex Transm Infect 1998;74:300–1.

de Gruijl TD, Bontkes HJ, Walboomers JM, Schiller JT, Stukart MJ, Groot BS, et al. Immunoglobulin G responses against human papillomavirus type 16 virus-like particles in a prospective nonintervention cohort study of women with cervical intraepithelial neoplasia. J Natl Cancer Inst 1997;89:630–38.

de Sanjosé S, Muñoz N, Bosch FX, Reimann K, Pedersen NS, Orfila J, et al. Sexually transmitted agents and cervical neoplasia in Colombia and Spain. Int J Cancer 1994;56:358–63.

de Villiers EM, Fauquet C, Broker TR, Bernard HU, zur Hausen H. Classification of papillomaviruses. Virology. 2004;324:17–27.

Dillner J, Lehtinen M, Bjorge T, Luostarinen T, Youngman L, Jellum E, et al. Prospective seroepidemiologic study of human papillomavirus infection as a risk factor for invasive cervical cancer. J Natl Cancer Inst 1997; 89:1293–99.

Dillner J, Wiklund F, Lenner P, Eklund C, Frederiksson-Shanazarian V, Schiller JT, et al. Antibodies against linear and conformational epitopes of human papillomavirus type 16 that independently associate with incident cervical cancer. Int J Cancer 1995;60:377–82.

Dosemeci M, Hayes RB, Vetter R, Hoover RN, Tucker M, Engin K, et al. Occupational physical activity, socioeconomic status, and risks of 15 cancer sites in Turkey. Cancer Causes Control 1993;4:313–21.

Eluf-Neto J, Booth M, Muñoz N, Bosch FX, Meijer CJ, Walboomers JM. Human papillomavirus and invasive cervical cancer in Brazil. Br J Cancer 1994;69:114–19.

Franco EL, Villa LL, Richardson H, Rohan T, Ferenczy A. Epidemiology of cervical human papillomavirus infection In: Franco E, Monsonego J (Ed): New Developments in Cervical Cancer Screening and Prevention. Oxford: Blackwell Science, 1997, pp 14–22.

Franco EL, Villa LL, Sobrinho JP, Prado JM, Rousseau M-C, Désy M, et al. Epidemiology of acquisition and clearance of cervical human papillomavirus infection in women from a high-risk area for cervical cancer. J Infect Dis 1999;180:1415–23

Franco EL, Cuzick J, Hildesheim A, de Sanjosé S. Chapter 20. Issues in planning cervical cancer screening in the era of HPV vaccination. Vaccine 2006;24:171–77.

Frisch M, Biggar RJ, Goedert JJ, for the AIDS-Cancer Match Registry Study Group. Human papillomavirus–associated cancers in patients with human immunodeficiency virus infection and acquired immunodeficiency syndrome. J Natl Cancer Inst 2000; 92:1500–10.

Galloway, DA. Serological assays for the detection of HPV antibodies. In: Muñoz N, Bosch FX, Shah, KV, Meheus A (Eds.). The Epidemiology of Cervical Cancer and Human Papillomavirus. Lyon, International Agency for Research on Cancer, 1992, pp. 147–61.

Garcia-Closas R, Castellsague X, Bosch X, Gonzalez CA. The role of diet and nutrition in cervical carcinogenesis: a review of recent evidence. Int J Cancer 2005;117:629–37.

Giuliano AR, Siegel EM, Roe DJ, Ferreira S, Baggio ML, Galan L, et al. Dietary intake and risk of persistent human papillomavirus (HPV) infection: the Ludwig-McGill HPV Natural History Study. J Infect Dis. 2003; 188:1508–16.

Goldie S, Gaffkin L, Goldhaber-Fiebert JD, Gordillo-Tobar A, Levin C, Mahe C, et al. Cost-effectiveness of cervical-cancer screening in five developing countries. N Engl J Med. 2005;353:2158–68.

Guerrero E, Daniel RW, Bosch FX, Castellsague X, Muñoz N, Gili M, et al. Comparison of ViraPap, Southern hybridization, and polymerase chain reaction methods for human papillomavirus identification in an epidemiological investigation of cervical cancer. J Clin Microbiol 1992;30:2951–59.

Gustafsson L, Pontén J, Zack M, Adami HO. International incidence rates of invasive cervical cancer after introduction of cytological screening. Cancer Causes Control 1997;8: 755–63.

Harper DM, Franco EL, Wheeler CM, Moscicki AB, Romanowski B, Roteli-Martibs CM, et al. Sustained efficacy up to 4.5 years of a bivalent L1 virus-like particle vaccine against human papillomavirus types 16 and 18: follow-up from a randomised control trial. Lancet 2006;367:1247–55.

Helland A, Olsen AO, Gjoen K, Akselsen HE, Sauer T, Magnus P, et al. An increased risk of cervical intra-epithelial neoplasia grade II–III among human papillomavirus positive patients with the HLA-DQA1*0102-DQB1* 0602 haplotype: a population-based case-control study of Norwegian women. Int J Cancer 1998;76:19–24.

Hemminki K, Vaittinen P. Familial risks in in situ cancer from the family-cancer database. Cancer Epidemiol Biomarkers Prev 1998; 7:865–68.

Herrero R. Epidemiology of cervical cancer. J Natl Cancer Inst Monogr 1996;21:1–6.

Hildesheim A, Mann V, Brinton LA, Szklo M, Reeves WC, Rawls WE. Herpes simplex virus type 2: a possible interaction with human papillomavirus types 16/18 in the development of invasive cervical cancer. Int J Cancer 1991;49:335–40.

Hildesheim A, Reeves WC, Brinton LA, Lavery C, Brenes M, De La Guardia ME, et al. Association of oral contraceptive use and human papillomaviruses in invasive cervical cancers. Int J Cancer 1990;45:860–64.

Hildesheim A, Schiffman M, Brinton LA, Fraumeni JF Jr, Herrero R, Bratti MC, et al. p53 polymorphism and risk of cervical cancer. Nature 1998;396:531–32.

Hildesheim A, Schiffman MH, Gravitt PE, Glass AG, Greer CE, Zhang T, et al. Persistence of type-specific human papillomavirus infection among cytologically normal women. J Infect Dis 1994;169:235–40.

Ho GYF, Burk RD, Klein S, Kadish AS, Chang CJ, Palan P, et al. Persistent genital human papillomavirus infection as a risk factor for persistent cervical dysplasia. J Natl Cancer Inst 1995;87:1365–71.

Ho GYF, Bierman R, Beardsley L, Chang CJ, Burk RD. Natural history of cervicovaginal papillomavirus infection in young woman. N Engl J Med 1998;338:423–28.

Holowaty P, Miller AB, Rohan T, To T. Natural history of dysplasia of the uterine cervix. J Natl Cancer Inst 1999;91;252–58.

Howley PM. Papillomavirnae: the viruses and their replication. In: Fields BN, Knipe DM, Howley PM (Eds): Fields Virology. Third Edition. Philadelphia, Lippincott-Raven, 1996, pp 2045–76.

International Agency for Research on Cancer. Human Papillomavirus. IARC Monographs on the Evaluation of Carcinogenic Risks to Humans. Vol. 64. Lyon, International Agency for Research on Cancer, 1995a.

International Agency for Research on Cancer. Dry Cleaning, Some Chlorinated Solvents and Other Industrial Chemicals. IARC Monographs on the Evaluation of Carcinogenic Risks to Humans. Vol. 63. Lyon, International Agency for Research on Cancer, 1995b.

International Agency for Research on Cancer. Human Immunodeficiency Viruses and Human T-Cell Lymphotropic Viruses. IARC Monographs on the Evaluation of Carcinogenic Risks to Humans. Vol. 67. Lyon, International Agency for Research on Cancer, 1996a.

International Agency for Research on Cancer. Printing Processes and Printing Inks, Carbon Black and Some Nitro Compounds. IARC Monographs on the Evaluation of Carcinogenic Risks to Humans. Vol. 65. Lyon, International Agency for Research on Cancer, 1996b.

International Agency for Research on Cancer. Ionizing Radiation, Part 1: X- and Gamma (g)-Radiation, and Neutrons. IARC Monographs on the Evaluation of Carcinogenic Risks to Humans. Vol. 75. Lyon, International Agency for Research on Cancer, 2000.

International Collaboration of Epidemiological Studies of Cervical Cancer. Carcinoma of the cervix and tobacco smoking: Collaborative reanalysis of individual data on 13,541 women with carcinoma of the cervix and 23,017 women without carcinoma of the cervix from 23 epidemiological studies. Int J Cancer 2006;118:1481–95

Josefsson AM, Magnusson PK, Ylitalo N, Quarforth-Tubbin P, Pontén J, Adami HO, et al. p53 polymorphism and risk of cervical cancer. Nature 1998;396:531.

Josefsson AM, Magnusson PKE, Ylitalo N, Sørensen P, Qwarforth-Tubbin P, Andersen PK, et al. Viral load of human papilloma virus 16 as a determinant for development of cervical carcinoma in situ: a nested case-control study. Lancet 2000;355:2189–93.

Kirnbauer R, Hubbert NL, Wheeler CM, Becker TM, Lowy DR, Schiller JT. A virus-like particle enzyme-linked immunosorbent assay detects serum antibodies in a majority of women infected with human papillomavirus type 16. J Natl Cancer Inst 1994;86:494–99.

Kiviat NB, Critchcow CW, Kurman RJ. Reassessment of the morphological continuum of cervical intraepithelial lesions: does it reflect different stages in the progression to cervical carcinoma. In: Muñoz N, Bosch FX, Shah KV, Meheus A (Eds): The Epidemiology of Cervical Cancer and Human Papillomavirus. Lyon, International Agency for Research on Cancer, 1992, pp 59–66.

Kiviat NB, Koutsky LA. Specific human papillomavirus types as the causal agents of most cervical intraepithelial neoplasia: implications for current views and treatment. J Natl Cancer Inst 1993;85:934–35.

Kjaer SK, Brinton LA. Adenocarcinoma of the uterine cervix: the epidemiology of an increasing problem. Epidemiol Rev 1993;15:486–98.

Kjaer SK, Engholm G, Dahl C, Bock JE. Case-control study of risk factors for cervical squamous cell neoplasia in Denmark: role of smoking habits. Eur J Cancer Prev 1996a;5:359–65.

Konya J, Dillner J. Immunity to oncogenic human papillomaviruses. Adv Cancer Res 2001;82:205–38.

Koutsky LA, Galloway DA, Holmes KK. Epidemiology of genital human papillomavirus infection. Epidemiol Rev 1988;10:122–63.

Koutsky LA, Holmes KK, Critchlow CW, Stevens CE, Paavonen J, Beckmann AM, et al. A cohort study of the risk of cervical intraepithelial neoplasia grade 2 or 3 in relation to papillomavirus infection. N Engl J Med 1992;327:1272–78.

Koutsky LA, Ault KA, Wheeler CM, Brown DR, Barr E, Alvarez FB, et al. A controlled trial of a human papillomavirus type 16 vaccine. N Engl J Med. 2002;347:1645–51

Kyrgiou M, Kolipoulos P, Martin-Hirsch P, Arbyn M, Prendiville W, Paraskevaidis E. Obstetric outcomes after conservative treatment for intraepithelial or early invasive cervical lesions: systematic review and meta-analysis. Lancet 2006;367:489–98.

Lacey JV, Swanson CA, Brinton LA, Altekruse SF, Barnes WA, Grawitt PE, et al. Obesity as a potential risk factor for adenocarcinomas and squamous cell carcinomas of the uterine cervix. Cancer. 2003;98:814–21.

Lehtinen M, Dillner J, Knekt P, Luostarinen T, Aromaa A, Kirnbauer R, et al. Serologically diagnosed infection with human papillomavirus type 16 and risk for subsequent development of cervical carcinoma: nested case-control study. Br Med J 1996;312:537–39.

Lema C, Fuessel-Haws AL, Lewis LR, Rady PL, Lee P, Turbat-Herrera EA, et al. Association between HLA-DQB1 and cervical dysplasia in Vietnamese women. Int J Gynecol Cancer. 2006;16:1269–77.

Liaw KL, Glass AG, Manos MM, Greer CE, Scott DR, Sherman M, et al. Detection of human papillomavirus DNA in cytologically normal women and subsequent cervical squamous intraepithelial lesions. J Natl Cancer Inst 1999;91:954–60.

Lichtenstein P, Holm NV, Verkasalo PK, Iliadou A, Kaprio J, Koskenvua M, et al. Environmental and heritable factors in the causation of cancer—analyses of cohorts of twins from Sweden, Denmark, and Finland.N Engl J Med. 2000;343:78–85.

Lowy DR, Schiller JT. Papillomaviruses and cervical cancer: pathogenesis and vaccine development. Monogr Natl Cancer Inst 1998; 23:27–30.

Madeleine MM, Daling JR, Schwartz SM, Shera K, McKnight B, Carter JJ, et al. Human papillomavirus and long-term oral contraceptive use increased the risk of adenocarcinoma in situ of the cervix. Cancer Epidemiol Biomarkers Prev 2001;10:171–77.

Magnusson PK, Lichtenstein P, Gyllensten U. Heritability of cervical tumours. Int J Cancer. 2000;88:698–701.

McCann MF, Irwin DE, Walton LA, Hulka BS, Morton JL, Axelrad CM. Nicotine and cotinine in the cervical mucus of smokers, passive smokers, and nonsmokers. Cancer Epidemiol Biomarkers Prev 1992;1:125–29.

Mitchell MF, Tortolero-Luna G, Wright T, Sarkar A, Richards-Kortum R, Hong WK, et al. Cervical human papillomavirus infection and intraepithelial neoplasia: a review. J Natl Cancer Inst Monogr 1996;21:17–25.

Moreno V, Bosch FX, Muñoz N, Meijer CJL, Shah KV, Walboomers JMM, et al. Effect of oral contraceptives on risk of cervical cancer in women with human papillomavirus infection: the IARC multicentric case-control study. Lancet 2002;359:1085–92.

Muñoz N, Bosch FX. The causal link between HPV and cervical cancer and its implications for prevention of cervical cancer. Bull Pan Am Health Organ 1996;30:362–77.

Muñoz N, Bosch FX, de SanJosé S, Herrero R, Castellsagué X, Shah KV, et al. Epidemiologic classification of human papillomavirus types associated with cervical cancer. N Engl J Med 2003;348:518–27.

Muñoz N, Bosch FX, de SanJosé S, Vergara A, del Moral A, Muñoz MT, et al. Risk factors for cervical intraepithelial neoplasia grade III/carcinoma in situ in Spain and Colombia. Cancer Epidemiol Biomarkers Prev 1993;2: 423–31.

Muñoz N, Bosch FX, Kaldor JM. Does human papillomavirus cause cervical cancer? The state of the epidemiologic evidence. Br J Cancer 1988;57:1–5.

Muñoz N, Franceschi S, Bosetti C, Moreno V, Herrero R, Smith JS, et al. Role of parity and human papillomavirus in cervical cancer: the IARC multicentric case-control study. Lancet 2002;359:1093–101.

Muñoz N, Kato I, Bosch FX, de SanJosé S, Sundquist VA, Izarzugaza I, et al. Cervical cancer and herpes simplex virus type 2: case-control studies in Spain and Colombia, with special reference to immunoglobulin-G subclasses. Int J Cancer 1995;60:438–42.

Ngelangel C, Muñoz N, Bosch FX, Limson GM, Festin MR, Deacon J, et al. Causes of cervical cancer in the Philippines: a case-control study. J Natl Cancer Inst 1998;90:43–49.

Nonnenmacher B, Hubbert NL, Kirnbauer R, Shah KV, Muñoz N, Bosch FX, et al. Serologic response to human papillomavirus type 16 (HPV-16) virus-like particles in HPV-16 DNA-positive invasive cervical cancer and cervical intraepithelial neoplasia grade III patients and controls from Colombia and Spain. J Infect Dis 1995;172:19–24.

Olsen AO, Dillner J, Gj en K, Sauer T, Orstavik I, Magnus P. A population-based case-control study of human papillomavirus-type 16 seropositivity and incident high-grade dysplasia of the uterine cervix. Int J Cancer 1996;68:415–19.

Odunsi KO, Ganesan TS. The roles of the human major histocompatibility complex and human papillomavirus infection in cervical intraepithelial neoplasia and cervical cancer. Clin Oncol 1997;9:4–13.

Palefsky JM, Holly EA. Molecular virology and epidemiology of human papillomavirus and cervical cancer. Cancer Epidemiol Biomarkers Prev 1995;4:415–28.

Parkin DM, Bray F, Ferlay J, Pisani P. Global cancer statistics, 2002. CA Cancer J Clin 2005;55:74–108.

Plummer M, Herrero R, Franceschi S, Meijer CJ, Snijder P, Bosch FX, et al. Smoking and cervical cancer: pooled analysis of the IARC multi-centric case—control study. Cancer Causes Control 2003;14:805–14.

Pontén J, Adami HO, Bergstrom R, Dillner J, Friberg LG, Gustafsson L, et al. Strategies for global control of cervical cancer. Int J Cancer 1995;60:1–26.

Potischman N, Brinton LA. Nutrition and cervical neoplasia. Cancer Causes Control 1996; 7:113–26.

Ron E. Ionizing radiation and cancer risk: evidence from epidemiology. Radiat Res 1998; 150(Suppl):S30–S41.

Ronco G, Giorgi-Rossi P, Carozzi F, Dalla Palma P, Del Mistro A, De Marco L, et al. Human papillomavirus testing and liquid-based cytology in primary screening of women younger than 35 years: results at recruitment for a randomised controlled trial. Lancet Oncol 2006;7:545–53.

Rosenthal A, Ryan A, Al-Jehani RM, Storey A, Harwood CA, Jacobs IJ. p53 codon 72 polymorphism and risk of cervical cancer in UK. Lancet 1998;352:871–72.

Sala M, Dosemeci M, Zahm SH. A death certificate–based study of occupation and mortality from reproductive cancers among women in 24 U.S. states. J Occup Environ Med 1998;40:632–39.

Sanjeevi CB, Hjelmstrom P, Hallmans G, Wiklund F, Lenner P, Angstrom T, et al. Different HLA-DR-DQ haplotypes are associated with cervical intraepithelial neoplasia among human papillomavirus type-16 seropositive and seronegative Swedish women. Int J Cancer 1996;68:409–14.

Sasieni P, Adams J. Changing rates of adenocarcinoma and adenosquamous carcinoma of the cervix in England. Lancet 2001;357:1490–93.

Savitz DA, Andrews KW, Brinton LA. Occupation and cervical cancer. J Occup Environ Med 1995;37:357–61.

Schiffman MH. Recent progress in defining the epidemiology of human papillomavirus infection and cervical neoplasia. J Natl Cancer Inst 1992a;84:394–98.

Schiffman MH. Validation of hybridization assays. Correlation of filter in situ dot blot, and PCR with Southern blot. In: Muñoz N, Bosch FX, Shah KV, Meheus A (Eds): The Epidemiology of Cervical Cancer and Human Papillomavirus. Lyon, International Agency for Research on Cancer; 1992b, pp 169–79.

Schiffman MH, Bauer HM, Hoover RN, Glass AG, Cadell DM, Rush BB, et al. Epidemiologic evidence showing that human papillomavirus infection causes most cervical intraepithelial neoplasia. J Natl Cancer Inst 1993;85:958–64.

Schiffman MH, Brinton LA. The epidemiology of cervical carcinogenesis. Cancer 1995; 76(Suppl 10):1888–1901.

Schiffman M, Khan MJ, Solomon D, Herrero R, Wacholder S, Hildesheim A. A study of the impact of adding HPV types to cervical cancer screening and triage tests. J Natl Cancer Inst 2005;97:147–50.

Schiffman MH, Schatzkin A. Test reliability is critically important to molecular epidemiology: an example from studies of human papillomavirus infection and cervical neoplasia. Cancer Res 1994;54(Suppl 7):1944S–47S.

Schneider A, Koutsky LA. Natural history and epidemiologic features of genital HPV infection. In: Muñoz N, Bosch FX, Shah KV, Meheus A (Eds): The Epidemiology of Cervical Cancer and Human Papillomavirus. Lyon, International Agency for Research on Cancer, 1992, pp 25–52.

Sedjo RL, Roe DJ, Abrahamsen M, Harris RB, Craft N, Baldwin S, et al. Vitamin A, carotenoids, and risk of persistent oncogenic human papillomavirus infection. Cancer Epi Biomark Prev 2002;11:876–84.

Sherman ME, Schiffman MH, Strickler H, Hildesheim A. Prospects for a prophylactic HPV vaccine: rationale and future implications for cervical cancer screening. Diagn Cytopathol 1998;18:5–9.

Smith HO, Tiffany MF, Qualls CR, Key CR. The rising incidence of adenocarcinoma relative to squamous cell carcinoma of the uterine cervix in the United States—a 24-year population-based study. Gynecol Oncol 2000; 78:97–105.

Smith JS, Bosetti C, Muñoz N, Herrero R, Bosch FX, Eluf-Neto J, et al. Chlamydia trachomatis and invasive cervical cancer: a pooled analysis of the IARC multicentric case-control study. Int J Cancer. 2004;111:431–39.

Smith JS, Green J, Berrington de Gozalez A, Appleby P, Peto J, Plummer M, et al. Cervical cancer and use of hormonal contraceptives: a systematic review. Lancet 2003;361:1159–67.

Sonoda Y, Saigo PE, Boyd J. p53 and genetic susceptibility to cervical cancer. J Natl Cancer Inst 1999;91:557.

Southern SA, Herrington CS. Molecular events in uterine cervical cancer. Sex Transm Inf 1998;74:101–9.

Storey A, Thomas M, Kalita A, Harwood C, Gardiol D, Mantovani F, et al. Role of a p53 polymorphism in the development of human papillomavirus–associated cancer. Nature 1998;393:229–34.

Trottier H, Franco EL. The epidemiology of genital human papillomavirus infection. Vaccine. 2006 Mar 30;24 Suppl 1:S1-15. Review.

Ursin G, Peters RK, Henderson BE, d'Ablaing G, Monroe KR, Pike MC. Oral contraceptive use and adenocarcinoma of cervix. Lancet 1994;344:1390–94.

Ursin G, Pike M, Preston-Martin S, d'Ablaing G, Peters RK. Sexual, reproductive, and other risk factors for adenocarcinoma of the cervix: results from a population-based case-control study (California, United States). Cancer Causes Control 1996;7:391–401.

Vernon SD, Hart CE, Reeves WC, Icenogle JP. The HIV-1 tat protein enhances E2-dependent human papillomavirus 16 transcription. Virus Res 1993;27:133–45.

Villa LL, Ault KA, Giuliano AR, Costa RLR, Petta CA, Andrade RP, et al. Immunologic responses following administration of a vaccine targeting human papillomavirus types 6,11,16 and 18. Vaccine 2006;24:5571–83.

Viscidi R, Sun Y, Tsuzaki B, Bosch FX, Muñoz N, Shah KV. Serologic response in human papillomavirus–associated invasive cervical cancer. Int J Cancer 1993;55:780–84.

Vizcaino AP, Moreno V, Bosch FX, Muñoz N, Barros-Dios XM, Parkin DM. International trends in the incidence of cervical cancer: adenocarcinoma and adenosquamous cell carcinomas. Int J Cancer 1998;75:536–45.

von Knebel Doeberitz M. Papillomaviruses in human disease: part I. Pathogenesis and epidemiology of human papillomavirus infections. Eur J Med 1992;1:415–23.

von Knebel Doeberitz M, Spitkovsky D, Ridder R. Interactions between steroid hormones and viral oncogenes in the pathogenesis of cervical cancer. Verh Dtsch Ges Pathol 1997; 81:233–39.

Wallin KL, Wiklund F, Luostarinen T, Angstrom T, Anttila T Bergman F, et al. A population-based prospective study of Chlamydia trachomatis infection and cervical carcinoma. Int J Cancer 2002;101:371–74.

Wank R, Thomssen C. High risk of squamous cell carcinoma of the cervix for women with HLA-DQw3. Nature 1991;352:723–25.

Wideroff L, Schiffman MH, Nonnenmacher B, Hubbert N, Kirnbauer R, Greer CE, et al. Evaluation of seroreactivity to human papillomavirus type 16 virus-like particles in an incident case-control study of cervical neoplasia. J Infect Dis 1995;172:1425–30.

Winer RL, Hughes JP, Feng Q, O'Reilly S, Kiviat NB, Holmes KK, et al. Condom use and the risk of genital human papillomavirus infection in young women. N Engl J Med 2006; 354:2645–54.

Winkelstein W Jr. Smoking and cancer of the cervix: hypothesis. Am J Epidemiol 1977;10: 257–59.

Winkelstein W Jr. Smoking and cervical cancer—current status: a review. Am J Epidemiol 1990;131:945–57.

World Cancer Research Fund. Food, Nutrition and the Prevention of Cancer: A Global Perspective. Washington, DC, American Institute for Cancer Research, 1997.

Ylitalo N, Josefsson A, Melbye M, Sörensen P, Frisch M, Kragh Andersen P, et al. A prospective study showing long-term infection with human papillomavirus 26 before the development of cervical carcinoma in situ. Cancer Res 2000a;60:6027–32.

Ylitalo N, Sørensen P, Josefsson A, Frisch M, Sparen P, Pontén J, et al. Smoking and oral contraceptives as risk factors for cervical carcinoma in situ. Int J Cancer 1999;81:357–65.

Ylitalo N, Sørensen P, Josefsson AM, Magnusson PKE, Andersen PK, Pontén J, et al. Consistent high viral load of human papillomavirus 16 and risk of cervical carcinoma in situ: a nested case-control study. Lancet 2000b;355:2194–98.

zur Hausen H. Human papillomaviruses and their possible role in squamous cell carcinomas. Curr Top Microbiol 1977;78:1–30.

zur Hausen H. Human genital cancer: synergism between two virus infections or synergism between a virus infection and initiating events? Lancet 1982;2:1370–72.

18

Endometrial Cancer

IMMACULATA DEVIVO, INGEMAR PERSSON,
AND HANS-OLOV ADAMI

Two of the most common cancers in women originate in the uterus, cancer of the cervix and endometrial cancer emanating from the corpus uteri. These malignancies differ drastically in terms of both etiology and clinical characteristics. Cervical cancer is a model of viral carcinogenesis, perhaps the only tumor with a necessary—albeit not sufficient—cause, namely, human papillomavirus. Similarly, endometrial cancer is a model of hormonal carcinogenesis. Indeed, the effect of estrogens is so direct and strong that widespread use of hormone therapy for menopausal symptoms increased the incidence of endometrial cancer in the United States almost epidemically in the 1970s. Endometrial cancer is also the only known malignancy for which cigarette smoking has been convincingly shown to confer protection.

Methodologically, epidemiologic studies of endometrial cancer are relatively straightforward. However, when diagnosed at advanced stages—which is still common in less developed countries—cancers originating from the corpus and cervix uteri can be difficult to distinguish. Obviously, this may distort incidence and mortality statistics. In analytic epidemiologic studies, the strong protective effect of oral contraceptive use and the even stronger adverse effect of postmenopausal hormone therapy may introduce important confounding because these exposures may be associated with a range of other potentially relevant lifestyle factors.

CLINICAL SYNOPSIS

Subgroups

Ninety-seven percent of tumors in the uterine body originate in the glands of the endometrium, which means they are endometrial cancers (also denoted cancers of the corpus uteri or uterine body); 3% are sarcomas (cancers of the myometrium). Endometrial cancers are classified, according to World Health Organization (WHO) standards, as endometroid adenocarcinomas (90% of all tumors), adenosquamous

468

cancers, clear-cell and uterine papillary serous carcinomas, or mucinous, squamous, and undifferentiated tumors (rare).

Symptoms

In postmenopausal women—80% of patients—menstruation-like bleedings or scanty, irregular bleedings are the key early symptoms, present in 90% of all patients. Premenopausal patients typically present with bleedings between menstruations or heavier periodic bleedings.

Diagnosis

The diagnosis is established through histopathologic examination of specimens obtained through curettage of the cervical epithelium and of the endometrium, separately.

Treatment

Established treatments include surgery, radiation therapy, endocrine therapy, and chemotherapy. A patient with low-risk stage I cancer would typically receive hysterectomy and oophorectomy together with postoperative vaginal irradiation; another patient with a high-risk cancer of the same stage would receive extensive surgery, external irradiation, and adjuvant cytostatic treatment. Stage II patients and those with more extensive tumors would get individualized combinations of intrauterine and external irradiation and subsequent surgery; and patients with the most advanced disease would receive cytotoxic drugs or endocrine therapy.

Prognosis

The 5-year survival rate is 70% to 80% overall in western countries, ranging from 90% for stage I patients to 20% for stage IV patients.

Progress

To improve clinical management, a number of procedures are being evaluated: radical surgery and hormonal treatment, timing and mode of radiation therapy, new virulence factors and methods to optimize staging, protocols for individualized treatments, assays of DNA ploidy and of nuclear morphology of hormone receptors, markers of proliferation, proteins related to P53 mutations, and oncogene mutations as prognosticators.

DESCRIPTIVE EPIDEMIOLOGY

In terms of incidence—approximately 136 000 women in developed countries and 63 000 in developing countries (2002) are diagnosed with endometrial cancer annually. Endometrial cancer is a frequent gynecologic cancer, but in terms of mortality it is not. In Europe the cumulative mortality rates have generally been three to four times lower than the incidence rates; in Canada and the United States, these rates have been about eight times lower (Ferlay et al, 2004).

Endometrial cancer accounts for 3.9% of all cancers in women worldwide (Parkin et al, 2002). Rates are highest in North America. In Asian countries they are considerably lower than in other parts of the world, although rising in successive birth cohorts, especially in Japan. Although a marked decrease in incidence was seen in European and North American women born around 1925 and some time thereafter (Waterhouse et al, 1992), which might partly be a result of an increasing use of replacement estrogens and of combined high-dose oral contraceptives (Persson et al, 1990), more recent data suggest that incidence rates among postmenopausal women are rising again (Bray et al, 2005). Changes over time in characterization, that is, fewer cases included in the subgroup "not otherwise specified," and in therapy, that is, increasing hysterectomy rates, must be considered when interpreting statistics on the incidence and mortality of endometrial cancer.

The incidence rates rise steadily 5 to 10 years before menopause and peak at ages 65 to 70. This has been observed in many countries, albeit at different levels (Fig. 18–1). In the US population, the age-specific incidence rates are higher among whites than among blacks and native Asian women (Fig. 18–2) (Sherman et al, 2005; Devesa

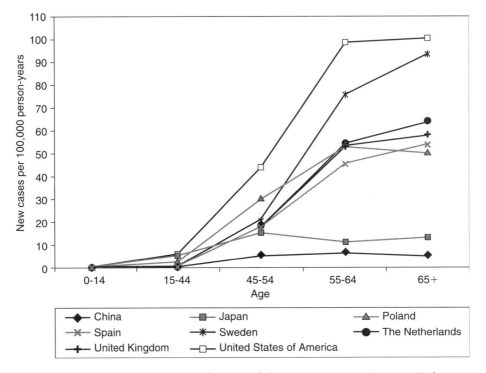

Figure 18–1. Age-specific incidence rates of cancer of the uterine corpus. (*Sources*: Ferlay et al, 2004)

et al, 1995a, 1995b). In contrast, mortality rates are lower, about 60%, among white women—and still lower among Asian women (Devesa et al, 1995b). A likely explanation is that black women on the average are diagnosed with more advanced tumors and have a treatment that is not optimal.

Data on mortality show consistent trends; rates are falling in most countries and age groups (Waterhouse et al, 1992). One exception is Japan, where mortality has doubled since the 1970s, with a significant increase in the youngest age groups. In North America the decline has been steady since the 1960s. The overall reduction in mortality suggests that endometrial cancers are detected earlier and/or treated more efficiently. Further, risk factors that have become more prevalent, such as hormone replacement therapy, may be associated predominantly with biologically less aggressive and, hence, more curable tumors (Grady et al, 1995; Weiderpass et al, 1999a).

GENETIC AND MOLECULAR EPIDEMIOLOGY

Inherited Susceptibility

Endometrial cancer is part of a family of hereditary cancers known as hereditary nonpolyposis colorectal cancer syndrome (HNPCC), attributable to the inheritance of rare, highly penetrant mutated DNA repair genes (Papadopoulos et al, 1994; Nicolaides et al, 1994). HNPCC is characterized by a familial predisposition to colorectal carcinoma and extracolonic cancers; endometrial cancer is the second most common malignancy (Risinger et al, 1993). Women with this inherited predisposition to endometrial neoplasia tend to develop the disease 15 years earlier than the general population (Vasen et al, 1994). The four major genes known to be involved in HNPCC are DNA mismatch repair (MMR) genes *MSH2, MLH1, PMS1*, and *PMS* (Papadopoulos et al, 1994; Nicolaides et al, 1994;

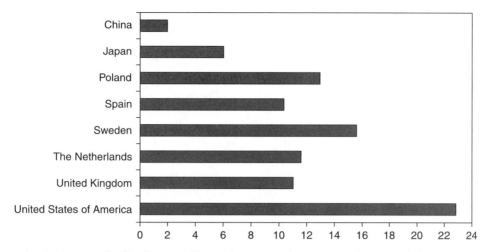

Figure 18–2. Age standardized (to world population) incidence rates of cancer of the uterine corpus. (*Source*: Ferlay et al, 2004)

Peltomaki et al, 1993; Aaltonen et al, 1993). Mutations in these genes are thought to be carried by considerably less than 1% of the general population. To date, extensive studies have not identified common low-penetrance polymorphisms in these genes as associated with endometrial cancer.

Given the small percentage (2%–5%) of endometrial cancers attributable to family cancer syndromes, other genetic factors may play a role in their development. A population-based case-control study has shown that a family history of endometrial cancer in a first-degree female relative increased the risk by nearly threefold (Gruber and Thompson, 1996). Those researchers concluded that family history is an important risk factor in the population at large. It has been hypothesized that other susceptibility genes carry low absolute risk, but potentially high population-attributable risk, especially when considered in combination with environmental exposures. Polymorphic variations in relevant genes are likely to confer only a modest increase in risk, or may confer increases in risk only in conjunction with carcinogen exposure; and therefore, they may not cause noticeable family aggregation. However, these polymorphisms can represent very common and even modest relative risks; when the polymorphism is

highly prevalent, they may account for a higher population-attributable risk than highly penetrant but rare gene mutations (Khoury et al, 1993). For endometrial cancer, genes involved in the steroidogenic pathway and related hormonal pathways are natural candidates in the search for polymorphisms that influence individual susceptibility. Though the long-term impact of genetic variation on endometrial cancer is unknown, studies in this area have increased dramatically aided in part by the deluge of genomic data and automation.

Hormone Metabolizing Genes

Cytochrome P450c1 (CYP17)
The *CYP17* gene encodes the rate-limiting enzyme in androgen production and has two catalytic actions: 17-alpha-hydrolase, which converts pregnenolone to 17-hydroxypregnenolone; and 17,20-lyase, which converts progesterone to 17-hydroxyprogesterone. The "A2" allele, which is hypothesized to result in increased transcription, has been shown to be associated with a significant decrease in endometrial cancer risk. Although these findings were replicated in independent Caucasian populations, the studies were small (Haiman et al, 2001; Berstein et al, 2002). Interestingly, the inverse association between the

A2 allele and endometrial cancer risk was stronger among women with a first-degree family history of endometrial and/or colorectal cancer (Haiman et al, 2001). Morever, modest elevations were observed for hormone fractions, estrone and estradiol (Haiman et al, 2001).

Cytochrome P45019 (*CYP19*) encodes aromatase, the main enzyme that catalyzes the final and rate-limiting step of estrogen biosynthesis, the aromatization of androstenedione and testosterone to estrone and estradiol, respectively (Means et al, 1989). After menopause, a woman's endogenous estrogen production shifts from a predominantly ovarian source to a peripheral (adipose) source. Several common genetic polymorphisms in *CYP19* have been described including the *TCT* insertion/deletion, the *(TTTA)n* repeat polymorphism, and a *3'UTR C/T* polymorphism (Siegelmann-Danieli and Buetow, 1999; Kristensen et al, 1998). Few studies have examined these variants in relation to endometrial cancer. Two published studies investigating the *CYP19 (TTTA)n* repeat polymorphism and endometrial cancer risk observed that possession of longer alleles were overrepresented in cases compared to controls (Berstien et al, 2001, 2004).

Recently, a haplotype-tagging approach, using SNPS to capture the genetic variation across the *CYP19* gene, has been implemented to assess associations (Haiman et al, 2003). The evaluation revealed that among American Caucasians a specific *CYP19* haplotype was associated with a twofold risk of endometrial cancer, and the haplotype was also significantly associated with the ratio of estrone to androstene dione, the product and substrate of the enzyme aromatase (Paynter et al, 2003).

HSD17B family (17β-Hydroxysteroid dehydrogenase)

17β-HSD is responsible for the interconversion of 17-ketosteroids (eg, androstenedione and estrone) and their corresponding 17β-hydroxysteroids (eg, testosterone and 17β-estradiol) (Labrie et al, 1997; Yang et al, 2001). In the endometrium, oxidation of estradiol to estrone is an important step in steroid metabolism, since estrone has a much lower potency for the activation of the estrogen receptor than estradiol (Tseng and Gurpide, 1975).

There are at least 11 17β-HSD isoenzymes, designated Types 1 through 11, that have individual cell-specific expression, substrate specificity, regulation mechanisms, and reductive or oxidative catalytic activity (Adamski and Jakob, 2001). 17β-HSD Type 1, Type 2, and Type 4 are specific to the uterus (Yang et al, 2001; Labrie et al, 1997; Husen et al, 2000). In a nested case-control study of endometrial cancer no overall association by SNP or haplotype analysis with endometrial cancer risk was observed. However, there was an association between *HSD17B1* and circulating estradiol levels (Setiawan et al, 2004).

Estrogen Metabolism and Detoxification

The cytochrome P450 enzymes, encoded by *CYP1A1* and *CYP1B1*, catalyze the hydroxylation of estrone (E1) and estradiol (E2), mainly at the C-2 and C-4 positions, resulting in the formation of catechol (2,4-(OH)) estrogens, which can be genotoxic. Two polymorphisms, *Leu432Val* and *Asn453Ser* in exon 3 of the *CYP1B1* gene have been evaluted in relation to endometrial cancer. The *Ser* allele of the *Asn453Ser* polymorphism is associated with a nonsignificant reduction in endometrial cancer risk (McGrath et al, 2004). Studies evaluating the association between the *Leu432-Val* and endometrial cancer risk have been inconsistent, possibly due to different study populations (McGrath et al, 2004; Doherty et al, 2005; Sasaki et al, 2003).

The catechol estrogens are further metabolized to the more neutral methoxy-estrogens by COMT. In addition to being nontoxic, the O-methylated estrogens may have unique antitumoral activities not mediated by ER-α, including the inhibition of cell proliferation and angiogenesis. A functional polymorphism within *COMT*, *Val158Met*, has been shown to impact its ability to detoxify estrogens. Those homozygous for the *Met* allele have a threefold decrease in enzymatic activity that may result in higher levels of catechol estrogen. Two studies have evaluated this polymorphism in relation to endometrial cancer risk and reported a null or nonsignificant reduction in endometrial cancer risk (McGrath et al, 2004; Doherty et al, 2005)

Steroid Receptors

AR (Androgen receptor)

Androgen receptors are expressed in 65% to 75% of endometrial tumors, and androgens display a direct inhibitory effect on human endometrial cell proliferation in vitro (Neulen et al, 1987; Rose et al, 1988). The functional polymorphic CAG repeat within exon 1, which encodes a polyglutamine chain, in the region of the AR, is related to DNA transcription (Carson-Jurica et al, 1990; McPhaul et al, 1993). In two recent small studies, both groups observed that endometrial cancer patients had longer alleles than normal healthy controls (Yaron et al, 2001; Sasaki et al, 2003b). In contrast, a larger study observed that longer alleles were associated with a decreased risk of endometrial cancer (McGrath et al, 2006).

ESR1 (Estrogen receptor α)

ESR1, a ligand-activated transcription factor, mediates hormonal responses such as proliferation in estrogen-sensitive tissues such as the endometrium. A Japanese study investigated six different ESR1 loci and detected an association between a codon 10 polymorphism in the NH2-terminal region and endometrial cancer (Sasaki et al, 2005). Several other polymorphisms, including PvuII and XbaI and a TA dinucleotide repeat in exon 1, have been associated with endometrial cancer in Swedish (Weiderpass et al, 2000a) and Japanese populations (Iwamoto et al, 2003).

ESR2 (Estrogen receptor β)

To date only one small study has evaluated the two SNPs in exon 5 and an intronic dinucleotide CA repeat and found no association with endometrial cancer (Setiawan et al, 2004).

PGR (Progesterone receptor)

Progesterone has proven antineoplastic effects in the uterus. The effects of progesterone are mediated through its receptor (PGR). The PGR gene contains several polymorphisms in the hormone-binding domain, three of which are 100% linked, a complex referred to as PROGINS, none of which have been associated with endometrial cancer. The recently discovered funtional polymorphism in the promoter region, +331 G/A, is associated with a significant twofold risk in endometrial cancer; the risk was fourfold among overweight women (De Vivo, 2002). These findings are based on a small sample size; therefore, replication in larger studies is warranted.

A brief summary of the polymorphisms, putative function, and association with endometrial cancer is provided in Table 18–1.

Somatic Events

Carcinogenesis in the endometrium is, in most cases, believed to be a process with a morphologic transition from normal to hyperplastic, atypically hyperplastic, and then neoplastic endometrial cells. This would be characteristic of so-called type I tumors, believed to be related primarily to estrogen influence (Deligdisch and Holinka, 1987). Estrogens, without an opposing antiestrogenic effect of progesterone or progestins, enhance the proliferation of the endometrial cells. This proliferation leads to a more frequent occurrence of spontaneous mutations, decreased time for mismatch repair, increased sensitivity to genotoxic agents, and expansion of transformed clones (Preston-Martin et al, 1990). For type I cancers, the resulting molecular alterations may involve mutations activating the K-ras oncogene, inactivation of the PTEN tumor-suppressor gene, silencing of mismatched repair genes by gene-promoter hypermethylation (Risinger et al, 2003), mutations in CTNNB1—a gene producing cell-adhesion molecules like Beta-catenin (Machin et al, 2002)—and, further, the dysregulated expression of growth factors like transforming growth factor alpha

Table 18–1. Genetic polymorphisms, their putative functional significance and association with endometrial cancer risk

Candidate gene	Polymorphism	Putative function	Association with endometrial cancer risk
Hormone metabolizing and detoxification genes			
CYP17	A2	Increased androgen production	A2 associated with decreased risk
CYP19	TCT insertion/deletion (TTTA)$_n$ repeat 3'UTR C/T polymorphism	Aromatization of androgens to estrogens	Longer alleles associated with increased risk
HSD17B	+1004C/T, +1322C/A, +1954A/G (Ser312Gly)	Conversion of 17-ketosteroids (e.g., androstenedione and estrone) to 17β-hydroxysteroids (e.g. testosterone and 17β-estradiol)	No association between HSD17B1 haplotypes and endometrial cancer risk but the +1954A/A genotype was associated with circulating estradiol levels in lean women
Estrogen metabolism and detoxification			
CYP1A1			
CYP1B1	Leu432Val, Asn453Ser	Catalyzes hydroxylation of E1 and E2	Non-significant reduction in risk
COMT	Val158Met	Decreased detoxification of estrogens	Non-significant reduction in risk
Steroid receptors			
AR	CAG repeat	Longer alleles associated with decreased androgenicity	Longer alleles associated with decreased endometrial cancer risk
ESR1	PvuII, XbaI, TA repeat	Mediates estrogenic effect	Homozygous variant genotypes associated with a reduction in risk
ESR2	CA repeat and two SNPs in exon 5	Mediates estrogenic effect	No association
PGR	PROGINS +331G/A	Increases expression of hPR-B isoform	A allele associated with increased risk

(TGF-a) in autocrine pathways and EGF1 and TGF-b in paracrine pathways (Boyd, 1996).

For type II endometrial cancers, assumed to be unrelated to estrogens, less is known about pathogenic events. Overexpression of the *ERBB-2* oncogene and inactivation of the *P53* tumor-suppressor gene are believed to be important steps late in the process (Boyd, 1996; Santin et al, 2002; Lax et al, 2000).

RISK FACTORS

Tobacco

The preponderance of evidence suggests that current cigarette smoking confers protection against endometrial cancer.

A protective effect of cigarette smoking was first suggested by Weiss et al (1980). Since then 23 case-control and 4 cohort studies have evaluted the association (reviewed in Terry et al, 2002b). In general, these studies showed a reduced risk for current smokers and a weak reduction or no reduction in risk for former smokers. A recent study of nurses followed for 24 years reported that the protective effect of smoking occurs early in adulthood and is long lasting (Viswanathan et al, 2005). In studies stratifying by menopausal status, the effect seems stronger in postmenopausal women. Among premenopausal women, the association is less consistent (Terry et al, 2002). Some (Terry et al, 2002b; Brinton et al, 2002b; Lawrence et al, 1987; Lesko et al, 1985; Stockwell and Lyman, 1987) but not all (Terry et al, 1999; Lawrence et al, 1989; Newcomer et al, 2001; Williams and Horm, 1977) that evaluated a dose effect observed a greater reduction in risk with increased intensity (cigs/day) or duration (years of smoking) among current smokers. However, no dose effect was observed among former smokers.

Data regarding the joint effect of hormonal replacement therapy (HRT) and smoking in relation to endometrial cancer risk is inconsistent. Two studies show an inverse association between smoking and endometrial cancer among HRT users (Franks et al, 1987; Levi et al, 1987) while two other studies show no association (Lawrence et al, 1987; Terry et al, 2002b). Similarly, the data regarding smoking and obesity in relation to endometrial cancer are mixed. Two studies show no difference in the smoking–endometrial cancer association by body weight while a third study showed a stronger association among women with a higher body weight (Elliott et al, 1990; Levi et al, 1987; Lawrence et al, 1987).

Because cigarette smoking is related to earlier age at menopause and increased risk of osteoporotic fractures, both of which reflect less exposure to endogenous estrogens, it has been hypothesized to act by diminishing estrogenic effects. The suggested mechanism is an upregulation of the 2-hydroxylation pathways, resulting in an increased level of 2-hydroxyestrone instead of 16alpha-hydroxyestrone and a net reduction in biologically active estradiol levels (Michnovicz et al, 1988; Barbieri et al,

1986). Several studies, however, found no reduction in serum estrogen levels among smokers compared to nonsmokers (Key et al, 1996). One suggested that elevated androgen levels might convey a protective effect (Khaw et al, 1988). In a report comparing estrone, estradiol, and estriol levels in urine samples from smokers and non-smokers, no difference was noted among premenopausal women, whereas among postmenopausal women, estriol excretion rates were about 20% lower in smokers than in nonsmokers (Key et al, 1996).

Diet

Overall, given the methodologic limitations of the reported studies and the inconsistencies of their results, no firm conclusions can be drawn about the possible association between diet and endometrial cancer risk.

Ecologic studies generally show a correlation between endometrial cancer risk and high fat intake (Prentice and Sheppard, 1990). Case-control studies provide inconsistent data on a positive association with intake of animal fat (Potischman et al, 1993; Shu et al, 1993; Littman et al, 2001), as well as protective effects of carotene (Barbone et al, 1993; Negri et al, 1996), of monounsaturated fat (Tzonou et al, 1996), complex carbohydrates (Kolonel et al, 1981), whole grains (Kasum et al, 2001), fatty fish (Terry et al, 2002c), and green vegetables (La Vecchia et al, 1986). One case-control study of the multiethnic population of Hawaii evaluated the effects of over 250 food items on endometrial cancer risk (Goodman et al, 1997a). Independently of other risk factors, diets low in fat, high in fiber, and rich in legumes (especially soybeans), whole-grain foods, vegetables, and fruits were associated with a reduced risk of endometrial cancer; diets rich in soy products and fiber reduced the risk by over 50%. A Swedish case-control study showed that calcium supplements lower endometrial cancer risk but iron supplements increase risk (Terry et al, 2002d). A recent diet-intervention trial concluded that a change in fiber, increased intake, was related to reduced bioavailable estrogen (Rock et al, 2004).

A protective effect of plant-based diets is deemed biologically credible since the component phytoestrogens genestain and daidzen compete with more potent estrogens for the estrogen receptor, causing an antiestrogenic effect in the target organ. Further, a high-fiber diet may decrease endogenous estrogen levels by reducing enterohepatic recirculation of ovarian estrogens; it is postulated that prevalent food habits may explain part of the lower rates of endometrial cancer in Asian countries compared to western countries (Goodman et al, 1997b). A possible link between diet, mostly intake of fat, and estrogen levels has been explored in several studies (Hill and Austin, 1996). Studies of vegetarians suggest that a low-fat diet may reduce estrogen levels; vegetarians have 45% lower estradiol levels than nonvegetarians (Barbosa et al, 1990; Goldin et al, 1986). Four randomized intervention trials, however, noted conflicting results—three of them showing no change in the levels of available estrogens in relation to fat intake (Bennett and Ingram, 1990)—as did three epidemiologic studies. One study reported an elevation of bound but not free estradiol in relation to high fat intake (Prentice et al, 1990), while the two other large studies showed null effects (Katsouyanni et al, 1991; London et al, 1991).

Alcohol

Data regarding alcohol consumption and endometrial cancer risk have been inconsistent. Although most studies report a nonsignificant decrease in risk with alcohol consumption (Weiderpass et al, 2001b; Austin et al, 1993; Garpstur et al, 1993; Kalandidi et al, 1996; Kato et al, 1989; Swanson et al, 1993b), others have observed a significant increase (LaVecchia, 1986) or a significant decrease (Webster and Weiss, 1989) with alcohol consumption. Surprisingly, a study of 37 000 alcoholics showed a 24% reduction in endometrial cancer risk compared to the general population (Weiderpass et al, 2001). These

results are contrary to expected since alcohol is associated with increased estrogen levels (Hankinson et a1,1995; Reichman et al, 1993).

Reproductive Factors

It is clear from epidemiologic data that the hormonal exposures associated with childbearing and progesterone produced in regular menstrual cycles confer substantial protection against endometrial cancer.

Under the hypothesis that estrogens increase the incidence of endometrial cancer, all factors reflecting ovarian, placental, or adrenal sex hormone production may influence the risk of endometrial cancer. Thus, aspects of menstruation and reproduction have been explored extensively in numerous epidemiologic studies (Garte et al, 1997). No consistent association with age at menarche has been observed, although some studies found an increased risk with early menarche (Brinton et al, 1992), sometimes limited to premenopausal (La Vecchia et al, 1984) or obese women (Henderson et al, 1983). In most studies, late age at menopause was a risk factor (Kvale et al, 1988). A history of regular menstruations was more common in cases than in controls (Henderson et al, 1983). Many cycles without opposing progesterone (unovulatory cycles in fertile women or in those with irregular periods) or cycles without interrupting pregnancies (nulliparity, late menopause) increased the risk (Key et al, 1988).

Nulliparity has been consistently associated with a two- to threefold elevated risk, the parity dependent reduction of risk was mostly related to the number of children (Brinton et al, 1992). Age at first birth appears to be of no importance (Brinton et al, 1992). In some studies, pregnancy at a relatively advanced age was linked to a lower risk; thus, last birth at age 35 to 40 versus before 20 to 25 conferred a 50% reduced risk (Parazzini et al, 1991), a result corroborated by subsequent findings of a decreasing risk with decreasing time since last birth (Parazzini et al, 1998). The hypothesized mechanism was either shedding and removal of malignant or premalignant cells after each delivery (Kvale et al, 1992) or elimination of hyperplasia through atrophy of the endometrium due to high levels of placentally produced progesterone. Infertility, defined as unsuccessful attempts to become pregnant during a 3-year period, or seeking medical advice because of inability to become pregnant, was associated with an up to threefold increased risk (Henderson et al, 1983; Brinton et al, 1992).

Hormones

Exposure to excessive estrogens of endogenous as well as exogenous origin entailing continued stimulation of the endometrium appears to be the key mechanism in endometrial carcinogenesis, perhaps a common denominator for most of the established risk factors.

Endogenous Estrogens

Convincing evidence indicates that a crucial pathway for most endometrial cancers is excessive exposure to unopposed estrogens. In postmenopausal women, the main mechanism for estrogen production is the conversion of androstenedione to estrone. Other pathogenic mechanisms, such as hyperinsulinemia, have also been suggested (see following). Benign granulosa and theca cell tumors of the ovary entail excessive production of estrogens in postmenopausal patients; these women are at a substantially increased risk of endometrial cancer (Björkholm and Pettersson, 1980). The same is true for young women with the polycystic ovary syndrome (Grady and Ernster, 1996), which involves chronic hyperstimulation of the ovary through persistently elevated levels of luteinizing hormone, resulting in anovulation and increased production of androstenedione, which is converted to estrone through aromatization.

Higher levels of estrogens and/or androgens were associated with endometrial cancer in some clinical studies (Pettersson et al, 1986; Nyholm et al, 1993) but not in others (Nisker et al, 1980; Davidson et al, 1981). In three case-control studies (Austin et al, 1991; Potischman et al, 1996; Sher-

man et al, 1997), a consistently increased risk of endometrial cancer emerged with high levels of total and free estrone, and of estradiol and androstenedione and with low levels of sex hormone-binding globulin (SHBG), associations that were independent of body size. Regarding premenopausal women, one of the studies showed that only high androstenedione levels, not high estrogen levels, were associated with an increased risk (Potischman et al, 1996).

Exogenous Hormones

Oral contraceptives

The epidemiologic literature provides convincing evidence that combined estrogen-progestin contraceptives convey substantial and long-lasting protection against endometrial cancer. This protective effect is now also becoming discernible on a population level through decreasing incidence rates among young women (see the section "Descriptive Epidemiology"). Data on the modern low-dose combined oral contraceptives are, however, still too sparse, and follow-up is too short, to allow any reliable conclusions.

In the early 1970s, epidemiologic studies revealed an increased risk of endometrial cancer in premenopausal women who used sequential oral contraceptives characterized by a high dose of synthetic estrogen and then added low-dose progestin for part of the treatment cycle (Henderson et al, 1983). The evidence of this adverse effect led to the removal of sequential contraceptive compounds from the market. The use of combined oral contraceptives (COCs), on the other hand, with formulations containing a high-potency synthetic estrogen (ethinyl estradiol or mestranol) for 3 of the cycle's 4 weeks, always combined with a potent synthetic progestin, has been consistently found to markedly reduce the risk in a large number of epidemiologic studies (IARC, 1999). The protective effect, noticeable after 3 years, may persist for many years (Schlesselman, 1991) and is independent of several other risk factors. A large case-control study provided further evidence that the protective effect may persist for at least 20 years after cessation of COC use and may be similar for all degrees of tumor differentiation and invasiveness (Weiderpass et al, 1999c). A few studies showed protective effects from progestin-only contraceptives (mini-pills and injectible compounds), but data are insufficient to allow any firm conclusions (IARC, 1999).

Replacement with estrogens alone
Numerous epidemiological studies have established a strong link between long-term use of replacement estrogens alone (ie, without the concomitant use of a progestin, denoted unopposed treatment) and an excess risk of endometrial cancer. This link is stronger for early stage and low-grade tumors.

The first evidence that exogenous estrogens may cause endometrial cancer emanates from studies in the 1970s. They showed that young women with inherited gonadal insufficiency who received synthetic estrogens for replacement (MacMahon, 1974) and breast cancer patients treated with high-dose estrogens (Hoover et al, 1976) developed endometrial cancer more often than expected. Further, following a fourfold increase in the prescriptions for replacement estrogens during the 1960s and early 1970s in the United States, an epidemic rise in endometrial cancer incidence was noted (Kennedy et al, 1985). Since 1975, at least 12 cohort studies and over 40 case-control studies have analyzed the associations between unopposed estrogens and endometrial cancer risk. Publications by the IARC (1999) and Grady et al (1995) provided a complete tabulation of studies and their reported results. In addition, the findings of 29 eligible studies, published through April 1994, were summarized in a meta-analysis (Table 18–2).

These aggregated data demonstrate the definite risk increase for ever-users of estrogens shown in both case-control and cohort studies, the possible dose–risk relationship, and the obvious duration–risk relationship. Risk estimates were at least tenfold elevated after more than 10 years of

continuous estrogen intake (Fig. 18–3). The risk was higher for current or recent intake but persisted and remained, with a twofold increase for 5 years or more, after cessation of treatment. No clear differences in risk-elevating effects were seen between treatment regimens—intermittent or cyclic versus daily—or types of estrogen—conjugated equine estrogens versus estradiol. A notable gradient in the magnitude of the excess risk with tumor stage has been observed: a sixfold increase for noninvasive cancers, a fourfold increase for invasive stage I tumors, and a slight and nonsignificant increase for stage II or more advanced tumors. The meta-analysis by Grady et al (1995) also provides evidence, based on three of the studies, that estrogen users may also be at increased risk of dying from endometrial cancer. However, survival in endometrial cancer subjects exposed to exogenous estrogens has been observed to be higher than in nonusers (Chu et al, 1982).

The possibility of effect modification by other factors has been addressed by Brinton and colleagues (1993b), who examined subgroups of women with regard to parity, hypertension, diabetes, smoking, and COC use. However, the findings were inconclusive; there were indications that the risk-enhancing effect of replacement therapy was confined to lean women and was more pronounced in smokers than in nonsmokers.

A large case-control study in Sweden provided data on the effects of orally (estriol, 1 or 2 mg) and vaginally (estriol or dienoestrol) administered low potency estrogens prescribed chiefly for treatment or prevention of urogenital symptoms related to atrophy of the estrogen-dependent urogenital epithelium (Weiderpass et al, 1999b). Oral intake increased the risk in a duration-dependent manner, with a threefold increased risk after more than 5 years of intake; the highest risk estimates involved low-grade tumors (Fig. 18–3). Risk estimates for locally applied low-potency estrogens were close to unity.

Table 18–2. Relative risk estimates from a meta-analysis of epidemiologic studies of hormone replacement therapy and endometrial cancer risk

	RR	95% CI	No. of studies
Ever-use of estrogens			
All eligible studies	2.3	2.1–2.5	29
Cohort studies	1.7	1.3–2.1	4
Case-control studies	2.4	2.2–2.6	25
Conjugated estrogen dose (mg)			
0.3	3.9	1.6–9.5	3
0.625	3.4	2.0–5.6	4
≥1.25	5.8	4.5–7.5	9
Duration of use (years)			
<1	1.4	1.0–1.8	9
1–5	2.8	2.3–3.5	12
5–10	5.9	4.7–7.5	10
>10	9.5	7.4–12.3	10
Regimen			
Intermittent and cyclic	3.0	2.4–3.8	8
Continuous	2.9	2.2–3.8	
Type of estrogen			
Conjugated equine	2.5	2.1–2.9	9
Synthetic*	1.3	1.1–1.6	7
Time since last use (years)			
≤1	4.1	2.9–5.7	3
1–4	3.7	2.5–5.5	3
≥5	2.3	1.8–3.1	5
Stage/invasiveness			
Stage 0–1	4.2	3.1–5.7	3
Stage 2–4	1.4	0.8–2.4	3
Noninvasive	6.2	4.5–8.4	4
Invasive	3.8	2.9–5.1	6
Death from endometrial cancer	2.7	0.9–8.0	3

*Synthetic estrogens include primarily ethinyl estradiol, estradiol valerate, estriol, and unspecified other estrogens; diethylstilbestrol and estrogen combined with androgen excluded, except in cases where such use was lumped together with all synthetic estrogens.

RR, relative risk; CI, confidence interval.

Source: Grady et al. 1995.

In the IARC report (1999), studies published through 1998 were included. The qualitative review in this report concluded that the vast majority of epidemiologic studies show an association between use of postmenopausal estrogens and an increased risk of endometrial cancer, a risk increasing with duration of use and declining after cessation of use but remaining for at least 10 years.

Replacement with combined estrogen-progestin regimens

Epidemiologic data show that unopposed estrogens, even orally administered low-potency estrogens, cause an excess risk of en-

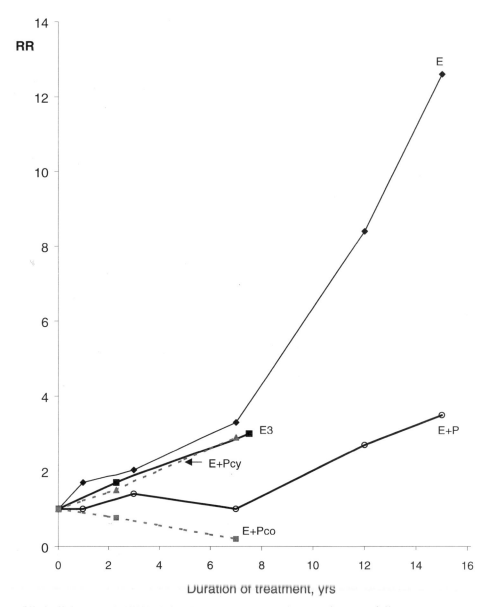

Figure 18–3. Relative risk (RR) of developing invasive endometrial cancer following post-menopausal hormone replacement with weak estrogens (E3-estriol, 1–2 mg/day) and medium-potency estrogens alone (E) or combined with progestins (E+P). In the latter category, separate analyses were also carried out for estrogens combined with progestins cyclically for less than 16 days per cycle (E+Pcy) or continuously (E+Pco). (*Source*: Weiderpass et al, 1999a, 1999b)

dometrial cancer. In order to prevent the endometrium from developing premalignant and malignant lesions during estrogen treatment, progestins are added. The use of these opposed regimens has become stan-

dard. In a cyclic regimen, progestin is usually added during 10 to 12 days of the monthly cycle, producing withdrawal bleeding. In a continuous combined regimen, progestin is added during all days of the cycle. This regimen is commonly recommended to women who are a few years beyond menopause to avoid bleeding.

Data on the effect of added progestins have been available only since the 1990s. The results of one cohort study and five case-control studies are shown in Tables 18–2 and 18–3. In the cohort study (Persson et al, 1989), the risk for women ever using unopposed estrogens was increased by 40%, whereas for women exposed to a cyclic combined regimen, it was at baseline. In a follow-up study of the same cohort (Persson et al, 1999), 6 years or less of progestin-combined use conferred no change in risk compared to nonuse or short-term use—less than 1 year—whereas a combined regimen with a duration longer than 6 years yielded a slight but nonsignificant risk increase. Two case-control studies from the United States (Brinton et al, 1993b; Jick et al, 1993) found some evidence that adding progestins to conjugated estrogens increased the risk less than unopposed treatment (Table 18–3). The interpretation of these early studies is hampered by the small number of participants and by missing data for duration categories.

A protective effect of added progestins is biologically plausible, since progesterone as well as synthetic progestins counteract the estrogenic proliferative effect by downregulating estrogen receptor levels, enhancing the metabolic inactivation of estradiol, and decreasing DNA synthesis (Graham and Clarke, 1997). In clinical trials, the addition of progestins during at least 12 days per cycle significantly reduced the occurrence of endometrial hyperplasia (The Writing Group for the PEPI Trial, 1996). Epidemiologic data still leave uncertain the optimal length of progestin addition, as well as the type and dose of the compound necessary to completely eliminate an adverse effect on the endometrium by long-term estrogen-replacement treatment. Three cases-control studies of opposed regimens reported that added progestins do reduce the risk. The more days they are added in the cycle, the greater the reduction in risk.

Pike et al (1997), in a study of invasive endometrial cancer, reported that women exposed to estrogens alone increased their risk of endometrial cancer about twofold for each 5-year period of medication. Those women who had used a cyclic combined regimen with addition of less than 10 days of progestin per cycle had a doubled risk after 5 years of treatment. If the addition was for 10 days or longer per cycle, no excess risk was noted. The women who had received a continuous combined regimen showed no change in risk pattern.

In the second case-control study, by Beresford et al (1997), treatment with estrogens alone was associated with a fourfold risk increase. When progestins were added

Table 18–3. Summary of cohort studies on estrogen-progestin combined replacement and endometrial cancer risk

Reference	Study base	Design: cohort, follow-up	RR (95% CI)
Persson (1989)	Six counties in Sweden, 1977–83	23,244 women ≥35 years of age. Follow-up through record linkage	E + P,* ever; 0.9 (0.4–2.0) Duration: ≤36 months 1.4 (0.5–3.6) 37 + months 1.2 (0.3–5.5)
Persson (1999)	Same as above, 1987–93	Subset of cohort, 8438 women. Follow-up through record linkage. Nested case-control study	E + P* analyses[†] E + P 1–6 yr 1.1 (0.4–3.1) ≥6 yr 1.4 (0.6–3.3)

*Combined estrogen-progestin regimens, estradiol 2 mg combined with the progestins levonogestrel or norethisterone acetate, either cyclically or continuously.

[†]Nested case-control analyses; women with no exposure or less than 1 year of exposure used as references.

RR, relative risk; CI, confidence interval.

Table 18–4. Summary of recent case-control studies on estrogen-progestogen combined hormone replacement therapy and endometrial cancer risk

Reference	Study base	Design; cases and controls	Regimen	RR (95% CI)
Jick (1993)	Washington state, USA, 1979–89, 50–64 yrs of age	Members of HMO: 172/1720	Any E+P*	1.9 (0.9–3.8)
			Duration, <3 yrs:	2.2 (0.7–7.3)
			≥3 yrs:	1.3 (0.5–3.4)
Brinton (1993)	Five U.S. areas, 1987–90, 20–74 yrs of age	General population: 300/207	Any E+P use ≥3 months[†]	1.8 (0.6–4.9)
Pike (1997)	California, USA, 1987–93, 50–74 yr of age	General population: 833/791	Any E+P[‡,§] <10 days/cycle	
			Per 5 yrs:	1.9 (1.3–2.7)
			Any E+P, P ≥10 days/cycle	
			Per 5 yrs:	1.1 (0.8–1.4)
			Any E+P, P all days/cycle	
			Per 5 yrs:	1.1 (0.8–1.4)
Beresford (1997)	Washington state, USA, 1985–91, 45–74 yrs of age	General population: 832/1154	Any E+P:	1.4 (1.0–1.9)
			P ≤10 days/cycle	
			6–35 months:	2.1 (0.9–4.7)
			36–59 months:	1.4 (0.3–5.4)
			≥60 months:	3.7 (1.7–8.2)
			P >10 days/cycle;	
			6–35 months:	0.8 (0.4–1.8)
			36–59 months:	0.6 (0.2–1.6)
Weiderpass (1998)	Sweden, 1993–99, 50–74 yrs of age	General population: 709/3368	Cyclic E+P[i]	
			Duration <5 yrs:	0.8 (0.5–1.3)
			≥5 yrs:	2.9 (1.8–4.6)
			Continuous (28 days/cycle):	
			Duration <5 yrs:	0.8 (0.5–1.3)
			≥5 yrs:	0.2 (0.1–0.8)

* Estrogens1progestins.

[†] No data on duration.

[‡] Estrogen: conjugated estrogens 0.625 or 1.25 mg; progestin: medroxy progesterone acetate (MPA).

[§] Number of days of added progestins.

[i] Estrogens: two-thirds of women used estradiol, one-third conjugated estrogens. Progestins (predominantly levonorgestrel and norethisterone acetate, in a minor proportion MPA): 65% of women used cyclic regimens (80% with 10 days addition/cycle) and 35% used a continuous regimen.

for less than 10 days of the cycle, the risk was increased threefold; when they were added for 10 days or more, no significant risk increase was observed. For women who used combined treatments for 5 years or more, the risk was increased about three-fold, regardless of the number of days progestins were added.

In the third study (Weiderpass et al, 1999a), Swedish women taking estrogens alone had a 17% risk increase per year of use, with an about eightfold increase after 10 to 14 years of treatment. This excess risk seemed to persist for at least 5 years. Women who had used any type of combined regimen for more than 10 years had an overall threefold greater risk than those who had no treatment. Cyclic addition, mainly during 10 days of the cycle, conferred an average risk increase of 10% per year of intake, whereas continuous addition reduced the risk by 14% per year of use compared with nontreated women (Fig. 18–3).

Anthropometric Measures

Obesity is a well-established risk factor for endometrial cancer in both pre- and postmenopausal women.

High body mass index (BMI) was consistently reported as a risk factor for endometrial cancer, assessed in 11 follow-up and case-control studies reviewed by Garte and colleagues (1997). The adverse effect on the endometrial cancer risk has been reported mostly for currently obese women, with a two- to threefold excess risk for women in the highest versus lowest BMI categories. A high BMI at a young age, reported in one study, did not affect the risk (Olson et al, 1995). In a few studies, the risk has also been related to an increase in body weight over time and to a high waste/hip circumference ratio (Swanson et al, 1993a). Conversely, weight loss has been associated with risk reduction (Trentham-Dietz 2006). Observations that the effects may be greatest among older postmenopausal women and are present only for currently obese women indicate that obesity may influence carcinogenesis at a late stage (Garte et al, 1997).

A causal link is biologically plausible, as a greater amount of fat tissue entails a higher efficiency of conversion from androstenedione to estrone and lower levels of SHBG, which in turn leads to higher serum levels of bioavailable estrone and estradiol (MacDonald et al, 1978). Further, in premenopausal women, obesity has been associated with an increase in the frequency of anovulatory menstrual cycles (Key et al, 1988).

The relationship between obesity, body fat patterns, and serum levels of sex hormones, however, seems complex. Abdominal obesity (a high waist/hip ratio) has been associated with elevated levels of testosterone and lower levels of SHBG, as well as with higher levels of estradiol. These discrepancies may be explained by the difficulty of measuring these hormone levels accurately (Garte et al, 1997). A further complexity involves the finding that increased levels of estrogens measured in endometrial cancer patients may be independent of BMI levels, that is, hypothetically produced through means other than estrogen production in fat tissue—for example,

through hyperinsulinemia per se (Potischman et al, 1996; Troisi et al, 1997). Recently, adiponectin, a protein that decreases with hyperinsulinemia, was found to be inversely associated with endometrial cancer risk, lending support to the role of hyperinsulinemia in endometrial carcinogenesis (Soliman et al, 2006).

Infections

A possible role for oncogenic human papillomaviruses, an established cause of cervical cancer (Leminen et al, 1991), has been suggested in endometrial cancer etiology, but data are sparse and controversial. No other infections have attracted interest.

Physical Activity

Evidence for a link between physical activity and endometrial cancer risk is scanty, but there are indications that persistent, vigorous physical exercise may reduce the risk.

The hypothesis behind the testing of physical activity is that it reduces the risk by acting indirectly—through other risk factors such as BMI level, age at menarche or menopause, or prevalence of anovulation—or directly by lowering the levels of ovarian hormones. Supportive of a true effect is the finding of lowered concentrations of circulating estrogens in physically active versus sedentary women (Sturgeon et al, 1993). Participation in sports and other vigorous exercise, particularly in the late teenage years, has been associated with a somewhat lower risk; studies examining the effects of walking have produced less consistent results (Olson et al, 1992). In a large Swedish study, the risk of endometrial cancer was 40% higher for women with a sedentary lifestyle compared to those with a high-/very high physical activity level; among sedentary women 50 to 69 years old at follow-up, a corresponding 60% increased risk was noted (Moradi et al, 1998, 2000).

Ionizing Radiation

There are no reported data linking ionizing radiation to the risk of endometrial cancer.

Occupation

Data from a large Finnish study using census data showed no association between job titles and endometrial cancer risk. However, women with sedentary jobs and women exposed to animal dust (ie, furriers) had a significantly increased risk of endometrial cancer risk (Weiderpass et al, 2001a). As for other possible correlates of socioeconomic status, the level of education had a strong inverse relationship to the risk of endometrial cancer in an Italian case-control study (La Vecchia et al, 1992).

Medical Conditions and Treatment

Most case-control studies have established diabetes mellitus and abnormal glucose tolerance as risk factors for endometrial cancer (Grady et al, 1995). The pathogenic mechanism behind this linkage was long assumed to be obesity, associated with excessive estrogen levels. However, detailed analyses revealed that the effect of diabetes on the risk of endometrial cancer may be independent of BMI (Brinton et al, 1992). This observation led to the hypothesis that the risk increase in women with noninsulin-dependent diabetes mellitus (NIDDM) is actually caused by an increased level of insulin. A case-control study (Shoff and Newcomb, 1998) indicated an effect of NIDDM on the endometrial cancer risk independent of obesity. The authors suggested that insulin itself may be causally related, by acting as a mitogen on the endometrium directly, or by enhancing the level of insulin like growth factor and lowering the level of SHBG or stimulating local tissue growth factors. However, a previous study (Troisi et al, 1997) had found no evidence that increased insulin levels, estimated from C-peptide levels, mediated the effect of NIDDM on the endometrial cancer risk in obese women.

Due to contradictory findings, there is a need to study the crucial endocrine and local determinants in endometrial carcinogenic pathways in relation to documented risk factors such as obesity and diabetes

and perhaps also the polycystic ovary syndrome.

Hypertension

Hypertension has likewise been reported in the majority of studies to be a risk factor for endometrial cancer (Grady et al, 1995). Whether the relationship is confounded by other risk factors, such as estrogen use or high BMI, is unclear. In one study that adjusted for these and other potential confounding factors, no increase in risk emerged (Brinton et al, 1992). In some women, hypertension may be part of a metabolic syndrome involving hyperinsulinemia and other endocrine abnormalities (Kaaks, 1996).

Other Risk Factors

Environmental xenoestrogens

Concern has been raised that some persistent environmental pollutants, such as dichlorodiphenyltrichloroethane (DDT) and polychlorinated biphenyls (PCBs), may exert hormonal effects and thereby affect the risk of endometrial cancer. When levels of 3 DDT compounds and 10 PCB congeners were studied in relation to endometrial cancer risk, comparisons of the highest and the lowest levels of dichlorodiphenyldichloroethylene (DDE) or total PCBs did not indicate any associations (Sturgeon et al, 1998). A large case-control study that analyzed serum concentrations of 10 chlorinated pesticides and 10 PCB congeners—both individually and grouped according to their putative estrogenic and antiestrogenic effects—revealed no associations with levels of the studied compounds (Weiderpass et al, 2000b).

Given that the endometrium is sensitive to even low levels of estrogens, the null results of these two studies provide reassuring evidence that the observed blood levels of organochlorins do not have a measurable effect on endometrial cancer risk.

Tamoxifen

Tamoxifen is a nonsteroidal compound with both a partially estrogenic and an an-

Table 18–5. Summary of risk factors for endometrial cancer

Risk factors	Effect	Strength	Comment
Early menarche	↑	(+)	
Late menopause	↑	+	
Anovulation	↑	++	
Nulliparity	↑	++	
Infertility	↑	(+)	
Obesity	↑	++	
"Metabolic syndrome"	↑	+	Obesity, diabetes, hypertension
Smoking	↓	+	
Alcohol	↑	(+)	
Physical activity	↓	(+)	
Endogenous estrogens	↑	+	
Combined Oral Contraceptives	↓	+++	
Estrogen-only replacement	↑	+++	
Estrogen-progestin combined replacement	↑ ~ ↓	(+)	Depending on the number of days progestins are added
Tamoxifen	↑	+	

↑ Factor increasing the risk.

↓ Factor decreasing the risk.

↑ ~ ↓ Factor increasing or decreasing the risk.

+ Weak effect.

++ Intermediate effect.

+++ Strong effect.

ticstrogenic effect, depending on the target tissues. After its introduction in the 1970s, tamoxifen was mainly used to treat advanced breast cancer. Extensive clinical trials in the 1980s established its efficacy as adjuvant therapy both in reducing the risk of recurrence or contralateral breast cancer and in improving survival in postmenopausal women with early stage, receptor-positive tumors (Early Breast Cancer Trialist's Collaborative Group, 1988). Tamoxifen is also being evaluated as adjuvant therapy in premenopausal women and for primary chemoprevention of breast cancer in high-risk groups.

In view of the partially agonistic estrogenic property of tamoxifen, its potential to stimulate tumor growth, and its ability to form DNA adducts, a causal association with endometrial cancer has been considered plausible. However, there is still controversy concerning the magnitude of the adverse ef-

fect on the endometrium, the impact of dose and duration, and the biological behavior of tamoxifen-associated endometrial tumors (Rutqvist, 1998). Six randomized trials have evaluated the efficacy and side effects of treatment. Four of them reported a three- to sevenfold increase in the risk of endometrial cancer, while two smaller studies failed to find an association (Early Breast Cancer Trialist's Collaborative Group, 1988; Grady et al, 1995). A pooled analysis based on a median follow-up period of 9 years yielded a fourfold increased risk (Rutqvist et al, 1995). Evaluation of available evidence for an association with an increased risk of endometrial cancer prompted the IARC to classify tamoxifen as a carcinogen (IARC, 1996). Efforts to evaluate the rationale for using tamoxifen for chemoprevention of breast cancer in healthy or high-risk women obviously need to take into consideration its substantial adverse effects.

CONCLUSION

In western countries, endometrial cancer is a common malignancy that occurs mostly after menopause and has an excellent prognosis. The age-standardized incidence varies at least tenfold across countries, suggesting the strong influence of modifiable risk factors (summarized in Table 18–5). Among these, estrogens and progestins emerge as central in malignant transformation of the endometrium. Hence, it is conceivable that risk reduction conferred by current smoking, past oral contraceptive use, childbearing, and, tentatively, physical actvity is mediated by hormones. This may also pertain to the risk increase associated with obesity—which increases peripheral production of estrogens—and with diabetes mellitus. The most compelling evidence that hormones determine the risk of endometrial cancer comes from studies of hormone therapy following menopause. Use of estrogens alone for 10 years or more increases the risk about tenfold. This excess risk may be counteracted substantially by combined use of estrogens and progestins. Continuous use throughout the treatment cycle may confer an even lower risk than nonuse of exogenous hormones. Hence, it should be possible to prevent a substantial fraction of all endometrial cancers through modification of lifestyle, maintaining normal weight, and optimal use of oral contraceptives and postmenopausal hormones.

REFERENCES

Aaltonen L, Peltomaki P, Leach F, Sistonen P, Pylkkanen L, Mecklin J, Jarvinen H, Powell S, Jen J, Hamilton S, Petersen G, Kinszler K, Vogelstein B, de le Chapelle A. Clues to the pathogenesis of familial colorectal cancer. Science 1993;260:812–16.

Adamski J, Jakob FJ. A guide to 17beta-hydroxysteroid dehydrogenases. Mol Cell Endocrin01.2001;171(1–2):1–4.

Austin H, Austin JM Jr, Partridge EE, Hatch KD, Shingleton HM. Endometrial cancer, obesity, and body fat distribution. Cancer Res 1991;51:568–72.

Austin H, Drews C, Partridge EE. A case-control study of endometrial cancer in relation to cigarette smoking, serum estrogen levels, and alcohol use. Am J Obstet Gynecol. 1993 Nov; 169(5):1086–91.

Barbieri RL, McShane PM, Ryan KJ. Constituents of cigarette smoke inhibit human granulosa cell aromatase. Fertil Steril 1986; 46:232–36.

Barbosa JC, Shultz TD, Filley SJ, et al. The relationship among adiposity, diet, and hormone concentrations in vegetarian and and nonvegetarian postmenopausal women. Am J Clin Nutr 1990;51(5):798–803.

Barbone F, Austin H, Partridge EE. Diet and endometrial cancer: a case–control study. Am J Epidemiol 1993;137:393–403.

Bennett FC, Ingram DM. Diet and female sex hormone concentrations: an intervention study for the type of fat consumed. Am J Clin Nutr 1990;52;808–12.

Beresford SA, Weiss NS, Voigt LF, McKnight B. Risk of endometrial cancer in relation to use of oestrogen combined with cyclic progestagen therapy in postmenopausal women. Lancet 1997;349:458–61.

Berstein LM, Imyanitov EN, Gamajunova VB, Kovalevskij AJ, Kuligina Esh, Belogubova EV, Buslov KG, Karpova MB, Togo AV, Volkov ON, Kovalenko IG. CYP17 genetic polymorphism in endometrial cancer: are only steroids involved? Cancer Lett 2002 Jun 6;180(1):47–53.

Berstein LM, Imyanitov EN, Kovalevskij AJ, et al. CYP19 gene polymorphism in endometrial cancer patients. J CAncer Res Clin Oncol 2001;127:135–38.

Berstein LM, Imyanitov EN, Kovalevskij AJ, et al. CYP17 and CYP19 genetic polymorphisms in endometrial cancer: association with intratumoral aromatase activity. Cancer Lett 2004;207:191–96.

Björkholm E, Pettersson F. Granulosa-cell and theca-cell tumors. The clinical picture and long-term outcome for the Radiumhemmet series. Acta Obstet Gynecol Scand 1980;59: 161–63.

Boyd J. Estrogen as a carcinogen: the genetics and molecular biology of human endometrial carcinoma. Prog Clin Biol Res 1996; 394: 151–73.

Bray F, Dos Santos Silva I, Moller H, Weiderpass E. Endometrial cancer incidence trends in Europe: underlying determinants and prospects for prevention. Cancer Epidemiol Biomarkers Prev 2005 May;14(5):1132–42.

Brinton LA, Barrett RJ, Berman ML, Mortel R, Twiggs LB, Wilbanks GD. Cigarette smoking and the risk of endometrial cancer. Am J Epidemiol. 1993 Feb 1;137

Brinton LA, Berman ML, Mortel R, Twiggs LB, Barrett RJ, Wilbanks GD, et al. Reproductive, menstrual, and medical risk factors for endometrial cancer: results from a case-control study. Am J Obstet Gynecol 1992; 167:1317–25.

Brinton LA, Hoover RN. Estrogen replacement therapy and endometrial cancer risk: unresolved issues. The Endometrial Cancer Collaborative Group. Obstet Gynecol 1993;81: 265–71.

Carson-Jurica MA, Schrader WT, O'Malley BW. Steroid receptor family: structure and functions. Endocr Rev 1990;11(2):201–20.

Cauley JA, Gutai JP, Kuller LH, LeDonne D, Powell JG. The epidemiology of serum sex hormones in postmenopausal women. Am J Epidemiol 1989;129:1120–31.

Chu J, Schweid AI, Weiss NS. Survival among women with endometrial cancer: a comparison of estrogen users and nonusers. Am J Obstet Gynecol 1982;143:569–73.

Cust AE, Armstrong BK, Friedenreich CM, Slimani N, Bauman A. Physical activity and endometrial cancer risk: a review of the current evidence, biologic mechanisms and the quality of physical activity assessment methods. Cancer Causes Control 2007 Apr;18(3):243–58. Epub 2007 Jan 8.

Davidson BJ, Gambone JC, Lagasse LD, Castaldo TW, Hammond GL, Siiteri PK, et al. Free estradiol in postmenopausal women with and without endometrial cancer. J Clin Endocrinol Metab 1981;52:404–8.

Deligdisch L, Holinka CF. Endometrial carcinoma: two diseases? Cancer Detect Prev 1987;10:237–46.

d'Errico A, Malats N, Vineis P, Boffetta P. Review of studies of selected metabolic polymorphisms and cancer. In: Veneis P, Malats N, Lang M, d'E rrico A, Caporaso N, Cuzick J, Bofetta P (Eds): Metabolic Polymorphisms and Susceptibility to Cancer. IARC Sci. Pub. No. 148. Lyon, International Agency for Research on Cancer, 1999, pp 323–93.

Jick SS. Combined estrogen and progesterone use and endometrial cancer. Epidemiology 1993 Jul;4(4):384.

Devesa SS, Blot WJ, Stone BJ, Miller BA, Tarone RE, Fraumeni JF Jr. Recent cancer trends in the United States. J Natl Cancer Inst 1995a; 87:175–82.

Devesa SS, Donaldson J, Fears T. Graphical presentation of trends in rates. Am J Epidemiol 1995b;141:300–4.

De Vivo I, Huggins GS, HAnkinson SE, Lescault PJ, Boezen M, Coldotz GA, Hunter DJ: A functional polymorphism in the promoter of the progesterone receptor gene associated with endometrial cancer risk. Proc Natl Acad Sci USA 2002;99:12263–68.

Doherty JA, Weiss NS, Freeman RJ, Dightman DA, Thornton PJ, Houck JR, Voigt LF, Rossing MA, Schwartz SM, Chen C. Genetic factors in catechol estrogen metabolism in relation to the risk of endometrial cancer. Cancer Epidemiol Biomarkers Prev 2005 Feb;14(2):357–66.

Early Breast Cancer Trialists' Collaborative Group. Effects of adjuvant tamoxifen and of cytotoxic therapy on mortality in early breast cancer. An overview of 61 randomized trials among 28,896 women. N Engl J Med 1988; 319:1681–92.

Elliott EA, Matanoski GM, Rosenshein NB, Grumbine FC, Diamond EL. Body fat patterning in women with endometrial cancer. Gynecol Oncol 1990;39:253–58.

Esteller M, Garcia A, Martinez-Palones JM, Xercavins J, Reventos J. Germ line polymorphisms in cytochrome-P450 1A1 (C4887 CYP1A1) and methylenetetrahydrofolate reductase (MTHFR) genes and endometrial cancer susceptibility. Carcinogenesis 1997 Dec; 18(12):2307–11.

Ferlay J, Bray F, Pisani P, Parkin DM. GLOBOCAN 2000: Cancer Incidence, Mortality and Prevalence Worldwide. International Agency for Research on Cancer, Lyon, 2001.

Fornasarig M, Campagnutta E, Talamini R, Franceschi S, Boz G, Scarabelli C, et al. Risk factors for endometrial cancer according to familial susceptibility. Int J Cancer 1998 July 3;77(1):29–32.

Franks AL, Kendrick JS, Tyler CW Jr. Postmenopausal smoking, estrogen replacement therapy, and the risk of endometrial cancer. Am J Obstet Gynecol 1987 Jan;156(1):20–23.

Garte S, Zocchetti C, Taioli E. Gene–environment interactions in the application of biomarkers of cancer susceptibility in epidemiology. In: Toniolo P, Bofetta P, Shuker DEG, Rothman N, Hulka B, Pearce N (Eds): Application of Biomarkers in Cancer Epidemiology. IARC Sci. Pub. No. 142. Lyon, International Agency for Research on Cancer, 1997, pp 251–64.

Garpstur SM, Potter JD, Sellers TA, Kushi LH, Folsom AR. Alcohol consumption and postmenopausal endometrial cancer: results from the Iowa Women's Health Study. Cancer Causes Control. 1993 Jul;4(4):323–29.

Goldin BR, Adlercreutz H, Sherwood L, Woods MN, Dwyer, JT, Conlon, T, et al. The relationship between estrogen levels and diets of Caucasian American and Oriental immigrant women. Am J Clin Nutr 1986;44:945–53.

Goodman MT, Hankin JH, Wilkens LR, Lyu LC, McDuffie K, Liu LQ, et al. Diet, body size, physical activity, and the risk of endometrial cancer. Cancer Res 1997a;57:5077–85.

Goodman MT, Wilkens LR, Hankin JH, Lyu LC, Wu AH, Kolonel LN. Association of soy and fiber consumption with the risk of endometrial cancer. Am J Epidemiol 1997b; 146:294–306.

Grady D, Ernster V. Endometrial cancer. In: Cancer Epidemiology and Prevention, 2nd ed. New York, Oxford University Press, 1996, pp 1058–89.

Grady D, Gebretsadik T, Kerlikowske K, Ernster V, Petitti D. Hormone replacement therapy and endometrial cancer risk: a meta-analysis. Obstet Gynecol 1995;85:304–13.

Graham JD, Clarke CL. Physiological action of progesterone in target tissues. Endocrinol Rev 1997;18:502–19.

Gruber S, Thompson W: A population-based study of endometrial cancer and familial risk in younger women. Cancer Epidemiol Bomarkers Prev 1996;5:411–17.

Haiman CA, Hankinson SE, Colditz GA, Hunter DJ, De Vivo I. A polymorphism in CYP17 and endometrial cancer risk. Cancer Res 2001;61:3955–60.

Haiman CA, Hankinson SE. De Vivo I, Guillemette C, Ishibe N, Hunter DJ, Byrne C. Polymorphisms in steroid hormone pathway genes and mammographic density. Breast Cancer Res Treat 2003;77:27–36.

Hankinson SE, Willet WC, Manson JE, Hunter DJ, Colditz GA, Stampfer MJ, Longcope C, Speizer FE. Alcohol height, and andiposity in relation to estrogen and prolactin levels in postmenopausal women. J Natl Cancer Inst 1995 Sep 6;87(17):1297–302.

Henderson BE, Casagrande JT, Pike MC, Mack T, Rosario I, Duke A. The epidemiology of endometrial cancer in young women. Br J Cancer 1983;47:749–56.

Hill HA, Austin H. Nutrition and endometrial cancer. Cancer Causes Control 1996;7:19–32.

Hoover R, Fraumeni JF, Everson R. Cancer of the uterine corpus after hormonal treatment for breast cancer. Lancet 1976;1:885.

Husen B, Psonka N, Jacob-Meisel M, Keil C, Rune GM. Differential expression of 17beta-hydroxysteroid dehydrogenases types2 and 4 in human endometrial epithelial cell lines. J Mol Endocrinol 2000;24(1):135–44.

International Agency for Research on Cancer. Some hormones. IARC Monographs on the Evaluation of Carcinogenic Risks to Humans: Some Pharmaceutical Drugs. Vol. 66. Lyon, IARC, 1996.

International Agency for Research on Cancer. Some hormones. IARC Monographs on the Evaluation of Carcinogenic Risks to Humans: Postmenopausal Hormone Therapy and Hormonal Contraception. Vol. 72. Lyon, IARC, 1999.

Iwamoto I, Fujino T, Douchi T, Nagata Y. Association of estrogen receptor alpha and

beta3-adrenergic receptor polymorphisms with endometrial cancer.Obstet Gynecol 2003 Sep;102(3):506–11.

Jick SS. Combined estrogen and progesterone use and endometrial cancer. Epidemiology 1993 Jul;4(4):384.

Jick SS, Walker AM, Jick H. Estrogens, progesterone, and endometrial cancer. Epidemiology 1993;4:20–24.

Kaaks R. Nutrition, hormones and breast cancer: is insulin the missing link? Cancer Causes Control 1996;7:605–25.

Kalandidi A, Tzonou A, Lipworth L, Gamatsi I, Filippa D. A case-control study of endometrial cancer in relation to reproductive, somatometric, and life-style variables. Oncology 1996 Sep-Oct;53(5):354–59.

Kasum CM, Nicodemus K, Harnack LJ, Jacobs DR, Folsom AR. Whole grain intake and incident endometrial cancer. the Iowa Women's Health Study. Nutr Cancer 2001; 39(2):180–86.

Kato I, Tominaga S, Terao C. Alcohol consumption and cancers of hormone-related organs in females. Jpn J Clin Oncol 1989 Sep;19(3):202–7.

Katsouyanni K, Boyle P, Trichopoulos D. Diet and urine estrogens among postmenopausal women. Oncology 1991;48:490–94.

Kelsey JL, LiVolsi VA, Holford TR, Fischer DB, Mostow ED, Schwartz PE, et al. A case-control study of cancer of the endometrium. Am J Epidemiol 1982;116:333–42.

Kennedy DL, Baum C, Forbes MB. Noncontraceptive estrogens and progestins: use patterns over time. Obstet Gynecol 1985;65: 441–46.

Key TJ, Pike MC. The dose–effect relationship between "unopposed" estrogens and endometrial mitotic rate: its central role in explaining and predicting endometrial cancer risk. Br J Cancer 1988;57:205–12.

Key TJ, Pike MC, Brown JB, Hermon C, Allen DS, Wang DY. Cigarette smoking and urinary oestrogen excretion in premenopausal and post-menopausal women. Br J Cancer 1996;74:1313–16.

Khaw K, Taude S, Barrett-Connor E. Cigarette smoking and levels of adrenal androgens in postmenopausal women. N Engl J Med 1988;318:1705–9.

Khoury M, Beaty T, Cohen B. Fundamentals of Genetic Epidemiology. New York, Oxford University Press, 1993.

Kolonel LN, Hankin JH, Lee J, Chu SY, Nomura AMY, Hinds MW. Nutrient intakes in relation to cancer incidence in Hawaii. Br J Cancer 1981;44:332–39.

Koumantaki Y, Tzonou A, Koumantakis E, Kaklamani E, Arvantinos D, Trichopoulos D. A case-control study of cancer of the endometrium in Athens. Int J Cancer 1989 May 15;43(5):795–99.

Kristensen V, Andersen T, Lindbolm A, Erikstein B, Magnus P, Borresen-Dale A-L. A rare CYP19(aromatase) variant may increase the risk of breast cancer. Pharmacogenetics 1998;8:43–48.

Kvale G, Heuch I, Ursin G. Reproductive factors and risk of the uterine corpus: a prospective study. Cancer Res 1988;48:6217–21.

Kvale G, Heuch I, Nilssen S. Endometrial cancer and age at last delivery: evidence for an association [letter]. Am J Epidemiol 1992;135:453–55.

Labrie F, Luu-The V, Lin S-X, et al. The key role of 17B-hydroxysteroid dehydrogenases in sex steroid biology. Steroids 1997;62;148–58.

La Vecchia C, Decarli A, Fasoli M, Gentile A. Nutrition and diet in the etiology of endometrial cancer. Cancer 1986;57:1248–53.

La Vecchia C, Francheschi S, Decarli A, Gallus G, Tognoni G. Risk factors for endometrial cancer in different ages. J Natl Cancer Inst 1984;73:667–71.

La Vecchia C, Negri E, Franceschi S. Education and cancer risk. Cancer 1992;70:2935–41.

Lawrence C, Tessaro I, Durgerian S, Caputo T, Richart R, Jacobson H, Greenwald P. Smoking, body weight, and early-stage endometrial cancer. Cancer. 1987 May 1; 59(9):1665–69.

Lawrence C, Tessaro I, Durgerian S, Caputo T, Richart RM, Greenwald P. Advanced-stage endometrial cancer: contributions of estrogen use, smoking, and other risk factors. Gynecol Oncol 1989 Jan;32(1):41–45.

Lax SF, Kendall B, Tashiro H, Slebos RJ, Hedrick L. The frequency of p53, K-ras mutations, and microsatellite instability differs in uterine endomtrioid and serous carcinoma: evidence of distinct molecular genetic pathways. Cancer 2000;88:814–24.

Leminen A, Paavonen J, Vesterinen E, Wahlstrom T, Rantala I, Lehtinen M. Human papillomavirus types 16 and 18 in adenocarcinoma of the uterine cervix. Am J Clin Pathol 1991;95:647–52.

Lesko SM, Rosenberg L, Kaufman DW, Helmrich SP, Miller DR, Strom B, Schottenfeld D, Rosenshein NB, Knapp RC, Lewis J, et al. Cigarette smoking and the risk of endometrial cancer.N Engl J Med 1985 Sep 5; 313(10):593–96.

Levi F, la Vecchia C, Declari A. Cigarette smoking and the risk of endometrial cancer. Eur J Cancer Clin Oncol 1987 Jul;23(7): 1025–29.

Lichtenstein P, Holm NV, Verkasalo PK, Iliadou A, Kaprio J, Koskenvuo M, et al. Environmental and heritable factors in the causation of cancer. Analyses of cohorts of twins from Sweden, Denmark and Finland. N Engl J Med 2000 July 13;343(2):78–85.

Littman AJ, Beresford SA, White E. The association of dietary fat and plant foods with endometrial cancer (United States). Cancer Causes Control 2001 Oct;12(8):691–702.

London S, Willett W, Longcope C, McKinlay S. Alcohol and other dietary factors in relation to serum hormone concentrations in women at climacteric. Am J Clin Nutr 1991;53:166–71.

Lynch HT, Krush AJ, Larsen AL, Magnuson CW. Endometrial carcinoma: multiple primary malignancies, constitutional factors, and heredity. Am J Med Sci 1966 Oct; 252(4):381–90.

MacDonald PC, Edman CD, Hansell DL, Porter SC, Siteri PK. Effect of obesity on conversion of plasma androstenedione to estrone in postmenopausal women with and without endometrial cancer. Am J Obstet Gynecol 1978;130:448–55.

Machin P, Catasus L, Pons C, Munoz J, Matias-Guiu X, Prat J. CTNNB1 mutations and beta-catenin expression in endometrial carcinomas. Hum Pathol 2002 Feb;33(2):206–12.

MacMahon B. Risk factors for endometrial cancer. Gynecol Oncol 1974;2:122–29.

McGrath M, Lee IM, Hankinson SE, Kraft P, Hunter DJ, Buring J, De Vivo I. Androgen receptor polymorphisms and endometrial cancer risk. Int J Cancer 2006 Mar 1;118(5): 1261–68.

McGrath M, Hankinson SE, Arbeitman L, Colditz GA, Hunter DJ, De Vivo I. Cytochrome P450 1B1 and catechol-O-methyltransferase polymorphisms and endometrial cancer susceptibility. Carcinogenesis 2004;25:559–65.

McPhaul MJ, Marcelli M, Zoppi S, Griffin JE, Wilson JD. Genetic basis of endocrine disease. The spectrum of mutations in the androgen receptor gene that causes androgen resistance. J Clin Endocrinol Metab 1993; 76(1):17–23.

Means G, Mahendroo M, Corbin C, Mathis J, Powell F, Mendelson C, Simpson E. Structural analysis of the gene encoding human aromatase cytochrome P-450, the enzyme responsible for estrogen biosynthesis. J Biol Chem 1989;264:19385–91.

Michnovicz JJ, Naganuma H, Hershcopf RJ, Bradlow HL, Fishman J. Increased urinary catechol estrogen excretion in female smokers. Steroids 1988;1–2:69–83.

Moradi T, Nyrén O, Bergstrom R, Gridley G, Linet M, Wolk A, et al. Risk for endometrial cancer in relation to occupational physical activity: a nationwide cohort study in Sweden. Int J Cancer 1998;76:665–70.

Moradi T, Weiderpass E, Signorello LB, Persson I, Nyren O, Adami HO. Physical activity and postmenopausal endometrial cancer risk (Sweden). Cancer Causes Contol 2000 Oct;11(9):829–37.

Negri E, La Vecchia C, Franceschi S, Levi F, Parazzini F. Intake of selected micronutrients and the risk of endometrial carcinoma. Cancer 1996;77:917–23.

Nelson CL, Sellers TA, Rich SS, Potter JD, McGovern PG, Kushi LH. Familial clustering of colon, breast, uterine, and ovarian cancers as assessed by family history. Genet Epidemiol 1993;10(4):235–44.

Neulen J, Wagner B, Runge M, Breckwoldt M. Effect of progestins, androgens estrogens and antiestrogens on 3H-thymidine uptake by human endometrial and endosalpinx cells in vitro. Arch Gynecol 1987;240(4):255–32.

Newcomb PA, Trentham-Dietz A, Storer BE. Alcohol consumption in relation to endometrial cancer risk. Cancer Epidemiol, Biomarkers Prev 1997 Oct 6(10):775–78.

Newcomer LM, Newcomb PA, Trentham-Dietz A, Storer BE. Hormonal risk factors for endometrial cancer: modification by cigarette smoking (United States). Cancer Causes Control 2001 Nov;12(9):829–35.

Nicolaides N, Papadopoulous N, Liu B, Wei Y, Carter K, Ruben S, Rosen C, Haseltine W, Fleischmann R, Fraser C. Mutations in two PMS homologues in hereditary nonpolyposis colon cancer. Nature 1994;371:75–80.

Nisker JA, Hammond GL, Davidson BJ, Frumar AM, Takaki NK, Judd HL, et al. Serum sex hormone-binding globulin capacity and the percentage of free estradiol in postmenopausal women with and without endometrial carcinoma. A new biochemical basis for the association between obesity and endometrial carcinoma. Am J Obstet Gynecol 1980; 138:637–42.

Nordlund LA, Carstensen JM, Pershagen G. Cancer incidence in female smokers: a 26-year follow-up. Int J Cancer 1997 Nov 27;73(5):625–28.

Nyholm HC, Nielsen AL, Lyndrup J, Dreisler A, Hagen C, Haug E. Plasma oestrogens in postmenopausal women with endometrial cancer. Br J Obstet Gynaecol 1993;100:1115–19.

Olson SH, Kelsey JL, Pearson TA, Levin B. Evaluation of random digit dialing as a method of control selection in case-control studies. Am J Epidemiol 1992;135:210–22.

Olson SH, Trevisan M, Marshall JR, Graham S, Zielezny M, Vena JE, et al. Body mass index, weight gain, and risk of endometrial cancer. Nutr Cancer 1995;23:141–49.

Papadopoulos N, Nicolaides N, Wei Y, Ruben S, Carter K, Rosen C, Haseltine W, Fleischmann R, Fraser C, Adams M. Mutation of a mutl homolog in hereditary colon cancer. Science 1994;263:1625–29.

Parazzini F, La Vecchia C, Negri E, Fidele L, Barlotta F. Reproductive factors and risk of endometrial cancer. Am J Obstet Gynecol 1991;164:522–27.

Parazzini F, Negri E, La Vecchia C, Benzi G, Chiaffarino F, Polatti A, et al. Role of reproductive factors on the risk of endometrial cancer. Int J Cancer 1998;76:784–86.

Parkin DM. Epidemiology of cancer: global patterns and trends. Toxicol Lett 1998 Dec 28:102–103:227–34.

Parkin DM, Bray F, Ferlay J, Pisani P. Global cancer statistics, 2002. CA Cancer J Clin 2005 Mar-Apr;55(2):74–108.

Paynter RA, Hankinson SE, Colditz GA, Kraft P, Hunter DJ, De Vivo I. CYP19 (aromatase) haplotypes and endometrial cancer risk. Int J Cancer 2005 Aug 20;116(2):267–74.

Peltomaki P, Aaltonen L, Sistonen P, Pylkkanen L, Mecklin J, Marvinen H, Green J, Jass J, Weber J, Leach F, Petersen G, Hamilton S, de le Chapelle A, Vogelstein B. Genetic mapping of a locus predisposing to human colorectal cancer. Science 1993;260:810–12.

Persson I, Adami HO, Bergkvist L, Lindgren A, Pettersson B, Hoover R, et al. Risk of endometrial cancer after treatment with oestrogens alone or in conjunction with progestogens: results of a prospective study. Br Med J 1989;298:147–51.

Persson I, Schmidt M, Adami HO, Bergström R, Pettersson B, Sparen P. Trends in endometrial cancer incidence and mortality in Sweden, 1960–84. Cancer Causes Control 1990;1:201–8.

Persson I, Weiderpass E, Bergkvist L, Bergström L, Schairer C. Risks of breast and endometrial cancer after estrogen and estrogen-progestin replacement. Cancer Causes Control 1999;10:253–60.

Pettersson B, Bergström R, Johansson ED. Serum estrogens and androgens in women with endometrial cancer. Gynecol Oncol 1986;25:223–33.

Pike MC, Peters RK, Cozen W, Probst-Hensch NM, Felix JC, Wan PC, et al. Estrogen-progestin replacement therapy and endometrial cancer. J Natl Cancer Inst 1997;89:1110–16.

Potischman N, Hoover RN, Brinton LA, Siiteri P, Dorgan JF, Swanson CA, et al. Case-control study of endogenous steroid hormones and endometrial cancer. J Natl Cancer Inst 1996;88:1127–35.

Potischman N, Swanson CA, Brinton LA, McAdams M, Barrett RJ, Berman ML, et al. Dietary associations in a case-control study of endometrial cancer. Cancer Causes Control 1993;4:239–50.

Prentice RL, Sheppard L. Dietary fat and cancer: consistency of the epidemiologic data, and disease prevention that may follow from a practical reduction in fat consumption. Cancer Causes Control 1990;1:81–97.

Prentice R, Thomson D, Clifford C, Gorbach S, Goldin B, Byar D. Dietary fat reduction and plasma estradiol concentration in healthy postmenopausal women. J Natl Cancer Inst 1990;82:129–34.

Preston-Martin S, Pike MC, Ross RK, Jones PA, Henderson BE. Increased cell division as a cause of human cancer. Cancer Res 1990; 50:7415–21.

Reichman ME, Judd JT, Longcope C, Schatzkin A, Clevidence BA, Nair PP, Campbell WS, Taylor PR. Effects of alcohol consumption on plasma and urinary hormone concentrations in premenopausal women. J Natl Cancer Inst 1993 May 5;85(9):722–27.

Risinger J, Berchuck A, Kohler M, Watson P, Lynch H, Boyd J. Genetic instability of microsatellites in endometrial cancer carcinoma. Cancer Res 1993;53:5100–3.

Risinger JI, Maxwell GL, Berchuck A, Barrett JC. Promoter hypermethylation as an epigenetic component in Type I and Type II endometrial cancers. Ann N T Acad Sci 2003; 983:208–12.

Rock CL, Flatt SW, Thomson CA, Stefanick ML, Newman VA, Jones LA, Natarajan L, Ritenbaugh C, Hollenbach KA, Pierce JP, Chang RJ. Effects of a high-fiber, low-fat diet intervention on serum concentrations of reproductive steroid hormones in women with history of breast cancer. J Clin Oncol 2004 Jun 15;22(12):2379–87.

Rose GL, Dowsett M, Mudge JE, White JO, Jeffcoate SL. The inhibitory effects of danazol, danazol metabolites, gestrinone, and testosterone on the growth of human endometrial cells in vitro. Fertil Steril 1988;49(2): 224–28.

Rutqvist LE. Controversial issues in adjuvant systemic therapy of early breast cancer. Acta Oncol 1998;37:421–30.

Rutqvist LE, Johansson H, Signomklao T, Johansson U, Fornander T, Wilking N. Adjuvant tamoxifen therapy for early stage breast cancer and second primary malignancies. Stockholm Breast Cancer Study Group. J Natl Cancer Inst 1995;87:645–51.

Sasaki M, Tanaka Y, Kaneuchi M, Sakuragi N, Dahiya R. Alleles of polymorphic sites that correspond to hyperactive variants of CYP1B1 protein are significantly less frequent in Japanese as compared to American and German populations.Hum Mutat 2003a Jun;21(6):652.

Sasaki M, Sakuragi N, Dahiya R: The CAG repeats in exon 1 of the androgen receptor gene

are significantly longer in endometrial patients. Biochem Biophys Res Commun 2003b;305:1105–8; Sasaki M, Tanaka Y, Kaneuchi M, Sakuragi N, Dahiya R. Polymorphisms of estrogen receptor alpha gene in endometrial cancer. Biochem Biophys Res Commun 2002 Sept 27; 297(3):558–64.

Santin AD, Bellone S, Gokden M, Palmieri M, Dunn D, Agha J, Roman JJ, Hutchins L, Pecorelli S, O'Brien T, Cannon MJ, Parham GP. Overexpression of HER-2/neu in uterine serous papillary cancer. Clin Cancer Res 2002;8:1271–79.

Schlesselman JJ. Oral contraceptives and neoplasia of the uterine corpus. Contraception 1991;43:557–79.

Setiawan VW, Hankinson SE, Colditz GA, Hunter DJ, De Vivo, I. HSD17B1 gene polymorphisms and risk of endometrial and breast cancer. Cancer Epidemiol Biomarkers Prev 2004;13(2):213–19.

Sherman ME, Carreon JD, Lacey JV Jr, Devesa SS. Impact of hysterectomy on endometrial carcinoma rates in the United States. J Natl Cancer Inst 2005 Nov 16;97(22):1700–2.

Sherman ME, Sturgeon S, Brinton LA, Potischman N, Kurman RJ, Berman ML, et al. Risk factors and hormone levels in patients with serous and endometrioid uterine carcinomas. Mod Pathol 1997;10:963–68.

Shoff SM, Newcomb PA. Diabetes, body size, and risk of endometrial cancer. Am J Epidemiol 1998;148:234–40.

Shu XO, Zheng W, Potischman N, Brinton LA, Hatch MC, Gao YT, et al. A population-based case–control study of dietary factors and endometrial cancer in Shanghai, People's Republic of China. Am J Epidemiol 1993; 137:155–65.

Siegelmann-Danieli N, Buetow KH. Constitutional genetic variation at the human aromatase gene (Cyp19) and breast cancer risk. Br J Cancer 1999 Feb;79(3–4):456–63.

Soliman PT, Wu D, Tortolero-Luna G, Schumeler KM, Slomovitz BM, Bray MS, Gershenson DM, Lu KH. Association between adiponectin, insulin resistance, and endometrial cancer. Cancer 2006 Jun 1;106(11): 2376–81.

Stockwell HG, Lyman GH. Cigarette smoking and the risk of female reproductive cancer. Am J Obstet Gynecol. 1987 Jul; 157(1):35–40.

Sturgeon SR, Brinton LA, Berman ML, Mortel R, Twiggs LB, Barrett RJ, et al. Past and present physical activity and endometrial cancer risk. Br J Cancer 1993;68:584–89.

Sturgeon SR, Brock JW, Potischman N, Needham LL, Rothman N, Brinton LA, et al. Serum concentrations of organochlorine compounds and endometrial cancer risk

(United States). Cancer Causes Control 1998;9:417–24.

Swanson CA, Potischman N, Wilbanks GD, Twiggs LB, Mortel R, Berman ML, et al. Relation of endometrial cancer risk to past, contemporary body size and body fat distribution. Cancer Epidemiol Biomarkers Prev 1993a;2:321–27.

Swanson CA, Wilbanks GD, Twiggs LB, Mortel R, Barrett RJ, Brinton LA. Moderate alcohol consumption nd the risk of endometrial cancer. Epidemiology 1993b Nov; 4(6):530–36.

Terry P, Baron JA, Weiderpass E, Yuen J, Lichtenstein P, Nyren O. Lifestyle and endometrial cancer risk: a cohort study from the Swedish Twin Registry. Int J Cancer 1999 Jul 2;82(1):38–42.

Terry PD, Miller AB, Rohan TE. A prospective cohort study of cigarette smoking and the risk of endometrial cancer. Br J Cancer 2002a May 6;86(9);1430–35.

Terry PD, Rohan TE, Franceschi S, Weiderpass E. Cigarette smoking and the risk of endometrial cancer. Lancet Oncol 2002b Aug; 3(8):470–80.

Terry P, Vainio H, Wolk A, Weiderpass E. Dietary factors in relation to endometrial cancer: a nationwide case-control study in Sweden. Nutr Cancer 2002c;42(1):25–32.

Terry P, Wolk A, Vainio H, Weiderpass E. Fatty fish consumption lowers the risk of endometrial cancer: a nationwidw case-control study in Sweden. Cancer Epidemiol Biomarkers Prev 2002d Jan;11(1): 143–45.

The Writing Group for the PEPI Trial. Effects of hormone replacement therapy on endometrial histology in postmenopausal women. The Postmenopausal Estrogen/Progestin Interventions (PEPI) Trial. JAMA 1996;275: 370–75.

Trentham-Dietz A, Nichols HB, Hampton JM, Newcomb PA. Weight change and risk of endometrial cancer. Int J Epidemiol 2006 Feb,35(1).151–58.

Tseng L, Gurpide E. Induction of human endometrial dehydrogenase by progestins. Endocrinolgy 1975;97:825–29.

Troisi R, Potischman N, Hoover RN, Siiteri P, Brinton LA. Insulin and endometrial cancer. Am J Epidemiol 1997;146:476–82.

Tzonou A, Lipworth L, Kalandidi A, Trichopoulou A, Gamatsi I, Hsieh CC, et al. Dietary factors and the risk of endometrial cancer: a case-control study in Greece. Br J Cancer 1996;73:1284–90.

Vasen H, Watson M, Mecklin J, Jass J, Green J, Nomizu T, Muller H, Lynch H. The epidemiolgy of endometrial cancer in hereditary nonpolyposis colorectal cancer.Anticancer Res 1994;14:1675–78.

Viswanathan AN, Feskanich D, De Vivo I, Hunter DJ, Barbeieri RL, Rosner B, Colditz GA, Hankinson SE. Smoking and the risk of endometrial cancer: results from the Nurses' Health Study. Int J Cancer 2005 May 10;114(6):996–1001.

Waterhouse J, Muir C, Correa P. Cancer Incidence in Five Continents. IARC Sci Pub. No. 143. Lyon International Agency for Research on Cancer, 1992, p 120.

Webster LA, Weiss NS. Alcohol beverage consumption and the risk of endometrial cancer. Cancer and Steroid Hormone Study Group. Int J Epidemiol 1989 Dec;18(4):786–91.

Weiderpass E, Adami HO, Baron JA, Magnusson C, Bergström R, Lindgren A, et al. Risk of endometrial cancer following estrogen replacement with and without progestins. J Natl Cancer Inst 1999a;91:1131–37.

Weiderpass E, Adami HO, Baron JA, Magnusson C, Lindgren A, Persson I. Use of oral contraceptives and endometrial cancer risk (Sweden). Cancer Causes Control 1999c;10: 277–84.

Weiderpass E, Adami HO, Baron JA, Wicklund-Glynn A, Aune M, Atuma S, et al. Organochlorines and endometrial cancer risk. Cancer Epidemiol Biomarkers Prev 2000b;9: 487–93.

Weiderpass E, Baron JA, Adami HO, Magnusson C, Lindgren A, Bergstrom R et al. Low-potency oestrogen and risk of endometrial cancer: a case-control study. Lancet 1999b; 353:1824–28.

Weiderpass E, Persson I, Melhus H, Wedrén S, Kindmark A, Baron JA. Estrogen receptor a gene polymorphisms and endometrial cancer risk. Carcinogenesis 2000a;21:623–27.

Weiderpass E, Pukkala E, Vasama-Neuvonen K, Kauppinen T, Vainio H, Paakkulainen H, Boffetta P, Partanen T. Occupational exposures and cancers of the endometrium and cervix uteri in Finland. Am J Ind Med. 2001a Jun;39(6):572–80.

Weiderpass E, Ye W, Mucci LA, Nyren O, Trichopoulos D, Vainio H, Adami HO. Alcoholism and risk for endometrial cancer. Int J Cancer 2001b Jul 15;93(2):299–301.

Weiss NS, Farewell VT, Szekely DR, English DR, Kiviat N. Oestrogens and endometrial cancer: effect of other risk factors on the association. Maturitas 1980;2:185–90.

Williams RR, Horm JW. Association of cancer sites with tobacco and alcohol consumption and socioeconomic status of patients: interview study from the Third National Cancer Survey. J Natl Cancer Inst 1977;58:525–47.

Yang S, Fang Z, Gurates B, Tamura M, Miller J, Ferrer K, SE B. Stromal PRs mediate induction of 17B-hydroxysteroid type 2 expression in human endometrial epithelium: a paracrine mechanism for inactivation of E2. Mol Endocrinol 2001;15:2093–2105.

Yaron M, Levy T, Chetrit A, Levavi H, Sabah G, Schneider D, Halperin R, Ben-Rafael Z, Friedman E: The polymorphic CAG repeat in androgen receptor gene in Jewish Israeli women with endometrial carcinoma. Cancer 2001;92:1190–94.

19

Ovarian Cancer

PENELOPE WEBB, DOROTA GERTIG,
AND DAVID HUNTER

Among the malignancies originating in the female reproductive organs, cancer of the ovary is an outlier for several reasons: No precursor lesion is established, there is no screening tool with documented efficacy, and clinical presentations often occur at a late stage. As a corollary, the prognostic outlook is poor. While the etiology of cancers of the cervix uteri and endometrium is well understood, less is known about the causes of ovarian cancer. Admittedly, epidemiologists have been relatively successful in defining the relationship between reproductive factors, notably higher parity, and interventions, such as oral contraceptive use and tubal ligation, in protecting against the disease. Because few other associations are established, long-term oral contraceptive use, tubal ligation, or oophorectomy are presently the only realistic options to achieve primary prevention and these are not practical for implementation at the population level. Several plausible biological mechanisms have been proposed to explain the relationship between these factors and the

carcinogenic process, although convincing molecular evidence for these mechanisms is lacking.

CLINICAL SYNOPSIS

Subgroups

Ovarian tumors are classified according to their tissue of origin as epithelial (90%), sex-cord stromal (6%), or germ-cell (3%) tumors. Malignant epithelial tumors may be classified as either borderline (low malignant potential) or malignant. Epithelial ovarian cancers are believed to arise from the surface epithelium of the ovary, which is derived from the celomic epithelium of the embryonic gonadal ridge—that is, the Mullerian duct—and therefore has the potential to differentiate into the types of epithelium that derive from this duct. Consequently, serous ovarian tumors are histologically similar to fallopian tube epithelium, mucinous tumors resemble the endocervix, and endometrioid ovarian tumors have the appearance of endometrial tissue.

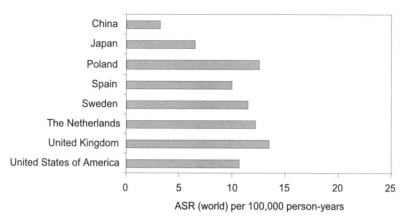

Figure 19–1. Age-standardized (to the world population) incidence rates of ovarian cancer among women. (*Source*: Ferlay et al, 2004)

Symptoms

Ovarian cancer is usually insidious, with most patients presenting when their disease has reached an advanced stage. Symptoms include abdominal pain or discomfort, abdominal swelling, or other nonspecific symptoms due to pelvic pressure such as urinary frequency. An abdominal mass is frequently present on examination.

Diagnosis

A laparotomy is essential for diagnosis, staging, and treatment of the tumor. Diagnostic imaging is also performed to exclude other causes of a pelvic mass.

Treatment

Surgical removal of the tumor is usually necessary, followed by combination chemotherapy.

Prognosis

Overall 5-year survival rates are 40% to 45%, with little change over time. A good response to treatment is seen if the cancer is confined to the ovaries (only about a quarter of cases); however, population-based screening for detection of early tumors is not available at present.

DESCRIPTIVE EPIDEMIOLOGY

The incidence of ovarian cancer varies widely among countries. In general, incidence rates are higher in developed than in less developed countries. Northern European countries like Poland, the United Kingdom, and Sweden have the highest age-standardized rates, (11–13 cases/100 000 women), Spain and other southern European countries have somewhat lower rates (9–10/100 000), and Asian countries, such as China and Japan, have the lowest rates (< 7/100 000) (Fig. 19–1). Differences in completeness of cancer surveillance may explain some of this international variation, as may variation in hysterectomy rates among countries, since fewer women are at risk of ovarian cancer in countries with higher rates of hysterectomy and oophorectomy. Other lifestyle, reproductive, dietary, and environmental factors are also likely to play a major role.

In most developed countries, incidence rates have remained relatively stable over the past 25 years. However, there is a suggestion that rates may be increasing among older women and declining among younger women. The declining trends may be explained in part by the protective effects (see following) of widely used oral contraceptives among younger women. In the United States, white women have approximately 40% higher rates of ovarian cancer than African-American and Hispanic women, and this difference has persisted in both pre- and postmenopausal women (Tortolero-Luna et al, 1994). In low-risk countries, incidence

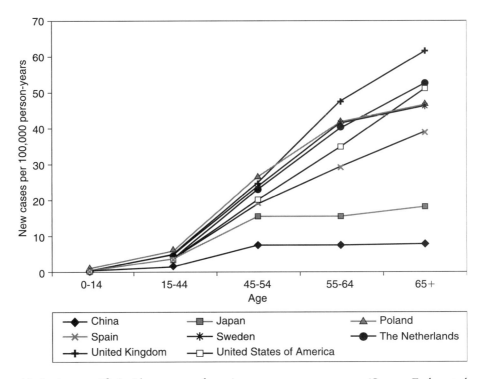

Figure 19–2. Age-specific incidence rates of ovarian cancer among women. (*Source*: Ferlay et al, 2004)

rates of ovarian cancer have increased modestly over the past 25 years.

Studies of women emigrating from low-risk countries to the United States, and studies of the descendants of these women, suggest that women born in Asia generally maintain a lower incidence of ovarian cancer than women born in the United States. However, rates are higher among younger Chinese and Japanese women born in the United States than among their Asian-born counterparts and are more similar to rates among white women in the United States (Herrinton et al, 1994).

Ovarian cancer is rare in women under 40 years of age. The risk increases sharply after about age 40 and peaks between the ages of 65 and 79 years (Fig. 19–2). Germ-cell tumors account for more than 90% of ovarian cancers in women under 40, while epithelial tumors account for about 90% of tumors overall. Most epidemiologic studies of ovarian cancer have therefore focused on epithelial cancer, the most common cancer for which data are available.

GENETIC AND MOLECULAR EPIDEMIOLOGY

Ovarian tumors are believed to result from a multistep process that involves accumulation of mutations in a number of genes, including tumor-suppressor genes and proto-oncogenes. As with other cancers, this accumulation of genetic lesions may result from progressive transformation of benign or borderline tumors although this seems a more likely model for the mucinous subtype of ovarian cancer than for the more common high-grade serous subtype (Shih and Kurman, 2004).

Inherited Susceptibility

Although the percentage of ovarian cancers explained by a positive family history is relatively small, family history has consistently emerged as a risk factor for ovarian cancer in most case-control studies, with relative risks ranging from two- to more than tenfold (Parazzini et al, 1991). The data are less consistent regarding ovarian cancer risk and a family history of breast cancer, with only about half of case-control studies showing positive associations. Familial aggregation of ovarian cancer has been described in numerous kindreds, as have a variety of heritable syndromes involving an increased risk of ovarian cancer.

Germline mutations

Germline mutations in genes associated with ovarian cancer occur in two recognized hereditary syndromes, which together account for at least 10% of all ovarian cancers (Boyd, 2003).

Breast-ovarian cancer syndrome. This syndrome accounts for about 90% of hereditary ovarian cancers. Affected families have an excess of both breast and ovarian cancer. A wide variety of germline mutations in *BRCA1*, located on chromosome 17q, and *BRCA2*, located on chromosome 13q, account for the majority of hereditary breast-ovarian cancer syndromes. The location of mutations within the *BRCA1* and *BRCA2* genes may influence the development of breast or ovarian cancer. Mutations in the 3′ untranslated region of *BRCA1* and in exon 11 of *BRCA2* have been associated with an increased risk of ovarian cancer (Gayther et al, 1995, 1997), although these observations require confirmation.

Women carrying mutations in *BRCA1* have an estimated 40% to 50% risk of developing ovarian cancer by age 70. For *BRCA2* mutation carriers, the risk is lower, about 10% to 20% (Boyd, 2003). The majority of ovarian cancers associated with germline *BRCA1* or *BRCA2* mutations are high-grade serous tumors. *BRCA1* and *BRCA2* mutations have rarely been found in sporadic breast and ovarian tumors, leading to speculation that mutations in these genes may not play a role in sporadic ovarian cancers, although allelic deletions

in chromosomes 17q and 13q frequently occur in ovarian tumors.

Site-specific ovarian cancer. In site-specific ovarian cancer, which accounts for about 10% to 15% of hereditary ovarian cancers, the ovaries are the only site involved. This syndrome is considered a variant of the hereditary breast-ovarian cancer syndrome, as most affected families have germline *BRCA1* or *BRCA2* mutations (Liede et al, 1998).

Hereditary nonpolyposis colon cancer (HNPCC) or Lynch syndrome. HNPCC is an autosomal dominant disorder that is associated with an increased risk of colorectal and other cancers, including endometrial and ovarian cancers. Ovarian cancer occurs in about 5% to 10% of female HNPCC patients. Germline mutations in genes involved in DNA mismatch repair, including *MSH2*, *MLH1*, *PMS1*, and *PMS2*, predispose to the syndrome (Lynch et al, 1998).

Rare hereditary disorders. Rare hereditary disorders predispose to the development of ovarian tumors other than epithelial tumors. Peutz-Jeghers syndrome is an autosomal dominant condition characterized by intestinal hamartomas and mucocutaneous pigmentation, as well as an increase in the frequency of sex-cord stromal tumors and epithelial ovarian tumors. Germ-cell tumors, in particular gonadoblastomas, occur with increased frequency in phenotypic females with an XY karyotype and dysgenetic gonads.

Gene polymorphisms

Common variation in genes involved in metabolism of carcinogens, hormonal pathways, and DNA repair may increase susceptibility to ovarian cancer. However, while many studies have suggested associations between various polymorphisms and ovarian cancer risk, these have rarely been confirmed in subsequent studies.

Both androgens and progestins have been implicated in the etiology of ovarian cancer. Thus it is plausible that polymorphisms in the androgen or progesterone receptor genes might influence ovarian cancer risk. A variant of the progesterone receptor gene known as *PROGINS* is characterized by an Alu insertion in intron 7 and two single nucleotide polymorphisms (SNPs) in exons 4 and 5. This variant has been associated with breast cancer risk and an early study suggested a link with ovarian cancer although subsequent studies did not consistently confirm this (Modugno, 2004). Haplotype analysis suggested that although genetic variation in the progesterone receptor was associated with risk, this was not related to the *PROGINS* variant (Pearce et al, 2005). The androgen receptor gene contains a highly polymorphic CAG repeat in exon 1, but data regarding an association with ovarian cancer risk are again inconsistent (Modugno, 2004). Similarly, polymorphisms in estrogen metabolizing genes, such as *CYP1A1*, *CYP1B1* and *CYP17*, have not been associated with risk of ovarian cancer (Spurdle et al, 2000; Goodman et al, 2001).

Somatic mutations of the *p53* gene are a relatively common event in ovarian cancer (see following). A common polymorphism in codon 72 of the *p53* gene has been well studied but no consistent association has been reported between this polymorphism and ovarian cancer risk. Mutant alleles of the highly polymorphic *HRAS1* microsatellite locus, located just downstream from the proto-oncogene H-*ras*-1, have been associated with risk of a number of cancers including ovarian cancer (Weitzel et al, 2000). Other candidate genes studied include those involved in DNA repair (for example, *XRCC2*, *XRCC3*, *RAD51*, *RAD52*, *BRCA2*), carcinogen metabolism (the glutathione S-transferases *GST-M1*, *GST-T1*, *GST-P1*, microsomal epoxide hydrolase), and inflammation (interleukins and interleukin receptor antagonists). Typically the studies have been small, often with suboptimal control groups, and initial positive findings have not been confirmed. The glutathione S-transferase polymor-

phisms have also been studied in relation to ovarian cancer survival because they may affect metabolism of chemotherapeutic agents making them less efficacious. A number of studies have reported improved outcomes among women with genotypes associated with lower GST activity (Beeghly et al, 2006) but the studies have been small, and others have found no independent association between GST genotype and survival.

Somatic Events

Ovarian carcinogenesis involves damage to oncogenes and tumor-suppressor genes within ovarian surface epithelial cells. Structural changes in chromosomes, such as translocations, insertions, and deletions, can result in oncogene activation. Tumor-suppressor genes may be inactivated in a number of ways, including loss of heterozygosity (LOH), deletions, or point mutation. The structural changes associated with abnormalities in both oncogenes and tumor-suppressor genes have been observed in numerous chromosomes in ovarian tumor cells. DNA amplification is seen in about 50% of tumors and occurs in a wide variety of genes and chromosomal locations. Most commonly, sites on chromosomes 8q, 3q, and 20q are amplified; other common sites are 7q, 17q, and 19q (Lynch et al, 1998). Loss of alleles for specific markers in ovarian epithelial tumors is observed throughout every chromosome and, together with the frequent LOH in genomic segments, suggests the presence of tumor-suppressor genes in these regions (Lynch et al, 1998). At least 30% of tumors show LOH at high frequency in chromosomes 17p,q, 18q, 6q, and 11q,p.

The *p53* gene, located on the short arm of chromosome 17, is the most frequently mutated gene in human tumors including ovarian cancer. It has been proposed that the epithelial proliferation that occurs after ovulation to repair the ovarian epithelium might increase DNA damage and consequently the risk of *p53* mutation and thus cancer. However, while one study found that women who had undergone a greater lifetime number of ovulatory cycles were more likely to have tumors that over-expressed p53 protein (Schildkraut et al, 1998), this was not confirmed in a second study (Webb et al, 1998). Although *p53* mutation is more common in advanced-stage ovarian cancers it does not appear to be an independent predictor of poorer prognosis (Hall et al, 2004).

While *p53* mutations are common in high-grade serous cancers they are less common in low-grade serous cancers and rare in borderline tumors. Over-expression of *Her2/neu* (c-ErbB-2), a cell-surface glycoprotein homologous to the epidermal growth factor receptor, and *AKT2*, a serine-threonine protein kinase, is also seen in high-grade serous cancers but rarely in borderline tumors (Shih and Kurman, 2004). Conversely, approximately one-third of borderline and low-grade invasive serous ovarian cancers carry a mutation in either *KRAS* or *BRAF*, but these mutations are rarely seen in the more common high-grade serous cancers (Singer et al, 2003). This suggests that while low-grade serous cancers may arise via progression from borderline tumors, high-grade cancers develop via a different pathway.

KRAS but not *BRAF* mutations have also been observed in up to one-half of borderline and invasive mucinous ovarian cancers (Gemignani et al, 2003). Identical mutations have been reported in benign, borderline, and invasive areas within the same tumor, suggesting that *KRAS* mutations are early events in the development of mucinous tumors via an adenoma-carcinoma sequence (Garrett et al, 2001). *KRAS* mutations are lesss common in clear cell cancers and rare in endometrioid tumors, which are more often associated with abnormalities in *PTEN* or *CTNNB1*, the gene that codes β-catenin. Both clear cell and endometrioid tumors are also associated with microsatellite instability, although this is rarely seen in serous and mucinous tumors (Shih and Kurman, 2004).

Two novel candidate tumor-suppressor genes, *OVCA1* and *OVCA2,* are located on chromosome 17p. Expression of these highly conserved genes is reduced or absent in ovarian tumors but their function and role in ovarian carcinogenesis remains unclear (Jensen and Helin, 2004).

RISK FACTORS

Tobacco

Tobacco smoking appears to increase risk of the mucinous subtype of ovarian cancer only, with little association seen for serous ovarian cancers and a possible inverse association with the endometrioid and clear cell subtypes. The relationship of tobacco use with reproductive cancers is potentially complex, as the effects of cigarette smoking on ovarian function may be both direct and indirect. Cigarette smokers have reduced levels of urinary estradiol (Westhoff et al, 1996), which may result in elevated gonadotropin levels and, on average, smokers have an earlier onset of menopause than nonsmokers (McKinlay, 1996). Postmenopausal smokers also have elevated levels of androgens compared to nonsmokers (Khaw et al, 1988). Although the vast majority of early studies found no association between cigarette smoking and ovarian cancer risk, recent case-control and cohort studies have fairly consistently shown a two- to threefold increased risk of mucinous ovarian cancer among smokers (Marchbanks et al, 2000; Green et al, 2001; Terry et al, 2003; Jordan et al, 2007). The risks increase with increasing pack-years of smoking and return to baseline within 20 to 30 years of smoking cessation. In contrast, smoking does not appear to increase risk of serous cancers and results from a pooled analysis of 10 case-control studies suggest that it may be inversely associated with the endometrioid and clear cell subtypes of ovarian cancer (Kurian et al, 2005). This latter observation is consistent with the observed reduction in risk of endometrial cancer among smokers (U.S. Department of Health and Human Services, 2004).

Diet

The initial suggestions of a potential link between ovarian cancer and dietary factors came from international correlations between national ovarian cancer incidence and mortality rates and per capita dietary consumption data. Positive correlations between ovarian cancer mortality rates and intake of total fat in various countries were noted by Armstrong and Doll (1975) (r = 0.79) and by Rose et al (1986) (r = 0.67). Positive correlations were highest for milk and meats and weaker for eggs. Strong inverse correlations were observed between mortality rates for ovarian cancer and vegetable availability. An association between increased westernization of the Japanese diet—that is, increases in the intake of fat-rich foods—and increased mortality from ovarian cancer has also been noted (Kato et al, 1987).

Dairy foods and lactose/galactose

High intake of lactose-containing foods may slightly increase a woman's risk of ovarian cancer although the data are not consistent. The strong correlation between ovarian cancer and per capita milk consumption led to the hypothesis that consumption of lactose may be a risk factor for ovarian cancer. Dietary lactose is hydrolysed to glucose and galactose and Cramer and colleagues (1989) proposed that galactose may be a risk factor for ovarian cancer, as galactose is toxic to oocytes. Hypergonadotropic hypogonadism and early ovarian failure occur in women with reduced activity of the enzyme galactose-1-phosphate uridyltransferase (GALT), which converts galactose to glucose. Subsequent increases in gonadotropin-releasing hormones may stimulate neoplastic changes in the ovary (Cramer et al, 1989).

Case control studies that have examined lactose intake—milk consumption in particular—and the risk of ovarian cancer have given mixed results but, overall, do not support any substantial association (Larsson et al, 2006). The results of three published cohort studies are more consistent and a meta-analysis of these based on 728 cases suggested a significant 13% increase in risk of ovarian cancer for every additional 10g of lactose consumed per day (Larsson et al, 2006). However, a more comprehensive pooled analysis that included both pub-lished and unpublished data from 12 cohort studies with a total of 2132 cases reported a more modest effect with a nonsignificant 4% increase in risk per 10g of lactose (Genkinger et al, 2006a). Women who consumed more than 30g of lactose per day (equivalent to 3 glasses of milk) were, however, at significantly higher risk than those consuming less than 10g (RR = 1.2). The results did not vary appreciably for the different subtypes of ovarian cancer. Studies evaluating the relation between vitamin D and calcium intake and ovarian cancer risk have reported mixed results. The pooled cohort analysis found no association with calcium intake but reported a modest but statistically significant increase in risk with increasing dietary vitamin D intake (pooled RR = 1.06 per 100 IU vitamin D per day) although no association was seen for total vitamin D including supplements (Genkinger et al, 2006a).

In an early case-control study GALT activity measured in erythrocytes was inversely related to ovarian cancer (Cramer et al, 1989). The protective effect of oral contraceptives was limited to women with high lactose consumption in a secondary analysis of this study, suggesting that oral contraceptives might counter the hypergonadotropic effect of galactose (Harlow et al, 1991). Subsequent studies have not, however, confirmed the association with low GALT activity (Fung et al, 2003).

Coffee and tea

Evidence regarding the association between coffee and tea drinking and ovarian cancer risk is currently inconsistent. While coffee drinking has been associated with an approximately twofold increased risk of ovarian cancer in some case-control studies (Whittemore et al, 1988; Kuper et al, 2000), most studies have not found a dose–response association and others have detected no elevation in risk (Jordan et al, 2004; Larsson and Wolk, 2005a). The mechanism for a potential association between coffee drinking and ovarian cancer is unclear. Caffeine may be associated with menstrual cycle abnormalities (Fenster et al, 1999) and coffee drinking has been reportedly linked with decreased maternal pregnancy estrogen levels (Petridou et al, 1992) and early follicular estrogen levels (Lucero et al, 2001). However, there is little evidence for a direct role of estrogens in ovarian cancer, and coffee has not been associated with either breast or endometrial cancer, both of which are more strongly associated with increased estrogen levels.

In 2002, Zhang and colleagues reported that tea drinking, particularly green tea, was associated with a significant 70% reduction in risk of ovarian cancer in a Chinese case-control study (Zhang et al, 2002a). In contrast, most studies conducted in non-Asian populations where black tea is more common have not reported any association between tea drinking and ovarian cancer risk (Kuper et al, 2000; Jordan et al, 2004). An exception is a recent cohort study from Sweden that reported a significant inverse association between tea consumption and ovarian cancer risk (Larsson and Wolk, 2005b). An association is biologically plausible as both black and green tea contain abundant polyphenols that have been shown to inhibit carcinogenesis in in vitro and animal studies (Yang et al, 2002).

Dietary fat and eggs
Fat intake has not been consistently linked with ovarian cancer. Case-control studies in several countries have reported an association between ovarian cancer risk and intake of saturated or animal fat, but not of vegetable fat or polyunsaturated fat (Cramer et al, 1984; Shu et al, 1989; Risch et al, 1994a). However, there was no association between intake of animal fat or saturated fat and ovarian cancer in two published cohort studies (Kushi et al, 1999; Bertone et al, 2002). A meta-analysis that included one cohort and seven case-control studies with a total of 2314 cases found a positive association for total fat intake (RR = 1.24) as well as for saturated fat (RR = 1.20) and animal fat (RR = 1.70) (Huncharek and Kupelnick, 2001). However, a pooled analysis of 12 cohort studies that included 2132 cases reported a significant association only

for saturated fat (RR = 1.29), and this was only seen at the highest decile of intake (Genkinger et al, 2006b).

A number of case-control and cohort studies have reported a significant association between egg consumption and ovarian cancer risk (Pirozzo et al, 2002), but in a pooled analysis of cohort studies the risk of ovarian cancer did not differ significantly between women who consumed more than about one egg per day or less than one per week (Genkinger et al, 2006b).

Fruit and vegetables
Overall it seems unlikely that fruit and vegetable intake have any major effect on ovarian cancer risk although vegetables or their components may have a modest protective effect. An inverse association between ovarian cancer and intake of green vegetables, carrots, and certain micronutrients, for example, vitamins A and E, has been noted in some case-control studies (Cramer et al, 2001; Zhang et al, 2002b), while a meta-analysis of five case-control studies found a significant inverse association for beta-carotene (Huncharek et al, 2001). Recent cohort studies including a pooled analysis of 12 cohort studies have, however, found no association between either vegetable or fruit intake and ovarian cancer risk (Fairfield et al, 2001; Koushik et al, 2005; Schulz et al, 2005). The only exception is a Swedish study that reported a significant inverse association with increasing vegetable intake but not for fruit (Larsson et al, 2004b).

Cohort studies have also reported null results for micronutrients including vitamins A, C, and E (Kushi et al, 1999; Fairfield et al, 2001), and a pooled analysis of 10 cohort studies found no association with any of the major carotenoids (Koushik et al, 2006). Increasing folate intake has been associated with a reduced risk of ovarian cancer, particularly among women with higher alcohol intake, in some (Kelemen et al, 2004; Larsson et al, 2004a) but not all (Tworoger et al, 2006) studies. Vitamin E intake was associated with increased survival in one study (Nagle et al, 2003).

Alcohol

Alcohol intake, at least at moderate levels, does not appear to increase risk of ovarian cancer. Alcohol affects the reproductive system and is, therefore, potentially a risk factor for ovarian cancer. It could be a direct ovarian toxin and may also act on the hypothalamic-pituitary axis. In alcohol-fed rats, functional and histologic ovarian failure has been demonstrated, with an absence of corpora lutea and developing follicles, as well as a decrease in estradiol concentration and an increase in estrone concentration (Van Thiel et al, 1978). Alcoholism is associated with menstrual abnormalities, reproductive problems, and changes in secondary sex characteristics. In studies of moderate long-term alcohol intake by healthy women, there are inconsistencies in the degree of alteration in hormone levels. Hankinson et al (1995) noted a positive association between long-term alcohol intake and postmenopausal plasma levels of estrogen and estrone sulfate, but other studies yielded contradictory results (London et al, 1991).

Results of epidemiologic studies have been inconsistent. A meta-analysis of population-based studies reported a 30% reduction in risk of ovarian cancer among women with the highest intake of alcohol (Webb et al, 2004), but more recent pooled analyses of data from 10 US-based case-control studies (Kurian et al, 2005) and 10 cohort studies (Genkinger et al, 2006c) reported no association between alcohol intake and ovarian cancer risk. Similarly, while some studies have reported inverse associations between wine consumption and ovarian cancer (Kelemen et al, 2004; Webb et al, 2004), no such association was seen in the pooled cohort analysis (Genkinger et al, 2006c).

In a prospective study of alcoholic women in Sweden, an overall deficit of cases of ovarian cancer of about 14% was noted. This deficit was particularly strong and statistically significant among alcoholic women below 60 years of age (Lagiou et al, 2001) and is compatible with the reported reduction of gonadotropin levels among alcoholic women below age 60 and with the hypothesis invoking these gonadotropins in the etiology of ovarian cancer.

Reproductive Factors

Parity

Nulliparity is a well-established risk factor for ovarian cancer. Almost all studies have found a lower risk of ovarian cancer among women who have had at least one child than among nulliparous women (Whittemore et al, 1992a; Adami et al, 1994; Risch et al, 1994b). The large Swedish study by Adami and colleagues (1994) also observed a nearly 60% decrease in risk among women with more than five births compared to women with only one birth (RR = 0.44). The protective effect of parity applied to all invasive ovarian cancers, including epithelial, germ cell, and stromal tumors, but was less pronounced for borderline tumors.

Several large studies have demonstrated significant trends toward increasing protection with each birth, with a decrease in risk of approximately 20% for each subsequent live birth (Negri et al, 1991; Whittemore et al, 1992a; Adami et al, 1994; Risch et al, 1994b). However, the potential role of difficulty in conceiving must be considered in order to distinguish the effects of nulliparity from those of infertility (Weiss, 1988). In studies addressing this issue, a significant inverse association between parity and ovarian cancer was noted, even among women with no history of infertility (Whittemore et al, 1992a; Risch et al, 1994b).

There is conflicting evidence regarding the effect of age at first pregnancy on ovarian cancer risk. Several case-control studies found a higher risk of ovarian cancer with older age at first birth, while other studies, including one prospective study, found no such association after adjustment for parity (Parazzini et al, 1991). Similarly, some studies have observed a lower risk among women who were older at the time of their last birth (Whiteman et al, 2003), but others have not confirmed this.

One explanation for the protective effect of parity is the interruption of ovulation due to pregnancy, consistent with the incessant ovulation hypothesis, which states that repeated trauma to ovarian surface epithelium from repeated ovulation increases the risk of ovarian cancer. Alternatively, pregnancy may exert long-lasting effects on gonadotropin secretion. However, differences in gonadotropin concentration according to parity or age at first pregnancy have not been consistently observed. Pregnancy is also associated with high levels of progesterone, which may reduce ovarian cancer risk (Risch, 1998). Evidence to support this latter hypothesis comes from observations that, although they have higher gonadotropin levels and are more likely to double ovulate than women with only singleton births, mothers of twins do not have an elevated risk ovarian cancer. Instead women who have twins appear to have a slightly lower risk of ovarian cancer and this has been attributed to the higher progesterone levels associated with twin pregnancies (Whiteman et al, 2000).

On the basis of these hypotheses, failed pregnancies (miscarriages, abortions, or ectopic pregnancies) would be predicted to confer less protection against ovarian cancer than full-term pregnancies. Indeed, such an effect has been observed, particularly among parous women.

Infertility and fertility drugs

There is growing concern about the possible role of fertility drugs in ovarian cancer. Over the past 20 years, the use of fertility drugs has increased substantially because indications for their use have expanded. Clomiphene citrate—an estrogen antagonist—human chorionic gonadotropin, and gonadotropin-releasing hormone agonists are used to induce ovulation in infertile women. To varying degrees, all of these agents increase the number of ovulations per cycle, the number of follicles developed, and the number of oocytes obtained. They may also be associated with raised levels of endogenous hormones, particularly estrogen and progesterone.

The evidence linking infertility and ovarian cancer is inconsistent. Studies have been limited by imprecise definitions of infertility,

difficulties in distinguishing associations with treatment from confounding by indications for treatment, and small numbers of cases. Aside from numerous case reports of ovarian cancer following treatment with fertility drugs, several case-control and cohort studies have studied the relationship between use of infertility drugs and risk of ovarian cancer (Brinton et al, 2005). The largest cohort study, carried out among women undergoing in vitro fertilization, revealed no excess risk among women treated with ovarian stimulation (Venn et al, 1999). However, an increased risk of ovarian cancer more than 15 years after treatment and among subgroups of women with prolonged use or who remain nulliparous cannot be excluded (Whittemore et al, 1992a; Ness et al, 2002; Brinton et al, 2004). Most studies show little or no increase in risk of invasive ovarian cancer in infertile women (Venn et al, 2003), although increased risk has been reported for specific causes of infertility including endometriosis (see "Medical Conditions and Treatment," following).

Tubal ligation and hysterectomy

The relationship between tubal ligation and reduced risk of ovarian cancer is well established, with the majority of epidemiologic studies showing an inverse association with relative risks varying between 0.2 and 0.9 (Hankinson et al, 1993). Studies examining hysterectomy and ovarian cancer risk have demonstrated similar inverse associations (Kreiger et al, 1997). Surgical sterilization is a relatively common procedure in some countries, notably the United States, and is often considered together with hysterectomy in regard to ovarian cancer risk on the assumption that these procedures act via similar mechanisms.

The proposed biological rationale for these procedures in preventing ovarian cancer is threefold. First, both types of surgery may prevent potential carcinogens from ascending the reproductive tract, via the fallopian tubes, to the ovaries. Indeed, Cramer and colleagues (1982) hypothesized that potential environmental carcinogens gain access to the ovarian surface epithelium via the genital tract, leading to tumor formation. Second, both tubal ligation and hysterectomy may affect ovarian circulation or plasma hormone levels, although there is no convincing empirical evidence for this theory. Finally, there may be differences in menstrual cycle regularity following tubal ligation (Dennerstein et al, 1997).

The timing of surgery may be a relevant factor. If a lag period is required to achieve the protective effect then women who had their surgery several years prior to the study period may be more likely to be protected than women who had more recent surgery. Furthermore, women undergoing these procedures have their ovaries screened for abnormalities; women whose ovaries are found to be normal at the time of surgery will be less likely to develop ovarian cancer than women who have not had the opportunity to be examined—a "healthy screenee effect" (Irwin et al, 1991). If the reduced risk were due only to screening, this effect would diminish once enough time had elapsed after surgery for new malignant lesions to develop. Thus far, studies addressing this question have shown that the reduced risk appears to persist for at least 10 years following surgery (Kjaer et al, 2004).

Tubal ligation was also associated with a reduced risk of ovarian cancer among *BRCA1* mutation carriers, suggesting this may be a feasible option for high-risk women who have completed their family to reduce their risk of ovarian cancer (Narod et al, 2001).

Breast feeding

Lactation may reduce risk of ovarian cancer by suppressing ovulation. Most studies have found that women who have ever breast-fed are at lower risk of ovarian cancer than parous women who never breast-fed, and a trend toward decreasing risk with an increasing number of months of breast-feeding has been observed (Rosenblatt and Thomas, 1993; Kurian et al, 2005). Because the suppression of ovulation is stronger in the early postnatal period than after a lon-

ger duration of breast-feeding, the reduction in risk would be expected to be greatest during the first few months after birth. Rosenblatt and Thomas (1993) demonstrated a reduction in risk with short-term lactation, but this effect was not apparent for women who had breast-fed for longer durations. In a pooled analysis of 12 case-control studies, Whittemore et al (1992b) estimated that the reduction in risk per year of anovulation associated with breast-feeding was 8.5% for women less than 55 years of age—that is, smaller than the estimated 28% reduction in risk associated with pregnancy (which suppresses ovulation more effectively than does lactation).

Hormones

Oral contraceptive use

Oral contraceptive use is widely accepted as being inversely associated with the risk of ovarian cancer. A lower risk among women using oral contraceptives has been consistently observed in the majority of studies, and the summary relative risk based upon 20 epidemiologic studies through 1991 was estimated as 0.64 for ever use of oral contraceptives (Hankinson et al, 1992). Other pooled analyses also revealed a 30% to 40% reduction in ovarian cancer risk for ever users compared with never users (Whittemore et al, 1992a; Kurian et al, 2005).

The protective effect of oral contraceptives increases with the duration of use, the reduction in risk being about 10% per year (Hankinson et al, 1992). Furthermore, the protective effect appears to persist up to 30 years after discontinuation of use (Ness et al, 2000b). Short-term use may also provide some benefit; in the Cancer and Steroid Hormone Study, risk decreased even among women who used oral contraceptives for only 3 to 6 months (Anonymous, 1987). Similar reductions have also been reported for women who carry BRCA mutations in most studies that have evaluated this (Whittemore et al, 2004).

There may be differences among the associations between oral contraceptive use and different histologic types of ovarian tumors. The risk of nonepithelial ovarian tumors in the Cancer and Steroid Hormone Study was elevated with oral contraceptive use, although the number of tumors was small (Anonymous, 1987). An Australian study found that the protective effects of parity and oral contraceptive use were greater for nonmucinous than mucinous tumors (Purdie et al, 2001b), but others have found similar effects for all subtypes (Kurian et al, 2005).

The mechanism of protection by oral contraceptives may relate to suppression of plasma pituitary gonadotropins or inhibition of ovulation. Higher-dose preparations cause greater suppression of gonadotropins than more recent lower-dose preparations. However, few studies have specifically considered the effect of dose of ethinyl estradiol or progesterone. In one study, high-dose preparations were not associated with a greater reduction in risk than preparations containing lower doses of estradiol and progesterone (Ness et al, 2000b); however, a second study has reported greater protection for high-progestin formulations (Schildkraut et al, 2002). Furthermore, use of progestin-only contraceptives, which do not consistently inhibit ovulation, also appears to be associated with a reduced risk of ovarian cancer (Anonymous, 1987).

Postmenopausal hormone use

Use of hormone replacement therapy has been directly associated with ovarian cancer risk although there is currently limited information regarding the effects of different formulations. Positive but not uniformly significant associations for ever versus never use of estrogen or estrogen plus progestin replacement therapy have been seen in several but not all case-control studies. A meta-analysis of studies published through 1997 estimated a significant summary relative risk for ever use of 1.15, with the greatest risk for a duration of use of more than 10 years (Garg et al, 1998). In a reanalysis of four European case-control studies, Negri et al (1999) reported a 70% elevation in ovarian cancer risk with ever use of hormone replacement therapy, which declined with time since last use.

Only limited data exist comparing estrogen-only and combined estrogen and progestin formulations in relation to ovarian cancer. The strong protective effect of pregnancy, which is associated with high progesterone levels, suggests that adding progestins might mitigate any potential adverse effects of estrogen as is seen for endometrial cancer. The results of one large case-control study support this as the use of estrogens and sequential progestins conferred about the same modest excess risk as estrogens alone, but no association was seen for estrogens with continuous addition of progestins (Riman et al, 2002). More recently, however, a US-based cohort study reported that use of estrogen plus continuous progestins was associated with a significant increase in risk of ovarian cancer, similar in magnitude to that seen for estrogen alone, while an even stronger effect was seen for estrogen plus sequential progestins (Lacey et al, 2006). The Women's Health Initiative trial also reported a nonsignificant 60% increase in risk of ovarian cancer among women assigned to estrogen plus continuous progestin (Anderson et al, 2003).

The various histologic tumor subtypes may differ in estrogen responsiveness. In particular, endometrioid tumors, which resemble endometrial tissue, may be more responsive to estrogen than other types. An increase in the risk of endometrioid ovarian cancers associated with ever use of estrogen replacement therapy compared with never use has been observed in some (Purdie et al, 1999; Riman et al, 2002) but not all studies (Kurian et al, 2005).

Despite the relatively strong evidence for a role of pituitary or sex hormones in ovarian cancer etiology—in particular, the consistent inverse relationship of ovarian cancer with parity and oral contraceptive use—the role of estrogen replacement therapy remains incompletely understood. Estrogens administered during menopause decrease pituitary hormone levels through negative feedback and, under the gonadotropin hypothesis, this effect would be expected to protect against ovarian cancer (Table 19–1) but, overall, use of postmenopausal estrogen appears if anything to increase risk.

Lifetime number of ovulatory cycles
Women who have experienced higher numbers of ovulations are at increased risk of ovarian cancer. The number of a woman's lifetime ovulatory cycles is primarily determined by parity and by duration of oral contraceptive use, as well as the onset and cessation of menses. The ovulatory hypothesis predicts that longer periods of anovulation would protect against ovarian cancer. In addition to the large body of ev-

idence supporting the inverse association of parity and oral contraceptive use with ovarian cancer, studies have specifically examined the association of calculated number of lifetime ovulatory cycles and ovarian cancer. These studies observed a reduction in the risk of ovarian cancer among women with fewer lifetime ovulatory cycles compared to women with a greater number of cycles (Schildkraut et al, 1998; Webb et al, 1998). Whittemore et al (1992b) examined the percentage reduction of invasive epithelial ovarian cancer due to different causes of anovulation. Pregnancy

Table 19–1. Mechanisms proposed for ovarian cancer pathogenesis

Hypothesis	Mechanisms proposed for ovarian cancer pathogenesis	Epidemiologic evidence consistent with hypotheses	Epidemiologic evidence inconsistent with hypotheses
Incessant ovulation	Damage to ovarian epithelium from repeated ovulation leads to neoplasia.	Reduced risk with parity, breast-feeding and oral contraceptive use. Increased risk with increased lifetime ovulatory cycles.	No clear protective effect of late menarche or early menopause.
Excess gonadotropin stimulation	Excess gonadotropin secretion leads to increased estrogen stimulation of ovarian epithelium.	Reduced risk with parity and oral contraceptive use.	Hormone replacement therapy (HRT) has been associated with increased risk but HRT reduces gonatropin levels. Lactation increases gonadotropins but has been associated with decreased risk.
Pregnancy clearance	High levels of progesterone in pregnancy clear the ovaries of transformed cells.	Reduced risk with increasing parity and possibly with higher age at first / lower age at last pregnancy; this effect diminishes with time.	
Exogenous carcinogens	Environmental carcinogens gain access to ovaries through reproductive tract.	Tubal ligation reduces risk. Perineal talc use associated with risk of ovarian cancer in some studies.	
Inflammation	Local inflammation and inflammatory cytokines damage the ovarian epithelium leading to neoplasia.	Factors associated with inflammation such as ovulation, talc use, endometriosis associated with increased risk.	Anti-inflammatory drugs not clearly associated with reduced risk.

appeared to confer the greatest protection against ovarian cancer among younger women, and oral contraceptive use was most protective for women over 55 years of age.

Age at menarche and age at menopause are determining factors of reproductive duration; however, neither is clearly associated with ovarian cancer risk (Riman et al, 2004b). A possible explanation for this lack of association comes from an examination of the timing of ovulation and ovarian cancer. Ovulations around the age of menarche and menopause, which are more likely to be anovulatory, were less strongly associated with ovarian cancer risk than those in the peak reproductive years (20–29 years of age) (Purdie et al, 2003).

Although the number of ovulations appears to play a role in the etiology of ovarian cancer, it is not sufficient to explain the pathogenesis of ovarian cancer. This is because the reduction in risk associated with factors such as parity and oral contraceptive use is much greater than would be predicted simply from their suppression of ovulation (Risch, 1998).

Proposed hormonal mechanisms
A number of theories have been put forward to explain the pathogenesis of ovarian cancer (Table 19–1). Fathalla (1971) proposed that incessant ovulation causes repeated minor trauma to the epithelial surface of the ovary, leading to proliferation of ovarian epithelium and repair of the ovulatory wound. Entrapment of surface epithelium within the ovarian stroma occurs when inclusion cysts are formed during ovulation. This event is of potential importance, as these cysts break down the normal barrier between the hormonally active stroma and the surface epithelium, resulting in proliferation due to excess stimulation of the entrapped epithelium by hormonal factors and possibly an increased risk of ovarian cancer.

An alternative hypothesis, originally proposed by Stadel (1975), relates to exposure of ovarian surface epithelium to high levels of circulating pituitary gonadotropins, particularly follicle-stimulating hormone (FSH). Animal studies have shown that high gonadotropin levels are associated with ovarian cancer, although animal tumors are usually stromal in origin and may not appropriately represent the epithelial cancers of humans. Gonadotropins also stimulate growth of human ovarian cancer cell lines (Simon et al, 1983). Furthermore, secretion of gonadotropins increases with age, peaking after menopause. This pattern resembles that of ovarian cancer incidence, although the latter peak occurs approximately 15 years after the peak in FSH levels (Cramer and Welch, 1983).

Lastly, Adami et al (1994) suggested that pregnancy may clear ovaries from cells in various stages of malignant transformation and, more recently, it has been proposed that this effect may be mediated by the high progesterone levels seen in pregnancy. Data to support this hypothesis come from a primate study in which oral contraceptives containing progestin were found to stimulate apoptosis in the ovarian epithelium (Rodriguez et al, 1998). Androgen concentrations are higher than estrogen levels during the follicular phase of the menstrual cycle, thus androgens may also be relevant to the etiology of ovarian cancer (Risch, 1998).

Anthropometric Measures

The evidence regarding a relationship between obesity and ovarian cancer risk is contradictory. Increased risks of ovarian cancer among overweight or obese women have been reported from both prospective and case-control studies (Purdie et al, 2001a; Schouten et al, 2003), but others have observed no such association (Fairfield et al, 2002b). The results of a meta-analysis suggested a modest association between obesity and ovarian cancer with a significant 40% increase in risk seen for the heaviest compared to the lightest women in population-based case-control studies and a 20% increase among cohort studies (Purdie et al, 2001a). Given the strong association between obesity and risk of endometrial cancer it might be expected that any association with ovarian cancer would be strongest for the endometrioid subtype. However, while stronger risks have been reported for endometrioid ovarian tumors in some studies (Farrow et al, 1989), this has not been consistent (Purdie et al, 2001a).

Obesity affects sex-steroid hormone levels via several pathways: It increases the peripheral conversion of androgens to estrogens in adipose tissue by aromatization, it increases free estradiol levels by reducing sex hormone-binding globulin capacity, and it increases androgen secretion in the adrenal gland (Farrow et al, 1989). Postmenopausal obesity has been associated with an increased risk of hormone-related cancers, particularly breast and endometrial cancers. Premenopausal obesity may lead to an increased number of anovulatory menstrual cycles, which would potentially reduce the ovarian cancer risk. The effects of obesity on ovarian cancer risk may, therefore, differ by menopausal status and may be modified by whether a woman is taking postmenopausal hormones. In the postmenopausal period, when peripheral conversion of androgens is the main source of estrogens, the effect of obesity may be "overwhelmed" in the analysis by the much higher levels of estrogens ingested through taking postmenopausal hormones. Stratification by histologic subtype may also be important.

Physical Activity

Findings regarding physical activity and risk of ovarian cancer are contradictory. Vigorous physical activity can lead to anovulation, luteal-phase insufficiency, and amenorrhea (Ellison et al, 1993). Thus, during the reproductive years, vigorous activity may decrease ovarian cancer risk due to an increase in anovulatory cycles. Alternatively, serum estrogen levels have been inversely correlated with physical activity in postmenopausal women, possibly leading to an increase in gonadotropins via hypothalamic feedback and potentially increasing the ovarian cancer risk.

Several case-control studies have reported an inverse association between recreational physical activity and ovarian cancer risk (Riman et al, 2004a; Pan et al, 2005). In contrast, no inverse association was observed in several large prospective studies in the United States and Scandinavia (Bertone et al, 2001; Patel et al, 2006; Weiderpass et al, 2006); rather a modest increase in risk with frequent vigorous activity was found in some studies (Bertone et al, 2001). Studies of occupational physical activity have also shown inconsistent results (Zheng et al, 1993; Pukkala et al, 1993), but sedentary behavior has been associated with increased ovarian cancer risk (Patel et al, 2006).

Infections

Evidence regarding an assoiation between mumps infection and ovarian cancer risk is inconsistent. Mumps virus has an affinity for glandular tissue, including the ovaries, and premature menopause has occasionally been documented following mumps parotitis or oophoritis. Some studies have indicated an inverse association of ovarian cancer with a history of mumps parotitis, with cases less likely to report past infection than controls (Menczer et al, 1979; Cramer et al, 1983). Others have, however, reported no association and a small Chinese case-control study documented significantly higher mumps antibody titers in cases (Chen et al, 1992). Late infection with Epstein-Barr virus (Littman et al, 2003) and past or chronic persistent infection with *Chlamydia trachomatis* (Ness et al, 2003) have also been associated with increased risk of ovarian cancer, but these results have yet to be confirmed.

Ionizing Radiation

Ionizing radiation appears to modestly increase the risk of ovarian cancer; however, because of the small percentage of women exposed, the population-attributable risk is likely to be low. Follow-up studies of female survivors of the atomic bomb explosions in Hiroshima and Nagasaki suggest that the incidence of ovarian cancer was increased twofold among women exposed to more than 100 rads over that among women who had not been exposed (Tokuoka et al, 1987).

The increase was particularly prominent among women who were of reproductive age at the time of the detonation and was not seen until 20 years after exposure.

The incidence of ovarian cancer has also been found to increase following radiation treatment for cancers and a variety of other disorders. Radiation therapy for benign pelvic conditions was associated with an 80% increase in the risk of ovarian cancer in two studies (Doll and Smith, 1968; Wagoner, 1984). Among 150 000 women who received radiation therapy for cervical cancer, the incidence of ovarian cancer was increased after 10 years (RR = 1.4) (Boice et al, 1988). In a small case-control study in New York, a history of pelvic x-rays was associated with a nonsignificant 30% increase in risk of ovarian cancer overall with a significant excess risk seen for women of Jewish ancestry (Harlap et al, 2002). In contrast, no excess of ovarian cancer was observed in a study of Chinese diagnostic x-ray workers (Wang et al, 1988) and a British study found no elevation in risk among women irradiated for ankylosing spondylitis (Darby et al, 1987).

Occupation

A potential link between ovarian cancer and asbestos exposure was first reported in 1960 in a case series of women with asbestosis who also had a diagnosis of ovarian cancer (Keal, 1960). Follow-up studies of female workers employed in asbestos-related industries have documented excess deaths from ovarian cancer (Wignall and Fox, 1982). An excess of mortality from ovarian cancer has been noted among employees in health care industries that may entail exposure to hazardous substances such as radiation and chemotherapeutic drugs (Sala et al, 1998). Potential problems with these studies are that peritoneal mesotheliomas and ovarian cancer may be difficult to distinguish and that histologic material was not available for all cases. Some studies have suggested an increased risk of ovarian cancer among hairdressers and beauticians, but the data are inconclusive (Shen et al, 1998).

Medical Conditions and Treatment

The association between ovarian cancer risk and infertility, use of fertility drugs, and surgical procedures such as tubal ligation and hysterectomy has already been described. Other medical conditions related to hormonal imbalances have also been evaluated for their potential role in ovarian cancer etiology. Polycystic ovarian syndrome (PCOS) occurs in about 1% to 5% of the population and is characterized by androgen excess and an elevated LH (luteinizing hormone) to FSH ratio. In the Cancer and Steroid Hormone Study, an elevated risk of ovarian cancer was seen among women diagnosed with PCOS (RR = 2.5), but the study included only seven cases with PCOS (Schildkraut et al, 1996). A history of endometriosis has consistently been linked to an increased risk of ovarian cancer, particularly the endometrioid and clear cell subtypes (Brinton et al, 1997; Ness et al, 2000a). Some studies have oberved an association between pelvic inflammatory disease and ovarian cancer (Ness and Cottreau, 1999).

Use of nonsteroidal anti-inflammatory drugs (NSAIDs) has been considered as a possible protective factor for ovarian cancer but the results are inconsistent. Some studies have reported significant inverse associations between use of aspirin (Schildkraut et al, 2006) or other NSAIDs (Fairfield et al, 2002a) and ovarian cancer risk. In contrast, others have observed no association for NSAIDs, but signficant reductions in risk for long-term or regular use of acetaminophen (Cramer et al, 1998; Moysich et al, 2001).

The potential link between inflammatory medical conditions, use of anti-inflammatory medications, and ovarian cancer risk led Ness and Cottreau (1999) to propose a possible role for ovarian epithelial inflammation in the development of ovarian cancer (Table 19–1).

Other Risk Factors

Talcum powder

There is lack of agreement regarding the relationship between perineal talc use and ovarian cancer. Talc is a natural mineral fiber similar in composition to asbestos, which has been linked to ovarian cancer. The hypothesis for the association of talc and ovarian cancer is based on the ability of talc fibers to migrate up the female genital tract and lodge in the ovaries. Indeed, talc fibers have been detected in benign and malignant ovarian tissue, although no relation between reported levels of talc exposure and ovarian talc counts has been discerned (Heller et al, 1996). The few relevant studies of talc exposure in animals have not demonstrated a consistent increase in ovarian cancer among animals subjected to chronic aerosol talc exposure (Boorman and Seely, 1995). However, these data should be interpreted cautiously, given the anatomic and physiologic differences between rodents and humans.

The first case-control study linking talc and ovarian cancer, published in 1982, showed an almost twofold increase in the risk of ovarian cancer with any perineal talc use (Cramer et al, 1982). Most subsequent case-control studies found positive associations with talc use, although not all were statistically significant and the magnitude of the observed risks was modest, ranging from 1.2 to 2.0 with a pooled estimate of 1.4 from a meta-analysis (Huncharek et al, 2003). While some studies demonstrated a marginally significant increasing trend in risk with increased frequency of use, duration of use, and "total lifetime applications" (Harlow et al, 1992; Cramer et al, 1999), other studies detected no significant dose–response association (Whittemore et al, 1988; Mills et al, 2004). Case-control studies are potentially limited by recall bias, which might account for the observed positive associations. The only prospective study to address this question found no overall association between talc use and ovarian cancer, but information on duration of use was not available (Gertig et al, 2000).

The association between talc use and ovarian cancer may be limited to serous ovarian cancers as the strongest associations have generally been reported for this sub-type (Cramer et al, 1999; Gertig et al, 2000; Mills et al, 2004). It would be expected that any association between talc and ovarian cancer would be restricted to women with a patent genital tract in whom talc could conceivably migrate up to the ovaries. However, while some have reported stronger associations among women who have not undergone tubal sterilization (Mills et al, 2004), others have reported no such differences (Gertig et al, 2000).

CONCLUSION

Older age and family history have strong positive associations with risk of ovarian cancer, while oral contraceptive use, increased parity, breast-feeding, and tubal ligation are inversely associated with risk. These factors provide evidence for more than one proposed mechanism of ovarian cancer pathogenesis (Table 19–1). Oral contraceptive use and parity provide support for both the incessant ovulation hypothesis and the gonadotropin hypothesis. Both factors induce anovulation and are associated with decreases in gonadotropin concentrations.

The association between breast-feeding and ovarian cancer is consistent with the incessant ovulation hypothesis, but this and the assocation with postemenopausal hormone use contradict the gonadotropin hypothesis. Use of postmenopausal hormones decreases circulating levels of LH and FSH and thus would be expected to decrease the ovarian cancer risk. Lactation increases FSH, but studies have generally observed an inverse association of lactation with ovarian cancer. The biological mechanism for the effects of tubal ligation is unclear and may involve decreased access of environmental carcinogens, changes in the hormonal milieu, or changes in blood flow to the ovaries.

Ovarian tumors are histologically heterogeneous, resembling different epithelial surfaces of the reproductive tract. Different histologic subtypes of epithelial ovarian cancer may thus have different etiologies. The inability of many studies to stratify tumors by subtype due to insufficient numbers of cases of the less common subtypes may explain the lack of consistent findings for some risk factors among studies.

Apart from oral contraceptive use, there are few readily modifiable risk factors for ovarian cancer. There is contradictory evidence for a possible increase in risk with lactose consumption, saturated fat intake, and talc use and for a decrease in risk with vegetable intake, while smoking appears to increase risk of mucinous ovarian tumors only. It is unclear whether obesity and/or physical activity influence ovarian cancer risk. Together with the lack of procedures available for population-based routine screening, the lack of modifiable risk factors underscores the need for further research on preventable causes of ovarian cancer in addition to advances in treatment.

REFERENCES

Adami HO, Hsieh CC, Lambe M, Trichopoulos D, Leon D, Persson I, et al. Parity, age at first childbirth, and risk of ovarian cancer. Lancet 1994;344:1250–54.

Anderson GL, Judd HL, Kaunitz AM, Barad DH, Beresford SA, Pettinger M, et al. Effects of estrogen plus progestin on gynecologic cancers and associated diagnostic procedures: the Women's Health Initiative randomized trial. JAMA 2003;290:1739–48.

Anonymous. The reduction in risk of ovarian cancer associated with oral-contraceptive use. The Cancer and Steroid Hormone Study of the Centers for Disease Control and National Institutes of Health and Human Development. N Engl J Med 1987;316:650–55.

Armstrong B, Doll R. Environmental factors and cancer incidence and mortality in different countries with special reference to dietary practices. Int J Cancer 1975;15:617–31.

Beeghly A, Katsaros D, Chen H, Fracchioli S, Zhang Y, Massobrio M, et al. Glutathione S-transferase polymorphisms and ovarian cancer treatment and survival. Gynecol Oncol 2006;100:330–37.

Bertone ER, Rosner BA, Hunter DJ, Stampfer MJ, Speizer FE, Colditz GA, et al. Dietary fat intake and ovarian cancer in a cohort of US women. Am J Epidemiol 2002;156:22–31.

Bertone ER, Willett WC, Rosner BA, Hunter DJ, Fuchs CS, Speizer FE, et al. Prospective study of recreational physical activity and ovarian cancer. J Natl Cancer Inst 2001;93:942–48.

Boice J, Engholm G, Kleiner R, Blettner M, Stovall M, Lisco H, et al. Radiation dose and second cancer risk in patients treated for cancer of the cervix. Radiation Res 1988;116:3–55.

Boorman GA, Seely JC. The lack of an ovarian effect of lifetime talc exposure in F344/N rats and B6C3F1 mice. Regulatory Toxicol Pharmacol 1995;21:242–43.

Boyd J. Specific keynote: hereditary ovarian cancer: what we know. Gynecol Oncol 2003;88:S8–S10.

Brinton LA, Gridley G, Persson I, Baron J, Bergqvist A. Cancer risk after a hospital discharge diagnosis of endometriosis. Am J Obstet Gynecol 1997;176:572–79.

Brinton LA, Lamb EJ, Moghissi KS, Scoccia B, Althuis MD, Mabie JE, et al. Ovarian cancer risk after the use of ovulation-stimulating drugs. Obstet Gynecol 2004;103:1194–203.

Brinton LA, Moghissi KS, Scoccia B, Westhoff CL, Lamb EJ. Ovulation induction and cancer risk. Fertil Steril 2005;83:261–74.

Chen Y, Wu PC, Lang JH, Ge WJ, Hartge P, Brinton LA. Risk factors for epithelial ovarian cancer in Beijing, China. Int J Epidemiol 1992;21:23–29.

Cramer DW, Harlow BL, Titus-Ernstoff L, Bohlke K, Welch WR, Greenberg ER. Over-the-counter analgesics and risk of ovarian cancer. Lancet 1998;351:104–7.

Cramer DW, Harlow BL, Willett WC, Welch WR, Bell DA, Scully RE, et al. Galactose consumption and metabolism in relation to the risk of ovarian cancer. Lancet 1989;2:66–71.

Cramer DW, Kuper H, Harlow BL, Titus-Ernstoff L. Carotenoids, antioxidants and ovarian cancer risk in pre- and postmenopausal women. Int J Cancer 2001;94:128–34.

Cramer D, Liberman RF, Titus-Ernstoff L, Welch W, Greenberg ER, Baron JA, et al. Genital talc exposure and risk of ovarian cancer. Int J Cancer 1999;81:351–56.

Cramer DW, Welch WR. Determinants of ovarian cancer risk. II. Inference regarding pathogenesis. J Natl Cancer Inst 1983;71:717–21.

Cramer DW, Welch WR, Cassells S, Scully RE. Mumps, menarche, menopause, and ovarian cancer. Am J Obstet Gynecol 1983;147:1–6.

Cramer DW, Welch WR, Hutchison GB, Willett WC, Scully RE. Dietary animal fat in relation to ovarian cancer risk. Obstet Gynecol 1984;63:833–38.

Cramer DW, Welch WR, Scully RE, Wojciechowski CA. Ovarian cancer and talc: a case-control study. Cancer 1982;50:372–76.

Darby SC, Doll R, Gill SK, Smith PG. Long term mortality after a single treatment course with X-rays in patients treated for ankylosing spondylitis. Br J Cancer 1987;55:179–90.

Dennerstein L, Gotts G, Brown JB. Effects of age and non-hormonal contraception on menstrual cycle characteristics. Gynecol Endocrinol 1997;11:127–33.

Doll R, Smith PG. The long-term effects of x irradiation in patients treated for metropathia haemorrhagica. Br J Radiol 1968; 41362–68.

Ellison P, Panter-Brick C, Lipson SF, O'Rourke MT. The ecological context of human ovarian function. Hum Reprod 1993;8:2248–58.

Fairfield KM, Hankinson SE, Rosner BA, Hunter DJ, Colditz GA, Willett WC. Risk of ovarian carcinoma and consumption of vitamins A, C, and E and specific carotenoids: a prospective analysis. Cancer 2001;92:2318–26.

Fairfield KM, Hunter DJ, Fuchs CS, Colditz GA, Hankinson SE. Aspirin, other NSAIDs, and ovarian cancer risk (United States). Cancer Causes Control 2002a;13:535–42.

Fairfield KM, Willett WC, Rosner BA, Manson JE, Speizer FE, Hankinson SE. Obesity, weight gain, and ovarian cancer. Obstet Gynecol 2002b;100:288–96.

Farrow DC, Weiss NS, Lyon JL, Daling JR. Association of obesity and ovarian cancer in a case-control study. Am J Epidemiol 1989; 129:1300–4.

Fathalla MF. Incessant ovulation—a factor in ovarian neoplasia? Lancet 1971;2:163.

Fenster L, Quale C, Waller K, Windham G, Elkin E, Benowitz N, et al. Caffeine consumption and menstrual function. Am J Epidemiol 1999;149:550–57.

Ferlay J, Bray F, Pisani P, Parkin DM. GLOBOCAN 2002: Cancer Incidence, Mortality and Prevalence Worldwide, Version 2.0. International Agency for Research on Cancer, Lyon, 2004.

Fung WL, Risch H, McLaughlin J, Rosen B, Cole D, Vesprini D, et al. The N314D polymorphism of galactose-1-phosphate uridyl transferase does not modify the risk of ovarian cancer. Cancer Epidemiol Biomarkers Prev 2003;12:678–80.

Garg P, Kerlikowske K, Subak L, Grady D. Hormone replacement therapy and the risk of epithelial ovarian carcinoma: a meta-analysis. Obstet Gynecol 1998;92:472–79.

Garrett AP, Lee KR, Colitti CR, Muto MG, Berkowitz RS, Mok SC. k-ras mutation may be an early event in mucinous ovarian tumorigenesis. Int J Gynecol Pathol 2001;20: 244–51.

Gayther SA, Mangion J, Russell P, Seal S, Barfoot R, Ponder BAJ, et al. Variation of risks of breast and ovarian cancer associated with different germline mutations of the BRCA2 gene. Nat Genet 1997;15:103–5.

Gayther SA, Warren W, Mazoyer S, Russell PA, Harrington PA, Chiano M, et al. Germline mutations of the BRCA1 gene in breast and ovarian cancer families provide evidence for a genotype–phenotype correlation. Nature Genet 1995;11:428–33.

Gemignani ML, Schlaerth AC, Bogomolniy F, Barakat RR, Lin O, Soslow R, et al. Role of KRAS and BRAF gene mutations in mucinous ovarian carcinoma. Gynecol Oncol 2003;90:378–81.

Genkinger JM, Hunter DJ, Spiegelman D, Anderson KE, Arslan A, Beeson WL, et al. Dairy products and ovarian cancer: a pooled analysis of 12 cohort studies. Cancer Epidemiol Biomarkers Prev 2006a;15:364–72.

Genkinger JM, Hunter DJ, Spiegelman D, Anderson KE, Beeson WL, Buring JE, et al. A pooled analysis of 12 cohort studies of dietary fat, cholesterol and egg intake and ovarian cancer. Cancer Causes Control 2006b;17: 273–85.

Genkinger JM, Hunter DJ, Spiegelman D, Anderson KE, Buring JE, Freudenheim JL, et al. Alcohol intake and ovarian cancer risk: a pooled analysis of 10 cohort studies. Br J Cancer 2006c;94:757–62.

Gertig D, Hunter D, Cramer D, Colditz G, Speizer F, Willett W, et al. A prospective study of talc use and ovarian cancer. J Natl Cancer Inst 2000;92:249–52.

Goodman MT, McDuffie K, Guo C, Terada K, Donolon T. CYP17 genotype and ovarian cancer: a null case-control study. Cancer Epidemiol Biomarkers Prev 2001;5:563–64.

Green A, Purdie D, Bain C, Siskind V, Webb PM. Cigarette smoking and risk of epithelial ovarian cancer (Australia). Cancer Causes Control 2001;12:713–19.

Hall J, Paul J, Brown R. Critical evaluation of p53 as a prognostic marker in ovarian cancer. Expert Rev Mol Med 2004;2004:1–20.

Hankinson SE, Colditz GA, Hunter DJ, Spencer TL, Rosner B, Stampfer MJ. A quantitative assessment of oral contraceptive use and risk of ovarian cancer. Obstet Gynecol 1992;80: 708–14.

Hankinson SE, Hunter DJ, Colditz GA, Willett WC, Stampfer MJ, Rosner B, et al. Tubal ligation, hysterectomy, and risk of ovarian cancer. JAMA 1993;270:2813–18.

Hankinson SE, Willett WC, Manson JE, Hunter DJ, Colditz GA, Stampfer MJ, et al. Alcohol, height, and adiposity in relation to estrogen and prolactin levels in postmenopausal women. J Natl Cancer Inst 1995;87:1297–302.

Harlap S, Olson SH, Barakat RR, Caputo TA, Forment S, Jacobs AJ, et al. Diagnostic x-rays and risk of epithelial ovarian carcinoma in Jews. Ann Epidemiol 2002;12:426–34.

Harlow BL, Cramer DW, Bell DA, Welch WR. Perineal exposure to talc and ovarian cancer risk. Obstet Gynecol 1992;80:19–26.

Harlow BL, Cramer DW, Geller J, Willett WC, Bell DA, Welch WR. The influence of lactose consumption on the association of oral contraceptive use and ovarian cancer risk. Am J Epidemiol 1991;134:445–53.

Heller DS, Westhoff C, Gordon RE, Katz N. The relationship between perineal cosmetic talc usage and ovarian talc particle burden. Am J Obstet Gynecol 1996;174:1507–10.

Herrinton LJ, Stanford JL, Schwartz SM, Weiss NS. Ovarian cancer incidence among Asian migrants to the United States and their descendants. J Natl Cancer Inst 1994;86:1336–39.

Huncharek M, Geschwind JF, Kupelnick B. Perineal application of cosmetic talc and risk of invasive epithelial ovarian cancer: a meta-analysis of 11,933 subjects from sixteen observational studies. Anticancer Res 2003;23:1955–60.

Huncharek M, Klassen H, Kupelnick B. Dietary beta-carotene intake and the risk of epithelial ovarian cancer: a meta-analysis of 3,782 subjects from five observational studies. In Vivo 2001;15:339–43.

Huncharek M, Kupelnick B. Dietary fat intake and risk of epithelial ovarian cancer: a meta-analysis of 6,689 subjects from 8 observational studies. Nutr Cancer 2001;40:87–91.

Irwin KL, Weiss NS, Lee NC, Peterson HB. Tubal sterilization, hysterectomy, and the subsequent occurrence of epithelial ovarian cancer. Am J Epidemiol 1991;134:362–69.

Jensen MR, Helin K. OVCA1: emerging as a bona fide tumor suppressor. Genes Dev 2004;18:245–48.

Jordan SJ, Purdie DM, Green AC, Webb PM. Coffee, tea and caffeine and risk of epithelial ovarian cancer. Cancer Causes Control 2004;15:359–65.

Jordan SJ, Whiteman DC, Purdie DM, Green AC, Webb PM. Smoking is associated with mucinous ovarian cancer: a systematic review and meta-analysis. Gynecol Oncol 2006;103:1122–29

Kato I, Tominaga S, Kuroishi T. Relationship between westernization of dietary habits and mortality from breast and ovarian cancers in Japan. Jpn J Cancer Res 1987;78:349–57.

Keal E. Asbestosis and abdominal neoplasms. Lancet 1960;2:1211–16.

Kelemen L, Sellers T, Vierkant R, Harnack L, Cerhan J. Association of folate and alcohol with risk of ovarian cancer in a prospective study of postmenopausal women. Cancer Causes and Control 2004;15:1085–93.

Khaw K, Tazuke S, Barrett-Connor E. Cigarette smoking and levels of adrenal androgens in postmenopausal women. New Engl J Med 1988;318:1705–9.

Kjaer SK, Mellemkjaer L, Brinton LA, Johansen C, Gridley G, Olsen JH. Tubal sterilization

and risk of ovarian, endometrial and cervical cancer. A Danish population-based follow-up study of more than 65 000 sterilized women. Int J Epidemiol 2004;33:596–602.

Koushik A, Hunter DJ, Spiegelman D, Anderson KE, Arslan AA, Beeson WL, et al. Fruits and vegetables and ovarian cancer risk in a pooled analysis of 12 cohort studies. Cancer Epidemiol Biomarkers Prev 2005;14:2160–67.

Koushik A, Hunter DJ, Spiegelman D, Anderson KE, Buring JE, Freudenheim JL, et al. Intake of the major carotenoids and the risk of epithelial ovarian cancer in a pooled analysis of 10 cohort studies. Int J Cancer 2006;119:2148–54.

Kreiger N, Sloan M, Cotterchio M, Parsons P. Surgical procedures associated with risk of ovarian cancer. Int J Epidemiol 1997;26:710–15.

Kuper H, Titus-Ernstoff L, Harlow BL, Cramer DW. Population based study of coffee, alcohol and tobacco use and risk of ovarian cancer. Int J Cancer 2000;88:313–18.

Kurian AW, Balise RR, McGuire V, Whittemore AS. Histologic types of epithelial ovarian cancer: have they different risk factors? Gynecol Oncol 2005;96:520–30.

Kushi LH, Mink PJ, Folsom AR, Anderson KE, Zheng W, Lazovich D, et al. Prospective study of diet and ovarian cancer. Am J Epidemiol 1999;149:21–31.

Lacey Jr JV, Brinton LA, Leitzmann MF, Mouw T, Hollenbeck A, Schatzkin A, et al. Menopausal hormone therapy and ovarian cancer risk in the National Institutes of Health—AARP Diet and Health Study Cohort. J Natl Cancer Inst 2006;98:19:1397–405.

Lagiou P, Ye W, Wedren S, Ekbom A, Nyrén O, Trichopoulos D, et al. Incidence of ovarian cancer among alcoholic women: a cohort study in Sweden. Int J Cancer 2001;91:264–66.

Larsson S, Orsini N, Wolk A. Milk, milk products and lactose intake and ovarian cancer risk: a meta-analysis of epidemiological studies. Int J Cancer 2006;118:431–41.

Larsson SC, Giovannucci E, Wolk A. Dietary folate intake and incidence of ovarian cancer: the Swedish Mammography Cohort. J Natl Cancer Inst 2004a;96:396–402.

Larsson SC, Holmberg L, Wolk A. Fruit and vegetable consumption in relation to ovarian cancer incidence: the Swedish mammography cohort. Br J Cancer 2004b;90:2167–70.

Larsson SC, Wolk A. Coffee consumption is not associated with ovarian cancer incidence. Cancer Epidemiol Biomarkers Prev 2005a;14:2273–74.

Larsson SC, Wolk A. Tea consumption and ovarian cancer risk in a population-based cohort. Arch Intern Med 2005b;165:2683–86.

Liede A, Tonin PN, Sun CC, Serruya C, Daly MB, Narod SA, et al. Is hereditary site-specific ovarian cancer a distinct genetic condition? Am J Med Genet 1998;75:55–58.

Littman AJ, Rossing MA, Madeleine MM, Tang MT, Yasui Y. Association between late age at infectious mononucleosis, Epstein-Barr virus antibodies, and ovarian cancer risk. Scand J Infect Dis 2003;35:728–35.

London S, Willett W, Longcope C, McKinlay S. Alcohol and other dietary factors in relation to serum hormone concentrations in women at climacteric. Am J Clin Nutr 1991; 53:166–71.

Lucero J, Harlow BL, Barbieri RL, Sluss P, and Cramer DW. Early follicular phase hormone levels in relation to patterns of alcohol, tobacco and coffee use. Fertil Steril 2001;76: 723–29.

Lynch HT, Casey M, Lynch J, Tacey EK. Genetics and ovarian carcinoma. Semin Oncol 1998;25:265–80.

Marchbanks PA, Wilson H, Bastos E, Cramer DW, Schildkraut JM, Peterson HB. Cigarette smoking and epithelial ovarian cancer by histologic type. Obstet Gynecol 2000;2:255–60.

McKinlay SM. The normal menopause transition: an overview. Maturitas 1996;23:137–45.

Menczer J, Modon M, Ranon L. Possible role of mumps virus in the etiology of ovarian cancer. Cancer 1979;43:1375.

Mills PK, Riordan DG, Cress RD. Epithelial ovarian cancer risk by invasiveness and cell type in the Central Valley of California. Gynecol Oncol 2004;95:215–25.

Modugno F. Ovarian cancer and polymorphisms in the androgen and progesterone receptor genes: a HuGE review. Am J Epidemiol 2004;159:319–35.

Moysich KB, Mettlin C, Piver MS, Natarajan N, Menezes RJ, Swede H. Regular use of analgesic drugs and ovarian cancer risk. Cancer Epidemiol Biomarkers Prev 2001;10:903–6.

Nagle CM, Purdie DM, Webb PM, Green A, Harvey PW, Bain CJ. Dietary influences on survival after ovarian cancer. Int J Cancer 2003;106:264–69.

Narod SA, Sun P, Ghadirian P, Lynch H, Isaacs C, Garber J, et al. Tubal ligation and risk of ovarian cancer in carriers of BRCA1 or BRCA2 mutations: a case-control study. Lancet 2001;357:1467–70.

Negri E, Franceschi S, Tzonou A, Booth M, La Vecchia C, Parazzini F, et al. Pooled analysis of 3 European case-control studies: I. Reproductive factors and risk of epithelial ovarian cancer. Int J Cancer 1991;49:50–56.

Negri E, Tzonou A, Beral V, Lagiou P, Trichopoulos D, Parazzini F, et al. Hormonal therapy for menopause and ovarian cancer in a collaborative re-analysis of European studies. Int J Cancer 1999;80, 848–51.

Ness R, Cottreau C. Possible role of ovarian epithelial inflammation in ovarian cancer. J Natl Cancer Inst 1999;91:1459–67.

Ness R, Grisso J, Cottreau C, Klapper J, Vergona R, Wheeler J, et al. Factors related to inflammation of the ovarian epithelium and risk of ovarian cancer. Epidemiology 2000a; 11:111–17.

Ness R, Grisso J, Klapper J, Schlesselman J, Silberzweig S, Vergona R, et al. Risk of ovarian cancer in relation to estrogen and progestin dose and use characteristics of oral contraceptives. Am J Epidemiol 2000b;152: 233–41.

Ness RB, Cramer DW, Goodman MT, Kjaer SK, Mallin K, Mosgaard BJ, et al. Infertility, fertility drugs, and ovarian cancer: a pooled analysis of case-control studies. Am J Epidemiol 2002;155:217–24.

Ness RB, Goodman MT, Shen C, Brunham RC. Serologic evidence of past infection with Chlamydia trachomatis, in relation to ovarian cancer. J Infect Dis 2003;187:1147–52.

Pan SY, Ugnat AM, Mao Y. Physical activity and the risk of ovarian cancer: a case-control study in Canada. Int J Cancer 2005;117:300–7.

Parazzini F, Franceschi S, La Vecchia C, Fasoli M. The epidemiology of ovarian cancer. Gynecol Oncol 1991;43:9–23.

Patel AV, Rodriguez C, Pavluck AL, Thun MJ, Calle EE. Recreational physical activity and sedentary behavior in relation to ovarian cancer risk in a large cohort of US women. Am J Epidemiol 2006;163:709–16.

Pearce CL, Hirschhorn JN, Wu AH, Burtt NP, Stram DO, Young S, et al. Clarifying the PROGINS allele association in ovarian and breast cancer risk: A haplotype-based analysis. J Natl Cancer Inst 2005;97:51–59.

Petridou E, Katsouyanni K, Spanos E, Skalkidis Y, Panagiotopoulou K, Trichopoulos D. Pregnancy estrogens in relation to coffee and alcohol intake. Ann Epidemiol 1992;2:241–47.

Pirozzo S, Purdie D, Kuiper-Linley M, Webb P, Harvey P, Green A, et al. Ovarian cancer, cholesterol, and eggs: a case-control analysis. Cancer Epidemiol Biomarkers Prev 2002;11: 1112–14.

Pukkala E, Poskiparta M, Apter D, Vihko V. Life-long physical activity and cancer risk among Finnish female teachers. Eur J Cancer Prev 1993;2:369–76.

Purdie DM, Bain CJ, Siskind V, et al. Hormone replacement therapy and risk of epithelial ovarian cancer. Br J Cancer 1999;81:559–63.

Purdie DM, Bain CJ, Siskind V, Webb PM, Green AC. Ovulation and risk of epithelial ovarian cancer. Int J Cancer 2003;104:228–32.

Purdie DM, Bain CJ, Webb PM, Whiteman DC, Pirozzo S, Green AC. Body size and ovarian cancer: case-control study and systematic review (Australia). Cancer Causes Control 2001a;12:855–63.

Purdie DM, Siskind V, Bain CJ, Webb PM, Green AC. Reproduction-related risk factors for mucinous and nonmucinous epithelial ovarian cancer. Am J Epidemiol 2001b;153: 860–64.

Riman T, Dickman PW, Nilsson S, Correia N, Nordlinder H, Magnusson CM, et al. Hormone replacement therapy and the risk of invasive epithelial ovarian cancer in Swedish women. J Natl Cancer Inst 2002;94:497–504.

Riman T, Dickman PW, Nilsson S, Nordlinder H, Magnusson CM, Persson IR. Some lifestyle factors and the risk of invasive epithelial ovarian cancer in Swedish women. Eur J Epidemiol 2004a;19:1011–19.

Riman T, Nilsson S, Persson IR. Review of epidemiological evidence for reproductive and hormonal factors in relation to the risk of epithelial ovarian malignancies. Acta Obstet Gynecol Scand 2004b;83:783–95.

Risch HA. Hormonal etiology of epithelial ovarian cancer, with a hypothesis concerning the role of androgens and progesterone. J Natl Cancer Inst 1998;90:1744–86.

Risch HA, Jain M, Marrett LD, Howe GR. Dietary fat intake and risk of epithelial ovarian cancer. J Natl Cancer Inst 1994a;86: 1409–15.

Risch HA, Marrett LD, Howe GR. Parity, contraception, infertility, and the risk of epithelial ovarian cancer. Am J Epidemiol 1994b; 140:585–97.

Rodriguez G, Walmer D, Cline M, Krigman H, Lessey B, Whitaker R, et al. Effect of progestin on the ovarian epithelium of Macaques: cancer prevention through apoptosis? J Soc Gynecol Invest 1998;5:271–76.

Rose DP, Boyar AP, Wynder EL. International comparisons of mortality rates for cancer of the breast, ovary, prostate, and colon, and per capita food consumption. Cancer 1986; 58:2363–71.

Rosenblatt KA, Thomas DB. Lactation and the risk of epithelial ovarian cancer. The WHO Collaborative Study of Neoplasia and Steroid Contraceptives Int J Epidemiol 1993;22: 192–97.

Sala M, Dosemeci M, Zahm S. A death certificate–based study of occupation and mortality from reproductive cancers among women in 24 US states. J Occup Environ Med 1998; 40:632–39.

Schildkraut J, Bastos E, Berchuck A. Relationship between lifetime ovulatory cycles and overexpression of mutant p53 in epithelial ovarian cancer. J Natl Cancer Inst 1998;90: 1729–34.

Schildkraut JM, Calingaert B, Marchbanks PA, Moorman PG, Rodriguez GC. Impact of progestin and estrogen potency in oral contraceptives on ovarian cancer risk. J Natl Cancer Inst 2002;94:32–38.

Schildkraut JM, Moorman PG, Halabi S, Calingaert B, Marks JR, Berchuck A. Analgesic drug use and risk of ovarian cancer. Epidemiology 2006;17:104–7.

Schildkraut JM, Schwingl PJ, Bastos E, Evanoff A, Hughes C. Epithelial ovarian cancer risk among women with polycystic ovary syndrome. Obstet Gynecol 1996;88:554–59.

Schouten LJ, Goldbohm RA, van den Brandt PA. Height, weight, weight change, and ovarian cancer risk in the Netherlands cohort study on diet and cancer. Am J Epidemiol 2003; 157:424–33.

Schulz M, Lahmann PH, Boeing H, Hoffmann K, Allen N, Key TJA, et al. Fruit and vegetable consumption and risk of epithelial ovarian cancer: the European prospective investigation into cancer and nutrition. Cancer Epidemiol Biomarkers Prev 2005;14:2531–35.

Shen N, Weiderpass E, Antilla A, Goldberg MS, Vasama-Neuronenk KM, Boffetta P, et al. Epidemiology of occupational and environmental risk factors related to ovarian cancer. Scand J Work, Environ Health 1998;24: 175–82.

Shih I-M, Kurman RJ. Ovarian tumorigenesis: a proposed model based on morphological and molecular genetic analysis. Am J Pathol 2004;164:1511–18.

Shu XO, Gao YT, Yuan JM, Ziegler RG, Brinton LA. Dietary factors and epithelial ovarian cancer. Br J Cancer 1989;59:92–96.

Simon WE, Albrecht M, Hansel M, Dietel D, Hotzel F. Cell lines derived from human ovarian carcinomas. Growth stimulation by gonadotrophic and steroid hormones. J Natl Cancer Inst 1983;70:839–45.

Singer G, Oldt R, III, Cohen Y, Wang BG, Sidransky D, Kurman RJ, et al. Mutations in BRAF and KRAS characterize the development of low-grade ovarian serous carcinoma. J Natl Cancer Inst 2003;95:484–86.

Spurdle AB, Chen X, Abbazadegan M, Martin N, Khoo SK, Hurst T, et al. CYP17 promotor polymorphism and ovarian cancer risk. Int J Cancer 2000;86:436–39.

Stadel BV. The etiology and prevention of ovarian cancer [letter]. Am J Obstet Gynecol 1975;123:772–73.

Terry PD, Miller AB, Jones JG, Rohan TE. Cigarette smoking and the risk of invasive epithelial ovarian cancer in a prospective cohort study. Eur J Cancer 2003;39:1157–64.

Tokuoka S, Kawai K, Shimizu Y, Inai K, Ohe K, Fujikura T, et al. Malignant and benign ovarian neo-plasms among atomic bomb survivors, Hiroshima and Nagasaki, 1950–80. J Natl Cancer Inst 1987;79:47–57.

Tortolero-Luna G, Mitchell MF, Rhodes-Morris HE. Epidemiology and screening of ovarian cancer. Obstet Gynecol Clin North Am 1994;21:1–23.

Tworoger SS, Hecht JL, Giovannucci E, Hankinson SE. Intake of folate and related nutrients in relation to risk of epithelial ovarian cancer. Am J Epidemiol 2006;163:1101–11.

US Department of Health and Human Services (2004). The health consequences of smoking: a report of the Surgeon General. Atlanta, GA, US Department of Health and Human Services, Centers for Disease Control and Prevention, National Center for Chronic Disease Prevention and Health Promotion, Office on Smoking and Health.

Van Thiel D, Gavaler J, Lester R. Alcohol-induced ovarian failure in the rat. J Clin Invest 1978;61:624–63.

Venn A, Healy D, McLachlan R. Cancer risks associated with the diagnosis of infertility. Best Pract Res Clin Obstet Gynaecol 2003; 17:343–67.

Venn A, Watson L, Bruinsma F, Giles G, Healy D. Risk of cancer after use of fertility drugs with in-vitro fertilisation. Lancet 1999;354: 1586–90.

Wagoner J. Leukaemia and Other Malignancies Following Radiation Therapy for Gynecologic Disorders. New York, Raven Press, 1984.

Wang J-X, Boice J, Li B-X, Zhang J-Y, Fraumeni JF. Cancer among medical diagnostic X-ray workers in China. J Natl Cancer Inst 1988; 80:344–50.

Webb PM, Green A, Cummings MC, Purdie DM, Walsh MD, Chevenix-Trench G. Relationship between number of ovulatory cycles and accumulation of mutant p53 in epithelial ovarian cancer. J Natl Cancer Inst 1998;90:1729–34.

Webb PM, Purdie DM, Bain CJ, Green AC. Alcohol, wine, and risk of epithelial ovarian cancer. Cancer Epidemiol Biomarkers Prev 2004;13:592–99.

Weiderpass E, Margolis KL, Sandin S, Braaten T, Kumle M, Adami H-O, et al. Prospective study of physical activity in different periods of life and the risk of ovarian cancer. Int J Cancer 2006;118:3153–60.

Weiss NS. Measuring the separate effects of low parity and its antecedents on the incidence of ovarian cancer. Am J Epidemiol 1988;128: 451–55.

Weitzel JN, Ding S, Larson GP, Nelson RA, Goodman A, Grendys EC, et al. The HRAS1 minisatellite locus and risk of ovarian cancer. Cancer Res 2000;60:259–61.

Westhoff C, Gentile G, Lee J, Zacur H, Helbig D. Predictors of ovarian steroid secretion in reproductive age women. Am J Epidemiol 1996;144:381–88.

Whiteman DC, Murphy MF, Cook LS, Cramer DW, Hartge P, Marchbanks PA, et al. Multiple births and risk of epithelial ovarian cancer. J Natl Cancer Inst 2000;92:1172–77.

Whiteman DC, Siskind V, Purdie DM, Green AC. Timing of pregnancy and the risk of epithelial ovarian cancer. Cancer Epidemiol Biomarkers Prev 2003;12:42–46.

Whittemore AS, Balise RR, Pharoah PD, Dicioccio RA, Oakley-Girvan I, Ramus SJ, et al. Oral contraceptive use and ovarian cancer risk among carriers of BRCA1 or BRCA2 mutations. Br J Cancer 2004;91: 1911–15.

Whittemore AS, Harris R, Itnyre J. Characteristics relating to ovarian cancer risk: collaborative analysis of 12 U.S. case-control studies. II. Invasive epithelial ovarian cancers in white women. Collaborative Ovarian Cancer Group [see comments]. Am J Epidemiol 1992a;136:1184–203.

Whittemore AS, Harris R, Itnyre J. Characteristics relating to ovarian cancer risk: collaborative analysis of 12 US case-control studies. IV. The pathogenesis of epithelial ovarian cancer. Am J Epi 1992b;136:1212–20.

Whittemore AS, Wu ML, Paffenbarger RS Jr, Sarles DL, Kampert JB, Grosser S, et al. Personal and environmental characteristics related to epithelial ovarian cancer. II. Exposures to talcum powder, tobacco, alcohol, and coffee. Am J Epidemiol 1988;128:1228–40.

Wignall BK, Fox AJ. Mortality of female gas mask assemblers. Br J Indust Med 1982;39: 34–38.

Yang CS, Maliakal P, Meng X. Inhibition of carcinogenesis by tea. Annu Rev Pharmacol Toxicol 2002;42:25–54.

Zhang M, Binns CW, Lee AH. Tea consumption and ovarian cancer risk: a case-control study in China. Cancer Epidemiol Biomarkers Prev 2002a;11:713–18.

Zhang M, Yang ZY, Binns CW, Lee AH. Diet and ovarian cancer risk: a case-control study in China. Br J Cancer 2002b;86:712–17.

Zheng W, Shu XO, McLaughlin JK, Chow WH, Gao YT, Blot WJ. Occupational physical activity and the incidence of cancer of the breast, corpus uteri, and ovary in Shanghai. Cancer 1993;71:3620–24.

20

Prostate Cancer

LORELEI A. MUCCI, LISA B. SIGNORELLO,
AND HANS-OLOV ADAMI

There are two giants in the cancer landscape of women and men in western countries, each of them accounting for approximately one-fourth of all incident malignancies: breast cancer in women and prostate cancer in men. Breast cancer has been investigated in an overwhelming number of epidemiologic studies, beginning in the 1920s. Until rather recently, however, prostate cancer remained a hidden disease. Its causes were enigmatic, little epidemiologic research was being done, and no curative treatment could be offered. Starting in the 1980s, this situation changed dramatically. The number of scientific studies is now astounding, attempts to achieve early diagnosis and treatment are widespread, and several renowned men with prostate cancer have given this common malignancy an identity. Admittedly, convincing evidence for progress in the prevention and cure of prostate cancer is still scant, but a fascinating story of increasing complexity is emerging.

CLINICAL SYNOPSIS

Subgroups

Almost all (99%) prostate cancers are adenocarcinomas derived from the glandular epithelial cells. Autopsies have revealed, even at middle age, a high prevalence of the malignant precursor prostatic intraepithelial neoplasia (PIN) and small invasive cancers. The biological potential of these lesions to progress to clinical cancer is unknown.

Symptoms

The general clinical symptoms—which cannot be distinguished from those caused by benign prostatic hyperplasia—are urinary frequency, nocturia, and urgency caused by obstruction of the urethra. In some cases, initial symptoms come from painful skeletal metastases or, more rarely, from anemia due to bone marrow replacement. The majority of cases in the current clinical domain present without symptoms, however.

Diagnosis

Traditionally, prostate cancers were diagnosed by digital rectal examination alone. Modern individualized treatment, however, requires morphologic confirmation by core biopsy, fine-needle aspiration biopsy, or transurethral resection and staging. Staging is done by digital rectal examination, transrectal ultrasound, measurement of prostate-specific antigen (PSA) in the blood, skeletal scintigraphy, and the degree of differentiation and/or the Gleason score assessed from a tissue specimen. Since the late 1980s, an increasing proportion of prostate cancers in asymptomatic men has been detected through screening with PSA.

Treatment

Treatment of prostate cancer is controversial and complex, and differs greatly among doctors, hospitals, and countries. Options vary from active surveillance ("watchful waiting"), to radical local treatment in patients with localized and/or asymptomatic disease, to systemic palliative therapy with numerous forms of endocrine manipulation (including castration) in advanced disease. Treatment with a curative intent—radical prostatectomy or local irradiation—was introduced first during the 1980s without evidence of survival benefit from randomized trials. Recent trial data comparing radical prostatectomy versus watchful waiting has demonstrated a significant reduction in mortality associated with treatment. Local irradiation can effectively alleviate pain from skeletal metastases, whereas cytotoxic treatment plays a limited role.

Prognosis

Prognosis varies greatly among time periods and countries. Five-year relative survival among European men with prostate cancer diagnosed between 1985 and 1989 ranged between 37% and 72%; currently in the US, 5-year relative survival is 100%, which may reflect the lead time introduced by PSA screening. Mortality to incidence ratios range from 0.16 in US whites to 0.60 in Denmark. Because radical local treatment with a curative intent did not reach widespread use until the late 1980s—and then only in certain areas—this substantial variation in prognosis is unlikely to reflect differences in therapeutic efficacy. Rather, the detection of prostate cancer depends strongly on diagnostic intensity, with identification of preclinical disease through PSA screening as an extreme example. A high survival rate, and as a corollary a low mortality-to-incidence ratio, may therefore be due primarily to detection of many cancers unlikely to progress to advanced lethal disease.

Progress

Ongoing randomized trials are investigating whether early detection with PSA, radical local treatment, and/or novel forms of endocrine manipulation will reduce mortality in patients with prostate cancer. Moreover, molecular signatures are being evaluated that could distinguish lethal and indolent prostate cancer.

DESCRIPTIVE EPIDEMIOLOGY

Incidence

Prostate cancer is among the most common male cancers, with more than 679 000 cases diagnosed in 2002 (Ferlay et al, 2004). The burden of this disease shows remarkable worldwide variation, and it is the most frequently diagnosed male cancer in developed countries (Ferlay et al, 2004). Globally, however, it is only the third most common (world age-standardized incidence rate of 25 per 100 000) (Ferlay et al, 2004). Figure 20–1 shows the striking international disparity in prostate cancer incidence rates. Among countries with reliable cancer statistics, prostate cancer rates are highest in westernized countries such as the United States and western European countries and lowest in Asian countries. A 30-fold difference in incidence has been noted between population groups with the highest (African-American men in the United States) and the lowest (Japanese and Chinese men living in their native countries) prostate cancer burden (Muir et al, 1987).

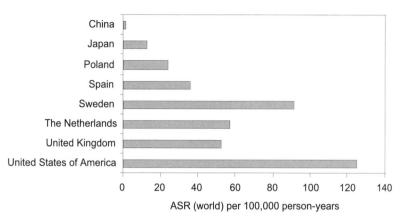

Figure 20–1. Age-standardized (to the world population) incidence rates of prostate cancer. (*Source*: Ferlay et al, 2004)

More than with any other cancer, prostate cancer incidence must be interpreted in the context of diagnostic intensity and screening behavior. The prevalence of latent prostate cancer is high; 15% to 30% of men over the age of 50 will have a prostatic adenocarcinoma that, while meeting the histopathologic criteria for malignacy, is thought to have low potential for growth and metastasis (Chan et al, 1998b). Screening by prostate specific antigen (PSA) has dramatically influenced the incidence and presentation of prostate cancer. PSA was first introduced in 1986 to monitor disease progression. Widespread opportunitistc screening by PSA has since been introduced in several western countries, allowing the detection of a significant proportion of latent lesions. Consequently, incidence rates in some countries, the United States being a prime example, reflect the sum of clinical disease and latent disease but in other countries only clinical disease. Nevertheless, geographic variation in prostate cancer incidence, although less extreme, was apparent in the pre-PSA era. Data from the 1970s and early 1980s reflect a country ranking of prostate cancer incidence similar to the current standings.

A secular trend of increasing worldwide incidence, on the order of about 3% per year, has been evident for the past several decades (Quinn and Babb, 2002). The United States first displayed a dramatic departure from this trend, beginning in the late 1980s, with the introduction of intensive PSA screening. Similar patterns of increase have occurred in other countries after introduction of screening (Fig. 20–2). PSA screening has also led to a shift in stage presentation, with concomitant increase in the ratio of localized to advanced disease cases and a decrease in the age at diagnosis (Brawley et al, 1998). The importance of cancers diagnosed through PSA screening is questionable, with estimates that 25% to 50% of prostate cancer cases may be overdiagnosed by PSA screening (Etzioni et al, 2002; Ciatto et al, 2005). The influence of screening on studies of prostate cancer epidemiology cannot be understated, and illustrate the importance of identifying risk factors for "clinically important" prostate cancer, or disease that represents the greatest potential for lethality.

Mortality

In 2002, 221 000 men died of prostate cancer worldwide. In developed countries, prostate cancer death is among the top three most common causes of cancer death among men (Stat bite, 2005), while mortality rates are much lower in many Asian countries, consistent with differences in incidence. Notwithstanding the considerable

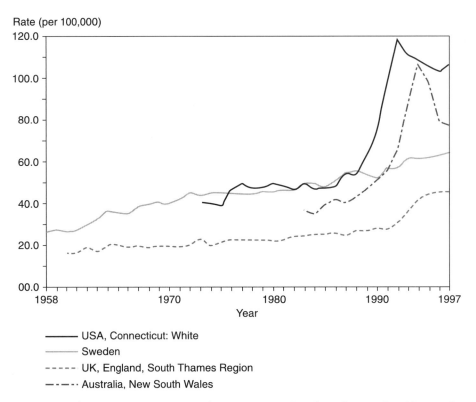

Figure 20–2. Trends in prostate cancer incidence over time in selected countries. (*Source*: International Agency for Research on Cancer.)

mortality associated with this disease, prostate cancer has a long and variable course. Natural history studies demonstrate that deaths from cancer can occur even 20 years after diagnosis (Johansson et al, 2004; Albertsen et al, 2005; Cuzick et al, 2006). On the other hand, most men die with and not from their cancers, and many harbor tumors that remain indolent even in the absence of therapy. This is shown clearly in the only randomized trial of prostatectomy versus watchful waiting, where 19 men had to be treated to save one from dying of cancer (Bill-Axelson et al, 2005). This trial predated PSA screening; the majority of cancer diagnosed in the PSA era are now localized to the prostate, at a stage with excellent survival.

Mortality rates have increased over the past several decades, although a small decline has been noted during the past several years in the United States and some other

developed countries (Quinn and Babb, 2002). The overall increase was seen predominantly in men over the age of 65 (Zaridze et al, 1984). Within younger age groups, mortality has been stable across decades (Doll and Peto, 1981; Zaridze et al, 1984). The fact that mortality rates in some population groups have not changed, despite large elevations in incidence and limited improvement in survival, has prompted speculation that the rise in the overall prostate cancer burden consists mostly of cancers detected incidentally during transurethral resection for benign prostatic hyperplasia or of PSA-detected indolent tumors that would never have come to clinical attention (Doll and Peto, 1981; Potosky et al, 1990; Catalona et al, 1993). The similar mortality rates in developed countries despite variation in incidence further support this.

The lack of a clear decline in mortality among populations that utilize PSA screening has also sparked a debate about the benefit of this screening tool (Etzioni et al, 1999; Feuer et al, 1999; Godley, 1999; Hankey et al, 1999). Since the advent of PSA screening in the United States, mortality rates have risen and then fallen back to their prescreening level (Feuer et al, 1999). Detailed analyses of these time trends suggest that PSA screening cannot be wholly responsible for the recent decrease in US mortality unless unusually short lead times are assumed (Etzioni et al, 1999). Screening trials of PSA are ongoing in the US (PLCO) and Europe (ERSPC) to evaluate its effectiveness in reducing cancer mortality.

Migrant Studies

Migrant studies have demonstrated that immigrants from low-risk countries manifest some excess prostate cancer incidence by moving to a high-risk country but that they typically do not assume the full risk profile of high-risk country natives. Such evidence has been found in studies of Japanese and Polish immigrants to the United States, whose prostate cancer risk is many times higher than that of their native counterparts yet still well below that of US white men (Lilienfeld et al, 1972; Shimizu et al, 1991). Although a shift toward higher incidence rates following migration to a high-risk country could reflect different or more widespread screening practices, the observation of similar changes in prostate cancer mortality does argue for an environmental cause.

Age

Age is the most well-documented risk factor for prostate cancer. The age-specific incidence curve provided in Figure 20–3 shows the exponential rise in prostate cancer incidence beginning at approximately age 50 to 55. This pattern is less evident in Asian countries, but in western countries it represents the steepest age-dependent incline of any cancer (Brawley et al, 1998). United States white males aged 75 to 79 have roughly 130 times the risk of prostate cancer of men aged 45 to 49 (Chan et al, 1998b). PSA screening has led to a shift in age-specific

incidence curves to a younger age at presentation in populations in which screening is common (Hemminki et al, 2005).

GENETIC AND MOLECULAR EPIDEMIOLOGY

Inherited Susceptibility

Data from twin studies suggest that prostate cancer has one of the strongest heritable components of any cancer, with an estimate of 30% to 40% of cancer risk explained by genetic factors (Lichtenstein et al, 2000; Baker et al, 2005). Epidemiologic studies have provided further strong evidence of a heritable component. Relying on self-reports of prostate cancer occurrence among study participants' fathers and brothers, data from both case-control (McLellan and Norman, 1995; Bratt et al, 1999b; Ghadirian et al, 1997; Lesko et al, 1996) and cohort (Grönberg et al, 1996; Cerhan et al, 1999; Schuurman et al, 1999c; Thompson et al, 2006) studies show that men with a first-degree relative with prostate cancer have a two- to four fold increased risk of disease.

It has been asserted that men with affected family members are more likely to seek prostate cancer screening. The identification (via PSA screening) of latent microscopic prostate cancers among this group of men could create or inflate an association between family history and prostate cancer incidence. Some studies indirectly support this argument by showing that the relationship between family history and prostate cancer risk is stronger for localized than for advanced disease (Lesko et al, 1996; Cerhan et al, 1999). Other studies, however, report the opposite (Schuurman et al, 1999), and still others show no effect modification by disease stage (Hayes et al, 1995). Recent evidence from the Prostate Cancer Prevention Trial (PCPT), a trial of the alpha-reductase inhibitor finasteride versus placebo (Thompson et al, 2003), may dispute this further. All men received annual testing by PSA and DRE, and all men were encouraged to undergo an end-of-study biopsy. In this

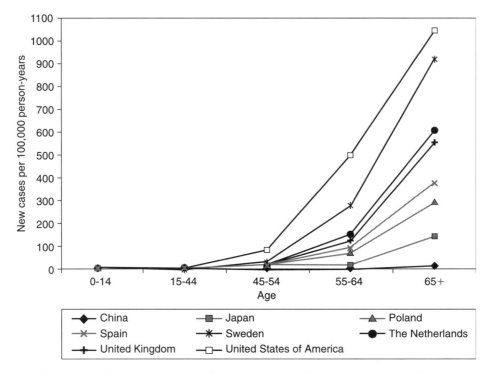

Figure 20–3. Age-specific incidence rates of prostate cancer. (*Source*: Ferlay et al, 2004)

cohort, family history was associated with relative risk of 1.31 (95% CI = 1.11 to 1.55), controlling for other clinical factors (Thompson et al, 2006).

A notable finding in some studies (Keetch et al, 1995; Whittemore et al, 1995b; Cerhan et al, 1999; Schuurman et al, 1999c) is that having an affected brother confers a stronger elevation in risk than does having an affected father. This pattern of risk could result from a greater degree of misclassification of the father's (as opposed to the sibling's) disease history but could also be suggestive of an X-linked or recessive model of inheritance (Monroe et al, 1995; Cerhan et al, 1999). In 1998, a prostate cancer susceptibility locus was localized to chromosome X, supporting this hypothesis (Xu et al, 1998). The androgen receptor gene for which polymorphisms have been associated with prostate cancer risk (Giovannucci et al, 1997b; Ingles et al, 1997; Stanford et al, 1997) is also located on the X chromosome.

Other important observations are the following:

1. Family history appears to be a stronger risk factor for men who develop the disease earlier in life (usually defined as younger than 70 years) (Lesko et al, 1996; Cerhan et al, 1999; Schuurman et al, 1999c). This is compatible with our understanding of the etiology of many cancer types—that genetically predisposed individuals will exhibit earlier onset of the disease.

2. A family history characterized by a male relative with early onset disease confers a higher risk than a family history characterized by a male relative with prostate cancer diagnosed later in life (after 70 years) (Whittemore et al, 1995b; Lesko et al, 1996).

3. The larger the number of affected first-degree relatives, the higher the prostate cancer risk (Whittemore et al, 1995b; Lesko et al, 1996; Rodriguez et al, 1997a).

Notwithstanding evidence of a strong heritable component in prostate cancer, there has been limited reproducibilities across studies in identifying a specific genetic factor.

Results of three complex segregation analyses are consistent with the hypothesis of an autosomal dominant susceptibility gene (Carter et al, 1992; Grönberg et al, 1997; Schaid et al, 1998), although the proposed models differed. Linkage analysis can be used to identify genes involved in the development of cancer, but due to the late age at which prostate cancer is diagnosed, it is rare to have DNA from men of families affected in more than one generation. As a result of studies of high-risk prostate cancer families in the United States and Sweden, the first prostate cancer susceptibility locus was reported in 1996; it was located on the long arm of chromosome 1 (HPC1) (Smith et al, 1996). Studies that confirm (Cooney et al, 1997; Neuhausen et al, 1999) and that do not confirm (McIndoe et al, 1997; Eeles et al, 1998) a linkage to markers in this region (1q24–25) have since been reported, and a study of 772 prostate cancer families found that HPC1 may only be associated with a small minority (10%) of hereditary prostate cancer cases (Xu, 2000). Several other possible prostate cancer susceptibility loci have been identified on chromosome 1 (Gibbs et al, 1999), chromosome 16 (Suarez et al, 2000), chromosome 20 (Berry et al, 2000), and chromosome X (Xu et al, 1998). Even though several chromosomal loci have been reported, no prostate cancer gene has been fully characterized.

8q24

The most compelling evidence for a role of genetic susceptibility and prostate cancer risk may be a common variant on chromosome 8q24, which was identified initially in an Icelandic family-based study using linkage analysis to identify a signal with a lod score of 2.11 (Amundadottir et al, 2006). Genotyping of additional markers in the region identified a variant allele at microsatellite DG8S737, associated with a 60% increased risk of prostate cancer among men of European ancestry from Iceland, Sweden, and the US, as well as an African American population. The frequency of the variant among controls in the European study was 4% to 8% in the European groups and 16% among African Americans. This initial finding has been consistently confirmed in several other studies in the US and Europe (Freedman et al, 2006; Schumacher et al, 2007). Currently, it is unknown whether 8q24 maps to a specific gene, and work is underway to characterize the function of 8q24. Interestingly, microarray analysis had previously identified amplification of the 8q24 region, which includes the oncogene c-myc, in prostate tumors (van Duinet al, 2005; Saramaki et al, 2006) and these somatic alterations portend a poor prognosis (Sato et al, 1999).

Numerous studies have examined low penetrance susceptibility polymorphisms in candidate genes in relation to prostate cancer risk. While significant findings have been reported, many of these associations could not be replicated in subsequent studies, suggesting the findings of earlier studies may have been due to chance or bias. Below are summarized the evidence for germline variation in selected genes.

Androgen receptor

Prostate cell division is strongly influenced by certain steroid hormones, including testosterone and dihydrotestosterone, the actions of which are mediated through the prostate cell androgen receptor. The transactivation region of the androgen receptor gene is polymorphic, and one particular polymorphism, a CAG repeat in exon 1, has been studied extensively with regard to prostate cancer risk (Kantoff et al, 1998). The normal range of the number of CAG repeats is thought to be between 9 and 30 (Ingles et al, 1997). Even within this normal range, in vitro studies have demonstrated that androgen receptor transactivation is inversely related to the number of CAG repeats (Beilin et al, 2000). Thus, it would be expected that fewer CAG repeats would predict an elevation in prostate cancer risk.

Several epidemiologic studies have in fact reported that androgen receptor short alleles (fewer than approximately 20 repeats) are linked to a risk elevation of 50% to 100% (Giovannucci et al, 1997b; Ingles et al, 1997; Stanford et al, 1997; Hsing et al, 2000b), and may also be associated with prostate cancer progression (Nam et al, 2000), a young age at diagnosis, and a poor response to endocrine therapy (Bratt et al, 1999a). At the same time, other studies have failed to find an association between CAG-length and prostate cancer risk (Beilin et al, 2001; Freedman et al, 2005). A meta-analysis of 19 case control studies reported a relative risk of 1.19 (1.07–1.31) comparing ≤ 21 CAG repeats to men with > 21 CAG repeats for total prostate cancer (Zeegers et al, 2004). Moreover, a haplotype analysis of systematic variation across the androgen receptor gene failed to find an association in a multiethnic cohort (Freedman et al, 2005). The average number of CAG repeats has also been found to vary in a race-specific manner that mirrors the ranking of race-specific prostate cancer risk (Chan et al, 1998b; Sartor et al, 1999).

Vitamin D receptor

The vitamin D receptor mediates the biologic actions of the vitamin D metabolites 1,25 dihydroxyvitamin D3 (1,25(OH)2D) and 25-hydroxyvitamin D3 (25(OH)D) on epithelial cells. Several polymorphisms in the gene encoding vitamin D receptor, including a translation initiation codon in exon 2 FokI, the variant f, which codes 3 additional amino acids, and has lower transcriptional activity than the wildtype allele. While a meta-analysis of four studies showed no association between FokI and risk, three subsequent studies showed an increased risk associated with the ff genotype (Bodiwala et al, 2004; Mishra et al, 2005; John et al, 2005; Ntais et al, 2003). In light of the role of the vitamin D receptor in mediating the effects of vitamin D metabolites, it may be relevant to examine polymorphisms in vitamin D receptor in combination with vitamin D levels.

IGF-I

Accumulating epidemiological evidence supports a role of the insulin-like growth factor-I (IGF) in prostate carcinogenesis (Renehan et al, 2004). Genetic variation in the gene encoding IGF-I has been characterized. A common (CA)n repeat sequence located upstream from the IGF1 transcription start site has been studied extensively. Inconsistent findings suggest positive associations between homozygosity for the (CA)19 repeat and prostate cancer risk (Nam et al, 2003; Tsuchiya et al, 2005)—an inverse association (Schildkraut et al, 2005; Friedrichsen et al, 2005), and no association (Li et al, 2004; Neuhausen et al, 2005). A more comprehensive genetic study sequenced IGF-I exons in germline DNA from 95 men with advanced prostate cancer and identified common haplotypes (Cheng et al, 2006). Furthermore, haplotype analysis among 2320 prostate cancer cases and 2290 controls from the Multiethnic Cohort revealed nominally significant associations with prostate cancer risk in each of the four haplotype blocks, with relative risks of 1.2 to 1.3 for total prostate cancer, with limited power to examine clinical subtypes. Because the study did not measure circulating IGF-I levels, the genotype-phenotype association remains to be further elucidated.

Genes involved in inflammation

Several lines of evidence support a role of chronic inflammation in the pathogenesis and progression of prostate cancer. Polymorphisms in genes involved in response to infection have been evaluated and are presented in the following.

RNASEL. The ribonuclease L (RNASEL) gene is one of two candidate prostate cancer susceptibility genes that play roles in innate immunity and inflammation (Carpten et al, 2002; Xu et al, 2002). RNASEL maps to hereditary prostate cancer 1 (HPC1) and is the terminal enzyme of the 2–5A system, a RNA degradation pathway that plays an important role in mediating the biologic effects of interferons, especially in response to viral infection (Carpten et al, 2002). R462Q, one of four germline mutations in HPC1/*RNASEL* observed in hereditary prostate cancer cases, is a common missense variant. This variant is associated with decreased activity compared to the wildtype enzyme (Casey et al, 2002), impaired induction of apoptosis in response to activation by 2–5A (Xiang et al, 2003), and may involve a functionally significant amino acid substitution (Rennert et al, 2005). Approximately 15% of Caucasians are homozygous for the R462Q variant (Packer et al, 2006). Association studies examining the role of the R462Q variant in prostate cancer risk have been mixed. On one hand, the *RNASEL* R462Q mutation was implicated in 13% of unselected prostate cancer cases in a sib-pair study (Casey et al, 2002). However, in a large Swedish population-based case-control study, the frequency of the homozygous variant was similar among controls (14%), sporadic prostate cancer cases (15%), and familial cases (15%) (Wiklund et al, 2004).

Toll-like receptors. The Toll-like receptors (TLRs) play an important role in innate immunity and reponse to infection. TLRs respond to key ligands found on host pathogens, which upon exposure leads to upregulation of pro-inflammatory cytokines and chemokines. At present, 10 members of the TLR family have been identified. Variants in the TLR genes could alter the inflammatory response to infection and inflammation, which could affect risk. A large Swedish case-control study sequenced the *TLR4* gene and identified variation in 8 markers, while haplotype analysis showed no association of *TLR4* variation and prostate cancer risk. However, variation in the TLR4_15844 allele corresponding to 11381G/C was associated with a 30% increased risk of prostate cancer (95% CI 1.0–1.6), and a somewhat stronger increased risk for early onset prostate cancer (Zheng et al, 2004). A large US nested study examined 20 variants in *TLR4*. While the study found no association of the TLR4_15844 allele, it identified two common haplotypes that were significantly associated with prostate cancer risk (Chen et al, 2005). Several of the variants were also more strongly associated with early onset disease. Variants in *TLR1*, *TLR6*, and *TLR10* appear also to be associated with risk of prostate cancer (Sun et al, 2006). Through a phylogenetic tree analysis, a *TLR6-TLR1-TLR10* gene cluster region was identified that was evolutionarily related and significantly associated with prostate cancer risk.

In summary, genetic predisposition likely plays an important role in prostate cancer risk and progression. It is unlikely that highly penetrant genes are responsible for the majority of disease. Instead, common but low penetrant susceptibility alleles are likely to play a role, but be associated with modest increases in relative risks. Future studies should be designed to accommodate the large sample sizes needed to detect the associations of the genes alone, or in combination with environmental factors. Recent collaborative efforts designed to pool cohorts certainly address issues of statistical power (Hunter et al, 2005). Given the influence of PSA screening in overdiagnosing prostate cancer, it becomes increasingly important to identify biologically relevant subtypes of disease, either pathologically or molecularly.

RISK FACTORS

Epidemiological studies have an important role to shed light on potential risk factors for prostate cancer, and toward understanding opportunities for prevention. It is becoming increasingly clear that prostate cancer is a disease of considerable heterogeneity. Researchers are beginning to make distinctions between prostate cancer that is of clinical significance versus indolent disease, and that these two entities may reflect different etiologies. Thus, it is critical in evaluating the epidemiological literature to consider the associations of various factors with respect to clinically advanced or high-grade disease, and also to explore the role of different exposures of prostate cancer progression.

Tobacco

Although strongly linked to a number of cancers, the role of cigarette smoking on prostate cancer is unclear. Limited evidence suggests that smoking can modulate the endocrine system to some degree—possibly by increasing circulating levels of testosterone or of the adrenal androgen androstenedione (Dai et al, 1988). Both of these hormones have been linked, albeit inconsistently, to prostate cancer risk (Nomura and Kolonel, 1991; Andersson et al, 1993; Gann et al, 1996). N-nitroso compounds (tobacco constituents) may induce prostate cancer, but this has been shown only in rodent models (Pour, 1983). Descriptive epidemiology provides evidence that geographically or racially varying prostate cancer incidence rates must be influenced by environmental promoters, and tobacco smoke is a well-known and potent promoter of carcinogenesis.

With few exceptions, epidemiologic studies have not supported a causal relationship between smoking and total prostate cancer incidence (Colditz, 1996; Lumey, 1996). The overwhelming majority of case-control studies (utilizing both population- and hospital-based control groups) and cohort studies have reported null associations with numerous measures of smoking: current/former/never smoking, number of cigarettes per day, number of years of smoking, age when started smoking, years since first smoked, and years since quitting (Lumey, 1996; Lumey et al, 1997). Some longitudinal studies, however, have noted an elevated risk as high as two- to threefold for smokers of more than one pack per day (Hiatt et al, 1994; Cerhan et al, 1997). Nevertheless, these few studies did not convincingly demonstrate a dose–response relationship, nor did they account for the confounding influence of diet in their analyses. Smokers are known to consume fewer vegetables and more animal fat, factors that are possibly related to prostate cancer risk.

The relationship between smoking and prostate cancer mortality has been documeted more consistently. Within several large cohort studies, investigators have established a link between cigarette smoking and development of lethal prostate cancer (Hsing et al, 1990b; Coughlin et al, 1996; Rodriguez et al, 1997b; Giovannucci et al, 1999). Cigarette smokers are estimated to be up to twice as likely as nonsmokers to die from prostate cancer. The majority of these studies did not document a risk gradient for either the number of cigarettes smoked per day or the duration of smoking. However, Giovannucci et al (1999) did find a convincing dose–response association for pack-years smoked during the previous decade. Former smokers do not appear to be at increased risk of dying from prostate cancer, although one study (Giovannucci et al, 1999) did note that this null relationship existed only after quitting for more than 10 years. While these findings for lethal prostate cancer could be attributed to residual confounding, these data also highlight the complexity of epidemiological studies of prostate cancer and emphasize that advanced and slow-growing cancers are likely to be different diseases (Willett, 2006).

Diet

Studies attempting to elucidate the nutritional etiology of prostate cancer are many, yet no definitive answers have emerged.

A western diet has long been regarded as a potentially important risk factor. This suspicion is based on international comparisons of prostate cancer mortality rates—largely regarded as the result of disparate rates of progression of initiated prostate cancer to advanced disease—and the observation that migrants from low- to high-risk geographic areas, as well as their offspring, assume the higher risk profile of their adopted countries. Both observations suggest that strong environmental factors are involved. Ecologic studies provided the basis for the initial hypotheses regarding diet and prostate cancer, demonstrating the striking disparity in animal product and fat consumption between high-risk (United

States, Sweden) and low-risk (Japan, China) countries (Rose et al, 1986). Ecologic study designs, however, cannot adequately control for the effect of confounders and are limited in their ability to isolate important single foods or nutrients.

Fat intake

Since the 1990s, a large number of analytic epidemiologic studies have been conducted to evaluate the nutritional etiology of prostate cancer. Dietary animal fat (from meat and dairy products) has with relative consistency been reported as a positive risk factor, but the interpretation of this finding remains controversial. A number of other dietary factors are known to covary with fat intake (Gann, 1998), such as total energy intake, which is often inadequately accounted for in epidemiologic analyses. For any given level of total energy intake, a proportionately high fat intake can be taken at face value or can be viewed as reflecting a proportionately low intake of other foods, some possibly protective against prostate cancer. Dairy foods contribute greatly to total animal fat intake in most western populations and most are also high in calcium, itself a proposed risk factor for prostate cancer.

There is no conclusive evidence regarding the effect of total calories per se on prostate cancer risk (Bosland et al, 1999). Interestingly, in a prostate cancer animal model, an energy-restricted diet led to reduced tumor angiogenesis and decreased tumor growth (Mukherjee et al, 1999), suggesting total energy may be important with respect to prognosis. Large studies that took fat intake and total energy intake simultaneously into account reached different conclusions, some finding a positive effect (Rohan et al, 1995; Andersson et al, 1996b) and others no effect of fat-adjusted energy intake (Whittemore et al, 1995a; Hayes et al, 1999). Likewise, findings relating to the effect of unsaturated lipid intake, primarily vegetable lipids, have been essentially null (Kolonel et al, 1999).

A large number of epidemiologic studies have evaluated the effect of animal (saturated) fat intake, or of food items high in animal fat content, with inconsistent results (Kolonel et al, 1999). A review of these studies suggests that when data collection allows for proper control of total energy intake, the results are less likely to implicate animal fat as a risk factor for prostate cancer. Investigations that focused on particular food items have been slightly more concordant in showing that high red meat or dairy product consumption may increase the risk anywhere between 50% and 150% (Kolonel et al, 1999). Some of them have even demonstrated within the same analysis no persuasive evidence for an effect of fat but significant positive associations with high red meat or milk intake (Mettlin et al, 1989; Giovannucci et al, 1993b). Thus, there is reason to suspect that some other constituents of high-animal-fat foods may be related to the risk of prostate cancer or that animal fat in conjunction with other nutrients may increase the risk.

Several prospective studies have evaluated intake of specific fatty acids, rather than total fat, in relation to prostate cancer. In western diets, alpha-Linolenic acid (ALA) is the principal dietary n–3 fatty acid while Linoleic acid (LA) is the most abundant n–6 fatty acid. Measured in prospective plasma samples, higher levels of ALA—from vegetable or animal sources—was associated with an increased risk of advanced prostate cancer, while increasing ratios of LA to ALA were associated with a lower risk of advanced disease (Gann et al, 1994). While these findings agree with other plasma-based and dietary-based prospective studies (Harvey et al, 1997; Leitzmann et al, 2004), others have reported no association (Koralek et al, 2006; Schuurman et al, 1999b). If the findings are replicated more consistently, it is intriguing that n–3 fatty acids mainly from terrestrial and those mainly from marine sources (see following) have potentially different effects.

Fish intake

Populations with a high consumption of fish, for example in Japan and among Eskimos in Alaska, have lower rates of prostate cancer than populations with Western food habits, where the fish intake in general is lower (Nutting et al, 1993; Zhang et al, 1999; Dewailly et al, 2003). Fish contain long-chain marine omega-3 fatty acids, which can modify inflammatory pathways and thereby affect prostate cancer risk and progression (Chan et al, 2005). However, inconsistent results emerge from analytic epidemiologic studies of prostate cancer risk in relation to frequency of fish intake (Andersson et al, 1995; Key et al, 1997; Terry et al, 2001). In a large prospective study from the United States, the intake of four or more servings per week was associated with a reduced risk of advanced prostate cancer. In this study, the association between intake of specific marine fatty acids was weaker than that for fish intake, suggesting that compounds in fish other than fatty acids are etiologically relevant (Augustsson et al, 2003).

An Australian study that measured biomarkers of two long-chain omega-3s—eicosapentaenoic acid and docosahexaenoic acid—among prostate cancer cases and controls observed significant reduced risks of prostate cancer associated with higher levels of the biomarkers (Norrish et al, 1999). A small study from Japan (Mishina et al, 1985) and a Swedish case-control study (Hedelin et al, 2006) provided further support for a protective effect of fish intake. There is also evidence that the effect of frequent fish intake may be modified by genetic variants in genes involved in fatty acid metabolism and inflammation (Hedelin et al, 2007). Moreover, assessment of fish intake after diagnosis was associated with a lower risk of prostate cancer progression (Chan et al, 2006). Two studies from Hawaii, however, were null for marine intake and cancer risk (Le Marchand et al, 1994; Severson et al, 1989).

Diary products, calcium, and vitamin D
Increased intake of dairy products has been associated with prostate cancer risk in several case-control studies and cohort studies (Chan et al, 1998a; Tseng et al, 2005; Rodriguez et al, 2003). Dairy products, in addition to containing a substantial amount of animal fat, are the most common dietary sources of calcium and vitamin D. The strong correlation between dairy foods and these nutrients create challenges in trying to disentangle the independent effects. One study found an approximate doubling of risk for high versus low calcium intake (Chan et al, 1998a). However, the high correlation (0.90) between dairy food consumption and calcium intake in this study warrants caution against the interpretation that calcium per se is the critical risk factor (Gann, 1998). Another large study found no change in prostate cancer risk among increasing quartiles of energy-adjusted calcium consumption (Hayes et al, 1999). A US cohort study, applying perhaps a more reliable method of quantifying the role of micronutrients in disease etiology, indicated that calcium supplement users were at increased risk of prostate cancer compared to nonusers (Giovannucci et al, 1998b). Moreover, very high intake of calcium through diet or supplementation was associated with significant excess risks (Rodriguez et al, 2003; Giovannucci et al, 2006; Tseng et al, 2005), particularly for advanced or lethal prostate cancer (Giovannucci et al, 2006).

Calcium has been proposed to increase the risk of prostate cancer by suppressing circulating levels of dihydroxyvitamin D (1,25(OH)2D), a possible protective factor for prostate cancer (Giovannucci et al, 1998b). This bioactive metabolite of vitamin D is a steroid hormone involved in regulating differentiation and proliferation of many cell types, including prostate epithelia, which express functional vitamin D receptors. There is some epidemiologic evidence linking high circulating levels of 1,25(OH)2D to low prostate cancer risk. However, enough contradictory findings have been published to render the etiologic relationship, at this point, equivocal (Giovannucci, 1998).

Lycopene and tomatoes
The relationship between tomatoes, lycopene—a carotenoid consumed princi-

pally from tomato products—and prostate cancer has received a great deal of attention (Giovannucci, 1999), as preliminary evidence suggesting a significant benefit associated with high intake of tomatoes or lycopene represents a possible avenue for prostate cancer prevention. There is reliable experimental evidence that cooked or processed tomato products, such as tomato sauce, tomato soup, and ketchup, offer more readily bioavailable sources of lycopene than fresh tomatoes (Tonucci et al, 1995; Gartner et al, 1997). Accordingly, some epidemiologic studies have found significant inverse effects for tomato sauce while reporting weaker results for raw tomato intake and no significant influence for tomato juice (Giovannucci, 1999). Four cohort studies have assessed tomato product intake or dietary lycopene and subsequent risk of prostate cancer (Giovannucci, 1999; Giovannucci, 2002). All found a risk reduction of approximately 30% to 50% for various measures of high versus low tomato intake or dietary lycopene. Case-control studies have been less persuasive with some reporting lower risks, no effect, or even increased risks.

The correlation between dietary estimates of lycopene based on food frequency questionnaires and circulating levels measured in blood are relatively low, ranging from 0 to 0.47 (Giovannucci, 2002). To date, the results of three studies of blood levels of lycopene and prostate cancer risk have been published. Two prospective studies reported an inverse association with higher lycopene levels (Hsing et al, 1990a; Gann et al, 1999), but not other carotenoids (only one was statistically significant— Gann et al, 1999). Another reported a null association when comparing the highest to the lowest intake, although plasma levels in this cohort were substantially lower than in other populations (Nomura et al, 1997). In a large cohort of men with prostate cancer, higher intake of tomato products after diagnosis was associated with a lower risk of disease progression (Chan et al, 2006).

Although not definitive, the available data suggest that increased consumption of tomato and tomato-based products may be associated with lower prostate cancer risk and progression. A trial is currently underway to examine whether tomato oil capsules among men with high-grade prostatic intraepithelial neoplasia, a potential cancer precursor, reduce subsequent risk of prostate cancer.

Soy/Phytoestrogens

Given the substantially lower incidence of prostate cancer in Asia, epidemiological attention has turned to dietary practices that are characteristic of these low-risk populations. Traditional Asian diets are notably high in phytoestrogens chiefly from soy-based products, which may be cancer preventative (Messina et al, 1994; Tham et al, 1998). Dietary phytoestrogens, naturally occurring constituents of plants, are divided into two main categories: lignants and isoflavonoids. While lignants occur in wholegrain bread, seeds, berries, vegetables, and tea, the main source of isoflavonoids is soy beans and soy products. Notwithstanding the intriguing ecologic correlation between high intake of phytoestrogens and low incidence of prostate cancer, data from analytic epidemiologic studies are inconclusive. The investigation by Severson et al (1989) of Japanese men residing in Hawaii and the case-control study by Lee et al (1998) of dietary risk factors for prostate cancer in China both reported nonsignificant inverse associations between soy products and prostate cancer incidence. The Chinese study showed remarkably high soy intake among the controls (an average of 11.7 servings of soy per week).

Unfortunately, low exposure has been a serious obstacle to research efforts in western populations. Jacobsen et al (1998) circumvented this problem by studying Adventist men in California, who regularly consume soy milk. In this study, men who drank soy milk more than once per day exhibited a 70% reduction in prostate cancer risk. A recent multiethnic case-control study also showed a trend of decreasing prostate cancer risk with increasing intake of legumes, including soy products (Kolonel et al, 2000). In a Swedish case-control study, higher phytoestrongen intake, in which legumes were a major source, was associated with a reduced risk of prostate cancer, while no association was observed for isoflavenoids (Hedelin et al, 2006). Circulating levels of enterolactone, a phytoestrogen produced from dietary lignants, has been studied, with one retrospective study reporting a protective effect (Hedelin et al, 2006) and a prospective study reporting no association (Stattin et al, 2004). More work on phytoestrogens is warranted, notably since animal studies have suggested several possible mechanisms for a preventive effect. Phytoestrogens may for example be estrogenic, inhibit angiogenesis, exert antioxidant activity (Messina et al, 1994; Adlercreutz and Mazur, 1997), stimulate apoptosis, and inhibit cell growth (Bylund et al, 2000; Kyle et al, 1997).

Selenium

Selenium is a biological trace element, with body stores derived mainly from the dietary intake of food grown in selenium-rich soil. It is thought to be essential for physiologic processes ranging from skeletal muscle and immune system function to spermatogenesis and normal functioning of the prostate gland. Dietary intake of selenium varies greatly among geographic areas, and ecologic studies have suggested an inverse association between selenium content in the local soil and prostate cancer incidence (Rayman, 2000). Experimental studies have shown that selenium strongly inhibits growth and stimulates apoptosis in human prostate cancer cell lines, and that cancer cells show greater sensitivity to the growth-inhibitory effects of selenium than nonmalignant cells (Redman et al, 1998; Menter et al, 2000).

Quantification of dietary selenium intake cannot be validly accomplished by methods other than biological sampling, because the selenium content of the soil in which foods are grown is unknowable and can vary substantially even for similar items grown and/or consumed in the same geographic region. Epidemiological studies have thus focused on measuring selenium levels in blood or toe nails. Four prospective studies have reported a significant inverse association between higher levels of selenium, measured in blood or toe nails, and prostate cancer risk (Yoshizawa et al, 1998; Nomura et al, 2000; Li et al, 2004), particularly for advanced disease (Yoshizawa et al, 1998; Nomura et al, 2000; Li et al, 2004). Not all studies have reported this protective effect, however (Hartman et al, 1998a; Goodman et al, 2001). The strongest evidence for selenium comes from one randomized placebo-controlled clinical trial, which found selenium supplementation associated with a 63% prostate cancer reduction (Clarke et al, 1996). Intriguingly, a nationwide program in Finland to supplement soil with selenium has documented no reduction in prostate cancer incidence or mortality (http://www.mtt.fi/english/press/050902.html).

Overall, the evidence suggests that selenium inhibits prostate carcinogenesis, but more study is needed before selenium supplementation can be confidently suggested as a means of primary chemoprevention. One large randomized intervention trial with selenium and vitamin E (SELECT trial) is now underway in the United States.

Vitamin E

Vitamin E is a fat-soluble vitamin with the ability to reduce DNA damage and inhibit malignant transformation of cells due to its potent antioxidant capacity (Meydani, 1995). This, in addition to its stimulatory effect on the immune system, has prompted many investigators to study the potential role of vitamin E—or alpha-tocopherol, the most biologically active of the naturally occurring forms of vitamin E and the most common source of dietary vitamin E (Meydani, 1995)—in preventing several forms of cancer. Experimental results have shown that vitamin E derivatives inhibit growth and induce apoptosis in prostate cancer cell lines (Israel et al, 1995; Gunawardena et al, 2000). Vitamin E adjuvant to traditional cancer treatment enhances therapeutic effects in human prostate cancer cells in vitro (Ripoll et al, 1986) and animal prostate tumors in vivo (Drago et al, 1988).

Findings of epidemiologic studies are equivocal, however (Patterson et al, 1997). A Finnish intervention trial (Heinonen et al, 1998) suggested that male smokers randomized to alpha-tocopherol supplements were at significantly decreased risk of both incidence (32% reduction) and mortality (41% reduction), an association that had been observed in previous analyses from the same cohort (Alpha-Tocopherol, Beta-Carotene Cancer Prevention Study Group, 1994; Albanes et al, 1995). The generalizability of the Finnish finding is questionable, given the select population of older male smokers. Another follow-up study also found an inverse association between plasma vitamin E and prostate cancer risk preferentially among those who smoked (Eichholzer et al, 1996). Nested case-control studies (Hsing et al, 1990a; Nomura et al, 1997), including one (Hartman et al, 1998a) using baseline blood specimens from the Finnish cohort mentioned previously, have thus far not supported the striking findings of the intervention trial. Reported vitamin E supplement use was associated with a lower risk of lethal prostate cancer among current or former smokers (Chan et al, 1999), however, in line with the Finnish trial. Furthermore, there is preliminary evidence that the role of vitamin E may be modified by polymorphisms in genes involved in oxidative stress (Li et al, 2005). It could be that the prostate cancer protection conferred by vitamin E in more general populations is weak. In any case, the Finnish trial results are sufficiently intriguing and of potentially enormous public health significance to merit more study.

Summary of evidence for diet

The apparently inconsistent findings in many studies can probably be attributed to the workings of often unavoidable epidemiologic bias. When dealing with diet–disease associations, the measurement error inherent in dietary assessment instruments and laboratory analyses can obscure findings to the point where their interpretation becomes dubious. Cohort studies that attempt to link prediagnostic dietary exposures to disease often assess exposure at just one arbitrary point in time, years before diagnosis, and cannot account for changing exposure over time. Case-control studies are, to varying extents, always susceptible to recall bias. Still, the present body of work concerning diet and prostate cancer has provided important clues that will direct future investigations. Table 20–1 summarizes the current state of knowledge for dietary factors and prostate cancer where the greatest evidence lies.

Alcohol

Over the past decades, more than 30 epidemiologic studies have addressed the role of alcohol drinking as a possible modifiable

Table 20–1. Summary of evidence of nutritional factors for prostate cancer incidence and mortality. Adapted from Chan J et al, J Clin Oncol, 2005

Dietary Factor	Quality of evidence	Direction of association	
		Prostate cancer incidence	Prostate Cancer Mortality
Selenium	Strong	Inverse	Inverse
Tomatoes/lycopene	Good	Inverse	Inverse
Vitamin E	Good	Inverse	Inverse
Vitamin D	Fair to Good	Inverse	—
Calcium and dairy	Good	Positive	Positive
Fish intake	Fair to Good	Inverse	—
Fat intake	Fair	Positive	—
Phytoestrogens	Fair	Inverse	—

risk factor for prostate cancer (comprehensively reviewed by Breslow and Weed, 1998). Some biological basis for an association between alcohol and cancer, in general, does exist. A metabolite of alcohol, acetaldehyde, is itself a carcinogen, and alcohol is known to affect cell-membrane integrity, enhance production of free radicals, impair immune function, and reduce levels of DNA repair enzymes (Jensen et al, 1996). Overwhelmingly, however, the evidence indicates that alcohol drinking, in moderation, is not associated with cancer of the prostate.

Two studies among cohorts of alcoholics have provided limited evidence that very heavy drinking may increase the risk of prostate cancer (Adami et al, 1992; Tonnesen et al, 1994). One group of investigators found a significantly elevated risk for their total alcoholic population compared to the general population (Tonnesen et al, 1994); the other group found a similar effect, but only among alcoholics aged 50 to 64 (Adami et al, 1992). Yet, to the extent that heavy drinkers in population-based studies can be considered comparable to alcoholics, there is little other epidemiologic evidence to support these findings (Dennis, 2000). In a large US cohort study, men who consumed more than five alcoholic drinks per day had exactly the same risk as men who consumed less than one drink per day after adjusting for age, smoking, race, and education (Hiatt et al, 1994). This finding has been replicated in some cohort studies (Platz et al, 2004; Baghetto et al, 2006), while others have reported an increased risk of prostate cancer associated with high intake of alcohol (Schuurman et al, 1999a; Putnam et al, 2000).

It could be that men in the alcoholic cohorts also suffer from liver cirrhosis, which may modify cancer risk by altering hormone levels and impairing metabolism of carcinogens. A nationwide follow-up study of liver cirrhosis patients in Denmark, however, concluded that these patients had the same risk of prostate cancer as the general Danish male population (Sorensen et al, 1998). Perhaps the proposed elevated risk among alcoholics is mediated by some mechanism other than cirrhosis. It is also possible that population-based studies have contained too few subjects with exposure levels as high as those of the alcoholic cohorts and therefore were unable to document any effect.

Reproductive Factors

See "Infections" for a discussion of sexual activity in relation to prostate cancer risk.

Hormones

Androgens

There is a long-standing suspicion—based on a convincing array of circumstantial and experimental, but not epidemiologic, evidence—that endogenous hormones play a role in the etiology of prostate cancer. Androgens, particularly testosterone and dihydrotestosterone, are essential for the normal growth and functioning of the prostate. Testosterone diffuses into prostate cells, where 90% is irreversibly converted to dihydrotestosterone, the more active intracellular androgen, by an enzyme, 5-alpha-reductase. Both testosterone and dihydrotestosterone bind to a cytoplasmic androgen receptor. The complex of androgen to androgen receptor then binds to specific DNA sites, resulting in increased transcriptional activity and cell division (Coffey, 1979). The reliance on androgens for normal prostatic growth, the fact that the presence of functioning testes also appears to be essential for the development of prostate cancer, the observation that bilateral orchiectomy can result in prostate cancer remission, and the finding that androgens can induce prostate cancer in experimental animals all implicate androgens as, at the very least, important permissive factors for prostate cancer.

Most epidemiologic evidence does not strongly support the hypothesis that high levels of circulating androgens correspond to an increased risk of prostate cancer (Nomura and Kolonel, 1991; Eaton et al, 1999). The relevant case-control studies have received critical commentary regarding the possibility that prostate cancer may alter levels of circulating hormones. This would preclude studies that used post-diagnostic case sera from discussing findings in a causal context. However, very little evidence has emerged that would indicate a change in circulating sex hormone levels resulting from this particular disease process. Moreover, many other studies have utilized frozen prediagnostic sera collected from large cohorts and still have detected no substantial difference in the levels of a number of circulating androgens between men with and without prostate cancer (Eaton et al, 1999).

A summary of the epidemiologic evidence, showing that testosterone, dihydrotestosterone, dehydroepiandrosterone sulfate (an adrenal androgen), and androstenedione (another adrenal androgen) have been positively, negatively, and not associated with prostate cancer leaves investigators with few promising avenues to pursue. Several studies have measured both free and total testosterone, with the expectation that the former, a readily bioavailable form, would turn out to be more closely related to the risk. This was not found to be the case in most of these studies (Nomura et al, 1996; Guess et al, 1997; Dorgan et al, 1998). Similarly, some investigators have measured sex hormone-binding globulin, in order to assess the potential impact of high or low levels of androgen binding, with no remarkable findings (Signorello et al, 1997; Dorgan et al, 1998). The ratio of testosterone to dihydrotestosterone in blood has also been examined as a possible risk factor. Some findings have suggested a positive association (Nomura et al, 1988; Hsing and Comstock, 1993; Gann et al, 1996; Dorgan et al, 1998) (only the Gann et al finding reaching statistical significance), but on the whole, the results have been unremarkable (Nomura et al, 1996; Vatten et al, 1997).

Interest in androgens has sparked again with the recent identification of a novel translocation in prostate cancer (Tomlins et al, 2005). Through a bioinformatics approach, researchers identified a common gene fusion between the highly androgen regulated gene *TMPRSS2* and members of the ETS family of transcription factors. The *TMPRSS2*:ETS fusion occurs in prostate cancer, where it is present in 30% to 60% of cases, as well as high-grade PIN, but has not been observed in benign prostate tissue. Higher expression levels of the gene fusion is associated with poor prostate cancer prognosis (Demichelis et al, 2007). The role of hormones on prostate cancer risk and progression may therefore be modified according to presence or absence of the translocation.

5-alpha reductase

5-alpha reductase in the prostate works to convert testosterone to the more potent dihydrotestosterone, which, by binding to the androgen receptor, initiates a chain of molecular events that induces prostate cell division. Ross et al (1992) found that young Japanese men display lower 5-alpha reductase activity than young Caucasian or African American men. Consequently, there has been considerable speculation that 5-alpha reductase activity could be related to prostate cancer risk and could also partially account for the low rate of prostate cancer observed in the Japanese population. 5-alpha reductase activity is reflected by serum biomarkers, including 3-alpha-androstenediol glucuronide and androsterone glucuronide, which are downstream products of dihydrotestosterone metabolism.

Epidemiologic studies have offered no compelling evidence that these markers of 5-alpha reductase activity are related to prostate cancer risk (Gann et al, 1996; Nomura et al, 1996; Guess et al, 1997; Vatten et al, 1997). It has been suggested that these null findings may be due to our current inability to measure type I and type II 5-alpha reductase activity separately (Guess et al, 1997; Vatten et al, 1997). Type II is the predominant intraprostatic isoenzyme, type I the predominant extraprostatic isoenzyme. Serum levels of biomarkers of 5-alpha reductase activity would reflect the total amount of type I and type II activity, leading to measurement error of unpredictable magnitude. The results of a large, randomized trial of finasteride, a 5-alpha reductase inhibitor, demonstrated a 25% reduction in risk of prostate cancer over 7 years of follow-up (Thompson et al, 2003). At the same time, the men randomized to finasteride were at greater risk of high-grade disease, a finding that has yet to be explained. Whether finasteride should be considered as a wide-scale chemopreventive agent has been discussed, although currently is unlikely to be cost-effective (Svatek et al, 2006).

Estrogens

Estrogens are produced within the prostate through the aromatization of testosterone. Although the role of estrogen within the gland has not been clearly elucidated, some investigators have speculated that these hormones have the ability to increase prostate cell sensitivity to androgens, these deductions following from observations that increasing estradiol can upregulate androgen receptors in the prostates of dogs (Trachtenberg et al, 1980). The epidemiologic literature on estrogens in relation to prostate cancer does not provide any clear-cut messsage regarding risk implications, although the weight of the evidence suggests a null effect (Barrett-Connor et al, 1990; Hsing and Comstock, 1993; Dorgan et al, 1998) or, at most, a slight protective effect (Andersson et al, 1993; Gann et al, 1996; Signorello et al, 1997).

Insulin-like growth factor 1 and Insulin-like growth factor binding proteins

One promising advance in our understanding of prostate cancer etiology involves the peptide hormone insulin-like growth factor 1 (IGF-1), a major growth-regulating molecule that is known to be a potent mitogen that can also inhibit apoptosis. It is secreted mainly by the liver but is also produced in several other tissues, including the prostate, in response to growth hormone. IGF-1 is present in large concentrations in circulation, which can have systemic or local effects on cell behavior. In circulation, 80% of IGF-1 is bound in a ternary complex with its binding protein-3 and the glycoprotein acid-labile subunit. IGF-1 exerts its effect by binding with IGF-1 receptors, expressed on prostate cells, leading to induction of cellular proliferation. The ability of IGF-1 to cross the endothelial barrier and exert its effects is directly dependent on IGF availability and is modulated by IGFBP-3 binding proteins. Until the late 1990s, there was little epidemiologic literature regarding the association between serum levels of IGF-1 and prostate, or in fact any, cancer.

However, a succession of studies from different countries found similar and strong effects of IGF-1 on prostate cancer risk, and has now provided compelling evidence that IGF-1 may be a key risk factor for the disease (Mantzoros et al, 1997; Chan et al, 1998c; Wolk et al, 1998; Djavan et al, 1999; Harman et al, 2000; Stattin et al, 2000). Even within the normal range of variation of IGF-1, an increase of 60 to 100 ng/ml may double the risk of prostate cancer (Mantzoros et al, 1997; Chan et al, 1998c; Wolk et al, 1998). Both case-control investigations (using postdiagnostic blood samples) and prospective cohorts (using blood samples taken years prior to the cancer diagnosis) are in relative agreement about the effect of IGF-1. A meta-analysis in 2003 reported a summary odds ratio of 2.4 (95% CI 1.1–5.3) comparing high and low IGF-1 levels (Renehan et al, 2004). Taken together, the experimental and epidemiologic evidence linking IGF-1 to prostate cancer is compelling and should be further developed to clarify the role of IGF-1 in prostate cancer detection, progression, and mortality.

Because of their central role in the regulation of bioavailable IGF-1, the insulin-like growth factor binding proteins (IGFBPs) have also come under scrutiny as potential mediators of prostate cancer risk (Drivdahl et al, 1995; Nunn et al, 1997; Figueroa et al, 1998). There is some debate concerning which, if any, of the IGFBPs may be relevant. Epidemiologically, IGFBP-3 has been examined the most thoroughly, with evidence of an inverse association with prostate cancer risk from one prospective (Chan et al, 1998c) and one retrospective study (Chokkalingam et al, 2001) that is not supported by other investigations (Wolk et al, 1998; Harman et al, 2000; Stattin et al, 2000; Platz et al, 2005). Insulin-like growth factor binding protein 3 has received the most attention primarily because over 95% of circulating IGF-1 is bound to this protein (Jones and Clemmons, 1995). However, it is IGFBP-1 that effectively shuttles IGF-1 across blood vessel membranes (Lewitt et al, 1993), and if serum IGFBP-1 levels are predictive of the amount of circulating IGF-1 available to prostate tissue, they may consequently be predictive of prostate cancer risk. One study has found that high serum IGFBP-1 levels were strongly predictive of prostate cancer risk (Signorello et al, 1999), but another study found no such association (Stattin et al, 2000).

Methodologic issues
Studying endogenous hormones in relation to prostate cancer risk is challenging for a number of reasons. First, the concentration of many circulating hormones has a circadian rhythm, and not all epidemiologic studies have properly accounted for this by either matching on blood sampling timing or restricting blood draws to a narrow time-of-day window. Second, within-person variation in circulating hormone levels, coupled with unavoidable laboratory measurement error, can introduce exposure misclassification of unpredictable magnitude. It is generally assumed, however, that these errors are nondifferential with respect to cases and noncases, therefore biasing results toward the null. Still, the resulting overly conservative and highly imprecise relative risks are difficult to draw etiologic inferences from.

A single blood measurement is probably not sufficiently reliable to characterize an individual's typical hormonal profile (Nomura et al, 1996) and may explain why the multitude of relevant studies have not been able to detect consistent differences between the average sex hormone levels of prostate cancer patients and healthy com-

parison men. Moreover, serum hormone levels may not accurately reflect tissue levels, which cannot be determined in standard epidemiologic studies because of the invasiveness and risk involved in collecting the necessary samples. Alternatively, it may be that sex hormones are merely permissive factors. In their presence, prostate cancer can arise in response to cellular events not yet explainable, but in their absence (ie, through castration), the mechanisms by which the disease develops are blocked.

Anthropometric Measures
Body mass index
Because body mass and/or composition can influence endogenous levels of sex hormones (Pasquali et al, 1991; Mantzoros and Georgiadis, 1995), body mass index (BMI), has been studied as a possible influential factor in many epidemiologic studies. With few exceptions, adult BMI has been found to be unrelated to prostate cancer risk in case-control studies (Kolonel, 1996; Lee et al, 1998; Hayes et al, 1999). Prospective studies of incidence and mortality are more supportive of a positive association (Garfinkel, 1986; Severson et al, 1988; Thompson et al, 1989; Putnam et al, 2000) but are not in total agreement (Giovannucci, 1997a).

It remains unclear whether a positive association between BMI and prostate cancer, if one indeed exists, reflects an effect of adiposity or of lean muscle mass. Body mass index typically does not distinguish well between the two and often reflects the latter, considering that muscle tissue is denser than fat tissue. Thus, for any given height, a higher relative amount of muscle mass will result in a higher BMI. One prospective study of Japanese-American men found that prostate cancer risk was in fact related to arm muscle mass and not arm fat area (Severson et al, 1988). This finding may have biological plausibility and indirect support from other epidemiologic studies: Arm muscle mass has been found to correlate with the testosterone/dihydrotestosterone ratio in serum (Henderson, 1990); some epidemiologic data indicate that this hormone ratio is positively associated with prostate cancer (Gann et al, 1996), and a large Swedish study found prostate cancer risk to be more strongly associated with lean body mass than with BMI (Andersson et al, 1997).

Alternatively, adiposity may play some role. Prostate cancer has been positively associated with abdominal obesity, as measured by the waist-to-hip ratio (Hsing et al, 2000a). Also, in a cohort study, men given a hospital discharge diagnosis of obesity experienced a significant 30% elevation in the risk of prostate cancer compared with the general population (Moller et al, 1994). These results may reflect the effect of the cohort's dietary practices, but dietary data were not collected.

Few investigators have been able to characterize the relationship between BMI at different stages of life and prostate cancer. Indeed, at this point, the relevant exposure period is unknown. Two US studies, one cohort (Cerhan et al, 1997) and one case-control (Hayes et al, 1999), demonstrated no association between BMI at age 25 and subsequent risk of prostate cancer. In contrast, one cohort study from the Netherlands did report a significant trend of increasing prostate cancer risk with increasing BMI at age 20 (Schuurman et al, 2000). Childhood obesity, on the other hand, has been inversely related to future prostate cancer risk, notably for advanced metastatic cancer, where the relative risk for the highest compared to the lowest quintile of BMI at age 10 was 0.38 (Giovannucci et al, 1997a). In this same study, several measures of adult obesity were unrelated to the risk of prostate cancer. Adiposity is known to increase estrogen and decrease androgen serum concentrations in men (Pasquali et al, 1991). Hence, a childhood hormonal milieu characterized by low exposure to the stimulating effect of androgens on the prostate might protect against the disease.

Weight change

In a US prospective study, the investigators found no association between BMI at the time of cohort enrollment (average age 73.5 years) and risk of prostate cancer, but they did note a significant trend of increasing risk with the percent change in BMI from age 50 to age at enrollment (Cerhan et al, 1997). The effect was modest (a 30% increase in risk for a more than 10% increase in BMI over this time period). A weight loss of at least 10% after the age of 50, however, corresponded to a 60% reduction in risk. The investigators did not observe any association with percentage change in BMI from age 25 to enrollment age. While the interpretation of these results is not clear, the data suggest that weight change in late adult life may be a critical factor.

Height

The current data relating height to prostate cancer risk are conflicting. Adult height has been found to be unrelated to risk in several investigations (Kolonel, 1996; Hsieh et al, 1999; Hsing et al, 2000a), but some studies (Le Marchand et al, 1994; Andersson et al, 1997; Giovannucci et al, 1997a; Hebert et al, 1997) have reported an increase in risk of 15% to 100% for taller men—the highest height categories varying from 173 cm to 180 cm. Male adult height can reflect nutritional status in early life and is determined in part by circulating growth factors and other hormones during puberty. It is possible that men who attain greater height might have had higher exposure to pubertal levels of androgens at a time when the prostate gland is commencing its normal development and function (Giovannucci et al, 1997a). In preadolescent boys, the production of testosterone markedly increases the level of plasma IGF-1 (Keenan et al, 1993), and adult height has been positively correlated with serum IGF-1 levels (Signorello et al, 2000). Thus, it may be exposure to high circulating levels of IGF-1, more than to androgens, that is driving the observed positive associations, given that IGF-1 has been found to be a strong risk factor. Tall height may also simply be a marker for large organ size, where the larger number of cells at risk would contribute to a positive association (Trichopoulos and Lipworth, 1995).

Infections

A growing body of epidemiologic, genetic, and molecular pathological data points to the role of chronic inflammation in the pathogenesis and progression of prostate cancer (Nelson et al, 2004). The pathways involved in chronic inflammation induce cellular damage and compensatory cellular proliferation (Kuper et al, 2000). Clinical prostatitis has been associated with prostate cancer risk (Palapattu et al, 2004), and poor outcomes among men with disease (Irani et al, 1999). Infectious agents are likely targets involved in the initiation and exacerbation of chronic inflammation. Infectious agents may also have direct effects on carcinogenesis through the transformation of cells via incorporation of active oncogenes into the host genome, inhibition of tumor suppressors, stimulation of proliferation signals, or through immune suppression. To date, however, no specific infectious agent has clearly emerged as a causative agent.

Sexually transmitted diseases

The suspicion that correlates of sexual behavior may influence prostate cancer risk has prompted numerous investigations of individual infectious agents. Originally, this research effort focused principally on gonorrhea, syphilis, chlamydia, and the herpes simplex virus. Gonorrhea infection has been linked to prostate cancer, with evidence from ecologic data (Heshmat et al, 1975) and a population-based case-control study that reported a relative risk of 1.6 among men who reported a history of either gonorrhea or syphilis (Hayes et al, 2000). Another study showed a significant threefold increase in risk among men with a history of syphilis but no association with arsenical drugs (an early treatment for syphilis) (Lees et al, 1985). However, many of the studies have been limited by a small sample size, retrospective exposure assessment, reliance on self-reported data on infections, and consideration of exposure to only a limited number of STIs.

Seroepidemiologic study has generally detected no differences in the presence of chlamydia antibodies between case and control subjects (Dillner et al, 1998), but has demonstrated an excess prostate cancer risk among men with serologic evidence of syphilis (Hayes et al, 2000). In prostate tissue, herpes simplex virus type-2 (HSV-2) is no more prevalent among cases of prostate cancer than among controls (Boldogh et al, 1983; Haid and Sharon, 1984), but there is limited evidence that serum antibodies to HSV-2 may predict prostate cancer risk weakly (Baker et al, 1981; Luleci et al, 1981).

Human papillomavirus

A major shift in focus occurred when the human papillomavirus (HPV) emerged as a strong causal factor for other genitourinary cancers. Whether this oncogenic virus contributes to the development of prostate cancer remains debated, because epidemiologic results have been radically divergent. Researchers have attempted to compare HPV detection rates in the prostate tissue of cancer cases to those in the prostate tissue of men with benign prostatic hyperplasia; prostate tissue from nondiseased subjects is typically unavailable. The results of various studies argue against HPV as an important risk factor for prostate cancer (Tu et al, 1994; Wideroff et al, 1996; Noda et al, 1998; Strickler et al, 1998) and even suggest that HPV infection in the prostate may be very rare (Tu et al, 1994; Strickler et al, 1998). Others have implicated HPV type 16 (Moyret-Lalle et al, 1995; Suzuki et al, 1996; Serth et al, 1999), the HPV type known to be most strongly linked to anogenital cancers. In quite a few studies, however, HPV DNA was detected more often in nonmalignant tissue than in prostate cancer tissue. A combined analysis of several studies estimated that 32%, 49%, and 9% of prostate cancer, benign prostatic hyperplasia, and normal prostate tissue, respectively, were HPV DNA positive (Cuzick, 1995). This observation raises the question of whether benign prostatic hyperplasia tissue is an appropriate control group if, in fact, HPV infection is implicated in its own etiology.

Seroepidemiologic studies have not appreciably clarified the situation. While some data reveal serologic evidence of HPV infection to be the same among cases and controls (Strickler et al, 1998), one study found that those with antibodies against HPV types 16 or 18 had 2.5-fold greater risk of prostate cancer (Dillner et al, 1998). This same study reported no association between HPV types 11 and 13 and prostate cancer. An important contributing factor to the conflicting results may lie in the laboratory analyses. It has been shown that HPV analyses in the relevant studies can be quite dependent on the assay, primer sets, or even annealing temperature utilized (Sinclair et al, 1993; Terris and Peehl, 1997). Moreover, viral detection can be variable in different specimens from the same patient's tissue (Terris and Peehl, 1997).

A history of sexually transmitted infections (STIs) has been associated with prostate cancer, but no specific pathogen has yet emerged as an important risk factor. Epidemiological studies have shown associations between prostate cancer and several indicators of sexual activity, such as number of partners, relations with prostitutes, and age at first marriage (Andersson et al, 1996). Contradictory reports have also been published, however, including one that noted no deficit of prostate cancer mortality among Catholic priests (Ross et al, 1983; Ewings and Bowie, 1996; Hsieh et al, 1999).

T. vaginalis

The parasitic protozoan *T. vaginalis* is the most common nonviral STI (Petrin et al, 1998), with a prevalence of 5% to 20% among US young adults (Plitt et al, 2005) and globally affecting 170 million each year. Typically the infection is asymptomatic (Petrin et al, 1998) and does not clear such that infection can be detected several years after initial exposure. *T. vaginalis* has received considerably less attention in prostate cancer research than infections such as chlamydia or gonorrhea. In men, *T. vaginalis* has been associated with an increased risk of nongonococcal urethritis

(Krieger et al, 1993) and clinical prostatitis (Sutcliffe et al, 2006). Trichomonads can infect and elicit a strong inflammatory response within the prostate (Gardner et al, 1986; Van Laarhoven et al, 1967).

T. vaginalis adhesion to epithelial cells upregulates expression of anti-apoptopic genes including defenders against cell death and cycloxygenase-2, as well as proinflammatory genes such as interleukin-8 and monocyte chomoattractant protein (Kucknoor et al, 2005). *T. vaginalis* is adept at evading the host's immune system through a number of mechanisms, and reinfection does not confer immunity in humans. Nevertheless, antibodies to *T. vaginalis* can be detected in the serum of infected patients.

A large nested case-control study of *T. vaginalis* seroprevalence and prostate cancer found a 43% increase in the odds of total prostate cancer (95% CI: 1.00–2.03) and 76% increase in the odds of high-grade prostate cancer (95% CI: 0.97–3.18) among men who were seropositive (Sutcliffe et al, 2006). The only other study that has investigated the role of *T. vaginalis* in prostate cancer used self-reported history of infection and found no association (Checkoway et al, 1987). However, because the infection is most frequently asymptomatic in men and because of the high self-reported frequency of other STIs in the study population, exposure ascertainment was potentially biased.

XMRV virus

Using a viral-detection microarray, researchers recently identified the xenotropic MuLV-related virus (XMRV), a novel pathogen isolated from the prostates of men undergoing radical prostatectomy (Urisman et al, 2006). The arrays contained oligonucleotides homologous to over 5050 different viruses, and a gammaretrovirus signature, now called XMRV, was detected. Intriguingly, detection of XMRV differed according to *RNASEL* R462Q genotype, which is involved in viral clearance, described previously. XMRV was detected in tumors of only 1/52 (2%) men who were homozygous wildtypes and 0/14 men who were heterozygous (0%), but 8/20 (40%) of men who were homozygous variants. FISH studies established that XMRV is confined to stromal cells adjacent to neoplastic glands. If etiologically related to cancer, XMRV may be acting through modification of the cross-talk occurring between stromal and epithelial cells. While these initial data are intriguing, they need to be replicated in additional settings and the role of XMRV in prostate carcinogenesis needs to be explored.

Physical Activity

At this stage, physical activity should not be considered a definite risk factor for prostate cancer.

Physical activity is suspected to reduce the risk of several types of cancer via biological mechanisms that, although poorly understood, may involve, for example, enhanced immune system function (Lee, 1995), changes in the endogenous hormonal milieu, or reduced obesity (Simopoulos, 1990). For prostate cancer, studies that have focused on the effect of leisure and/or occupational physical activity have thus far produced inconsistent results (Oliveria and Lee, 1997). Many suggest at least a small reduction in prostate cancer risk with increasing activity (Lee et al, 1992; Hsing et al, 1994; Thune and Lund, 1994; Hartman et al, 1998b; Clarke and Whittemore, 2000), but others are essentially null (Whittemore et al, 1995a; Giovannucci et al, 1998a; Liu et al, 2000; Putnam et al, 2000), and some even report an increased risk (Le Marchand et al, 1991; Ilic et al, 1996).

The reported positive associations between activity level and prostate cancer could be artifacts generated by residual confounding. For example, heavy laborers may be more highly exposed to occupational carcinogens than sedentary professional workers (Ilic et al, 1996). Moreover, men who engage in regular recreational physical activity are more likely to engage in other health-conscious behaviors, such as cancer screening (Patterson et al, 1998).

Physical activity is also known to sharply, albeit transiently, increase serum levels of PSA in men (Oremek and Seiffert, 1996), which could result in a higher probability of PSA-diagnosed, otherwise occult, prostate cancers.

The assessment of long-term physical activity levels is challenging. Study participants are often asked to report on the type, intensity, and duration of their average physical activity, both currently and in the past. The resulting misclassification may be responsible for the weak and often nonsignificant findings. Subgroups less prone to measurement error, such as, men who engage in a serious and regular regimen of vigorous activity, may offer the best chance of detecting a relationship between exercise and prostate cancer if one exists. In fact, results of two prospective studies conducted in the United States (Lee et al, 1992; Giovannucci et al, 1998a) found a significant reduction (50% to 90%) in prostate cancer risk among men in the highest category of vigorous activity. These two studies did not, however, provide evidence that moderate or even moderately high levels of activity have an appreciable impact on risk.

Ionizing Radiation

Prostate cancer is exceptional in that it is among the few malignancies plainly unrelated to radiation exposure (Boice et al, 1996). Routes of ionizing radiation exposure include medical treatment (eg, radiation therapy for cancer), occupational contact (eg, workers at nuclear facilities), and military exposures (eg, atomic bomb survivors). There is no evidence of excess prostate cancer incidence or death among even highly exposed populations (Boice et al, 1996).

Occupation

Prostate epithelial cells contain the highest concentration of zinc in the human body (Untergasser et al, 2000). This essential trace element has been implicated in the normal regulation of cell growth and may play a critical role in DNA and RNA repair (Chan et al, 1998b). Cadmium is known to be a zinc antagonist, and as such has been hypothesized to disrupt normal cell-cycle regulation and increase the risk of neoplastic changes to prostate cells (Kolonel and Winkelstein, 1977; Feustel and Wennrich, 1984; Brys et al, 1997). For this reason, occupational cadmium exposure has been extensively studied with regard to prostate cancer risk.

Early occupational studies that addressed this issue were hindered by small numbers of both expected and observed prostate cancer cases, and they reported modest excesses for cadmium-exposed workers (Lemen et al, 1976; Kolonel and Winkelstein, 1977). These men were engaged in a variety of occupations including smelting, alkaline battery manufacturing, welding, and electroplating. A later study that was population based and that identified prostate cancer cases using a cancer registry did not find any positive association with occupations involving potential cadmium exposure (Ross et al, 1979). Further studies have also not corroborated the early reports from the small occupational cohorts (Chan et al, 1998b).

Again, early in the study of prostate cancer etiology, many reports emerged linking farming to high risk (Chan et al, 1998b). More recent studies, however, have been notably inconsistent, and no specific etiologic agent (eg, a specific pesticide) has been recognized to account for the positive findings, which supports the probability of a noncausal explanation. The reported prostate cancer excess among farmers is even more dubious given the relatively consistent reports of higher risk associated with urban, rather than rural, living (Andersson et al, 1995; Hsieh et al, 1999).

Medical Conditions and Treatment

Vasectomy

Considering the evidence as a whole, vasectomy is unlikely to play a causal role in prostate carcinogenesis.

Results of several epidemiologic studies during the past decade have generated the suspicion that vasectomy may increase the risk of prostate cancer (Bernal-Delgado et al, 1998). The most commonly offered biological explanation for the involvement of vasectomy in the etiology of prostate cancer is the potential for this surgery to alter endocrine function (Howard, 1993). Longitudinal data from small numbers of men followed after vasectomy overall reveal no consistent effect on circulating sex hormone concentrations (Richards et al, 1981). One noteworthy population-based and multiethnic study measured testosterone, dihydrotestosterone, and sex hormone-binding globulin in a group of 850 healthy men with normal PSA levels (John et al, 1995). Within this group, the vasectomized men had a lower serum concentration of sex hormone-binding globulin and a higher ratio of dihydrotestosterone to testosterone. These findings imply higher prostate tissue availability of sex hormones, and particularly of the more biologically active intracellular androgen, dihydrotestosterone. Overall, there is some evidence that vasectomy somewhat alters the hormonal profile. Nevertheless, given the largely circumstantial nature of the evidence linking sex hormones to prostate cancer, this evidence falls short of satisfying the basis for a biological and causative claim for the association.

Alternatively, bias may have led to positive findings. Detection bias may be likely to blame, since vasectomized men may be more likely to visit a urologist subsequently and would therefore be at higher risk of cancer detection by routine prostate screening than are men who do not have the motive to visit a urologist. In a number of studies (Giovannucci et al, 1993a; Rosenberg et al, 1994), a stronger association was noted preferentially among the subset of cases with early stage prostate cancer, which reinforced doubts that heightened physician surveillance could underlie the incidental identification of occult cancer in these men.

Many studies, including one conducted within a health maintenance organization and able to account for medical care utilization (Zhu et al, 1996), have found no evidence of a link between vasectomy and prostate cancer (DerSimonian et al, 1993; Bernal-Delgado et al, 1998). A meta-analysis of 14 studies (5 cohort and 9 case-control, with relative risks ranging from 0.44 to 6.70) estimated a pooled relative risk of 1.23 (Bernal-Delgado et al, 1998). However, the authors concluded that their estimate was quite sensitive to study base, study design, and the possibility of certain biases and was probably subject to the influence of publication bias. Another review of the literature concluded that most studies had been deficient in avoiding detection bias and in obtaining accurate vasectomy histories from study participants (DerSimonian et al, 1993).

Perinatal Factors

Ecologic data, including observations that circulating steroid levels are markedly different in pregnant African American and Chinese versus white women (Henderson et al, 1988; Lipworth et al, 1999), that populations with higher average birth weights have a higher incidence of prostate cancer (Wang et al, 1994; Lawson, 1998), and that the secular trend of increasing worldwide prostate cancer incidence was preceded by a corresponding increase in average birth weight (Ekbom et al, 1996), provide some support for the hypothesis that in utero exposures may influence the future risk of prostate cancer. Direct testing through analytic epidemiologic investigation, however, has not demonstrated a relationship between factors such as birth weight, birth length, placental weight, or maternal age and prostate cancer risk, although an inverse association with increasing duration of gestation has been reported (Ekbom et al, 2000).

CONCLUSION

Although the genetic component may be larger for prostate cancer than for most other malignancies, notably among patients diagnosed at an early age, the evidence that environmental factors are important is also overwhelming; the substantial geographic variation and changing incidence among migrants demonstrate this. However, the unusual natural history of this malignancy complicates interpretation of both descriptive and analytic studies. This complication arises due to the high prevalence of subclinical cancers—(detectable at autopsy)—among elderly men. Such lesions may now be diagnosed even in asymptomatic men, for example by means of PSA testing. Hence, diagnostic intensity may substantially influence the observed incidence of prostate cancer and thereby confound comparisons among geographic areas and among different time periods.

In analytic epidemiologic studies, it may be hard or impossible to tell whether identified risk factors play a role in malignant transformation or merely in progression from indolent to clinically significant cancer. To deal with this problem, epidemiologists more and more often analyze localized and advanced cancers separately. A stronger association with advanced cancers would then suggest a promoting rather than an initiating effect of the particular risk factor. Presently, age, area of residence, ethnic background, and family history remain the only established risk factors for prostate cancer. Hence, no intervention strategy exists that could predictably reduce the incidence of prostate cancer.

However, since prostate cancer began to attract more epidemiologic interest in the 1980s, numerous etiologic clues have been identified, and areas are now emerging as promising in the search for causes of prostate cancer. Besides genetic studies, exposures belonging to the broad categories of nutritional and hormonal factors are now being intensively investigated by epidemiologists. Obviously, these areas are not mutually exclusive since dietary factors may act via hormonal pathways. Among nutritional factors, a protective effect of lycopene, selenium, vitamin E, and perhaps phytoestrogens and fish oil appear particularly promising, although no definite answers have yet emerged. Hormonal influences are also biologically plausible. While studies of steroid hormones, chiefly androgens, have not produced consistent results, a positive association between serum levels of IGF-1 and prostate cancer appears convincing.

REFERENCES

Adami HO, McLaughlin JK, Hsing AW, Wolk A, Ekbom A, Holmberg L, et al. Alcoholism and cancer risk: a population-based cohort study. Cancer Causes Control 1992;3:419–25.

Adlercreutz H, Mazur W. Phyto-oestrogens and Western diseases. Ann Intern Med 1997; 29:95–120.

Albanes D, Heinonen OP, Huttunen JK, Taylor PR, Virtamo J, Edwards BK, et al. Effect of alpha-tocopherol and beta-carotene supplements on cancer incidence in the Alpha-tocopherol Beta-Carotene Cancer Prevention Study. Am J Clin Nutr 1995;62:1427S–1430S.

Albertsen PC, Hanley JA, Fine J. 20-year outcomes following conservative management of clinically localized prostate cancer. JAMA. 2005;293(17):2095–101.

Alpha-Tocopherol, Beta-Carotene Cancer Prevention Study Group. The effect of vitamin E and beta carotene on the incidence of lung cancer and other cancers in male smokers. The Alpha-Tocopherol, Beta Carotene Cancer Prevention Study Group. N Engl J Med 1994;330:1029–35.

Amundadottir LT, Sulem P, Gudmundsson J, Helgason A, Baker A, Agnarsson BA, Sigurdsson A, Benediktsdottir KR, Cazier JB, Sainz J, Jakobsdottir M, Kostic J, Magnusdottir DN, Ghosh S, Agnarsson K, Birgisdottir B, Le Roux L, Olafsdottir A, Blondal T, Andresdottir M, Gretarsdottir OS, Bergthorsson JT, Gudbjartsson D, Gylfason A, Thorleifsson G, Manolescu A, Kristjansson K, Geirsson G, Isaksson H, Douglas J, Johansson JE, Balter K, Wiklund F, Montie JE, Yu X, Suarez BK, Ober C, Cooney KA, Gronberg H, Catalona WJ, Einarsson GV, Barkardottir RB, Gulcher JR, Kong A, Thorsteinsdottir U, Stefansson K. A common variant associated with prostate cancer in European and African populations. Nat Genet. 2006; 38(6):652–58. Epub 2006 May 7.

Andersson SO, Adami HO, Bergström R, Wide L. Serum pituitary and sex steroid hormone levels in the etiology of prostatic cancer—a population based case-control study. Br J Cancer 1993;68:97–102.

Andersson SO, Baron J, Wolk A, Lindgren C, Bergström R, Adami HO. Early life risk factors for prostate cancer: a population-based case-control study in Sweden. Cancer Epidemiol Biomarkers Prev 1995;4:187–92.

Andersson SO, Baron J, Bergstrom R, Lindgren C, Wolk A, Adami HO. Lifestyle factors and prostate cancer risk: a case-control study in Sweden. Cancer Epidemiol Biomarkers Prev 1996a;5(7):509–13.

Andersson SO, Wolk A, Bergström R, Adami HO, Engholm G, Englund A, et al. Body size and prostate cancer: a 20-year follow-up study among 135006 Swedish construction workers. J Natl Cancer Inst 1997;89:385–89.

Andersson SO, Wolk A, Bergström R, Giovannucci E, Lindgren C, Baron J, et al. Energy, nutrient intake and prostate cancer risk: a population-based case-control study in Sweden. Int J Cancer 1996b;68:716–22.

Augustsson K, Michaud D, Rimm E, Leitzmann M, Stampfer M, Willett WC, et al. A prospective study of intake of fish and marine fatty acids and prostate cancer. Cancer Epidemiol Biomarkers Prev 2003; 12:64–67.

Baglietto L, Severi G, English DR, Hopper JL, Giles GG. Alcohol consumption and prostate cancer risk: results from the Melbourne collaborative cohort study. Int J Cancer 2006 Sep 15;119(6):1501–4

Baker LH, Mebust WK, Chin TD, Chapman AL, Hinthorn D, Towle D. The relationship of herpesvirus to carcinoma of the prostate. J Urol 1981;125:370–74.

Baker SG, Lichtenstein P, Kaprio J, Holm N. Genetic susceptibility to prostate, breast, and colorectal cancer among Nordic twins. Biometrics 2005;61:55–63.

Barrett-Connor E, Garland C, McPhillips JB, Khaw KT, Wingard DL. A prospective, population-based study of androstenedione, estrogens, and prostatic cancer. Cancer Res 1990;50:169–73.

Beilin J, Ball EM, Favaloro JM, Zajac JD. Effect of the androgen receptor CAG repeat polymorphism on transcriptional activity: specificity in prostate and non-prostate cell lines. J Mol Endocrinol 2000;25:85–96.

Beilin J, Harewood L, Frydenberg M, Mameghan H, Martyres RF, Farish SJ, et al. A case-control study of the androgen receptor gene CAG repeat polymorphism in Australian prostate carcinoma subjects. Cancer 2001; 92:941–49.

Bernal-Delgado E, Latour-Perez J, Pradas-Arnal F, Gomez-Lopez LI. The association between vasectomy and prostate cancer: a systematic review of the literature. Fertil Steril 1998; 70:191–200.

Berry R, Schroeder JJ, French AJ, McDonnell SK, Peterson BJ, Cunningham JM, et al. Evidence for a prostate cancer–susceptibility locus on chromosome 20. Am J Hum Genet 2000;67:82–91.

Bill-Axelson A, Holmberg L, Ruutu M, Haggman M, Andersson SO, Bratell S, Spangberg A, Busch C, Nordling S, Garmo H, Palmgren J, Adami HO, Norlen BJ, Johansson JE; Scandinavian Prostate Cancer Group Study No. 4. N Engl J Med. 2005;352:1977–84.

Bodiwala D, Luscombe CJ, French ME, Liu S, Saxby MF, Jones PW, Fryer AA, and Strange RC. Polymorphisms in the vitamin D receptor gene, ultraviolet radiation, and susceptibility to prostate cancer. Environ Mol Mutagen 2004;43:121–27.

Boice JD Jr, Land CE, Preston DL. Ionizing radiation. In: Schottenfeld D, Fraumeni JR Jr (Eds): Cancer Epidemiology and Prevention, 2nd ed. New York, Oxford University Press, 1996, pp 319–54.

Boldogh I, Baskar JF, Mar EC, Huang ES. Human cytomegalovirus and herpes simplex type 2 virus in normal and adenocarcinomatous prostate glands. J Natl Cancer Inst 1983;70:819–26.

Bosland MC, Oakley-Girvan I, Whittemore AS. Dietary fat, calories, and prostate cancer risk. J Natl Cancer Inst 1999;91:489–91.

Bratt O, Borg A, Kristoffersson U, Lundgren R, Zhang QX, Olsson H. CAG repeat length in the androgen receptor gene is related to age at diagnosis of prostate cancer and response to endocrine therapy, but not to prostate cancer risk. Br J Cancer 1999a;81: 672–76.

Bratt O, Kristoffersson U, Lundgren R, Olsson H. Familial and hereditary prostate cancer in southern Sweden. A population-based case-control study. Eur J Cancer 1999b;35: 272–77.

Brawley OW, Knopf K, Merrill R. The epidemiology of prostate cancer part I: descriptive epidemiology. Semin Urol Oncol 1998;16: 187–92.

The Breast Cancer Linkage Consortium. Cancer risks in BRCA2 mutation carriers. J Natl Cancer Inst 1999;91:1310–16.

Breslow RA, Weed DL. Review of epidemiologic studies of alcohol and prostate cancer: 1971–1996. Nutr Cancer 1998;30:1–13.

Brys M, Nawrocka AD, Mickos E, Zydek C, Foksinski M, Barecki A, et al. Zinc and cadmium analysis in human prostate neoplasms. Biol Trace Elem Res 1997;59:145–52.

Bylund A, Zhang JX, Bergh A, Damber JE, Widmark A, Johansson A, et al. Rye bran and soy protein delay growth and increase apoptosis of human LNCaP prostate adenocarcinoma in nude mice. Prostate 2000; 42:304–14.

Carpten JD, Nupponen N, Isaacs SD, et al. Germline mutations in the ribonuclease L gene in families showing linkage with HPC1. Nature Genetics 2002;30:181–84.

Carter BS, Beaty TH, Steinberg GD, Childs B, Walsh PC. Mendelian inheritance of familial prostate cancer. Proc Natl Acad Sci USA 1992;89:3367–71.

Casey G, Neville PJ, Plummer SJ, et al. RNASEL Arg462Gln variant is implicated in up to 13% of prostate cancer cases. Nat Genet 2002;32(4):581–83.

Catalona WJ, Smith DS, Ratliff TL, Basler JW. Detection of organ-confined prostate cancer is increased through prostate-specific antigen-based screening. JAMA 1993;270:948–54.

Cerhan JR, Parker AS, Putnam SD, Chiu B C-H, Lynch CF, Cohen MB, et al. Family history and prostate cancer risk in a population-based cohort of Iowa men. Cancer Epidemiol Biomarkers Prev 1999;8:53–60.

Cerhan JR, Torner JC, Lynch CF, Rubenstein LM, Lemke JH, Cohen MB, et al. Association of smoking, body mass, and physical activity with risk of prostate cancer in the Iowa 651 Rural Health Study (United States). Cancer Causes Control 1997;8:229–38.

Chan JM, Giovannucci E, Andersson SO, Yuen J, Adami HO, Wolk A. Dairy products, calcium, phosphorous, vitamin D, and risk of prostate cancer (Sweden). Cancer Causes Control 1998a;9:559–66.

Chan JM, Stampfer MJ, Giovannucci EL. What causes prostate cancer? A brief summary of the epidemiology. Semin Cancer Biol 1998b;8:263–73.

Chan JM, Stampfer MJ, Giovannucci E, Gann PH, Ma J, Wilkinson P, et al. Plasma insulin-like growth factor-I and prostate cancer risk: a prospective study. Science 1998c;279:563–66.

Chan JM, Stampfer MJ, Ma J, Rimm EB, Willett WC, Giovannucci EL. Supplemental vitamin E intake and prostate cancer risk in a large cohort of men in the United States. Cancer Epidemiol Biomarkers Prev 1999 Oct;8(10): 893–99.

Chan JM, Gann PH, Giovannucci EL. Role of diet in prostate cancer development and progression. J Clin Oncol 2005 Nov 10; 23(32):8152–60. Review.

Chan JM, Holick CN, Leitzmann MF, Rimm EB, Willett WC, Stampfer MJ, Giovannucci EL. Diet after diagnosis and the risk of prostate cancer progression, recurrence, and death (United States). Cancer Causes Control 2006 Mar;17(2):199–208.

Checkoway H, DiFerdinando G, Hulka BS, Mickey DD. Medical, lifestyle, and occupational risk factors for prostate cancer. Prostate 1987;10:79–88.

Chen YC, Giovannucci E, Lazarus R, Kraft P, Ketkar S, Hunter DJ. Sequence variants of

Toll-like receptor 4 and susceptibility to prostate cancer. Cancer Res 2005 Dec 15; 65(24):11771–78.

Cheng I, Stram DO, Penney KL, Pike M, Le Marchand L, Kolonel LN, Hirschhorn J, Altshuler D, Henderson BE, Freedman ML. Common genetic variation in IGF1 and prostate cancer risk in the Multiethnic Cohort. J Natl Cancer Inst 2006; 98(2):123–34.

Chokkalingam AP, Pollak M, Fillmore CM, Gao YT, Stanczyk FZ, Deng J, Sesterhenn IA, Mostofi FK, Fears TR, Madigan MP, Ziegler RG, Fraumeni JF Jr, Hsing AW. Insulin-like growth factors and prostate cancer: a population-based case-control study in China. Cancer Epidemiol Biomarkers Prev 2001 May;10(5):421–27.

Ciatto S, Gervasi G, Bonardi R, Frullini P, Zendron P, Lombardi C, Crocetti E, Zappa M. Determining overdiagnosis by screening with DRE/TRUS or PSA (Florence pilot studies, 1991–1994). Eur J Cancer 2005; 41(3):411–15.

Clarke G, Whittemore AS. Prostate cancer risk in relation to anthropometry and physical activity: the National Health and Nutrition Examination Survey I Epidemiological Follow-up Study. Cancer Epidemiol Biomarkers Prev 2000;9:875–81.

Clarke LC, Coombs GF, Turnbull BW, Slate EH, Chalker DK, Chow J, et al. Effects of selenium supplementation for cancer prevention in patients with carcinoma of the skin. A randomized trial. JAMA 1996;276:1957–63.

Coffey DS. Physiological control of prostate growth. An overview. In: Prostate Cancer. UICC Technical Report Series. Vol. 48. Geneva, International Union Against Cancer, 1979.

Colditz G. Consensus conference: smoking and prostate cancer. Cancer Causes Control 1996;7:560–62.

Cooney KA, McCarthy JD, Lange E, Huang L, Miesfeldt S, Montie JE, et al. Prostate cancer susceptibility locus on chromosome 1q: a confirmatory study. J Natl Cancer Inst 1997;89:955–59.

Coughlin SS, Neaton JD, Sengupta A. Cigarette smoking as a predictor of death from prostate cancer in 348,874 men screened for the Multiple Risk Factor Intervention Trial. Am J Epidemiol 1996;143:1002–6.

Cuzick J. Human papillomavirus infection of the prostate. Cancer Surv 1995;23:91–95.

Cuzick J, Fisher G, Kattan MW, Berney D, Oliver T, Foster CS, Moller H, Reuter V, Fearn P, Eastham J, Scardino P; Transatlantic Prostate Group. Long-term outcome among men with conservatively treated localised prostate cancer. Br J Cancer 2006;95:1186–94.

Dai WS, Gutai JP, Kuller LH, Cauley JA for the MRFIT Research Group. Cigarette smoking and serum sex hormones in men. Am J Epidemiol 1988;128:796–805.

Demichelis F, Fall K, Perner S, Andrén O, Schmidt D, Setlur SR, Hoshida Y, Mosquera JM, Pawitan Y, Lee C, Adami HO, Mucci LA, Kantoff PW, Andersson SO, Chinnaiyan AM, Rubin MA. TMPRSS2:ERG Gene Fusion Associated with Lethal Prostate Cancer in a Watchful Waiting Cohort. Oncogene 2007; 26:4596–9.

Dennis LK. Meta-analysis for combining relative risks of alcohol consumption and prostate cancer. Prostate 2000;42:56–66.

DerSimonian R, Clemens J, Spirtas R, Perlman J. Vasectomy and prostate cancer risk: methodological review of the evidence. J Clin Epidemiol 1993;46:163–72.

Dewailly E, Mulvad G, Sloth Pedersen H, Hansen JC, Behrendt N, Hart Hansen JP. Inuit are protected against prostate cancer. Cancer Epidemiol Biomarkers Prev 2003 Sep;12(9): 926–27.

Dillner J, Knekt P, Boman J, Lehtinen M, Af Geijersstam V, Sapp M, et al. Sero-epidemiological association between human-papillomavirus infection and risk of prostate cancer. Int J Cancer 1998;75:564–67.

Djavan B, Bursa B, Seitz C, Soeregi G, Remzi M, Basharkhah A, et al. Insulin-like growth factor 1 (IGF-1), IGF-1 density, and IGF-1/PSA ratio for prostate cancer detection. Urology 1999;54:603–6.

Doll R, Peto R. The Causes of Cancer: Quantitative Estimates of Avoidable Risks of Cancer in the United States Today. New York, Oxford University Press, 1981.

Dorgan JF, Albanes D, Virtamo J, Heinonen OP, Chandler DW, Galmarini M, et al. Relationships of serum androgens and estrogens to prostate cancer risk: results from a prospective study in Finland. Cancer Epidemiol Biomarkers Prev 1998;7:1069–74.

Drago JR, Nesbitt JA, Badalament RA, Smith J. Chemotherapy and vitamin E in treatment of Nb rat prostate tumors. In Vivo 1988;2: 399–401.

Drivdahl RH, Loop SM, Andress DL, Ostenson RC. IGF-binding proteins in human prostate tumor cells: expression and regulation by 1,25-dihydroxyvitamin D3. Prostate 1995; 26:72–79.

Eaton NE, Reeves GK, Appleby PN, Key TJ. Endogenous sex hormones and prostate cancer: a quantitative review of prospective studies. Br J Cancer 1999;80:930–34.

Eeles RA, Durocher F, Edwards S, Teare D, Badzioch M, Hamoudi R, et al. Linkage analysis of chromosome 1q markers in 136 prostate cancer families. The Cancer Research Campaign/British Prostate group U.K. Familial Prostate Cancer Study Collaborators. Am J Hum Genet 1998;62:653–58.

Eichholzer M, Stahelin HB, Gey KF, Ludin E, Bernasconi F. Prediction of male cancer mortality by plasma levels of interacting vitamins: 17-year follow-up of the prospective Basel study. Int J Cancer 1996;66:145–50.

Ekbom A, Hsieh CC, Lipworth L, Wolk A, Ponten J, Adami HO, et al. Perinatal characteristics in relation to incidence of and mortality from prostate cancer. Br Med J 1996;313:337–41.

Ekbom A, Wuu J, Adami HO, Lu CM, Lagiou P, Trichopoulos D, et al. Duration of gestation and prostate cancer risk in offspring. Cancer Epidemiol Biomarkers Prev 2000;9:221–23.

Etzioni R, Legler JM, Feuer EJ, Merrill RM, Cronin KA, Hankey BF. Cancer surveillance series: interpreting trends in prostate cancer—part III: quantifying the link between population prostate-specific antigen testing and recent declines in prostate cancer mortality. J Natl Cancer Inst 1999;91:1033–39.

Etzioni R, Penson DF, Legler JM, di Tommaso D, Boer R, Gann PH, Feuer EJ. Overdiagnosis due to prostate-specific antigen screening: lessons from U.S. prostate cancer incidence trends. J Natl Cancer Inst 2002; 94(13):981–90.

Ewings P, Bowie C. A case-control study of cancer of the prostate in Somerset and east Devon. Br J Cancer 1996;74:661–66.

Ferlay J, Bray F, Pisani P, Parkin DM. GLOBOCAN 2002: Cancer Incidence, Mortality and Prevalence Worldwide. International Agency for Research on Cancer, Lyon, 2004.

Feuer EJ, Merrill RM, Hankey BF. Cancer surveillance series: interpreting trends in prostate cancer—part II: cause of death misclassification and the recent rise and fall in prostate cancer mortality. J Natl Cancer Inst 1999;91:1025–32.

Feustel A, Wennrich R. Zinc and cadmium in cell fractions of prostate cancer tissues of different histological grading in comparison to BPH and normal prostate. Urol Res 1984;12:147–50.

Figueroa JA, De Raad S, Tadlock L, Speights VO, Rinehart JJ. Differential expression of insulin-like growth factor binding proteins in high versus low Gleason score prostate cancer. J Urol 1998;159:1379–83.

Freedman ML, Pearce CL, Penney KL, Hirschhorn JN, Kolonel LN, Henderson BE, Altshuler D. Systematic evaluation of genetic variation at the androgen receptor locus and risk of prostate cancer in a multiethnic cohort study. Am J Hum Genet 2005;76(1):82–90.

Freedman ML, Haiman CA, Patterson N, McDonald GJ, Tandon A, Waliszewska A, Penney K, Steen RG, Ardlie K, John EM, Oakley-Girvan I, Whittemore AS, Cooney KA, Ingles SA, Altshuler D, Henderson BE, Reich D. Admixture mapping identifies 8q24 as a prostate cancer risk locus in African-American men. Proc Natl Acad Sci USA 2006;103(38):14068–73.

Friedrichsen DM, Hawley S, Shu J, Humphrey M, Sabacan L, Iwasaki L, Etzioni R, Ostrander EA, Stanford JL. IGF-I and IGFBP-3 polymorphisms and risk of prostate cancer. Prostate 2005;65(1):44–51.

Gann PH, Hennekens CH, Sacks FM, Grodstein F, Giovannucci EL, Stampfer MJ. Prospective study of plasma fatty acids and risk of prostate cancer. J Natl Cancer Inst 1994;86:281–86.

Gann PH. Diet and prostate cancer risk: the embarrassment of riches. Cancer Causes Control 1998;9:541–43.

Gann PH, Hennekens CH, Ma J, Longcope C, Stampfer MJ. Prospective study of sex hormone levels and risk of prostate cancer. J Natl Cancer Inst 1996;88:1118–26.

Gann PH, Ma J, Giovannucci E, Willett W, Sacks FM, Hennekens CH, Stampfer MJ. Lower prostate cancer risk in men with elevated plasma lycopene levels: results of a prospective analysis. Cancer Res 1999; 59:1225–30.

Gardner WA, Culberson DE, Bennett BD. *Trichomonas vaginalis* in the prostate gland. Archives of Pathology and Laboratory Medicine 1986;110:430–32.

Garfinkel L. Overweight and mortality. Cancer 1986;58:1826–29.

Gartner C, Stahl W, Sies H. Lycopene is more bioavailable from tomato paste than from fresh tomatoes. Am J Clin Nutr 1997;66:116–22.

Ghadirian P, Howe GR, Hislop TG, Maisonneuve P. Family history of prostate cancer: a multi-center case-control study in Canada. Int J Cancer 1997;70:679–81.

Gibbs M, Stanford JL, McIndoe RA, Jarvik GP, Kolb S, Goode EL, et al. Evidence for a rare prostate cancer–susceptibility locus at chromosome lp36. Am J Hum Genet 1999;64:776–87.

Giovannucci E. Dietary influences of 1,25(OH)2 vitamin D in relation to prostate cancer: a hypothesis. Cancer Causes Control 1998;9:567–82.

Giovannucci E. Tomatoes, tomato-based products, lycopene, and cancer: review of the epidemiologic literature. J Natl Cancer Inst 1999;91:317–31.

Giovannucci E, Ascherio A, Rimm EB, Colditz GA, Stampfer MJ, Willett WC. A prospective cohort study of vasectomy and prostate cancer in U.S. men. JAMA 1993a;269:873–77.

Giovannucci E, Leitzmann M, Spiegelman D, Rimm EB, Colditz GA, Stampfer MJ, et al. A prospective study of physical activity and prostate cancer in male health professionals. Cancer Res 1998a;58:5117–22.

Giovannucci E, Rimm EB, Ascherio A, Colditz G, Spiegelman D, Stampfer MJ, et al. Smoking and risk of total and fatal prostate cancer in United States health professionals. Cancer Epidemiol Biomarkers Prev 1999;8:277–82.

Giovannucci E, Rimm EB, Stampfer MJ, Colditz GA, Willett WC. Height, body weight, and risk of prostate cancer. Cancer Epidemiol Biomarkers Prev 1997a;6:557–63.

Giovannucci E, Rimm EB, Colditz GA, Stampfer MJ, Ascherio A, Chute CC, et al. A prospective study of dietary fat and risk of prostate cancer. J Natl Cancer Inst 1993b;85:1571–79.

Giovannucci E, Rimm EB, Wolk A, Ascherio A, Stampfer MJ, Colditz GA, et al. Calcium and fructose intake in relation to risk of prostate cancer. Cancer Res 1998b;58:442–47.

Giovannucci E, Stampfer MJ, Krithivas K, Brown M, Brufsky A, Talcott J, et al. The CAG repeat within the androgen receptor gene and its relationship to prostate cancer. Proc Natl Acad Sci USA 1997b;94:3320–23.

Giovannucci E. A review of epidemiologic studies of tomatoes, lycopene, and prostate cancer. Exp Biol Med (Maywood). 2002 Nov;227(10):852–59. Review.

Giovannucci E, Liu Y, Stampfer MJ, Willett WC. A prospective study of calcium intake and incident and fatal prostate cancer. Cancer Epidemiol Biomarkers Prev 2006;15(2):203–10.

Godley PA. Prostate cancer screening: promise and peril—a review. Cancer Detect Prev 1999;23:316–24.

Goodman GE, Schaffer S, Barnhan DD, Thorhos MP, Omenn GS. Predictors of serum selenium in cigarette smokers and the lack of association with lung and prostate cancer risk. Cancer Epidemiol Biomarkers Prev 2001;10:1069–76.

Grönberg H, Damber L, Damber JE. Familial prostate cancer in Sweden. A nationwide register cohort study. Cancer 1996;77:138–43.

Grönberg H, Damber L, Damber JE, Iselius L. Segregation analysis of prostate cancer in Sweden: support for dominant inheritance. Am J Epidemiol 1997;146:552–57.

Guess HA, Friedman GD, Sadler MC, Stanczyk FZ, Vogelman JH, Imperato-McGinley J, et al. 5 Alpha-reductase activity and prostate

cancer: a case-control study using stored sera. Cancer Epidemiol Biomarkers Prev 1997;6:21–24.

Gunawardena K, Murray DK, Meikle AW. Vitamin E and other antioxidants inhibit human prostate cancer cells through apoptosis. Prostate 2000;44:287–95.

Haid M, Sharon N. Immunofluorescent evidence of prior herpes simplex virus type-2 infection in prostate carcinoma. Urology 1984;24:623–25.

Hankey BF, Feuer EJ, Clegg LX, Hayes RB, Legler JM, Prorok PC, et al. Cancer Surveillance series: interpreting trends in prostate cancer—part I: evidence of the effects of screening in recent prostate cancer incidence, mortality, and survival rates. J Natl Cancer Inst 1999;91:1017–24.

Harman SM, Metter EJ, Blackman MR, Landis PK, Carter HB. Serum levels of insulin-like growth factor I (IGF-I), IGF-II, IGF-binding protein-3, and prostate-specific antigen as predictors of clinical prostate cancer. J Clin Endocrinol Metab 2000;85:4258–65.

Hartman TJ, Albanes D, Pietinen P, Hartman AM, Rautalahti M, Tangrea JA, et al. The association between baseline vitamin E, selenium, and prostate cancer in the alpha-to-copherol beta-carotene cancer prevention study. Cancer Epidemiol Biomarkers Prev 1998a;7:335–40.

Hartman TJ, Albanes D, Rautalahti M, Tangrea JA, Virtamo J, Stolzenberg R, et al. Physical activity and prostate cancer in the Alpha-Tocopherol, Beta-Carotene (ATBC) Cancer Prevention Study (Finland). Cancer Causes Control 1998b;9:11–18.

Harvey S, Bjerve KS, Tretli S, Jellum E, Robsahm TE, Vatten L. Prediagnostic level of fatty acids in serum phospholipids: omega-3 and omega-6 fatty acids and the risk of prostate cancer. Int J Cancer 1997;71:545–51.

Hayes RB, Liff JM, Pottern LM, Greenberg RS, Schoenberg JB, Schwartz AG, et al. Prostate cancer risk in U.S. blacks and whites with a family history of cancer. Int J Cancer 1995;60:361–64.

Hayes RB, Pottern LM, Strickler H, Rabkin C, Pope V, Swanson GM, et al. Sexual behaviour, STDs and risks for prostate cancer. Br J Cancer 2000;82:718–25.

Hayes RB, Ziegler RG, Gridley G, Swanson C, Greenberg RS, Swanson GM, et al. Dietary factors and risks for prostate cancer among blacks and whites in the United States. Cancer Epidemiol Biomarkers Prev 1999;8:25–34.

Hebert PR, Ajani U, Cook NR, Lee IM, Chan KS, Hennekens CH. Adult height and incidence of cancer in male physicians (United

States). Cancer Causes Control 1997;8:591–97.

Hedelin M, Klint A, Chang ET, Bellocco R, Johansson JE, Andersson SO, Heinonen SM, Adlercreutz H, Adami HO, Gronberg H, Balter KA. Dietary phytoestrogen, serum enterolactone and risk of prostate cancer: the cancer prostate Sweden study (Sweden). Cancer Causes Control 2006 Mar;17(2):169–80.

Hedelin M, Chang ET, Wiklund F, Bellocco R, Klint A, Adolfsson J, Shahedi K, Xu J, Adami HO, Gronberg H, Balter KA. Association of frequent consumption of fatty fish with prostate cancer risk is modified by COX-2 polymorphism. Int J Cancer 2007 Jan 15;120(2):398–405.

Heinonen OP, Albanes D, Virtamo J, Taylor PR, Huttunen JK, Hartman AM, et al. Prostate cancer and supplementation with alpha-tocopherol and beta-carotene: incidence and mortality in a controlled trial. J Natl Cancer Inst 1998;90:440–46.

Hemminki K, Rawal R, Bermejo JL. Prostate cancer screening, changing age-specific incidence trends and implications on familial risk. Int J Cancer 2005;113:312–15.

Henderson BE. Summary report of the sixth symposium on cancer registries and epidemiology in the Pacific Basin. J Natl Cancer Inst 1990;82:1186–90.

Henderson BE, Bernstein L, Ross RK, Depue RH, Judd HL. The early in utero oestrogen and testosterone environment of blacks and whites: potential effects on male offspring. Br J Cancer 1988;57:216–18.

Heshmat MY, Kovi J, Herson J, Jones GW, Jackson MA. Epidemiologic association between gonorrhea and prostatic carcinoma. Urology 1975;6:457–60.

Hiatt RA, Armstrong MA, Klatsky AL, Sidney S. Alcohol consumption, smoking, and other risk factors, and prostate cancer in a large health plan cohort in California (United States). Cancer Causes Control 1994;5:66–72.

Howard SS. Possible biological mechanisms for a relationship between vasectomy and prostatic cancer. Eur J Cancer 1993;29A:1060–62.

Hsieh CC, Thanos A, Mitropoulos D, Deliveliotis C, Mantzoros CS, Trichopoulos D. Risk factors for prostate cancer: a case-control study in Greece. Int J Cancer 1999;80:699–703.

Hsing AW, Comstock GW. Serological precursors of cancer: serum hormones and risk of subsequent prostate cancer. Cancer Epidemiol Biomarkers Prev 1993;2:27–32.

Hsing AW, Comstock GW, Abbey H, Polk BF. Serologic precursors of cancer. Retinol, carotenoids, and tocopherol and risk of prostate cancer. J Natl Cancer Inst 1990a;82:941–46.

Hsing AW, Deng J, Sesterhenn IA, Mostofi FK, Stanczyk FZ, Benichou J, et al. Body size and prostate cancer: a population-based case-control study in China. Cancer Epidemiol Biomarkers Prev 2000a;9:1335–41.

Hsing AW, Gao YT, Wu G, Wang X, Deng J, Chen YL, et al. Polymorphic CAG and CGN repeat lengths in the androgen receptor gene and prostate cancer risk: a population-based case-control study in China. Cancer Res 2000b;60:5111–16.

Hsing AW, McLaughlin JK, Schuman LM, Bjelke E, Gridley G, Wacholder S, et al. Diet, tobacco use, and fatal prostate cancer: results from the Lutheran Brotherhood Cohort Study. Cancer Res 1990b;50:6836–40.

Hsing AW, McLaughlin JK, Zheng W, Gao YT, Blot WJ. Occupation, physical activity, and risk of prostate cancer in Shanghai, People's Republic of China. Cancer Causes Control 1994;5:136–40.

Hunter DJ, Riboli E, Haiman CA, Albanes D, Altshuler D, Chanock SJ, Haynes RB, Henderson BE, Kaaks R, Stram DO, Thomas G, Thun MJ, Blanche H, Buring JE, Burtt NP, Calle EE, Cann H, Canzian F, Chen YC, Colditz GA, Cox DG, Dunning AM, Feigelson HS, Freedman ML, Gaziano JM, Giovannucci E, Hankinson SE, Hirschhorn JN, Hoover RN, Key T, Kolonel LN, Kraft P, Le Marchand L, Liu S, Ma J, Melnick S, Pharoah P, Pike MC, Rodriguez C, Setiawan VW, Stampfer MJ, Trapido E, Travis R, Virtamo J, Wacholder S, Willett WC; National Cancer Institute Breast and Prostate Cancer Cohort Consortium. A candidate gene approach to searching for low-penetrance breast and prostate cancer genes. Nat Rev Cancer 2005;5:977–85.

Ilic M, Vlajinac H, Marinkovic J. Case-control study of risk factors for prostate cancer. Br J Cancer 1996;74:1682–86.

Ingles SA, Ross RK, Yu MC, Irvine RA, La Pera G, Haile RW, et al. Association of prostate cancer risk with genetic polymorphisms in vitamin D receptor and androgen receptor. J Natl Cancer Inst 1997;89:166–70.

Irani J, Goujon J-M, Ragni E, et al. High-grade inflammation in prostate cancer as a prognostic factor for biochemical recurrence after radical prostatectomy. Urology 1999;54:467–72

Israel K, Sanders BG, Kline K. RRR-alpha-tocopheryl succinate inhibits the proliferation of human prostatic tumor cells with defective cell cycle/differentiation pathways. Nutr Cancer 1995;24:161–69.

Jacobsen BK, Knutsen SF, Fraser GE. Does high soy milk intake reduce prostate cancer incidence? The Adventist Health Study (United States). Cancer Causes Control 1998;9:553–57.

Jensen OM, Paine SL, McMichael AJ, Ewertz M. Alcohol. In: Schottenfeld D, Fraumeni JF (Eds): Cancer Epidemiology and Prevention, 2nd ed. New York, Oxford University Press, 1996, pp 290–318.

Johansson JE, Andren O, Andersson SO, Dickman PW, Holmberg L, Magnuson A, Adami HO. Natural history of early, localized prostate cancer. JAMA. 2004 Jun 9;291(22):2713–19.

John EM, Whittemore AS, Wu AH, Kolonel LN, Hislop TG, Howe GR, et al. Vasectomy and prostate cancer: results from a multiethnic case-control study. J Natl Cancer Inst 1995;87:662–69.

John EM, Schwartz GG, Koo J, Van Den Berg D, and Ingles SA. Sun exposure, vitamin D receptor gene polymorphisms, and risk of advanced prostate cancer. Cancer Res 2005;65:5470–79.

Jones JI, Clemmons DR. Insulin-like growth factors and their binding proteins: Biological actions. Endocrinol Rev 1995;16:3–34.

Kantoff P, Giovannucci E, Brown M. The androgen receptor CAG repeat polymorphism and its relationship to prostate cancer. Biochem Biophys Acta 1998;1378:C1–C5.

Keenan BS, Richards GE, Ponder SW, Dallas FS, Nagamani M, Smith ER. Androgen-stimulated pubertal growth: the effects of testosterone and dihydrotestosterone on growth hormone and insulin-like growth factor-1 in the treatment of short stature and delayed puberty. J Clin Endocrinol Metab 1993;76:996–1001.

Keetch DW, Rice JP, Suarez BK, Catalona WJ. Familial aspects of prostate cancer: a case control study. J Urol 1995;154:2100–2.

Key TJA, Silcocks PB, Davey GK, Appleby PN, Bishop DT. A case-control study of diet and prostate cancer. Br J Cancer 1997;76:678–87.

Kolonel LN. Nutrition and prostate cancer. Cancer Causes Control 1996;7:83–94.

Kolonel LN, Hankin JH, Whittemore AS, Wu AH, Gallagher RP, Wilkens LR, et al. Vegetables, fruits, legumes and prostate cancer: a multiethnic case-control study. Cancer Epidemiol Biomarkers Prev 2000;9:795–804.

Kolonel LN, Nomura AMY, Cooney RV. Dietary fat and prostate cancer: current status. J Natl Cancer Inst 1999;91:414–28.

Kolonel L, Winkelstein W Jr. Cadmium and prostatic carcinoma. Lancet 1977;2:566–67.

Koralek DO, Peters U, Andriole G, Reding D, Kirsh V, Subar A, Schatzkin A, Hayes R,

Leitzmann MF. A prospective study of dietary alpha-linolenic acid and the risk of prostate cancer (United States). Cancer Causes Control. 2006;17(6):783–91.

Krieger JN, Verdon M, Siegel N, Holmes KK. Natural history of urogenital trichomoniasis in men. Journal of Urology 1993;149:1455–58.

Kucknoor A, Mundodi V, Alderete JF. Trichomonas vaginalis adherence mediates differential gene expression in human vaginal epithelial cells. Cellular Microbiology 2005;7:887–97.

Kuper H, Adami HO, Trichopoulos D. Infections as a major preventable cause of human cancer. Journal of Internal Medicine 2000;248:171–83.

Kyle E, Neckers L, Takimoto C, Curt G, Bergan R. Genistein-induced apoptosis of prostate cancer cells is preceded by specific decrease in focal adhesion kinase activity. Molecular Pharmacology 1997;51:193–200.

Lawson JS. Prostate cancer, birthweight, and diet. Epidemiology 1998;9:217.

Le Marchand L, Kolonel LN, Wilkens LR, Myers BC, Hirohata T. Animal fat consumption and prostate cancer: a prospective study in Hawaii. Epidemiology 1994;5:276–82.

Le Marchand L, Kolonel LN, Yoshizawa CN. Lifetime occupational physical activity and prostate cancer risk. Am J Epidemiol 1991;133:103–11.

Lee IM. Exercise and physical health: cancer and immune function. Res Q Exerc Sport 1995;66:286–91.

Lee IM, Paffenbarger RS Jr, Hsieh CC. Physical activity and risk of prostatic cancer among college alumni. Am J Epidemiol 1992;135:169–79.

Lee MM, Wang R-T, Hsing AW, Gu F-L, Wang T, Spitz M. Case-control study of diet and prostate cancer in China. Cancer Causes Control 1998;9:545–52.

Lees RE, Steele R, Wardle D. Arsenic, syphilis, and cancer of the prostate. J Epidemiol Commun Health 1985;39:227–30.

Leitzmann MF, Stampfer MJ, Michaud DS, Augustsson K, Colditz GC, Willett WC, Giovannucci EL. Dietary intake of n-3 and n-6 fatty acids and the risk of prostate cancer. Am J Clin Nutr 2004;80(1):204–16.

Lemen RA, Lee JS, Wagoner JK, Blejer HP. Cancer mortality among cadmium production workers. Ann Ny Acad Sci 1976;271:273–79.

Lesko SM, Rosenberg L, Shapiro S. Family history and prostate cancer risk. Am J Epidemiol 1996;144:1041–47.

Lewitt MS, Saunders H, Cooney GJ, Baxter RC. Effect of human insulin-like growth factor binding protein-1 on the half life and action of administered insulin-like growth factor in rats. J Endocrinol 1993;136:253–60.

Li H, Stampfer MJ, Giovannucci EL, Morris JS, Willett WC, Gaziano JM, Ma J. A prospective study of plasma selenium levels and prostate cancer risk. J Natl Cancer Inst 2004 May 5;96(9):696–703.

Li H, Kantoff PW, Giovannucci E, Leitzmann MF, Gaziano JM, Stampfer MJ, Ma J. Manganese superoxide dismutase polymorphism, prediagnostic antioxidant status, and risk of clinical significant prostate cancer. Cancer Res 2005 Mar 15;65(6):2498–504.

Li L, Cicek MS, Casey G, Witte JS. No association between genetic polymorphisms in IGF-I and IGFBP-3 and prostate cancer. Cancer Epidemiol Biomarkers Prev 2004; 13(3): 497–98.

Lichtenstein P, Holm NV, Verksalo PK, Iliadou A, Kapriou J, Koskenvuo M, et al. Environmental and heritable factors in the causation of cancer—analyses of cohorts of twins from Sweden, Denmark and Finland. N Engl J Med 2000;343:78–85.

Lilienfeld AM, Levin ML, Kessler II. Cancer in the United States. APHA Monograph. Cambridge, Harvard University Press, 1972.

Lipworth L, Hsieh CC, Wide L, Ekbom A, Yu SZ, Yu GP, et al. Maternal pregnancy hormone levels in areas with high incidence (Boston, USA) and low incidence (Shanghai, China) of breast cancer. Br J Cancer 1999; 79:7–12.

Liu S, Lee IM, Linson P, Ajani U, Buring JE, Hennekens CH. A prospective study of physical activity and risk of prostate cancer in US physicians. Int J Epidemiol 2000;29:29–35.

Luleci G, Sakizli M, Gunalp A, Erkan I, Remzi D. Herpes simplex type 2 neutralization antibodies in patients with cancers of the urinary bladder, prostate, and cervix. J Surg Oncol 1981;16:327–31.

Lumey LH. Prostate cancer and smoking: a review of case-control and cohort studies. Prostate 1996;29:249–60.

Lumey LH, Pittman B, Zang EA, Wynder EL. Cigarette smoking and prostate cancer: no relation with six measures of lifetime smoking habits in a large case-control study among U.S. whites. Prostate 1997;33:195–200.

Mantzoros CS, Georgiadis EI. Body mass and physical activity are important predictors of serum androgen concentrations in young healthy men. Epidemiology 1995;6:433–35.

Mantzoros CS, Tzonou A, Signorello LB, Stampfer MJ, Trichopoulos D, Adami HO. Insulin-like growth factor 1 in relation to prostate cancer and benign prostatic hyperplasia. Br J Cancer 1997;76:1115–18.

McIndoe RA, Stanford JL, Gibbs M, Jarvik GP, Brandzel S, Neal CL, et al. Linkage analysis of 49 high-risk families does not support a common familial prostate cancer–susceptibility gene at lq24–25. Am J Hum Genet 1997;61: 347–53.

McLellan DL and Norman RW. Hereditary aspects of prostate cancer. Can Med Assoc J 1995;153:895–900.

Menter DG, Sabichi AL, Lippman SM. Selenium effects on prostate cell growth. Cancer Epidemiol Biomarkers Prev 2000;9:1171–82.

Messina MJ, Persky V, Setchell KDR, Barnes S. Soy intake and cancer risk: a review of the in vitro and in vivo data. Nutr Cancer 1994;21: 113–31.

Mettlin C, Selenskas S, Natarajan N, Huben R. Beta-carotene and animal fats and their relationship to prostate cancer risk. A case-control study. Cancer 1989;64:605–12.

Meydani M. Vitamin E. Lancet 1995;345:170–75.

Mishina T, Watanabe H, Araki H, Nakao M. Epidemiological study of prostate cancer by matched-pair analysis. Prostate 1985;6:423–36.

Mishra DK, Bid HK, Srivastava DS, Mandhani A, and Mittal RD. Association of vitamin D receptor gene polymorphism and risk of prostate cancer in India. Urol Int 2005;74: 315–18.

Moller H, Mellemgaard A, Lindvig K, Olsen JH. Obesity and cancer risk: a Danish record-linkage study. Eur J Cancer 1994;30A:344–50.

Monroe KR, Yu MC, Kolonel LN, Coetzee GA, Wilkins LR, Ross RK, et al. Evidence of an X-linked or recessive genetic component to prostate cancer risk. Nat Med 1995;1:827–29.

Moyret-Lalle C, Marcais C, Jacquemier J, Moles JP, Daver A, Soret JY, et al. ras, p53 and HPV status in benign and malignant prostate tumors. Int J Cancer 1995;64:124–29.

Muir C, Waterhouse J, Mack T, et al (Eds): Cancer Incidence in Five Continents, Vol V. International Agency for Research on Cancer, Lyon, IARC Press, 1987.

Mukherjee P, Sotnikov AV, Mangian HJ, Zhou JR, Visek WJ, Clinton SK. Energy intake and prostate tumor growth, angiogenesis, and vascular endothelial growth factor expression. J Natl Cancer Inst 1999;91(6):512–23.

Nam RK, Elhaji Y, Krahn MD, Hakimi J, Ho M, Chu W, et al. Significance of the CAG repeat polymorphism of the androgen receptor gene in prostate cancer progression. J Urol 2000;164:567–72.

Nam RK, Zhang WW, Trachtenberg J, Jewett MA, Emami M, Vesprini D, Chu W, Ho M, Sweet J, Evans A, Toi A, Pollak M, Narod

SA. Comprehensive assessment of candidate genes and serological markers for the detection of prostate cancer. Cancer Epidemiol Biomarkers Prev 2003;12(12):1429–37.

Nelson WG, De Marzo AM, DeWeese TL, Isaacs WB. The role of inflammation in the pathogenesis of prostate cancer. J of Urol2004;172:S6-S12.

Neuhausen SL, Farnham JM, Kort E, Tavtigian SV, Skolnick MH, Cannon-Albright LA. Prostate cancer susceptibility locus HPC1 in Utah high-risk pedigrees. Hum Mol Genet 1999;8:2437–42.

Neuhausen SL, Slattery ML, Garner CP, Ding YC, Hoffman M, Brothman AR. Prostate cancer risk and IRS1, IRS2, IGF1, and INS polymorphisms: strong association of IRS1 G972R variant and cancer risk. Prostate 2005 Jul 1;64(2):168–74.

Noda T, Sasagawa T, Dong Y, Fuse H, Namiki M, Inoue M. Detection of human papillomavirus (HPV) DNA in archival specimens of benign prostatic hyperplasia and prostatic cancer using a highly sensitive nested PCR method. Urol Res 1998;26:165–69.

Nomura AMY, Heilbrun LK, Stemmermann GN, Judd HL. Prediagnostic serum hormones and the risk of prostate cancer. Cancer Res 1988;48:3515–17.

Nomura AMY, Lee J, Stemmermann GN, Combs GF. Serum selenium and subsequent risk of prostate cancer. Cancer Epidemiol Biomarkers Prev 2000;9:883–87.

Nomura AMY and Kolonel LN. Prostate cancer: a current perspective. Epidemiol Rev 1991; 13:200–27.

Nomura AMY, Stemmermann GN, Chyou PH, Henderson BE, Stanczyk FZ. Serum androgens and prostate cancer. Cancer Epidemiol Biomarkers Prev 1996;5:621–25.

Nomura AMY, Stemmermann GN, Lee J, Craft NE. Serum micronutrient and prostate cancer in Japanese Americans in Hawaii. Cancer Epidemiol Biomarkers Prev 1997;6:487–91.

Norrish AE, Skeaff CM, Arribas CL, Sharpe SJ, Jackson RT. Prostate cancer risk and consumption of fish oils: a dietary biomarker-based case-control study. Br J Cancer 1999; 81(7):1238–42.

Ntais C, Polycarpou A, and Ioannidis JP. Vitamin D receptor gene polymorphisms and risk of prostate cancer: a meta-analysis. Cancer Epidemiol Biomarkers Prev 2003;12:1395–402.

Nunn SE, Gibson TB, Rajah R, Cohen P. Regulation of prostate cell growth by the insulin-like growth factor binding proteins and their proteases. Endocrinology 1997;7:115–18.

Nutting PA, Freeman WL, Risser DR, Helgerson SD, Paisano R, Hisnanick J, et al. Cancer incidence among American Indians and Alaska Natives, 1980 through 1987. Am J Public Health 1993;83:1589–98.

Oliveria SA, Lee IM. Is exercise beneficial in the prevention of prostate cancer? Sports Med 1997;23:271–78.

Oremek GM, Seiffert UB. Physical activity releases prostate-specific antigen (PSA) from the prostate gland into blood and increases serum PSA concentrations. Clin Chem 1996;42:691–95.

Packer BR, Yeager M, Burdett L, et al. SNP500Cancer: a public resource for sequence validation, assay development, and frequency analysis for genetic variation in candidate genes. Nucleic Acids Res Jan 1 2006;34(Database issue):D617–D621.

Palapattu GS, Sutcliffe S, De Marzo AM, Isaacs WB, Nelson WG. Prostate carcinogenesis and inflammation: emerging insights. Carcinogenesis 2004;26:1170–81.

Pasquali R, Casimirri F, Cantobelli S, Melchionda N, Morselli Labate AM, Fabbri R, et al. Effect of obesity and body fat distribution on sex hormones and insulin in men. Metabolism 1991;40:101–4.

Patterson RE, Neuhouser ML, White E, Hunt JR, Kristal AR. Cancer-related behavior of vitamin supplement users. Cancer Epidemiol Biomarkers Prev 1998;7:79–81.

Patterson RE, White E, Kristal AR, Neuhouser ML, Potter JD. Vitamin supplements and cancer risk: the epidemiologic evidence. Cancer Causes Control 1997;8:786–802.

Petrin D, Delgaty K, Bhatt R, Garber G. Clinical and microbiological aspects of *Trichomonas vaginalis*. Clinical Microbiology Reviews 1998;11:300–17.

Platz EA, Leitzmann MF, Rimm EB, Willett WC, Giovannucci E. Alcohol intake, drinking patterns, and risk of prostate cancer in a large prospective cohort study. Am J Epidemiol. 2004 Mar 1;159(5):444–53.

Platz EA, Pollak MN, Leitzmann MF, Stampfer MJ, Willett WC, Giovannucci E.Plasma insulin like growth factor 1 and binding protein-3 and subsequent risk of prostate cancer in the PSA era. Cancer Causes Control. 2005 Apr;16(3):255–62.

Plitt SS, Garfein RS, Gaydos CA, Strathdee SA, Sherman SG, Taha TE. Prevalence and correlates of chlamydia trachomatis, neisseria gonorrhoeae, trichomonas vaginalis infections, and bacterial vaginosis among a cohort of young injection drug users in Baltimore, Maryland. Sexually Transmitted Diseases 2005;32:446–53.

Potosky AL, Kessler L, Gridley G, Brown CC, Horm JW. Rise in prostatic cancer incidence associated with increased use of transurethral resection. J Natl Cancer Inst 1990; 82:1624–28.

Pour P. Prostatic cancer induced in MRC rats by N-nitroso-bis(2-oxopropyl)amine and N-nitroso-bis(2-hydroxypropyl)amine. Carcinogenesis 1983;4:49–55.

Putnam SD, Cerhan JR, Parker AS, Bianchi GD, Wallace RB, Cantor KP, et al. Lifestyle and anthropometric risk factors for prostate cancer in a cohort of Iowa men. Ann Epidemiol 2000;10:361–69.

Quinn M and Babb P. Patterns and trends in prostate cancer incidence, survival, prevalence and mortality: Part I: international comparisons. BJU International 2002;90:162–73.

Rayman MP. The importance of selenium to human health. Lancet 2000;356:233–41.

Redman C, Scott JA, Baines AT, Basye JL, Clark LC, Calley C, et al. Inhibitory effect of selenomethionine on the growth of three selected human tumor cell lines. Cancer Lett 1998; 125:103–10.

Renehan AG, Zwahlen M, Minder C, O'Dwyer ST, Shalet SM, Egger M. Insulin-like growth factor (IGF)-I, IGF binding protein-3, and cancer risk: systematic review and meta-regression analysis. Lancet 2004 Apr 24; 363(9418):1346–53. Review.

Rennert H, Zeigler-Johnson CM, Addya K, et al. Association of susceptibility alleles in ELAC2/HPC2, RNASEL/HPC1, and MSR1 with prostate cancer severity in European American and African American men. Cancer Epidemiol Biomarkers Prev 2005;14(4): 949–57.

Richards IS, Davis FE, Lubell I. Current status of endocrinologic effects of vasectomy. Urology 1981;18:1–6.

Ripoll EA, Rama BN, Webber MM. Vitamin E enhances the chemotherapeutic effects of adriamycin on human prostatic carcinoma cells in vitro. J Urol 1986;136:529–31.

Rodriguez C, Calle EE, Miracle McMahill HL, Tatham LM, Wingo PA, Thun MJ, et al. Family history and risk of fatal prostate cancer. Epidemiology 1997a;8:653–57.

Rodriguez C, Tatham LM, Thun MJ, Calle EE, Heath CW Jr. Smoking and fatal prostate cancer in a large cohort of adult men. Am J Epidemiol 1997b;145:466–75.

Rodriguez C, McCullough ML, Mondul AM, Jacobs EJ, Fakhrabadi-Shokoohi D, Giovannucci EL, Thun MJ, Calle EE. Calcium, dairy products, and risk of prostate cancer in a prospective cohort of United States men. Cancer Epidemiol Biomarkers Prev 2003; 12(7):597–603.

Rohan TE, Howe GR, Burch JD, Jain M. Dietary factors and risk of prostate cancer: a case-control study in Ontario, Canada. Cancer Causes Control 1995;6:145–54.

Rose DP, Boyer AP, Wynder EL. International comparisons of mortality rates for cancer of the breast, ovary, prostate, and colon, and per capita food consumption. Cancer 1986;58:2363–71.

Rosenberg L, Palmer JR, Zauber AG, Warshauer ME, Strom BL, Harlap S, et al. The relation of vasectomy to risk of cancer. Am J Epidemiol 1994;140:431–38.

Ross RK, Bernstein L, Lobo RA, Shimizu H, Stanczyk FZ, Pike M, et al. 5-Alpha-reductase activity and risk of prostate cancer among Japanese and U.S. white and black males. Lancet 1992;339:887–89.

Ross RK, McCurtis JW, Henderson BE, Menck HR, Mack TM, Martin SP. Descriptive epidemiology of testicular and prostatic cancer in Los Angeles. Br J Cancer 1979;39:284–92.

Ross RK, Paganini-Hill A, Henderson BE. The etiology of prostate cancer: what does the epidemiology suggest? Prostate 1983;4: 333–44.

Saramaki OR, Porkka KP, Vessella RL, Visakorpi T. Genetic aberrations in prostate cancer by microarray analysis. Int J Cancer 2006;119(6):1322–29.

Sartor O, Zheng Q, Eastham JA. Androgen receptor gene CAG repeat length varies in a race-specific fashion in men without prostate cancer. Urology 1999;53:378–80.

Sato K, Qian J, Slezak JM, Lieber MM, Bostwick DG, Bergstralh EJ, Jenkins RB. Clinical significance of alterations of chromosome 8 in high-grade, advanced, nonmetastatic prostate carcinoma. J Natl Cancer Inst 1999; 91(18):1574–80.

Schaid DJ, McDonnell SK, Blute ML, Thibodeau SN. Evidence for autosomal dominant inheritance of prostate cancer. Am J Hum Genet 1998;62:1425–38.

Schildkraut JM, Demark-Wahnefried W, Wenham RM, Grubber J, Jeffreys AS, Grambow SC, Marks JR, Moorman PG, Hoyo C, Ali S, Walther PJ. IGF1 (CA)19 repeat and IGFBP3 -202 A/C genotypes and the risk of prostate cancer in Black and White men. Cancer Epidemiol Biomarkers Prev 2005;14(2): 403–8.

Schumacher FR, Feigelson HS, Cox DG, Haiman CA, Albanes D, Buring J, Calle EE, Chanock SJ, Colditz GA, Diver WR, Dunning AM, Freedman ML, Gaziano JM, Giovannucci E, Hankinson SE, Hayes RB, Henderson BE, Hoover RN, Kaaks R, Key T, Kolonel LN, Kraft P, Le Marchand L, Ma J, Pike MC, Riboli E, Stampfer MJ, Stram DO, Thomas G, Thun MJ, Travis R, Virtamo J, Andriole G, Gelmann E, Willett WC, Hunter DJ. A common 8q24 variant in prostate and breast cancer from a large nested case-control study. Cancer Res 2007;67:2951-6.

Schuurman AG, Goldbohm RA, van den Brandt PA. A prospective cohort study on consumption of alcoholic beverages in relation to prostate cancer incidence (The Netherlands). Cancer Causes Control 1999a Dec;10(6):597–605.

Schuurman AG, van den Brandt PA, Dorant E, Brants HA, Goldbohm RA. Association of energy and fat intake with prostate carcinoma risk: results from The Netherlands Cohort Study. Cancer 1999b;86:1019–27.

Schuurman AG, Zeegers MPA, Goldbohm RA, van den Brandt PA. A case-cohort study on prostate cancer risk in relation to family history of prostate cancer. Epidemiology 1999c; 10:192–95.

Schuurman AG, Goldbohm RA, Dorant E, van den Brandt PA. Anthropometry in relation to prostate cancer risk in the Netherlands Cohort Study. Am J Epidemiol 2000;151:541–49.

Serth J, Panitz F, Paeslack U, Kuczyk MA, Jonas U. Increased levels of human papillomavirus type 16 DNA in a subset of prostate cancers. Cancer Res 1999;59:823–25.

Severson RK, Grove JS, Nomura AM, Stemmermann GN. Body mass and prostatic cancer: a prospective study. Br Med J 1988;297: 713–15.

Severson RK, Nomura AMY, Grove JS, Stemmermann GN. A prospective study of demographics, diet, and prostate cancer among men of Japanese ancestry in Hawaii. Cancer Res 1989;49:1857–60.

Shimizu H, Ross RK, Bernstein L, Yatani R, Henderson BE, Mack TM. Cancers of the prostate and breast among Japanese and white immigrants in Los Angeles County. Br J Cancer 1991;63:963–66.

Signorello LB, Brismar K, Bergstrom R, Andersson SO, Wolk A, Trichopoulos D, et al. Insulin-like growth factor-binding protein-1 and prostate cancer. J Natl Cancer Inst 1999;91:1965–67.

Signorello LB, Kuper H, Lagiou P, Wuu J, Mucci LA, Trichopoulos D, et al. Lifestyle factors and insulin like growth factor 1 levels among elderly men. Eur J Cancer Prev 2000;9:173–78.

Signorello LB, Tzonou A, Mantzoros CS, Lipworth L, Lagiou P, Hsieh CC, et al. Serum steroids in relation to prostate cancer risk in a case-control study (Greece). Cancer Causes Control 1997;8:632–36.

Simopoulos AP. Energy imbalance and cancer of the breast, colon and prostate. Med Oncol Tumor Pharmacother 1990;7:109–20.

Sinclair AL, Nouri AM, Oliver RT, Sexton C, Dalgleish AG. Bladder and prostate cancer screening for human papillomavirus by polymerase chain reaction: conflicting results using different annealing temperatures. Br J Biomed Sci 1993;50:350–54.

Smith JR, Freije D, Carpten JD, Gronberg H, Xu J, Isaacs SD, et al. Major susceptibility locus for prostate cancer on chromosome 1 suggested by a genome-wide search. Science 1996;274:1371–74.

Sorensen HT, Friis S, Olsen JH, Thulstrup AM, Mellemkjaer L, Linet M, et al. Risk of liver and other types of cancer in patients with cirrhosis: a nationwide cohort study in Denmark. Hepatology 1998;28:921–25.

Stanford JL, Just JJ, Gibbs M, Wicklund KG, Neal CL, Blumenstein BA, et al. Polymorphic repeats in the androgen receptor gene: molecular markers for prostate cancer risk. Cancer Res 1997;57:1194–98.

Stat Bite: Estimated worldwide cancer mortality among men, 2002. J Natl Cancer Inst 2005; 97(19):1402.

Stattin P, Bylund A, Rinaldi S, Biessy C, Dechaud H, Stanman UH, et al. Plasma insulin-like growth factor-1, insulin-like growth factor-binding proteins, and prostate cancer risk: a prospective study. J Natl Cancer Inst 2000;92:1910–17.

Stattin P, Bylund A, Biessy C, Kaaks R, Hallmans G, Adlercreutz H. Prospective study of plasma enterolactone and prostate cancer risk (Sweden). Cancer Causes Control 2004 Dec;15(10):1095–102.

Strickler HD, Burk R, Shah K, Viscidi R, Jackson A, Pizza G, et al. A multifaceted study of human papillomavirus and prostate carcinoma. Cancer 1998;82:1118–25.

Suarez BK, Lin J, Burmester JK, Broman KW, Weber JL, Banerjee TK, et al. A genome screen of multiplex sibships with prostate cancer. Am J Hum Genet 2000;66:933–44.

Sun J, Wiklund F, Hsu FC, Balter K, Zheng SL, Johansson JE, Chang B, Liu W, Li T, Turner AR, Li L, Li G, Adami HO, Isaacs WB, Xu J, Gronberg H. Links Interactions of sequence variants in interleukin-1 receptor-associated kinase4 and the toll-like receptor 6–1–10 gene cluster increase prostate cancer risk. Cancer Epidemiol Biomarkers Prev 2006; 15(3):480–85.

Sutcliffe S, Giovannucci E, Alderete JF, et al. Plasma antibodies against Trichomonas vaginalis and subsequent risk of prostate cancer. Cancer Epidemiology Biomarkers and Prevention 2006;15:939–45.

Suzuki H, Komiya A, Aida S, Ito H, Yatani R, Shimazaki J. Detection of human papillomavirus DNA and p53 gene mutations in human prostate cancer. Prostate 1996;28: 318–24.

Svatek RS, Lee JJ, Roehrborn CG, Lippman SM, Lotan Y. The cost of prostate cancer chemoprevention: a decision analysis model. Cancer Epidemiol Biomarkers Prev 2006; 15(8):1485–89.

Terris MK, Peehl DM. Human papillomavirus detection by polymerase chain reaction in benign and malignant prostate tissue is dependent on the primer set utilized. Urology 1997;50:150–56.

Terry P, Lichtenstein P, Feychting M, Ahlbom A, Wolk A. Fatty fish consumption and risk of prostate cancer. Lancet 2001;357:1764–66.

Tham MD, Gardner DC, Haskell LW. Potential Health benefits of dietary phytoestrogens: A review of the clinical epidemiological, and mechanistic evidence. J Clin Endoc and Metab 1998;83:2223–35.

Thompson IM, Goodman PJ, Tangen CM, Lucia MS, Miller GJ, Ford LG, Lieber MM, Cespedes RD, Atkins JN, Lippman SM, Carlin SM, Ryan A, Szczepanek CM, Crowley JJ, Coltman CA Jr. The influence of finasteride on the development of prostate cancer. N Engl J Med. 2003;349(3):215–24.

Thompson IM, Ankerst DP, Chi C, Goodman PJ, Tangen CM, Lucia MS, Feng Z, Parnes HL, Coltman CA Jr. Assessing prostate cancer risk: results from the Prostate Cancer Prevention Trial. Natl Cancer Inst 2006;98(8):529–34.

Thompson MM, Garland C, Barrett-Connor E, Khaw K, Friedlander NJ, Wingard DL. Heart disease risk factors, diabetes and prostatic cancer in an adult community. Am J Epidemiol 1989;129:511–17.

Thune I, Lund E. Physical activity and the risk of prostate can testicular cancer: a cohort study of 53,000 Norwegian men. Cancer Causes Control 1994;5:549–56.

Tomlins SA, Rhodes DR, Perner S, Dhanasekaran SM, Mehra R, Sun XW, Varambally S, Cao X, Tchinda J, Kuefer R, Lee C, Montie JE, Shah RB, Pienta KJ, Rubin MA, Chinnaiyan AM. Recurrent fusion of TMPRSS2 and ETS transcription factor genes in prostate cancer. Science. 2005;310(5748):644–48.

Tonnesen H, Moller H, Andersen JR, Jensen E, Juel K. Cancer morbidity in alcohol abusers. Br J Cancer 1994;69:327–32.

Tonucci LH, Holden JM, Beecher GR, Khachik F, Davis CS, Mulokozi G. Carotenoid content of thermally processed tomato-based food products. J Agric Food Chem 1995; 43:579–86.

Trachtenberg J, Hicks LL, Walsh PC. Androgen- and estrogen-receptor content in spontaneous and experimentally induced canine prostatic hyperplasia. J Clin Invest 1980;65: 1051–59.

Trichopoulos D, Lipworth L. Is cancer causation simpler than we thought, but more intractable? Epidemiology 1995;6:347–49.

Tseng M, Breslow RA, Graubard BI, Ziegler RG. Dairy, calcium, and vitamin D intakes and prostate cancer risk in the National Health and Nutrition Examination Epidemiologic Follow-up Study cohort. Am J Clin Nutr 2005;81(5):1147–54.

Tsuchiya N, Wang L, Horikawa Y, Inoue T, Kakinuma H, Matsuura S, Sato K, Ogawa O, Kato T, Habuchi T. CA repeat polymorphism in the insulin-like growth factor-I gene is associated with increased risk of prostate cancer and benign prostatic hyperplasia. Int J Oncol 2005;26(1):225–31.

Tu H, Jacobs SC, Mergner WJ, Kyprianou N. Rare incidence of human papillomavirus types 16 and 18 in primary and metastatic human prostate cancer. Urology 1994;44: 726–31.

Untergasser G, Rumpold H, Plas E, Witkowski M, Pfister G, Berger P. High levels of zinc ions induce loss of mitochondrial potential and degradation of antiapoptotic Bcl-2 protein in in vitro cultivated human prostate epithelial cells. Biochem Biophys Res Commun 2000;279:607–14.

Urisman A, Molinaro RJ, Fischer N, Plummer SJ, Casey G, Klein EA, Malathi K, Magi-Galluzzi C, Tubbs RR, Ganem D, Silverman RH, DeRisi JL. Identification of a novel Gammaretrovirus in prostate tumors of patients homozygous for R462Q RNASEL variant. PLoS Pathog 2006 Mar;2(3):e25.

van Duin M, van Marion R, Vissers K, Watson JE, van Weerden WM, Schroder FH, Hop WC, van der Kwast TH, Collins C, van Dekken H. High-resolution array comparative genomic hybridization of chromosome arm 8q: evaluation of genetic progression markers for prostate cancer. Genes Chromosomes Cancer 2005;44(4):438–49.

Van Laarhoven PHA. Trichomonas vaginalis, a pathogen of prostatitis. Archivum Chirurgicum Neerlandicum 1967;19:263–73.

Vatten LJ, Ursin G, Ross RK, Stanczyk FZ, Lobo RA, Harvei S, et al. Androgens in serum and the risk of prostate cancer: a nested case-control study from the Janus Serum Bank in Norway. Cancer Epidemiol Biomarkers Prev 1997;6:967–69.

Wang X, Guyer B, Paige DM. Differences in gestational age-specific birthweight among Chinese, Japanese and white Americans. Int J Epidemiol 1994;23:119–28.

Whittemore AS, Kolonel LN, Wu AH, John EM, Gallagher RP, Howe GR, et al. Prostate cancer in relation to diet, physical activity, and body size in blacks, whites, and Asians in the United States and Canada. J Natl Cancer Inst 1995a;87:652–61.

Whittemore AS, Wu AH, Kolonel LN, John EM, Gallagher RP, Howe GR, et al. Family history and prostate cancer risk in black, white, and Asian men in the United States and Canada. Am J Epidemiol 1995b;141:732–40.

Wideroff L, Schottenfeld D, Carey TE, Beals T, Fu G, Sakr W, et al. Human papillomavirus DNA in malignant and hyperplastic prostate tissue of black and white males. Prostate 1996;28:117–23.

Wiklund F, Jonsson BA, Brookes AJ, et al. Genetic analysis of the RNASEL gene in hereditary, familial, and sporadic prostate cancer. Clin Cancer Res 2004;10(21):7150–56.

Willett W. Split Prostate Cancer Four Ways. J. Natl. Cancer Inst 2006; 98:959–60.

Wolk A, Mantzoros CS, Andersson SO, Bergstrom R, Signorello LB, Lagiou P, et al. Insulin-like growth factor 1 and prostate cancer risk: a population-based, case-control study. J Natl Cancer Inst 1998;90:911–15.

Xiang Y, Wang Z, Murakami J, et al. Effects of RNase L mutations associated with prostate cancer on apoptosis induced by 2,'5'-oligoadenylates. Cancer Res 2003;63(20):6795–6801.

Xu J. Combined analysis of hereditary prostate cancer linkage to lq24–25: results from 772 hereditary prostate cancer families from the International Consortium for Prostate Cancer Genetics. Am J Hum Genet 2000;66:945–57.

Xu J, Zheng SL, Komiya A, et al. Germline mutations and sequence variants of the macrophage scavenger receptor 1 gene are associated with prostate cancer risk. Nature Genetics 2002;32:321–25.

Xu J, Meyers D, Freije D, Isaacs S, Wiley K, Nusskern D, et al. Evidence for a prostate cancer susceptibility locus on the X chromosome. Nat Genet 1998;20:175–79.

Yoshizawa K, Willett WC, Morris SJ, Stampfer MJ, Spiegelman D, Rimm EB, Giovannucci E. Study of prediagnostic selenium level in toenails and the risk of advanced prostate cancer. J Natl Cancer Inst 1998;90(16):1219–24.

Zaridze DG, Boyle P, Smans M. International trends in prostatic cancer. Int J Cancer 1984;33:223–30.

Zeegers MP, Kiemeney LA, Nieder AM, Ostrer H. How strong is the association between CAG and GGN repeat length polymorphisms in the androgen receptor gene and prostate cancer risk? Cancer Epidemiol Biomarkers Prev. 2004 Nov;13(11 Pt 1):1765–71.

Zhang J, Sasaki S, Amano K, Kesteloot H. Fish consumption and mortality from all causes, ischemic heart disease, and stroke: an ecological study. Prev Med 1999;28:520–29.

Zheng SL, Augustsson-Balter K, Chang B, Hedelin M, Li L, Adami HO, Bensen J, Li G, Johnasson JE, Turner AR, Adams TS, Meyers DA, Isaacs WB, Xu J, Gronberg H. Sequence variants of toll-like receptor 4 are associated with prostate cancer risk: results from the CAncer Prostate in Sweden Study. Cancer Res 2004;64(8):2918–22.

Zhu K, Stanford JL, Daling JR, McKnight B, Stergachis A, Brawer MK, et al. Vasectomy and prostate cancer: a case-control study in a health maintenance organization. Am J Epidemiol 1996;144:717–22.

21

Testicular Cancer

LORENZO RICHIARDI, RULLA TAMIMI,
AND HANS-OLOV ADAMI

Cancer of the testis should not be confused, as sometimes happens, with scrotal cancer, a malignancy of the scrotal skin that killed young chimney sweeps in the United Kingdom 2 centuries ago and that has been largely eliminated. Testicular cancer offers real challenges due to its unique descriptive epidemiology and unknown etiology. Albeit rare and highly curable, it is the most common cancer among young men. Moreover, the incidence of testicular cancer has been increasing to epidemic proportions throughout the world since the beginning of the twentieth century. Very little is known about its etiology, and risk factors responsible for the rise in incidence remain enigmatic. The occurrence of this malignancy now doubles every 15 to 25 years in many developed countries, and preventive measures are urgently needed.

Methodologically, descriptive and analytic studies of testicular cancer are uncomplicated. The organ is visible and palpable, and the origin of the tumor and the need for treatment are obvious, notably among the typically young to middle-aged

men who are stricken by the disease. Hence, both misclassification and underascertainment are probably less common than for most other malignancies. A real difficulty in analytic studies, however, is measurement of the etiologically relevant exposures since they are likely to operate early in life, perhaps even in utero.

CLINICAL SYNOPSIS

Subgroups

Testicular cancer occurs in two main histopathologic types, seminomas and non-seminomas, the latter being predominantly teratomas. Although these two types have different clinical characteristics, they have a similar descriptive epidemiology and most likely share the main risk factors. Therefore, we will consider them together unless otherwise stated.

Symptoms

A painless palpable mass usually perceived as an enlargement of the testicle is the cardinal symptom of testicular cancer.

Diagnosis

Traditionally, orchidectomy with histopathologic examination, sometimes frozen section examination from an open biopsy, serve both diagnostic and therapeutic purposes. Nowadays, ultrasound and in some settings needle biopsy may establish the diagnosis, so that unnecessary surgery is avoided.

Treatment

Orchidectomy remains the standard treatment. Complementary radiotherapy is used routinely in the primary management of seminomas, whereas treatment of nonseminomas often include a cisplatinumbased chemotherapy regimen. In more advanced stages retroperitoneal lymph node dissection may be necessary. In patients with metastatic disease, chemotherapy is the cornerstone of clinical management.

Prognosis

In the 1960s and early 1970s, the 5-year relative survival rate was approximately 70%, with the majority of deaths occurring among patients with nonseminoma cancer. By the end of the twentieth century, the rate had increased to 95% in areas where state-of-the-art technology is available, such as the United States and most of Europe. Because few cancer-related deaths occur later, these encouragingly high rates approach the proportion of cures.

Progress

Introduction of ciplatinum-based therapy during the 1970s is one of the success stories of modern oncology. Suddenly, many young men with an otherwise highly lethal nonseminoma cancer could be cured.

DESCRIPTIVE EPIDEMIOLOGY

The incidence of testicular cancer is low before puberty. After puberty there is a dramatic increase in incidence, which peaks at around age 30 and declines to almost zero by age 60 (Fig. 21–1). Because the disease

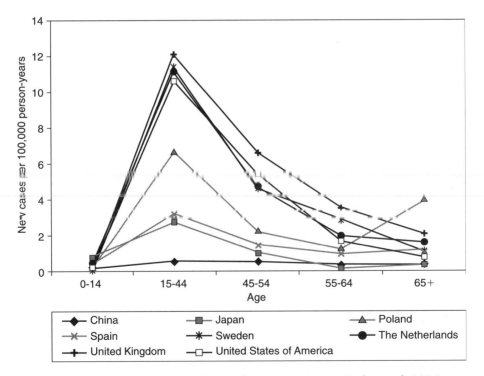

Figure 21.1. Age-specific incidence rates of testicular cancer. (*Source*: Ferlay et al, 2004)

occurs primarily in young men and is virtually nonexistent in older men, it is generally believed that early life exposures play a role in the development of testicular cancer (Richiardi et al, 2004c; McGlynn et al, 2005; Bray et al, 2006b). The considerable increase in incidence rates after puberty has been interpreted by some to indicate that adult hormones are necessary for the growth and progression of testicular tumors (Moss et al, 1986; Moller and Skakkebaek, 1996; Weir et al, 1998). The age-specific incidence patterns for nonsemimonas and seminomas are different, with nonseminomas having a peak at around ages 25 to 30, whereas for seminomas, peak incidence occurs at around age 35 (Richiardi et al, 2004c).

The geographic variation in age-adjusted incidence rates of testicular cancer worldwide is considerable (Fig. 21–2). The incidence is highest in western European populations, with Norway leading at 10.6 per 100 000 person-years (Ferlay et al, 2004). The lowest rates are observed in Asian populations, with age-standardized rates estimated to be 0.5–1 per 100 000 person-years. There is little information on the incidence rates in Africa, although they are estimated to be well below 1.0 per 100 000 person-years.

Globally, the incidence rates for testicular cancer have been increasing dramatically over the past century, beginning as early as the 1920s. An annual increase of 2% to 7% has been reported from several European countries, the US white population, Australia, Japan, and New Zealand (Pearce et al, 1987; dos Santos Silva et al, 1999; Bray et al, 2006b; Purdue et al, 2005; McGlynn et al, 2005). The increase has been largely the same for seminomas and nonseminomas, suggesting that the two histological types may have similar causes (Richiardi et al, 2004c; Bray et al, 2006a).

Age-period-cohort analysis reveals that birth cohort is a strong determinant of testicular cancer (Richiardi et al, 2004c; Bray et al, 2006b). Figure 21–3 demonstrates the remarkable age-period-cohort effect in six European countries (Bergström et al, 1996). In the former East Germany, the incidence rates for men born around 1965 are 11 times greater than for men born at the beginning of the twentieth century; in Sweden, a similar comparison reveals a fourfold difference. Such impressive cohort effects suggest that recently introduced environmental factors play a role in the dramatic rise in incidence. Interestingly, in the Scandinavian countries, the dramatic increases are slowed in cohorts born between the late 1930s and early 1940s (Moller, 1993; Bergström et al, 1996; Richiardi et al, 2004c). This time period corresponds to the years immediately leading up to and during World War II. It is possible that altered access to and consumption of certain goods and foods as a consequence of the war may

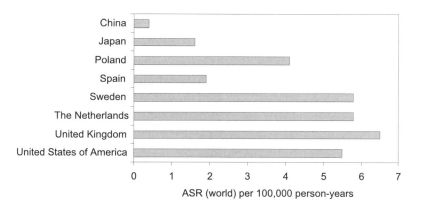

Figure 21–2. Age-standardised incidence rates of testicular cancer. (*Source*: Ferlay et al, 2004)

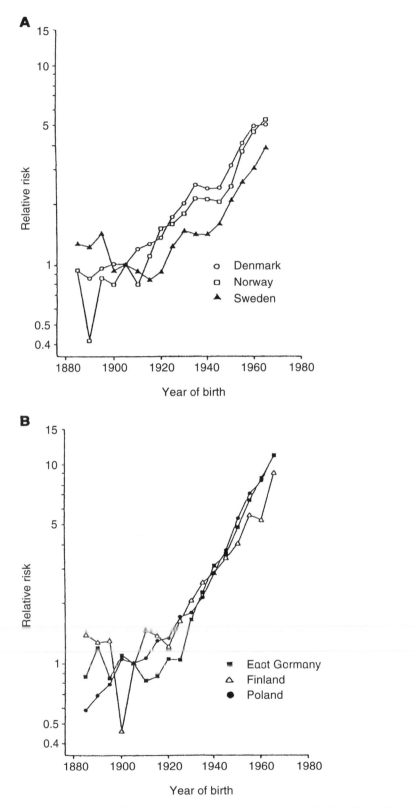

Figure 21–3. Observed age-specific incidence of testicular cancer in selected birth cohorts by country. (*Source*: Bergström et al, 1996)

be responsible for the interruption in the increasing trend.

There are, however, a few notable exceptions to this otherwise universal trend. The US black population have had, at least until 1990, stable low incidence rates (McGlynn et al, 2005), whereas the canton of Vaud in Switzerland has stable yet high incidence rates (Levi et al, 2003). In The United States, testicular cancer incidence in the white population is around six times that of the black population (McGlynn et al, 2005). The large geographic variations in testicular cancer incidence makes migration studies of great interest. Some studies observed that migrants tend to maintain the baseline risk of their country of origin, as shown by migrants moving from Asia to Australia (Grulich et al, 1995); by Asians, Africans, and Europeans moving to Israel (Parkin and Iscovich, 1997); and by Finns migrating to Sweden (Ekbom et al, 2003). The latter have been found to be at lower risk regardless of their age at immigration and duration of stay (Ekbom et al, 2003). Two studies found that offspring of immigrants experience rates that tend to approach those of the host population (Parkin and Iscovich, 1997; Montgomery et al, 2005). These patterns suggest that environmental factors are fundamental in the development of testicular cancer and should play a role early in life, perhaps in utero.

GENETIC AND MOLECULAR EPIDEMIOLOGY

Inherited Susceptibility

The early age of onset among familial cases found in some studies (Dong et al, 2001; Forman et al, 1992), and the high proportion of bilateral testicular cancer (Heimdal et al, 1996), suggest that, apart from shared environmental factors, there is an important genetic component to the disease. Cancer family databases have found a tenfold increased risk of testicular cancer among brothers and a two- to fourfold increased risk among fathers/sons of testicular cancer patients (Dong et al, 2001;

Westergaard et al, 1996; Forman et al, 1992).

The negative findings from linkage analyses suggest a role for moderate risk genes, although few association studies have been conducted so far. A genome-wide linkage analysis has recently been carried out on 237 pedigrees included in an international collaborative project that collected families with at least two cases of testicular cancer. The authors did not find clear evidence of susceptibility at any locus (Crockford et al, 2006). In particular, they could not confirm their previous finding of a region of susceptibility on chromosome Xq27, called *testicular germ cell tumor cell 1* (*TGCT1*). An increased risk for testicular cancer has been detected among carriers of the "*gr/gr*" deletion, a 1.6-Mb deletion of the Y chromosome that removes part of the AZFc region and is associated with spermatogenic failure (Nathanson et al, 2005). Higher *CYP1A2* activity among men and their mothers has been associated with a decreased risk of testicular cancer in a population-based case-parent study, although estimates did not reach statistical significance (Starr et al, 2005).

Testicular cancer is associated with a number of genetic disorders usually involving abnormalities in the Y chromosome, such as Klinefelter's syndrome (47,XXY), Turner's syndrome, male pseudohermaphroditism, testicular feminization, gonadal dysgenesis, Down's syndrome, and recessive X-linked icthyosis (Hill et al, 2003; Lutke Holzik et al, 2003).

Somatic Events

An isochromosome of the short arm of chromosome 12 has been identified in carcinoma in situ and in 80% of all testicular tumors, regardless of histology (Skotheim and Lothe, 2003). The etiologic relevance of this is unclear.

RISK FACTORS

Very little is known about the etiology of testicular cancer. As summarized in Table 21–1 there are few well-established risk

Table 21–1. Epidemiology of testicular cancer: risk factor summary

Risk factors

Well-Confirmed Risk Factors
Age*
Area of residence**
Contralateral testicular cancer
Cryptorchidism
Ethnic group***
Family history

Probable Relationship Exists, based on Substantial Data
Early puberty
Tallness
Subfertility

Weak, if Any, Relationship Exists, Based on Substantial Data
Tobacco
Alcohol
Vasectomy

Possible, but Results are Conflicting or Limited Studies to Date
Endocrine disruptors
Fetal exposure to maternal sex hormones
Intake of milk and diary products
Hypospadias
Infection (e.g., mumps, rubella, EBV)
Immunosuppression
Perinatal characteristics (including: low birth order, high maternal age, short gestational duration, low birth weight)

* After puberty there is a dramatic increase in incidence, which peaks at around age 30 and declines to almost zero by age 60.

** The rates are highest in some Northern European populations and lowest in Asian populations.

*** In the US, the rate of testicular cancer is about 6 times greater in whites as compared with blacks.

factors and the causal mechanisms of these exposures remain to be elucidated.

Tobacco

Studies of tobacco smoking and subsequent risk of testicular cancer have been consistently null (Henderson et al, 1979; Brown et al, 1987; United Kingdom Testicular Cancer Study Group, 1994a; Thune and Lund, 1994; Gallagher et al, 1995).

Diet

The role of diet in testicular cancer has not been adequately evaluated in large analytical studies. However, an ecological study including 42 countries showed a high correlation between incidence of testicular cancer and per capita consumption of cheese, milk, and animal fat (Ganmaa et al, 2002). In addition, a few case-control studies have fairly consistently reported that diets high in dairy products, milk, or fat are associated with an increased risk (Davies et al, 1996; Sigurdson et al, 1999; Garner et al, 2003; Stang et al, 2006; McGlynn et al, 2007). In a cohort of around 45 000 Swedish men followed-up for a maximum of 25 years, baseline high serum cholesterol level was associated with an increased risk of testicular cancer, with evidence of a dose–response relationship (Wirehn et al, 2005).

Alcohol

Studies of alcohol in relation to testicular cancer have been consistently null (Henderson et al, 1979; Brown et al, 1987; United Kingdom Testicular Cancer Study Group, 1994a).

Reproductive Factors and Hormones

Testicular cancer rarely occurs in boys before puberty, which suggests that hormones influence the development of this cancer. Because testicular cancer is probably preceded by carcinoma in situ and occurs relatively early in life, it has been proposed that hormones play a role in tumor progression (Skakkebaek et al, 1987). Reports that the risk of testicular cancer decreases with increasing age at puberty have been fairly consistent (Depue et al, 1983; Moss et al, 1986; Swerdlow et al, 1989; United Kingdom Testicular Cancer Study Group, 1994b; Gallagher et al, 1995; Moller and Skakkebaek, 1996; Weir et al, 1998; McGlynn et al, 2007). In addition, men with Kallman's syndrome (hypogonadotropic hypogonadism) experience puberty very late, if at all, and have a low risk of developing testicular cancer despite the high prevalence of cryptorchidism in these men (Rajpert-De Meyts and Skakkebaek, 1993).

Baldness has been used as a proxy for increased androgen levels. One study found a reduced risk of testicular cancer with increasing degree of baldness (Petridou et al, 1997). Severe acne is another proxy for increased androgen exposure (Pochi, 1982). Studies of severe acne and the risk of testicular cancer have been conflicting, with most of the studies reporting a null association (Henderson et al, 1979; Brown et al, 1987; United Kingdom Testicular Study Group, 1994a).

Semen Quality and Fertility

Impaired fertility has consistently been associated with an increased risk of testicular cancer; however, the mechanism underlying this association is not known. It has been hypothesized that perhaps a growing tumor may affect fertility or that there may be a common etiological link between subfertility and testicular cancer. Several questionnaire-based case-control studies have found an association between different indicators of subfertility—including prior diagnosis of infertility, number of children, time to pregnancy—and testicular cancer risk (Haughey et al, 1989; Swerdlow et al, 1989; United Kingdom Testicular Cancer Study Group, 1994b; Moller and Skakkekaek, 1999; Doria-Rose et al, 2005; Baker et al, 2005). Register-based studies in Denmark, Norway, and Sweden revealed that men with testicular cancer father less children than population controls and this association is apparent several years prior to the cancer diagnosis (Jacobsen et al, 2000b; Fossa and Kravdal, 2000; Richiardi et al, 2004b).

Jacobsen et al (2000a) conducted a study to assess more directly the effect of subfertility on testicular cancer by utilizing prospectively conducted semen analysis. Overall, men in couples with fertility problems had a 60% increased risk of testicular cancer compared to the general population. Men classified with low sperm concentra-

tions, poor motility, or a high percentage of abnormal sperm had a significant two- to threefold increased risk of testicular cancer. In contrast, men within normal ranges for these semen characteristics had a risk similar to that of the general population.

Recently, a register-based Swedish study found that brothers, but not sisters, of testicular cancer patients might have an impaired fertility, measured as decreased number of children and decreased frequency of opposite-sex twins among the children (Richiardi and Akre, 2005). Genetic or shared environmental factors may explain this finding.

During the past few decades, a pattern of decreasing fertility and semen quality has been reported by some investigators (Swan et al, 2000). However, the reports of declining fertility have not been convincing (Safe, 2000) and have been met with criticism. It is unclear how semen quality fits in with the descriptive epidemiology of testicular cancer.

Anthropometric Measures

Height

Studies of height have tended to show either positive or null associations with testicular cancer (Dicckmann and Pichlmeier, 2002). Evidence of an increased risk of testicular cancer among tall men has been found in Norway (Akre et al, 2000), Sweden (Richiardi et al, 2003), Germany (Dieckmann and Pichlmeier, 2002), Canada (Gallagher et al, 1995), and the US (McGlynn et al, 2007). Height is believed to be a risk factor with a number of potential mechanisms. Testicular cancer risk and postpubertal height might have common intrauterine determinants. Birth weight and gestational duration, on the one hand, and adult height, on the other hand, may, however, act as independent risk factors (Rasmussen et al; 2003; Richiardi et al, 2003). Nutritional factors affecting prepubertal growth may be implicated in the development of testicular cancer and, finally, height may be a marker of insulin-like growth factor 1 exposure, which has been found to be associated with a number of cancers.

Body mass index

Body mass index (BMI) does not appear to be associated with testicular cancer risk (Dieckmann and Pichlmeier, 2002). Two studies, however, reported some evidence of an inverse association (Petridou et al, 1997; Akre et al, 2000).

Infections

Based on epidemiological similarities with Hodgkin's lymphoma, it has been suggested that testicular cancer may be associated with infection at later ages (Newell et al, 1984). The elevated risk of testicular cancer observed among patients with acquired immunodeficiency syndrome (AIDS) (Frisch et al, 2001) and renal transplant patients (Adami et al, 2003) provide evidence of an etiologic role of the immune system and a possible infectious etiology. Most of the studies conducted on the role of infection in testicular cancer etiology are, however, null.

There is some evidence that orchitis and mumps orchitis increase the risk of testicular cancer (Brown et al, 1987; Swerdlow et al, 1987a; Stone et al, 1991; United Kingdom Testicular Cancer Study Group, 1994a; Moller and Skakkebek, 1999). The majority of these studies have been small, retrospective, and suffered from potential recall bias. Studies on mumps infection and other common childhood infections, including rubella, chicken pox, pertussis, and measles, have in general found no association with testicular cancer risk (Henderson et al 1979; Brown et al, 1987; Swerdlow et al, 1987a; Prener et al, 1992; United Kingdom Testicular Cancer Study Group, 1994a; Petridou al, 1997). Two studies have reported that men with a positive history of sexually transmitted diseases were at an increased risk of testicular cancer (United Kingdom Testicular Cancer Study Group, 1994a; Gallagher et al, 1995).

Epstein-Barr virus (EBV) is the most frequently studied infectious agent in relation to testicular cancer. Results of the studies are conflicting and, as EBV is ubiquitous, infection alone is not sufficient to cause cancer. One case-control study on viral infections and testicular cancer was based on prospectively collected serum specimens. No clear evidence of association was found with seroactivity against EBV, cytomegalovirus (CMV) (Akre et al, 1999), and human parvovirus B19 (Tolfvenstam et al, 2002).

Physical Activity

Only a few studies have looked at physical activity and testicular cancer, with little consistency in results. Positive (Srivastava and Kreiger, 2000) as well as inverse (Gallagher et al, 1995) and null (Thune and Lund, 1994) associations have been reported. There are, however, limitations in those studies, both in the assessment of physical activity through questionnaires and in the choice of the relevant period in life to be investigated.

Ionizing Radiation

Little research has looked at the association between ionizing radiation and the risk of testicular cancer. Although animal studies suggest that radiation may cause testicular tumors (Berdjis, 1964; Hulse, 1980), human studies do not support any association (National Academy of Sciences Advisory Committee on the Biological Effects of Ionizing Radiations, 1980).

Occupation

A number of studies have reported an association between occupation and the risk of testicular cancer, yet initial findings have been seldom replicated; therefore, no occupational exposure has emerged as a strong candidate risk factor. Studies have reported an association between aircraft mechanics and an increased risk of testicular cancer (Garland et al, 1988; Foley et al, 1995). Other studies have found an increased risk among petroleum workers (Mills et al, 1984), metal workers (Rhomberg et al, 1995), and their sons (Kardaun et al, 1991). Associations have also been observed among men in the leather industry (Marshall et al, 1990), and among fire fighters (LeMasters et al, 2006; Bates et al, 2007). A null association has been found with occupational exposure to electromagnetic fields (Baumgardt-Elms et al, 2002). An exploratory analysis carried out on 43 chemical agents and around 400 occupations in Finland found some evidence of an association with testicular cancer for exposure to pesticides, textile dust, and some organic solvents (Guo et al, 2005).

Medical Conditions and Treatment

Cryptorchidism

Cryptorchidism, that is, undescended testes, is a well-established risk factor for testicular cancer. Most studies investigating the association between cryptorchidism and testicular cancer have reported relative risks of 2 to 10 (United Kingdom Testicular Cancer Study Group, 1994b; Moller and Skakkebaek, 1996; Weir et al, 2000). A meta-analysis of 20 published case-control studies has estimated a pooled odds ratio of 4.8 (95% confidence interval: 4.0–5.7), based on approximately 6000 cases and 8000 controls (Dieckmann and Pichlmeier, 2004). Cohort studies may produce more valid estimates of the effect of cryptorchidism, as they are not affected by recall bias. Relative risks of 7.5 have been estimated in cohorts of cryptorchid men in the UK (Swerdlow et al, 1997b) and Sweden (Pinczowski et al, 1991). Although the association is strong and well established, it is unclear whether the ectopic position of the testis itself is a cause of testicular cancer or whether the two conditions have a common etiology. These two mechanisms are, however, not mutually exclusive.

Normally, the testes descend from the groin to the scrotum during the third trimester of pregnancy. In infants born with undescended testes, they may descend spontaneously during the first months after birth, and occasionally later on during childhood. Some studies have found that spontaneously descending testicles are not associated with an increased risk of testicular cancer (Moller et al, 1996; Prener et al, 1996).

The risk is greater in the maldescended than in the contralateral testis (Strader et al, 1988; United Kingdom Testicular Cancer Study Group, 1994b; Moller et al, 1996), supporting the hypothesis of an effect of the ectopic position. In addition, surgical correction at an earlier age has been associated with a protective effect against cancer (Strader et al, 1988; United Kingdom Testicular Cancer Study Group, 1994b; Moller et al, 1996; Herrinton et al, 2003). It is not clear, however, at what age orchidopexy should be carried out, and if an early correction may entirely prevent the excess risk associated with cryptorchidism. Data from a large cohort study based on about 17 000 patients who underwent orchidopexy show that there is a baseline twofold increased risk for testicular cancer that increases to fourfold if orchidopexy is carried out after puberty (Pettersson et al, 2007b). This implies that the association between cryptorchidism and testicular cancer is explained by both shared etiology and the ectopic position. Moreover, it seems that there are two relevant windows of susceptibility for testicular cancer development: The first one is the fetal life and the second one is puberty.

Both cryptorchidism and testicular cancer have similarities in their descriptive epidemiology and perhaps share some risk factors, suggesting a possible common etiology for disease. A study estimated that the prevalence of cryptorchidism at birth is 9% in Denmark and 2.4% in Finland (Boisen et al, 2004). Three months after birth, these figures were 1.9% and 1.0%, respectively. The age-standardized incidence of testicular cancer in Denmark is three times that observed in Finland (Ferlay et al, 2004).

Hypospadias

Hypospadias (a condition in which the urethral opening is located along the underside rather than at the tip of the penis), has been associated with an increased risk of testicular cancer, yet this finding was based on studies with very small numbers (Swerdlow et al, 1987a; United Kingdom Testicular Cancer Study Group, 1994b; Prener et al, 1996). Because hypospadias is extremely rare, its possible association with testicular cancer has been difficult to determine.

There is some evidence that cryptorchidism and hypospadias have been increasing in prevalence over time, although reports are controversial (Paulozzi, 1999; Boisen et al, 2004). Despite the fact that hypospadias is not a well-established risk factor for testicular cancer, it is often grouped in the literature with cryptorchidism in an effort to illustrate that the potential increases in these two malformations are consistent with the increases in testicular cancer and may in fact represent a shared etiology.

Inguinal hernia

Inguinal hernia has often been associated with testicular cancer risk, but this finding should be interpreted with much caution, since inguinal hernia is strongly associated with cryptorchidism and the majority of the studies did not control for its confounding effect. Besides, difference in recall between cases and controls is a likely source of bias in retrospective studies. As a corollary, studies restricted to men without cryptorchidism found a convincing null association between inguinal hernia and testicular cancer (Pinczowski et al, 1991; Moller et al, 1996).

Hydrocele

There has been contradictory evidence regarding hydrocele—fluid accumulation around the testicle—with some studies finding a positive association with testicular cancer and others finding none (Swerdlow et al, 1987a; Gershman and Stolley, 1988; United Kingdom Testicular Cancer Study Group, 1994b; Gallagher et al, 1995). These studies do have potential recall bias. It is also unclear if hydrocele may be an early sign of cancer development.

Other Risk Factors

Prenatal exposures

The early age at diagnosis and birth cohort patterns of testicular cancer, in conjunction with the increased risk observed in the contralateral testis of cryptorchid men and in animal studies, suggest that early life and perhaps in utero exposures may be causally related to testicular cancer (Henderson et al, 1979; Walker et al, 1990; Moller, 1993; Sharpe and Skakkebaek, 1993).

Maternal smoking during pregnancy. Since it has been observed that the increasing rates of smoking in women parallel the increasing rates of testicular cancer, maternal smoking during pregnancy has been hypothesized to be a cause of testicular cancer (Clemmesen, 1997; Pettersson et al, 2004). However, questionnaire-based case-control studies on maternal smoking have been consistently null (Henderson et al, 1979; Brown et al, 1986; Moller and Skakkebaek, 1996; Swerdlow et al, 1987b; Weir et al, 2000; Coupland et al, 2004; McGlynn et al, 2006). Results of these studies have been questioned on the basis of the potential bias introduced by assessing maternal smoking during pregnancy 20 to 50 years after the child's birth. A recent register-based case-control study with prospectively collected information on smoking has, however, confirmed the null association (Pettersson et al, 2007a).

Neonatal jaundice. Neonatal jaundice has been reported to be a risk factor for cryptorchidism (Davies et al, 1986), but only a few studies have examined it as a risk factor for testicular cancer. Although an association between neonatal jaundice and testicular cancer has been suggested in two independent studies, updates of these studies found a null association (Richiardi et al, 2002; Aschim et al, 2006).

Birth weight and gestational duration. Low birth weight has been associated with an increased risk of testicular cancer in a number of studies (Depue et al, 1983; Brown et al, 1986; Moller and Skakkebaek, 1997; Richiardi et al, 2002; Coupland et al, 2004), although several other studies did not support the association (Moss et al, 1986; Petridou et al, 1997; Sabroe and Olsen, 1998; Weir et al, 2000; English et al, 2003; Aschim et al, 2006). A few studies also report an association between high birth weight and increased risk of testicular cancer (Richiardi et al, 2002; Aschim et al, 2006). It has been debated whether the possible effect of low birth weight differs between seminomas and nonseminonas (Akre et al, 1996). Most of the studies investigating the two histological groups separately, however, did not find clear evidence of heterogeneity (Moller and Skakkebek, 1997; Sabroe and Olsen, 1998; Richiardi et al, 2002; English et al, 2003).

Gestational duration has been examined as a risk factor for testicular cancer both as an indicator of fetal growth and of exposure to pregnancy hormones, because women who deliver preterm are reported to have higher levels of circulating pregnancy estrogens (McGregor et al, 1995). Some studies report a significant increase in risk of testicular cancer for preterm births and/or a decrease in risk for posterm births, compared to that of babies born at term (Brown et al, 1986; Weir et al, 2000; Richiardi et al, 2002; English et al, 2003; Coupland et al, 2004). Other studies found no effect of gestational duration (Moller and Skakkebaek, 1997; Sabroe and Olsen, 1998)

Some studies combined information on gestational duration and birth weight to investigate the effect of being born small for gestational age, which is a better proxy of retarded fetal growth (Brown et al, 1986; Richiardi et al, 2002; English et al, 2003). However, the combination of these two variables has some methodological difficulties and would require larger sample sizes to be correctly interpreted.

Hormones. Since the end of the 1970s it has been suggested that the hormonal milieu during gestation may play a role in testicular cancer etiology, although evidence for an effect of fetal exposure to hormones remains conflicting. The hypothesis of an etiological role of maternal sex hormones, known as the *estrogen hypothesis*, was formalized at the beginning of the 1990s by Sharpe and Skakkebaek (1993). A number of factors associated with pregnancy hormone levels have been used as surrogate measures of in utero exposure to sex hormones and many of the findings on prenatal

characteristics have been interpreted on the basis of the estrogen hypothesis.

Nausea during pregnancy occurs at the end of the first trimester, when there is an escalation in pregnancy hormones. Severe nausea during pregnancy has been attributed to increased levels of estrogens and chorionic gonadotropin (Depue et al, 1987) and has been associated with an increased risk of testicular cancer in some (Henderson et al, 1979; Moss et al, 1986; Brown et al, 1986; Petridou et al, 1997), but not all studies (Moller and Skakkebaek, 1997; Coupland et al, 2004).

Twin pregnancies, dizygotic more so than monozygotic, have higher estrogen and chorionic gonadotropin levels than single pregnancies. A number of small studies reported a positive association of being a twin, compared to being a singleton, with the risk of testicular cancer (Depue et al, 1983; Swerdlow et al, 1987b; Braun et al, 1995; Aschim et al, 2006). Another study reported that dizygotic twins had a 50% greater risk of developing testicular cancer than monozygotic twins (Swerdlow et al, 1997a).

Studies examining the role of exogenous hormones during pregnancy as risk factors for testicular cancer have reported conflicting results (Brown et al, 1986; Prener et al, 1992; Moller and Skakkebaek, 1996; Weir et al, 2000; Coupland et al, 2004). The relative risk estimates varied from less than one to an almost fivefold increased risk. Because exposure had not been validated in these studies, recall bias is a potential problem. A cohort study on fetal exposure to diethylstilbrestol (DES)—a nonsteroidal estrogen that has been used in the past to prevent abortions and pregnancy complications and is strongly associated with the risk of adenocarcinoma of the vagina—found a threefold increased risk for testicular cancer, albeit it was based on only seven cases (Strohsnitter et al, 2001).

Birth order. The association between birth order and testicular cancer risk has been investigated in a great number of studies, several of which found an increased risk among firstborns (Depue et al, 1983;

Swerdlow et al, 1987b; Prener et al, 1992; Moller and Skakkebaek, 1996, 1997; Sabroe and Olsen, 1998; Richiardi et al, 2002; English et al, 2003; Richiardi et al, 2004a; Aschim et al, 2006). There are possible interpretations for this finding. First, there is evidence that first pregnancies are associated with higher levels of circulating estrogens than subsequent pregnancies (Panagiotopoulou et al, 1990). Second, firstborns tend to be exposed to specific micro-organisms at older ages compared to laterborns. Finally, birth order correlates with sibship size that is a (weak) indicator of parental fertility. The latter mechanism is supported by some studies that found no effect of birth order within each category of sibship size (Moller and Skakebbaek, 1996; Richiardi et al, 2004a).

Maternal age. Studies on maternal age tend to show either positive (Henderson et al, 1979; Moller and Skakkebaek 1996; Petridou et al, 1997; Sabroe and Olsen, 1998; Richiardi et al, 2004a) or null associations (Brown et al, 1986; Swerdlow et al, 1987a; Petridou et al, 1997; Weir et al, 2000). One study also reported an inverse association (Aschim et al, 2006). It has been suggested that maternal age is associated with sex hormone levels (Panagiotopoulou et al, 1990), although this hypothesis has not been confirmed (Kaijser et al, 2002). Because of the conflicting results and the lack of a strong biological basis, the role of maternal age in testicular cancer etiology remains unclear.

Testicular dysgenesis syndrome and endocrine disruptors. Although reports of increases in cryptorchidism and hypospadias (Paulozzi, 1999) and decreases in semen quality (Safe, 2000) are in part controversial, these potential trends, in addition to the increasing rates of testicular cancer, have led to the hypothesis that they all may have similar etiologies. Indeed, it has been suggested that these four conditions are all part of a syndrome with a prenatal etiology. The syndrome has been named by Skakkebaek and colleagues (2001) *Testicular Dysgenesis Syndrome* (TDS). Studies have shown that geographical variations in incidence of testicular cancer between Denmark—a high-incidence country—Sweden—an intermediate-incidence country—and Finland—a low-incidence country—are paralleled by similar differences in prevalence of cryptorchidism between Denmark and Finland (Boisen et al, 2004) and in sperm quality between Denmark, Sweden, and Finland (Jørgensen et al, 2002).

It has been suggested that fetal exposure to agents with estrogenic or antiandrogenic effect—endocrine disruptors—is a major cause of TDS (Skakkebaek et al, 2001; Toppari 1996; Hardell et al, 2004). Normal development and function of the male reproductive system requires hormonal input at critical stages during development (Sharpe, 2001). According to the endocrine disruptor hypothesis, any interference with this hormonal signaling could result in abnormal development or reduced function of the reproductive system—hence, in TDS.

The endocrine disruptor hypothesis has been challenged mainly on the basis of lack of empirical evidence (Joffe, 2001). Similarly, the hypothesis of the existence of a TDS remains speculative and more data will be needed for confirmation. The TDS hypothesis, however, indicates that better and perhaps broader definition of the case phenotype might be valuable for future etiologic research.

Trauma

Several case-control studies have found a positive association between testicular trauma and the risk of cancer. Despite the consistency of study results, however, it is most likely that the observed positive association can be attributed to recall bias (Merzenich et al, 2000). The United Kingdom Testicular Cancer Group (1994b) observed that a greater fraction of cases, compared to controls, reported injuries to the testis that could not be medically confirmed.

Vasectomy

Vasectomy has convincingly been ruled out as a potential risk factor for testicular cancer (Moss et al, 1986; Moller et al, 1994; United Kingdom Testicular Cancer Study Group, 1994b).

Socioeconomic status

High socioeconomic status has been associated fairly consistently with an increased risk of testicular cancer starting in the early twentieth century (Brown et al, 1987; Pearce et al, 1987; Haughey et al, 1989; Prener et al, 1992). The effect of socioeconomic status has probably decreased over time (Richiardi et al, 2004a). This has been well described by a Finnish study: In the early 1970s testicular cancer incidence in Finland was five times greater in the highest social class compared with the lowest, but this disparity decreased to a less than two-fold difference in the 1990s (Pukkala and Weiderpass, 2002).

CONCLUSION

Only age, area of residence, ethnic group, cryptorchidism, contralateral testicular cancer, and family history are undoubted determinants of testicular cancer risk. While analytic epidemiologic research has provided numerous etiologic clues, all of them remain tentative. Many studies are hampered by small sample size and by retrospective assessment of exposures that may be difficult to recall and/or are susceptible to bias. Overwhelming evidence indicates the fundamental importance of environmental factors in the etiology of this enigmatic cancer. Moreover, by means of its many salient features, the descriptive epidemiology of this malignancy provides a unique benchmark for testing novel etiologic hypotheses. For example, the decisive influence of exposures early in life is strongly indicated by the age-incidence curve, the apparent birth-cohort pattern, analyses in migrants, and some early data from analytic studies. However, testicular cancer has also

a strong genetic component, which has been poorly studied so far.

In order to further explain geographic, ethnic, and temporal patterns, we must consider exposures that differ markedly even within limited geographic areas, that strike whites much more than blacks in the United States, and that have become increasingly prevalent over the last century. To identify factors that tally with this pattern is a formidable and exciting scientific challenge. None of the risk factors so far seriously considered appear to be promising candidates to explain the occurrence pattern of testicular cancer. Detailed ecologic studies in areas with reliable incidence data appear to be still a resource to generate novel hypotheses. Analytical studies based on international collaboration to compare risk factors in different countries, reach an adequate sample size, and solve inconsistencies between previous findings will be highly informative.

REFERENCES

Adami J, Gäbel H, Lindelöf B, Ekström K, Rydh B, Glimelius B, et al. Cancer risk following organ transplantation: a nationwide cohort study in Sweden. Br J Cancer 2003;89:1221–27.

Akre O, Ekbom A, Hsieh CC, Trichopoulos D, Adami HO. Testicular nonseminoma and seminoma in relation to perinatal characteristics. J Natl Cancer Inst 1996;88:883–89.

Akre O, Lipworth L, Tretli S, Linde A, Engstrand L, Adami HO, et al. Epstein-Barr virus and cytomegalovirus in relation to testicular-cancer risk: a nested case-control study. Int J Cancer 1999;82:1–5.

Akre O, Ekbom A, Sparen P, Tretli S. Body size and testicular cancer. J Natl Cancer Inst 2000;92:1093–96.

Aschim EL, Haugen TB, Tretli S, Daltveit AK, Grotmol T. Risk factors for testicular cancer—differences between pure non-seminoma and mixed seminoma/non-seminoma? Int J Androl 2006;29:458–67.

Bates MN. Registry-based case-control study of cancer in California firefighters. Am J Ind Med 2007;50:339–44.

Baumgardt-Elms C, Ahrens W, Bromen K, Boikat U, Stang A, Jahn I, Stegmaier C, Jockel H. Testicular cancer and electromagnetic fields

(EMF) in the workplace: results of a population-based case-control study in Germany. Cancer Causes Control 2002;13:895–902.

Baker JA, Buck GM, Vena JE, Moysich KB. Fertility patterns prior to testicular cancer diagnosis. Cancer Causes Control 2005; 16:295–99.

Berdjis CC. Testicular tumors in normal and irradiated rats. Oncologie 1964;17:197–220.

Bergström R, Adami HO, Mohner M, Zatonski W, Storm H, Ekbom A, et al. Increase in testicular cancer incidence in six European countries: a birth cohort phenomenon. J Natl Cancer Inst 1996;88:727–33.

Boisen KA, Kaleva M, Main KM, Virtanen HE, Haavisto A-M, Schmidt IM, Chellakooty M, Damgaard I N, Mau C, Reunanen M, Skakkebaek N E, Toppari J. Difference in prevalence of congenital cryptorchidism in infants between two Nordic countries. Lancet 2004;363:1264–69.

Braun MM, Ahlbom A, Floderus B, Brinton LA, Hoover RN. Effect of twinship on incidence of cancer of the testis, breast, and other sites (Sweden). Cancer Causes Control 1995;6:519–24.

Bray F, Richiardi L, Ekbom A, Forman D, Pukkala E, Cuminkova M, Moller H. Do testicular seminoma and nonseminoma share the same etiology? Evidence from an age-period-cohort analysis of incidence trends in eight European countries. Cancer Epidemiol Biomarkers Prev 2006a;15:652–58.

Bray F, Richiardi L, Ekbom A, Pukkala E, Cuminkova M, Moller H. Trends in testicular cancer incidence and mortality in 22 European countries: continuing increases in incidence and declines in mortality. Int J Cancer 2006b;118:3099–11.

Brown LM, Pottern LM, Hoover RN. Prenatal and perinatal risk factors for testicular cancer. Cancer Res 1986;46:4812–16.

Brown LM, Pottern LM, Hoover RN. Testicular cancer in young men: the search for causes of the epidemic increase in the United States. J Epidemiol Commun Health 1987;41:349–54.

Clemmesen J. Is pregnancy smoking causal to testis cancer in sons? A hypothesis. Acta Oncol 1997;36:59–63.

Coupland CAC, Forman D, Chilvers CED, Davey G, Pike MC, Oliver RTD. Maternal risk factors for testicular cancer: a population-based case-control study (UK). Cancer Causes Control 2004;15:277–83.

Crockford GP, Linger R, Hockley S, Dudakia D, Johnson L, Huddart R, et al. Genome-wide linkage screen for testicular germ cell tumour susceptibility loci. Hum Mol Genet 2006; 15:443–51.

Davies TW, Williams DR, Whitaker RH. Risk factors for undescended testis. Int J Epidemiol 1986;15:197–201.

Davies TW, Palmer CR, Ruja E, Lipscombe JM. Adolescent milk, dairy product and fruit consumption and testicular cancer. Br J Cancer 1996;74:657–60.

Depue RH, Bernstein L, Ross RK, Judd HL, Henderson BE. Hyperemesis gravidarum in relation to estradiol levels, pregnancy outcome, and other maternal factors: a seroepidemiologic study. Am J Obstet Gynecol 1987;156:1137–41.

Depue RH, Pike MC, Henderson BE. Estrogen exposure during gestation and risk of testicular cancer. J Natl Cancer Inst 1983;71: 1151–55.

Dieckmann KP, Pichlmeier U. Is risk of testicular cancer related to body size? Eur Urol 2002;42:564–69.

Dieckmann KP, Pichlmeier U. Clinical epidemiology of testicular germ cell tumors. World J Urol 2004;22:1–14.

Dong C, Lönnstedt I. Hemminki K. Familial testicular cancer and second primary cancers in testicular cancer patients by histological type. Eur J Cancer 2001;15:1878–85.

Doria-Rose VP, Biggs ML, Weiss NS. Subfertility and the risk of testicular germ cell tumors (United States). Cancer Causes Control 2005;16:651–56.

Dos Santos Silva I, Swerdlow AJ, Stiller CA, Reid A. Incidence of testicular germ-cell malignancies in England and Wales: trends in children compared with adults. Int J Cancer 1999;83:630–34.

Ekbom A, Richardi L, Akre O, Montgomery S, Sparén P. Testicular cancer risk among Finnish immigrants: Perinatal influences. J Natl Cancer Inst 2003;95:1238–40.

English PB, Goldberg DE, Wolff C, Smith D. Parental and birth characteristics in relation to testicular cancer risk among males born between 1960 and 1995 in California (United States). Cancer Causes Control 2003;14: 815–25.

Ferlay J, Bray F, Pisani P, Parkin DM. GLOBOCAN 2002: Cancer Incidence, Mortality and Prevalence Worldwide. IARC CancerBase No. 5. version 2.0, IARCPress, Lyon, 2004.

Foley S, Middleton S, Stitson D, Mahoney M. The incidence of testicular cancer in Royal Air Force personnel. Br J Urol 1995;76:495–96.

Forman D, Oliver RT, Brett AR, Marsh SG, Moses JH, Bodmer JG, et al. Familial testicular cancer: a report of the UK family register, estimation of risk and an HLA class 1 sibpair analysis. Br J Cancer 1992;65:255–62.

Fossa SD, Kravdal O. Fertility in Norwegian testicular cancer patients. Br J Cancer 2000; 82:737–41.

Frisch M, Biggar RJ, Engels EA, Goedert JJ, AIDS-Cancer Match Registry Study Group. Association of cancer with AIDS-related immunosuppression in adults. JAMA 2001; 285:1736–45.

Gallagher RP, Huchcroft S, Phillips N, Hill GB, Coldman AJ, Coppin C, et al. Physical activity, medical history, and risk of testicular cancer (Alberta and British Columbia, Canada). Cancer Causes Control 1995;6:398–406.

Ganmaa D, Li XM, Wang J, Qin LQ, Wang PY, Sato A. Incidence and mortality of testicular and prostatic cancers in relation to world dietary practices. Int J Cancer 2002;98:262–67.

Garland FC, Gorham ED, Garland CF, Ducatman AM. Testicular cancer in U.S. Navy personnel. Am J Epidemiol 1988;127:411–14.

Garner MJ, Birkett NJ, Johnson KC, Shatenstein B, Ghadirian P, Krerwski D, Canadian Cancer Registries Epidemiology Research Group. Dietary risk factors for testicular carcinoma. Int J Cancer 2003;106:934–41.

Gershman ST, Stolley PD. A case-control study of testicular cancer using Connecticut tumour registry data. Int J Epidemiol 1988;17: 738–42.

Grulich AE, McCredie M, Coates M. Cancer incidence in Asian migrants to New South Wales, Australia. Br J Cancer 1995;71:400–408.

Guo J, Pukkala E, Kyyrönen P, Lindbohm ML, Heikkilä P, Kauppinen T. Testicular cancer, occupation and exposure to chemical agents among Finnish men. Cancer Cause Control 2005;16:97–103.

Hardell L, Van Bavel B, Lindstrom G, Carlberg M, Eriksson M, Dreifaldt AC, Wijkstrom H, Starkhammar H, Hallquist A, Kolmert T. Concentrations of polychlorinated biphenyls in blood and the risk for testicular cancer. Int J Androl 2004;27:282–90.

Haughey BP, Graham S, Brasure J, Zielezny M, Sufrin G, Burnett WS. The epidemiology of testicular cancer in upstate New York. Am J Epidemiol 1989;130:25–36.

Heimdal K, Olsson H, Tretli S, Flodgren P, Borresen AL, Fossa SD. Familial testicular cancer in Norway and southern Sweden. Br J Cancer 1996;73:964–69.

Henderson BE, Benton B, Jing J, Yu MC, Pike MC. Risk factors for cancer of the testis in young men. Int J Cancer 1979;23:598–602.

Herrinton LJ, Zhao W, Husson G. Management of cryptorchidism and risk of testicular cancer. Am J Epidemiol 2003;157:602–5.

Hill DA, Gridley G, Canattingius S, Mellemkjaer L, Linet M, Adami HO, et al. Mortality and cancer incidence among individuals with Down syndrome. Arch Intern Med 2003; 163:705–11.

Hulse EV. Tumour incidence and longevity in neutron and gamma-irradiated rabbits, with an assessment of r.b.e. Int J Radiat Biol Relat Stud Phys Chem Med 1980;37:633–52.

Jacobsen R, Bostofte E, Engholm G, Hansen J, Skakkebaek NE, Moller H. Fertility and offspring sex ratio of men who develop testicular cancer: a record linkage study. Hum Reprod 2000b;15:1958–61.

Jacobsen R, Bostofte E, Engholm G, Hansen J, Olsen JH, Skakkebaek NE, et al. Risk of testicular cancer in men with abnormal semen characteristics: cohort study. Br Med J 2000a;321:789–92.

Joffe M. Are problems with male reproductive health caused by endocrine diruption? Occup Environ Med 2001;58:281–88.

Jørgensen N, Carlsen E, Nermoen I, Punab M, Suominen J, Andersen A-E, et al. East-West gradient in semen quality in the Nordic-Baltic area: a study of men from the general population in Denmark, Norway, Estonia and Finland. Hum Reprod 2002;17:2199–208.

Kaijser M, Jacobsen G, Granath F, Cnattingius S, Ekbom A. Maternal age, anthropometrics and pregnancy oestriol. Paediatr Perinat Epidemiol 2002;16:149–53.

Kardaun JW, Hayes RB, Pottern LM, Brown LM, Hoover RN. Testicular cancer in young men and parental occupational exposure. Am J Ind Med 1991;20:219–27.

LeMasters GK, Genaidy AM, Succop P, Deddens J, Sobeih T, Barriera-Viruet H, Dunning K, Lockey J. Cancer risk among firefighters: a review and meta-analysis of 32 studies. J Occup Environ Med 2006;48:1189-202.

Levi F, Te VC, Radimbison L, La Vecchia C. Trends in testicular cancer incidence in Vaud, Switzerland. Eur J Cancer Prev 2003; 12:347–49.

Lutke Holzik MF, Sijmons RH, Sleijfer DT, Sonneveld DJ, Hoekstra-Weebers JE, van Echten-Arends J, Hoekstra HJ. Syndromic aspects of testicular carcinoma. Cancer 2003;97:984–92.

Marshall EG, Melius JM, London MA, Nasca PC, Burnett WS. Investigation of a testicular cancer cluster using a case-control approach. Int J Epidemiol 1990;19:269–73.

McGlynn KA, Devesa SS, Graubard BI, Castle PE. Increasing incidence of testicular germ cell tumors among black men in the United States. J Clin Oncol 2005;23:5757–61.

McGlynn KA, Sakoda LC, Rubertone MV, Sesterhenn IA, Lyu C, Graubard BI, Erickson

RL. Body size, dairy consumption, puberty, and risk of testicular germ cell tumors. Am J Epidemiol 2007;165:355-63.

McGlynn KA, Zhang Y, Sakoda LC, Rubertone MV, Erickson RL, Graubard BI. Maternal smoking and testicular germ cell tumors. Cancer Epidemiol Biomarkers Prev 2006; 15:1820-24.

McGregor JA, Jackson GM, Lachelin GC, Goodwin TM, Artal R, Hastings C, et al. Salivary estriol as risk assessment for preterm labor: a prospective trial. Am J Obstet Gynecol 1995;173:1337-42.

Merzenich H, Ahrens W, Stang A, Baumgardt-Elms C, Jahn I, Stegmaier C, et al. Sorting the hype from the facts in testicular cancer: is testicular cancer related to trauma? J Urol 2000;164:2143-44.

Mills PK, Newell GR, Johnson DE. Testicular cancer associated with employment in agriculture and oil and natural gas extraction. Lancet 1984;1:207-10.

Moller H, Knudsen LB, Lynge E. Risk of testicular cancer after vasectomy: cohort study of over 73,000 men. Br Med J 1994;309:295-99.

Moller H. Clues to the aetiology of testicular germ cell tumours from descriptive epidemiology. Eur Urol 1993;23:8-15.

Moller H, Prener A, Skakkebaek NE. Testicular cancer, cryptorchidism, inguinal hernia, testicular atrophy, and genital malformations: case-control studies in Denmark. Cancer Causes Control 1996;7:264-74.

Moller H, Skakkebaek NE. Risks of testicular cancer and cryptorchidism in relation to socioeconomic status and related factors: case-control studies in Denmark. Int J Cancer 1996;66:287-93.

Moller H, Skakkebaek NE. Testicular cancer and cryptorchidism in relation to prenatal factors: case-control studies in Denmark. Cancer Causes Control 1997;8:904-12.

Moller H, Skakkebaek NE. Risk of testicular cancer in subfertile men: case control study. Br Med J 1999;318:559-62.

Montgomery SM, Granath F, Ehlin A, Sparen P, Ekbom A. Germ-cell testicular cancer in offspring of Finnish immigrants to Sweden. Cancer Epidemiol Biomarkers Prev 2005;14:280-82

Moss AR, Osmond D, Bacchetti P, Torti FM, Gurgin V. Hormonal risk factors in testicular cancer. A case-control study. Am J Epidemiol 1986;124:39-52.

National Academy of Sciences Advisory Committee on the Biological Effects of Ionizing Radiations. The Effects on Populations of Exposure to Low Levels of Ionizing Radiation. Washington, DC, National Academy Press, 1980, pp 266-67.

Nathanson KL, Kanetsky PA, Hawes R, et al. The Y deletion gr/gr and susceptibility to testicular germ cell tumor. Am J Hum Genet 2005;77:1034-43.

Newell GR, Mills PK, Johnson DE. Epidemiologic comparison of cancer of the testis and Hodgkin's disease among young males. Cancer 1984;54:1117-23.

Panagiotopoulou K, Katsouyanni K, Petridou E, Garas Y, Tzonou A, Trichopoulos D. Maternal age, parity, and pregnancy estrogens. Cancer Causes Control 1990;1:119-24.

Parkin DM, Iscovich J. Risk of cancer in migrants and their descendants in Israel: II. Carcinomas and germ-cell tumours. Int J Cancer 1997;70:654-60.

Paulozzi LJ. International trends in rates of hypospadias and cryptorchidism. Environ Health Perspect 1999;107:297-302.

Pearce N, Sheppard RA, Howard JK, Fraser J, Lilley BM. Time trends and occupational differences in cancer of the testis in New Zealand. Cancer 1987;59:1677-82.

Petridou E, Roukas KI, Dessypris N, Aravantinos G, Bafaloukos D, Efraimidis A, et al. Baldness and other correlates of sex hormones in relation to testicular cancer. Int J Cancer 1997;71:982-85.

Pettersson A, Kaijser M, Richiardi L, Ekbom A, Akre O. Women smoking and testicular cancer: one epidemic causing another? Int J Cancer 2004;109:941-44.

Pettersson A, Akre O, Richiardi L, Ekbom A, Kaijser M. Maternal smoking and the epidemic of testicular cancer-a nested case-control study. Int J Cancer 2007a;120:2044-46.

Pettersson A, Richiardi L, Nordenskjold A, Kaijser M, Akre O. Age at surgery for undescended testis and risk of testicular cancer. N Engl J Med 2007b;356:1835-41.

Pinczowski D, McLaughlin JK, Lackgren G, Adami HO, Persson I. Occurrence of testicular cancer in patients operated on for cryptorchidism and inguinal hernia. J Urol 1991;146:1291-94.

Pochi PE. Acne: endocrinologic aspects. Cutis 1982;30:212-14.

Prener A, Engholm G, Jensen OM. Genital anomalies and risk for testicular cancer in Danish men. Epidemiology 1996;7:14-19.

Prener A, Hsieh CC, Engholm G, Trichopoulos D, Jensen OM. Birth order and risk of testicular cancer. Cancer Causes Control 1992; 3:265-72.

Pukkala E, Weiderpass E. Socio-economic differences in incidence rates of cancers of the male genital organs in Finland, 1971-95. Int J Cancer 2002;102:643-48.

Purdue MP, Devesa SS, Sigurdson AJ, McGlynn KA. International patterns and trends in testis cancer incidence. Int J Cancer 2005; 115:822–27.

Rajpert-De Meyts E, Skakkebaek NE. The possible role of sex hormones in the development of testicular cancer. Eur Urol 1993; 23:54–61.

Rasmussen F, Gunnell D, Ekbom A, Hallqvist J, Tynelius P. Birth weight, adult height, and testicular cancer: cohort study of 337,249 Swedish young men. Cancer Cause Control 2003;14:595–98.

Rhomberg W, Schmoll HJ, Schneider B. High frequency of metal workers among patients with seminomatous tumors of the testis: a case-control study. Am J Ind Med 1995; 28:79–87.

Richiardi L, Akre O, Bellocco R, Ekbom A. Perinatal determinants of germ-cell testicular cancer in relation to histological subtypes. Br J Cancer 2002;87:545–50.

Richiardi L, Askling J, Granath F, Akre O. Body size at birth and adulthood and the risk for germ-cell testicular cancer. Cancer Epidemiol Biomarkers Prev 2003;12:669–73.

Richiardi L, Akre O, Lambe M, Granath F, Montgomery SM, Ekbom A. Birth order, sibship size, and risk for germ-cell testicular cancer. Epidemiology 2004a;15:323–29.

Richiardi L, Akre O, Montgomery SM, Lambe M, Kvist U, Ekbom A. Fecundity and twinning rates as measures of fertility before diagnosis of germ-cell testicular cancer. J Natl Cancer Inst 2004b;96:145–47.

Richiardi L, Bellocco R, Adami H-O, Torrång A, Barlow L, Hakulinen T, et al. Testicular cancer incidence in eight Northern European countries: secular and recent trend. Cancer Epidemiol Biomarkers Prev 2004c;13:2157–66.

Richiardi L, Akre O. Fertility among brothers of patients with testicular cancer. Cancer Epidemiol Biomarkers Prev 2005;14:2557–62.

Sabroe S, Olsen J. Perinatal correlates of specific histological types of testicular cancer in patients below 35 years of age: a case-cohort study based on midwives' records in Denmark. Int J Cancer 1998;78:140–43.

Safe SH. Endocrine disruptors and human health—is there a problem? An update. Environ Health Perspect 2000;108:487–93.

Sharpe RM. Hormones and testis development and the possible adverse effects of environmental chemicals. Toxicol Lett 2001; 120:221–32.

Sharpe RM, Skakkebaek NE. Are estrogens involved in falling sperm counts and disorders of the male reproductive tract? Lancet 1993;341:1392–95.

Sigurdson AJ, Chang S, Annegers JF, Duphoren CM, Pillow PC, Amato RJ, et al. A case-control study of diet and testicular carcinoma. Nutr Cancer 1999;34:20–26.

Skakkebaek NE, Berthelsen JG, Giwercman A, Muller J. Carcinoma-in-situ of the testis: possible origin from gonocytes and precursor of all types of germ cell tumours except spermatocytoma. Int J Androl 1987;10:19–28.

Skakkebaek, NE, Rajpert-De Meyts E, & Main, KM. Testicular dysgenesis syndrome: an increasingly common developmental disorder with environmental aspects. Hum Reprod 2001;16:972–78.

Skotheim RI, Lothe RA. The testicular germ cell tumour genome. APMIS 2003;111:136–50.

Srivastava A, Kreiger N. Relation of physical activity to risk of testicular cancer. Am J Epidemiol 2000;151:78–87.

Stang A, Ahrens W, Baumgardt-Elms C, Stegmaier C, Merzenich H, de Vrese M, Schrezenmeir J, Jockel KH. Adolescent milk fat and galactose consumption and testicular germ cell cancer. Cancer Epidemiol Biomarkers Prev 2006;15:2189–95.

Starr JR, Chen C, Doody DR, Hsu L, Ricks S, Weiss NS, Schwartz SM. Risk of testicular germ cell cancer in relation to variation in maternal and offspring cytochrome p450 genes involved in catechol estrogen metabolism. Cancer Epidemiol Biomarkers Prev 2005;14:2183–90.

Stone JM, Cruickshank DG, Sandeman TF, Matthews JP. Laterality, maldescent, trauma and other clinical factors in the epidemiology of testis cancer in Victoria, Australia. Br J Cancer 1991;64:132–38.

Strader CH, Weiss NS, Daling JR, Karagas MR, McKnight B. Cryptorchidism, orchiopexy and the risk of testicular cancer. Am J Epidemiol 1988;127:1013–18.

Strohsnitter WC, Noller KL, Hoover RN, Robboy SJ, Palmer JR, Titus-Ernstoff L, et al. Cancer risk in men exposed in utero to diethylstilbestrol. J Natl Cancer Inst 2001; 93:545–51

Swan SH, Elkin EP, Fenster L. The question of declining sperm density revisited: an analysis of 101 studies published 1934–1996. Environ Health Perspect 2000;108:961–66.

Swerdlow AJ, Huttly SR, Smith PG. Testicular cancer and antecedent diseases. Br J Cancer 1987a;55:97–103.

Swerdlow AJ, Huttly SR, Smith PG. Prenatal and familial associations of testicular cancer. Br J Cancer 1987b;55:571–77.

Swerdlow AJ, Huttly SRA, Smith PG. Testis cancer: post-natal hormonal factors, sexual behaviour and fertility. Int J Cancer 1989; 43:549–53.

Swerdlow AJ, De Stavola BL, Swanwick MA, Maconochie NES. Risks of breast and testicular cancers in young adult twins in England and Wales: evidence on prenatal and genetic aetiology. Lancet 1997a;350:1723–28.

Swerdlow AJ, Higgins CD, Pike MC. Risk of testicular cancer in boys with cryptorchidism. Br Med J 1997b;314:1507–11.

Thune I, Lund E. Physical activity and the risk of prostate and testicular cancer: a cohort study of 53,000 Norwegian men. Cancer Causes Control 1994;5:549–56.

Tolfvenstam T, Papadogiannakis N, Andersen A, Akre O. No association between human parvovirus B19 and testicular germ cell cancer. J Gen Virol 2002;83:2321–24.

Toppari J, Larsen JC, Christiansen P, Giwercman A, Grandjean P, Guillette LJ Jr, et al. Male reproductive health and environmental xenoestrogens. Environ Health Perspect 1996;104 (Suppl 4):741–803.

United Kingdom Testicular Cancer Study Group. Social, behavioural and medical factors in the aetiology of testicular cancer: results from the U.K. study. Br J Cancer 1994a; 70:513–20.

United Kingdom Testicular Cancer Study Group. Aetiology of testicular cancer: association with congenital abnormalities, age at puberty, infertility, and exercise. Br Med J 1994b;308:1393–99.

Walker AH, Bernstein L, Warren DW, Warner NE, Zheng X, Henderson BE. The effect of in utero ethinyl oestradiol exposure on the risk of cryptorchid testis and testicular teratoma in mice. Br J Cancer 1990;62:599–602.

Weir HK, Kreiger N, Marrett LD. Age at puberty and risk of testicular germ cell cancer (Ontario, Canada). Cancer Causes Control 1998;9:253–58.

Weir HK, Marrett LD, Kreiger N, Darlington GA, Sugar L. Pre-natal and peri-natal exposures and risk of testicular germ-cell cancer. Int J Cancer 2000;87:438–43.

Westergaard T, Olsen JH, Frisch M, Kroman N, Nielsen JW, Melbye M. Cancer risk in fathers and brothers of testicular cancer patients in Denmark. A population-based study. Int J Cancer 1996;66:627–31.

Wirehn AB, Tornberg S, Carsten J. Serum chiolosterol and testicular cancer incidence in 45 000 men followed for 25 years. Br J Cancer 2005;92:1785–86.

22

Urinary Bladder Cancer

MANOLIS KOGEVINAS, MONTSERRAT GARCIA-CLOSAS,
AND DIMITRIOS TRICHOPOULOS

Bladder cancer occupies an important place in the history of epidemiology, particularly occupational epidemiology. The highest cumulative incidence of any cancer ever reported is for bladder cancer among workers in the dye industry. This is also the first human cancer for which powerful evidence about its infectious aetiology (*Schistosoma haematobium*) was obtained, even though this dubious distinction is usually attached to liver cancer in relation to the hepatitis viruses. Finally, bladder cancer is one of the first cancers for which interactions between environmental exposures and genetic polymorphisms were demonstrated.

Transitional cell cancer, the predominant histopathologic type, arises in the renal pelvis and ureters as well as in the bladder. Therefore, most of the risk factors described in this chapter for transitional cell cancers of the bladder are relevant to these sites as well, although the associations may differ in strength.

CLINICAL SYNOPSIS

Subgroups and Staging

In industrialized countries, transitional cell carcinomas constitute 93% to 95% of malignant tumors in the urinary bladder. The 5% to 7% nontransitional cell carcinomas include squamous cell carcinomas, adenocarcinomas, undifferentiated carcinomas, and other rare histologic types such as small-cell carcinomas and lymphomas. About 70% of all tumors occur in the lateral and posterior wall and near the trigone, about 20% in the trigone, and 10% in the dome. Among urothelial (transitional cell) neoplasms of the urinary bladder, around 75% present as superficial disease and the remaining as muscle-invasive. Among superficial tumors, most appear as low-grade superficial lesions (Ta), and less than 10% as carcinoma in situ, which is generally high grade.

Symptoms

A visible but painless bleeding (hematuria) is the cardinal symptom of bladder cancer, sometimes accompanied by urgency, other voiding problems, or urinary obstruction.

Diagnosis

Diagnosis is confirmed through visual inspection by a cystoscope, combined with histopathologic examination of a biopsy specimen or resected tumor tissue. Cytologic examination of urine may provide additional information. In advanced stages, palpation under general anaesthesia is required for local staging, and x-ray examination of the upper urinary tract reveals obstruction of the ureters.

Treatment

Surgery is the predominant curative treatment. Depending on the stage of disease, such treatment ranges from transurethral resection to radical cystectomy, followed by various approaches to restore the urinary conduit. Radiotherapy and various chemotherapy regimen are used both as an adjuvant to surgical treatment and for palliation in patients with advanced disease. Occasionally, radiotherapy or chemotherapy alone may be curative.

Prognosis

Overall 5-year survival rates are now approaching 80%—balancing the excellent prognosis for patients with low-grade superficial tumors against the substantially poorer outcome for those with locally advanced or metastatic tumors.

Progress

In the United States, overall 5-year relative survival rose from 72% in the mid-1970s to 83% in cases diagnosed after 1995. Chemotherapy has turned out to be curative in a small number of patients even if they have metastases. Moreover, urinary diversion with continent reservoirs has led to a better quality of life for patients receiving radical cystectomy.

DESCRIPTIVE EPIDEMIOLOGY

The incidence of urinary bladder cancer is highest in Western Europe and North America and considerably lower in most of Asia (Figs. 22–1 to 22–4). Part of the international variation in incidence may be due to different practices in the registration of low-grade superficial tumors. This bias is also likely to affect time trends. Generally, the incidence of urinary bladder cancer has been increasing moderately in industrialized countries during the last decades. Mortality has somewhat decreased over time, particularly among men. In Europe, the highest mortality rates have been seen among men in cohorts born between 1920 and 1940 (La Vecchia and Airoldi, 1999), that is, the generations most heavily exposed to tobacco smoke and to industrial carcinogens. The pattern for women is similar but less consistent.

The incidence of bladder cancer rises steeply with age in both genders after age 50 (Figs. 22–1 and 22–2). In most industrialized countries, bladder cancer is approximately three times more frequent in men than in women, attributed in part to differences in smoking habits. In southern European countries the male to female ratio in incidence is higher (Samanic et al, 2006). Although hormonal factors have also been implicated in the gender difference, the gender ratio for bladder cancer closely follows that for lung cancer in all countries, indicating smoking as the more relevant factor.

Incidence rates are generally higher in urban than in rural areas. White men in the United States have approximately twice the rate of black men, while the difference is less pronounced for women. Studies in migrants, from Japan and China to the United States, and from Asia and New Zealand to the United Kingdom, invariably show that the risk of bladder cancer in migrants approximates that in the host country with increasing duration of stay. The higher prevalence of smoking among lower socioeconomic levels and the preponderance of jobs entailing a high risk of bladder cancer among

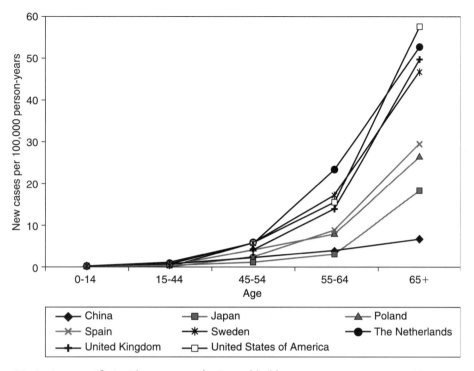

Figure 22–1. Age-specific incidence rates of urinary bladder cancer among women. (*Source*: Ferlay et al, 2004)

manual workers would have led to the assumption that the incidence is higher in lower than in upper social classes, but neither male nor female mortality data suggest a consistent social class gradient (Faggiano et al, 1997).

GENETIC AND MOLECULAR EPIDEMIOLOGY

Inherited Susceptibility

High-penetrance genes
Familial clustering of bladder cancer has been reported over the last 40 years (Kiemeney and Schoenberg, 1996) and several of these studies point to an early age of onset, compatible with a genetic component. However, there are no established high-penetrance genes for bladder cancer to date. Studies examining familial aggregation have found relative risks ranging from 1.2 to 4.0 (Plna and Hemminki, 2001). On the basis of these results, the attributable fraction

of familial aggregation in bladder cancer can be estimated to be around 1%. A recent follow-up study identified an increased bladder cancer risk among hereditary retinoblastoma cases (Fletcher et al, 2004). Segregation analyses argue against the existence of a major hereditary subtype of bladder cancer. The role of genetic susceptibility in bladder carcinogenesis has been demonstrated principally in relation to metabolic polymorphisms rather than to monogenic, high-penetrance conditions.

Genetic polymorphisms
Given the relative homogeneity in bladder cancer histology, the well-known environmental causes and the substantial interindividual variation in carcinogen-metabolizing processes and in the repair of DNA damage caused by these compounds, bladder carcinogenesis is an excellent model for the evaluation of genetic susceptibility and gene–environment interactions. Although many

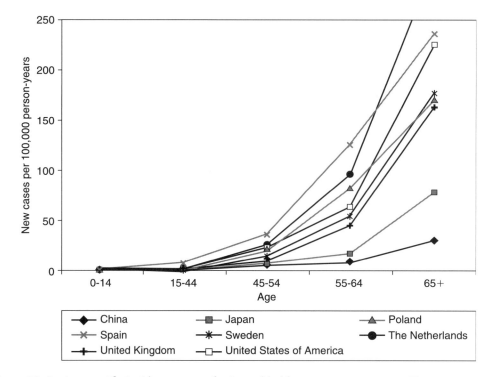

Figure 22–2. Age-specific incidence rates of urinary bladder cancer among men. (*Source*: Ferlay et al, 2004)

studies have evaluated genetic polymorphism and bladder cancer risk, most lack the statistical power to detect moderate to weak associations, or to evaluate gene–environment interactions (Deitz et al, 2004). Therefore, meta-analyses and pooled analyses of data from individual studies have become an important approach to identify associations unlikely to be false positives.

Figure 22–5 shows some of the likely etiologic pathways that have been evaluated.

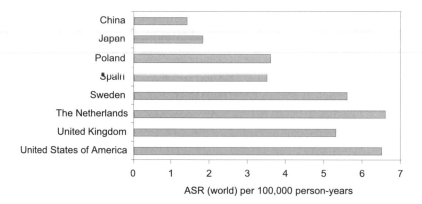

Figure 22–3. Age-standardized (to the world population) incidence rates of cancer of the urinary bladder among women. (*Source*: Ferlay et al, 2004)

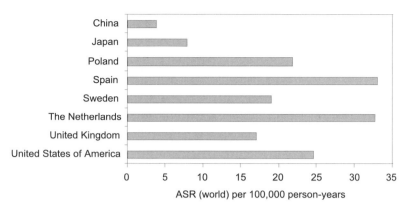

Figure 22–4. Age-standardized (to the world population) incidence rates of cancer of the urinary bladder among men. (*Source*: Ferlay et al, 2004)

Precarcinogens in tobacco smoke undergo metabolism that can result in either activation or detoxification of chemicals. Activated chemicals can cause DNA damage, leading to mutations and initiation of the carcinogenic process. Reactive oxygen species generated during metabolic reactions may also cause DNA damage. DNA repair and cell-cycle checkpoints are two primary defense mechanisms against DNA damage.

Candidate genes include also those frequently affected by somatic alterations in bladder tumors. Although most studies to date have evaluated only a few variants in each candidate gene, advances in genotyping technology and single nucleotide polymorphism (SNP) databases are allowing more comprehenvise evaluations of common variants in pathways of interest, as well as genome-wide association studies.

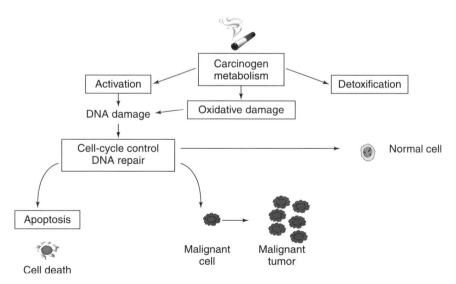

Figure 22–5. Key etiologic pathways that have been evaluated in studies on genetic susceptibility to bladder cancer.

Carcinogen metabolism

The capacity to detoxify by N-acetylation aromatic monoamines, including 4-aminobiphenyl implicated in tobacco-related bladder carcinogenesis, is polymorphic in human populations. About 50% of Caucasian and a lower percentage of African (30%) and Asian (15%) populations are homozygous for a mutated N-acetyl transferase gene (*NAT2*), responsible for decreased enzyme activity (slow acelylators) (Weber, 1987;Vatsis et al, 1991; Hein, 2002). Pooling and meta-analyses of relatively small studies (average size of about 100 cases per study) found evidence for an increased risk of bladder cancer among *NAT2* slow acetylators (Marcus et al, 2000). Although concerns had been raised about

publication bias and heterogeneity of results across studies, these findings were confirmed in a large case-control study and an updated meta-analysis (Garcia-Closas et al, 2005). *NAT2* slow acetylators had an about 40% increased risk for developing bladder cancer, and a higher risk from tobacco smoking than *NAT2* rapid or intermediate acetylators (Fig. 22–6).

This gene–environment interaction has strong biological plausibility; *NAT2* slow acetylators have a decreased capacity to detoxify aromatic monoamines (Hein, 2002), tobacco smoking is a primary source of exposure to aromatic amines in the general population, aromatic amines are suspected of being the primary bladder carcinogen in tobacco smoke, and smokers with the *NAT2*

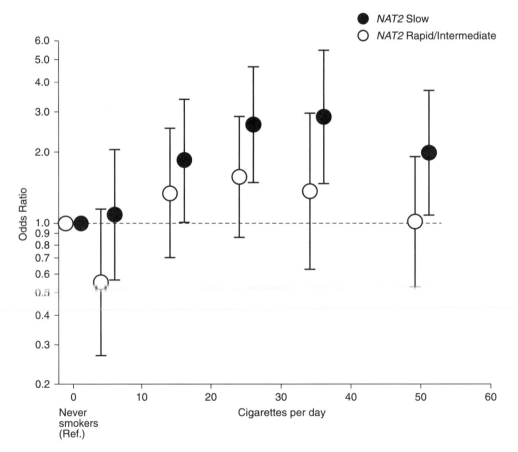

Figure 22–6. Association between smoking intensity (average number of cigarettes per day in categories of 10 cigarettes) and bladder-cancer risk compared with never smokers, stratified by NAT2 acetylation genotype. Bars indicate 95% confidence intervals. (*Source*: Garcia-Closas et al, 2005)

slow polymorphism have higher levels of the hemoglobin adduct of 4-aminobiphenyl than smokers with the *NAT2* rapid polymorphism (Yu et al, 1994). The evidence for an effect of *NAT2* slow acetylation on bladder cancer risk comes mainly from studies in European Caucasian populations, and additional evidence is needed to confirm this association in other populations, as well as to evaluate differences in the *NAT2* effect by other factors such as tobacco type (black/blond tobacco), intensity of smoking, and gender.

Most studies discussed previously were conducted in the general population, without specific occupational or environmental exposures to bladder carcinogens. Studies among subjects occupationally exposed to aromatic amines also tend to show associations between *NAT2* slow acetylation and increased bladder cancer risk (eg, Vineis et al, 2001; Weber et al, 1983). Studies of workers exposed to the carcinogenic aromatic amine, benzidine, have not shown excess of slow acetylators among subjects with bladder cancer (eg, Carreon et al, 2006), indicating that the association between *NAT2* polymorphisms and bladder cancer risk may depend on the exposure to specific aromatic amines.

The *NAT1* gene codes for an enzyme involved in the activation of aromatic amines by O-acetylation (Hein, 2002). There is inconsistent evidence for an association between bladder cancer risk and *NAT1*10* allele alone or in combination with *NAT2* slow acetylation (eg, Garcia-Closas et al, 2005; Gu et al, 2005).

The *GSTM1* gene codes for glutathione S-transferase M1, an enzyme involved in detoxification of a range of carcinogens, including polycyclic aromatic hydrocarbons (PAHs) and reactive oxygen species. This gene presents a polymorphism associated with lack of enzyme activity due to homozygous deletion (null genotype), which is present in about 50% of Caucasians. As for *NAT2*, meta-analyses suggested that the *GSTM1* null genotype increases the risk of bladder cancer (Engel et al, 2002), and these findings were recently confirmed in a large

study in Spain, as well as in an updated meta-analysis (Garcia-Closaset al, 2005). In this report, the increased risk for *GSTM1* null genotype and bladder cancer was similar for smokers and never smokers, suggesting that the *GSTM1* activity protects equally against tobacco-related and nontobacco-related bladder cancers. It appears that *GSTM1* may reduce the risk of bladder cancer through mechanisms that are not specific to the detoxification of PAHs in tobacco smoke. Other mechanisms of action for *GSTM1* could be protection from oxidative damage through metabolism of reactive oxygen species (Hayes and Strange, 2000). Associations between bladder cancer risk and polymorphisms in other glutathione S-transferase genes, eg, *GSTT1*, *GSTP1*, have been less frequently explored with inconsistent results across studies.

The cytochrome P-450 *CYP1A2* is involved in the activation of aromatic amines by N-hydroxylation, and is polymorphic in human populations; however, the functional relevance of the genetic variants is not well characterized (Landi et al, 1999), and to date it is unclear whether they play a role in bladder cancer. Other enzymes that depend on polymorphisms that could affect the risk of bladder cancer include other cytochrome P-450 enzymes such as *CYP1A1*, *CYP1B1*, *CYP2C19*, *CYP2D6*, and *CYP2E1*; sulfotransferases involved in the activation of aromatic amines; and microsomal epoxide hydrolase involved in the metabolism of epoxides formed during oxidative metabolism of xenobiotic substances such as PAHs.

DNA repair
A complex network of complementary DNA repair mechanisms prevent the detrimental consequences of DNA damage caused by exogenous chemicals. The main pathway involved in the repair of bulky chemical adducts produced by aromatic amines and other carcinogens in tobacco smoke is the nucleotide excision repair (NER) pathway. Epidemiological studies suggest that genetic variation in NER genes could affect bladder cancer risk (eg, Sanyal et al, 2004;

Garcia-Closas et al, 2006; Sak et al, 2005; Schabath et al, 2005); however, additional evidence is needed to establish these associations. Polymorphic genes are also involved in the base excision repair (BER) pathway, mainly affecting the removal of minor base damage induced by alkylating and oxidating agents (eg, Andrew et al, 2006; Wu et al, 2006), and in the double strand break (DSB) repair, implicated in maintaining genomic stability, (eg, Wu et al, 2006); these genes have also been evaluated in relation to bladder cancer risk with promising but unconfirmed findings.

Assays that measure the capacity to repair DNA after exposure to carcinogens in cultured peripheral lymphocytes have been used as an integrative measure of susceptibility to carcinogenic exposures. Thus, bladder cancer cases have been found to be more susceptible than controls to the effects of benzo(a)pyrene diol epoxide (Schabath et al, 2003), and to have decreased capacity to repair DNA damage induced by 4-aminobiphenyl (Lin et al, 2005). Measures of chromosomal telomere length have also been used as a marker for genetic stability and susceptibility to cancer. There are reports for an association between shorter telomeres and increased bladder cancer risk (Wu et al, 2003; Broberg et al, 2005).

Somatic Events

Tumor markers have been used to distinguish between bladder tumor subtypes with different prognosis and response to treatment. Epidemiological studies are increasingly using such markers to classify bladder tumors into potentially distinct etiological groups. Bladder cancer is caused by the accumulation of genetic and epigenetic alterations in tumor-suppressor genes and oncogenes. Alterations in proteins coded by these genes have been evaluated with regard to prognosis and response to treatment (eg, tumor suppressors p53, Rb, *WAF1/p21*, *p16INK4*, and oncogenes *FGFR3*, *c-erbB-2*, *bcl-2*), as well as other proteins such as telomerase involved in genomic stability and the E-cadherin binding protein. RNA and protein microarray analyses of bladder tumors are now being used to explore expression of a wider range of tumor markers.

Other approaches to characterize tumors include global and gene-specific epigenetic changes and cytogenetic changes. Several studies have proposed that superficial/papillary and invasive tumors proceed along two different, but overlapping, molecular pathways (Knowles, 1998); deletions of chromosome 9 are more commonly found in superficial/papillary tumors. In contrast, *TP53* mutations and loss of heterozygosity on chromosome 17 are more frequent in high-grade carcinomas, flat carcinoma in situ, and muscle-invading tumors. p53 alterations have been proposed to be associated with poor prognosis (Esrig et al, 1994), but overall the evidence is not consistent (Malats et al, 2005). Recent reports have proposed that *FGFR3* mutations are associated with low risk of recurrence of superficial tumors.

RISK FACTORS

Tobacco

Cigarette smoking

Cigarette smoking is the most important cause of bladder cancer, particularly among men. The association between bladder cancer and cigarette smoking has been examined in more than 40 case-control and more than 20 cohort studies (Hartge et al, 1987; Doll et al, 1994; Brennan et al, 2000; IARC, 2004a). Nearly all of them showed excess risks among smokers, on average a twofold risk of bladder cancer in ever smokers compared to nonsmokers. Among smokers of more than 20 cigarettes per day, the relative risk estimates are around 5 in studies in Europe but tend to be lower in studies in North America.

The effect of smoking appears to be similar among men and women (Puente et al, 2006) although a higher level of ABP (aminobiphenyl) haemoglobin adducts were found in women compared to men who smoked a similar amount of cigarettes (Castelao et al, 2001). Differences in tobacco smoking–bladder cancer risk gradients among ethnic groups are compatible

Table 22–1. Case-control studies examining the risk of bladder cancer tobacco in persons smoking black tobacco (air-cured) or blond tobacco (flue-cured)

Reference	Relative Risk (95% CI)	Comments
Vineis et al. (1984), Italy	1.8 (0.8–4.2)	Blond tobacco smokers vs. nonsmokers
	4.0 (2.2–7.3)	Black tobacco smokers vs. nonsmokers
Iscovich et al. (1987), Argentina	2 to 3	Black vs. blond tobacco smokers; exact value not provided.
Clavel et al. (1989), France	1.9 (1.2–2.9)	Blond tobacco smokers vs. nonsmokers
	4.4 (2.3–8.3)	Black tobacco smokers vs. nonsmokers
D'Avanzo et al. (1990), Italy	2.7 (1.8–4.0)	Blond tobacco smokers vs. nonsmokers
	3.8 (2.0–7.4)	Black tobacco smokers vs. nonsmokers
De Stefani et al. (1991), Uruguay	2.7 (1.3–5.4)	Black vs. blond tobacco smokers
Momas et al. (1994), France	1.6 (0.7–3.6)	Black vs. blond tobacco smokers
Samanic et al. (2006), Spain	5.8 (3.4–10.0)	Blond vs. never smokers
	7.3 (4.9–10.9)	Black vs. never smokers

CI, confidence interval

with chance variation. There is considerable variation among studies in the risk gradient with number of cigarettes smoked daily, which may be due to different study designs, different ways of smoking, or different types of tobacco smoked (IARC, 2004a).

The risk of bladder cancer increases with both the number of years of smoking and the average number of cigarettes a person has smoked (Doll et al, 1994; Brennan et al, 2000). The excess risk may, however, level off at high tobacco-consumption levels. In a pooled analysis the risk of bladder cancer for those who smoked 15 to 19 cigarettes per day was similar to the risk of those who smoked more than 20 per day (Brennan et al, 2000). The levelling off in the exposure–response pattern may be interpreted as an effect of measurement error if heavy smokers tend to underestimate their consumption, or could reflect the interaction between genes and the environment or saturation of enzymes (Vineis et al, 2000).

The age at which a person starts smoking may affect the risk of bladder cancer. A higher risk among smokers starting before age 20 compared to those starting after age 20 has been found by some investigators. However, duration of smoking, age at start, and age at stopping smoking are strongly correlated variables and few studies have

tried to disentangle them. Former smokers are at lower risk than current smokers. Following cessation of smoking, the relative risk of bladder cancer has, in most studies, been found to fall by 20% to 30% within the first 5 years. In long-term ex-smokers, however, 20 years after quitting the risk seems to remain higher than in never smokers (IARC, 2004a; Brennan et al, 2000).

Blond tobacco (flue-cured) is the standard tobacco type in northern Europe and North America, while in southern Europe and South America black tobacco (air-cured) is still widely consumed. Studies comparing the two types of tobacco have found an approximately twofold risk associated with black tobacco compared to blond tobacco (Table 22–1). The smoke condensate from black tobacco contains a higher concentration of aromatic amines such as 4-aminobiphenyl, b-naphthylamine, and o-toluidine than the smoke condensate from blond tobacco. Levels of 4-aminobiphenyl haemoglobin adducts have been found to be approximately twice as high in smokers of black compared to smokers of blond tobacco with the same amount of smoking. Moreover, black tobacco smokers have been found to excrete a 1.8-fold higher level of urinary mutagens than blond tobacco smokers (Malaveille et al, 1989).

Smoking unfiltered cigarettes may be associated with a 30% to 50% increase in the risk of bladder cancer as compared to the risk of subjects who smoke only filtered cigarettes; a similar pattern is observed for subjects who inhale into the throat as compared to those who do not inhale deeply (IARC, 2004a; Hartge et al, 1987; Samanic et al, 2006).

Most studies examining exposure to environmental tobacco smoke (ETS) in relation to bladder cancer have not found an increasing risk with number of years of ETS exposure.

Pipes, cigars, and other forms of smoking
The epidemiologic data on pipe, cigar, and other forms of smoking in relation to bladder cancer is more equivocal (IARC, 2004a; Shapiro et al, 2000). In general, the data support a small excess risk of bladder cancer among heavy pipe and heavy cigar smokers. The few reports on other forms of smoking such as snuff and chewing tobacco are mostly negative, but the relative risk estimates were based on small numbers of exposed cases and controls.

The effect of tobacco on bladder cancer risk may be mediated through its effect on urine mutagenicity. Increased concentrations of mutagens in the urine have been observed in smokers compared to nonsmokers and in smokers of black tobacco compared to those of blond tobacco or nonsmokers. Higher levels of smoking-related DNA adducts have been detected in bladder tissues among smokers compared to nonsmokers (IARC, 2004a).

Diet

Except for the relatively consistent finding of a protective effect of fruits and vegetables, there is little evidence for an association of other foods with bladder cancer risk.

Fruits, fruit juices, and vegetables such as carrots, cruciferous vegetables, and dark-green vegetables have, in numerous studies, appeared to protect against bladder cancer. In a meta-analysis (Steinmaus et al, 2000), increased risk of bladder cancer was found for diets low in fruit intake (RR = 1.4,

95% CI 1.1–1.8), or low in vegetable intake (RR = 1.2, 95% Cl 1.0–1.3). In one cohort study, the strongest effect was seen for cruciferous vegetables (Michaud et al, 1999b). With respect to specific micronutrients some studies seem to support that supplemental or dietary intake of vitamin A, vitamin C, and dietary intake of folate and carotenoids are protective against this cancer (Knekt et al, 1990; Michaud et al, 1999b); but, overall, results are inconsistent (Zeegers et al, 2001a; Steinmaus et al, 2000). An inverse association with long-term intake of vitamin E has been observed in some studies. A moderate inverse association with selenium intake has also been observed in several studies, including large cohort studies, but results are not entirely consistent (Brinkman et al, 2006).

An increased risk of bladder cancer with increased consumption of meat or even poultry and fish has been reported, but the overall evidence is inconclusive (Steinmaus et al, 2000). Diets low in fat may be associated with a decreased risk (Steinmaus et al, 2000). There is no converging evidence to support or refute a role for dairy products, other major food groups, specific macronutrients (lipids, proteins, carbohydrates), or total energy intake. Cooking may modify the effect of some dietary items. In particular, heterocyclic amines, potent mutagenic and carcinogenic agents in animals, are formed mainly through grilling or frying of meat. The International Agency for Research on Cancer (IARC) has classified one heterocyclic amine (IQ) as a probable human carcinogen and several others (MeIQ, MeIQx, PhIP) as possible carcinogens (IARC, 1993). While two studies found a twofold increased risk of bladder cancer among subjects with high consumption of fried foods or fried/grilled meat or fish, another found no significant excess risk in subjects with the highest intake of heterocyclic amines compared to those with the lowest (Augustsson et al, 1999). A population-based study in Sweden did not find an increased risk for dietary exposure to acrylamide (Mucci et al, 2003).

A role for dietary factors in the etiology of bladder cancer is plausible. First, fruits and vegetables have been consistently associated with a protective effect for bladder cancer similar to several other cancers. Second, people who consume large amounts of cooked meats, and thus heterocyclic amines, have higher levels of urinary mutagens. Third, flavonoids, associated with dietary intake of foods such as onions, lettuce, apples, and red wine, inhibit the bacterial mutagenicity of aromatic and heterocyclic amines in vitro (Malaveille et al, 1998). Finally, urine acidity, which is altered by dietary factors, has been shown in experimental studies to influence the metabolism of carcinogens in the urine and the formation of DNA adducts. An acidic urine results from high consumption of cheese and meat products, whereas alkaline urine is associated with consumption of fruits and vegetables.

Coffee and tea

Since the first reports in 1971 of an increased risk of bladder cancer from coffee consumption, numerous studies have examined this association. Although the results vary across studies, the data as a whole suggest a weak positive association between coffee consumption and bladder cancer. An IARC working group (1991) concluded that coffee is possibly carcinogenic to the human urinary bladder. Exposure–response relationships for both duration and amount of coffee consumed have been found, with the highest risk often observed among subjects with the heaviest consumption.

The confounding effect of cigarette smoking, a habit closely related to coffee consumption in some settings, introduces one of the major difficulties in the evaluation of coffee consumption as an independent risk factor for bladder cancer. Residual confounding may bias the results even when adjustment for smoking is done. To avoid such confounding, coffee consumption has been examined among nonsmokers. Most of the data support an elevated risk of bladder cancer among heavy coffee drinkers (Sala et al, 2000; Zeegers et al, 2001b).

The same IARC working group (1991) evaluated the association between tea consumption and the risk of bladder cancer and considered the evidence inadequate; most of the reviewed cohort and case-control studies had found either no or an inverse association. Studies published since that evaluation (Michaud et al, 1999a) and a meta-analysis (Zeegers et al, 2001b) do not support an association between tea consumption and bladder cancer. Animal studies have shown that compounds in tea may have inhibitory effects on bladder tumor growth possibly due to antioxidative and antiproliferative effects of polyphenol compounds present in green tea, but also found in black teas.

Total fluid intake

Prolonged exposure of the bladder urothelium to carcinogens in the urine has been suggested to affect the development of bladder cancer and perhaps also to influence the site distribution of tumors within the bladder. In an attempt to test this hypothesis, epidemiologic studies have evaluated the risk of bladder cancer in relation to quantity of fluid intake.

Contrary to expectations, many epidemiologic studies have found a slight excess risk in subjects with high total fluid intake, although the results have not been consistent (Moller-Jensen et al, 1986; Michaud et al, 1999a; Geoffroy-Perez and Cordier, 2001). The strongest evidence of a protective effect comes from the Health Professionals follow-up study. In this large cohort of US men, a 240 ml increase in total fluid intake decreased the risk significantly by 7% after adjusting for types of beverages (Michaud et al, 1999a). Subjects consuming more than 2531 ml/day of total fluids had a 49% lower risk than those drinking less than 1290 ml/day. A pooled analysis of six case-control studies of bladder cancer found an increased risk with intake of tap water while no increased risk was observed for the same intake of nontap water (Villanueva et al, 2006).

High fluid intake could reduce the contact of carcinogens with the urothelium by diluting the urine or increasing the frequency of urination, whereas there are no plausible biological hypotheses explaining how high total fluid intake could increase the risk. The positive associations in some studies may be attributed to the types of fluid consumed, such as coffee or tap water, which may contain carcinogenic constituents. Findings may vary between studies also due to differences in the definition of total fluid intake.

Sweeteners

Saccharin, a nonnutritive sweetener, is absorbed slowly, remains unmetabolized, and is excreted through the kidneys. In experimental studies, bladder cancer incidence is higher in rats exposed to high doses of saccharin in utero and during weaning (Schoenig et al, 1985). While one epidemiologic study found an excess risk in men consuming artificial sweeteners (saccharin and cyclamate), the results of most subsequent studies did not support this association (Elcock and Morgan, 1993).

Alcohol

Epidemiologic evidence has, on the whole, not supported a role for alcohol in the etiology of bladder cancer (IARC, 1988). A meta-analysis of case-control and cohort studies found that alcohol consumption slightly increases bladder cancer risk in men (OR 1.35, 95% CI 0.96–1.9) but not in women. Furthermore, no statistically significant dose-response trends were identified (Zeegers et al, 2001c). Results for specific alcoholic beverages and bladder cancer risk are inconsistent.

Reproductive Factors and Hormones

The difference in incidence between men and women seen in most countries, although not in some African countries, led to the hypothesis that hormonal factors play a role in the occurrence of bladder cancer (Hartge et al, 1990). Only indirect epidemiologic evidence and limited experimental data support this hypothesis. Some epidemiologic studies found an inverse association of parity with bladder cancer.

Anthropometric Measures

Anthropometric measures have not been evaluated in relation to bladder cancer in humans. Obesity has mainly been evaluated in relation to prognosis, with overweight patients having worse prognosis and more perioperative complications.

Infections

Inflammation of the bladder, by either infections or stones, may affect the development of cancer in the bladder. The evidence is strongest for squamous cell carcinoma in relation to infection by *S. Haematobium-bilharziasis* (see "Nontransitional Cell Carcinomas").

A positive relationship between cystitis or nonspecific infections of the urinary tract and bladder cancer risk has been consistently reported, including reports from patients with spinal cord injury. Possible mechanisms include increased absorption of carcinogenic substances, chronic inflammation, and the role of bacteria in the endocystic formation of N-nitroso compounds. The varying results point to the difficulties in studying this association because early symptoms of bladder cancer are similar to those of cystitis. Also, patients may recall urinary conditions better than controls.

The prevalence of human papillomavirus (HPV) in bladder cancer biopsy specimens is around 5% or less (Gillison and Shah, 2003), indicating that HPV is not a major factor in the aetiology of the disease. There is some evidence linking HPV with the occurrence of bladder cancer caused by *S. haematobium* (Yang et al, 2005). An excess risk in subjects reporting condylomata acuminata (produced by noncarcinogenic HPV types) has been reported. Recent studies have associated Polyomaviruses (BKV and JCV) infection with bladder cancer (Weinreb et al, 2006).

Physical Activity

There is limited evidence on the association of physical activity with bladder cancer risk.

Ionizing Radiation

Convincing evidence for a link between bladder cancer and exposure to ionizing radiation originates from studies of medically exposed subjects, of atomic bomb

Table 22–2. Occupational carcinogens, occupations and industries that have been associated with bladder cancer, classified by the strength of the evidence. Included are definite (Group 1) and probable (Group 2A), as well as selected possible carcinogens (2B) as classified by IARC (adapted from Siemiatycki et al, 2004)

Strong evidence

- Aluminium production;
- 4-aminobiphenyl;
- Auramine manufacture;
- Benzidine;
- Coal gasification;
- Magenta manufacture;
- 2-napththylamine;
- Rubber industry

Suggestive evidence

- Benz[a]anthracene;
- Benzidine-based dyes;
- Benzo[a]pyrene;
- Boot and shoe manufacture and repair;
- 4-chloro-ortho-toluidine;
- Coal tars and pitches;
- Coke production;
- Dibenz[a,h]anthracene;
- Diesel engine exhaust;
- Dry cleaning (Group 2B)
- Hairdressers and barbers;
- 4,4′methylene bis(2-chloroaniline);
- Mineral oils, untreated and mildly treated;
- Ortho-toluidine;
- Painters;
- Petroleum refining
- Printing processes (Group 2B)
- Tetrachloroethylene
- Textile manufacturing industry (Group 2B)

survivors, and of occupational groups. X-ray treatment for patients with ankylosing spondylitis substantially increased mortality from various neoplasms including bladder cancer (Weiss et al, 1994). The risk of bladder cancer was increased fourfold in women receiving radiotherapy for benign gynocologic conditions (Boice et al, 1988). An excess risk was also observed among atomic bomb survivors, workers of nuclear installations, and participants in the UK nuclear weapon testing programs conducted in Australia and the Pacific Ocean (McGeoghegan and Binks, 2000).

Occupation

After smoking, specific occupational exposures have been jointly identified as the second most important risk factor category for bladder cancer in both men and women. Studies in the 1980s and 1990s suggest that certain high-risk occupations may be responsible for 4% to 10% of bladder cancer cases in men (Kogevinas et al, 2003) and a lower percentage in women (Mannetje et al, 1999). Aromatic amines, PAHs, and diesel engine exhaust are the exposures most consistently found to increase the risk. The occupational exposures classified by the IARC as being associated with a higher risk of bladder cancer are listed in Table 22–2.

Among blue-collar workers, the occupations linked most consistently with bladder cancer are those of painter, machinist, mechanic, work in the metal industry such as sheet metal work and blacksmithing, work in the textile industry, leather work and shoemaking, hairdressing, dry cleaning, and transport work. These occupational relationships reflect, in part, past exposure to chemicals not currently used, such as benzidine or b-naphthylamine, but also more current exposures, possibly to aromatic amines, PAHs, cutting oils, and solvents. Various studies have also observed excess risks in white-collar occupations such as sales workers, even after adjusting for potential confounding variables, an observation compatible with the socioeconomic pattern of this disease. These excess risks are difficult to attribute directly to exposures in the workplace and may be more likely related to general lifestyle factors.

An open question is whether occupational exposures in industries identified in the past as high risk can still be linked to an excess risk of bladder cancer. In a pooled analysis (Kogevinas et al, 2003), attributable risks were higher for subjects first employed in a high-risk occupation before the 1950s than for those employed later. The attributable risk was also related to age, with higher estimates for people younger than 50 years.

Aromatic amines

The first large occupational epidemiology study directly examining aromatic amines was conducted among dyestuff manufacturing workers in the United Kingdom in 1954 (Case et al, 1993). Exposure to b-naphthylamine entailed a 90-fold and to benzidine a 14-fold excess risk of bladder cancer. Numerous other studies of dyestuff manufacture workers confirmed these findings (Vineis and Pirastu, 1997) and provided analyses of the exposure–response patterns for these chemicals. Among workers manufacturing aromatic amines, including b-naphthylamine, benzidine, 4-aminobiphenyl, and 4-o-toluidine, relative risks ranging from 6 to 70 have been found. Findings for users of dyes are less consistent (IARC, 1994a).

An excess risk of bladder cancer identified in the rubber industry in the early 1950s was associated with the use of an antioxidant containing b-naphthylamine (Veys, 2004). The withdrawal of this compound in the rubber industry led to a reduction of bladder cancer risk among rubber workers, although an excess risk in the order of 50% appears to persist (Kogevinas et al, 1998).

Aromatic amines are present in lower quantities in many other occupations including aluminium production, hairdressing, painting, printing, and shoemaking. The extent to which these compounds contribute to the excess risk of bladder cancer observed in these occupations has not been adequately examined.

Polyaromatic hydrocarbons and diesel engine exhaust

Heavy exposure to PAHs, particularly from coal tars and pitches, and to diesel exhaust entails a moderately increased risk of bladder cancer (Boffetta and Silverman, 2001), although the evidence is not entirely consistent. Exposure to PAH is high for workers in several industries such as the potrooms in aluminium production, coal gasification, roofing, road paving, and the transport industry. Many case-control studies provided evidence of excess risk among transport workers exposed to engine exhausts including diesel exhausts (Silverman et al, 1986). Cohort studies among workers exposed to diesel engine exhaust, such as taxi and truck drivers and operators of heavy equipment, however, have not confirmed a positive relationship between exposure to PAHs or diesel exhausts and bladder cancer risk.

Metal workers are exposed to a heterogeneous group of potential carcinogens including cuttings oils—a category including numerous agents—PAHs, metal fumes, and dusts, as well as combustion gases and vapors. In European Union countries, metal workers appear to be the largest occupational group associated with increased bladder cancer risk (Kogevinas et al, 2003). An excess risk associated with metal working, although only moderately high, is among the most consistent epidemiologic findings. An elevated risk of bladder cancer has frequently been found among aluminium smelter workers, blacksmiths, foundry workers, furnace operators, machinists, welders, and others (Silverman et al, 1990; Gaertner et al, 2004).

Less consistent are the findings for persons in numerous other occupations such as construction worker, electrical fitter, engine driver, food processor and preserver, garage worker, plumber and welder, railway worker, slaughterer and meat processor, cook, and waiter.

Hair dyes

Epidemiologic studies have examined bladder cancer risk in hairdressers, barbers, and users of hair dyes. The IARC (1994a) evaluated hairdressing and barbering as occupations entailing exposures that are probably carcinogenic to humans; personal use of hair colorants could not be evaluated in terms of its carcinogenicity. The prevalence of use of hair dyes is high among women in industrialized countries with more than a third of women above age 18 applying hair dyes in Europe and the US (IARC 1994a). Consumers use all major types of hair colorants, which may contain aromatic amines, nitro-substituted aromatic amines, high molecular weight complexes, metal salts, and other chemicals. A recent exposure study identified small amounts of the bladder carcinogen 4-aminobiphenyl (4-ABP), an aromatic amine, in 8 out of the 11 hair dyes tested (Turesky et al, 2003). Although an excess risk has been seen in some studies that included information on personal use of permanent hair dyes and bladder cancer risk (Gago-Dominguez et al, 2001), the overall results are not converging (Hartge et al, 1982; Henley and Thun, 2001; Kogevinas et al, 2006). A recent meta-analysis yielded a pooled relative risk of 1.01 (Takkouche et al, 2005)

Medical Conditions and Treatment

Medical conditions

Urinary tract stones and cancer of the renal pelvis are medical conditions associated with an increased risk of bladder cancer.

Urinary tract stones may cause chronic irritation and infection or they may be markers of an underlying chronic infection. The strongest evidence for an association with bladder cancer comes from a Swedish population-based cohort of 61 144 patients hospitalized for kidney or ureter stones followed for up to 25 years (Chow et al, 1997). A significantly increased risk of bladder cancer was observed, higher among women than among men and higher among patients with than without a diagnosis of urinary tract infection. The evidence from case-control studies is inconsistent; some studies found an approximately twofold risk, one found an excess risk only in women, and three found no association.

Several studies of patients with cancer of the renal pelvis have found increased relative risks, ranging from 3 to 40, of a second primary bladder cancer. In one study (McCredie et al, 1996), about half of the second primary tumors were detected within 2 months, and the excess risk decreased with time since the initial tumor diagnosis. This pattern is indicative of a shared etiology of the tumors (eg, tobacco smoking or use of phenacetin). Moreover, the initial increase and subsequent decrease in bladder cancer risk over time could reflect increased medical surveillance shortly after diagnosis of

a first tumor or a concomitant decrease in exposure to specific risk factors such as smoking.

An excess risk of bladder cancer has also been reported among patients with cancers of the prostate, renal parenchyma, testis, and skin (nonmelanocytic). There are no identified common risk factors between these neoplasms and bladder cancer, except perhaps of smoking for renal cancer, and the excess occurrence of second cancers may be related to treatment, diagnostic surveillance, or other yet unidentified influences. Studies of diabetics in various countries have found no excess risk of bladder cancer. Patients with Wagener's granulomatosis may have an increased bladder cancer risk irrespective of their treatment with cyclophosphamide (Knight et al, 2004).

Medication

Analgesics and anti-inflammatory drugs, cyclophosphamide, and barbiturates are the main medications associated with an increased or, in the case of barbiturates and NSAIDS, decreased risk for bladder cancer.

Analgesics. Heavy use of phenacetin provokes chronic interstitial nephropathy. Therefore, this widely used analgesic has been gradually withdrawn from the market. Since the 1960s, a number of reports have associated use of phenacetin with tumors of the renal pelvis, the ureter, and, later, the urinary bladder, with a two- to sixfold increased risk in abusers of drugs containing phenacetin (Piper et al, 1985). Since the withdrawal of phenacetin, the sale of paracetamol (acetaminophen), an aromatic amine metabolite of phenacetin, has increased. Evaluations have associated paracetamol with, at most, a small, nonsignificant excess risk of bladder cancer in heavy users (Derby and Jick, 1996; Fortuny et al, 2006). However, use of paracetamol has become widespread only recently, so possible long-term effects on cancer risk may not yet be possible to document. Aspirin and other NSAIDs have been associated with reduced risks of several cancers, mainly of the gastrointestinal tract. The effect of

NSAIDs on bladder cancer has been less studied. Some studies found an inverse association but, overall, results are inconclusive (Fortuny et al, 2006).

Cyclophosphamide. Cyclophosphamide is mainly used, as a single drug or in combination, for treatment of non-Hodgkin's lymphoma, other neoplasias, and some nonneoplastic diseases (Knight et al, 2004); it is estimated to be prescribed to about half a million patients annually worldwide. Clinical studies have revealed a high risk of bladder cancer in patients treated with cyclophosphamide; among those with non-Hodgkin's lymphoma, the cumulative risk was 10.7% at 12 years of follow-up (Pedersen-Bjergaard et al, 1988) and the risk may be higher with longer follow-up. It is not known which of the three major DNA-binding metabolites of cyclophosphamide produces the carcinogenic effect.

Barbiturates. In two cohort studies of patients prescribed anticonvulsants (phenobarbital, phenytoin, and others) for the treatment of epilepsy, the risk of bladder cancer was lower than expected (Olsen et al, 1989). The hypothesis that treatment interacts negatively with smoking has received some epidemiologic support. Moreover, experimental studies indicate that phenobarbital induces drug-metabolizing enzymes in the liver and may deactivate bladder carcinogens such as 4-aminobiphenyl, found in tobacco smoke.

Other drugs. Chlornaphazine, an antineoplastic drug no longer used, has occasionally been associated with an excess risk of bladder cancer, as have the tuberculosis drug isoniazid and some laxatives.

Other Risk Factors

Contaminants in drinking water

Chlorination by-products in drinking water have been associated with bladder cancer risk in some well-conducted epidemiologic studies (see following). Arsenic contamination of water is a localized problem. IARC

(2004b) classified the evidence that arsenic in drinking water causes cancer of the urinary bladder as sufficient.

Chlorination by-products. Chlorination of drinking water is used in most industrialized countries for disinfection. During chlorination, chlorine reacts with organic matter in water to produce a mixture of by-products, including trihalomethanes and numerous other compounds. The levels of these compounds depend mainly on the amount of chlorine added and the water source. Trihalomethanes are mutagenic to bacteria, and some are carcinogenic to animals. Epidemiologic studies have used trihalomethanes as indicators of the level of chlorination by-products. However, other compounds such as the MX (3-chloro-4-(dichloromethyl)-5-hydroxy-2(5H)-furanone), iodomethanes (produced during chloramination), or halonitromethanes may contribute to the toxicity of drinking water to a larger extent than trihalomethanes.

The early epidemiological evidence was inadequate to classify chlorinated drinking water as a human carcinogen. One of the main problems was the limitations of the epidemiologic studies in assessing exposure to chlorination by-products. Since then, several studies have examined long-term exposure to chlorination by-products by combining residents' information from questionnaires with information from water utilities. Positive associations between bladder cancer and chlorinated drinking water have been reported (Cantor et al, 1987). A study examining ozoniation, an alternative to chlorination, found a decreased risk in subjects administered ozonated water compared to those using chlorinated water (Chevrier et al, 2004). A pooled analysis of case-control studies identified a 50% increased risk among subjects with long-term exposure to disinfection by-products at levels around 50 micrograms/L, which are levels currently observed in many industrialized countries (Villanueva et al, 2004).

Exposure to chlorinated by-products in water through inhalation and dermal absorption contribute to the total exposure to trihalomethanes more than exposure through ingestion. Only one epidemiological study has examined these routes of exposure and identified increased risks for exposure in showers and baths and for swimming in pools (Villanueva et al, 2007).

Arsenic and other contaminants. The evidence linking arsenic to bladder cancer comes mainly from studies of drinking water. Additional evidence is found in small follow-up studies of patients treated with Fowler's solution (potassium arsenite), in subjects with arsenic poisoning in Japan, and in studies of occupationally exposed subjects (Cantor, 1997).

Studies have been conducted in areas with high levels of arsenic in drinking water in Cordoba, Argentina, and in northern Chile. Average exposure to arsenic varied, and in some of those areas it was reported to be as high as 870 mg/1. Excess bladder cancer mortality was identified in both countries in the high-exposure areas compared to the low-exposure areas (Hopenhayn-Rich et al, 1996; Smith et al, 1998).

A series of studies were conducted in the blackfoot disease–endemic area in a Taiwanese population highly exposed to arsenic through consumption of artesian well water, with arsenic concentration ranging from 350 to 1100 mg/1. The typical content of arsenic in unpolluted surface and ground waters are in the range of 1 to 10 mg/1. Excess risks of bladder cancer—and other cancers—have been consistently found in both genders, with an exposure–response relationship by years of consumption and by level of arsenic in well water (Chiou et al, 2001). A progressive decrease in bladder cancer mortality was observed in a high arsenic-exposure area in southwestern Taiwan after the installation of a tap-water supply system. No studies are available for Bangladesh, which has some of the most exposed populations worldwide.

The excess incidence of bladder cancer in New England, United States, has been attributed, in part, to high arsenic content of well water (Karagas et al, 2004). Overall, however, findings from studies in Europe and the United States, conducted in areas with relatively low levels of arsenic, are not consistent. Arsenic does not directly damage DNA, and several other mechanisms for its carcinogenicity have been proposed (IARC, 2004b), including the inhibition of DNA repair mechanisms and a high arsenic-methylation ability.

Few ecologic or case-control studies have examined other water contaminants such as nitrates, certain metals (cadmium, nickel), radionucleotides, and tetrachloroethylene in relation to bladder cancer risk, and the epidemiologic evidence for excess risk is limited (Cantor, 1997).

Voiding frequency and Urine pH

Voiding frequency, which affects the retention time of the urine in the bladder, has not been examined in epidemiologic studies. However, experimental evidence has associated low voiding frequency with higher formation of DNA adducts to 4-aminobiphenyl, an aromatic amine (Kadlubar et al, 1991).

Urine acidity has been shown in experimental studies to influence the metabolism of carcinogens and the formation of DNA adducts. Among workers exposed to benzidine (Rothman et al, 1997), low urine pH was associated with higher levels of free urinary benzidine and tenfold higher levels of DNA adducts in urothelial cells. In one case-control study, subjects with acidic urine had higher risk of bladder cancer compared to those with urine pH above 6.0. Furthermore urine acidity was associated with bladder cancer risk mainly among smokers. Hence, urine acidity may act as an effect modifier of the risk conveyed by smoking (Alguacil et al, 2003).

NONTRANSITIONAL CELL CARCINOMAS

In western countries, nontransitional cell carcinomas (NTCCs) of the urinary bladder represent approximately 6% of all bladder tumors: 3% squamous cell carcinomas, 2% adenocarcinomas, and 1% undifferentiated carcinomas, small-cell carcinomas, and lymphomas. The suggested risk factors for squamous cell carcinoma are schistosomiasis, smoking, and mechanical and chemical irritation, although epidemiologic evidence exists only for *S. haematobium* and smoking.

The vast majority of studies in industrialized countries have not treated separately NTCC of the bladder, mainly because of few subjects. One small study in the United States (Kantor et al, 1988) and a slightly larger, pooled analysis in Europe (Fortuny et al, 1999) identified smoking as an important cause of squamous cell carcinomas. In the European study, current smoking was significantly associated with NTCC, the risk increasing with increasing number of pack-years.

In east African and Middle Eastern countries, squamous cell carcinoma is much more common than in Europe and North America, a pattern associated with a high prevalence of infection with *S. haematobium*. The World Health Organization has estimated that in the early 1990s, approximately two hundred million people were infected by *S. haematobium*, an infection that is endemic in Africa and the eastern Mediterranean. The first case reports, many from the Nile Delta, suggesting a link between *S. haematobium* infection and bladder cancer date back to the early 1900s (IARC, 1994b). In areas with a high prevalence of *S. haematobium* in southern Iraq, more than 50% of all bladder cancers are of the squamous cell type; in northern Iraq, where the infection is less common, this proportion is lower. An ecologic correlation between the prevalence of *S. haematobium* infection and death from bladder cancer has been noted in several African countries (IARC, 1994b).

Based on studies in Africa, the relative risk of NTCC of the bladder among those infected with *S. haematobium* is about fivefold (Vizcaino et al, 1994). According to an Egyptian study, a clinical history of urinary schistosomiasis could explain some 16%

of bladder cancer cases in this population (Bedwani et al, 1998).

CONCLUSION

Bladder cancer is common among men but less frequent in women. Transitional cell carcinoma is the dominant histologic type in industrialized countries, while squamous cell carcinoma is a common histologic form in developing countries with a high prevalence of *S. haematobium*. Tobacco is by far the main cause of bladder cancer, responsible for about one-third to two-thirds of all bladder cancers in different parts of the world. Black, in comparison to blond, tobacco smoking has been associated with a higher risk.

Occupational exposure, particularly to aromatic amines and possibly to PAHs, may play a substantial role in perhaps 10% of bladder cancers. Subjects with mutated N-acetyl transferase gene (*NAT2*) have a lower capacity to detoxify aromatic amines (slow acelylators) and have consistently been shown to have an about 40% increased risk for developing bladder cancer. *NAT2* slow acetylators have a higher relative risk from tobacco smoking than *NAT2* rapid acetylators. Consistent findings have also been found for the *GSTM1* gene that codes for glutathione S-transferase M1, an enzyme involved in detoxification of a range of carcinogens. Subjects with the *GSTM1* null genotype have an increased risk of bladder cancer. Associations between several other variants of metabolising genes and bladder cancer risk are not consistent.

Consumption of fresh fruits and vegetables and increased total fluid intake may be important protective factors in this cancer. Heavy coffee consumption is possibly associated with a modest excess risk, but the evidence is inconclusive. There is clear evidence that artificial sweeteners are not associated with an excess risk.

With regard to specific medications, both the suggested decreased risk with barbiturates, certain analgesics, and anti-inflammatory drugs, and the detrimental role of other analgesics, in particular acetaminophen, await confirmation. Cyclophosphamide, most commonly used as an anticancer agent, has been associated with an increased risk. An infectious aetiology of bladder cancer is suggested by the excess risk associated with cystitis, with nonspecific urinary tract infections, and with *S. haematobium*. Finally, some studies suggest that chlorinated by-products in water and arsenic in drinking water could increase the risk of bladder cancer.

REFERENCES

Alguacil J, Kogevinas M, Silverman D, Fortuny J, Rivas M, Malats N, García-Closas M, Tardon A, García-Closas R, Carrato A, Serra C, Real FX, Dosemeci M, Rothman N. Urine pH and bladder cancer risk in the Spanish Bladder Cancer Study. AACR special conference on Molecular and Genetic Epidemiology. Proceedings of the molecular and genetic epidemiology of cancer conference B52. Waikota, Hawaii, 2003.

Andrew AS, Nelson HH, Kelsey KT, Moore JH, Meng AC, Casella DP, Tosteson TD, Schned AR, Karagas MR. Concordance of multiple analytical approaches demonstrates a complex relationship between DNA repair gene SNPs, smoking, and bladder cancer susceptibility. Carcinogenesis 2006;27: 1030–37.

Augustsson K, Skog K, Jagerstad M, Dickman PW, Steineck G. Dietary heterocyclic amines and cancer of the colon, rectum, bladder, and kidney: a population-based study. Lancet 1999;353:703–7.

Bedwani R, Renganathan E, El Kwhsky F, Braga C, Abu Seif HH, Abul Azm T, et al. Schistosomiasis and the risk of bladder cancer in Alexandria, Egypt. Br J Cancer 1998;77: 1186–89.

Boffetta P, Silverman DT. A meta-analysis of bladder cancer and diesel exhaust exposure. Epidemiology 2001;12:125–30.

Boice JD Jr, Engholm G, Kleinerman RA, Blettner M, Stovall M, Lisco H, et al. Radiation dose and second cancer risk in patients treated for cancer of the cervix. Radiat Res 1988;116:3–55.

Brennan P, Bogillot O, Cordier S, Greiser E, Schill W, Vineis P, et al. Cigarette smoking and bladder cancer in men: a pooled analysis of 11 case-control studies. Int J Cancer 2000;86:289–94.

Brinkman M, Buntinx F, Muls E, Zeegers MP. Use of selenium in chemoprevention of bladder cancer. Lancet Oncol 2006;7:766–74.

Broberg K, Bjork J, Paulsson K, Hoglund M, Albin M. Constitutional short telomeres are strong genetic susceptibility markers for bladder cancer. Carcinogenesis 2005;26:1263–71.

Cantor KP, Hoover R, Hartge P, Mason TJ, Silverman DT, Altman R, et al. Bladder cancer, drinking water source, and tap water consumption: a case-control study. J Natl Cancer Inst 1987;79:1269–79.

Cantor KP. Drinking water and cancer. Cancer Causes Control 1997;8:292–308.

Carreon T, Ruder AM, Schulte PA, Hayes RB, Rothman N, Waters M, Grant DJ, Boissy R, Bell DA, Kadlubar FF, Hemstreet GP, III, Yin S, LeMasters GK. NAT2 slow acetylation and bladder cancer in workers exposed to benzidine. Int J Cancer 2006;118:161–68

Case RA, Hosker ME, McDonald DB, Pearson JT. Tumours of the urinary bladder in workmen engaged in the manufacture and use of certain dyestuff intermediates in the British chemical industry. Part I. The role of aniline, benzidine, alpha-naphthylamine, and beta-naphthylamine. 1954. Br J Ind Med 1993; 50:389–411.

Castelao JE, Yuan JM, Skipper PL, Tannenbaum SR, Gago-Dominguez M, Crowder JS, Ross RK, Yu MC. Gender- and smoking-related bladder cancer risk. J Natl Cancer Inst 2001; 93:538–45.

Chevrier C, Junod B, Cordier S. Does ozonation of drinking water reduce the risk of bladder cancer? Epidemiology 2004;15:605–14.

Chiou HY, Chiou ST, Hsu YH, Chou YL, Tseng CH, Wei ML, Chen CJ. Incidence of transitional cell carcinoma and arsenic in drinking water: a follow-up study of 8,102 residents in an arseniasis-endemic area in northeastern Taiwan. Am J Epidemiol 2001;153:411–18.

Chow WH, Lindblad P, Gridley G, Nyrén O, McLaughlin JK. Linet MS, et al. Risk of urinary tract cancers following kidney or ureter stones. J Natl Cancer Inst 1997;89:1453–57.

Clavel J, Cordier S, Boccon-Gibod L, Hemon D. Tobacco and bladder cancer in males: increased risk for inhalers and smokers of black tobacco. Int J Cancer 1989;44:605–10.

D'Avanzo B, Negri E, La Vecchia C, Gramenzi A, Bianchi C, Franceschi S, Boyle P. Cigarette smoking and bladder cancer. Eur J Cancer 1990;26:714–18.

Deitz AC, Rothman N, Rebbeck TR, Hayes RB, Chow WH, Zheng W, Hein DW, Garcia-Closas M. Impact of Misclassification in Genotype-Exposure Interaction Studies: Example of N-Acetyltransferase 2 (NAT2), Smoking, and Bladder Cancer. Cancer Epidemiol Biomarkers Prev. 2004;13:1543–46

Derby LE, Jick H. Acetaminophen and renal and bladder cancer. Epidemiology 1996;7:358–62.

De Stefani E, Correa P, Fierro L, Fontham E, Chen V, Zavala D. Black tobacco, mate, and bladder cancer. A case-control study from Uruguay. Cancer 1991;15:536–40.

Doll R, Peto R, Wheatley K, Gray R, Sutherland I. Mortality in relation to smoking: 40 years' observations on male British doctors. Br Med J 1994;309:901–11.

Elcock M, Morgan RW. Update on artificial sweeteners and bladder cancer. Regul Toxicol Pharmacol 1993;17:35–43.

Esrig D, Elmajian D, Groshen S, Freeman JA, Stein JP, Chen SC, et al. Accumulation of nuclear p53 and tumour progression in bladder cancer. N Engl J Med 1994;331:1259–64.

Engel LS, Taioli E, Pfeiffer R, Garcia-Closas M, Marcus PM, Lan Q, Boffetta P, Vineis P, Autrup H, Bell DA, Branch RA, Brockmoller J, Daly AK, Heckbert SR, Kalina I, Kang D, Katoh T, Lafuente A, Lin HJ, Romkes M, Taylor JA, Rothman N. Pooled analysis and meta-analysis of glutathione S-transferase M1 and bladder cancer: a HuGE review. Am J Epidemiol 2002;156:95–109. (Erratum in: Am J Epidemiol 2002;156:492).

Faggiano F, Partanen T, Kogevinas M, Boffetta P. Socioeconomic differences in cancer incidence and mortality. In: Kogevinas M, Pearce N, Susser M, Boffetta P (Eds).: Social Inequalities in Cancer. IARC Sci. Pub. No. 138. Lyon, International Agency for Research on Cancer, 1997, pp 65–176.

Ferlay J, Bray F, Pisani P, Parkin DM. GLOBOCAN 2002: Cancer Incidence, Mortality and Prevalence Worldwide. IARC CancerBase No. 5, version 2.0, IARCPress, Lyon, 2004.

Fletcher O, Easton D, Anderson K, et al: Lifetime risks of common cancers among retinoblastoma survivors. J Natl Cancer Inst 2004;96:357–63.

Fortuny J, Kogevinas M, Chang-Claude J, Gonzalez CA, Hours M, Jockel KH, et al. Tobacco, occupation and non-transitional-cell carcinoma of the bladder: an international case-control study. Int J Cancer 1999; 801:44–46.

Fortuny J, Kogevinas M, Garcia-Closas M, Real FX, Tardon A, Garcia-Closas R et al. Use of analgesics and NSAIDs, genetic predisposition and bladder cancer risk in Spain. Cancer Epidemiol Biomarkers Prev 2006;15:1696–1702.

Gaertner RR, Trpeski L, Johnson KC; Canadian Cancer Registries Epidemiology Research Group. A case-control study of occupational risk factors for bladder cancer in Canada. Cancer Causes Control 2004;15:1007–19.

Gago-Dominguez M, Castelao JE, Yuan JM, Yu MC, Ross RK. Use of permanent hair dyes and bladder cancer risk. Int J Cancer 2001; 91:575–79.

Garcia-Closas M, Malats N, Real FX, Welch R, Kogevinas M, Chatterjee N, Pfeiffer R, Silverman D, Dosemeci M, Tardon A, Serra C, Carrato A, Garcia-Closas R, Castaño-Vinyals G, Chanock S, Yeager M, Rothman N. Genetic variation in the nucleotide excision repair pathway and bladder cancer risk. Cancer Epidemiol Biomarkers Prev 2006; 15:536–42.

Garcia-Closas M, Malats N, Silverman D, Dosemeci M, Kogevinas M, Hein DW, Tardon A, Serra C, Carrato A, Garcia-Closas R, Lloreta J, Castaño-Vinyals G, Yeager M, Welch R, Chanock S, Chatterjee N, Wacholder S, Samanic C, Tora M, Fernandez F, Real FX, Rothman N. NAT2 slow acetylation, GSTM1 null genotype, and risk of bladder cancer: results from the Spanish Bladder Cancer Study and meta-analyses. Lancet 2005;366:649–59.

Geoffroy-Perez B, Cordier S. Fluid consumption and the risk of bladder cancer: results of a multicenter case-control study. Int J Cancer 2001;93:880–87.

Gillison ML, Shah KV. Role of mucosal human papillomavirus in nongenital cancers. J Natl Cancer Inst Monogr 2003;31:57–65.

Gu J, Liang D, Wang Y, Lu C, Wu X. Effects of N-acetyl transferase 1 and 2 polymorphisms on bladder cancer risk in Caucasians. Mutat Res 2005;581:97–104.

Hartge P, Harvey EB, Linehan WM, Silverman DT, Sullivan JW, Hoover RN, et al. Unexplained excess risk of bladder cancer in men. J Natl Cancer Inst 1990;82:1636–40.

Hartge P, Hoover R, Altman R, Austin DF, Cantor KP, Child MA, et al. Use of hair dyes and risk of bladder cancer. Cancer Res 1982;42:4784–87.

Hartge P, Silverman D, Hoover R, Schairer C, Altman R, Austin D, et al. Changing cigarette habits and bladder cancer risk: a case-control study. J Natl Cancer Inst 1987;78: 1119–25.

Hayes JD, Strange RC. Glutathione S-transferase polymorphisms and their biological consequences. Pharmacology 2000;61:154–66.

Hein DW. Molecular genetics and function of NAT1 and NAT2: role in aromatic amine metabolism and carcinogenesis. Mutat Res 2002;506–507:65–77.

Henley SJ, Thun MJ. Use of permanent hair dyes and bladder-cancer risk. Int J Cancer 2001; 94:903–6.

Hopenhayn-Rich C, Biggs ML, Fuchs A, Bergoglio R, Tello EE, Nicolli H, et al. Bladder cancer mortality associated with arsenic in drinking water in Argentina. Epidemiology 1996;7:117–24.

International Agency for Research on Cancer. Alcohol Drinking. IARC Monographs on the Evaluation of Carcinogenic Risks to Humans. Vol. 44. Lyon, IARC, 1988.

International Agency for Research on Cancer. Coffee, Tea, Mate, Methylxanthines and Methylglyoxal. IARC Monographs on the Evaluation of the Carcinogenic Risk of Chemicals to Humans. Vol. 51. Lyon, IARC, 1991.

International Agency for Research on Cancer. Occupational Exposures of Hairdressers and Barbers and Personal Use of Hair Colourants; Some Hair Dyes, Cosmetic Colourants, Industrial Dyestuffs and Aromatic Amines. IARC Monographs on the Evaluation of Carcinogenic Risks to Humans. Vol. 57. Lyon, IARC, 1994a.

International Agency for Research on Cancer. Schistosoma, Liver Flukes and Helicobacter pylori. IARC Monographs on the Evaluation of Carcinogenic Risks to Humans. Vol. 61. Lyon, IARC, 1994b.

International Agency for Research on Cancer. Some Naturally Occuring Substances: Food Items and Constituents, Heterocyclic Aromatic Amines and Mycotoxins. IARC Monographs on the Evaluation of Carcinogenic Risks to Humans. Vol. 56. Lyon, IARC, 1993.

International Agency for Research on Cancer. Some drinking water disinfectants and contaminants, including arsenic. Vol. 84. Lyon: IARC monographs on the evaluation of carcinogenic risks to humans, 2004b.

International Agency for Research on Cancer. Tobacco smoke and involuntary smoking. IARC Monographs on the Evaluation of Carcinogenic Risks to Humans. Vol. 83. Lyon, IARC, 2004a.

Iscovich J, Castelletto R, Esteve J, Munoz N, Colanzi R, Coronel A, et al. Tobacco smoking, occupational exposure and bladder cancer in Argentina. Int J Cancer 1987;40: 734–40.

Kadlubar FF, Dooley KL, Teitel CH, Roberts DW, Benson RW, Butler MA, et al. Frequency of urination and its cffccts on mctabolism, pharmacokinetics, blood haemoglobin adduct formation, and liver and urinary bladder DNA adduct levels in beagle dogs given the carcinogen 4-aminobiphenyl. Cancer Res 1991;51:4371–77.

Kantor AF, Hartge P, Hoover RN, Fraumeni JF Jr. Epidemiological characteristics of squamous cell carcinoma and adenocarcinoma of the bladder. Cancer Res 1988;48:3853–55.

Karagas MR, Tosteson TD, Morris JS, Demidenko E, Mott LA, Heaney J, Schned A. Incidence of transitional cell carcinoma of the bladder and arsenic exposure in New Hampshire. Cancer Causes Control 2004;15: 465–72.

Kiemeney LA, Schoenberg M. Familial transitional cell carcinoma. J Urol 1996;156:867–72.

Knekt P, Aromaa A, Maatela J, Aaran RK, Nikkari T, Hakama M, et al. Serum vitamin A and subsequent risk of cancer: cancer incidence follow-up of the Finnish Mobile Clinic Health Examination Survey. Am J Epidemiol 1990;132:857–70.

Knight A, Askling J, Granath F, Sparen P, Ekbom A. Urinary bladder cancer in Wegener's granulomatosis: risks and relation to cyclophosphamide. Ann Rheum Dis 2004;63: 1307–11.

Knowles MA. Molecular genetics of bladder cancer: pathways of development and progression. Cancer Surv 1998;31:49–76.

Kogevinas M, 't Mannetje A, Cordier S, Ranft U, González CA, Vineis P, Chang-Claude J, Lynge E, Wahrendorf J, Tzonou A, Jöckel KH, Serra C, Porru S, Hours M, Greiser E, Boffetta P. Occupation and bladder cancer among men in Western Europe. Cancer Causes Control 2003;14:907–14.

Kogevinas M, Fernandez F, Garcia-Closas M, Tardon A, Garcia-Closas R, Serra C, Carrato A, Castaño-Vinyals G, Yeager M, Chanock SJ, Lloreta J, Rothman N, Real FX, Dosemeci M, Malats N, Silverman D. Hair dye use is not associated with risk for bladder cancer: Evidence from a case-control study in Spain. Eur J Cancer 2006;42:1448–54.

Kogevinas M, Sala M, Boffetta P, Kazerouni N, Kromhout H, Hoar-Zahm S. Cancer risk in the rubber industry. A review of the recent epidemiological evidence. Occup Environ Med 1998;55:1–12.

La Vecchia C, Airoldi L. Human bladder cancer: epidemiological, pathological and mechanistic aspects. In: Capen CC, Dybing E, Rice JM, Wilbourn JD (Eds): Species Differences in Thyroid and Urinary Bladder Carcinogenesis. IARC Sci. Pub. No. 147. Lyon, International Agency for Research on Cancer, 1999, pp 139–57.

Landi MT, Sinha R, Lang NP, Kadlubar FF. Human cytochrome P4501A2. IARC Sci Publ 1999;173–195.

Lin J, Kadlubar FF, Spitz MR, Zhao H, Wu X. A modified host cell reactivation assay to measure DNA repair capacity for removing 4-aminobiphenyl adducts: a pilot study of bladder cancer. Cancer Epidemiol Biomarkers Prev 2005;14:1832–36.

Malats N, Bustos A, Nascimento CM, Fernandez F, Rivas M, Puente D, Kogevinas M, Real FX. P53 as a prognostic marker for bladder cancer: a meta-analysis and review. Lancet Oncol 2005;6:678–86.

Malaveille C, Hautefeuille A, Pignatelli B, Talaska G, Vineis P, Bartsch H. Antimutagenic dietary phenolics as antigenotoxic substances in urothelium of smokers. Mutat Res 1998; 18:219–24.

Malaveille C, Vineis P, Esteve J, Ohshima H, Brun G, Hautefeuille A, et al. Levels of mutagens in the urine of smokers of black and blond tobacco correlate with their risk of bladder cancer. Carcinogenesis 1989;10: 577–86.

Mannetje A, Kogevinas M, Chang-Claude J, Cordier S, Gónzalez CA, Hours M, et al. Occupation and bladder cancer in European women. Cancer Causes Control 1999;10: 209–17.

Marcus PM, Vineis P, Rothman N. NAT2 slow acetylation and bladder cancer risk: a meta-analysis of 22 case-control studies conducted in the general population. Pharmacogenetics 2000;10:115–22.

McCredie M, Macfarlane GJ, Stewart J, Coates M. Second primary cancers following cancers of the kidney and prostate in New South Wales (Australia), 1972–91. Cancer Causes Control 1996;7:337–44.

McGeoghegan D, Binks K. The mortality and cancer morbidity experience of workers at the Capenhurst uranium enrichment facility 1946–95. J Radiol Prot 2000;20:381–401.

Michaud DS, Spiegelman D, Clinton SK, Rimm EB, Curhan GC, Willett WC, et al. Fluid intake and the risk of bladder cancer in men. N Engl J Med 1999a;340:1390–97.

Michaud DS, Spiegelman D, Clinton SK, Rimm EB, Willett WC, Giovannucci EL. Fruit and vegetable intake and incidence of bladder cancer in a male prospective cohort. J Natl Cancer Inst 1999b;91:605–13.

Moller-Jensen O, Wahrendorf J, Knudsen JB, Sorensen BL. The Copenhagen case–control study of bladder cancer. II. Effect of coffee and other beverages. Int J Cancer 1986;15: 577–82.

Momas I, Daures JP, Festy B, Bontoux J, Gremy F. Bladder cancer and black tobacco cigarette smoking. Some results from a French case-control study. Eur J Epidemiol 1994;10:599–604.

Mucci LA, Dickman PW, Steineck G, Adami HO, Augustsson K. Dietary acrylamide and cancer of the large bowel, kidney, and bladder: absence of an association in a population-based study in Sweden. Br J Cancer. 2003;88:84–89.

Olsen JH, Boice JD Jr, Jensen JP, Fraumeni JF Jr. Cancer among epileptic patients exposed to anticonvulsant drugs. J Natl Cancer Inst 1989;81:803–8.

Pedersen-Bjergaard J, Ersboll J, Hansen VL, Sorensen BL, Christoffersen K, Hou-Jensen K, et al. Carcinoma of the urinary bladder after treatment with cyclophosphamide for non-Hodgkin's lymphoma. N Engl J Med 1988;318:1028–32.

Plna K, Hemminki K. Familial bladder cancer in the national Swedish family cancer database. J Urol 2001;166:2129–33.

Piper JM, Tonascia J, Matanoski GM. Heavy phenacetin use and bladder cancer in women aged 20 to 49 years. N Engl J Med 1985; 313:292–95.

Puente D, Hartge P, Greiser E, Cantor KP, King WD, González CA, Cordier S, Vineis P, Lynge E, Chang-Claude J, Porru S, Tzonou A, Jöckel KH, Serra C, Hours M, Lynch CF, Ranft U, Wahrendorf J, Silverman D, Fernandez F, Boffetta P, Kogevinas M. A pooled analysis of bladder cancer case-control studies evaluating smoking in men and women. Cancer Causes Control 2006;17:71–79.

Rothman N, Talaska G, Hayes RB, Bhatnagar VK, Bell DA, Lakshmi VM, et al. Acidic urine pH is associated with elevated levels of free urinary benzidine and N-acetylbenzidine and urothelial cell DNA adducts in exposed workers. Cancer Epidemiol Biomarkers Prev 1997;6:1039–42.

Sak SC, Barrett JH, Paul AB, Bishop DT, Kiltie AE. The polyAT, intronic IVS11–6 and Lys939Gln XPC polymorphisms are not associated with transitional cell carcinoma of the bladder. Br J Cancer 2005;92:2262–65.

Sala M, Cordier S, Chang-Claude J, Donato F, Escolar-Pujolar A, Fernandez F, et al. Coffee consumption and bladder cancer in non-smokers: a pooled analysis of case-control studies in European countries. Cancer Causes and Control 2000;11:925–31.

Samanic C, Kogevinas M, Dosemeci M, Malats N, Real FX, Garcia-Closas M, Serra C, Carrato A, Garcia-Closas R, Sala M, Lloreta J, Tardon A, Rothman N, Silverman D. Smoking and Bladder Cancer in Spain: Effects of Tobacco Type, Timing, Environmental Tobacco Smoke, and Gender. Cancer Epidemiol Biomarkers Prev 2006;15:1348–54.

Sanyal S, Festa F, Sakano S, Zhang Z, Steineck G, Norming U, Wijkstrom H, Larsson P, Kumar R, Hemminki K. Polymorphisms in DNA repair and metabolic genes in bladder cancer. Carcinogenesis 2004;25:729–34.

Schabath MB, Delclos GL, Grossman B, Wang Y, Lerner SP, Chamberlain RM, Spitz MR, Wu X. Polymorphism in XPD exons 10 and 23 and bladder cancer risk. Cancer Epidemiol Biomarkers Prev 2005;14:878–84.

Schabath MB, Spitz MR, Grossman HB, Zhang K, Dinney CP, Zheng PJ, Wu X. Genetic instability in bladder cancer assessed by the comet assay. J Natl Cancer Inst 2003;95: 540–47.

Schoenig GP, Goldenthal EI, Geil RG, Frith CH, Richter WR, Carlborg FW. Evaluation of the dose response and in utero exposure to saccharin in the rat. Food Chem Toxicol 1985; 23:475–90.

Shapiro JA, Jacobs EJ, Thun MJ. Cigar smoking in men and risk of death from tobacco-related cancers. J Natl Cancer Inst 2000;92: 333–37.

Siemiatycki J, Richardson L, Straif K, et al. Listing occupational carcinogens. Environ Health Perspect 2004;112:1447–59.

Silverman DT, Hoover RN, Mason TJ, Swanson GM. Motor exhaust–related occupations and bladder cancer. Cancer Res 1986;46: 2113–16.

Silverman DT, Levin L, Hoover RN. Occupational risks of bladder cancer among white women in the United States. Am J Epidemiol 1990;132:453–61.

Smith AH, Goycolea M, Haque R, Biggs ML. Marked increase in bladder and lung cancer mortality in a region of northern Chile due to arsenic in drinking water. Am J Epidemiol 1998;147:660–69.

Steinmaus CM, Nunez S, Smith AH. Diet and bladder cancer: a meta-analysis of six dietary variables. Am J Epidemiol 2000;151: 693–702.

Takkouche B, Etminan M, Montes-Martínez A. Personal Use of Hair Dyes and Risk of Cancer. A Meta-analysis. JAMA 2005;293:2516–25

Turesky RJ, Freeman JP, Holland RD, Nestorick DM, Mille DL, Ratnasinghe DL, Kadlubar FF. Identification of 4-aminobiphenyl in commercial hair dyes. Chem Res Toxicol 2003;16:1162–73.

Vatsis KP, Martell KJ, Weber WW. Diverse point mutations in the human gene for polymorphic N-acetyltransferase. Proc Natl Acad Sci USA 1991;88:6333–37

Veys CA. Bladder tumours in rubber workers: a factory study 1946–1995. Occup Med (Lond) 2004;54:322–29.

Villanueva CM, Cantor KP, Cordier S, Jaakkola JJ, King WD, Lynch CF, Porru S,Kogevinas M. Disinfection byproducts and bladder cancer: a pooled analysis. Epidemiology 2004; 15:357–67.

Villanueva CM, Cantor KP, Grimalt JO, Malats N, Silverman D, Tardon A, Garcia-Closas R, Serra C, Carrato A, Castaño-Vinyals G, Marcos R, Rothman N, Real FX, Dosemeci M, Kogevinas M. Bladder cancer and exposure to water disinfection by-products through ingestion, bathing, showering and swimming pool attendance. Am J Epidemiol Am J Epidemiol 2007; 165: 148–56

Villanueva CM, Cantor KP, King WD, Jaakkola JJK, Cordier S, Lynch CF, Porru S, Kogevinas M. Total and specific fluid consumption as determinants of bladder cancer risk. Int J Cancer 2006;118:2040–47.

Vineis P, Estève J, Terracini B. Bladder cancer and smoking in males: types of cigarettes, age at start, effect of stopping and interaction with occupation. Int J Cancer 1984;34:165–70.

Vineis P, Kogevinas M, Simonato L, Bogillot O, Brennan P, Boffetta P. Levelling-of the risk of lung and bladder cancer in heavy smokers: an analysis based on multicentric case-control studies and a metabolic interpretation. Mutat Res 2000;463:103–10.

Vineis P, Marinelli D, Autrup H, Brockmoller J, Cascorbi I, Daly AK, Golka K, Okkels H, Risch A, Rothman N, Sim E, Taioli E. Current smoking, occupation, N-acetyltransferase-2 and bladder cancer: a pooled analysis of genotype-based studies. Cancer Epidemiol Biomarkers Prev 2001;10:1249–52.

Vineis P, Pirastu R. Aromatic amines and cancer. Cancer Causes Control 1997;8:346–55.

Vizcaino AP, Parkin DM, Boffetta P, Skinner ME. Bladder cancer: epidemiology and risk factors in Bulawayo, Zimbabwe. Cancer Causes Control 1994;5:517–22.

Weber WW. The acetylator gene and drug response. Oxford University Press, New York, 1987.

Weber WW, Hein DW, Litwin A, Lower GM, Jr. Relationship of acetylator status to isoniazid toxicity, lupus erythematosus, and bladder cancer. Fed Proc 1983;42:3086–97.

Weinreb DB, Desman GT, Amolat-Apiado MJ, Burstein DE, Godbold JH Jr, Johnson EM. Polyoma virus infection is a prominent risk factor for bladder carcinoma in immuno-competent individuals. Diagn Cytopathol 2006;34:201–3.

Weiss HA, Darby SC, Doll R. Cancer mortality following X-ray treatment for ankylosing spondylitis. Int J Cancer 1994;59:327–38.

Wu X, Amos CI, Zhu Y, Zhao H, Grossman BH, Shay JW, Luo S, Hong WK, Spitz MR. Telomere dysfunction: a potential cancer predisposition factor. J Natl Cancer Inst 2003;95:1211–18.

Wu X, Gu J, Grossman HB, Amos CI, Etzel C, Huang M, Zhang Q, Millikan RE, Lerner S, Dinney CP, Spitz MR. Bladder cancer predisposition: a multigenic approach to DNA-repair and cell-cycle-control genes. Am J Hum Genet 2006;78:464–79.

Yang H, Yang K, Khafagi A, Tang Y, Carey TE, Opipari AW, Lieberman R, Oeth PA,Lancaster W, Klinger HP, Kaseb AO, Metwally A, Khaled H, Kurnit DM. Sensitive detection of human papillomavirus in cervical, head/-neck, and schistosomiasis-associated bladder malignancies. Proc Natl Acad Sci USA 2005; 102:7683–88.

Yu MC, Skipper PL, Taghizadeh K, Tannenbaum SR, Chan KK, Henderson BE, Ross RK.

Acetylator phenotype, aminobiphenyl-hemoglobin adduct levels, and bladder cancer risk in white, black, and Asian men in Los Angeles, California. J Natl Cancer Inst 1994;86:712–16.

Zeegers MP, Goldbohm RA, Brandt PA. Are retinol, vitamin C, vitamin E, folate and carotenoids intake associated with bladder cancer risk? Results from the Netherlands Cohort Study. Br J Cancer 2001a;85:977–83.

Zeegers MP, Tan FE, Goldbohm RA, van den Brandt PA. Are coffee and tea consumption associated with urinary tract cancer risk? A systematic review and meta-analysis. Int J Epidemiol 2001b;30:353–62.

Zeegers MP, Volovics A, Dorant E, Goldbohm RA, van den Brandt PA. Alcohol consumption and bladder cancer risk: results from The Netherlands Cohort Study. Am J Epidemiol 2001c;153:38–41.

23

Kidney Cancer

EUNYOUNG CHO, PER LINDBLAD,
AND HANS-OLOV ADAMI

The malignancy addressed in this chapter was earlier called *hypernephroma* because Grawitz suggested in 1883 that it arises from the adrenal gland (hypernephroid tissue), located adjacent to the kidney. Although this theory was disproved a few years later, the battle about the cancer's origin continued for many years. It is now established that the predominant malignancy of the kidney arises from the epithelium of the renal tubules; hence it is called *renal cell cancer*. We use the term *kidney cancer* in this chapter for convenience, although it covers both renal cell cancer, that is, cancer of the renal parenchyma—and cancer of the renal pelvis. The etiology of the latter resembles that of bladder cancer and is not reviewed here. Neither Wilms' tumor nor nephroblastoma, a malignant kidney tumor of embryonal origin occurring primarily among children are discussed. Only the etiology of renal cell cancer, which represents about 80% to 90% of all malignant kidney tumors in adults, is addressed.

CLINICAL SYNOPSIS

Subgroups

Renal malignancies comprise a heterogeneous class of tumors arising from different cell types within the nephron. Advances in our understanding of the genetics underlying the pathogenesis of renal cell neoplasms have led to a histopathologic classification of tumors of the kidney into five subgroups: conventional (clear cell) renal cell carcinoma, also called nonpapillary (75% to 80%); papillary (chromophilic) renal cell carcinoma (10% to 15%); chromophobe renal cell carcinoma; collecting duct carcinoma; and unclassified renal cell carcinoma.

Symptoms

General symptoms are hematuria (50% to 60% of the patients), abdominal pain (40%), and a palpable abdominal or flank mass (30% to 40%). Common nonspecific symptoms and signs (10% to 40%) are hypertension, weight loss, fever, malaise, night sweats, hypercalcemia, erythrocytosis, thrombocytosis, and hepatic dysfunction.

Diagnosis

Intravenous urography is often used initially for the evaluation of hematuria and function of the contralateral kidney. Additional tools for diagnosis and staging are contrast-enhanced computed tomography (CT), ultrasound, and magnetic resonance imaging. Widespread use of modern high-sensitivity imaging techniques such as CT might entail detection of small tumors with a low malignant potential.

Treatment

Radical or partial nephrectomy is the only curative treatment. Surgery is also used as palliative treatment of metastatic disease, as is radiotherapy. The success of chemotherapy in treating kidney cancer has been poor. Recently, the understanding of novel molecular pathways in angiogenesis have led to new promising targeted therapies.

Prognosis

The clinical course is extremely variable. In patients with apparently localized disease, 50% ultimately develop distant metastases after removal of the primary tumor. Five-year survival rates over all stages are 40% to 50%. With appropriate treatment, the 5-year survival for patients with localized disease (stages I and II) is between 80% and 95%. About one-third of patients have detectable metastatic spread at the time of diagnosis. Disease progression is variable even in metastatic disease.

Progress

There has been only a small, if any, improvement in cure rates over the past decades. Further refinements in the treatment of kidney cancer with immunotherapy, gene-therapy techniques to modify tumor cells, creating tumor vaccines, and anti-angiogenesis modalities are needed.

DESCRIPTIVE EPIDEMIOLOGY

During the late twentieth century, when the burden of cancer began to be better characterized, the incidence of and mortality from renal cell cancer increased in many parts of the world. In 2002, kidney cancer was estimated to afflict about 200 000 individuals worldwide, accounting for 2% of all malignant diseases (Ferlay et al, 2004).

The global variation in incidence is more than tenfold (Figs. 23–1 and 23–2). The rates are highest in northern, western, and eastern Europe, Australia, and North America, intermediate in southern Europe and Japan, and low elsewhere in Asia, Africa, and the Pacific (Figs. 23–3 and 23–4, Table 23–1) (Ferlay et al, 2004). In the United States, incidence rates are somewhat higher among the black than the white population. The estimated numbers of new kidney cancers in 2002 were about 40 000 in North America and 59 000 in the European Union (Ferlay et al, 2004).

The geographic variation has been ascribed to differences in diagnostic intensity and autopsy rates, as well as to environmental factors that are likely to play an important role in renal cell carcinogenesis. The increasing incidence observed in almost all areas of the world can also be explained in part by the increased diagnostic intensity following the introduction of new imaging methods such as ultrasound and CT—although declining autopsy rates may have counteracted this trend. The incidence rates are highest in the sixth and seventh decades (Figs. 23–1 and 23–2). Kidney cancer is more common in men than in women, male-to-female ratios are generally between 1.5:1 and 2.5:1.

Trends in mortality have accurately paralleled trends in incidence, with rises in almost all countries. However, it has recently been shown in some European countries that rates have levelled off (Levi et al, 2004). The estimated worldwide mortality rates were about 100 000 in 2002— that is, 1.5% of all cancer deaths (Ferlay et al, 2004). The age-adjusted rates for men in Europe varied

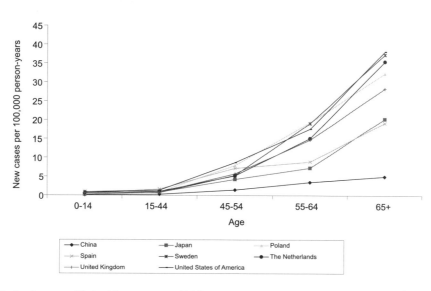

Figure 23–1. Age-specific incidence rates of kidney cancer among women. (*Source*: Ferlay et al, 2004)

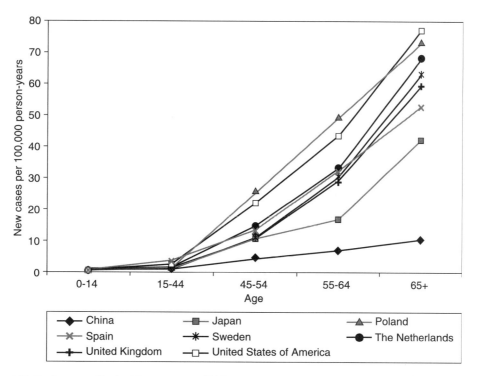

Figure 23–2. Age-specific incidence rates of kidney cancer among men. (*Source*: Ferlay et al, 2004)

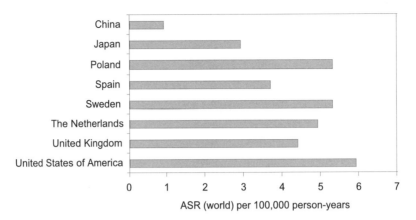

Figure 23–3. Age-standardized (to the world population) incidence rates of kidney cancer among women. (*Source*: Ferlay et al, 2004)

between just over 2 per 100 000 in some southern countries and 10 per 100 000 in some eastern countries. On average they were three to four times higher in more developed than less developed countries (Ferlay et al, 2004). There is a high mortality to incidence ratio for kidney cancer compared to other urologic malignancies.

GENETIC AND MOLECULAR EPIDEMIOLOGY

Inherited Susceptibility

Although most kidney cancers are sporadic, several genetic diseases are associated with kidney cancer, including von Hippel-Lindau

(VHL) syndrome, hereditary papillary renal carcinoma, and Birt-Hogg-Dube syndrome (Kim and Kaelin, 2004). The genes underlying each of these conditions have been cloned, and germline mutations in affected patients have been identified (Table 23–2). Strong correlations have been found between some of these genes involved in the pathogenesis of renal tumors and the histopathological and clinical features.

Von Hippel-Lindau syndrome is a dominantly inherited multisystemic disorder associated with significant morbidity. Patients are at risk of developing tumors in a number of organs: kidneys—often multiple, bilateral tumors—pancreas, adrenal glands,

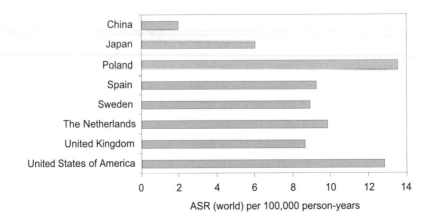

Figure 23–4. Age-standardized (to the world population) incidence rates of kidney cancer among men. (*Source*: Ferlay et al, 2004)

Table 23–1. Range of incidence within some areas in 2002.

Area	ASR (World), per 100,000	
	Men	Women
Northern Europe	8.3–17.3	4.3–8.4
Western Europe	8.2–12.3	4.6–6.8
Eastern Europe	5.1–21.1	2.0–10.2
Southern Europe	5.5–11.5	2.7–5.2
North America		
USA	12.8	5.9
Canada	11.4	5.8
Australia	11.6	6.5

Source: Ferlay et al, 2004.

epididymis, eyes, spine, and cerebellum (Choyke et al, 1995). The cumulative risk of kidney cancer is more than 70% by the age of 60, and renal cell cancer is the most common cause of death (Maher, 1996).

The VHL tumor-suppressor gene, located on chromosome 3p, is involved in both spontaneous and hereditary kidney cancer and is inactivated via several mechanisms, including mutation and silencing by DNA methylation (Kim and Kaelin, 2004). This gene is exclusively involved in the conventional (clear-cell) carcinoma, consistent with the hypothesis that distinct molecular etiologies may exist for different types of kidney cancer. Loss of VHL gene function correlates with increased expression of angiogenetic factors such as vascular endothelial growth factor. Overexpression of endothelial growth factor in vascularized tumors such as kidney cancer may promote its growth and progression (Jacobsen et al,

2004). The VHL tumor-suppressor protein (pVHL) plays a central role also in the mammalian oxygen-sensing pathway through hypoxia-inducible factor (HIF) (Kim and Kaelin, 2004). In the absence of pVHL, HIF induces the expression of several genes that are related to regulation of angiogenesis, cell growth, or cell survival. Other genetic abnormalities associated with kidney cancer progression include loss of heterozygosity of chromosome 14q (Van Poppel et al, 2000).

Hereditary papillary renal cell carcinoma is characterized by, among other things, multifocal and bilateral tumor. This syndrome has an autosomal dominant inheritance pattern, distinct from that of other hereditary kidney cancers. It is caused by a germline mutation of the c-MET proto-oncogene on chromosome 7q or loss-of-function mutations of Fumarate Hydratase gene. Apart from that, there is no loss of alleles of the short arm of chromosome 3 in papillary renal cell carcinoma; trisomies mainly of chromosomes 7, 16, and 17 and, in men, loss of chromosome Y are found. Fumarate Hydratase mutations are also associated with an increased risk of cutaneous leiomyomata and uterine fibroids. Birt-Hogg-Dube (BHD) syndrome, caused by germline loss-of-function mutations of the BHD gene, is characterized by fibrofolliculomas, lung cysts, and a spectrum of renal carcinomas of varying histological subtypes (chromophobe, oncocytoma, clear-cell, or papillary) (Van Poppel et al, 2000; Kim and Kaelin, 2004).

Families with kidney cancer have also been characterized by constitutionally balanced

Table 23–2. Genes predisposing to inherited renal cell carcinoma

Inherited disease			
Hereditary papillary renal cell carcinoma	Papillary (Type I)	c-MET	7q31
Hereditary leiomyomata and renal cell carcinoma	Papillary (Type II)	Fumarate hydratase (FH)	1q42
Birt-Hogg-Dube syndrome	All (esp chromophobe)	BHD	17p11

Source: Kim, 2004.

translocations between chromosomes 3 and 6 or 8 and between chromosomes 2 and 3 (Van Poppel et al, 2000).

Few analytical epidemiologic studies have reported on a family history of kidney cancer. One study found a 60% increased risk, and another a 2.5-fold increased risk of kidney cancer if a first-degree relative was affected with the disease (Schlehofer et al, 1996; Gago-Dominguez et al, 2001), whereas no association was found in a smaller study (Kreiger et al, 1993).

Somatic Events

Somatic mutation of *VHL* gene explains about 50% of sporadic clear-cell kidney cancer and methylation of the gene explains another 10% to 20% of the cancer (Kim and Kaelin, 2004). One report identified a "hotspot" for mutations of the *VHL* gene associated with exposure to trichloroethylene (Brauch et al, 1999). Little information is available on the relationships between *VHL* gene inactivation and major established environmental risk factors in kidney cancer.

RISK FACTORS

Tobacco

While the International Agency for Research on Cancer (IARC) has found "sufficient evidence" for a carcinogenic role of tobacco smoking in cancer of the renal pelvis, the evidence for a causal relation with kidney cancer was not considered sufficient when the evaluation was done in 1986 (IARC Working Group on the Evaluation of the Carcinogenic Risk of Chemicals to Humans, 1986). However, subsequent epidemiologic studies have convincingly demonstrated that cigarette smoking is a cause of renal cell cancer also.

Both case-control (Hu and Ugnat, 2005; Yuan et al, 1998c; McLaughlin et al, 1995b) and cohort studies (Chow et al, 2000; Coughlin et al, 1997; Flaherty et al, 2005; Heath et al, 1997; McLaughlin et al, 1990) have linked kidney cancer to tobacco smoke. Relative risks are generally moder-

ate, but the dose–response relationship reported in both men and women is often strong. This observation, together with the decline in risk following cessation, supports a causal interpretation of the association between cigarette smoking and kidney cancer (Yuan et al, 1998c; McLaughlin et al, 1995b) (Table 23–3). One case-control study reported a positive association with passive smoking also (Hu and Ugnat, 2005). Among studies reporting on tobacco products other than cigarettes, only a few have found an association with smokeless tobacco or a positive association with cigar and pipe smoking (Kreiger et al, 1993, Muscat et al, 1995); one found a significantly increased risk for heavy cigar smoking (Yuan et al, 1998c).

Most of the constituents in cigarette smoke are metabolized or excreted through the urinary tract. It is not clear which constituents are responsible for kidney cancer, but nitroso compounds, especially N-nitrosodimethylamine, found in tobacco smoke, have caused kidney cancer in several animal species (Hamilton, 1975; IARC Working Group on the Evaluation of the Carcinogenic Risk of Chemicals to Humans, 1986). The possible role of nitroso compounds has gained support from a study in which N-nitrosodimethylamine-induced rat clear-cell renal tumors were identified with *VHL* mutations. This was the first experiment that linked *VHL* gene mutations to chemical exposure, thereby providing a possible molecular pathway from tobacco smoking to kidney cancer (Gnarra, 1998; Shiao et al, 1998). A study found gene–environment interaction with N-acetyl transferase 2 (NAT2), an enzyme involved in metabolism of products from tobbaco smoke, and smoking; the association between smoking and kidney cancer was much stronger among slow acetylators of NAT2 (Semenza et al, 2001).

The proportion of kidney cancers that could be attributed to cigarette smoking is between 21% and 30% among men and between 9% and 24% among women (McLaughlin et al, 1995b; McLaughlin et al, 1984; Yuan et al, 1998c), depending on the

Table 23–3. Main result of the two large case-control studies investigating the association between cigarette smoking and kidney cancer

Location publ. year	Number of cases/controls	Risk estimates	Observations	
Australia, Denmark, Germany, Sweden, USA (1995) (McLaughlin et al, 1995b)	1732/2309	Ever: 1.3 Current: 1.4 Former: 1.2 Heavy smokers: 2.1	Trend with intensity: + Decreased risk following cessation: 25% >15 years after quitting	Attributable risk Men: 24% Women: 9%
California, USA 1998 (Yuan et al, 1998c)	1204/1204	Ever: 1.35 Current: 1.53 Former: 1.24 Heavy smokers: 1.90	Trend with intensity: + Decreased risk following cessation: 30% >10 years after quitting	Attributable risk Men: 21% Women: 11%

prevalence of smoking in the population studied.

Diet

Several of the prevailing nutritional hypotheses have been generated from ecologic studies. Positive correlations with kidney cancer were found for per capita consumption of milk, fats, sugar, and meat and, on the nutritional level, of protein, fat, and calories; a negative correlation was found in one study for protein and calories from plant products. Results of analytic, mostly case-control, studies suggest that diet may have a role in the development of kidney cancer, although no link between any specific food item or nutrient and the risk of kidney cancer has yet been established (Wolk et al, 1996b).

Foods

Several analytic epidemiologic studies have shown a positive association with meat, milk and margarine, oils, or butter (Hu et al, 2003). Several case-control studies found a protective effect of vegetables and/or fruits, which is especially strong for dark-green and cruciferous vegetables (Hu et al, 2003; Wolk et al, 1996a; Wolk et al,

1996b; Yuan et al, 1998b). However, prospective data have been sparse and inconclusive (Fraser et al, 1990; Nicodemus et al, 2004; Rashidkhani et al, 2005b; van Dijk et al, 2005; Weikert et al, 2006). In a prospective study from European countries, no associations between fruit and vegetable consumption and kidney cancer risk were observed (Weikert et al, 2006). A weak inverse association was observed for root vegetables only. In another prospective study in the U.S., inverse association was found between fruit and vegetable consumption and kidney cancer in men (Lee JE et al, 2006). Two studies have examined dietary pattern and kidney cancer; one study found an inverse association with the Drinker pattern (Rashidkhani et al, 2005a) and the other study found a positive association with high-fat and high-protein diets (Handa and Kreiger, 2002).

Nutrients

Analyses of specific nutrients and their relation to kidney cancer have linked elevated risks to protein and dietary fat (Chow et al, 1994) and decreased risks to carotenes (Mclure and Willett, 1990; Yuan et al, 1998b), vitamin C (Lindblad et al, 1997;

Yuan et al, 1998b; Hu et al, 2003), and vitamin E (Hu et al, 2003; Lindblad et al, 1997; Nicodemus et al, 2004).

Total energy intake was analyzed in a few studies (van Dijk et al, 2004), and in some a positive association with the risk of kidney cancer was found (Mellemgaard et al, 1996; Wolk et al, 1996a). Adjustment for total energy intake strengthened several of the negative associations between vegetables and antioxidants and the risk of kidney cancer. It is problematic to disentangle the individual effects of protein and fat and the risk of kidney cancer because these energy-driving nutrients are so highly correlated with each other. The question is if the increased risk is confined to total energy intake rather than related to individual energy sources (Wolk et al, 1996a).

Several mechanisms have been suggested to explain how meat and protein might increase the risk of kidney cancer. Possible mediators could be nitrites and nitrates in meat; animal models have produced evidence that nitrosamines can induce renal cell tumors (Hamilton, 1975; Nogueira et al, 1993). Or, the increased risk could be due to heterocyclic amines formed when meat is cooked at high-temperature and long-duration (Friedman, 1991). Experimental models with heterocyclic amines demonstrated DNA adducts in different organs, including the kidney (Munro et al, 1993). The method of cooking and the degree of doneness affected the risk increase in one (Wolk et al, 1996b) but not in another case-control study (Chow et al, 1994). The association of estimated intake of hetero cyclic amines with increased risk of kidney cancer (De Stefani et al, 1998) was not supported by a study using a validated questionnaire to estimate the intake of heterocyclic amines (Augustsson et al, 1999).

Coffee and tea
Neither coffee nor tea drinking has been convincingly associated with kidney cancer despite numerous studies (Wolk et al, 1996b; Yuan et al, 1998b). However, a pooled analysis of 13 prospective studies suggested that coffee and tea consumption

may be associated with a lower risk of kidney cancer (Lee JE et al, 2007a).

Drinking water "contamination"
Carcinogenic and mutagenic compounds found in chlorinated drinking water have raised concern over the potential long-term effect of chlorination (IARC, 1991; Morris, 1995). A cohort study from the United States found no excess rates of kidney cancer in a population supplied with chlorinated surface water compared with a population with deep, unchlorinated wells (Wilkins and Comstock, 1981). However, a Finnish case-control study that used information on past drinking sources and past residence—combined with information from waterworks on the water supply, quality, and treatment practices—found a significant excess risk of kidney cancer among men (Koivusalo et al, 1998). In areas with chronic exposure to arsenic from drinking water, studies from Taiwan (Chen et al, 1992) and Argentina (Hopenhayn-Rich et al, 1998) showed a dose-related association with an increased risk of kidney cancer.

Artificial sweeteners
The possible role of saccharine and other artificial sweeteners has been addressed in five case-control studies. Four of them indicated no association with a kidney cancer risk, while one found a positive association for men (Wolk et al, 1996b).

Alcohol

Although alcohol intake is related to elevated risk of several cancer sites, such as oral cavity, esophagus, and breast, some case-control (Goodman et al, 1986; Hu et al, 2003; Wolk et al, 1996; Parker et al, 2002; Greving et al, 2007) and cohort (Mahabir et al, 2005; Nicodemus et al, 2004; Rashidkhani et al, 2005) studies suggest that alcohol intake is associated with a reduced risk of kidney cancer. Overall, it is quite convincing that alcohol intake does not increase risk of kidney cancer (Lee JE et al, 2007b). Because alcohol consumption enhances insulin sensitivity and is inversely associated with diabetes risk, alcohol may benefit through the pathway (Davies et al, 2002; Facchini et al, 1994).

Reproductive Factors and Hormones

Gender difference in kidney cancer incidence suggest a role of hormonal factors. However, expression of steroid hormone receptors in kidney cancer was not detected or is low (Langner et al, 2004).

Generally, studies have found little evidence that reproductive factors are important in relation to kidney cancer (McLaughlin et al, 1984; Talamini et al, 1990; Wynder et al, 1974; Yu et al, 1986).

Positive associations—albeit weak—have been reported occasionally for oral contraceptives (McLaughlin et al, 1992) and for use of replacement estrogens in some (Asal et al, 1988; McLaughlin et al, 1992; Nicodemus et al, 2004) but not all studies (Adami et al, 1989; McLaughlin et al, 1984). In contrast, a multicenter case-control study (Lindblad et al, 1995) found a significantly reduced risk of kidney cancer following oral contraceptive use among women who did not smoke, with a suggestion of increased reduction with duration of use. Furthermore, some studies have found an increased risk associated with number of births (Chow et al, 1995; Kreiger et al, 1993; Lambe et al, 2002; Lindblad et al, 1995; Nicodemus et al, 2004). Therefore, although the findings of the relatively few investigations dealing with reproductive and hormonal factors remain enigmatic and inconsistent, there is some evidence that certain hormone-related factors are associated with the risk of kidney cancer.

Anthropometric Measures

The most consistent finding in epidemiologic studies of kidney cancer is the excess risk among subjects who are overweight or obese, generally measured as body mass index (BMI) (Wolk et al, 1996b). About 30 mostly case-control studies have investigated the relationship and found an association, with a few exceptions, stronger and more consistent among women; several observed a dose–effect trend. The results of prospective cohort studies are in most instances in agreement with those of the case-control studies (Bergstrom et al, 2001b; Chow et al, 2000; Flaherty et al, 2005; Nicodemus et al, 2004; Tulinius et al, 1997).

A quantitative review of published studies (Bergstrom et al, 2001a) (Fig. 23–5) shows that increased BMI is equally strongly associated with an increased risk of kidney cancer among men and women, in spite of the fact that weight has been measured at different ages in the various studies and in spite of differences in controlling for confounding factors.

Few studies have examined waist circumference or waist-to-hip ratio (WHR) in relation to kidney cancer risk. A cohort study among postmenopausal women found a positive association between WHR and kidney cancer risk independent of maximum weight (Nicodemus et al, 2004). Recently, a European cohort study with 287 kidney cancer cases found that measured waist circumference, hip circumference, and WHR were each related to an elevated risk of kidney cancer in women but not in men (Pischon et al, 2005). However, overall results were much attenuated after adjusting for body weight.

Mellemgaard and colleagues (1995) also evaluated weight changes over time. Positive associations, confined to women, became nonsignificant after simultaneous adjustment for BMI, rate of weight change, and number of weight changes in the analyses. A separate analysis of the Swedish data indicated, however, that women who had decreased their weight by 5 kg or more two or more times had an increased risk of kidney cancer independent of BMI (Lindblad et al, 1994). A study from the Netherlands found that adult weight gain was associated with increased risk of kidney cancer (van Dijk et al, 2004).

The mechanisms by which obesity influences renal carcinogenesis are not clear, but there are several plausible biological explanations. Obesity may affect sex steroid hormone levels, especially in women. Sex steroid hormones may stimulate renal cell proliferation and growth by direct

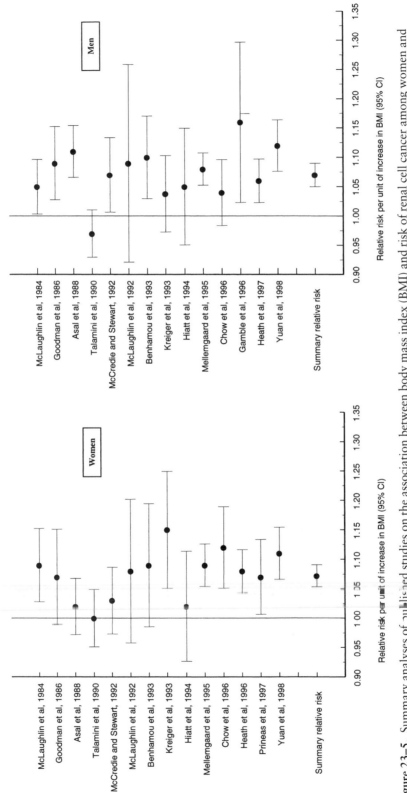

Figure 23–5. Summary analyses of published studies on the association between body mass index (BMI) and risk of renal cell cancer among women and among men. Relative risk per unit of increase in BMI (kg/m²) and 95% confidence intervals (CI). (*Source:* Bergström et al, 2001a)

endocrine receptor–mediated effects, by regulation of receptor concentrations, or through paracrine growth factors such as epidermal growth factor. Further, obesity is related to a number of endocrine disorders such as decreased levels of sex hormone-binding globulin and progesterone, anovulation, insulin resistance, and increased levels of biologically active insulin-like growth factor (IGF-I). Thus, the risk might be mediated via insulin and IGF-I. Epidemiologic studies indicate that patients with diabetes have an increased risk of renal cell cancer (Lindblad et al, 1999), which further support this biological pathway. Moreover, hypertension that may be an intermediate step in the causal pathway between obesity and kidney cancer could induce renal damage or could be associated with metabolic or functional changes within the renal tubules that increase the kidney's susceptibility to carcinogenes or cancer-promoting agents.

The cumulative evidence from analytic epidemiologic studies is most consistent for obesity as a risk factor for kidney cancer in both women and men. The attributable risk of obesity was estimated to be 21% in the United States (Benichou et al, 1998), 13% in Australia (McCredie et al, 1992), and about 25% in the European Union (Bergstrom et al, 2001b).

Studies have examined height and kidney cancer (Bjorge et al, 2004; Chow et al, 2000; Pischon et al, 2005; Tulinius et al, 1997; van Dijk et al, 2004). Some (Bjorge et al, 2004; Tulinius et al, 1997; van Dijk et al, 2004) of the studies, but not others (Chow et al, 2000, Pischon et al, 2005), found a positive association between height and kidney cancer risk.

Infections

Viruses have been implicated in animal experimental models as etiologic factors in kidney carcinoma, but no oncogenic viruses have been associated with kidney cancer in humans (Newsom and Vugrin, 1987). On the other side, there is no unique excess of kidney cancer in patients with acquired immunodeficiency syndrome (Selik and Rabkin, 1998).

See under "Medical Conditions and Treatment" for discussion of urinary tract infections.

Physical Activity

A role of physical activity in the development of kidney cancer is plausible, since energy expenditure is an important determinant of adult weight and obesity, but reports are not consistent and the mechanism is unclear.

The impact of occupational and/or recreational physical activity on the risk of kidney cancer has been reported in several case-control (Goodman et al, 1986; Lindblad et al, 1994; Mellemgaard et al, 1994; Menezes et al, 2003; Mellemgaard et al, 1995) and cohort studies (Bergstrom et al, 1999; Bergstrom et al, 2001c; Mahabir et al, 2004; Nicodemus et al, 2004; Paffenbarger et al, 1987; van Dijk et al, 2004). Some studies found that either occupational (Bergstrom et al, 1999) or recreational (Bergstrom et al, 2001c; Menezes et al, 2003) physical activity was associated with reduced risk of kidney cancer. It is not entirely clear whether the association is independent of obesity.

Ionizing Radiation

Various types of ionizing radiation have been associated with an excess risk of kidney cancer. Women with cervical cancer treated with radiotherapy experienced a small but significantly increased risk (Kleinerman et al, 1995), as did men treated for testicular cancer (Travis et al, 1997). Among patients with ankylosing spondylitis who had received x-ray treatment, the mortality from kidney cancer was significantly increased (Weiss et al, 1994). Thorotrast, an alpha-emitting contrast medium, has been linked to kidney cancer in patients who had undergone retrograde pyelography with thorotrast; however, the cancers are mostly urothelial cancers of the renal pelvis (Oyen et al, 1988). Only one case-control study (Asal et al, 1988) found a significant positive association among women between any lifetime radiation therapy received and kidney cancer.

Occupation

Except for asbestos, no occupational exposure or occupation has been consistently associated with kidney cancer (Mandel et al, 1995), and even asbestos is unlikely to be responsible for any important increase in kidney cancer risk (Sali and Boffetta, 2000).

Kidney cancer, in contrast to bladder cancer, is generally not considered an occupation-related cancer, but associations have been reported with asbestos in several studies (Enterline et al, 1987; Maclure, 1987; Mandel et al, 1995; Mattioli et al, 2002; Selikoff et al, 1979), with gasoline and other petroleum products in some (Lynge et al, 1997; Mandel et al, 1995; Partanen et al, 1991) but not all (McLaughlin, 1993; Wong et al, 1999) studies, and further with hydrocarbons (Boffetta et al, 1997; Kadamani et al, 1989; Sharpe et al, 1989), lead (Cocco et al, 1997; Pesch et al, 2000), cadmium (Kolonel, 1976; Mandel et al, 1995; Pesch et al, 2000), and work or exposure related to dry cleaning and laundry (Duh and Asal, 1984; Mandel et al, 1995).

The IARC has considered both trichloroethylene—used mainly in metal degreasing—and tetrachloroethylene—used in dry cleaning—as carcinogenic to animals and probably also to humans. However, critical reviews of both cohort and case-control studies concluded that there is no convincing evidence that these solvents pose a risk to humans; findings from cohort studies argue against a causal relationship (McLaughlin and Blot, 1997). Another review has a different view, and finds the evidence supporting an association between trichloroethylene and kidney cancer stronger than for any other cancer site, and that there is supporting evidence of an association between incidence of kidney cancer among workers exposed to degreasing agents and solvents and to those in both iron and steel and dry cleaning and laudry work industries; although, direct causality cannot be assesed (Bruning et al,

2003; Wartenberg et al, 2000). Kidney cancer patients who had been exposed to trichloroethylene certainly showed frequent somatic *VHL* mutations (Brauch et al, 1999), but this finding needs further confirmation.

Medical Conditions and Treatment

A number of medical conditions have been associated with kidney cancer, but the evidence is consistent for only a few of them. A major concern in the case-control studies is recall bias, especially in regard to urinary tract conditions.

End-stage renal disease

Acquired cystic kidney disease, which occurs in end-stage renal disease with progressive development of cysts in a poorly functioning or nonfunctioning kidney, is strongly associated with the development of kidney cancer. Acquired cystic kidney disease has been observed in 7% to 22% of patients with end-stage renal disease prior to dialysis, but the proportion increases to 90% after 10 years of dialysis. A notable sex difference has been observed, men having a higher incidence and more severe cystic change than women (Ishikawa, 1991; Marple et al, 1994).

The incidence of kidney cancer in patients with end-stage renal disease has been reported to be up to 40 to 100-times higher than in the general population (Denton et al, 2002; Ishikawa, 1991; Maisonneuve et al, 1999; Marple et al, 1994). An increased risk has also been seen in native kidneys after renal transplantation (Doublet et al, 1997; Khem et al, 1997). While proliferation of proximal tubular epithelial cells has been identified as the major pathogenetic mechanism of cyst formation, hormones (eg, estrogens) and growth factors and their receptors may stimulate cell proliferation and promote carcinogenesis. This mechanism may also explain, in part, the onset of multiple renal adenomas and bilateral carcinomas that develop in patients with acquired cystic kidney disease (Concolino et al, 1993).

Urologic disorders

Kidney stones have been found to increase the risk of kidney cancer in several studies (Asal et al, 1988; Maclure and Willett, 1990; McCredie and Stewart, 1992; McLaughlin et al, 1984; Schlehofer et al, 1996; Talamini et al, 1990), except one cohort study (Chow et al, 1997). Also, kidney infections (Hiatt et al, 1994; McLaughlin et al, 1984; Schlehofer et al, 1996), lower urinary tract infection (McCredie and Stewart, 1992; Parker et al, 2004; Talamini et al, 1990), and unspecified urinary tract infections in women (Kreiger et al, 1993) have been positively associated with kidney cancer. For the reported possible associations between kidney cancer and thyroid disease (Rosenberg et al, 1990; Schlehofer et al, 1996), thyroid cancer (Tucker et al, 1985), and lymphoid malignancies (Barista, 1997), the evidence is weak.

Diabetes mellitus

Results of studies that investigated the role of diabetes mellitus in the etiology of kidney cancer are not consistent. Some case-control studies found no increased risk (La Vecchia et al, 1994; McLaughlin et al, 1992; Wynder et al, 1974; Yuan et al, 1998b), while others showed a nonsignificantly elevated risk (Asal et al, 1988; McCredie and Stewart, 1992). The risk increase was often confined to women (McLaughlin et al, 1984; O'Mara et al, 1985; Goodman et al, 1986; Kreiger et al, 1993; Mellemgaard et al, 1994), but was also—in one large study (Schlehofer et al, 1996)—seen in both women and men. Reports from cohort studies are equally inconsistent; a significantly increased incidence of kidney cancer was found among diabetic women (Adami et al, 1991), among both women and men (Wideroff et al, 1997; Lindblad et al, 1999), or no association was reported (Kessler, 1970; Coughlin et al, 1997). Elevated levels of growth factors and growth factor receptors may mediate the possible relationship between diabetes and kidney cancer (Lindblad et al, 1999).

Hypertension, antihypertensives, and diuretics

Difficulties have arisen in isolating the possible effects of antihypertensive medication from those of hypertension, which itself has been linked to kidney cancer (Fraser et al, 1990; McLaughlin et al, 1995; Gamble et al, 1996; Coughlin et al, 1997; Heath et al, 1997; Yuan et al, 1998a; Shapiro et al, 1999; Chow et al, 2000; Flaherty et al, 2005), because they are highly correlated.

An increased risk of kidney cancer has been reported following diuretic use in many epidemiologic studies, but the magnitude of the risk has varied substantially, especially for women (Yu et al, 1986; McLaughlin et al, 1988; Fraser et al, 1990; Finkle et al, 1993; Hiatt et al, 1994; Heath et al, 1997; Prineas et al, 1997). Excess risk, to a lesser degree, has also been reported for men (Kreiger et al, 1993; Weinmann et al, 1994). However, several studies reported that the association disappeared once hypertension was accounted for (McLaughlin et al, 1995a; Yuan et al, 1998a; Shapiro et al, 1999; Flaherty et al, 2005). Therefore, diuretics may be a marker of hypertension and may not be an independent risk factor for kidney cancer.

Nondiuretic antihypertensive use has been investigated in relation to kidney cancer. McCredie and Stewart (1992) found an association, particularly with beta-blockers, while in the multicenter study by McLaughlin et al (1995a), the excess risk was not confined to any specific drug. The risk was reduced after adjustment for hypertension but remained significant. A similar reduced effect of nondiuretic antihypertensive medication after adjustment for hypertension was reported by Shapiro et al (1999). In a large case-control study (Yuan et al, 1998a), regular nondiuretic medication increased the risk of kidney cancer, but the risk increase was not greater among hypertensive subjects and it was not seen among normotensive regular users.

The use and type of antihypertensive medication could be an indication of severity of hypertension, but high blood pressure was also associated with an increased risk among men and women who never took antihypertensive medication (Shapiro et al, 1999). Another explanation could be that kidney cancer may sometimes cause hypertension. However, many of the studies have also restricted analysis of hypertension to 5 to 10 or more years prior to cancer diagnosis and have still found an association between hypertension and kidney cancer, which makes hypertension unlikely to be a consequence of the cancer. It seems more likely that hypertension is an independent risk factor in the etiology of kidney cancer (Yu and Ross, 2001), but the difficulty of separating the effect of hypertension and its medical treatment hampers definite conclusions.

Analgesics

Phenacetin-containing analgesics have been implicated in the etiology of renal pelvic cancer (IARC, 1987); their role in the etiology of kidney cancer is less clear. A number of studies have associated a moderately elevated risk with regular or long-term use (McLaughlin et al, 1984; Maclure and MacMahon, 1985; McLaughlin et al, 1985; McCredie et al, 1988; McLaughlin et al, 1992; Kreiger et al, 1993; McCredie et al, 1993). A large case-control study showed an elevated risk associated with all major types of analgesics (Gago-Dominguez et al, 1999); in contrast, the international multicenter study by McCredie et al (1995) found no association with any type of analgesic (paracetamol, phenacetin, pyrazolones, and salicylates, mainly aspirin), notwithstanding detailed assessment of drug use and extensive analyses. This study, however, had limited power to evaluate phenacetin because the drug had been unavailable for many years in most of the participating countries.

Diet pills

Use of diet pills containing amphetamines for primarily pharmacologic treatment of obesity has been reported in a few studies. An association with an increased risk of kidney cancer has been found (Yu et al, 1986; Mellemgaard et al, 1995; Yuan et al, 1998). Sometimes this association appeared to be independent of obesity, although it is difficult to separate the effects of amphetamine use from those of obesity and its consequences. One study found a significant dose–response relationship (Yuan et al, 1998a).

Other Risk Factors

Educational or socioeconomic level has sometimes been associated with kidney cancer. In case-control studies, no major differences have been found (Wynder et al, 1974; McLaughlin et al, 1984; Goodman et al, 1986; Yu et al, 1986; Talamini et al, 1990; McCredie and Stewart, 1992; Krieger et al, 1993; De Stefani et al, 1998), although others have found an inverse relationship (Asal et al, 1988; Kadamani et al, 1989; Hiatt et al, 1994; Lindblad et al, 1997; Maclure and Willett, 1990; Mandel et al, 1995, Yuan et al, 1998a).

CONCLUSION

The increasing incidence of kidney cancer in most populations may be due in part to incidental detection with new imaging modalities. Further, the increase is not only restricted to small local tumors but also includes more advanced tumors, which may help explain the still high mortality rates. The variation in incidence among populations may have several other explanations. Traditionally, the starting point has been to consider environmental exposures (Table 23–4). Cigarette smoking and obesity may account for approximately 40% of cases in high-risk countries. Genetic variations may also be important as a cause of the difference among populations. Continued research in kidney cancer is needed since nearly 50% of the patients die within 5 years after diagnosis. With the aim of prevention, the continued search for environmental causes should take into account the fact that kidney

Table 23–4. Risk factors for RCC

Established	Needing further study or controversial	Dietary factors
Cigarette smoking	Alcohol	Vegetables and fruit—protective
Obesity	Physical activity	Protein and/or dietary fat
Acquired cystic kidney disease	Hypertension and/or antihypertensive medication	
Inherited susceptibility (e.g. VHL)	Analgesics	
	Reproductive factors and hormones (e.g. parity, oral contraceptives)	
	Occupational exposures (e.g. asbestos, cadmium, hydrocarbons, gasoline, trichloroethylene)	

cancer consists of different types with specific genetic molecular characteristics. In some cases, these genetic alterations have been purportedly associated with specific exposures. Furthermore, genetic polymorphisms may have a modulating effect on metabolic activation and detoxification enzymes. Thus, better understanding of the genetic and molecular processes involved in kidney cancer may help analyzing exposure associations that are important in both its initiation and progression.

REFERENCES

Adami HO, Persson I, Hoover R, Schairer C, Bergkvist L. Risk of cancer in women receiving hormone replacement therapy. Int J Cancer 1989;44:833–39.

Adami HO, McLaughlin J, Ekbom A, Berne C, Silverman D, Hacker D, et al. Cancer risk in patients with diabetes mellitus. Cancer Causes Control 1991;2:307–14.

Asal NR, Geyer JR, Risser DR, Lee ET, Kadamani S, Cherng N. Risk factors in renal cell carcinoma. II. Medical history, occupation, multivariate analysis, and conclusions. Cancer Detect Prev 1988;13:263–79.

Augustsson K, Skog K, Jagerstad M, Dickman PW, Steineck G. Dietary heterocyclic amines and cancer of the colon, rectum, bladder, and kidney: a population-based study. Lancet 1999;353:703–7.

Barista I. An association between renal cell carcinoma and lymphoid malignancies: a case series of eight patients. Cancer 1997;80:1004–5; author reply 6–7.

Benichou J, Chow WH, McLaughlin JK, Mandel JS, Fraumeni JF Jr. Population attributable risk of renal cell cancer in Minnesota. Am J Epidemiol 1998;148:424–30.

Bergstrom A, Moradi T, Lindblad P, Nyren O, Adami HO, Wolk A. Occupational physical activity and renal cell cancer: a nationwide cohort study in Sweden. Int J Cancer 1999;83:186–91.

Bergstrom A, Hsieh CC, Lindblad P, Lu CM, Cook NR, Wolk A. Obesity and renal cell cancer—a quantitative review. Br J Cancer 2001a;85:984–90.

Bergstrom A, Pisani P, Tenet V, Wolk A, Adami HO. Overweight as an avoidable cause of cancer in Europe. Int J Cancer 2001b;91:421–30.

Bergstrom A, Terry P, Lindblad P, Lichtenstein P, Ahlbom A, Feychting M, et al. Physical activity and risk of renal cell cancer. Int J Cancer 2001c;92:155–57.

Bjorge T, Tretli S, Engeland A. Relation of height and body mass index to renal cell carcinoma in two million Norwegian men and women. Am J Epidemiol 2004;160:1168–76.

Boffetta P, Jourenkova N, Gustavsson P. Cancer risk from occupational and environmental exposure to polycyclic aromatic hydrocarbons. Cancer Causes Control 1997;8:444–72.

Brauch H, Weirich G, Hornauer MA, Storkel S, Wohl T, Bruning T. Trichloroethylene exposure and specific somatic mutations in patients with renal cell carcinoma. J Natl Cancer Inst 1999;91:854–61.

Bruning T, Pesch B, Wiesenhutter B, Rabstein S, Lammert M, Baumuller A, et al. Renal cell cancer risk and occupational exposure to trichloroethylene: results of a consecutive case-control study in Arnsberg, Germany. Am J Ind Med 2003;43:274–85.

Chen CJ, Chen CW, Wu MM, Kuo TL. Cancer potential in liver, lung, bladder and kidney due to ingested inorganic arsenic in drinking water. Br J Cancer 1992;66:888–92.

Chow WH, Gridley G, McLaughlin JK, Mandel JS, Wacholder S, Blot WJ, et al. Protein intake and risk of renal cell cancer. J Natl Cancer Inst 1994;86:1131–39.

Chow WH, McLaughlin JK, Mandel JS, Blot WJ, Niwa S, Fraumeni JF, Jr. Reproductive factors and the risk of renal cell cancer among women. Int J Cancer 1995;60:321–24.

Chow WH, Lindblad P, Gridley G, Nyren O, McLaughlin JK, Linet MS, et al. Risk of urinary tract cancers following kidney or ureter stones. J Natl Cancer Inst 1997;89:1453–57.

Chow WH, Gridley G, Fraumeni JF, Jr., Jarvholm B. Obesity, hypertension, and the risk of kidney cancer in men. N Engl J Med 2000;343:1305–11.

Choyke PL, Glenn GM, Walther MM, Patronas NJ, Linehan WM, Zbar B. von Hippel-Lindau disease: genetic, clinical, and imaging features. Radiology 1995;194:629–42.

Cocco P, Hua F, Boffetta P, Carta P, Flore C, Flore V, et al. Mortality of Italian lead smelter workers. Scand J Work Environ Health 1997;23:15–23.

Concolino G, Lubrano C, Ombres M, Santonati A, Flammia GP, Di Silverio F. Acquired cystic kidney disease: the hormonal hypothesis. Urology 1993;41:170–75.

Coughlin SS, Neaton JD, Randall B, Sengupta A. Predictors of mortality from kidney cancer in 332,547 men screened for the Multiple Risk Factor Intervention Trial. Cancer 1997;79:2171–77.

Davies MJ, Baer DJ, Judd JT, Brown ED, Campbell WS, Taylor PR. Effects of moderate alcohol intake on fasting insulin and glucose concentrations and insulin sensitivity in postmenopausal women: a randomized controlled trial. JAMA 2002;287:2559–62.

De Stefani E, Fierro L, Mendilaharsu M, Ronco A, Larrinaga MI, Balbi JC, et al. Meat intake, 'mate' drinking and renal cell cancer in Uruguay: a case-control study. Br J Cancer 1998;78:1239–43.

Denton MD, Magee CC, Ovuworie C, Mauiyyedi S, Pascual M, Colvin RB, et al. Prevalence of renal cell carcinoma in patients with ESRD pre-transplantation: a pathologic analysis. Kidney Int 2002;61:2201–9.

Doublet JD, Peraldi MN, Gattegno B, Thibault P, Sraer JD. Renal cell carcinoma of native kidneys: prospective study of 129 renal transplant patients. J Urol 1997;158:42–44.

Duh RW, Asal NR. Mortality among laundry and dry cleaning workers in Oklahoma. Am J Public Health 1984;74:1278–80.

Enterline PE, Hartley J, Henderson V. Asbestos and cancer: a cohort followed up to death. Br J Ind Med 1987;44:396–401.

Facchini F, Chen YD, Reaven GM. Light-to-moderate alcohol intake is associated with enhanced insulin sensitivity. Diabetes Care 1994;17:115–19.

Ferlay J, Bray F, Pisani P, Parkin DM. GLOBOCAN 2002: Cancer Incidence, Mortality, and Prevalence Worldwide. Lyon, France: International Agency for Research on Cancer; 2004.

Finkle WD, McLaughlin JK, Rasgon SA, Yeoh HH, Low JE. Increased risk of renal cell cancer among women using diuretics in the United States. Cancer Causes Control 1993;4:555–58.

Flaherty KT, Fuchs CS, Colditz GA, Stampfer MJ, Speizer FE, Willett WC, et al. A prospective study of body mass index, hypertension, and smoking and the risk of renal cell carcinoma (United States). Cancer Causes Control 2005;16:1099–1106.

Fraser GE, Phillips RL, Beeson WL. Hypertension, antihypertensive medication and risk of renal carcinoma in California Seventh-Day Adventists. Int J Epidemiol 1990;19:832–38.

Friedman M. Prevention of adverse effects of food browning. Adv Exp Med Biol 1991;289:171–215.

Gago-Dominguez M, Yuan JM, Castelao JE, Ross RK, Yu MC. Regular use of analgesics is a risk factor for renal cell carcinoma. Br J Cancer 1999;81:542–48.

Gago-Dominguez M, Yuan JM, Castelao JE, Ross RK, Yu MC. Family history and risk of renal cell carcinoma. Cancer Epidemiol Biomarkers Prev 2001;10:1001–4.

Gamble JF, Pearlman ED, Nicolich MJ. A nested case-control study of kidney cancer among refinery/petrochemical workers. Environ Health Perspect 1996;104:642–50.

Gnarra JR. von Hippel-Lindau gene mutations in human and rodent renal tumors—association with clear cell phenotype. J Natl Cancer Inst 1998;90:1685–87.

Goodman MT, Morgenstern H, Wynder EL. A case-control study of factors affecting the development of renal cell cancer. Am J Epidemiol 1986;124:926–41.

Greving JP, Lee JE, Wolk A, Lukkien C, Lindblad P, Bergstrom A. Alcoholic beverages and risk of renal cell cancer. Br J Cancer 2007; 97:429-33.

Hamilton JM. Renal carcinogenesis. Adv Cancer Res 1975;22:1–56.

Handa K, Kreiger N. Diet patterns and the risk of renal cell carcinoma. Public Health Nutr 2002;5:757–67.

Heath CW, Jr., Lally CA, Calle EE, McLaughlin JK, Thun MJ. Hypertension, diuretics, and antihypertensive medications as possible risk factors for renal cell cancer. Am J Epidemiol 1997;145:607–13.

Hiatt RA, Tolan K, Quesenberry CP, Jr. Renal cell carcinoma and thiazide use: a historical, case-control study (California, USA). Cancer Causes Control 1994;5:319–25.

Hopenhayn-Rich C, Biggs ML, Smith AH. Lung and kidney cancer mortality associated with arsenic in drinking water in Cordoba, Argentina. Int J Epidemiol 1998;27:561–69.

Hu J, Mao Y, White K. Diet and vitamin or mineral supplements and risk of renal cell carcinoma in Canada. Cancer Causes Control 2003;14:705–14.

Hu J, Ugnat AM. Active and passive smoking and risk of renal cell carcinoma in Canada. Eur J Cancer 2005;41:770–78.

IARC Working Group on the Evaluation of the Carcinogenic Risk of Chemicals to Humans. Tobacco smoking. Lyon, France: World Health Organization, International Agency for Research on Cancer 1986.

IARC. Phenactin and analgesic mixtures containing phenacetin. Monographs on the evaluation of the carcinogenic risk of chemicals to humans. An updating of IARC Monographs. IARC Monographs 1987;1–42:310–12.

IARC. Chlorinated drinking-water; chlorination by-products; some other halogenated compounds; cobalt and cobalt compounds. International Agency for Research on Cancer (IARC) Working Group, Lyon, 12–19 June 1990. IARC Monogr Eval Carcinog Risks Hum 1991;52:1–544.

Ishikawa I. Uremic acquired renal cystic disease. Natural history and complications. Nephron 1991;58:257–67.

Jacobsen J, Grankvist K, Rasmuson T, Bergh A, Landberg G, Ljungberg B. Expression of vascular endothelial growth factor protein in human renal cell carcinoma. BJU Int 2004;93:297–302.

Kadamani S, Asal NR, Nelson RY. Occupational hydrocarbon exposure and risk of renal cell carcinoma. Am J Ind Med 1989;15:131–41.

Kessler II. Cancer mortality among diabetics. J Natl Cancer Inst 1970;44:673–86.

Kim WY, Kaelin WG. Role of VHL gene mutation in human cancer. J Clin Oncol 2004;22:4991–5004.

Kleinerman RA, Boice JD, Jr., Storm HH, Sparen P, Andersen A, Pukkala E, et al. Second primary cancer after treatment for cervical cancer. An international cancer registries study. Cancer 1995;76:442–52.

Kliem V, Kolditz M, Behrend M, Ehlerding G, Pichlmayr R, Koch KM, et al. Risk of renal cell carcinoma after kidney transplantation. Clin Transplant 1997;11:255–58.

Koivusalo M, Hakulinen T, Vartiainen T, Pukkala E, Jaakkola JJ, Tuomisto J. Drinking water mutagenicity and urinary tract cancers: a population-based case-control study in Finland. Am J Epidemiol 1998;148:704–12.

Kolonel LN. Association of cadmium with renal cancer. Cancer 1976;37:1782–87.

Kreiger N, Marrett LD, Dodds L, Hilditch S, Darlington GA. Risk factors for renal cell carcinoma: results of a population-based case-control study. Cancer Causes Control 1993;4:101–10.

La Vecchia C, Negri E, Franceschi S, D'Avanzo B, Boyle P. A case-control study of diabetes mellitus and cancer risk. Br J Cancer 1994;70:950–53.

Lambe M, Lindblad P, Wuu J, Remler R, Hsieh CC. Pregnancy and risk of renal cell cancer: a population-based study in Sweden. Br J Cancer 2002;86:1425–29.

Langner C, Ratschek M, Rehak P, Schips L, Zigeuner R. Steroid hormone receptor expression in renal cell carcinoma: an immunohistochemical analysis of 182 tumors. J Urol 2004;171:611–14.

Lee JE, Giovannucci E, Smith-Warner SA, Spiegelman D, Willett WC, Curhan GC. Intakes of fruits, vegetables, vitamins A, C, and E and carotenoids and risk of renal cell cancer. Cancer Epidemiol Biomarkers Prev 2006;15:2445–52.

Lee JE, Hunter DJ, Spiegelman D, Adami HO, Bernstein L, van den Brandt PA, Buring JE, Cho E, English D, Folsom AR, Freudenheim JL, Gile GG, Giovannucci E, Horn-Ross PL, Leitzmann MF, Marshall JR, Mannisto S, McCullough ML, Miller AB, Parker AS, Pietinen P, Rodriguez C, Rohan TE, Schatzkin A, Schouten LJ, Willett WC, Wolk A, Zhang SM, Smith-Warner SA. Intakes of coffee, tea, milk, soda and juice and renal cell cancer in a pooled analysis of 13 prospective studies. Int J Cancer 2007a;121:2246–53.

Lee JE, Hunter DJ, Spiegelman D, Adami HO, Albanes D, Bernstein L, van den Brandt PA, Buring JE, Cho E, Folsom AR, Freudenheim JL, Giovannucci E, Graham S, Horn-Ross PL, Leitzmann MF, McCullough ML, Miller AB, Parker AS, Rodriguez C, Rohan TE, Schatzkin A, Schouten LJ, Virtanen M, Willett WC, Wolk A, Zhang SM, Smith-Warner SA. Alcohol intake and renal cell cancer in a pooled analysis of 12 prospective studies. J Natl Cancer Inst 2007b;99:801–10.

Levi F, Lucchini F, Negri E, La Vecchia C. Trends in mortality from major cancers in the European Union, including acceding countries, in 2004. Cancer 2004;101:2843–50.

Lindblad P, Wolk A, Bergstrom R, Persson I, Adami HO. The role of obesity and weight fluctuations in the etiology of renal cell cancer: a population-based case-control study. Cancer Epidemiol Biomarkers Prev 1994;3:631–39.

Lindblad P, Mellemgaard A, Schlehofer B, Adami HO, McCredie M, McLaughlin JK, et al. International renal-cell cancer study. V. Reproductive factors, gynecologic operations and exogenous hormones. Int J Cancer 1995;61:192–98.

Lindblad P, Wolk A, Bergstrom R, Adami HO. Diet and risk of renal cell cancer: a population-based case-control study. Cancer Epidemiol Biomarkers Prev 1997;6:215–23.

Lindblad P, Chow WH, Chan J, Bergstrom A, Wolk A, Gridley G, et al. The role of diabetes mellitus in the aetiology of renal cell cancer. Diabetologia 1999;42:107–12.

Lynge E, Andersen A, Nilsson R, Barlow L, Pukkala E, Nordlinder R, et al. Risk of cancer and exposure to gasoline vapors. Am J Epidemiol 1997;145:449–58.

Maclure M, MacMahon B. Phenactin and cancer of urinary tract. N Engl J Med 1985:1479.

Maclure M. Asbestos and renal adenocarcinoma: a case-control study. Environ Res 1987;42:353–61.

Maclure M, Willett W. A case-control study of diet and risk of renal adenocarcinoma. Epidemiol 1990;1:430–40.

Mahabir S, Leitzmann MF, Pietinen P, Albanes D, Virtamo J, Taylor PR. Physical activity and renal cell cancer risk in a cohort of male smokers. Int J Cancer 2004;108:600–5.

Mahabir S, Leitzmann MF, Virtanen MJ, Virtamo J, Pietinen P, Albanes D, et al. Prospective study of alcohol drinking and renal cell cancer risk in a cohort of finnish male smokers. Cancer Epidemiol Biomarkers Prev 2005;14:170–75.

Maher ER. Inherited renal cell carcinoma. Br J Urol 1996;78:542–45.

Maisonneuve P, Agodoa L, Gellert R, Stewart JH, Buccianti G, Lowenfels AB, et al. Cancer in patients on dialysis for end-stage renal disease: an international collaborative study. Lancet 1999;354:93–99.

Mandel JS, McLaughlin JK, Schlehofer B, Mellemgaard A, Helmert U, Lindblad P, et al. International renal-cell cancer study. IV. Occupation. Int J Cancer 1995;61:601–5.

Marple JT, MacDougall M, Chonko AM. Renal cancer complicating acquired cystic kidney disease. J Am Soc Nephrol 1994;4:1951–56.

Mattioli S, Truffelli D, Baldasseroni A, Risi A, Marchesini B, Giacomini C, et al. Occupa-

tional risk factors for renal cell cancer: a case–control study in northern Italy. J Occup Environ Med 2002;44:1028–36.

McCredie M, Ford JM, Stewart JH. Risk factors for cancer of the renal parenchyma. Int J Cancer 1988;42:13–16.

McCredie M, Stewart JH. Risk factors for kidney cancer in New South Wales, Australia. II. Urologic disease, hypertension, obesity, and hormonal factors. Cancer Causes Control 1992;3:323–31.

McCredie M, Stewart JH, Day NE. Different roles for phenacetin and paracetamol in cancer of the kidney and renal pelvis. Int J Cancer 1993;53:245–49.

McCredie M, Pommer W, McLaughlin JK, Stewart JH, Lindblad P, Mandel JS, et al. International renal-cell cancer study. II. Analgesics. Int J Cancer 1995;60:345–49.

McLaughlin JK, Mandel JS, Blot WJ, Schuman LM, Mehl ES, Fraumeni JF, Jr. A population—based case—control study of renal cell carcinoma. J Natl Cancer Inst 1984;72:275–84.

McLaughlin JK, Blot WJ, Mehl ES, Fraumeni JF, Jr. Relation of analgesic use to renal cancer: population-based findings. Natl Cancer Inst Monogr 1985;69:217–22.

McLaughlin JK, Blot WJ, Fraumeni JF, Jr. Diuretics and renal cell cancer. J Natl Cancer Inst 1988;80:378.

McLaughlin JK, Hrubec Z, Heineman EF, Blot WJ, Fraumeni JF, Jr. Renal cancer and cigarette smoking in a 26-year followup of U.S. veterans. Public Health Rep 1990;105:535–37.

McLaughlin JK, Gao YT, Gao RN, Zheng W, Ji BT, Blot WJ, et al. Risk factors for renal-cell cancer in Shanghai, China. Int J Cancer 1992;52:562–65.

McLaughlin JK. Renal cell cancer and exposure to gasoline: a review. Environ Health Perspect 1993;101 Suppl 6:111–14.

McLaughlin JK, Chow WH, Mandel JS, Mellemgaard A, McCredie M, Lindblad P, et al. International renal-cell cancer study. VIII. Role of diuretics, other anti-hypertensive medications and hypertension. Int J Cancer 1995a;63:216–21.

McLaughlin JK, Lindblad P, Mellemgaard A, McCredie M, Mandel JS, Schlehofer B, et al. International renal-cell cancer study. I. Tobacco use. Int J Cancer 1995b;60:194–98.

McLaughlin JK, Blot WJ. A critical review of epidemiology studies of trichloroethylene and perchloroethylene and risk of renal-cell cancer. Int Arch Occup Environ Health 1997;70:222–31.

Mellemgaard A, Engholm G, McLaughlin JK, Olsen JH. Risk factors for renal-cell carcinoma in Denmark. III. Role of weight, physical activity and reproductive factors. Int J Cancer 1994;56:66–71.

Mellemgaard A, Lindblad P, Schlehofer B, Bergstrom R, Mandel JS, McCredie M, et al. International renal-cell cancer study. III. Role of weight, height, physical activity, and use of amphetamines. Int J Cancer 1995; 60:350–54.

Mellemgaard A, McLaughlin JK, Overvad K, Olsen JH. Dietary risk factors for renal cell carcinoma in Denmark. Eur J Cancer 1996;32A:673–82.

Menezes RJ, Tomlinson G, Kreiger N. Physical activity and risk of renal cell carcinoma. Int J Cancer 2003;107:642–46.

Morris RD. Drinking water and cancer. Environ Health Perspect 1995;103 Suppl 8:225–31.

Munro IC, Kennepohl E, Erickson RE, Portoghese PS, Wagner BM, Easterday OD, et al. Safety assessment of ingested heterocyclic amines: initial report. Regul Toxicol Pharmacol 1993;17:S1–S109.

Muscat JE, Hoffmann D, Wynder EL. The epidemiology of renal cell carcinoma. A second look. Cancer 1995;75:2552–57.

Nanus DM, Lynch SA, Rao PH, Anderson SM, Jhanwar SC, Albino AP. Transformation of human kidney proximal tubule cells by a src-containing retrovirus. Oncogene 1991;6:2105–11.

Newsom GD, Vugrin D. Etiologic factors in renal cell adenocarcinoma. Semin Nephrol 1987;7:109–16.

Nicodemus KK, Sweeney C, Folsom AR. Evaluation of dietary, medical and lifestyle risk factors for incident kidney cancer in postmenopausal women. Int J Cancer 2004;108:115–21.

Nogueira E, Cardesa A, Mohr U. Experimental models of kidney tumors. J Cancer Res Clin Oncol 1993;119:190–98.

O'Mara BA, Byers T, Schoenfeld E. Diabetes mellitus and cancer risk: a multisite case-control study. J Chronic Dis 1985;38:435–41.

Oyen RH, Gielen JL, Van Poppel HP, Verbeken EK, Van Damme BJ, Baert LV, et al. Renal thorium deposition associated with transitional cell carcinoma: radiologic demonstration in two patients. Radiology 1988;169:705–7.

Paffenbarger RSJ, Hyde RT, Wing AL. Physical activity and incidence of cancer in diverse populations: a preliminary report. Am J Clin Nutr 1987;45 (Suppl):312–17.

Parker AS, Cerhan JR, Lynch CF, Ershow AG, Cantor KP. Gender, alcohol consumption, and renal cell carcinoma. Am J Epidemiol 2002;155:455–62.

Parker AS, Cerhan JR, Lynch CF, Leibovich BC, Cantor KP. History of urinary tract infection and risk of renal cell carcinoma. Am J Epidemiol 2004;159:42–48.

Partanen T, Heikkila P, Hernberg S, Kauppinen T, Moneta G, Ojajarvi A. Renal cell cancer and occupational exposure to chemical agents. Scand J Work Environ Health 1991; 17:231–39.

Pesch B, Haerting J, Ranft U, Klimpel A, Oelschlagel B, Schill W. Occupational risk factors for renal cell carcinoma: agent-specific results from a case-control study in Germany. MURC Study Group. Multicenter urothelial and renal cancer study. Int J Epidemiol 2000;29:1014–24.

Pischon T, Lahmann PH, Boeing H, Tjonneland A, Halkjaer J, Overvad K, et al. Body size and risk of renal cell carcinoma in the European Prospective Investigation into Cancer and Nutrition (EPIC). Int J Cancer 2005.

Prineas RJ, Folsom AR, Zhang ZM, Sellers TA, Potter J. Nutrition and other risk factors for renal cell carcinoma in postmenopausal women. Epidemiology 1997;8:31–36.

Rashidkhani B, Akesson A, Lindblad P, Wolk A. Major dietary patterns and risk of renal cell carcinoma in a prospective cohort of Swedish women. J Nutr 2005a;135:1757–62.

Rashidkhani B, Lindblad P, Wolk A. Fruits, vegetables and risk of renal cell carcinoma: a prospective study of Swedish women. Int J Cancer 2005b;113:451–55.

Rosenberg AG, Dexeus F, Swanson DA, von Eschenbach AC. Relationship of thyroid disease to renal cell carcinoma. An epidemiologic study. Urology 1990;35:492–98.

Sali D, Boffetta P. Kidney cancer and occupational exposure to asbestos: a meta-analysis of occupational cohort studies. Cancer Causes Control 2000;11:37–47.

Schlehofer B, Pommer W, Mellemgaard A, Stewart JH, McCredie M, Niwa S, et al. International renal-cell-cancer study. VI. the role of medical and family history. Int J Cancer 1996;66:723–26.

Selik RM, Rabkin CS. Higher rates of death with non-AIDS-defining cancers among HIV-infected persons in the USA. *International Conference on AIDS* 1998.

Selikoff IJ, Hammond EC, Seidman H. Mortality experience of insulation workers in the United States and Canada, 1943—1976. Ann N Y Acad Sci 1979;330:91–116.

Semenza JC, Ziogas A, Largent J, Peel D, Anton-Culver H. Gene-environment interactions in renal cell carcinoma. Am J Epidemiol 2001; 153:851–59.

Shapiro JA, Williams MA, Weiss NS, Stergachis A, LaCroix AZ, Barlow WE. Hypertension, antihypertensive medication use, and risk of renal cell carcinoma. Am J Epidemiol 1999; 149:521–30.

Sharpe CR, Rochon JE, Adam JM, Suissa S. Case-control study of hydrocarbon exposures in patients with renal cell carcinoma. Cmaj 1989;140:1309–18.

Shiao YH, Rice JM, Anderson LM, Diwan BA, Hard GC. von Hippel-Lindau gene mutations in N-nitrosodimethylamine-induced rat renal epithelial tumors. J Natl Cancer Inst 1998;90:1720–23.

Talamini R, Baron AE, Barra S, Bidoli E, La Vecchia C, Negri E, et al. A case-control study of risk factor for renal cell cancer in northern Italy. Cancer Causes Control 1990;1:125–31.

Travis LB, Curtis RE, Storm H, Hall P, Holowaty E, Van Leeuwen FE, et al. Risk of second malignant neoplasms among long-term survivors of testicular cancer. J Natl Cancer Inst 1997;89:1429–39.

Tucker MA, Boice JD, Jr., Hoffman DA. Second cancer following cutaneous melanoma and cancers of the brain, thyroid, connective tissue, bone, and eye in Connecticut, 1935–82. Natl Cancer Inst Monogr 1985;68:161–89.

Tulinius H, Sigfusson N, Sigvaldason H, Bjarnadottir K, Tryggvadottir L. Risk factors for malignant diseases: a cohort study on a population of 22,946 Icelanders. Cancer Epidemiol Biomarkers Prev 1997;6:863–73.

van Dijk BA, Schouten LJ, Kiemeney LA, Goldbohm RA, van den Brandt PA. Relation of height, body mass, energy intake, and physical activity to risk of renal cell carcinoma: results from the Netherlands Cohort Study. Am J Epidemiol 2004;160:1159–67.

van Dijk BA, Schouten LJ, Kiemeney LA, Goldbohm RA, van den Brandt PA. Vegetable and fruit consumption and risk of renal cell carcinoma: results from the Netherlands cohort study. Int J Cancer 2005;117:648–54.

Van Poppel H, Nilsson S, Algaba F, Bergerheim U, Dal Cin P, Fleming S, et al. Precancerous lesions in the kidney. Scand J Urol Nephrol Suppl 2000:136–65.

Wartenberg D, Reyner D, Scott CS. Trichloroethylene and cancer: epidemiologic evidence. Environ Health Perspect 2000;108 Suppl 2:161–76.

Weikert S, Boeing H, Pischon T, Olsen A, Tjonneland A, Overvad K, et al. Fruits and vegetables and renal cell carcinoma: findings from the European prospective investigation into cancer and nutrition (EPIC). Int J Cancer 2006;118:3133–39.

Weinmann S, Glass AG, Weiss NS, Psaty BM, Siscovick DS, White E. Use of diuretics and other antihypertensive medications in relation to the risk of renal cell cancer. Am J Epidemiol 1994;140:792–804.

Weiss HA, Darby SC, Doll R. Cancer mortality following X-ray treatment for ankylosing spondylitis. Int J Cancer 1994;59:327–38.

Wideroff L, Gridley G, Mellemkjaer L, Chow WH, Linet M, Keehn S, et al. Cancer incidence in a population-based cohort of patients hospitalized with diabetes mellitus in Denmark. J Natl Cancer Inst 1997;89:1360–65.

Wilkins JR, 3rd, Comstock GW. Source of drinking water at home and site-specific cancer incidence in Washington County, Maryland. Am J Epidemiol 1981;114:178–90.

Wolk A, Gridley G, Niwa S, Lindblad P, McCredie M, Mellemgaard A, et al. International renal cell cancer study. VII. Role of diet. Int J Cancer 1996a;65:67–73.

Wolk A, Lindblad P, Adami HO. Nutrition and renal cell cancer. Cancer Causes Control 1996b;7:5–18.

Wong O, Trent L, Harris F. Nested case-control study of leukaemia, multiple myeloma, and kidney cancer in a cohort of petroleum workers exposed to gasoline. Occup Environ Med 1999;56:217–21.

Wynder EL, Mabuchi K, Whitmore WF, Jr. Epidemiology of adenocarcinoma of the kidney. J Natl Cancer Inst 1974;53:1619–34.

Yu MC, Mack TM, Hanisch R, Cicioni C, Henderson BE. Cigarette smoking, obesity, diuretic use, and coffee consumption as risk factors for renal cell carcinoma. J Natl Cancer Inst 1986;77:351–56.

Yu MC, Ross RK. Obesity, hypertension, and renal cancer. N Engl J Med 2001;344:531–32.

Yuan JM, Castelao JE, Gago-Dominguez M, Ross RK, Yu MC. Hypertension, obesity and their medications in relation to renal cell carcinoma. Br J Cancer 1998a;77:1508–13.

Yuan JM, Gago-Dominguez M, Castelao JE, Hankin JH, Ross RK, Yu MC. Cruciferous vegetables in relation to renal cell carcinoma. Int J Cancer 1998b;77:211–16.

Yuan JM, Castelao JE, Gago-Dominguez M, Yu MC, Ross RK. Tobacco use in relation to renal cell carcinoma. Cancer Epidemiol Biomarkers Prev 1998c; 7:429–33.

24

Brain Cancer

DAVID A. SAVITZ AND DIMITRIOS TRICHOPOULOS

Despite their relative rarity, brain cancers have drawn wide attention because of the fear inspired by their location, the young age at which they sometimes occur, the generally poor prognosis, and their perceived tendency to appear in clusters. Nevertheless, few cancers have proven as etiologically puzzling as brain cancer. The reasons why we have made so little progress are unclear, but there are several plausible explanations. Brain cancer occurs in an unusually diverse array of histologic types, with little certainty regarding the extent to which they share an etiology. Except for high doses of ionizing radiation, a nearly universal carcinogen, we lack clear, identified causal agents that can guide future research.

The distinction between the occurrence of brain tumors in children and adults in regard to the histology of tumors and presumed time period of development suggests that the epidemiologic considerations also be separated since there may well be different etiologies in the two groups. Given how little is currently known about etiology, however, it is not yet certain whether

the causes of brain tumors differ between children and adults. In the discussion that follows, the focus is largely on adult brain tumors, which are quantitatively dominant in the population and the focus of the vast majority of studies.

The epidemiology of brain tumors is challenging to summarize, even at the simple descriptive level. Unlike most other cancers, both benign and malignant brain tumors are of concern because their distinct anatomic location makes even benign tumors a serious threat to health and survival. An additional challenge to researchers is the difficulty of making comprehensive diagnoses because of the inaccessible location of these tumors. While advanced disease becomes apparent at some point in its clinical course, identification of subclinical disease or of tumors showing only nonspecific symptoms depends on advanced technology. As a result, comparing incidence rates across settings, populations, or time periods in which the diagnostic methods are unequally available or utilized is problematic. Last, the case-control investigation based on direct interview, a powerful tool in revealing the etiology of most forms of cancer, is of limited use with respect to brain tumors because of their effects on mental function.

CLINICAL SYNOPSIS

Subgroups

Although primary brain tumors occur in a wide variety of histopathologic types (Table 24–1), the two broad groups are gliomas arising from neuroepithelial cells and meningiomas, which are histopathologically benign (albeit frequently life threatening). The clinical features and management of these two types differ substantially.

Symptoms

Clinical manifestations arise through two mechanisms. First, there are different focal symptoms—related to the anatomic location and local infiltration of the tumor—such as seizures; changes in personality, mood, initiative, or memory; hemiplegia; aphasia; and visual aberrations. Second, general symptoms dominated by headache are due chiefly to high intracranial pressure.

Diagnosis

Neuroimaging through magnetic resonance imaging and computed tomography is the hallmark of diagnosis, in certain situations complemented with angiography—for example to delineate a vascular malformation or to determine the blood supply to a meningioma.

Treatment

The goal of surgery is complete resection of the tumor, although this is not possible in most gliomas and in certain meningiomas. Substantial palliation can be achieved through reduction of tumor volume, however, and acquisition of tissue for histopathologic examination may guide subsequent adjuvant or palliative radiation therapy and/or chemotherapy. While these modalities play an important role in the management of many brain tumors, their optimal use is complex and depends on the clinical and histopathologic features of the tumor.

Prognosis

In European countries, the overall relative 5-year survival rate is approximately 20%, with limited variation between countries. The corresponding rate in the United States is around 30%.

Progress

No therapeutic breakthroughs or any substantial improvement in long-term cure due to more extensive use of radiotherapy have been documented. Nevertheless, in the United States, 10-year relative survival, a good indicator of long-term cure, almost doubled from 13% in 1973 to 25% in 1984. Changes in diagnostic criteria and the use of more sensitive, modern imaging techniques resulting in the detection of smaller or slower-growing tumors may have contributed to this apparent progress.

DESCRIPTIVE EPIDEMIOLOGY

Benign tumors constitute about 25% of all brain tumors (Preston-Martin and Mack, 1996). Epidemiologic studies vary in the extent to which these tumors are considered in conjunction with malignant ones. A detailed histologic classification of brain tumors is given in Table 24–1.

Assessment of temporal trends in adults has been extremely controversial (Inskip et al, 1995), largely because a true increase in incidence is so difficult to distinguish from an apparent increase due to improved diagnosis. During the period between 1973 and 1987, a 23% increase in incidence and a 9.4% increase in mortality were reported in the United States (Stephens, 1991). Against these modest increments, the incidence doubled in persons over age 75 between 1968 and 1985 (Davis and Schwartz, 1988). While some fraction of that marked increase in the elderly may be real, it also seems likely that improvements in diagnostic technology have led to diagnoses of brain tumors that would not have been recognized as such in earlier periods. In locations and time periods in which accurate diagnoses are uncertain, the large number of tumors that originate in

Table 24–1. Distribution and incidence rates, per 100,000 person-years, of primary brain and central nervous system tumors by histology (United States, Central Brain Tumor Registry of the United States, 1998–2002)

Histology	% of all reported brain tumors	Mean age at diagnosis	Age-Adjusted incidence rate*
TUMORS OF NEUROEPITHELIAL TISSUE	43.6	53	6.42
Pilocytic astrocytoma	2.3	12	0.33
Diffuse astrocytoma	0.7	46	0.10
Anaplastic astrocytoma	3.2	51	0.47
Unique astrocytoma variants	0.5	37	0.08
Astrocytoma, not otherwise specified	3.1	45	0.46
Glioblastoma	20.3	64	3.05
Oligodendroglioma	2.5	41	0.35
Anaplastic oligodendroglioma	1.2	48	0.18
Ependymoma/anaplastic ependymoma	1.8	39	0.26
Ependymoma variants	0.5	39	0.07
Mixed glioma	1.1	42	0.16
Glioma malignant, NOS	2.6	43	0.38
Choroid plexus	0.3	2	0.04
Neuroepithelial, NOS	0.1	52	0.02
Benign and malignant neuronal/glial, neuronal, and mixed	1.5	26	0.21
Pineal parenchymal	0.2	22	0.03
Embryonal/primitive/medulloblastoma	1.7	9	0.24
TUMORS OF CRANIAL AND SPINAL NERVES	8.0	52	1.17
TUMORS OF MENINGES	31.4	63	4.70
Meningioma	30.1	64	4.52
Other mesenchymal, benign and malignant	0.4	44	0.06
Hemangioblastoma	0.9	46	0.12
LYMPHOMAS AND HEMOPOIETIC NEOPLASMS	3.1	60	0.46
GERM CELL TUMORS AND CYSTS	0.6	16	0.09
TUMORS OF THE SELLAR REGION	7.1	48	1.03
Pituitary	6.3	49	0.92
Craniopharyngioma	0.7	33	0.11
LOCAL EXTENSIONS FROM REGIONAL TUMORS			
Chordoma/chondrosarcoma	0.2	48	0.03
UNCLASSIFIED TUMORS	6.1	68	0.91
Hemangioma	0.6	43	0.08
Neoplasm, unspecified	5.5	71	0.82
ALL OTHER	0.0	48	0.01
TOTAL	100.0	57	14.80

Source: Central Brain Tumor Registry of the United States (2005).

other sites, such as the lung or breast, and metastasize to the brain create the potential for misclassification of metastatic as primary brain cancers. Since increases were more pronounced in countries with the most advanced medical care systems, and were concentrated in the elderly, who may well have previously been misdiagnosed as having stroke or degenerative neurologic disease, Inskip et al (1995) inferred that much, perhaps all, of the increase may be due to improved completeness of diagnosis.

Although the absolute incidence of brain tumors differs across geographic areas, the shape of the age–incidence curve is similar (Figs. 24–1 and 24–2). Considering malignant tumors only of the brain, cranial nerves, and cranial meninges, data from nine Surveillance, Epidemiology, and End Results (SEER) areas between 1975 and 1991 show an annual incidence ranging from around 4 per 100 000 in young adults to around 20 per 100 000 in those over age 60 (Inskip et al, 1995). Whether the apparent leveling off or decline in incidence at around age 75 is due to true stabilization of rates or is a reflection of underascertainment in the elderly is unknown. Analysis of age patterns for malignant brain tumors only (Inskip et al, 1995) indicates a peak in childhood (prior to age 10), a decline between ages 10 and 20, and then a rise through adulthood, with a decline after age 70. This is also the age pattern for astrocytic tumors, but rarer subtypes follow a variety of different age–incidence curves.

The proportions of the various types of brain tumors differ markedly by gender and,

to some extent, by race. Among men, approximately 60% of all tumors are malignant gliomas, 20% are meningiomas, and 8% are nerve sheath tumors, the latter two of which are histologically benign. Among women, approximately 40% of all tumors are malignant gliomas and 35% are meningiomas; the proportion of nerve sheath tumors is similar to that among men. Approximately 80% of all gliomas are astrocytomas or glioblastomas multiforme (Preston-Martin and Mack, 1996). Data from the US Central Brain Tumor Registry are given in Table 24–1.

International comparisons show elevated—and similar—rates of brain tumors in North American and western European whites, somewhat lower rates in eastern Europe, and notably lower rates in Asia and South America (Figs. 24–3 and 24–4). However, the four- or fivefold global variation in incidence is far more modest than for more common cancers such as those of the breast, lung, colon, liver, and

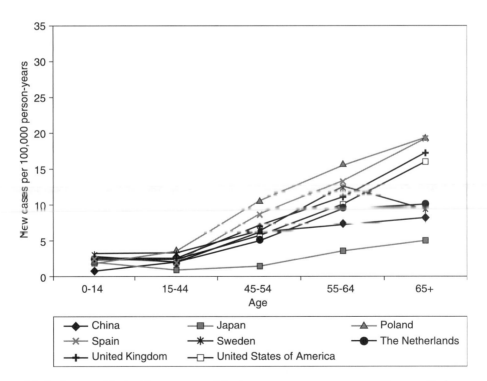

Figure 24–1. Age-specific incidence rates of brain cancer among women. (*Source*: Ferlay, 2004)

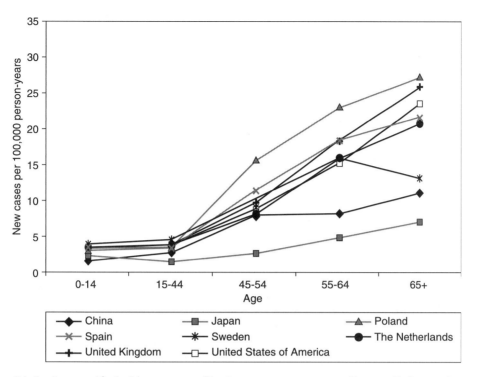

Figure 24–2. Age-specific incidence rates of brain cancer among men. (*Source*: Ferlay et al., 2004)

cervix. Again, the question of completeness must be considered as a partial explanation of this pattern of lower risk in less medically advanced settings, with the true extent of international variation possibly being even lower than has been reported.

Within the United States, whites have higher rates of glioma than blacks, whereas blacks show an excess of meningiomas. Asians and Hispanics in Lost Angeles had lower rates of both glioma and meningioma (Parkin et al, 2005). Other isolated findings on the descriptive epidemiology of brain cancer suggest a higher rate of meningioma among Jews (Newill, 1961), a higher rate of all brain cancers among Mormons (Lyon

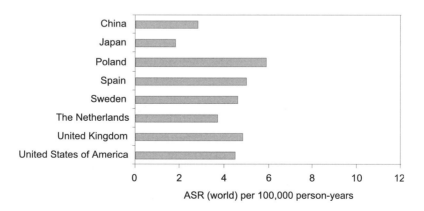

Figure 24–3. Age-standardized (to the world population) incidence rates of brain cancer among women. (*Source*: Ferlay et al, 2004)

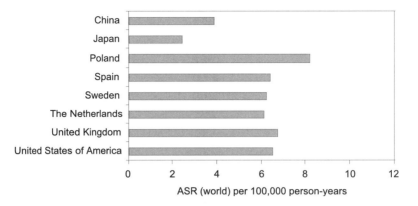

Figure 24–4. Age-standardized (to the world population) incidence rates of brain cancer among men. (*Source*:Ferlay et al, 2004)

et al, 1976), an increase among single men and women (Ernster et al, 1979), and some tendency toward increased rates in urban areas and among higher social classes (Demers et al, 1991; Preston-Martin et al, 1993). None of these findings are striking, and some are susceptible to differential completeness of diagnosis.

GENETIC AND MOLECULAR EPIDEMIOLOGY

Studies of inherited genetic influences on the occurrence of brain tumors and of the distribution and determinants of somatic genetic alterations in these tumors are both active avenues of investigation. One well-documented example of a hereditary predisposition is the Li-Fraumeni syndrome, which includes brain cancer as well as cancer of the breast and other sites. Nevertheless, known genes account for less than 1% of the cases and familial syndromes for less than 4% (Wrensch and Barger, 1990).

The increase in risk associated with having a relative with cancer is modest for gliomas (Burch et al, 1987; Preston-Martin et al, 1989a; Wrensch and Barger, 1990; Cicuttini et al, 1997), with relative risks of 1.6 or below, and in some studies very close to null (Wrensch et al, 1997a). A history of brain tumors in relatives was associated with a twofold increased risk in one study (Wrensch et al, 1997a). In the 1960s, an association

between blood type A and increased risk of brain tumors was reported (Yates and Pearce, 1960; Strang et al, 1966), but the results are not consistent (Ryan et al, 1992a; Schlehofer et al, 1992). What has not been identified to date is common genetic variation in susceptibility that might contribute to gene–environment interactions and that could account for a more substantial proportion of cases. Studies on glutathione S-Tranferases (GSTs) in relation to gliomas and meningiomas were synthesized in a meta-analysis, with the collective evidence suggesting no consistent association with any of the GST variants (Lai et al, 2005).

Somatic tumor characteristics have also been studied in an effort to identify etiologically distinctive subtypes. Glioblastomas show losses at chromosomes 17p, 10q, 13q, 22q, 19q, and 9p and gains at chromosome 7 (Inskip et al, 1995). An evaluation of mutations in the tumor-suppressor gene p53 demonstrated a high frequency of transversion mutations (Li et al, 1998).

RISK FACTORS

Our understanding of the causes of brain cancer based on epidemiologic studies is at an early stage of development.

Tobacco

Tobacco is not associated with brain tumors based on the evidence gathered thus far. A modest literature has accumulated in this area on both active smoking and environmental tobacco smoke. Active smoking was associated with the incidence of brain tumors in general in one study (Burch et al, 1987) but not with gliomas in two others (Preston-Martin et al, 1989a; Ryan et al, 1992a). Unfiltered cigarette use was associated with an increased risk of brain tumors, with some indication of a duration–response gradient (Lee et al, 1997). One study reported a strong association between environmental tobacco smoke and deaths from brain tumor (Hirayama, 1984), but this has not been replicated.

Findings of an association between tobacco smoking and meningiomas have been mixed; active and passive smoking were associated strongly with risk in one study (Ryan et al, 1992a). In another study, however, only a weak association was found among women (Preston-Martin et al, 1980), and no association at all was evident among men (Preston-Martin et al, 1983).

Diet

Compared to the promising data for other cancer sites, the evidence supporting dietary influences on the etiology of adult brain tumors is weak overall. There is some support for a positive association with cured meats and fish and an inverse association with fruit and vegetable intake (Giles, 1997).

The most extensively studied category of foods is cured meats and fish, motivated by a hypothesized etiologic pathway in which nitrites are converted to n-nitrosamines, established carcinogens in animal systems. In most case-control studies of gliomas—but not in all (Kaplan et al, 1997a), and not always equally for both sexes (Giles et al, 1994; Lee et al, 1997)—consumption of cured meats or fish was associated with an increased risk (Burch et al, 1987; Boeing et al, 1993; Giles et al, 1994; Blowers et al, 1997; Lee et al, 1997). Evidence supporting an association of cured-meat consumption with meningioma has also been reported (Preston-Martin et al, 1980; Preston-Martin and Mack, 1991). Attempts to examine nitrate and nitrite consumption directly in these same studies have not strengthened the pattern of association and, in many cases, these compounds have shown weaker associations than those found for cured meats (Boeing et al, 1993; Giles et al, 1994). Only when nitrosamine indices were constructed did the associations become stronger, with the highest tertiles of consumption showing relative risks on the order of 1.5 to 3.0 (Boeing et al, 1993; Giles et al, 1994).

A recent meta-analysis considered nine studies that addressed dietary cured-meat intake and adult gliomas (Huncharek et al, 2003). In the aggregate, cured-meat intake was associated with a significantly elevated risk, with a somewhat stronger association for ham intake. While these findings are not compelling in implicating cured meat in the etiology of gliomas, they do encourage continued efforts to elucidate this possible etiologic pathway.

Studies of fruit and vegetable intake in relation to brain tumors in adults have been sparse, with some evidence of an inverse association for gliomas (Burch et al, 1987; Boeing et al, 1993; Giles et al, 1994; Lee et al, 1997; Hu et al, 1999). Mixed results have been reported for a possibly protective effect of vitamin E (Burch et al, 1987; Giles et al, 1994; Hu et al, 1999) and for vitamin C–containing foods (Lee et al, 1997; Hu et al, 1999). Evaluation of vitamin supplements has yielded results suggesting a reduced risk of gliomas (Preston-Martin and Mack, 1991; Blowers et al, 1997) and of brain tumors in the aggregate (Burch et al, 1987). Cholesterol levels were found to be positively associated with brain tumor occurrence (Abramson and Kark, 1985; Neugut et al, 1989), but the etiologic significance of this finding is unclear (Inskip et al, 1995).

Nitrates in drinking water have also been studied in relation to brain tumor occurrence, in the context of the same hypothesis of an etiologic pathway involving nitrosamines. A large US study considered water nitrate intake over a 20-year period in conjunction with dietary nitrate and nitrite intake; essentially no link with risk of gliomas, or evidence for effect modification in relation to vitamin C intake, was found (Ward et al, 2005).

Alcohol

Preliminary evaluations of alcohol use and brain cancer have provided little motivation for additional, more detailed study and support the conclusion that no association exists (Giles, 1997).

Alcohol in the aggregate—as well as beer, wine, and liquor separately—have been examined in relation to both adult gliomas and meningiomas. Total alcohol has been reported to be associated with both an increased risk (Burch et al, 1987; Hu et al, 1998) and a decreased risk (Choi et al, 1970b) of brain tumors. No association was found with meningiomas (Preston-Martin et al, 1983). Evidence for absence of an association between beer and liquor consumption and glioma is fairly consistent (Burch et al, 1987; Preston-Martin et al, 1989a; Ryan et al, 1992a; Lee et al, 1997). Wine has been inversely related to the risk of glioma in two studies (Preston-Martin et al, 1989a; Ryan et al, 1992a) and positively in one (Burch et al, 1987).

Reproductive Factors

Direct evidence on reproductive factors in relation to brain tumors is limited, with some evidence for an inverse relationship between parity and brain cancer risk in women (Inskip et al, 1995; Cicuttini et al, 1997). More promising evidence links reproductive factors with meningioma based on the pronounced excess risk among women (Preston Martin, 1989) and the reported reduced risk among those with artificial menopause (Schlehofer et al, 1992).

Hormones

Hormones have not been evaluated in relation to brain tumors. There are only indirect inferences based on the possible relationship between reproductive history and the risk of meningioma in women.

Anthropometric Measures

One report indicated that obesity was positively associated with the risk of meningi-oma (Bellur et al, 1983); but, in general, anthropometric measures have not been systematically evaluated in relation to adult brain tumors. Among children, however, head circumference at birth has been strongly positively associated with brain cancer risk, suggesting that brain pathology may originate during fetal life (Samuelsen et al, 2006).

Infections

The isolated findings to date fail to provide a sufficient basis for conclusions regarding a role for infections in the etiology of brain tumors.

In 1967, Schuman and colleagues reported an association between a serologically documented history of infection with Toxoplasma gondii and astrocytoma. Later attempts to evaluate this finding indicated no association with glioma but an imprecise doubling of the risk of meningioma (Ryan et al, 1993). Two studies suggested an association between positive tuberculosis skin-test results and gliomas (Ward et al, 1973; Mills et al, 1989). An inverse association has been reported for a history of varicella-zoster infection based on either a self-report of chicken pox or shingles (relative risk of 0.4–0.5) or serologic evidence of prior infection (relative risk of 0.6) (Wrensch et al, 1997b). To the extent that birth order may be indicative of some aspect of early life infection, the finding of an increased risk of glioma among first-born persons (Cicuttini et al, 1997) may be relevant.

Physical Activity

Physical activity has not been systematically evaluated in relation to brain tumors.

Ionizing Radiation

The only well-established exogenous cause of adult brain tumors is exposure to high doses of ionizing radiation. The direct link between localized exposure to the head and development of brain tumors is strongest for meningiomas but is also present for gliomas (Ron et al, 1988). The atomic bombs exploded in Hiroshima and Nagasaki resulted in exposure of a cross section of the population, including children, to high levels of radiation. A nearly fivefold increased risk was reported for male children exposed to doses of 100 rads or more (Seyama et al, 1979), but no association was evident for female children.

High doses of radiation were once used to treat tinea capitus (ringworm), and several of these patient cohorts have been followed for their cancer experience. Cohorts of treated children from Israel (Modan et al, 1974) and New York (Shore et al, 1976) have been found to experience an increased incidence of brain tumor, both benign and malignant, during adulthood. The magnitude of the association was greatest for nerve sheath tumors (relative risk of 33), intermediate for meningioma (relative risk around 10), and lowest for glioma (relative risk of 2.6) (Ron et al, 1988). The strength of the association was consistently greater for benign tumors (Little et al, 1998). The same pattern of association has been seen in adults treated for pituitary adenomas (Brada et al, 1992; Tsang et al, 1993), in infants treated with x-rays for thymic enlargement (Hildreth et al, 1985), and in children given x-ray therapy for tonsil hypertrophy (Schneider et al, 1985). These studies provide a clear indication that ionizing radiation is capable of causing both benign and malignant tumors of the brain, but the exact nature of the dose–response gradient is not clear.

A series of investigations by Preston-Martin and colleagues (1980, 1982, 1983, 1989a, 1989b) indicate fairly strong associations between dental x-rays and meningiomas, acoustic neuromas, and gliomas, with relative risk estimates on the order of 2 to 4. In contrast, Ryan et al (1992b) found an inverse association of diagnostic x-rays with adult gliomas, whereas other studies (Burch et al, 1987; Schlehofer et al, 1992) reported no association.

Occupational exposure to radiation has also been evaluated, with mixed results. Increases in risk have been found in a number of groups with the potential for elevated exposure to ionizing radiation (Wilkinson et al, 1987; Checkoway et al, 1988), but the large pooled studies of nuclear industry workers revealed no association (Gilbert et al, 1993; Carpenter et al, 1994).

The most informative and widely accepted exposure-response estimates relating ionizing radiation to brain cancer come from the follow-up study of atomic bomb survivors (Preston et al, 2002). This is a very large population (> 80 000 persons) with clearly quantified dose information and detailed cancer incidence data, although the nature of the acute, high-dose exposure and other aspects of this cohort may limit generalizability. For nervous system tumors in the aggregate, the excess relative risk per Sievert is 1.2 (95% CI 0.6 to 2.1). Corresponding estimates are 0.56 (95% CI -0.2 to 2.0) for gliomas, 0.64 (95% CI -0.01 to 1.8) for menigioma, a notably higher 4.5 (95% CI 1.9 to 9.2) for schwannomas, with some indication of greater effect among males for all tumor types.

The circumstances in which high doses of ionizing radiation are encountered are limited, which makes the overall contribution of high-dose ionizing radiation to brain tumor incidence modest, and of decreasing importance over time with the reduced use of radiation for benign conditions (Inskip et al, 1995). Whether low-dose exposures cause brain cancer is unclear, but it is unlikely to have a major influence on brain tumor etiology at the population level.

Occupation

A promising set of leads regarding exogenous factors is occupational exposure to solvents and electromagnetic fields. There is a large, somewhat diffuse literature on a wide range of occupations and occupational exposures in relation to brain tumors (Wrensch et al, 1993). An abundant number of studies with limited power have reported isolated associations with one job or another (eg, Olin et al, 1987; Brownson et al, 1990; Kaplan et al, 1997b; Cocco et al, 1999), and a critical review of the earlier studies has been published (Thomas and Waxweiler, 1986). The topics discussed in the following are those for which there is some convergence of the literature.

Vinyl chloride

Summarizing a series of studies, Thomas and Waxweiler (1986) reported positive associations between occupational exposure to vinyl chloride and brain tumor risk, with relative risks in the range of 1.5 to 5.0. Some, but not all, of the more recent studies tend to support a possible positive association (Hagmar et al, 1990; Simonato et al, 1991; Wong et al, 1991). Given experimental support for an effect of vinyl chloride and these generally positive epidemiologic findings, the possible role of this agent in the etiology of adult brain tumors warrants attention.

Petrochemical workers

Since the mid-1970s, at least 15 studies have evaluated cancer among workers in the petroleum refining and petrochemical industries. The primary focus in those occupational studies has been solvent exposure, an association addressed specifically in some community-based studies as well (Rodvall et al, 1996). Among the petrochemical industry studies are several that report positive but imprecise associations between the potential for chemical exposure and brain tumor incidence or mortality (Thériault and Goulet, 1979; Thomas et al, 1982; Austin and Schnatter, 1983; Waxweiler et al, 1983; Teta et al, 1991). A number of studies of roughly comparable quality, however, fail to corroborate this pattern (Wen et al, 1983; Wong et al, 1986; Marsh et al, 1991). The challenge in interpreting these studies is to identify whether there is some aspect of petrochemical industry employment or exposure that has an etiologic relationship with brain tumors in the aggregate or with subsets of brain cancer.

The difficulty in summarizing the evidence is that some association may be present, but little progress has been made toward pinpointing the exact exposure that could be responsible or the type of brain tumor most likely to be affected. Some reviewers draw a more reserved conclusion about the presence of an increased risk (Wong and Raabe, 1989). Reports vary markedly in whether they are based on a broad census grouping of occupations associated with petroleum and coal products (McLaughlin et al, 1987), refinery workers (Thériault and Goulet, 1979; Wen et al, 1983; Demers et al, 1991), or a mixture of refinery and related chemical workers (Thomas et al, 1980; Marsh et al, 1991; Teta et al, 1991). The lack of specificity in exposure makes it difficult to compare studies or for the research to build momentum toward elucidating an etiologic pathway.

Electrical workers

Conclusions by reviewers of this literature range from perceived support for a weak association between occupational electric and magnetic fields and brain tumors (Kheifets et al, 1995; Wrensch et al, 1993), to a more reserved interpretation of the overall evidence (Inskip et al, 1995). Regardless of the eventual conclusion, the reported relative risks rarely exceed 2.0 and are more often in the very ambiguous range of 1.2 to 1.5. In this range, the potential for some form of selection bias for employment in electrical occupations is difficult to exclude (Kheifets et al, 1995). Early studies were based largely on job titles on death certificates, cancer registries, or community-based case-control studies (Kheifets et al, 1995), often with no explicit effort to examine exposure to electromagnetic fields. However, the sophistication of exposure assessment has risen steadily in both occupational-cohort studies (Sahl et al, 1993; Thériault et al, 1994; Savitz and Loomis, 1995; Harrington et al, 1997) and case-control studies, primarily in Sweden (Floderus et al, 1993; Feychting et al, 1997) and in Canada (Villeneuve et al, 2002).

Early studies generated some strikingly positive findings (Lin et al, 1985; Speers et al, 1988), as well as null results (Pearce et al, 1989). Among the largest, most detailed studies, the findings continue to vary, with suggestions of an association in some (Savitz and Loomis, 1995; Thériault et al, 1994) but not all (Sahl et al, 1993; Harrington et al, 1997) of the cohort studies of electric utility workers. A pooled analysis of several of these studies identified a weak positive gradient in risk, with relative risk estimates rarely exceeding 2.0 even at the most elevated exposure levels (Kheifets et al, 1999).

The category of *electrical workers* is quite diverse, encompassing welders, construction electricians, electric utility linemen, and electrical equipment operators, and there is little consistency across studies in who is included under this rubric. Efforts to identify occupational risks of brain tumors could be more productive if specific jobs were evaluated. The diversity of exposures encountered within any one of these jobs, let alone among the aggregation of electrical workers, is extensive and includes a wide range of solvents and polychlorinated biphenyls. Despite the inability to determine whether electric and magnetic fields or some other aspect of the workplace of electrical workers is related to brain tumors, there are some clues encouraging the pursuit of this research area.

Polychlorinated biphenyls
Polychlorinated biphenyls were manufactured for a variety of industrial applications, and, because of their persistence in the environment and slow excretion in humans, their long-term health effects, including cancer, have been of concern. The epidemiologic evidence for occupational exposure to polychlorinated biphenyls and cancer, including brain cancer, was summarized by Longnecker et al (1997). Data from a series of occupational studies, all with nine or fewer cases, were pooled together, yielding a relative risk of 1.3 (95% CI 0.8–2.0), thus providing little evidence of an increased risk of brain cancer. However, at least one of the included studies observed 9 brain cancer cases compared to 2.9 expected (Yassi et al, 1994). The largest study to date of electric utility workers potentially exposed to polychlorinated biphenyls in transformer maintenance and repair (Loomis et al, 1997) found some support for an association between greater presumed exposure and an increased risk of dying from brain cancer—with relative

risks on the order of 1.6 to 1.8—although there were no cases in the uppermost exposure category.

Health professions
Health professionals, including physicians (McLaughlin et al, 1987; Preston-Martin, 1989), dentists (Ahlbom et al, 1986), pathologists (Hall et al, 1991), veterinarians (Blair and Hayes, 1980), and mixed groups of health care industry workers (Thomas et al, 1986; McLaughlin et al, 1987) have an increased incidence of brain tumors. Even if this increased incidence can be ascribed in part to the presumably better access of health care workers to health services, there must be a concern that it reflects incomplete diagnosis in the population at large. On the other hand, health care workers are likely to have higher exposure to ionizing radiation and to a wide range of potentially toxic agents such as anesthetics, solvents, and pharmaceuticals.

Agriculture and pesticides
Several investigators have reported an elevated risk of brain tumors among agricultural workers (Blair et al, 1985; Musicco et al, 1988; Reif et al, 1989). The magnitude of the increase is inconsistent and generally modest, but the replication of this finding suggests that a clue to the etiology may be present. A meta-analysis, including 33 studies published in the 1980s and 1990s (Khuder et al, 1998), found a 30% excess risk of brain tumors among farmers. There are many aspects of lifestyle and occupational exposure that could distinguish agricultural workers, such as reduced contact with some contagious infectious agents in rural areas, as well as a direct link to specific pesticides or some other occupational hazard. Several studies have focused more directly on specific pesticides (Musicco et al, 1982, 1988; Ahlbom et al, 1986), but much work is needed to pinpoint or exonerate specific agents.

Rubber and tire industry
A series of studies from the 1960s through the 1980s considered brain tumor incidence

and mortality among rubber industry workers. Several of them reported marked but extremely imprecise elevations in risk (Mancuso, 1963; Mancuso et al, 1968; Monson and Fine, 1978; Preston-Martin et al, 1989a), while other, methodologically similar studies found no support for an association (Fox et al, 1974; McLaughlin et al, 1987; Sorahan et al, 1989). As the technology and industrial hygiene of the rubber industry have changed, the older studies are of limited value in present-day evaluation of risks. As with petrochemical workers, the number of positive reports lends some credence to the hypothesis that agents encountered at some time in the past in the rubber industry may be a cause of brain tumors, but it is difficult to be more specific or to make progress beyond this general and vague conclusion.

Medical Conditions and Treatment

Several studies have indicated that persons with epilepsy and those who receive anticonvulsant drugs to treat their epilepsy are at increased risk of developing brain tumors (White et al, 1979; Shirts et al, 1986; Olsen et al, 1989; Schlehofer et al, 1992; Wrensch et al, 1997a). However, there is reason to suspect that epilepsy is a consequence rather than a cause of the brain tumor, particularly since the increased risk is most pronounced when a diagnosis of epilepsy and the development of brain cancer are close together in time.

Sporadic findings for other diseases in relation to brain cancer include a reduced risk among diabetics in some but not all studies (Schlehofer et al, 1992; Cicuttini et al, 1997), a reduced risk associated with reported infections and colds (Schlehofer et al, 1992), and an increased risk among patients with multiple sclerosis (Reagen and Freeman, 1973). Allergic diseases have been reported to be inversely associated with the risk of glioma (Ryan et al, 1992a; Schlehofer et al, 1992), but not in all studies (Cicuttini et al, 1997).

Meningiomas have been found to be positively associated with breast cancer (Helseth et al, 1989; Knuckey et al, 1989),

suggesting a possible role of hormones in the etiology of this nonmalignant brain tumor, which would be consistent with the increased risk among women compared to men.

Other Risk Factors

Head trauma

Head trauma has been evaluated in a number of studies as a potential risk factor for the development of brain tumors, but a causal relationship seems unlikely.

Because of the impression among the public that a link between head trauma and brain cancer might exist, there is great concern about recall bias; brain tumor patients or their families might overreport or perhaps remember such events more completely than persons not affected by brain tumors. The strategy to minimize this potential bias has been to focus on more severe, documented head trauma, such as injury resulting in loss of consciousness or in medical treatment. When those stringent criteria are applied, an association, albeit modest, generally remains (Ahlbom et al, 1986; Burch et al, 1987; Choi et al, 1970a). Most studies have focused on malignant gliomas (Hu et al, 1998), but head trauma has also been associated with the risk of meningiomas (Preston-Martin et al, 1980, 1983). In a large prospective study of patients hospitalized due to brain injury in Sweden, however, the relative risk of all brain tumors was 1.0. Separate analyses by severity of trauma, duration of follow-up, and main histopathologic type consistently indicated a lack of association (Nygren et al, 2001).

One proposed biological mechanism for the speculative link between head traumas and the risk of brain tumors is that tissue repair after trauma requires increased cellular division, which could lead to an increased risk of genetic changes, with possible activation of cellular oncogenes (Preston-Martin et al, 1990). Another suggested mechanism is cocarcinogenic action through inflammation in conjunction with foreign material (Barnett et al, 1986). Along similar lines, an association between acoustic trauma in the form of loud noise and acoustic neuromas has been reported (Preston-Martin et al, 1989b).

Nonoccupational electric and magnetic field exposure

In contrast to the sizable and weakly positive results of occupational studies, there is little basis for further studies of residential magnetic fields and brain tumors.

Several studies has examined the role of magnetic fields encountered in homes and through the use of electric appliances in relation to brain cancer. While much of this research has focused on childhood brain tumors, a few studies have considered adult brain tumors. The review by Li et al (1996) identified only four studies of residential magnetic field exposure and adult brain tumors, two of which were too small to be informative. Of the other two, one reported a positive association between wire code and central nervous system tumors (Wertheimer and Leeper, 1982), and the other reported no association (Feychting and Ahlbom, 1994).

Drinking water disinfection by-products

Although most research on the possible carcinogenicity induced by the chlorination of public drinking water supplies has focused on bladder and colorectal cancers, there are studies that suggest a potential association with brain cancer as well (Cantor et al, 1978; Young et al, 1981; Gottlieb and Carr, 1982). A later study by Cantor et al (1999) provided perhaps the strongest evidence to date for such an association based on the quality of the methods and the observation of a dose–response gradient, although the association was limited to men.

Cellular telephones

It is unlikely that the use of cellular telephones causes brain tumors (Trichopoulos and Adami, 2001), with certainty tempered primarily by the short interval since such devices have become widely used and by the rapidly changing technology in this industry, which results in changing exposure characteristics. Cellular telephones emit low-power electromagnetic radiation in the radiofrequency range, which hypothetically could slightly increase the temperature of exposed tissue and through this mechanism impact human health. A possible role for cellular telephones in brain cancer stems mainly from anecdotal case reports that frequent users of cellular telephones happened to die from brain tumors. However, epidemiologic evidence did not support a causal association. In a large case-control study conducted in the United States, no association was found between cellular telephones, on the one hand, and the risk of glioma, meningioma, or acoustic neuroma, on the other (Inskip et al, 2001). Moreover, there was no indication of an effect on the risk of any brain tumor with either increasing daily use or cumulative use of cellular telephones. Microwave radiation is dispersed rapidly upon tissue entry, which would support specificity in the site of brain tumors if cellular telephones did indeed cause cancer. However, in this study there was no association between laterality of telephone use and laterality of the tumor. The findings of other large studies in the US and Europe also suggest lack of association between cellular telephone use and brain cancer risk (Muscat, 2000; Johansen et al, 2001; Auvinen et al, 2002).

RISK FACTORS FOR CHILDHOOD BRAIN TUMORS

As in adults, brain tumors in children include a diverse array of histologic types, with astrocytomas most common (around half of all tumors), followed by primitive neuroectodermal tumors, other gliomas, and ependymomas (Ries et al, 1999). As in adults, the only established risk factor is high-dose ionizing radiation to the head (Ron et al, 1988). Also, in parallel with studies of adult tumors, N-nitroso compounds in the form of cured meats and nitrosable drugs are of interest as potential contributors, with inconsistent support found in a small number of epidemiologic studies (Gurney et al, 2001). A sizable number of studies have evaluated pesticide exposure, magnetic fields, and parental occupational exposures, but in no case has there been clear support for an etiologic effect (Ross and Spector, 2006). Methodologic limitations, most notably regarding exposure assessment, hinder conclusions regarding environmental agents. Given the limited understanding of the etiology of brain tumors in both children and adults, the question of whether risk factors are shared or distinct remains unresolved.

CONCLUSION

The epidemiologic study of brain cancer faces distinct challenges due to the diverse histologic types and the possibility of incomplete diagnosis. Rates tend to be higher in North America and western Europe than in Asia and South America. Genetic syndromes account for a very small proportion of cases. Studies of such lifestyle factors as tobacco, alcohol, and diet have yielded inconsistent results and an overall impression that little or no association exists. The only established exogenous cause of brain cancer is ionizing radiation, as demonstrated in populations exposed to high doses by the atomic bomb or medical treatment, accounting for only a small proportion of cases. However, studies of populations with lower exposures incurred through occupation or diagnostic x-rays provide mixed findings regarding an increased risk of brain cancer.

A number of leads have been reported regarding associations with occupation, notably vinyl chloride exposure, petrochemical industry occupations, electrical industry occupations, polychlorinated biphenyl exposure, health professions, agriculture/pesticides, and the rubber and tire industry. In each instance, there is replicated evidence of an association with an increased risk of brain cancer, justifying continued research. Nonetheless, because of contradictory findings, small relative risks, and methodologic limitations, none of these associations with work setting or putative agent can be considered to have been established. Cellular telephones have come to

be of concern as a potential cause of brain cancer, but several large, well-designed studies have found no empirical evidence to suggest that the use of cell phones is associated with an increased risk. The literature on risk factors for childhood brain tumors has focused on N-nitroso compounds and selected environmental agents, with limited support for associations.

Hence, with the possible exception of a few leads from studies of occupational exposure to solvents, electromagnetic fields, and dietary nitrosamines, the epidemiologic study of brain cancer has not been successful in identifying modifiable causes that could prevent its occurrence. The reasons for this limited success may lie in the substantial diversity of subtypes of this tumor, as well as in the challenges of interviewing cases with a disease that has an impact on memory and communication. Perhaps with the continuing advances in noninvasive imaging technology, refinements in registration and resulting descriptive epidemiology, improved biological markers for infectious agents and other potential contributors, as well as unrelenting public concern, it will be possible to develop novel hypotheses accelerating the rate of progress.

REFERENCES

Abramson ZH, Kark JD. Serum cholesterol and primary brain tumours: a case-control study. Br J Cancer 1985;52:93–98.

Ahlbom A, Navier IL, Norell S, Olin R Spannare B. Nonoccupational risk indicators for astrocytomas in adults. Am J Epidemiol 1986; 124:334–37.

Austin SG, Schnatter AR. A case-control study of chemical exposures and brain tumors in petrochemical workers. J Occup Med 1983;25:313–20.

Auvinen A, Hietanen M, Luukkonen R, Koskela R-S. Brain tumors and salivary gland cancers among cellular telephone users. Epidemiology 2002; 13:356–59.

Barnett GH, Chou SM, Bay JW. Posttraumatic intracranial meningioma: a case report and review of the literature. Neurosurgery 1986; 18(1):75–78.

Bellur SN, Chandra V, Anderson RJ. Association of meningiomas with obesity [letter]. Ann Neurol 1983;13:346–47.

Blair A, Hayes HM Jr. Cancer and other causes of death among U.S. veterinarians. Int J Cancer 1980;25:181–85.

Blair A, Malker H, Cantor KP, Burmeister L, Wiklund K. Cancer among farmers: a review. Scand J Work Environ Health 1985;11:397–407.

Blowers L, Preston-Martin S, Mack WJ. Dietary and other lifestyle factors of women with brain gliomas in Los Angeles County (California, USA). Cancer Causes Control 1997; 8:5–12.

Boeing H, Schlehofer B, Blettner M, Wahrendorf J. Dietary carcinogens and the risk for glioma and meningioma in Germany. Int J Cancer 1993;53:561–65.

Brada M, Ford D, Ashley S, Bliss JM, Crowley S, Mason M. Risk of second brain tumour after conservative surgery and radiotherapy for pituitary adenoma. Br Med J 1992;304:1343–46.

Brownson RC, Reif JS, Chang JC, Davis JR. An analysis of occupational risks for brain cancer. Am J Public Health 1990;80:169–72.

Burch JD, Craib KJP, Choi BCK, Miller AB, Risch HA, Howe GR. An exploratory case-control study of brain tumors in adults. J Natl Cancer Inst 1987;78:601–9.

Cantor KP, Hoover R, Mason TJ, McCabe LJ. Associations of cancer mortality with halomethanes in drinking water. J Natl Cancer Inst 1978;61:979–85.

Cantor KP, Lynch CF, Hildesheim ME, Dosemeci M, Lubin J, Alavanja M, et al. Drinking water source and chlorination byproducts in Iowa. III. Risk of brain cancer. Am J Epidemiol 1999;150:552–60.

Carpenter L, Higgins C, Douglas A, Fraser P, Beral V, Smith P. Combined analyses of mortality in three United Kingdom nuclear industry workforces, 1946–1988. Radiat Res 1994;138:224–38.

Central Brain Tumor Registry of the United States. Statistical Report: Primary Brain Tumors in the United States, 1998–2002. Chicago, Central Brain Tumor Registry of the United States (pub.), 2005.

Checkoway H, Pearce N, Crawford-Brown DJ, Cragle DL. Radiation doses and cause-specific mortality among workers at a nuclear materials fabrication plant. Am J Epidemiol 1988;127:255–66.

Choi NW, Schuman LM, Gullen WH. Epidemiology of primary central nervous system neoplasms. I. Mortality from primary central nervous system neoplasms in Minnesota. Am J Epidemiol 1970a;91:238–59.

Choi NW, Schuman LM, Gullen WH. Epidemiology of primary central nervous system neoplasms. II. Case-control study. Am J Epidemiol 1970b;91:467–85.

Cicuttini FM, Hurley SF, Forbes A, Donnan GA, Salzberg M, Giles GG, et al. Association of adult glioma with medical conditions, family and reproductive history. Int J Cancer 1997; 71:203–7.

Cocco P, Heineman EF, Dosemeci M. Occupational risk factors for cancer of the central nervous system (CNS) among US women. Am J Ind Med 1999;36:70–74.

Davis DL, Schwartz J. Trends in cancer mortality: U.S. white males and females, 1968–83. Lancet 1988;1:633–36.

Demers PA, Vaughan TL, Schommer RR. Occupation, socioeconomic status, and brain tumor mortality: a death certificate-based case-control study. J Occup Med 1991;33:1001–6.

Ernster WL, Sacks ST, Selvin S, Petrakis NL. Cancer incidence by marital status: US Third National Cancer Survey. J Natl Cancer Inst 1979;63:567–85.

Feychting M, Ahlbom A. Magnetic fields, leukemia, and central nervous system tumors in Swedish adults residing near high-voltage power lines. Epidemiology 1994;5:501–9.

Feychting M, Forssén U, Floderus B: Occupational and residential magnetic field exposure and leukemia and central nervous system tumors. Epidemiology 1997;8:384–89.

Floderus B, Persson T, Stenlund C, Wennberg A, Ost A, Knave B. Occupational exposure to electromagnetic fields in relation to leukemia and brain tumors: a case-control study in Sweden. Cancer Causes Control 1993;4:465–76.

Fox AJ, Lindars DC, Owen R. A survey of occupational cancer in the rubber and cable-making industries: results of five year analysis, 1967–71. Br J Ind Med 1974;31:140–51.

Gilbert ES, Cragle DL, Wiggs LD. Updated analyses of combined mortality data for workers at the Hanford Site, Oak Ridge National Laboratory, and Rocky Flats Weapons Plant. Radiat Res 1993;136:408–21.

Giles GG. What do we know about risk factors for glioma? Cancer Causes Control 1997; 8:3–4.

Giles GG, McNeil JJ, Donnan G, Webley C, Staples MP, Ireland PD, et al. Dietary factors and the risk of glioma in adults: results of a case-control study in Melbourne, Australia. Int J Cancer 1994;59:357–62.

Gottleib MS, Carr JK. Case-control cancer mortality study and chlorination of drinking water in Louisiana. Environ Health Perspect 1982;46:169–77.

Gurney JG, Smith MA, Olshan AF, et al. Clues to the etiology of childhood brain cancer: N-nitroso compounds, polyomaviruses, and other factors of interest. Cancer Invest 2001; 19:630–40.

Hagmar L, Akesson B, Nielsen J, Andersson C, Linden K, Attewell R, et al. Mortality and cancer morbidity in workers exposed to low levels of vinyl chloride monomer at a polyvinyl chloride processing plant. Am J Ind Med 1990;17:553–65.

Hall A, Harrington JM, Aw TC. Mortality study of British pathologists. Am J Ind Med 1991; 20:83–89.

Harrington JM, McBride DI, Sorahan T, Paddle GM, van Tongeren M. Occupational exposure to magnetic fields in relation to mortality from brain cancer among electricity generation and transmission workers. Occup Environ Med 1997;54:7–13.

Helseth A, Mork SJ, Glattre E. Neoplasms of the central nervous system in Norway. V. Meningioma and cancer of other sites: an analysis of the occurrence of multiple primary neoplasms in meningioma patients in Norway from 1955 through 1986. APMAS 1989;97:738–44.

Hildreth NG, Shore RE, Hempelmann LH, Rosenstein M. Risk of extrathyroid tumors following radiation treatment in infancy for thymic enlargement. Radiat Res 1985;102:378–91.

Hirayama T. Cancer mortality in nonsmoking women with smoking husbands based on a large scale cohort study in Japan. Prev Med 1984;13:680–90.

Hu J, Johnson KC, Mao Y, Guo L, Zhao X, Jia X, et al. Risk factors for glioma in adults: a case-control study in northeast China. Cancer Detect Prev 1998;22:100–8.

Hu J, La Vecchia C, Negri E, Chatenoud L, Bosetti C, Jia X, et al. Diet and brain cancer in adults: a case-control study in northeast China. Int J Cancer 1999;81:20–23.

Huncharek M, Kupelnick B, Wheeler L. Dietary cured meat and the risk of adult glioma: a meta-analysis of nine observational studies. J Environ Pathol Toxicol Oncol 2003;22:129–37.

Inskip PD, Linet MS, Heineman EF. Etiology of brain tumors in adults. Epidemiol Rev 1995; 17:382–414.

Inskip PD, Tarone RE, Hatch EE, Wilcosky TC, Shapiro WR, Selker RG, et al. Cellular telephone use and brain tumors. N Engl J Med 2001;344:79–86.

Johansen C, Boice JD Jr, McLaughlin JK, Olsen JH. Cellular telephones and cancer—a nationwide cohort study in Denmark. J Natl Cancer Inst 2001;93:203–7.

Kaplan S, Etlin S, Novikov I, Modan B. Nutritional factors in the etiology of brain tumors. Potential role of nitrosamines, fat, and cholesterol. Am J Epidemiol 1997a;146:832–41.

Kaplan S, Etlin S, Novikov I, Modan B. Occupational risks for the development of brain tumors. Am J Ind Med 1997b;31:15–20.

Kheifets LI, Afifi AA, Buffler PA, Zhang ZW. Occupational electric and magnetic field exposure and brain cancer: a meta-analysis. J Occup Environ Med 1995;37:1327–41.

Kheifets LI, Gilbert ES, Sussman SS, Guénel P, Sahl JD, Savitz DA, Thériault G. Comparative analyses of the studies of magnetic fields and cancer in electric utility workers: studies from France, Canada, and the United States. Occup Environ Med 1999;56:567–74.

Khuder SA, Mutgi AB, Schaub EA. Meta-analyses of brain cancer and farming. Am J Ind Med 1998;34:252–60.

Knuckey NW, Stoll J Jr, Epstein MH. Intracranial and spinal meningiomas in patients with breast carcinoma: case reports. Neurosurgery 1989;25:112–17.

Lai R, Crevier L, Thabane L. Genetic polymorphisms of glutathione-S-transferases and the risk of adult brain tumors: a meta-analysis. Cancer Epidemiol Biomark Prev 2005;14:1784–90.

Lee M, Wrensch M, Miike R. Dietary and tobacco risk factors for adult onset glioma in the San Francisco Bay Area (California, USA). Cancer Causes Control 1997;8:13–24.

Li C-Y, Thériault G, Lin RS. Epidemiological appraisal of studies of residential exposure to power frequency magnetic fields and adult cancers. Occup Environ Med 1996;53:505–10.

Li Y, Millikan RC, Carozza S, Newman B, Liu E, Davis R, et al. p53 mutations in malignant glioma. Cancer Epidemiol Biomarkers Prev 1998;7:303–8.

Lin RS, Dischinger PC, Conde J, Farrell KP. Occupational exposure to electromagnetic fields and the occurrence of brain tumors: an analysis of possible associations. J Occup Med 1985;276:413–19.

Little MP, de Vathaire F, Shamsaldin A, Oberlin O, Campbell S, Grimaud E, et al. Risks of brain tumour following treatment for cancer in childhood: modification by genetic factors, radiotherapy and chemotherapy. Int J Cancer 1998;78:269–75.

Longnecker MP, Rogan WJ, Lucier G. The human health effects of DDT (dichlorodiphenyltrichloroethane) and PCBs (polychlorinated biphenyls) and an overview of organochlorines and public health. Annu Rev Public Health 1997;18:211–44.

Loomis D, Browning SR, Schenck AP, Gregory E, Savitz DA. Cancer mortality among electric utility workers exposed to polychlorinated biphenyls. Occup Environ Med 1997;54:720–28.

Lyon JL, Klauber MR, Gardner JW, Smart CR. Cancer incidence in Mormons and non-Mormons in Utah, 1966–70. N Engl J Med 1976;294:129–33.

Mancuso TF. Tumors of the central nervous system: industrial considerations. Acta UN Int Cancer 1963;19:488–89.

Mancuso TF, Ciocco A, El-Attar AA. An epidemiological approach to the rubber industry: a study based on departmental experience. J Occup Med 1968;10:213–32.

Marsh GM, Enterline PE, McCraw D. Mortality patterns among petroleum refinery and chemical plant workers. Am J Ind Med 1991; 19:29–42.

McLaughlin JK, Malker HSR, Blot W, Malker BK, Stone BJ, Weiner JA, et al. Occupational risks for intracranial gliomas in Sweden. J Natl Cancer Inst 1987;67:253–57.

Mills PK, Preston-Martin S, Annegers JF, Beeson WL, Phillips RL, Fraser GE. Risk factors for tumors of the brain and cranial meninges in Seventh-Day Adventists. Neuroepidemiology 1989;8:266–75.

Modan B, Baidatz D, Mart H, Steinitz R, Levin SG. Radiation induced head and neck tumors. Lancet 1974;1:277–79.

Monson RR, Fine LJ. Cancer mortality and morbidity among rubber workers. J Natl Cancer Inst 1978;61:1047–53.

Muscat JE, Malkin M, Thompson S, Shore RE, Stellman SD, McRee D, et al. Handheld cellular telephone use and risk of brain cancer. JAMA 2000;284:3001–7.

Musicco M, Filipini G, Bordo BM, Melotto A, Morello G, Berrino F. Gliomas and occupational exposure to carcinogens: case-control study. Am J Epidemiol 1982;116:782–90.

Musicco M, Sant M, Molinari S, Filippini G, Gatta G, Berrino F. A case-control study of brain gliomas and occupational exposure to chemical carcinogens: the risk to farmers. Am J Epidemiol 1988;128:778–85.

Neugut AI, Fink DJ, Radin D. Serum cholesterol and primary brain tumours: a case-control study. Int J Epidemiol 1989;18: 798–801.

Newill V. A distribution of cancer mortality among ethnic subgroups of the white population of New York City. J Natl Cancer Inst 1961;26:405–17.

Nygren C, Adami J, Ye W, Bellocco R, af Geijerstam JL, Borg J, et al. Primary brain tumors following traumatic brain injury—a population-based cohort study in Sweden. Cancer Causes Control 2001;12:733–37.

Olin RG, Ahlbom A, Lindberg-Navier I, Norell SE, Spännare B. Occupational factors associated with astrocytomas: a case-control study. Am J Ind Med 1987;11:615–25.

Olsen JH, Boice JD Jr, Jensen JPA, Frumeni JF Jr. Cancer among epileptic patients exposed to anticonvulsant drugs. J Natl Cancer Inst 1989;81:803–8.

Parkin DM, Whelan SL, Ferlay J, Storm H. Cancer Incidence in 5 Continents—CI5-ADDS version 1. 2005 IARCPress, Lyon, France.

Pearce N, Reig, J, Fraser J. Case-control studies of cancer in New Zealand electrical workers. Int J Epidemiol 1989;18:55–59.

Preston DL, Ron E, Yonehara S, Kobuke T, Fujii H, Kishikawa M, et al. Tumors of the nervous system and pituitary gland associated with atomic bomb radiation exposure. J Natl Cancer Inst 2002;94:1555–63.

Preston-Martin S. Descriptive epidemiology of primary tumors of the brain, cranial nerves and cranial meninges in Los Angeles County. Neuroepidemiology 1989;8:283–95.

Preston-Martin S, Lewis S, Winkelmann R, Borman B, Auld J, Pearce N. Descriptive epidemiology of primary cancer of the brain, cranial nerves, and cranial meninges in New Zealand, 1948–1988. Cancer Causes Control 1993;4:529–38.

Preston-Martin S, Mack W. Gliomas and meningiomas in men in Los Angeles County: investigation of exposures to n-nitroso compounds. In: O'Neill IK, et al (Eds): Relevance to Human Cancer of N-Nitroso Compounds, Tobacco Smoke and Mycotoxins. IARC Sci. Pub. No. 105. Lyon, International Agency for Research on Cancer, 1991, pp 1977–1203.

Preston-Martin S, Mack WJ. Neoplasms of the nervous system. In: Schottenfeld D, Fraumeni JF Jr (Eds): Cancer Epidemiology and Prevention, Second Edition. New York, Oxford University Press, 1996, pp 1231–81.

Preston-Martin S, Mack W, Henderson BE. Risk factors for gliomas and meningiomas in males in Los Angeles County. Cancer Res 1989a;49:6137–43.

Preston-Martin S, Paganini-Hill A, Henderson BE, Pike MC, Wood C. Case-control study of intracranial meningiomas in women in Los Angeles County, California. J Natl Cancer Inst 1980;65:67–73.

Preston-Martin S, Pike MC, Ross RK, Jones PA, Henderson BE. Increased cell division as a cause of human cancer. Cancer Res 1990;50(23)7415–21.

Preston-Martin S, Thomas DC, Wright WE, Henderson BE. Noise trauma in the aetiology of acoustic neuromas in men in Los Angeles County, 1978–1985. Br J Cancer 1989b;59: 783–86.

Preston-Martin S, Yu MC, Benton B, Henderson BE. N-nitroso compounds and childhood brain tumors: a case-control study. Cancer Res 1982;42:5240–45.

Preston-Martin S, Yu MC, Henderson BE, Roberts C. Risk factors for meningiomas in men in Los Angeles County. J Natl Cancer Inst 1983:70:863–66.

Reagen TJ, Freeman IS. Multiple cerebral gliomas in multiple sclerosis. J Neurol Neurosurg Psychiatry 1973;36:523–28.

Reif JS, Pearce N, Fraser J. Occupational risks for brain cancer: a New Zealand Cancer Registry-Based Study. J Occup Med 1989; 31:863–67.

Ries LA, Smith MA, Gurney JG, et al. Cancer Incidence and Survival among Children and Adolescents: United States SEER Program, 1975–1995. Bethesda, MD: National Cancer Institute, SEER Program. 1999.

Rodvall Y, Ahlbom A, Spännare B, Nise G. Glioma and occupational exposure in Sweden, a case-control study. Occup Environ Med 1996;53:526–32.

Ron E, Modan B, Boice JD, Alfandary E, Stovall M, Chetrit A, et al. Tumors of the brain and nervous system after radiotherapy in childhood. N Engl J Med 1988;319:1033–39.

Ross JA, Spector LG. Cancer in children. In: D Schottenfeld, JF Fraumeni Jr (Eds): Cancer Epidemiology and Prevention, Third Edition. New York, NY: Oxford University Press, 2006, pp 1251–68.

Ryan P, Hurley SF, Johnson AM, Salzberg M, Lee MW, North JB, et al. Tumours of the brain and presence of antibodies to Toxoplasma gondii. Int J Epidemiol 1993;22: 412–19.

Ryan P, Lee MS, North JB, McMichael AJ. Risk factors for tumors of the brain and meninges: results from The Adelaide Adult Brain Tumor Study. Int J Cancer 1992a;51:20–27.

Ryan P, Lee MW, North B, McMichael AJ. Amalgam fillings, diagnostic dental x-rays and tumors of the brain and meninges. Eur J Cancer 1992b;28B:91–95.

Sahl JD, Kelsh MA, Greenland S. Cohort and nested case-control studies of hematopoietic cancers and brain cancer among electric utility workers. Epidemiology 1993;4: 104–14.

Samuelsen SO, Bakketeig LS, Tretli S, Johannesen TB, Magnus P. Head circumference at birth and risk of brain cancer in childhood: a population-based study. Lancet Oncol. 2006;7:39–42.

Savitz DA, Loomis DP. Magnetic field exposure in relation to leukemia and brain cancer mortality among electric utility workers. Am J Epidemiol 1995;141:123–34.

Schlehofer B, Blettner M, Becker N, Martinsohn C, Wahrendorf J. Medical risk factors and the development of brain tumors. Cancer 1992;69:2541–47.

Schneider AB, Shore-Freedman E, Ryo UY, Bekerman C, Favus M, Pinsky S. Radiation-induced tumors of the head and neck following childhood irradiation. Medicine 1985;64:1–15.

Schuman LM, Choi NW, Gullen WH. Relationship of central nervous system neoplasms to Toxoplasma gondii infection. Am J Public Health 1967;57:848–56.

Seyama S, Ishimaru T, Iijima S, Mori K. Primary intracranial tumors among atomic bomb survivors and controls, Hiroshima and Nagasaki, 1961–1975. Radiat Effects Res Foundation Technical Reports 1979;15:1–19.

Shirts SB, Annegers JF, Houser WA, Kurland LT. Cancer incidence in a cohort of patients with severe seizure disorders. J Natl Cancer Inst 1986;77:83–87.

Shore RE, Albert RE, Pasternack BS. Follow-up study of patients treated by x-ray epilation for tinea capitis. Arch Environ Health 1976;31:17–24.

Simonato L, L-Abbe KA, Anderson A, Belli S, Comba P, Engholm G. A collaborative study of cancer incidence and mortality among vinyl chloride workers. Scand J Work Environ Health 1991;17:156–69.

Sorahan T, Parkes HG, Veys CA. Mortality in the British rubber industry, 1946–85. Br J Ind Med 1989;314:1010–15.

Speers MA, Dobbins JG, Miller VS. Occupational exposure and brain cancer mortality: a preliminary study of East Texas residents. Am J Ind Med 1988;13:629–38.

Stephens T. Special section: cancer. A mixed bag of cancer trends. J NIH Res 1991;3:71–72.

Strang RR, Tovi D, Lopez J. Astrocytomas and the ABO blood groups. J Med Genet 1966; 3:274–75.

Teta MJ, Ott MG, Schnatter AR. An update of mortality due to brain neoplasms and other causes among employees of a petrochemical facility. J Occup Med 1991;33:45–51.

Thériault G, Goldberg M, Miller AB, Armstrong B, Guénel P, Deadman J, et al. Cancer risks associated with occupational exposure to magnetic fields among electric utility workers in Ontario and Quebec, Canada, and France: 1970–1989. Am J Epidemiol 1994;139:550–72.

Thériault G, Goulet L. A mortality study of oil refinery workers. J Occup Med 1979;21: 367–70.

Thomas TL, DeCoufle P, Moure-Eraso R. Mortality among workers employed in petroleum refining and petrochemical plants. J Occup Med 1980;22:97–103.

Thomas TL, Waxweiler RJ. Brain tumors and occupational risk factors: a review. Scand J Work Environ Health 1986; 12:1–15.

Thomas TL, Waxweiler RJ, Moure-Eraso R, Itaya S, Fraumeni JF Jr. Mortality patterns among workers in three Texas oil refineries. J Occup Med 1982;24:135–41.

Trichopoulos D, Adami HO. Cellular telephones and brain tumors. N Engl J Med 2001; 344:133–34.

Tsang RW, Laperriere NJ, Simpson WJ, Brierley J, Panzarella T, Smyth HS. Glioma arising after radiation therapy for pituitary adenoma: a report of four patients and estimation of risk. Cancer 1993;72:2227–33.

Villeneuve PJ, Agnew DA, Johnson KC, Mao Y. Brain cancer and occupational exposure to magnetic fields among men: results from a Canadian population-based case-control study. Int J Epidemiol 2002;31:210–17.

Ward D, Mattison ML, Finn R. Association between previous tuberculosis infection and central glioma. Br Med J 1973;I:83–84.

Ward MH, Heineman EF, McComb RD, Weisenburger DD. Drinking water and dietary sources of nitrate and nitrite and risk of glioma. J Occup Environ Med 2005;47:1260–67.

Waxweiler RJ, Alexander V, Leffingwell SS, Haring M, Lloyd JW. Mortality from brain tumor and other causes in a cohort of petrochemical workers. J Natl Cancer Inst 1983;70:75–81.

Wen CP, Tsai SP, McClellan WA, Gibson RL. Long-term mortality study of oil refinery workers: 1. Mortality of hourly and salaried workers. Am J Epidemiol 1983;118:526–41.

Wertheimer N, Leeper E. Adult cancer related to electrical wires near the home. Int J Epidemiol 1982;11:345–55.

White SJ, McClean AEM, Howland C. Anticonvulsant drugs and cancer: a cohort study in patients with severe epilepsy. Lancet 1979;2:458–60.

Wilkinson GS, Tietjen GL, Wiggs LD, Galke WA, Acquavella JF, Reyes M, et al. Mortality among plutonium and other radiation workers at a plutonium weapons facility. Am J Epidemiol 1987;125:231–50.

Wong O, Morgan RW, Bailey WJ, Swencicki RE, Claxton K, Kheifets L. An epidemiologic study of petroleum refinery employees. Br J Ind Med 1986;43:6–17.

Wong O, Raabe GK. A critical review of cancer epidemiology in studies of petroleum industry employees, with a quantitative meta-analysis by cancer site. Am J Ind Med 1989; 15:283–310.

Wong O, Whorton MD, Foliart DE, Ragland D. An industry-wide epidemiologic study of vinyl chloride workers. Am J Ind Med 1991; 20:317–34.

Wrensch MR, Barger GR. Familial factors associated with malignant gliomas. Genet Epidemiol 1990;7:291–301.

Wrensch M, Bondy ML, Wiencke J, Yost M. Environmental risk factors for primary malignant brain tumors: a review. J Neuro-Oncol 1993;17:47–64.

Wrensch M, Lee M, Miike R, Newman B, Barger G, Davis R, et al. Familial and personal medical history of cancer and nervous system conditions among adults with glioma and controls. Am J Epidemiol 1997a;145:581–93.

Wrensch M, Weinberg A, Wiencke J, Masters H, Miike Ri, Barger G, et al. Does prior infection with varicella-zoster virus influence risk of adult glioma? Am J Epidemiol 1997b;145:594–97.

Yassi A, Tate R, Fish D. Cancer mortality in workers employed at a transformer manufacturing plant. Am J Ind Med 1994;25:425–37.

Yates O, Pearce KM. Recent changes in blood-group distribution of astrocytomas. Lancet 1960;1:194–95.

Young TB, Kanarek MS, Tsiatis AA. Epidemiologic study of drinking water chlorination and Wisconsin female cancer mortality. J Natl Cancer Inst 1981;67:1191–98.

25

Thyroid Cancer

PER HALL AND HANS-OLOV ADAMI

On April 26, 1986, a nuclear reactor at the Chernobyl nuclear power plant in Ukraine exploded, releasing enormous amounts of radioiodine into the environment. The most heavily contaminated areas were southern Belarus, northern Ukraine, and southwestern Russia. Protective actions were not taken immediately, so that individuals living in the heavily contaminated areas received high doses of ionizing radiation, mainly from short-lived radioiodines, to the thyroid gland.

The Chernobyl accident has probably brought thyroid cancer to the attention of epidemiologists and the lay public more than anything else has. As we will see in this chapter, the story behind the reports of an alarming thyroid cancer epidemic among the young is complex. The reason thyroid cancer has attracted limited epidemiologic interest is more obvious; overall, this malignancy is rare and comprises several distinct histopathologic entities, probably with different etiologies. These two features in combination have complicated epidemiologic studies of thyroid cancer, both descriptive and analytic.

CLINICAL SYNOPSIS

Subgroups

Approximately 90% of all thyroid cancers are epithelial. The most common histopathologic type is papillary carcinoma (50% to 80% of the cases), followed by the follicular type (15% to 20%). Medullary carcinoma accounts for less than 10% of all thyroid carcinomas, and a similar fraction comprises anaplastic carcinomas. The papillary, follicular, and anaplastic forms originate from the follicular cells, while medullary carcinoma derives from the parafollicular C cells that produce the hormone calcitonin. The epithelial thyroid carcinomas are also divided into highly differentiated (papillary, follicular, medullary) and poorly differentiated or anaplastic carcinoma.

Symptoms

Most differentiated thyroid cancers present as asymptomatic thyroid nodules. The first sign of thyroid cancer may also be hoarseness, cough, dysphagia, dyspnea, or a lymph node metastasis in the neck region.

636

Diagnosis

Usually a single malignant nodule is not clinically distinguishable from a benign tumor. A hard, irregular finding at palpation, including lymph nodes in the neck region, increases the likelihood of cancer. To confirm the diagnosis, fine-needle aspiration should be used, in selected cases combined with thyroid ultrasonography and thyroid scintigraphy. Sometimes, surgical removal with histopathologic examination of a suggestive tumor is required for definite diagnosis.

Treatment

The initial therapy for differentiated thyroid carcinomas is usually surgery, mostly total thyroidectomy, with or without removal of the regional lymph nodes. Preoperative radiotherapy combined with chemotherapy can be tried in selected patients with large and poorly differentiated carcinomas. To destroy any remaining thyroid tissue, including possible microcarcinomas, radioiodine therapy is occasionally given postoperatively to patients with papillary and follicular carcinomas.

Prognosis

Thyroid cancers range from indolent to extremely aggressive. The overall relative 5-year survival is over 90% in the United States. Mortality occurs mostly among elderly patients dying of anaplastic or poorly differentiated thyroid cancer.

Progress

Room for therapeutic progress exists chiefly for the anaplastic cancers due to their gloomy prognostic outlook following combinations of surgical, radiotherapeutic, and chemotherapeutic treatment. Unfortunately, no such progress is evident. Nor has the treatment of differentiated thyroid cancer changed appreciably over the last decades. There are, however, several ongoing randomized trials searching for the optimal surgery for differentiated thyroid cancer.

DESCRIPTIVE EPIDEMIOLOGY

Detailed understanding of the descriptive epidemiology of thyroid cancer is hampered by the fact that this malignancy comprises several distinct histopathologic entities (Table 25–1), which may have different etiologies, as suggested by the substantial proportional variation in different settings (Table 25–2). Overall, thyroid carcinomas are rare, but they are among the most common cancers in children and young adults. Globally, the incidence rates for thyroid cancer are approximately 1.2 per 100 000 person-years for males and 3.4 for females (http://www-dep.iarc.fr). There is substantial difference in the incidence between different parts of the world both among women (Fig. 25–1) and among men (Fig. 25–2). Thyroid cancer is also substantially more common in the developed compared to the less developed regions of the world (http://www-dep.iarc.fr). Indeed, a 20-fold difference in incidence can be found between developing and western countries, but there is a concern that the lowest reported incidence rates are underestimated due to low diagnostic intensity and/or under notification. An increasing incidence could be interpreted as a true increase in occurrence but may also reflect changing diagnostic criteria or increased diagnostic scrutiny. In the US, thyroid cancer incidence increased from 3.6 per 100 000 in 1973 to 8.7 in 2002 (Davies and Welch, 2006). This trend, completely confined to papillary thyroid cancers, might have arisen due to the changing recognition of nuclear morphological criteria rather than earlier defined architectural structures.

The indolent behavior of the tumor and the availability of health care and screening programs may explain some of the differences in incidence over time and across geographic areas. Changes in diagnostic criteria over time, as well as a high prevalence of differentiated tumors found at autopsy, could further affect the incidence rates.

Even within relatively small geographic regions, incidence varies substantially. In

Table 25–1. Classification and definitions of malignant thyroid tumors

Type of thyroid cancer	Definition
Epithelial Thyroid Cancer	
Papillary carcinoma	Evidence of follicular cell differentiation of papillary and follicular structures, as well as characteristic nuclear changes
Follicular carcinoma	Follicular cell differentiation without the diagnostic features of papillary carcinoma
Undifferentiated/anaplastic carcinoma	Highly malignant tumor composed totally or partly of undifferentiated cells
Medullary carcinoma	Originates from the parafollicular cells
Nonepithelial Thyroid Cancer	
Others	Composed of nonepithelial malignant tumors such as sarcoma, malignant lymphoma, and hemangioendothelioma, the last being highly malignant

the five Nordic countries a sixfold difference is seen among men and tenfold among women (Table 25–3). Rates are highest in Iceland and lowest in Denmark. Some differences in the female-to-male ratio within countries are also obvious (Table 25–3). No convincing explanation exists for this uneven distribution of thyroid cancers in the Nordic countries.

The varying distribution of histopathologic subtypes in different parts of the world (Table 25–2) may be related to differences in diagnostic abilities. Because papillary thyroid cancer is relatively easy to diagnose, its ascertainment is probably more complete than for follicular carcinoma. Difficulty in distinguishing follicular carcinoma from follicular adenoma might entail overreporting of the former entity. In a reevaluation of histophatologic specimens, only 54% of the initially diagnosed follicular carcinomas had a correct diagnosis, in contrast to 98% of the papillary carcinomas (Pettersson et al, 1991). The definition of

Table 25–2. Distribution of thyroid cancer by histopathologic type in selected populations

Study area	Study period	Total no.	Histology (%) Papillary	Follicular	Medullary	Anaplastic	Others
Iceland (Hrafnkelson et al. 1988)	1955–84	392	77	14	1	7	1
Hawaii, USA (Goodman et al. 1988)	1969–84	1,100	74	18	2	1	5
Connecticut, USA (Pottern et al. 1980)	1935–75	1,915	52	13	10	10	15
Sweden* (Pettersson et al. 1991)	1958–81	5,838	49	29	5	18	—

*Did not include nonepithelial thyroid cancers or autopsy cases.

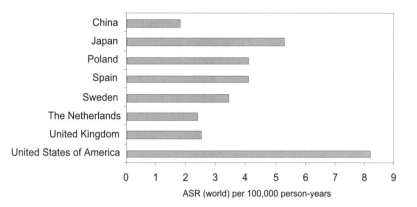

Figure 25–1. Age-standardized (to the world population) incidence rates of thyroid cancer among women. (*Source*: Ferlay et al, 2004)

papillary thyroid carcinoma has widened dramatically over the past years. Today cytologic criteria are more important than the previously used morphologic criteria. For instance, whereas a papillary growth pattern was previously required, tumors with a complete lack of papillae are now denoted papillary carcinomas if psammoma bodies or "ground-glass" nuclei are found.

Thyroid cancer has an unusual age distribution. While rare, it is one of the most common cancers below age 40 years and is diagnosed even before age 20 years. Among women, its incidence increases markedly throughout the reproductive period of life and levels off after age 50 (Fig. 25–3); among men the increase is seen across the life span (Fig. 25–4). This pattern suggests

an impact of hormonal factors, although direct evidence is lacking and other mechanisms have been suggested.

The age-specific incidence of thyroid cancer varies with the subtype. Papillary carcinomas have a wave-like appearance, with a peak incidence at 45 to 55 years for women, while the pattern is less pronounced for men (Ihre-Lundgren et al, 2003). The incidence of follicular carcinomas increases slowly with age and reaches its highest level at around 60 years of age for both men and women. Anaplastic carcinomas are uncommon before the age of 50 years, but their incidence increases with age with no notable difference between men and women.

The female predominance seen in follicular and papillary thyroid cancers peaks just

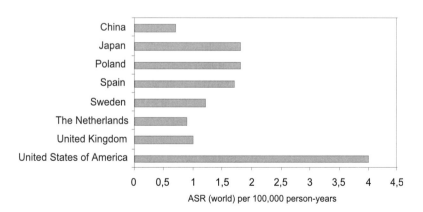

Figure 25–2. Age-standardized (to the world population) incidence rates of thyroid cancer among men. (Source: Ferlay et al, 2004)

Table 25–3. Thyroid cancer incidence rates (per 100,000 person-years) in the five Nordic countries by gender

	Denmark	Finland	Iceland	Norway	Sweden
Males	1.0	1.6	6.1	1.5	1.6
Females	1.6	4.2	15.7	4.2	3.9
Female-male ratio	1.6	2.6	2.6	2.8	2.4

Source: Möller Jensson et al, 1988.

after puberty. It persists as an approximately threefold difference during the fertile period of women and declines thereafter. Swedish data from 2004 (Cancer Incidence in Sweden, 2005) showed a female-to-male ratio of 3.1 during the first 50 years of life and 1.9 for the following period. This difference is not seen in medullary or anaplastic carcinomas (Franssila and Harach, 1986). In other words, the sex difference in overall thyroid cancer incidence seen before 50 years of age is less pronounced at older ages (Figs. 25–3 and 25–4).

GENETIC AND MOLECULAR EPIDEMIOLOGY

Inherited Susceptibility

The proportion of thyroid cancer accounted for by genetic factors was 53%, which is higher than for any other malignancy (Czene et al, 2002).

Several inherited syndromes increase thyroid cancer risk, including multiple endocrine neoplasia (MEN) types 2A and 2B, which is linked to medullary thyroid carcinoma. These syndromes, caused by germ-

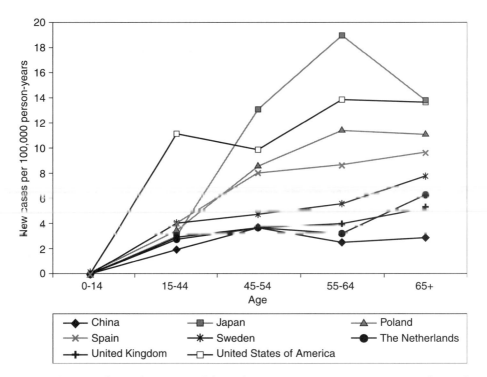

Figure 25–3. Age-specific incidence rates of thyroid cancer among women. (*Source*: Ferlay et al, 2004)

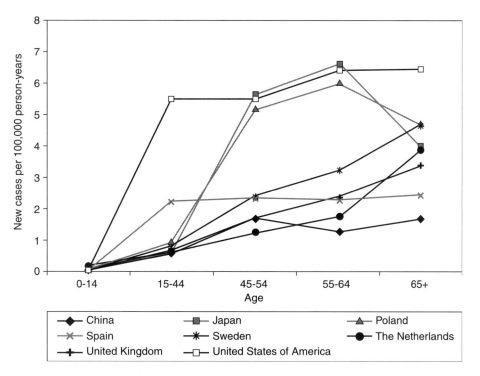

Figure 25–4. Age-specific incidence rates of thyroid cancer among men. (*Source*: Ferlay et al, 2004)

line mutations in the ret proto-oncogene, have an autosomal dominant mode of inheritance with high penetrance and variable expression. Approximately 20% of medullary thyroid cancers are attributed to MEN 2A/B or familial medullary thyroid cancer. Because the cumulative incidence of thyroid cancer among subjects with these syndromes is close to 100%, prophylactic thyroidectomies are often performed (Niccoli-Sire et al, 1999). Other rare familial syndromes associated with an excess risk of thyroid cancer include familial adenomatous polyposis (including Gardner's syndrome), Carney's and Werner's syndromes, and Cowden disease (Stratakis et al, 1997; Lindor et al, 1998). An approximately fivefold increased risk of thyroid cancer has been found among relatives to patients with nonmedullary thyroid cancer (Frich et al, 2001). Data from the Swedish Cancer and Multiple Generation Registries were used to further estimate the familial contri-

bution of thyroid cancer by histopathologic type (Hemminki and Dong, 2000). In the offspring of a thyroid cancer patient, the likelihood of being diagnosed with the same subtype was increased three- to eightfold for differentiated cancer, about 200-fold for anaplastic cancer, and several thousand times for medullary cancer (Table 25–4). The strong relationship for medullary cancer probably reflects the influence of MEN 2A/B and familial medullary thyroid cancer (see following). In addition, a nonsignificant increased risk of thyroid cancer has also been identified in relatives of patients with ataxia-teleangiectasia (Geoffrey-Perez et al, 2001).

Somatic Events

Advances in molecular biology have improved the understanding of the mechanisms of growth factors, growth factor receptors, oncogenes, and tumor-suppressor genes, but data are still conflicting. The

Table 25–4. Observed cases (Obs), standardized incidence rates (SIR), and 95% confidence intervals (CI) in offspring by concordant subgroup of thyroid cancer

Parental type of thyroid cancer	Son			Daughter		
	Obs	SIR	CI	Obs	SIR	CI
Adenocarcinoma*	11	7.8	3.9–13.2	13	2.8	1.5–4.5
Medullary carcinoma	4	3,580	932–7960	10	4520	2150–7760
Anaplastic cancer	6	239	86.2–469	7	168	66.4–315

*Papillary or follicular.

Source: Hemminki and Dong, 2000.

prevalence of genetic alterations in thyroid cancers varies substantially across studies, and the relationship between these changes and tumor characteristics and prognosis are unclear.

As all cancers do, thyroid cancers accumulate a number of genetic alterations. Chromosome instability has been identified in follicular adenomas and carcinomas, which are most often aneuploid with a high prevalence of loss of hetrozygosity involving multiple chromosomes (Castro et al, 2005). In contrast, papillary carcinomas that are most often diploid show less frequent loss of hetrozygosity (Sobrinho-Simões et al, 2005).

The proto-oncogene RET was the first activated receptor-tyrosine kinase to be identified in thyroid cancer. RET is normally expressed in the developing nervous systems. Oncogenic activation through RET includes several pathways, among them the mitogen-activated protein kinase (MAPK) signaling pathway that in turn activates other signaling pathways, cell-cycle regulators, and various adhesion molecules (Airaksinen and Saarma, 2002). The prevalence of the chimeric oncogene RET/PTC varies from 13% to 43% in papillary carcinomas depending on detection methods and study population and more than 15 different types of rearrangements have been described (Tallini and Asa, 2001).

A higher rate of RET/PTC has been found in cancers associated with ionizing radiation (Fugazzola et al, 1995; Klugbauer

et al, 1995; Ito et al, 1996; Williams et al, 1996b, Williams et al, 2004), although the associations have been questioned due to few cases and less stringent inclusion criteria. It was not possible to identify a gene expression signature for post-Chernobyl thyroid cancers when comparing possibly radiation associated cancers to sporadic (Detours et al, 2005).

The RAS proto-oncogene has been extensively studied in relation to thyroid carcinogenesis. A mutation in the ras gene probably represents an early event in the carcinogenic process, leading to alterations in its normal gatekeeper function (Kondo et al, 2006). Mutations in the RAS gene are found at similar frequencies in thyroid carcinomas and adenomas. Transgenic mice with RAS mutations show increased follicular cell proliferation and reduced expression of differentiation markers such as thyroglobulin. Moreover, follicular and papillary malignancies have been described in these animals (Santelli et al, 1993; Rochefort et al, 1996).

Although RET/PTC and RAS expression is associated with thyroid cancers in humans and mice (Powell et al, 1998), they probably represent an early event in cancer progression. Mutations in the BRAF proto-oncogene are the most recently identified effector of the MAPK pathway. Alterations are found in 30% to 60% of all papillary cancers, approximately 15% of all anaplastic cancers, but not in follicual cancers (Kondo et al, 2007). The prevalence of p53 mutations in differentiated thyroid cancer has not been studied extensively but seems to be rare in contrast to anaplastic thyroid carcinoma, where they are found more frequently (Fogelfeld et al, 1996).

Recently several genome wide studies on somatic alterations have been published, indicating a number of genes being differently regulated in malignant, compared to normal thyroid tissue (Kimmel et al, 2006; Wreesmann et al, 2004). Results are however conflicting probably due to small study samples.

RISK FACTORS

Tobacco

There is growing evidence that tobacco may lower the risk of differentiated thyroid cancer.

In women, smoking was associated with a 50% reduced risk of papillary thyroid cancer, although no clear dose–response relationship was observed with either number of years of smoking or pack-years (Rossing et al, 2000). Similar findings (RR 0.59) were observed in a Swedish case-control study, in which the lowest risk was seen for premenopausal women who started smoking before the age of 15 years (Galanti et al, 1996). A study of 14 pooled case-control studies found a more pronounced protective effect in current (OR = 0.6) compared to previous smokers (OR = 0.9; Mack et al, 2003). There were also significant trends of reduced risk with greater duration and frequency of smoking.

Conceivably, smoking might reduce the risk by lowering the level of thyroid stimulating hormone (TSH) secreted from the pituitary gland. This hormone stimulates follicular cell proliferation and may thereby increase the risk of thyroid cancer. Indeed, in one study, current male smokers had lower TSH levels than never smokers and former smokers (Fisher et al, 1997). Although the mechanism by which tobacco could influence TSH levels or activity is not understood, an antiestrogenic effect is plausible; estrogens have been suggested to in-fluence thyroid function, possibly through an effect on TSH (Henderson et al, 1982).

Diet

The role of diet in the pathogenesis of thyroid cancer has been intensively studied, but the data remain inconclusive. A high iodine intake may contribute to the high incidence of thyroid cancer observed among inhabitants of Hawaii, Iceland, and French Polynesia (Parkin et al, 1997), all consuming large amounts of iodine-rich fish and shellfish. These data are difficult to interpret, though, because the effects of iodine on risk might differ by type of thyroid cancer. Hence, a higher incidence of differentiated thyroid carcinomas, especially of the papillary subtype, has been observed in areas of adequate iodine intake (Franceschi et al, 1993), while, in contrast, an increased incidence of follicular thyroid cancer has been noted in iodine-deficient areas (Pettersson et al, 1991). However, in a large case-control study, a significantly decreased risk of papillary thyroid cancer was observed in patients with high dietary iodine intake but without any of the three best established risk factors: radiation to the head/neck, history of goiter, and family history of thyroid cancer (Horn-Ross et al, 2001). For patients with any of these risk factors, a nonsignificant increased risk, related to increased iodine intake, was noticed. An iodine-deficient diet will lead to a decreased level of thyroid hormones and consequently to reduced thyroid function followed by an increase in the TSH level.

Cruciferous vegetables contain substances with a goitrogenic effect that certainly increases TSH secretion, but also secretion of elements such as isothiocyanate that supposedly have a protective effect. The association between cruciferous and other vegetables and thyroid cancer risk was examined in a pooled analyses of 11 case-control studies conducted in the US, Asia, and Europe. A total of 2241 cases and 3716 controls were included. No consistent protective effect of high vegetable intake was found, nor any difference between cruciferous and noncruciferous vegetables (Bosetti et al, 2002).

One case-control study found an excess risk of differentiated thyroid cancer following high intake of starchy foods, cheese, butter, and oils other than olive oil (Franceschi et al, 1991). These results might, however, be confounded by deficiency of iodine and other nutrients such as vitamins and trace metals. The fact that, in this same study, ham and fish were significantly protective may reflect the high iodine content in fish and the high salt (potentially iodine-enriched) concentration in ham.

Thyroid cancer risk was not associated with consumption of coffee or tea. These findings were consistent in both gender-specific and histology-specific (papillary and follicular) analyses (Mack et al, 2003).

Alcohol

Theoretically, alcohol consumption may influence the TSH level and thus the risk of differentiated thyroid cancer. A substantially reduced risk of thyroid cancer was observed among current drinkers compared to nondrinkers, most markedly in postmenopausal women (Rossing et al, 2000). In contrast, a positive association between alcohol intake and thyroid cancer was found in a study based on detailed personal interviews. Other studies failed to show any relationship between alcohol and differentiated thyroid cancer (Franceschi et al, 1991). Consumption of wine and beer was significantly associated with thyroid cancer risk, but this trend disappeared after adjustment for current smoking (Mack et al, 2003).

Reproductive Factors

The sex and age distribution of thyroid cancer incidence indicates that female hormones might regulate thyroid cancer carcinogenesis. Indeed, follicular cells express the estrogen receptor and estrogen promotes the proliferation of these cells (Lee et al, 2005). However, there is still no clear evidence of a causal relationship between thyroid cancer and pregnancy or use of exogenous sex hormones (Haselkorn et al, 2003).

It has been hypothesized that female sex hormones act as promotors rather than initiators of malignant transformation because no gender difference is seen in subclinical tumors found at autopsy (Franssila and Harach, 1986). Although the thyroid gland is not as closely regulated by sex steroid hormones as, for example, the breast, uterus, and ovaries, the striking gender difference for thyroid cancers—as for most benign thyroid disorders—points to an influence of events or conditions related to reproductive parameters. Estrogens, pregnancy, and oral contraceptive use are all associated with an elevation of serum thyroxin and triiodothyronine levels. This might entail increased cell turnover and mutation rates. Further, estrogens are known to induce thyroid cancer in mice (Doniach, 1963; Miki et al, 1990), and estrogen receptors are found in papillary and follicular but not medullary carcinomas. Sex steroid hormones, and thus menstrual and reproductive factors, have therefore been suggested to play a role in thyroid cancer etiology, but the findings are inconsistent.

In a pooled analysis of 14 case-control studies, including 2247 thyroid cancer cases and 3699 controls (Negri et al, 1999), the thyroid cancer risk was weakly positively associated with late menarche and late age at first birth. The risk was higher during the first year after delivery and after artificial menopause. These associations were stronger in younger age groups. Contrary to previous findings, no relation to number of miscarriages was noted.

An increase in the risk of papillary carcinomas in particular was seen among current users of oral contraceptives (La Vecchia et al, 1999), whereas no such increase was evident among former users. Use of hormone replacement therapy or fertility drugs did not affect the risk of thyroid cancer.

Hormones

As already mentioned, elevated secretion of TSH from the pituitary gland has been discussed as a cause of thyroid cancer because it may increase mitotic activity in the follicular cells. According to the proposed mechanism, an elevated TSH level should increase the number of cells susceptible to malignant transformation and the proliferation of the follicular cells (Henderson et al, 1982; Williams, 1990).

A higher level of TSH could occur as a consequence of puberty, pregnancy and delivery, use of oral contraceptives, partial thyroidectomy for benign thyroid disorders, intake of goitrogens, and radiotherapy toward the head and neck area (Pacchiarotti et al, 1986; Williams, 1990). Molecular studies indicate that influences mediated by the TSH receptor may be involved in the carcinogenic process, but the possible pathogenic mechanisms have not been clarified.

Anthropometric Measures

Height and weight seem to moderately increase the risk of thyroid cancer, particularly among women (Dal Maso et al, 2000). A weak positive relationship of high body mass index and sudden weight gain with the risk of thyroid cancer, particularly in women, has been observed (Goodman et al, 1992), but the biological mechanism is unclear.

Physical Activity

No reliable information on the effect of physical activity on thyroid cancer risk has been published.

Ionizing Radiation

Ionizing radiation is the only definitely established cause of thyroid cancer in humans (UNSCEAR, 2000). The thyroid gland is indeed highly susceptible to ionizing radiation, presumably because of its superficial location, high level of oxygenation, and high cell-turnover rate. Doses as low as 0.1 Sievert (Sv) increase the risk of thyroid cancer. The exposure–response relationship seems to be linear below 4 Sv; above that level of radiation, cell killing probably outweighs the carcinogenic transformation (UNSCEAR, 2000). Protracted or fractionated exposure appears to be less carcinogenic than brief gamma exposure, but the

results are not entirely consistent. Further, the risk of thyroid cancer is highly dependent on age at exposure. The typical findings regarding radiation-associated thyroid cancer are summarized in Table 25–5.

Some of the earliest evidence for a role of ionizing radiation comes from observations following radiation treatment for benign disorders such as cervical lymphadenopathy, tonsillitis, enlarged thymus, and skin disorders. The extensive use of radiation treatments until the 1960 mirrors the increase in thyroid cancer incidence that was noted in the 1950s and reached a plateau in the 1980s (Pottern et al, 1980; Hrafnkelsson et al, 1988; Pettersson et al, 1991; Franceschi et al, 1993). In a birth cohort analysis, the incidence was low among those born between 1870 and 1910, increased among those born between 1920 and 1950, and declined among those born thereafter (Pottern et al, 1980). Epidemiologic investigations on the effects of radiation treatment include studies of children with ringworm of the scalp (tinea capitis), infants with supposedly enlarged thymus glands or hemangiomas, adolescents with enlarged tonsils, children with cancer, young adults with Hodgkin's disease, patients given whole-body irradiation, and women treated for cervical cancer (UNSCEAR, 2000).

Important additional evidence of a causal relationship between ionizing radiation and thyroid cancer comes from the study of Japanese atomic bomb survivors. The inci-

Table 25–5. Typical features of radiation-associated thyroid cancer

The relative risk is high.

A low dose (0.1 Sv) poses a hazard.

The dose–response relationship is linear.

The relative risk decreases with time.

The minimal latent period is 5–9 years.

Age dependency is profound.

Chronic exposure is somewhat less risky than brief exposure.

Women are more vulnerable than men.

There is a high fraction of papillary carcinomas.

dence of thyroid cancer among these survivors peaked 25 years after the exposure in 1945 (UNSCEAR, 2000). Occupational studies have also contributed to the understanding of the role of radiation in thyroid cancer. In addition, patients administered 131I because of hyperthyroidism are at excess risk (UNSCEAR, 2000).

No difference in excess relative risk between males and females in the atomic bomb survivor data (Table 25–6) was found, although previous findings indicated that the female thyroid gland is more susceptible to ionizing radiation. However, since the naturally occurring thyroid cancer is two to three times more common in women, the absolute radiation-induced risk was higher in women (Table 25–6).

A striking finding in radiation-associated thyroid cancers is the profound age dependency, which implies that the thyroid gland is especially sensitive to ionizing radiation in young people with rapid cell proliferation. The UNSCEAR report underlines the strong modifying effect of age at exposure, with no excess risk seen in individuals older than 20 years (Table 25–6). The highest relative and absolute risks ever measured for any radiation-associated cancer were

identified in the Israeli tinea capitis study (Table 25–6). A pooled analysis of seven studies revealed that thyroid cancer was induced even by low doses of brief external gamma radiation in childhood but rarely developed after exposure in adulthood (Ron et al, 1995). The same, pooled analysis also showed a latent period of 5 to 9 years; the relative risk was highest 15 to 29 years after exposure, and an excess risk remained until at least 40 years after exposure.

Following the Chernobyl accident, the first three cases of thyroid cancer in children were diagnosed in Ukraine 4 years later (Prisyazhniuk et al, 1991). Although a screening effect was seriously considered, it was postulated that "these thyroid cancers might represent the beginning of an epidemic. (p. 21)" One year later, Kazakov et al (1992) reported 131 cases of childhood thyroid cancer in Belarus. The geographic distribution suggested a relationship with the ionizing radiation caused by radionuclides released from the Chernobyl nuclear power plant. Fourteen years after the accident, approximately 1800 thyroid cancers among children younger than 15 years had been diagnosed in the three most contami-

Table 25–6. Risk estimates for thyroid cancer incidence from studies of radiation exposure

Study area	Observed cases	Expected cases	Mean dose (Sv)	Excess relative risk at 1 Sv	Excess absolute risk (10^4 PY/Sv)
Atomic bomb survivors					
Male	22	14.9	0.27	1.80	0.87
Female	110	79.4	0.26	1.40	2.32
Age at exposure					
0–9 years	24	7.6	0.21	10.25	4.21
10–19 years	35	14.6	0.31	4.50	3.46
20–29 years	18	17.5	0.28	0.10	0.13
>30 years	55	54.5	0.25	0.04	0.06
Other cohort studies of children, external exposure					
Israeli tinea capitis	43	10.7	0.1	34	13
Rochester thymic irradiation	37	2.7	1.4	9.5	3.0
Stockholm skin hemangioma	17	7.5	0.26	4.9	0.9

nated countries (UNSCEAR, 2000), compared to only 3 to 4 cases annually in the same age group and areas before the accident.

When the thyroid cancers diagnosed among children in Belarus and Ukraine were compared with those among children in England and Wales, differences were observed in the proportion of papillary tumors—approximately 98% in Belarus and Ukraine and 68% in England and Wales—but not in the aggressiveness of the tumors (Williams et al, 1996a). Somewhat surprisingly, no difference was seen in mutations in the examined oncogenes (ras, ret), the TSH receptor, or p53, the tumor-suppressor gene (Williams et al, 1996a).

The apparent increase in thyroid cancer within 5 years after the Chernobyl accident might be a result of improved detection and increased awareness rather than a genuine increase in incidence, because such a short latency period has previously not been reported—not even after childhood exposure to high doses of external radiotherapy (Thompson et al, 1994; Ron et al, 1995). To accommodate this concern, a well-conducted case-control study was recently conducted among Chernobyl-exposed individuals; the effect of ionizing radiation was evaluated in 276 patients with thyroid cancer diagnosed before 1998 and 1300 matched controls (Cardis et al, 2005). All participants were below 15 years at the time of the accident and individual doses were estimated for each subject based on their whereabouts, dietary habits, and likely stable iodine status at the time of the accident. A strong dose–response relationship was observed between radiation dose to the thyroid received in childhood and thyroid cancer risk. The risk of radiation-related thyroid cancer was three times higher in iodine-deficient areas than elsewhere. Administration of potassium iodide as a dietary supplement reduced this risk of radiation-related thyroid cancer by a factor of 3.

For the general population, diagnostic x-rays are the predominant source of exposure to ionizing radiation. Several studies have examined the relationship of x-ray examinations and thyroid cancer risk, but they all depended on recalled histories of examinations. However, in one case-control study, in which information on x-ray examinations was recorded prospectively from hospital charts, there was no evidence of an association between x-ray examinations and thyroid cancer risk (Inskip et al, 1995).

Occupation

Except for occupational studies of individuals exposed to ionizing radiation, such as military service personnel, nuclear industry workers, and individuals working in medical settings or underground miners (UNSCEAR, 2000), no data support a relationship between occupation and thyroid cancer.

Medical Conditions and Treatment

The possible relationship between benign thyroid disorders and thyroid cancer is methodologically difficult to investigate, because both the diagnostic workup and surgical treatment of presumably benign lesions will likely entail detection of indolent cancers that might never have become clinically significant. Although a number of studies related thyroid adenoma, goiter, and thyroiditis to an excess risk of thyroid carcinoma, other studies failed to support this relationship. Immunological factors might be involved in thyroid cancer progression because it has been shown that chronic lymphocytic thyroiditis harbors potential precursor lesions of malignancy (Gasbarri et al, 2004).

By analogy with thyroid carcinomas, benign thyroid disorders are hard to classify. The classification has been the focus of several reassessments following the availability of thyroid uptake tests, scintigraphy, ultrasound, fine-needle aspiration biopsies, and the possibility of measuring thyroid antibodies and thyroid hormones such as thyroxine, triiodothyronine, and TSH.

A history of hypothyroidism or hyperthyroidism has been associated with an increased risk of thyroid cancer only in a few reports. Two studies, however, indicated an increased risk in hyperthyroid patients treated with 131I (Ron et al, 1998; Franklyn et al, 1999). The short latent period suggests that the underlying condition rather than the ionizing radiation was the cause of the increased risk. In contrast, a pooled analysis of 12 case-control studies found no association between hypothyroidism and subsequent thyroid cancer, while a strong relationship with previous goiter, benign adenomas, and nodules was noted; the excess risk was 38-fold in men with a previous history of goiter (Franceschi et al, 1999). A positive association of thyroid cancer with Hashimoto's thyroiditis—an entity that could be followed by years of subclinical hypothyroidism and increased TSH secretion—has also been suggested but has received only weak support (Holm et al, 1985).

Because iodine is an essential part of the thyroid hormones and lack of iodine increases TSH secretion, the hypothesis that iodine deficiency/endemic goiter increases the risk of thyroid cancer lies near at hand and has also been tested repeatedly (Preston-Martin et al, 1987; Ron et al, 1987; Franceschi et al, 1989; Kolonel et al, 1990; Wingren et al, 1993). The association was generally strong, with relative risks between 5 and 10. Close medical surveillance, misclassification of the initial disease (reverse causality), and confounding by treatment could be part of the explanation. A true causal relationship, however, could not be ruled out given the number of investigations and the strength of the association. Other studies failed to show a relation between iodine deficiency and thyroid cancer, perhaps due to differences in histology, because follicular and anaplastic carcinomas are more common in endemic goiter areas (Doniach, 1971; Pettersson et al, 1991), whereas papillary carcinomas prevail in iodine-rich areas (Doniach, 1971; Williams et al, 1977).

The most consistent positive association with any other cancer was seen for cancer of the breast (Schottenfeld and Berg, 1971; Ron et al, 1984; Teppo et al, 1985; Tucker et al, 1985). Common risk factors such as oral contraceptive use and high radio-sensivity could explain the findings, although two Scandinavian studies failed to replicate them (Østerlind et al, 1985; Hall et al, 1990).

CONCLUSION

Thyroid cancer is one of the less common forms of cancer. It comprises four distinct entities—papillary, follicular, medullary, and anaplastic—with different etiologies, as suggested by their variation in age, sex, and geographic distribution. The indolent properties of many thyroid cancers, the availability of health care, changes in diagnostic criteria over time, the high prevalence of differentiated tumors found at autopsy, and screening programs may explain some of the differences.

In contrast to other cancers, the incidence of thyroid cancer is relatively high already before the age of 40 years. After the age of 50 years, the incidence of differentiated thyroid cancer levels off among women and continues to increase among men, a pattern particularly evident for papillary cancer. The suggestion that hormonal factors cause the gender difference lacks direct support, and other explanations have been suggested. Like benign thyroid lesions, thyroid cancer is more common in women.

Thyroid cancer seems to be one of the few cancers in which genetic factors account for a larger fraction that environmental factors. Approximately 20% of medullary thyroid cancers are attributed to MEN 2A/B or familial medullary thyroid cancer. There is still no firm evidence that specific somatic genetic alterations play a major role in the development of thyroid cancer.

The etiology of thyroid cancer has been studied in a number of relatively small (< 400 cases) case-control studies and some cohort studies. The only established cause is ionizing radiation. Except for red bone marrow and the premenopausal breast, the thyroid gland is the body tissue most susceptible to ionizing radiation. Doses of ionizing radiation as low as 0.1 Sv have been proven to increase the risk of thyroid cancer. The increased risk seems to be confined to exposure in childhood, as no study so far has found an association with adult exposure.

There are indications that diet, alcohol, reproductive factors, deficiency or excess of iodine, and changes in height and weight are causally related to the risk of thyroid cancer, but data are not consistent. An elevated level of TSH has been suggested as a causative risk factor since this hormone increases mitotic activity in the follicular cells and thus the risk of malignant transformation. There is, however, no firm proof of an influence of TSH on thyroid cancer incidence. The relationship between benign thyroid disorders and thyroid cancer is complex and methodologically difficult to investigate because increased medical surveillance will increase the likelihood of detecting indolent cancers that might never have become clinically significant.

REFERENCES

Airaksinen MS, Saarma M. The GDNF family: signalling, biological functions and therapeutic value. Nat Rev Neurosci 2002;5:383–94.

Bosetti C, Negri E, Kolonel L, Ron E, Franceschi S, Preston-Martin S, et al. A pooled analysis of case–control studies of thyroid cancer. VII. Cruciferous and other vegetables (International). Cancer Causes and Control 2002;13:765–75.

Cancer Incidence in Sweden 2004. The National Board of Health and Welfare, Stockholm, 2005.

Castro P, Eknæs M, Teixeira MR, Danielsen HE, Soares P, Lothe RA, et al. Adenomas and follicular carcinomas of the thyroid display two major patterns of chromosomal changes. J Pathol 2005;206:305–11.

Cardis E, Kesminiene A, Ivanov V, Malakhova I, Shibata Y, Khrouch V, et al Risk of Thyroid Cancer After Exposure to 131 I in Childhood. J Natl Cancer Inst 2005;97:724–32.

Czene K, Lichtenstein P, Hemminki K. Environmental and heritable causes of cancer among 9.6 million individuals in the Swedish Family Cancer Database. Int J Cancer 2002;99:260–66.

Dal Maso L, La Vecchia C, Franceschi S, Preston-Martin S, Ron E, Levi F, et al. A pooled analysis of thyroid cancer studies. V. An-

thropometric factors. Cancer Causes Control 2000;11:137–44.

Detours V, Wattel S, Venet D, Hutsebaut N, Bogdanova T, Tronko MD, et al. Absence of a specific radiation signature in post-Chernobyl thyroid cancers. British Journal of Cancer 2005;92:1545–52.

Doniach I. Aetiological considerations of thyroid cancer [abstract]. Br J Radiol 1971; 44:819.

Davies L, Welch HG. Increasing Incidence of thyroid cancer in the United States, 1973–2002. JAMA 2006;295:2164–67.

Doniach I. Effects including carcinogenesis of I-131 and x-rays on the thyroid of experimental animals—a review. Health Phys 1963;9:1357–62.

Ferlay J, Bray F, Pisani P, Parkin DM. GLOBOCAN 2000: Cancer Incidence, Mortality and Prevalence Worldwide. International Agency for Research on Cancer, Lyon, 2001.

Fisher CL, Mannino DM, Herman WH, Frumkin H. Cigarette smoking and thyroid hormone levels in males. Int J Epidemiol 1997; 26:972–77.

Fogelfeld L, Bauer TK, Schneider AB, Swartz JE, Zitman R. p53 gene mutations in radiation-induced thyroid cancer. J Clin Endocrinol Metab 1996;81:3039–44.

Franceschi S, Boyle P, Maisonneuve P, La Vecchia C, Burt AD, Kerr DJ, et al. The epidemiology of thyroid carcinoma. Crit Rev Oncogen 1993;4:25–53.

Franceschi S, Fassina A, Talamini R, Mazzolini A, Vianello S, Bidoli E, et al. Risk factors for thyroid cancer in nothern Italy. Int J Epidemiol 1989;18:578–84.

Franceschi S, Levi F, Negri E, Fassina A, La Vecchia C. Diet and thyroid cancer: a pooled analysis of four European case-control studies. Int J Cancer 1991;48:395–98.

Franceschi S, Preston-Martin S, Dal Maso L, Negri E, La Vecchia C, Mack WJ, et al. A pooled analysis of case-control studies of thyroid cancer. IV. Benign thyroid disease. Cancer Causes Control 1999;10:583–95.

Franklyn JA, Maisonneuve P, Sheppard M, Betteridge J, Boyle P. Cancer incidence and mortality after radioiodine treatment for hyperthyroidism: a population-based cohort study. Lancet 1999;353:2111–15.

Franssila KO, Harach HR. Occult papillary carcinoma of the thyroid in children and young adults. A systemic autopsy study in Finland. Cancer 1986;58:715–19.

Frich L, Glattre E, Akslen LA. Familial occurrence of nonmedullary thyroid cancer: a population-based study of 5,673 first-degree relatives of thyroid cancer patients from Norway. Cancer Epidemiol Biomarkers Prev 2001;10:113–17.

Fugazzola L, Pilotti S, Pinchera A, Vorontsova V, Mondellini P, Bongarzone I, et al. Oncogenic rearrangements of the RET proto-oncogene in papillary thyroid carcinomas from children exposed to the Tjernobyl nuclear accident. Cancer Res 1995;55:5617–20.

Galanti MR, Hansson L, Lund E, Bergström R, Grimelius L, Stalsberg H, et al. Reproductive history and cigarette smoking as risk factors for thyroid cancer in women: a population-based case-control study. Cancer Epidemiol Biomarkers Prev 1996;5:425–31.

Gasbarri A, Sciacchitano S, Marasco A, Papotti M, Di Napoli A, Marzullo A, et al. Detection and molecular characterisation of thyroid cancer precursor lesions in a specific subset of Hashimoto's thyroiditis. Br J Cancer 2004; 91:1096–1104.

Geoffrey-Perez B, Janin N, Ossian K, Lauge A, Croquette MF, Griscelli C, et al. Cancer risk in heterozygotes for ataxia-telangiectasia. Int J Cancer 2001;93:288–93.

Goodman MT, Kolonel LN, Wilkens LR. The association of body size, reproductive factors and thyroid cancer. Br J Cancer 1992; 66:1180–84.

Goodman MT, Yoshizawa CN, Kolonel LN. Descriptive epidemiology of thyroid cancer in Hawaii. Cancer 1988;61:1272–81.

Hall P, Holm L-E, Lundell G. Second primary tumors following thyroid cancer. A Swedish record-linkage study. Acta Oncol 1990; 29:869–73.

Haselkorn T, Stewart S L, Horn-Ross P L. Why are thyroid cancer rates so high in Southeast Asian women living in the United States? The Bay Area Thyroid Cancer Study. Cancer Epidemiology Biomarkers & Prevention 2003;12:144–150.

Hemminki K, Dong C. Familial relationship in thyroid cancer by histo-pathological type. Int J Cancer 2000;85:201–5.

Henderson BE, Ross RK, Pike MC, Casagrande JT. Endogenous hormones as a major factor in human cancer. Cancer Res 1982;42: 3232–39.

Holm L-E, Blomgren H, Löwhagen T. Cancer risks in patients with chronic lymphocytic thyroiditis. N Engl J Med 1985;312: 601–4.

Horn-Ross PL, Morris JS, Lee M, West DW, Whittemore AS, McDougall JR, et al. Iodine and thyroid cancer risk among women in a multiethnic population: The Bay Area Thyroid Cancer Study. Cancer Epidemiol Biomarkers Prev 2001;10:979–85.

Hrafnkelsson J, Joonasson JG, Sigurdsson G, Sigvaldason H, Tulinius H. Thyroid cancer in Iceland 1955–1984. Acta Endocrinol (Copenh) 1988;118:566–72.

Ihre-Lundgren C, Hall P, Ekbom A, Frisell J, Zedenius J, Dickman P W. Incidence and survival of Swedish patients with differentiated thyroid cancer. Int J Cancer 2003; 106:569–573.

Inskip PD, Ekbom A, Galanti MR, Grimelius L, Boice JD. Medical diagnostic x rays and thyroid cancer. J Natl Cancer Inst 1995; 87:1613–21.

Ito M, Yamashita S, Ashizawa K, Hara T, Namba H, Hoshi M. Histopathological characteristics of childhood thyroid cancer in Gomel, Belarus. Int J Cancer 1996;65:29–33.

Kazakov VS, Demidchik EP, Astakhova LN. Thyroid cancer after Tjernobyl. Nature 1992;359:21.

Kimmel RR, Zhao LP, Nguyen D, et al. Microarray Comparative Genomic Hybridization Reveals Genome-Wide Patterns of DNA Gains and Losses in Post-Chernobyl Thyroid Cancer. Radiat Res 2006;166:519–31.

Klugbauer S, Lengfelder E, Demidchik EP, Rabes HM. High prevalence of RET rearrangement in thyroid tumors of children from Belarus after the Tjernobyl reactor accident. Oncogene 1995;11:2459–67.

Kolonel LN, Hankin JH, Wilkens LR, Fukunaga FH, Hinds MW. An epidemiologic study of thyroid cancer in Hawaii. Cancer Causes Control 1990;1:223–34.

Kondo T, Ezzat S, Asa S L. Pathogenetic mechanisms in thyroid follicular-cell neoplasia. Nature Reviews Cancer 2006;6:292–306.

Kondo T, Zheng L, Liu W, et al. Epigenetically controlled fibroblast growth factor receptor 2 signaling imposes on the RAS/BRAF/mitogen-activated protein kinase pathway to modulate thyroid cancer progression. Cancer Res 2007;67:5461–70.

La Vecchia C, Ron E, Franceschi S, Dal Maso L, Mark SD, Chatenoud L, et al. A pooled analysis of case-control studies of thyroid cancer. III. Oral contraceptives, menopausal replacement therapy and other female hormones. Cancer Causes Control 1999;10:157–66.

Lee ML, Chen GG, Vlantis AC, Tse GMK, Leung, >BC>H, et al. Induction of Thyroid Papillary Carcinoma Cell Proliferation by Estrogen Is Associated with an Altered Expression of Bcl-xL. The Cancer Journal 2005;11:113–21.

Lindor N, Greene MH, and the Mayo Familial Cancer Program. The concise handbook of family cancer syndromes. Special article. J Natl Cancer Inst 1998;90:1039–71.

Mack W J, Preston-Martin S, Dal Maso L, Galanti R, Xiang M, Franceschi S, et al. A pooled analysis of case–control studies of thyroid cancer: cigarette smoking and consumption of alcohol, coffee, and tea. Cancer Causes and Control 2003;14:773–85.

Miki H, Oshimo K, Inoue H, Morimoto T, Monden Y. Sex hormone receptors in human thyroid tissues. Cancer 1990;66:1759–62.

Möller Jensson O, Carstensen B, Glattre E, Malker B, Pukkala E. Tulenius H. Atlas of Cancer Incidence in the Nordic Countries. A Collaborative Study of the Five Nordic Cancer Registries. Helsinki, 1988.

Negri E, Ron E, Franceschi S, Dal Maso L, Mark SD, Preston-Martin S, et al. A pooled analysis of case-control studies of thyroid cancer. I. Methods. Cancer Causes Control 1999;10:131–42.

Niccoli-Sire P, Murat A, Baudin E, Henry JF, Proye C, Bigorgne JC, et al. Early or prophylactic thyroidectomy in MEN 2/FMTC gene carriers: results in 71 thyroidectomized patients. The French Calcitonin Tumours Study Group (GETC). Eur J Endocrinol 1999;141:468–74.

Østerlind A, Olsson JH, Lynge E, Ewertz M. Second cancer following cutaneous melanoma and cancers of the brain, thyroid, connective tissue, bone, and eye in Denmark, 1943–80. Natl Cancer Inst Monogr 1985;68:361–88.

Pacchiarotti A, Martino E, Bartalena L, Buratti L, Mammoli C, Strigini F, et al. Serum thyrotropin by ultrasensitive immunoradiometric assay and serum free thyroid hormones in pregnancy. J Endocrinol Invest 1986;9:185–89.

Parkin DM, Whelan SL, Ferlay J, Raymond L, Young J. Cancer Incidence in Five Continents. Vol. VII. No. 143. International Agency for Research on Cancer. World Health Organization, Lyon, 1997.

Pettersson B, Adami HO, Wilander E, Coleman MP. Trends in thyroid cancer incidence in Sweden, 1958–1981, by histopathologic type. Int J Cancer 1991;48:28–33.

Pottern LM, Stone BJ, Day NE, Pickle LW, Fraumeni JF Jr. Thyroid cancer in Connecticut, 1935–1975: an analysis by cell type. Am J Epidemiol 1980;112:764–74.

Powell DJ Jr, Russell J, Nibu K, Li G, Rhee E, Liao M et al. The RET/PTC3 oncogene: metastatic solid-type papillary carcinomas in murine thyroids. Cancer Res 1998;58:5523–28.

Preston-Martin S, Bernstein L, Pike MC. Thyroid cancer among young women related to prior thyroid disease and pregnancy history. Br J Cancer 1987;55:191–95.

Prisyazhniuk A, Pjatak OA, Buzanov VA, Reeves GK, Beral V. Cancer in the Ukraine, post-Tjernobyl [letter]. Lancet 1991;338:1334–35.

Rochefort P, Caillou B, Michiels F-M, Ledent C, Talbot M, Schlumberger M, et al. Thyroid pathologies in transgenic mice expressing a human activated Ras gene driven by a thyroglobulin promoter. Oncogene 1996;12:111–18.

Ron E, Curtis R, Hoffman DA, Flannary JT. Multiple primary breast and thyroid cancer. Br J Cancer 1984;49:87–92.

Ron E, Doody MM, Becker DV, Brill AB, Curtis RE, Goldman MB, et al. Cancer mortality following treatment for adult hyperthyroidism. Cooperative Thyrotoxicosis Therapy Follow-up Study Group. JAMA 1998;280:347–55.

Ron E, Kleinerman RA, Boice JD Jr, LiVolsi VA, Flannery JT, Fraumeni JF Jr. A population-based case-control study of thyroid cancer. J Natl Cancer Inst 1987;79:1–12.

Ron E, Lubin JH, Shore RE, Mabuchi K, Modan B, Pottern LM, et al. Thyroid cancer after exposure to external radiation: a pooled analysis of seven studies. Radiat Res 1995; 141:259–77.

Rossing MA, Cushing K, Voight L, Wicklund K, Daling J. Risk of papillary thyroid cancer in women in relation to smoking and alcohol consumption. Epidemiology 2000;11:49–54.

Santelli G, de Franciscis V, Portella G, Chiappetta G, D'Alessio A, Califano D, et al. Production of transgenic mice expressing the Ki-ras oncogene under the control of a thyroglobulin promoter. Cancer Res 1993;53:5523–27.

Santoro M, Carlomagno F, Hay ID, Herrmann MA, Grieco M, Melillo R, et al. RET oncogene activation in human thyroid neoplasms is restricted to the papillary cancer subtype. J Clin Invest 1992;89:1517–22.

Santoro M, Sabino N, Ishizaka Y, Ushijima T, Carlomagno F, Cerrato A, et al. Involvement of RET oncogene in human tumours: specificity of RET activation to thyroid tumours. Br J Cancer 1993;68:460–64.

Schottenfeld D, Berg J. Incidence of multiple primary cancers. IV. Cancers of the female breast and genital organs. J Natl Cancer Inst 1971;46:161–70.

Sobrinho-Simões M, Preto A, Rocha AS, Castro P, Máximo V, Fonseca E et al. Virchows Arch 2005; 447:787–93.

Stratakis CA, Courcoutsakis NA, Abati A, Filie A, Doppman JL, Carney JA, et al. Thyroid gland abnormalities in patients with the syndrome of spotty skin pigmentation, myxomas, endocrine overactivity, and schwannomas (Carney complex). J Clin Endocrinol Metab 1997;82:2037–43.

Tallini G, Asa SL. RET oncogene activation in papillary thyroid carcinoma. Adv Anat Pathol 2001;6:345–54.

Teppo L, Pukkala E, Saxén E. Multiple cancer—an epidemiologic exercise in Finland. J Natl Cancer Inst 1985;75:207–17.

Thompson DE, Mabuchi K, Ron E, Soda M, Tokunaga M, Ochikubo S, et al. Cancer incidence in atomic bomb survivors. Part II: solid tumors, 1958–1987. Radiat Res 1994; 137:S17–S67.

Tucker MA, Boice JD Jr, Hoffman DA. Second cancer following cutaneous melanoma and cancers of the brain, thyroid, connective tissue, bone, and eye in Connecticut, 1935–82. Natl Cancer Inst Monogr 1985;68:161–89.

United Nations Scientific Committee on the Effects of Atomic Radiation (UNSCEAR). Sources and effects of ionizing radiation. UNSCEAR 2000 Report to the General Assembly, with Scientific Annexes. New York, United Nations, 2000.

Williams ED. TSH and thyroid cancer. Horm Metab Res (Suppl) 1990;23:72–75.

Williams ED, Cherstvoy E, Egloff B, Höfler H, Vecchio G, Bogdanova T, et al. Interaction of pathology and molecular characterization of thyroid cancers. In: Karaoglou A, Desmet G, Kelly GN, Menzel HG (Eds): The Radiological Consequences of the Tjernobyl Accident. Luxembourg, Office for Official Publications of the European Communities, 1996a, pp 699–714.

Williams ED, Doniach I, Bjarnason O, Michie W. Thyroid cancer in an iodide rich area. A histopathological study. Cancer 1977;39:215–22.

Williams GH, Rooney S, Thomas GA, Cummins G, Williams ED. RET activation in adult and childhood papillary thyroid carcinoma using a reverse transcriptase-n-polymerase chain reaction approach on archival-nested material. Br J Cancer 1996b;74:585–89.

Williams E D, Abrosimov A, Bogdanova T, Demidchik EP, Ito M, LiVolsi V et al. Thyroid carcinoma after Chernobyl latent period, morphology and aggressiveness. Br J Cancer 2004;90:2219–24.

Wingren G, Hatschek T, Axelson O. Determinants of papillary cancer of the thyroid. Am J Epidemiol 1993;138:482–91.

Wreesmann VB, Sleczka EM, Socci ND, et al. Genome-wide Profiling of Papillary Thyroid Cancer Identifies MUC1 as an Independent Prognostic Marker. Cancer Res 2004;64:3780–89.

26

Hodgkin Lymphoma

MADS MELBYE, HENRIK HJALGRIM,
AND HANS-OLOV ADAMI

Thomas Hodgkin (1798–1866), a British pathologist, philantropist, and traveler, who eventually died from dysentery in the Orient, gave name to the malignancy we will introduce now. First described by Hodgkin already in 1832 ("On some morbid appearances of the absorbent glands and spleen"), the disease became named after him in 1865. Nowadays, Hodgkin's disease or Hodgkin lymphoma, according to current terminology, represents approximately 10% of all malignant lymphomas. All others are grouped together under the category of non-Hodgkin lymphoma. Hodgkin lymphoma derives mostly from germinal center B cells and in rare cases (<2%) from peripheral T-cells. It has a unique histologic presentation, the tumor mass consisting of few Hodgkin and Reed-Sternberg (HRS) cells scattered among benign inflammatory cells suggesting that a specific immunologic reaction is important in Hodgkin lymphoma. Together with a characteristic clinical presentation and an epidemiologic pattern that indicates more than one etiologic pathway, this led to the speculation that Hodgkin lymphoma is

an unusual syndrome rather than a true neoplasm. However, with the finding that the HRS cell is a lymphoid cell of clonal origin, Hodgkin lymphoma is now considered a malignant lymphoma (Harris, 1999; Harris et al, 2000).

CLINICAL SYNOPSIS

Subgroups

According to the WHO classification, the disease occurs in two main forms, nodular lymphocyte predominant (~5%) and classical Hodgkin lymphoma (Table 27–1). The latter group is further divided into nodular sclerosis (the largest subgroup; ~70%), mixed cellularity (second largest subgroup; 20–25%), lymphocyte-rich (~5%), and lymphocyte-depleted (<5%) classical Hodgkin lymphoma.

Symptoms

The varying presenting signs and symptoms include painless enlargement of lymph nodes, coughing or shortness of breath, intermittent fever, night sweats, itching, fatigue, weight loss, and decreased appetite.

Diagnosis

Biopsy, usually from a lymph node, is necessary for microscopic identification of the neoplastic HRS cells. The extent of disease is characterized by imaging techniques (such as computed tomography or magnetic resonance imaging), bone marrow biopsy, and, in some cases, gallium scan or lymphangiogram.

Treatment

Radiation therapy and chemotherapy are the most common treatments. If the disease is localized, radiation therapy is sometimes used alone. In patients with relapsed disease bone marrow or peripheral stem cell transplantation in combination with high-dose chemotherapy has become standard salvage therapy. Also, various biological therapies are being evaluated in clinical trials.

Prognosis

Hodgkin lymphoma generally has a favorable prognosis. The 5-year relative survival rate improved from 40% in the beginning of the 1960s to more than 80% in the 1990s; the 10- and 15-year survival rates are 71% and 61%, respectively. The 5-year relative survival rates by stage of disease are 90% to 95% for stages I and II, 85% to 90% for stage III, and approximately 80% for stage

IV. Among children, the 5-year relative survival is 92%.

DESCRIPTIVE EPIDEMIOLOGY

Incidence

Internationally, the age-standardized (world) incidence of Hodgkin lymphoma varies considerably (Figs. 26–1 and 26–2), in recent data ranging from about 0.2 per 100,000 person-years in Chinese men and women to 3.2 in Jewish women in Israel and 4.0 in Swiss men (Parkin et al, 2002). Overall, Hodgkin lymphoma is 15% to 40% more common in males than in females in different settings. Among young adults, however, the incidence among females may equal or exceed that among males.

In contrast to the almost epidemic increase in non-Hodgkin lymphoma observed in the latter half of the 20th century, decreasing age-standardized incidence rates of Hodgkin lymphoma have been reported in several settings. To some extent this decline is spurious because some lymphomas previously considered to be Hodgkin lymphomas are now appropriately classified as non-Hodgkin lymphomas. However, this mechanism cannot explain increases in Hodgkin lymphoma occurrence documented among young adults in a number of industrialized countries in the same time period (Glaser and Swartz, 1990; Hartge et al, 1994; Chen et al, 1997; Hjalgrim et al,

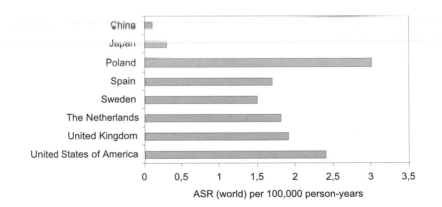

Figure 26–1. Age-standardized (to the world-population) incidence rates of Hodgkin lymphoma among women. (*Source*: Ferlay et al, 2004)

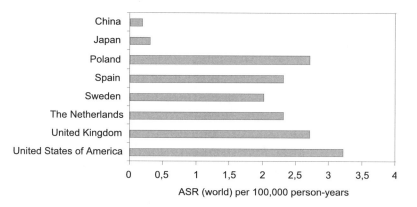

Figure 26–2. Age-standardized (to the world-population) incidence rates of Hodgkin lymphoma among men. (*Source*: Ferlay et al, 2004)

2001). The incidence patterns reveal substantial variation when examined by age, sex, ethnicity, social class, and histologic subtype. Because of the suggested strong influences of environmental factors in its etiology, this variation has made Hodgkin lymphoma an obvious candidate for analytic epidemiologic studies.

Age and Socioeconomic Patterns

In industrialized countries Hodgkin lymphoma is characterized by a bimodal age incidence curve (Figs. 26–3 and 26–4). This curve led MacMahon (1957, 1966) to suggest that it included two different disease entities, occurring in younger and older

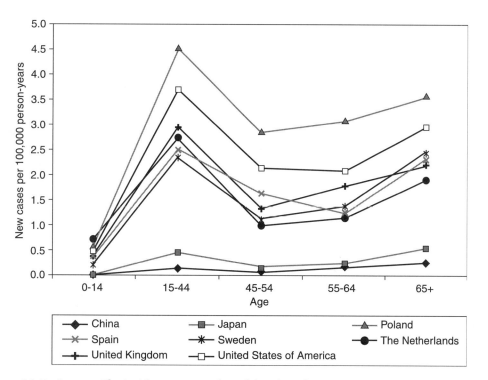

Figure 26–3. Age-specific incidence rates of Hodgkin lymphoma among women. (*Source*: Ferlay et al, 2004)

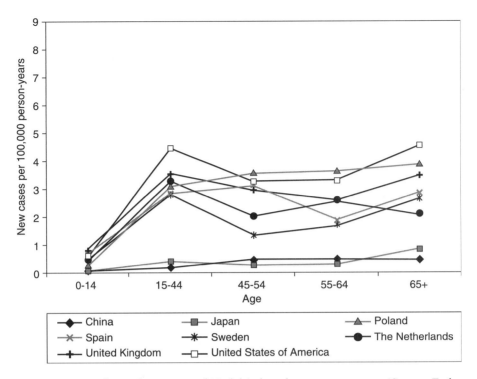

Figure 26–4. Age-specific incidence rates of Hodgkin lymphoma among men. (*Source*: Ferlay et al, 2004)

adults, respectively. Referring to this distribution as Pattern III, other age-specific patterns were reported in other geographical and ethnic settings. A Pattern I, which was seen in non-industrialized countries and socioeconomically deprived groups in industrialized countries, featured an incidence peak in boys, low incidence in young adults and increasing incidence in older adults (Correa and O'Conor, 1971; Gutensohn and Cole, 1977). As an intermediate between Patterns I and III, Pattern II displayed both a childhood and a young adult peak, observed in early industrialized and transitional societies such as India (Hartge et al, 1994; Correa and O'Conor, 1971; Gutensohn and Cole, 1977). Finally, a Pattern IV with low incidence in children and young adults has been observed in Asian populations.

Today, essentially all major populations of Europe and North America have a characteristic Pattern III profile. In the United States, a young adult peak is less prominent among Blacks than among Whites and barely visible among Hispanics and Asians. In contrast, a childhood peak is more common in Blacks and Hispanics than in Whites (Glaser and Jarrett, 1996). Data from Connecticut, which has one of the oldest cancer registries in the world, indicate that the bimodal distribution is becoming increasingly prominent over time, in particular with respect to the peak in young adult females (Fig. 26–5). In this age group, female rates have become as high as or higher than those in males, whereas among older people the rates are lower in females than in males (Chen et al, 1997; Hjalgrim et al, 2001).

Subtypes

The increasing incidence of Hodgkin lymphoma among young adults in Western societies is primarily explained by a marked increase in the incidence of the nodular sclerosis subtype. According to incidence data from the United States, nodular sclerosis

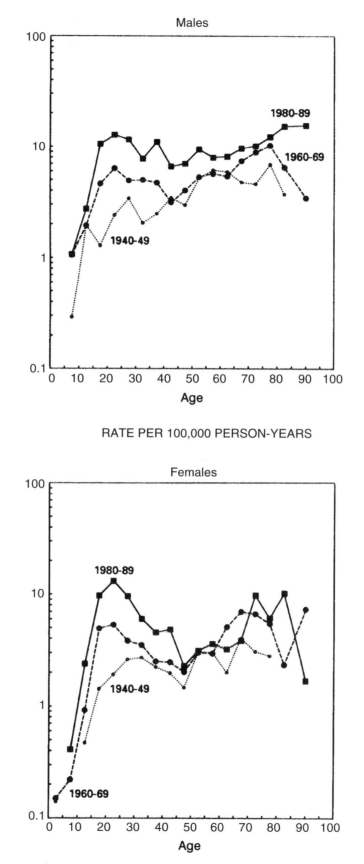

Figure 26–5. Age-specific incidence rates for Hodgkin lymphoma in different calendar periods, Connecticut, 1940–89. (*Source*: Hartge et al, 1994)

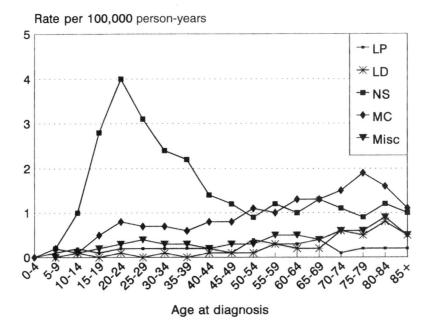

Figure 26–6. Age-specific incidence rates for Hodgkin lymphoma by histologic subtypes, all races, both sexes, SEER 1983–7, LP, lymphocytic predominance; LD, lymphocytic depletion; NS, nodular sclerosis; MC, mixed cellularity; Misc, miscellaneous. (*Source*: Medeiros and Greiner, 1995)

accounted for 40% of Hodgkin lymphomas in 1973–7 and 58% in 1983–7 (Medeiros and Greiner, 1995). Correspondingly, the proportion made up by the mixed cellularity subtype decreased slightly to 23% during the same period. As illustrated in Figure 26–6, the age-specific incidence of nodular sclerosis is essentially unimodal, with a peak in the 20 to 24 year age group. In contrast, the age-specific incidence pattern for the mixed cellularity subtype is bimodal, with the highest incidence in old age groups. While in industrialized countries nodular sclerosis Hodgkin lymphoma dominates, in non-industrialized countries Hodgkin lymphoma is primarily of the mixed cellularity or lymphocyte depleted subtypes.

Some authors in the Northern Hemisphere have suggested seasonality in the onset of Hodgkin lymphoma, with a low amplitude in the fall and a peak in February–April (Newell et al, 1985; Langagergaard et al, 2003; Chang et al, 2005a). This phenomenon, which needs confirmation, appears to be stronger among younger than among older patients.

GENETIC AND MOLECULAR EPIDEMIOLOGY

There is compelling evidence of familial clustering of Hodgkin lymphoma, in particular from register-based investigations (Goldin et al, 2004). Among siblings, reported excess risks have ranged from 3-fold to 7-fold. In a series of young adult siblings, those of the same gender as an affected person had twice the risk of gender-discordant siblings (Grufferman et al, 1977). While these observations could be explained by shared environmental factors, results of a twin study by Mack et al (1995) strongly imply a genetic component in the etiology as well. Specifically, the authors observed a 99-fold increased risk in siblings of monozygotic twins with Hodgkin lymphoma, much higher than among dizygotic twins. However, more than 90% of the monozygotic twins remained discordant, which suggests either that the overall penetrance of the susceptible genotype is low or that only a subgroup is genetically susceptible. Twin studies and studies of familial cases have consistently found an exceedingly high proportion of cases of the nodular sclerosis subtype. However, because this subtype is in general the most prevalent constituting nearly 60% of all cases, the observed pattern might not differ much from the expected.

Several observations suggest that genetic susceptibility to Hodgkin lymphoma relates to the immune system. Firstly, the disease is associated with certain human leukocyte antigen (HLA) types, notably HLA-A1, -B5, -B8, and -B18 (Diepstra et al, 2005a). Also, HLA-DPB1*0301 has been associated with elevated Hodgkin lymphoma risk, in particular the nodular sclerosis subtype (Diepstra et al, 2005a). Interestingly, some data indicate different heretability patterns for Epstein-Barr virus-negative and Epstein-Barr virus-positive lymphomas (Diepstra, 2005b). Secondly, abnormal cytokine production has been observed in affected patients (Gause et al, 1992). Lastly, immune deficiency has been described in family members of certain patients (Merk et al, 1990).

RISK FACTORS

Tobacco

Earlier studies provided little evidence of an association between Hodgkin lymphoma and tobacco, whether considering smoking status, number of cigarettes smoked, or duration of smoking (Briggs et al, 2002). However, recent studies have raised the possibility of an increased risk of certain types of Hodgkin lymphoma among current smokers (Briggs et al, 2002). Specifically, current smoking may be associated with an increased risk of mixed cellularity Hodgkin lymphoma and/or tumors harboring the Epstein-Barr virus (EBV) (Briggs et al, 2002; Chang et al, 2004a; Hjalgrim et al., 2007a).

Diet

There is no consistent evidence of an association between Hodgkin lymphoma and specific dietary products. A qualitative analysis of nine case-control studies suggested that children who were never breast-fed or breast-fed for a short period have a higher risk of developing Hodgkin lymphoma than those breast-fed for more than 6 months (Davis, 1998). However, the evidence appears weak.

Alcohol

A reduced risk of Hodgkin lymphoma has been reported with consumption of alcoholic beverages (eg, Besson et al, 2006). As yet, however, the evidence of an association between alcohol intake and Hodgkin lymphoma is not compelling, and no convincing dose-response pattern has been demonstrated.

Reproductive Factors and Hormones

The lower incidence among females after their childbearing years (Fig. 26–3) suggests an influence of hormones or reproductive factors on the development of Hodgkin lymphoma (Glaser, 1994). Alternatively, immunoregulatory changes during pregnancy may influence the risk of Hodgkin lymphoma through its association with immune dysfunction (Franceschi et al, 1994).

There is no convincing epidemiologic evidence that reproductive factors influence the risk of Hodgkin lymphoma. Both elevated and reduced risks in parous compared to nulliparous women have been reported (Olsson et al, 1990; Kravdal and Hansen, 1993; Zahm et al, 1995), as have findings of no effect (Kravdal and Hansen, 1996; Zwitter et al, 1996; Lambe et al, 1998). Limited evidence suggests a protective effect of parity restricted to the nodular sclerosis subtype (Kravdal and Hansen, 1993) and a positive association between late age at first birth and the risk of Hodgkin lymphoma (Olsson et al, 1990; Kravdal and Hansen, 1993; Lambe et al, 1998). Little or no information is available regarding the possible influence of age at menarche and menopause or time since last birth.

Anthropometric Measures

Reports based on limited numbers of subjects have indicated a positive association between measures of height at various ages and risk of Hodgkin lymphoma (Isager and Andersen, 1978; Gutensohn and Cole, 1981,

Glaser et al, 2002), whereas one large study found no association (Chang et al, 2005b).

Infections

An infectious origin of Hodgkin lymphoma has been suggested by several lines of reasoning. Firstly, its morphologic appearance resembles a chronic granulomatous infectious process. Secondly, its clinical course may include intermittent fever, night sweats, and weight loss, symptoms that are typical of infectious diseases. Lastly, the descriptive epidemiology of Hodgkin lymphoma shares similarities with paralytic poliomyelitis prior to the introduction of vaccines (Grufferman and Delzelle, 1984).

Considerable evidence has pointed to a role of EBV, a ubiquitous herpesvirus also associated with a variety of other malignancies, e.g. Burkitt lymphoma and nasopharyngeal carcinoma (IARC, 1997). Early case-control studies nested within large cohorts documented a particular antibody profile in prediagnostic sera obtained severeal years prior to Hodgkin lymphoma diagnosis (Evans, 1982; Mueller et al, 1989; Lehtinen et al, 1993). Typically, in adjusted analyses these subjects showed increased antibody responses to EBV nu-

clear antigens (EBNA) (Mueller et al, 1989; Lehtinen et al, 1993). Next, EBVgenome products may be demonstrated in the HRS cells in a proportion of Hodgkin lymphoma patients (Weiss et al, 1987). In these patients, EBV is consistently present in HRS cells in anatomically distinct sites at diagnosis, and patients whose tumors are EBV-positive at the time of diagnosis also appear to retain the virus in subsequent biopsy samples if they suffer from a relapse (IARC, 1997). Further supporting the direct involvement of EBV is the clonality of the virus with genomically identical EBV in different HRS cells from the same patient. This finding suggests that a single strain of EBV was present in the progenitor cells at the initial outgrowth of the tumor.

The proportion of EBV-positive lymphomas varies considerably between histologic subtypes. Among tumors of the mixed cellularity subtype, 60% to 80% contain EBV compared to 20% to 40% of those of the nodular sclerosis subtype (Glaser et al, 1997). Although the less common Hodgkin lymphoma subtypes have been less studied, the lymphocyte-predominant type appears to be little associated with EBV, whereas the lymphocyte depleted type shows a

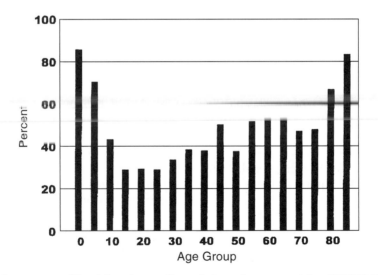

Figure 26–7. Percentage of Reed-Sternberg cells or their variants containing EBV DNA in Hodgkin lymphoma patients by age group. International collection of tumor materials from 1546 patients. (*Source*: Glaser et al, 1997)

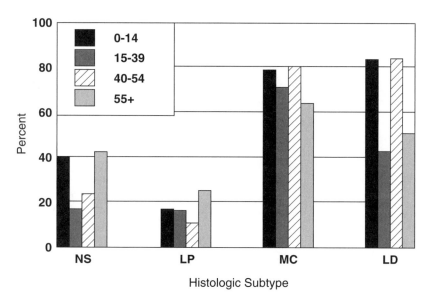

Figure 26–8. Percentage of Reed-Sternberg cells or their variants that contain EBV DNA in Hodgkin lymphoma patients by histologic subtype and age group. (*Source*: Glaser et al, 1997)

highly varied pattern. Given the difference in age and sex distribution of the mixed cellularity and nodular sclerosis subtypes, it is not surprising that the presence of EBV has a U-shaped relationship with age, with the highest proportion of cases being EBV-positive at the extremes of age and the lowest in young adulthood (Fig. 26–7). However, the distinct age distribution of EBV–positive cases persists after allowing for the effect of histologic subtype (Glaser et al, 1997; Armstrong et al, 1998). This pattern is particularly clear for nodular sclerosis (Fig. 26–8).

Both in developing and developed countries a high proportion (from 80% to more than 90%) of the tumors diagnosed in children below 10 years of age are EBV-positive (Armstrong et al, 1998; Ambinder et al, 1999; Flavell et al, 2001). The proportion of EBV-positive tumors decreases substantially thereafter, remaining below 20% to 30% up to the mid-40s (Fig. 26–7). At higher ages it rises gradually to exceed 80% among the oldest. For affected women in the age group 15 to 49 years, the likelihood of an EBV association is half of that among men (Glaser et al, 1997). Based on a limited number of studies, there is inconsistent ev-

idence of familial Hodgkin lymphoma EBV concordance (Mack et al, 1995; Lin et al, 1996; Kamper et al, 2005).

The data on EBV prevalence in tumor tissue strongly support the hypothesis that Hodgkin lymphomas have different etiologies in children, young adults, and older adults (MacMahon, 1966). The three-disease model, illustrated in Figure 26–9, describes the following entities (Jarrett, 2006; Armstrong et al, 1998):

1. EBV-related Hodgkin lymphoma that occurs predominantly, but not exclusively in children less than 10 years of age. It is typically of the mixed cellularity variant and occurs with a higher incidence in developing than developed countries and may be related to primary EBV infection.

2. The second entity, occuring mostly among those above 45 years of age, is also EBV-related and primarily of the mixed cellularity subtype. In contrast to the childhood equivalent, it is likely to be the result of reactivation of a latent EBV infection caused by an impaired immune response.

3. The third entity shows no evidence of EBV infection in HRS cells. The histologic subtype is primarily nodular sclerosis. This

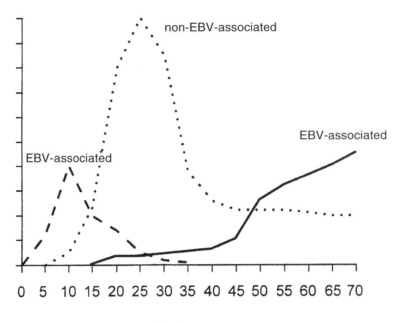

Figure 26–9. Schematic presentation of the three-disease model of Hodgkin lymphoma. (*Source*: Armstrong et al, 1998)

entity is most common in developed countries at ages 15–45 years, with a peak incidence in the mid-to-late 20s. The epidemiologic profile suggests a causal role of delayed infection or a delayed host response to an infection other than EBV.

Physical Activity

Two studies have evaluated the possible influence of physical activity on the risk of Hodgkin lymphoma (Paffenbarger et al, 1977; Keegan et al, 2006). Though both suggested that strenuous physical activity was associated with decreased Hodgkin lymphoma risk, the overall evidence of a causal association is considered to be weak.

Ionizing Radiation

Exposure to therapeutic and diagnostic radiation does not appear to increase the risk of Hodgkin lymphoma. Nor do results of the studies of atomic bomb survivors support an association with ionizing radiation (Ron, 1998).

Occupation

Occupation and occupational exposures play little if any role in the etiology of Hodgkin lymphoma. Two areas have previously attracted particular interest, namely wood-related industries and certain chemical exposures (Mueller and Grufferman, 2006), however, allowing no firm conclusions. The woodworking industry, with occupations such as sawmill and papermill work, has shown the most consistent link with an increased Hodgkin lymphoma risk, though reported risk estimates have varied considerably and data quality has been questioned. Increased risks have been reported with exposure to chemicals including chlorophenols and pesticides. Not all studies, however, have shown positive associations, and no single chemical has been consistently and unambiguously linked with the disease (McCunney, 1999). A meta-analysis of 30 studies that addressed a possible association between farming and Hodgkin lymphoma found this occupation to be associated with an overall 25% increased risk. However, the estimates that contributed to the overall result tended to be smallest in the more recent studies (Khuder et al, 1999).

Medical Conditions and Treatment

With the exception of infectious mononucleosis, certain immunodeficiency conditions and autoimmune disorders (discussed below), there is little evidence that medical conditions or treatments (e.g. chronic diseases, blood transfusions, chemotherapy, more common medications) influence the risk of Hodgkin lymphoma. A recent exception from this is the finding of decreased risk of Hodgkin lymphoma in regular users of aspirin and conversely, an increased risk in regular users of acetaminophen (Chang et al, 2004c). Furthermore, there is no consistent support for an association of vaccinations with Hodgkin lymphoma.

Infectious mononucleosis

Most, though not all, case-control studies report a weak but positive association between infectious mononucleosis and Hodgkin lymphoma, particularly in young adults. Seven cohort studies comprising more than 70,000 serologically confirmed cases of infectious mononucleosis, and all comparing observed with expected rates from the general population, documented 2- to 3-fold relative risks of Hodgkin lymphoma (summarized in IARC, 1997; Hjalgrim et al, 2000). The largest of these prospective studies reported a 2.5-fold increased risk; the risk remained elevated up to 20 years after diagnosis of infectious mononucleosis (Hjalgrim et al, 2000). Hodgkin lymphoma was the only cancer besides skin cancer (increased risk) and lung cancer (decreased risk) that could be linked to infectious mononucleosis, which suggests that this infection has a specific role in the etiology of Hodgkin lymphoma.

While the fact that EBV is the cause of most cases of infectious mononucleosis should further support its causal association with Hodgkin lymphoma, young adults were at particularly high risk of developing Hodgkin lymphoma following infectious mononucleosis in both case-control studies and prospective studies. Paradoxically, as already discussed, this age group generally has the lowest percentage of EBV-positive tumors (Glaser et al, 1997). Studies including information about tumor EBV status prior history of infectious mononucleosis provide conflicting findings. Infectious mononucleosis history was associated with particularly increased risk of EBV-positive Hodgkin lymphoma in case-control studies from the United Kingdom (Alexander et al, 2000) and Scandinavia (Hjalgrim et al., 2007b) and in a Scandinavian cohort study (Hjalgrim et al, 2003), whereas elevated risks were reported for both EBV-negative and EBV-positive Hodgkin lymphoma in another British investigation (Alexander et al, 2003). Still other studies have not observed an association between mononucleosis history and Hodgkin lymphoma risk, regardless of EBV status (Chang et al, 2004b; Glaser et al, 2005).

Altogether the present literature does not unambiguously support the idea that the role of infectious mononucleosis in Hodgkin lymphoma is simply as a marker of EBV exposure. An alternative explanation, that a history of infectious mononucleosis in young adults with Hodgkin lymphoma reflects an association with high social class and perhaps late exposure to other infectious agents, has found little support (Hjalgrim et al, 2002, 2007b). Again, however, conflicting data are available (Alexander et al, 2003). Perhaps instead the association reflects an individual ability among patients with infectious mononucleosis and Hodgkin lymphoma to immunologically hyperreact to certain stimuli, such as antigens.

Autoimmune diseases

One of the more interesting associations found for non-Hodgkin lymphoma is with different autoimmune and inflammatory conditions. An association with Hodgkin lymphoma is also apparent although not as strong and consistent. Two- to 5-fold increased risks of Hodgkin lymphoma following rheumatoid arthritis have been reported (Gridley et al, 1993; Kauppi et al, 1997;

Thomas et al, 2000; Landgren et al, 2006). Also, patients with systemic lupus erythematosus and immune thrombocytopenic purpura have been reported to have an excess risk of Hodgkin lymphoma (Mellemkjaer et al, 1997; Sultan et al, 2000; Landgren et al, 2006). In addition, a large population-based case-control study in Scandinavia reported a 14-fold increased risk with sarcoidosis (Landgren et al. 2006). Because of the historically significant classification problems with cases of non-Hodgkin lymphoma being misclassified as Hodgkin lymphoma, it is unclear to what extent the observed elevated risk estimates are real since the larger studies have been based on registry records rather than on manual identification and reclassification of cases.

Tonsillectomy

Evidence that tonsillectomy increases the risk of Hodgkin lymphoma remains inconclusive. Early studies focused on a possible association with removal of lymphoid tissue such as tonsillectomy (Mueller, 1987). Part of the interest was evoked by reported associations of tonsillectomy with poliomyelitis and multiple sclerosis, diseases that share epidemiologic characteristics with Hodgkin lymphoma. Case-control studies have generated inconsistent results. Some positive findings have been explained by the confounding effect of, for example, socioeconomic status and by potential effects of underlying disease (Mueller, 1987; Bonelli et al, 1990; Gledovic and Radovanovic, 1991; Liaw et al, 1997; Vineis et al, 2000). The large population-based study by Liaw et al. (1997) found no overall significant increase in Hodgkin lymphoma among patients with a history of tonsillectomy. Only those patients who had undergone tonsillectomy at a young age appeared to be at increased risk. However, in another study, tonsillectomy at young age was associated with a decreased risk (Bonelli et al, 1990).

Immunodeficiency

The risk of Hodgkin lymphoma is increased in patients with congenital immunodefi-

ciency and debatably in patients treated with immunosuppression following organ transplantation (Kinlen, 1992; Birkeland et al., 1995). Both follow-up studies among patients with acquired immune deficiency syndrome (AIDS) and large cohort studies among human immunodeficiency virus (HIV)–positive subjects have consistently documented an increased risk of Hodgkin lymphoma (Koblin et al, 1996; Goedert et al, 1998; Grulich et al, 1999; Frisch et al, 2001). In the largest of the studies from the United States, the overall excess risk was 11-fold, slightly lower among women (RR=8.3) than among men (RR=12.0). No difference was observed between ethnic groups or between the various groups at high risk of HIV exposure. The excess risk was particularly high for the mixed cellularity (RR=18.3) and lymphocytic depletion (RR=35.3) subtypes among AIDS patients (Frisch et al, 2001). In studies based on small numbers of subjects, the majority of tumor biopsy specimens from patients with HIV-associated Hodgkin lymphoma have been found to contain EBV. This resembles the situation for non-Hodgkin lymphoma, which is significantly more likely to be EBV-positive in patients with AIDS than those without.

Sibship Size and Social Class

Consistent with the ecologic association between socioeconomic status and age-specific incidence pattern of Hodgkin lymphoma, case-control and cohort studies have found Hodgkin lymphoma among young adults to be associated with high maternal educational level, small sibship size, low birth order, and less crowded housing (Mueller and Grufferman, 2006). This pattern has led to the suggestion that Hodgkin lymphoma in young adults may develop as a rare consequence of late infection with a common infectious agent (Gutensohn and Cole, 1977). This disease model is similar to that described for polio and EBV. Infection with polio and EBV viruses in early childhood is usually reported to be asymptomatic or mild. More severe disease manifestations, such as paralytic poliomyelitis and EBV-related infectious mononucleosis, are likely to occur when exposure is delayed until adolescence or young adult life (Evans and Niederman, 1989; Melnick, 1989).

In the context of a possible infectious etiology, sibship size may be a proxy for the overall probability of acquiring infection. Birth order may be important for the age at exposure to common infections, assuming that children of later birth order are more likely to be exposed to infectious agents at an earlier age via contact with their older siblings (Westergaard et al, 1997). In contrast to its occurrence in young adults, childhood Hodgkin lymphoma has been positively associated with sibship size in some studies but not in others. In particular, in a large Danish cohort analysis an increased risk of childhood Hodgkin lymphoma with increasing sib ship size was observed (Westergaard et al, 1997), whereas no such association was seen in similar Swedish data (Chang et al, 2004c). In the two investigations, risk of Hodgkin lymphoma in young adults, in contrast, was inversely correlated with number of older siblings (Chang et al, 2004c) or birth order (Westergaard et al, 1997). These results strongly indicate different risk factors for Hodgkin lymphoma in children and in young adults (Jarrett et al, 1996) (see also "Infections").

CONCLUSION

In contrast to what has been observed for non-Hodgkin lymphoma, the overall incidence of Hodgkin lymphoma has remained fairly stable in recent decades, however, with diverging trends observed in older (decreasing incidence) and younger (increasing incidence) adults. The descriptive epidemiology of Hodgkin lymphoma shows great variation by age, sex, social class, and histological subtype, which clearly indicates the importance of environmental factors in its etiology. In particular, EBV may be causally involved in Hodgkin lymphoma cases among children and older adults, whereas the lymphoma in young adults stands out as being different and with another etiology. For this particular group, factors associated with socio-economic affluence and small sibship size appear important. It has been suggested that a late infection with another common agent different from EBV could play a role. Besides EBV surprisingly few risk factors have been identified. These include immunodeficiency conditions (HIV-induced, for example) and certain autoimmune conditions. Thus, despite many years of research, the most intriguing associations pointing to possible etiologic factors involved in Hodgkin lymphoma are still those dictated by age, sex, social class, educational level, sibship size, and crowding. At present, one of the most obvious candidates as an etiologic factor in Hodgkin lymphoma, particularly among young adults, is another infectious agent yet to be identified.

REFERENCES

Alexander FE, Jarrett RF, Lawrence D, Armstrong AA, Freeland J, Gokhale DA, et al. Risk factors for Hodgkin's disease by Epstein-Barr virus (EBV) status: prior infection by EBV and other agents. Br J Cancer 2000; 82:1117–21.

Alexander FE, Lawrence DJ, Freeland J, Krajewski AS, Angus B, Taylor GM, et al. An epidemiologic study of index and family infectious mononucleosis and adult Hodgkin's disease (HD): evidence for a specific association with EBV+ve HD in young adults. Int J Cancer 2003;107(2):298–302.

Ambinder RF, Lemas MV, Moore S, Yang J, Fabian D, Krone C. Epstein-Barr virus and lymphoma. Cancer Treat Res 1999;99: 27–45.

Armstrong AA, Alexander FE, Cartwright R, Angus B, Krajewski AS, Wright DH, et al. Epstein-Barr virus and Hodgkin's disease: further evidence for the three disease hypothesis. Leukemia 1998;12:1272–76.

Besson H, Brennan P, Becker N, De SS, Nieters A, Font R, et al. Tobacco smoking, alcohol drinking and Hodgkin's lymphoma: a European multi-centre case-control study (EPILYMPH). Br J Cancer 2006;95:378–84.

Birkeland SA, Storm HH, Lamm LU, Barlow L, Blohmé I, Forsberg B, et al. Cancer risk after renal transplantation in the Nordic countries, 1964–1986. Int J Cancer 1995; 60:183–9.

Bonelli L, Vitale V, Bistolfi F, Landucci M, Bruzzi P. Hodgkin's disease in adults: association with social factors and age at tonsillectomy. A case-control study. Int J Cancer 1990;45:423–27.

Briggs NC, Hall HI, Brann EA, Moriarty CJ, Levine RS. Cigarette smoking and risk of Hodgkin's disease: a population-based case-control study. Am J Epidemiol 2002; 156(11):1011–20.

Chang ET, Blomqvist P, Lambe M. Seasonal variation in the diagnosis of Hodgkin lymphoma in Sweden. Int J Cancer 2005a;115: 127–30.

Chang ET, Hjalgrim H, Smedby KE, Akerman M, Tani E, Johnsen HE, et al. Body mass index and risk of malignant lymphoma in Scandinavian men and women. J Natl Cancer Inst 2005b;97:210–18.

Chang ET, Montgomery SM, Richiardi L, Ehlin A, Ekbom A, Lambe M. Number of siblings and risk of Hodgkin's lymphoma. Cancer Epidemiol Biomarkers Prev 2004c;13:1236–43.

Chang ET, Zheng T, Weir EG, Borowitz M, Mann RB, Spiegelman D, et al. Aspirin and the risk of Hodgkin's lymphoma in a population-based case-control study. J Natl Cancer Inst 2004b;96:305–15.

Chang ET, Zheng T, Lennette ET, Weir EG, Borowitz M, Mann RB, et al. Heterogeneity of risk factors and antibody profiles in epstein-barr virus genome-positive and -negative hodgkin lymphoma. J Infect Dis 2004a; 189:2271–81.

Chen YT, Zheng T, Chou MC, Boyle P, Holford TR. The increase of Hodgkin's disease incidence among young adults. Experience in Connecticut, 1935–1992. Cancer 1997;79: 2209–18.

Correa P, O'Conor GT. Epidemiologic patterns of Hodgkin's disease. Int J Cancer 1971;8: 192–201.

Davis MK. Review of the evidence for an association between infant feeding and childhood cancer. Int J Cancer 1998;11(S):29–33.

Diepstra A, Niens M, te Meerman GJ, Poppema S, van den BA. Genetic susceptibility to Hodgkin's lymphoma associated with the human leukocyte antigen region. Eur J Haematol Suppl 2005a;34–41.

Diepstra A, Niens M, Vellenga E, van Imhoff GW, Nolte IM, Schaapveld M, et al. Association with HLA class I in Epstein-Barr-virus-positive and with HLA class III in Epstein-Barr-virus-negative Hodgkin's lymphoma. Lancet 2005b;365:2216–24.

Evans AS. The clinical illness promotion factor: a third ingredient. Yale J Biol Med 1982;55: 193–99.

Evans AS, Niederman JC. Epstein-Barr virus. In: Evans AS (Ed): Viral Infections of Humans. Epidemiology and Control. New York, Plenum Medical, 1989, pp 265–92.

Ferlay J, Bray F, Pisani P, Parkin DM. GLOBOCAN 2000: Cancer Incidence, Mortality and Prevalence Worldwide. International Agency for Research on Cancer, Lyon, 2001.

Flavell KJ, Biddulph JP, Powell JE, Parkes SE, Redfern D, Weinreb M, et al. South Asian ethnicity and material deprivation increase the risk of Epstein-Barr virus infection in childhood Hodgkin's disease. Br J Cancer 2001;85:350–56.

Franceschi S, Bidoli E, La Vecchia C. Pregnancy and Hodgkin's disease. Int J Cancer 1994; 58:465–66.

Frisch M, Biggar RJ, Engels EA, Goedert JJ. Cancer among 302,834 adults with AIDS in the United States. JAMA 2001;285:1736–45.

Gause A, Keymis S, Scholz R, Schobert I, Jung W, Diehl V, et al. Increased levels of circulating cytokines in patients with untreated Hodgkin's disease. Lymphokine Cytokine Res 1992;11:109–13.

Glaser SL. Reproductive factors in Hodgkin's disease in women: a review. Am J Epidemiol 1994;139:237–46.

Glaser SL, Clarke CA, Nugent RA, Stearns CB, Dorfman RF. Social class and risk of Hodgkin's disease in young-adult women in 1988–94. Int J Cancer 2002; 98:110–17.

Glaser SL, Jarrett RF. The epidemiology of Hodgkin's disease. Baillieres Clin Haematol 1996;9:401–16.

Glaser SL, Keegan TH, Clarke CA, Trinh M, Dorfman RF, Mann RB, et al. Exposure to childhood infections and risk of Epstein-Barr virus—defined Hodgkin's lymphoma in women. Int J Cancer 2005;115:599–605.

Glaser SL, Lin RJ, Stewart SL, Ambinder RF, Jarrett RF, Brousset P, et al. Epstein-Barr virus–associated Hodgkin's disease: epidemiologic characteristics in international data. Int J Cancer 1997;70:375–82.

Glaser SL, Swartz WG. Time trends in Hodgkin's disease incidence. The role of diagnostic accuracy. Cancer 1990;66:2196–2204.

Gledovic Z, Radovanovic Z. History of tonsillectomy and appendectomy in Hodgkin's disease. Eur J Epidemiol 1991;7:612–15.

Goedert JJ, Cote TR, Virgo P, Scoppa SM, Kingma DW, Gail MH, et al. Spectrum of AIDS-associated malignant disorders. Lancet 1998;351:1833–39.

Goldin LR, Pfeiffer RM, Gridley G, Gail MH, Li X, Mellemkjaer L, et al. Familial aggregation of Hodgkin lymphoma and related tumors. Cancer 2004;100:1902–8

Gridley G, McLaughlin JK, Ekbom A, Klareskog L, Adami HO, Hacker DG, et al. Incidence of cancer among patients with rheumatoid arthritis. JNCI 1993;85:307–11.

Grufferman S, Cole P, Smith PG, Lukes RJ. Hodgkin's disease in siblings. N Engl J Med 1977;296:248–50.

Grufferman S, Delzelle E. Epidemiology of Hodgkin's disease. Epidemiol Rev 1984;6: 76–106.

Grulich AE, Wan X, Law MG, Coates M, Kaldor JM. Risk of cancer in people with AIDS. AIDS 1999;13:839–43.

Gutensohn N, Cole P. Epidemiology of Hodgkin's disease in the young. Int J Cancer 1977; 19:595–604.

Gutensohn N, Cole P. Childhood social environment and Hodgkin's disease. N Engl J Med 1981;304:135–40.

Gutensohn N, Li FP, Johnson RE, Cole P. Hodgkin's disease, tonsillectomy and family size. N Engl J Med 1975;292:22–25.

Harris NL. Hodgkin's lymphomas: classification, diagnosis, and grading. Semin Hematol 1999;36:220–32.

Harris NL, Jaffe ES, Diebold J, Flandrin G, Muller-Hermelink HK, Vardiman J, et al. The World Health Organization classification of neoplastic diseases of the haematopoietic and lymphoid tissues: Report of the Clinical Advisory Committee Meeting, Airlie House, Virginia, November 1997. Histopathology 2000;36:69–86.

Hartge P, Devesa SS, Fraumeni JF Jr. Hodgkin's and non-Hodgkin's lymphomas. Cancer Surv 1994;20:423–53.

Hjalgrim H, Askling J, Pukkala E, Hansen S, Munksgaard L, Frisch M. Increasing incidence of nodular sclerosis Hodgkin's disease among adolescents and young adults in the Nordic countries. Lancet 2001;358:297–98.

Hjalgrim H, Askling J, Sorensen P, Madsen M, Rosdahl N, Storm HH, et al. Risk of Hodgkin's disease and other cancers after infectious mononucleosis. J Natl Cancer Inst 2000;92:1522–28.

Hjalgrim H, Rostgaard K, Askling J, Madsen M, Storm H, Rabkin CS, Melbye M. Hematopoietic and lymphatic cancers in relatives of patients with infectious mononucleosis. J Natl Cancer Inst 2002;94:678–81.

Hjalgrim H, Askling J, Rostgaard K, Hamilton-Dutoit S, Frisch M, Zhang JS, Madsen M, Rosdahl N, Konradsen HB, Storm HH, Melbye M. Characteristics of Hodgkin's lymphoma after infectious mononucleosis. N Engl J Med 2003;349:1324–32.

Hjalgrim H, Smedby KE, Rostgaard K, Amini RM, Molin D, Hamilton-Dutoit S, Schollkopf C, Chang E, Ralfkiaer E, Adami HO, Glimelius B, Melbye M. Cigarette smoking and risk of Hodgkin lymphoma – a population-based case-control study. CEBP 2007a; 16(8):1561–6.

Hjalgrim H, Smedby KE, Rostgaard K, Molin D, Hamilton-Dutoit S, Chang E, Ralfkiaer E, Sundström C, Glimelius B, Adami HO, Melbye M. Infectious mononucleosis, childhood social environment and risk of Hodgkin lymphoma. Cancer Res 2007b;67(5): 2382–8.

International Agency for Research on Cancer. Epstein-Barr Virus and Kaposi's Sarcoma Herpesvirus/Herpesvirus 8. IARC Monographs on the Evaluation of Carcinogenic Risks to Humans. Lyon, IARC, 1997.

Isager H, Andersen E. Pre-morbid factors in Hodgkin's disease. I. Birth weight and growth pattern from 8 to 14 years of age. Scand J Haematol 1978;21:250–55.

Jarrett RF. Viruses and lymphoma/leukaemia. J Pathol 2006;208:176–86.

Jarrett RF, Armstrong AA, Alexander E. Epidemiology of EBV and Hodgkin's lymphoma. Ann Oncol 1996;7:5–10.

Kamper PM, Kjeldsen E, Clausen N, Bendix K, hamilton-Dutoit S, D'Amore F. Epstein-Barr virus-associated familial Hodgkin lymphoma: paediatric onset in three of five siblings. Br J Haematol 2005;129:615–17.

Kauppi M, Pukkala E, Isomaki H. Elevated incidence of hematologic malignancies in patients with Sjogren's syndrome compared with patients with rheumatoid arthritis. Cancer Causes Control 1997;8:201–4.

Keegan TH, Glaser SL, Clarke CA, Dorfman RF, Mann RB, DiGiuseppe JA et al. Body size, physical activity, and risk of Hodgkin's lymphoma in women. Cancer Epidemiol Biomarkers Prev 2006;15:1095–1101.

Khuder SA, Mutgi AB, Schaub EA, Tano BD. Meta-analysis of Hodgkin's disease among farmers. Scand J Work Environ Health 1999; 25:436–41.

Kinlen LJ. Immunosuppression and cancer. In: Vainio H, Magee PN, McGregor DB, McMichael AJ (Eds): Mechanisms of Carcinogenesis in Risk Identification. Lyon, International Agency for Research on Cancer, 1992, pp 237–53.

Koblin BA, Hessol NA, Zauber AG, Taylor PE, Buchbinder SP, Katz MH, et al. Increased incidence of cancer among homosexual men, New York City and San Francisco, 1978–1990. Am J Epidemiol 1996;144:916–23.

Kravdal O, Hansen S. Hodgkin's disease: the protective effect of childbearing. Int J Cancer 1993;55:909–14.

Kravdal O, Hansen S. The importance of childbearing for Hodgkin's disease: new evidence from incidence and mortality models. Int J Epidemiol 1996;25:737–43.

Lambe M, Hsieh CC, Tsaih SW, Adami J, Glimelius B, Adami HO. Childbearing and the risk of Hodgkin's disease. Cancer Epidemiol Biomarkers Prev 1998;7:831–34.

Landgren O, Engels E, Pfeiffer RM, Gridley G, Mellemkjaer L, Olsen JH, Kerstann KF, Wheeler W, Hemminki K, Linet MS, Goldin

LR. Autoimmunity and susceptibility to Hodgkin lymphoma: A population-based case-control study in Scandinavia. J Natl Cancer Inst 2006;98:1321–30.

Langagergaard V, Norgard B, Mellemkjaer L, Pedersen L, Rothman KJ, Sorensen HT. Seasonal variation in month of birth and diagnosis in children and adolescents with Hodgkin disease and non-Hodgkin lymphoma. J Pediatr Hematol Oncol 2003; 25:534–38

Lehtinen T, Lumio J, Dillner J, Hakama M, Knekt P, Lehtinen M, et al. Increased risk of malignant lymphoma indicated by elevated Epstein-Barr virus antibodies—a prospective study. Cancer Causes Control 1993;4:187–93.

Liaw KL, Adami J, Gridley G, Nyrén O, Linet MS. Risk of Hodgkin's disease subsequent to tonsillectomy: a population-based cohort study in Sweden. Int J Cancer 1997;72:711–13.

Lin AY, Kingma DW, Lennette ET, Fears TR, Whitehouse JM, Ambinder RF, et al.Epstein-Barr virus and familial Hodgkin's disease. Blood 1996; 88:3160–65.

Mack TM, Cozen W, Shibata DK, Weiss LM, Nathwani BN, Hernandez AM, et al. Concordance for Hodgkin's disease in identical twins suggesting genetic susceptibility to the young-adult form of the disease. N Engl J Med 1995;332:413–18.

MacMahon B. Epidemiological evidence of the nature of Hodgkin's disease. Cancer 1957; 10(5):1045–54.

MacMahon B. Epidemiology of Hodgkin's disease. Cancer Res 1966;26:1189–1201.

McCunney RJ. Hodgkin's disease, work, and the environment. A review. J Occup Environ Med 1999;4:36–46.

Medeiros LJ, Greiner TC. Hodgkin's disease. Cancer 1995;75:357–69.

Mellemkjaer L, Andersen V, Linet MS, Gridley G, Hoover R, Olsen JH. Non-Hodgkin's lymphoma and other cancers among a cohort of patients with lupus erythematosus. Arthritis Rheum 1997;40:761–68.

Melnick JL. Enteroviruses. In: AS Evans (Ed): Viral Infections of Humans. Epidemiology and Control. New York, Plenum Medical, 1989, pp 191–293.

Merk K, Bjorkholm M, Tullgren O, Mellstedt H, Holm G. Immune deficiency in family members of patients with Hodgkin's disease. Cancer 1990;66:1938–43.

Mueller NE. The epidemiology of Hodgkin's disease. In: Selby P, McElwain TJ (Eds): Hodgkin's Disease. Oxford, Blackwell Scientific, 1987, pp 68–93.

Mueller NE, Grufferman S. Hodgkin Lymphoma. In: Schottenfeld D, Fraumeni JF Jr (Eds): Cancer Epidemiology and Prevention. Oxford, Oxford University Press, 2006, pp 872–897.

Mueller NE, Evans A, Harris NL, Comstock GW, Jellum E, Magnus K, et al. Hodgkin's disease and Epstein-Barr virus. Altered antibody pattern before diagnosis. N Engl J Med 1989;320:689–95.

Newell GR, Lynch HK, Gibeau JM, Spitz MR. Seasonal diagnosis of Hodgkin's disease among young adults. J Natl Cancer Inst 1985; 74:53–56.

Olsson H, Olsson ML, Ranstam J. Late age at first full-term pregnancy as a risk factor for women with malignant lymphoma. Neoplasma 1990;37:185–90.

Paffenbarger RS Jr, Wing AL, Hyde RT. Characteristics in youth indicative of adult-onset Hodgkin's disease. J Natl Cancer Inst 1977; 58:1489–91.

Parkin DM, Whelan SL, Ferley J, Teppo L, Thomas DB (Eds):Cancer Incidence in Five Continents, Vol VIII. Lyon, IARC. IARC Scientific Publications No. 155, 2002.

Ron E. Ionizing radiation and cancer risk: evidence from epidemiology. Radiat Res 1998; 150:30–41.

Sultan SM, Ioannou Y, Isenberg DA. Is there an association of malignancy with systemic lupus erythematosus? An analysis of 276 patients under long-term review. Rheumatology 2000;39:1147–52.

Thomas E, Brewster DH, Black RJ, MacFarlane GJ. Risk of malignancy among patients with rheumatoid conditions. Int J Cancer 2000; 88:497–502.

Vineis P, Miligi L, Crosignani P, Fontana A, Masala G, Nanni O, et al. Delayed infection, family size and malignant lymphomas. J Epidemiol Commun Health 2000;54907–11.

Weiss LM, Strickler JG, Warnke RA, Purtilo DT, Sklar J. Epstein-Barr viral DNA in tissues of Hodgkin's disease. Am J Pathol 1987; 129:86–91.

Westergaard T, Melbye M, Pedersen JB, Frisch M, Olsen JH, Andersen PK. Birth order, sibship size and risk of Hodgkin's disease in children and young adults: a population-based study of 31 million person-years. Int J Cancer 1997;72:977–81.

Zahm SH, Hoover RN, Fraumeni JF Jr. Hodgkin's disease and parity. Int J Cancer 1995; 62:362–63.

Zwitter M, Zakelj MP, Kosmelj K. A case–control study of Hodgkin's disease and pregnancy. Br J Cancer 1996;73:246–51.

27

Non-Hodgkin Lymphoma

MADS MELBYE, KARIN EKSTRÖM SMEDBY, AND DIMITRIOS TRICHOPOULOS

Non-Hodgkin lymphoma (NHL) is unique among human malignancies for several reasons. First, it is distinguished as an entity by exclusion from a much less common group of lymphomas called Hodgkin lymphoma. Second—and more important—the incidence of NHL has been rising more rapidly than that of virtually any other human cancer in many parts of the world. Indeed, this increase has been considered almost epidemic and its causes remain enigmatic, though it suggests exposure to new causal agents that might be avoidable.

Finally, no other cancer entity comprises such a heterogeneous group of malignancies as does NHL. Originating from lymphocytes, NHL can develop from within organized lymphoid tissue, such as lymph nodes, or from other sites. Many lymphoid neoplasms pass through both solid tumor and circulating (leukemic) phases. Chronic lymphocytic leukemia and plasmocytoma/multiple myeloma now belong to the entity of NHL according to the widely accepted World Health Organization (WHO) classification (Jaffe et al, 2001), although they

are classified separately in the International Classification of Diseases (ICD). The diversity of NHL subgroups and the inconsistency in classification systems have complicated research on the causes of this cancer. In fact, only in recent years have studies begun to distinguish NHL by subtype.

CLINICAL SYNOPSIS

Subgroups

NHL, divided into B-cell and T-cell neoplasms based on their immunophenotypic characteristics, includes numerous specific entities that are often associated with particular karyotypic abnormalities. Due to the wide variety of disease entities, classification of NHL has been difficult, as reflected in the many taxonomies. In 2001, the WHO published a new classification (Jaffe et al, 2001) based on the previous Revised European-American Classification of Lymphoid Neoplasms (REAL). WHO recognizes B-cell neoplasms, T/NK-cell neoplasms, and Hodgkin lymphoma. The T- and B-cell neoplasms are divided into precursor lymphoblastic neoplasms (acute lymphoblastic leukemia/lymphoma), and mature neoplasms (Table 27–1).

Symptoms

The most common early signs are painless swelling of lymph nodes, fever, night sweats, and loss of weight. Poor appetite, excessive fatigue, bleeding and itchy skin, reddened patches on the skin, and bone pain may also be reported. Many cases of NHL are detected through routine procedures while still asymptomatic.

Diagnosis

Histopathologic diagnosis is based on biopsy material, mostly from lymph nodes. Detailed subgrouping requires immunohistochemistry, flow cytometry, cytogenetics, or molecular genetic studies. Clinical staging involves information on affected lymph nodes and spread to the bone marrow, spleen, or organs outside the lymphatic system. Imaging studies are used to determine the localization and extent of spread. Bone-marrow aspiration and biopsy are always used, sometimes with lumbar puncture as well.

Treatment

Disease localized to a group of lymph nodes or to an extranodal organ can be treated with radiotherapy. In more advanced stages, chemotherapy with or without radiation therapy is often used, depending on the type of NHL, symptoms, laboratory values, and location of the lymphoma. Many indolent lymphoma types are not treated until definite symptoms or other signs develop. New therapeutic regimens using monoclonal antibodies, with or without chemically bound radioactive isotope, directed at lymphoma cells, and high-dose chemotherapy with stem-cell transplantation are increasingly used in patients either at diagnosis or at relapse after standard treatment.

Prognosis and Progress

Because NHL is a heterogeneous malignancy, overall survival figures provide only crude information. The prognosis may vary from an aggressive course bringing death within a few weeks, to an indolent course even with no therapy for years or even decades. The 5-year relative survival rate improved from about 30% in the early 1960s to about 50% in the early 1990s, and has recently improved further with the addition of monoclonal antibody treatment. In children, relative 5-year survival approaches 80% to 90%, a great improvement from the mid-1970s, when few children were alive 5 years after diagnosis.

DESCRIPTIVE EPIDEMIOLOGY

Incidence

Worldwide, NHL constitutes the tenth most commonly diagnosed malignancy, whereas in the developed world it ranks seventh (Ferlay et al, 2004). The incidence of NHL varies from around 2 to 3 per 100 000 person-years in Thailand and China to about 14 per 100 000 person-years among whites in the United States and Canada. In general, the incidence is 40% to 70% higher among males than among females (Figs. 27–1 to 27–4) and is similarly higher among whites than among blacks, although these figures vary by subtype. For example, among whites the male-to-female ratio is greater than 2 for Burkitt leukemia/lymphoma, mantle cell lymphoma, and lymphoplasmacytoma, whereas it is close to 1 for marginal zone and follicular NHL (Morton et al, 2006b). For B-cell NHL the ratio of white-to-black age-adjusted incidence is between 2 and 3 for hairy cell leukemia, mantle cell and follicular lymphoma, and lymphoplasmacytoma. In contrast, peripheral T-cell NHL and plasma cell neoplasms are more common among blacks (Morton et al, 2006b).

As illustrated in Figures 27–1 and 27–2, the age-specific incidence pattern is different from that of Hodgkin lymphoma. The incidence increases steadily with age for almost all subtypes, except B- and T-cell lymphoblastic leukemia/lymphoma, which are diagnosed primarily in children.

Table 27–1. World Health Organization classification of lymphoid neoplasms

B-Cell Neoplasms

Precursor B-cell neoplasm
- Precursor B-lymphoblastic leukemia/lymphoma (precursor B-cell acute lymphoblastic leukemia)

Mature (peripheral) B-cell neoplasms*
- Chronic lymphocytic leukemia/small lymphocytic lymphoma
- B-cell prolymphocytic leukemia
- Lymphoplasmacytic lymphoma/waldenström macroglobulinemia
- Splenic marginal zone B-cell lymphoma (+/− villous lymphocytes)
- Hairy cell leukemia
- Plasmo cell neoplasm
- Extranodal marginal zone B-cell lymphoma of mucosa-associated lymphoid tissue (MALT lymphoma)
- Nodal marginal zone B-cell lymphoma (+/− monocytoid B cells)
- Follicular lymphoma
- Mantle cell lymphoma
- Diffuse large B-cell lymphoma
  - Mediastinal large B-cell lymphoma
- Primary effusion lymphoma
- Burkitt lymphoma/leukemia

T and NK-Cell Neoplasms

Precursor T-cell neoplasm
- Precursor T-lymphoblastic lymphoma/leukemia (precursor T-cell acute lymphoblastic leukemia)

Mature T-cell neoplasms†
- T-cell prolymphocytic leukemia
- T-cell large granular lymphocytic leukemia
- Aggressive NK-cell leukemia
- Adult T-cell leukemia/lymphoma
- Extranodal NK/T-cell lymphoma, nasal type
- Enteropathy-type T-cell lymphoma
- Hepatosplenic γδ T-cell lymphoma
- Subcutaneous panniculitis-like T-cell lymphoma
- Mycosis fungoides/Sézary syndrome
- Anaplastic large cell lymphoma, T/null cell, primary cutaneous type
- Peripheral T-cell lymphoma, not otherwise characterized
- Angioimmunoblastic T-cell lymphoma
- Anaplastic large cell lymphoma, T/null cell, primary systemic type

Hodgkin Lymphoma (Hodgkin's Disease)

- Nodular lymphocyte predominance Hodgkin lymphoma
- Classical Hodgkin lymphoma
- Nodular sclerosis Hodgkin lymphoma (grades 1 and 2)
- Lymphocyte-rich classic Hodgkin lymphoma
- Mixed cellularity Hodgkin lymphoma
- Lymphocyte depletion Hodgkin lymphoma

*B- and T/NK-cell neoplasms are grouped according to major clinical presentations (predominantly disseminated/leukemic, primary extranodal, predominantly nodel).

†Only major categories are included.

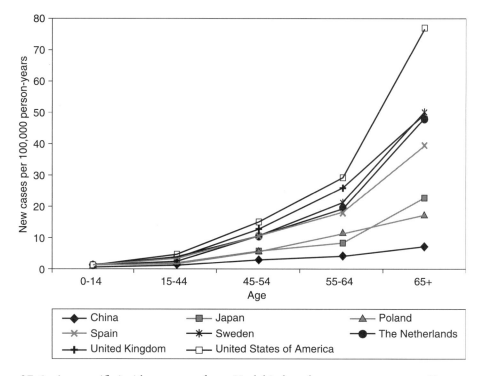

Figure 27–1. Age-specific incidence rates of non-Hodgkin lymphomas among women. (*Source*: Ferlay et al, 2004)

Time Trends

In the past decades, there has been a dramatic increase in the incidence of NHL in most western countries, on average 2% to 4% annually (Zheng et al, 1992; Devesa and Fears, 1992; Hjalgrim et al, 1996) (Fig. 27–5). This epidemic increase is among the most rapid observed for any cancer. An increase has also been observed in countries such as India, Japan, Brazil, and Singapore, as well as in Puerto Rico (Devesa and Fears, 1992). Changes in classification—cases previously diagnosed as Hodgkin lymphoma now classified as NHL—cannot explain the increase (Banks, 1992). Indeed, a number of detailed studies including pathologic reviews indicate that the increase is real (Hartge et al, 1994). According to figures from the United States and the Nordic countries, the long-lasting increase in incidence began to level off during the 1990s (Morton et al, 2006b; Sandin et al, 2006). The reasons for the past increase, as well as

for the recent apparent levelling off in some countries, remain unclear.

Subtype Trends

While the overall increase in NHL is unambiguous and indeed dramatic, our knowledge of incidence trends by subtype is limited. In the group of extranodal disease comprising 25% to 30% of all NHL, brain and skin disease show the highest proportional rise in incidence (Devesa and Fears, 1992; Groves et al, 2000). For NHL affecting the brain, the increase may partly be a result of improved diagnostic methods and, in some countries, may be caused by NHL secondary to human immunodeficiency virus (HIV) infection. In countries with substantial HIV spread, increases in immunoblastic and Burkitt-like NHL have also been striking (Devesa and Fears, 1992). Accordingly, the incidence of AIDS-associated NHL subtypes has decreased markedly in the developed world since the introduction of

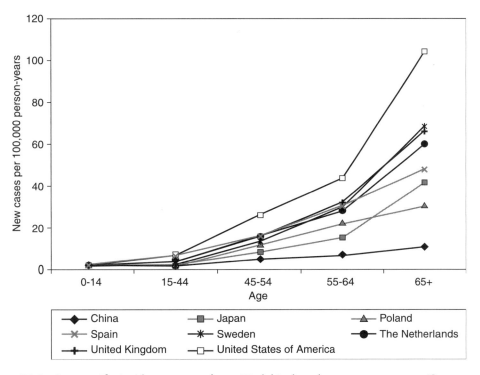

Figure 27–2. Age-specific incidence rates of non-Hodgkin lymphomas among men. (*Source*: Ferlay et al, 2004)

highly active antiretroviral therapy (HAART) (Eltom et al, 2002; Engels et al, 2006).

Analyses on incidence trends by histologic subtype are few. The Surveillance, Epidemiology, and End Results (SEER) program in the United States found high-grade NHL to have tripled among males and doubled among females between the periods 1978 to 1983 and 1990 to 1995. Immunoblastic NHL (a morphologic variant of diffuse large B-cell lymphoma, DLBCL) was the fastest-growing high-grade subtype (Groves et al, 2000). However, in a subsequent analysis for the period 1992 to 2002, overall

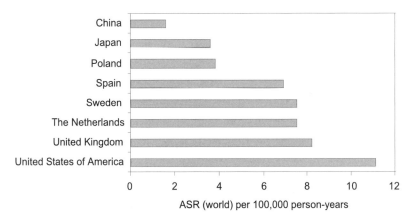

Figure 27–3. Age-standardized (to the world population) incidence rates of non-Hodgkin lymphomas among women. (*Source*: Ferlay et al, 2004)

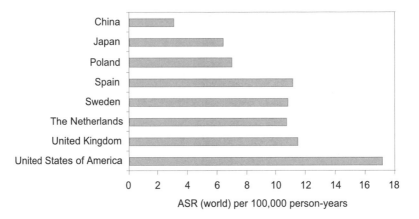

Figure 27–4. Age-standardized (to the world population) incidence rates of non-Hodgkin lymphomas among men. (*Source*: Ferlay et al, 2004)

incidence rates for DLBCL and chronic lymphocytic leukemia/small lymphocytic lymphoma declined, while rates for marginal zone, mantle cell, and peripheral T-cell lymphomas, as well as Burkitt leukemia/lymphoma, were still increasing (Morton et al, 2006b).

The B-cell phenotype of lymphomas dominates in most parts of the world. Our knowledge of the epidemiology of T-cell lymphomas is limited because available figures are often influenced by differences in classification. T-cell lymphomas are primarily of the peripheral T-cell type, whereas the cutaneous subtypes (e.g. Mycosis fungoides, Sézary syndrome) comprise only a small fraction. The geographic distribution of peripheral T-cell lymphoma varies greatly. In some parts of the Far East and the Caribbean, this is the dominant type. Hence, it comprises about 45% of NHL in different areas of Japan, 29% in Hong Kong, 39% in Taiwan, and at least 18% in mainland China (reviewed by Pallesen and Hamilton Dutoit, 1993). In contrast, corresponding figures for western countries reveal that only 5% to 15% of all NHLs are of the peripheral T-cell type.

Unexplained Increase

Following an extensive review of the literature, it was concluded in 1992 that known and suspected risk factors could not explain the dramatic increase in NHL (Banks, 1992; Hartge and Devesa, 1992; Obrams and O'Conor, 1992). After the likely effects of misdiagnosis of Hodgkin lymphoma, the inclusion of new entities, familial factors, HIV and other immune-suppressive conditions, drugs, and occupation were accounted for, it was estimated that 53% of the observed general increase among males over the past 40 years and 40% among males aged 0 to 64 years remained unexplained. An agent carrying a relative risk of 2 and rising in prevalence from 0% to 42% could account for the rise, but no such factor or factors have yet been identified.

GENETIC AND MOLECULAR EPIDEMIOLOGY

Non-Hodgkin lymphoma has repeatedly been reported to aggregate in certain families. Having close relatives with this disease or other hematolymphoproliferative malignancies increases the risk two to three fold (Paltiel et al, 2000; Chiu et al, 2004; Chang et al, 2005b). One study suggested that anticipation occurs in familial NHL, as shown by the lower age at onset in the child compared to the parent generation (Wiernik et al, 2000). Other studies have described a higher risk in siblings compared to parents and offspring of index persons with lymphoma or hematopoetic cancer (Paltiel et al, 2000; Chang et al, 2005b). This may indicate that both shared genetic and environmental factors contribute to the

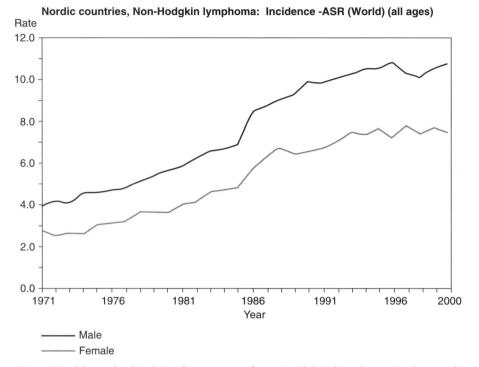

Figure 27–5. World-standardized incidence rates of non-Hodgkin lymphoma in the Nordic Countries 1971–2000.

observed overall association. In recent years, several studies of common genetic variation that could confer susceptibility to malignant lymphomas in the general population have been published. Examples of specific genes suggested to hold lymphoma susceptibility loci include those encoding for tumor necrosis factor alpha and other cytokines, DNA repair proteins, intermediates of the folate metabolism pathway, leptin and leptin receptors, and transcriptional factors (Skibola et al, 2007). Most promising so far are findings of associations with common variants in the interleukin-10 and tumor necrosis alpha genes and B-cell lymphomas, as reported in a large international pooled analysis (Rothman et al, 2006).

It is well known that many patients with certain inherited defects of immune function develop tumors, primarily B-cell lymphomas (Filipovich et al, 1992). These conditions include ataxia-telangiectasia, Wiskott-Aldrich syndrome, common variable immunodeficiency, severe combined immunodeficiency, X-linked lymphoproliferative disorder, Nijmegen breakage syndrome, hyper-IgM syndrome, and autoimmune lymphoproliferative syndrome (Jaffe et al, 2001). The mechanisms of lymphomagenesis are related to the underlying disorder and involve loss of T-cell control (Wiskott-Aldrich syndrome), apoptosis defects (autoimmune lymphoproliferative syndrome), abnormal DNA repair function (ataxia-telangiectasia, Nijmegen breakage syndrome), defective T-cell/B-cell interactions (hyper-IgM-syndrome), and perhaps chronic antigen stimulation (common variable immunodeficiency). However, these genetic disorders explain few new cases in the general population and cannot explain the strong temporal trends in incidence.

RISK FACTORS

Tobacco

Most large case-control and cohort studies have found no association between cigarette smoking and risk of overall NHL (Besson et al, 2006; Fernberg et al, 2006; Schollkopf et al, 2005; Zahm et al, 1997), although there are exceptions (Freedman et al, 1998; Morton et al, 2005a). It is at present unclear whether smoking causes an increase in specific NHL types. A cohort analysis of 253 000 members of a medical care program in the United States revealed a significant 1.9-fold increased risk of follicular lymphoma among smokers, but the strength of the association did not change with increasing duration or intensity of smoking (Herrinton and Friedman, 1998). In a large Danish-Swedish case-control study female but not male smokers were at increased risk of follicular lymphoma (Schollkopf et al, 2005). Another large international analysis of 6594 NHL cases and 8892 controls reported that current smokers, and in particular current heavy smokers, compared to nonsmokers, have an increased risk of follicular lymphoma (Morton et al, 2005a). The potential association is biologically interesting, because smoking may induce the chromosomal translocation t(14;18) (Bell et al, 1995; Schuler et al, 2003), which is found in 70% to 95% of follicular lymphomas (WHO, 2001). However, in the only study that so far has addressed this hypothesis, Schroeder and colleagues found no clear association between smoking and t(14;18)-positive NHL (Schroeder et al, 2002). Genetic variation is likely to explain possible important variations in the association between smoking and NHL risk but so far our knowledge is limited. In an evaluation of the role of aromatic and het erocyclic amines, which are metabolized by N-acetryltransferase (NAT) enzymes, cur rent cigarette smoking was associated with increased risk of NHL among NAT2 intermediate/rapid-acetylators (Morton et al, 2006a).

Diet

Research on the influence of dietary factors is complex per se and may be further complicated in NHL, if the different subgroups have different etiologies (Purdue et al, 2004). Intake of fruits, vitamin C, vegeta bles, lutein, zeaxanthin, and zinc has been inversely associated with NHL in some studies whereas results with respect to whole-grain foods have been mixed (Ward et al, 1994; Chang et al, 2005d; Kelemen et al, 2006; Talamini et al, 2006). The antioxidant or nitrosation-inhibiting properties of fruits and vegetables might be involved in reducing risk of NHL.

Dairy products have in many but not all studies been associated with an increased risk of NHL (Chiu et al, 1996; Zhang et al, 1999; Purdue et al, 2004; Zheng et al, 2004; Chang et al, 2005d; Talamini et al, 2006). Meat and in particular red meat consumption has been associated with an increased risk of NHL in some studies (De Stefani et al, 1998; Zhang et al, 1999; Chang et al, 2005d), whereas others have reported no association (Tavani et al, 2000b; Cross et al, 2006). Total fat and saturated fat intake has generally been associated with an increased risk of NHL (Chiu et al, 1996; Purdue et al, 2004; Zheng et al, 2004; Cross et al, 2006), whereas results on animal protein are conflicting (Ward et al, 1994; Zheng et al, 2004; Cross et al, 2006). The underlying mechanisms for the possible importance of certain meats and lipids are unknown. However, in addition to dietary carcinogens, it has been hypothesized that such products might lead to altered immunocompetence (Zhang et al, 1999; Zheng et al, 2004).

Nitrate in drinking water has been implicated as a possible risk factor for NHL. However, the evidence is limited and generally null (Freedman et al, 2000; Ward et al, 2006).

Alcohol

The literature describing the effects of alcohol on the risk of NHL is conflicting but in general does not support an important role for alcohol. Several studies found no association (Franceschi et al, 1989; Brown et al, 1992; Tavani et al, 1997; Chang et al, 2004; Willet et al, 2004), whereas one reported an inverse association between alcohol and the risk of NHL among women only (Nelson et al, 1997) and another among men only

(Besson, 2006). In a 9-year follow-up of 35 000 Iowa women, higher alcohol consumption was significantly associated with a decreased risk of NHL (Chiu et al, 1999). An international pooled analysis of nine case-control studies found that people who reported drinking alcohol had a lower risk of NHL than nondrinkers, but the inverse association did not increase with increasing alcohol consumption (Morton et al, 2005b).

Reproductive Factors

Because a pregnancy results in altered immunologic reactions and NHL is greatly influenced by immune dysregulation, it has been suggested that pregnancy could alter the incidence of NHL. However, there is no evidence of an association between a woman's reproductive history and risk of NHL (Adami et al, 1997b; Cerhan et al, 2002a).

Hormones

Notwithstanding the substantially higher incidence of NHL among men than among women, the possible role of hormones—endogenous or exogenous—has not been adequately investigated. The data on hormone replacement therapy are conflicting and based on small case-control studies (Nelson et al, 2001; Cerhan et al, 2002b; Beiderbeck et al, 2003a; Zhang et al, 2004c).

Anthropometric Measures

It has been speculated whether the obesity epidemic occurring in many parts of the world is linked to the the increasing incidence in NHL. In fact, several recent case-control studies have reported a positive association of body mass index (BMI) with risk of NHL (Holly et al, 1999; Cerhan et al, 2005; Willet et al, 2005; Pan et al, 2005). However, in one large study the association was only observed for the subtype of diffuse B-cell NHL (Cerhan et al, 2005), whereas in the Scandinavian lymphoma study (SCALE) encompassing more than 3000 cases, no overall association was found. A suggestive positive association with diffuse

large B-cell NHL was noted (Chang et al, 2005a). Recently, a prospective study based on Swedish construction workers did not confirm an association between high BMI and NHL (Fernberg et al, 2006). In one study, height was associated with increased risk of all NHL combined but also separately with diffuse B-cell lymphomas and follicular lymphomas (Cerhan et al, 2005). No consistent link has been found between birth weight and NHL in children or younger adults (Adami et al, 1996; Roman et al, 1997; Schuz et al, 1999).

Infections

Epstein-Barr virus

Epstein-Barr virus (EBV) is a ubiquitous human herpes virus that infects and persists in B lymphocytes of almost all humans without causing significant disease (Hjalgrim et al, 2006b). However, it encodes a number of genes that possess oncogenic potential by driving cell proliferation or conferring resistance to cell death (Ambinder, 2003). EBV was originally discovered in Burkitt lymphoma by investigators who believed that African Burkitt lymphoma was caused by a vectored virus (Epstein et al, 1964). The incidence of Burkitt lymphoma is highest among children in areas of Africa with holoendemic malaria, but sporadic cases occur at all ages in other parts of the world. It has been speculated that African Burkitt lymphoma might arise as a result of enhanced B-cell proliferation by early EBV infection interacting with the antigenic stimulatory effects of malaria.

Whereas EBV can be demonstrated in more than 95% of tumor biopsies of endemic cases in equatorial Africa, less than 20% of sporadic cases in developed countries are EBV-positive. Between 50% and 90% of Burkitt lymphomas in developing countries outside Africa are EBV-associated, but in regions with a temperate climate in South America, the EBV association is weaker than in tropical regions in the north of the continent (IARC, 1997).

Only a small fraction (usually less than 5%) of other B-cell NHL in immunocompetent patients contains EBV, and no consistent association between histologic type and EBV DNA has been evident. In contrast, EBV is often demonstrated in tumor material from T-cell lymphomas. These include in particular the extranodal NK/T-cell lymphoma of the nasal type, but also aggressive NK-cell leukemia (Nava and Jaffe, 2005) and possibly angioimmunoblastic T-cell lymphoma (Weiss et al, 1992; Chan et al, 1999) and extranodal enteropathy-type T-cell lymphoma (Huh et al, 1999). Sinonasal T-cell lymphomas, which are common in Asia but rare in Europe and the United States, are almost always EBV-associated. Between 18% and 70% of other peripheral T-cell lymphomas contain EBV (Pallesen et al, 1993). Increased incidence of NHL has been related to the X-linked lymphoproliferative syndrome, Wiskott-Aldrich syndrome, ataxia-telangiectasia, and other primary immunodeficiency syndromes. In those cases, EBV is almost always found (IARC, 1997). Epstein-Barr virus also appears to play a central role in most NHLs arising after organ transplantation. It is widely accepted that at least some of the tumors reflect in vivo outgrowth of EBV-immortalized lymphoblastoid cell lines as a consequence of failed immunosurveillance (Ambinder et al, 1999).

Among HIV-infected individuals, who suffer from a greatly increased risk of NHL (Engels et al, 2006), approximately half of the lymphomas contain monoclonal EBV. This percentage rises to nearly 100% if the central nervous system is affected. Although the incidence of Burkitt lymphoma is also significantly increased in HIV-infected individuals in Europe and the United States, the proportion being EBV-positive is only slightly higher compared to HIV-negative Burkitt lymphoma patients. Primary effusion lymphomas, almost exclusively reported in HIV-positive individuals, show dual infection with EBV and human herpes virus 8 (IARC, 1997).

Human T-cell leukemia/lymphoma virus 1
Several other infectious agents have been associated with NHL, primarily with rare subtypes. Thus, the etiologic fraction of non-EBV–infectious agents in overall NHL development is believed to be small. Nevertheless, human T-cell leukemia/lymphoma virus 1 (HTLV-I) is considered a cause of adult T-cell leukemia/lymphoma—a peripheral T-cell lymphoma type. This malignancy is particularly common in Japan and the Caribbean (IARC, 1997; Manns et al, 1999). In countries such as Japan, HTLV-1–induced human T-cell leukemia/lymphoma virus has become part of the definition of a case of adult T-cell leukemia/lymphoma. Although uncommon, other NHL types have also been found to be associated with the presence of HTLV-1 (Manns et al, 1999; Poiesz et al, 2001). The HTLV-2 virus was originally isolated from a patient with T-cell hairy cell leukemia, but at present there is little evidence to support a role for this virus in lymphoproliferative disorders.

Human herpes virus 8
Human herpes virus 8 (HHV8), primarily known for its association with Kaposi's sarcoma, is found in most patients with primary effusion lymphoma, a condition rarely seen and occurring almost exclusively among HIV-positive patients (Moore, 2000). Understanding the pathogenic role of HHV8 in primary effusion lymphoma is complicated by the fact that such lymphoma cells are often also infected with EBV. However, the lesions have been shown to be monoclonal expansions of a single infected cell. This finding suggests that HHV8 infection precedes tumor growth, which again supports an etiologic role of HHV8 in these proliferations (Judde et al, 2000).

Other infections
A high prevalence of hepatitis C virus (HCV) infection has been reported in B-cell NHL primarily from Mediterranean countries and Japan. For most other countries the association has been modest (2–4-fold increased) or absent (Gisbert et al, 2003; Negri et al, 2004; Giordano et al, 2007). In particular, it has been speculated that the E2 protein of HCV is one of the chronic antigenic stimuli involved in the lymphomagenetic process (De Re et al, 2000). The

role of HCV, however, is still unclear and needs to be substantiated by further studies.

It is well established that infection with *Helicobacter pylori* not only causes gastritis but also may lead to the development of low-grade mucosa-associated lymphoid tissue (MALT) lymphoma (Kusters et al, 2006). The bacterial infection may provide a chronic antigenic stimulation that elicits host immune responses capable of promoting clonal B-cell expansion. A causal link is substantiated by studies showing regression of the tumor in up to 75% of cases after elimination of the bacteria by antibiotic therapy (Guidoboni et al, 2006).

Infection with *Borrelia burgdorferi* may cause a lymphoproliferative condition, a pseudolymphoma, which responds to antibiotic treatment. In rare circumstances this condition might evolve into a primary cutaneous B-cell lymphoma (Willemze et al, 1997). Whereas an association between *Borrelia burgdorferi* and cutaneous B-cell lymphoma has been noted in several European countries, there is little evidence of an association in North America (Cerroni et al, 1997; Goodlad et al, 2000a, 2000b; Wood et al, 2001). This discrepancy is believed to be explained by genetic and phenotypic differences between *Borrelia burgdorferi* in Europe and North America (Wood et al, 2001).

Recently a case of immunoproliferative small intestinal disease (a rare MALT lymphoma) was shown to regress on antibiotic treatment and subsequent testing of archival tumor material from this and other patients showed evidence of infection with *Campylobacter jejuni* (Lecuit et al, 2004). In other recent studies patients with ocular adnexal lymphoma have been reported to have a high prevalence of *Clamydia psittaci* infection in both tumor tissue and PBMCs and to have responded to antibiotic therapy (Ferreri et al, 2004; Ferreri et al, 2005).

The previous observations indicate that there could be more infectious agents could be associated with this distinct category of infection-associated lymphoid malignancies, in which the agent does not directly infect and transform lymphoid cells, but rather indirectly increases the probability of lymphoid transformation by chronically stimulating the immune system. Studies addressing the effect of antibiotic therapy on tumor development and progression would appear to have some merit in this regard.

Physical Activity

Given the influence of immune dysfunction on the etiology of NHL, physical activity could be an important factor. Laboratory evidence suggests an effect of physical activity on immune status, but few studies have addressed this issue in the context of NHL. A case-control study by Zahm et al (1999) found no evidence that occupational physical activity plays a role, whereas two recent studies reported nonoccupational physical activity to be inversely associated with risk of NHL (Cerhan et al, 2005; Pan et al, 2005).

Ionizing Radiation

There is no evidence that ionizing radiation causes NHL (Boice, 1992). Low-dose radiation from diagnostic x-ray procedures or from occupational exposure has not been associated with an increased risk. Studies among atomic bomb survivors have also been negative (Ron, 1998). Associations have been found, albeit inconsistently, only among subjects who received nearly lethal doses of ionizing radiation. Under such circumstances, immunosuppression may play a role, perhaps through elimination of suppressor T cells. This depletion might lead to unregulated proliferation of B lymphocytes and, in rare circumstances, to NHL. Boice (1992) has remarked: "If radiation does not cause NHL, at least not by its accepted mechanism of action of breaking chromosomes, creating rearrangements, gene deletions, and mutations, perhaps other environmental mutagens and clastogens should not be considered likely causes of NHL."

Occupation

Reports on the association of NHL with occupational exposures are inconsistent (D'Amore et al, 1992; Scherr and Mueller,

1996). Excess risks have been reported among farmers, pesticide applicators, grain millers, wood and forestry workers, chemists, cosmetologists, machinists, printers, and workers in the petroleum, rubber, plastic, and synthetics industries.

Of these groups, farmers and general populations of rural communities have been most extensively studied, with inconsistent results (Waterhouse et al, 1996; Cerhan et al, 1998; Khuder et al, 1999; Lee et al, 2002; Zheng et al, 2002). In one meta-analysis of 36 studies, farmers had an overall 10% increased risk, with studies performed among farmers residing in the United States showing a more elevated risk. In general, male farmers were at higher risk than female farmers. The main hypothesis for the occupational risk of NHL focuses on exposure to pesticides, organic solvents, and allergens. Infectious zoonotic microorganisms have also been hypothesized to cause NHL, but evidence is lacking.

A number of studies have addressed more directly specific exposures that might be involved in the development of NHL. Case-control studies have suggested an increased risk in occupations using phenoxy acids and chlorophenol herbicides, particularly 2,4-dichlorophenoxyacetic acid. Exposure to pesticides has increased continuously since the 1940s. Independently of the effects of 2,4-dichlorophenoxyacetic acid, farmers who use organophosphate insecticides have also been reported to be at increased risk of NHL (Zahm et al, 1993). In a recent study, heptachlor epoxide was incriminated together with dieldrin, oxychlordane, and ss-benzene hexachloride (Quintana et al, 2004). The mechanism by which pesticides might increase the risk of NHL is not clear, but chromosomal rearrangements associated with pesticide application have been reported (Garry et al, 1989; Kirsch and Lipkowitz, 1992). In fact, Schroeder et al (2001) found NHL cases with t(14;18) translocation, but not without this translocation, to be associated with a range of agricultural pesticides.

In a literature review, d'Amore et al (1992) noted that a common feature in several of the industrial exposures identified is their capacity to alter the cell-mediated immune response. However, experimental evidence of pesticide-induced immunosuppression has not been substantiated in human studies. Indeed, when the exposure to Agent Orange (a mixture of two phenoxy herbicides) was investigated among Vietnam veterans, the highest incidence of lymphoma was found in ground troops stationed in areas of lowest exposure and among sailors in navy ships off the coast of Vietnam (Breslin et al, 1988; O'Brien et al, 1991).

Exposures to organic solvents and chemicals including benzene, styrene, 1,3-butadiene, trichlorethylene, perchlorethylene, creosote, lead arsenate, formaldehyde, and paint thinners have been suggested as possible risk factors for NHL, but the evidence is limited (Mueller, 1996). Benzene achieved early attention, but results have been inconclusive (Savitz and Andrews, 1997; Lamm et al, 2005). Solvents are also present in pesticides, and it has been proposed that immunotoxic effects of these agents may play a role as well (Vineis and D'Amore, 1992). Frequent translocations involving chromosome 14 at band q32 have been identified in studies of patients exposed to solvents (Brandt et al, 1989). In an exploratory analysis of occupational risk factors for various NHL subgroups, chemical solvent exposure was associated with small-cell diffuse lymphoma (Tatham et al, 1997).

Medical Conditions and Treatment

Immune modulation

The risk of NHL is strongly related to immune modulation. In fact, many researchers believe that the cause(s) of the worldwide increase in incidence is to be found among factors associated with immune modulation. Both primary, or genetic, disorders of immune dysfunction and acquired states of severe immunosuppression, including HIV/AIDS and organ transplantation, constitute strong and well-established risk factors for NHL, but explain few new cases in the general population. Clinical features shared by the majority of immunodeficiency-related lymphomas are diffuse large B-cell histology, extra-nodal location, aggressive clinical course, and an association with EBV.

A greatly increased risk of NHL in conjunction with potent immunosuppressive therapy following renal, liver, heart, or bone marrow transplantation has been reported consistently. The risk of NHL increases by about 10- to 20-fold in renal allograft recipients and up to about 200-fold in heart-transplant recipients, compared to the general population (Opelz and Dohler, 2004). Posttransplant lymphoproliferative disorders comprise a spectrum ranging from early EBV-driven polyclonal proliferations to EBV-positive (80%–90%) or EBV-negative NHL, predominantly of B-cell origin (Andreone et al, 2003). EBV-negative cases typically occur later than EBV-positive tumors: The majority of cases occurring more than 5 years after transplantation are EBV-negative. The pathogenesis of posttransplant lymphoproliferative disorders is most likely complex and multifactorial, although drug-induced impaired T-cell immune surveillance in combination with chronic antigenic stimulation exerted by the graft is believed to have a central role (Andreone et al, 2003). Modulating factors include donor and recipient EBV serologic status, type of transplanted organ, underlying disease, and type, duration, and intensity of the immunosuppressive treatment (Andreone et al, 2003).

In HIV-infected individuals, the relative risk of NHL is on average increased 100-fold, varying from 90- to 600-fold among children (Goedert et al, 1998; Frisch et al, 2000; Aboulafia et al, 2004). Among acquired immunodeficiency syndrome (AIDS) patients, this increase affects B-cell lymphomas more than T-cell lymphomas (Biggar et al, 2001), and the incidence of NHL increases with decreasing CD4 count, a measure of increasing immunosuppression. Another indication of the close association between level of immunocompetence and NHL comes from the treatment of AIDS patients. The introduction of highly active

antiretroviral therapy (HAART), which improves the immunocompetence of the patient and has markedly reduced the incidence of AIDS among HIV-infected individuals, has also lowered the incidence of and mortality from NHL in these patients (Engels et al, 2006; Navarro and Kaplan, 2006). Nevertheless, NHL still accounts for more than 20% of AIDS-related deaths in developed countries (Aboulafia et al, 2004).

The pathogenesis of AIDS-related lymphomas is complex and most likely varies according to NHL subtype. Nearly half of all AIDS-related lymphomas are associated with the presence of a gamma herpesvirus, EBV or HHV-8 (Wood and Harrington, 2005). B-cell proliferation driven by chronic anigenemia results in the induction of polyclonal, and ultimately monoclonal, lymphoproliferation. In addition, dysregulation of cytokine pathways (interleukin-6 and interleukin-10), coupled with *BCL6*, *P53*, and *MYC* mutations, has been implicated in the pathogenesis.

Blood transfusion
There is little evidence to support the hypothesis of an association between blood transfusion and NHL. Allogeneic blood transfusions can induce immunosuppression and increase susceptibility to infections, including infections caused by blood-borne organisms. Therefore, transfusions have been hypothesized to influence the risk of NHL. Several cohort studies have found a 1.6- to 3-fold increase in risk, whereas most case-control studies found no association (Chow and Holly, 2002; Zhang et al, 2004b). A large nested case-control study in Sweden that took advantage of information on exposure prior to disease outcome found no association overall with number of transfusions or types of blood transfusion products (Adami et al, 1997a). Analyses of close to 1 000 000 transfusion recipients in Denmark and Sweden showed a substantially increased risk immediately following the first transfusion, which then decreased sharply. This substantial risk increase with short follow-up most likely reflects reverse causality due to anemia in relation to incipient

NHL. A marginal risk increase was observed between 2 and 10 years of follow-up, but then disappeared (Hjalgrim et al, 2006a). Thus, although an association between NHL and blood transfusion is biologically plausible, the epidemiologic evidence is, at most, weak.

Autoimmune diseases

The association with several autoimmune disorders and NHL is well established. Rheumatoid arthritis, systemic lupus erythematosus, Sjogren's syndrome (Baecklund et al, 2006; Bernatsky et al, 2005b; Theander et al, 2006), celiac disease (Askling et al, 2002), dermatitis herpetiformis (Sigurgeirsson et al, 1994), and autoimmune thyroiditis (Holm et al, 1985) have all been consistently associated with an increased risk of NHL. Conversely, approximately 8% of NHL patients exhibit autoimmune phenomena (Gronbaek et al, 1995).

Although it cannot be excluded that immunosuppressive therapy or biological therapy with tumor necrosis factor antagonists, often given for autoimmune conditions, may cause an increase in the incidence of NHL, there is strong evidence to support a direct association with the underlying disease and its severity (Wolfe et al, 1998; Baecklund et al, 2006; Theander et al, 2006). Markers of severe Sjögren's syndrome, such as parotid enlargement, hypocomplementemia, palpable purpura, Ro/La antibody positivity, and low T CD4+ cell counts have been associated with a more pronounced risk of NHL (Ioannidis et al, 2002; Theander et al, 2006). In a large case-control study nested within a cohort of rheumatoid arthritis patients, medium overall disease activity was associated with an eightfold increase in lymphoma risk, and high activity with a 70-fold risk increase, compared to low disease activity when the confounding effect of treatment was taken into account in the analysis (Baecklund et al, 2006). Thus, the increased risk of lymphomas appears to be confined to a subset of patients with most severe disease. In celiac disease, highly increased lymphoma risks were reported already decades ago (Selby

and Gallagher, 1979), while recent studies have described lower, albeit still increased, risks (Catassi et al, 2002; Green et al, 2003). In the hitherto largest cohort study (Askling et al, 2002), the risk increase was restricted to patients diagnosed as adults. Whether the apparent risk-level discrepancy between old and new studies relates to an increasing recognition of mild or silent celiac disease (presumably at lower risk of NHL), patients diagnosed at an earlier age, or to better management of diagnosed patients, is yet unknown. Although attractive, the hypothesis that early total compliance to gluten-free diet therapy may protect against lymphomas in celiac disease is mostly supported by indirect evidence and small studies (Holmes et al, 1989).

With regard to lymphoma subtypes, there is evidence to suggest specific associations of Sjogren's syndrome, rheumatoid arthritis, and systemic lupus erythematosus, with the NHL subtype diffuse large B-cell lymphoma (Bernatsky et al, 2005a; Baecklund et al, 2006; Smedby et al, 2006; Theander et al, 2006), in addition to the well-established link between Sjogren's syndrome and mucosa-associated lymphoid tissue (MALT) lymphoma in the parotid gland (Voulgarelis et al, 1999). Traditionally, celiac disease has been linked to an uncommon form of T-cell lymphoma in the small intestine, referred to as enteropathy-type T-cell lymphoma (ETTL) in the WHO classification (Jaffe et al, 2001). However, in both celiac disease and dermatitis herpetiformis, other and more common types of NHL, such as nonintestinal T cell and B cell NHL, may also occur more often than expected (Hervonen et al, 2005; Smedby et al, 2005a).

Chronic infectious diseases

Chronic infections may lead to prolonged antigen stimulation and lymphocyte proliferation. Although the reasons are not fully understood, certain subjects are more susceptible to such conditions than others. Considering the overwhelming evidence of an association between NHL and conditions that affect the immune system, it is not inconceivable that persons susceptible to certain chronic infections might also be at higher risk of NHL. In fact, certain chronic infectious diseases such as tuberculosis, malaria, herpes zoster, chronic ear infection, bronchitis, and pyelonephritis have in some, but not all, studies been associated with an increased risk of NHL (Cartwright et al, 1988; Franceschi et al, 1989; Bernstein and Ross, 1992; Doody et al, 1992; La Vecchia et al, 1992; Askling and Ekbom, 2001). Observations of increased lymphoma risks in association with frequent antibiotic use could reflect similar mechanisms (Chang et al, 2005c). NHL may arise as a direct result of chronic antigenic stimulation of, for example, B cells by a chronic infection. Another possibility is that subjects particularly susceptible to chronic infections are also more susceptible to NHL development, because both conditions primarily arise in persons who, compared to the general population, are distinct in their immunologic response to certain exposures. Thus, our ability today to treat diseases that previously might have been lethal, such as tuberculosis and other chronic infections, may have led to an increasing pool of subjects at higher risk of NHL development. If this is true, such a situation might explain, to a certain extent, the observed worldwide increasing incidence of NHL.

Vaccinations

Bacille Calmette-Guérin (BCG) vaccination has in some but not other studies been associated with a moderately increased risk of NHL (Bernard et al, 1984; Bernstein and Ross, 1992; Tavani et al, 2000a; Becker et al, 2004). Other vaccinations such as attenuated live polio, cholera, yellow fever, and influenza vaccinations have, if anything, been associated with a decreased risk of NHL (Bernstein and Ross, 1992; Holly et al, 1999; Tavani et al, 2000a; Becker et al, 2004). However, with respect to both the possible influence of childhood vaccinations and vaccinations in adults, primarily travel vaccinations, the evidence must be regarded as preliminary and inconclusive.

Prior use of medication

The existing literature concerning use of different drugs and NHL risk is contradictory. Several studies have found a significantly elevated risk of lymphoma in association with use of antibiotics, nonsteroidal anti-inflammatory drugs (NSAIDs) and other analgesics, corticosteroids, statins, histamine2-receptor antagonists, psychotropic drugs, anticonvulsants, estrogen replacement therapy, antidepressants or anti-anxiety drugs, amphetamines, and digitalis or digitoxin (Bernstein and Ross, 1992; Holly et al, 1999; Kato et al, 2002; Iwata et al, 2006). Conversely, perhaps just as many studies have detected no or even an inverse association between risk of NHL and these same medications (Beiderbeck et al, 2003a; Beiderbeck et al, 2003a; Zhang et al, 2004c; Chang et al, 2005c; Fortuny et al, 2006). As several diseases, including acquired immunosuppression, autoimmune disorders, allergies, and infections also appear to be associated with NHL risk, it is difficult to determine whether apparent associations between medications and lymphoma risk are due to the effects of the medications themselves, or rather the underlying disorder.

Allergy

Three large case-control studies—one among HIV-positive men (Holly and Lele, 1997)—have found a 35% to 70% reduced risk of NHL among subjects with self-reported allergic rhinitis, hay fever, or food allergies (Holly and Lele 1997; Holly et al, 1999; Grulich et al, 2005). In general, however, most studies have not found allergic conditions to be statistically significantly associated with NHL, though many have reported odds ratios close to or below one. A large Scandinavian case-control study found patients with NHL to be significantly less likely to mount IgE antibodies against specific allergens. However, a causal interpretation of these results was challenged by further findings of a statistically significant inverse association between the dissemination of NHL disease at time of blood drawing and seropositivity to specific IgE. These latter results indicated that persons with widespread lymphoma of B-cell but not T-cell origin might have a reduced ability to mount a response to allergens. A subsequent prospective investigation in a Finnish maternity cohort revealed that, with the exception of specimens taken in the years immediately preceding the cancer diagnosis, there was no indication that persons with allergen-specific IgE antibodies were at different risk of developing NHL compared to seronegative subjects (Melbye et al, 2006). Thus, the findings suggest that the previously reported association may be explained by reverse causality—as a consequence of the disease rather than reflecting an etiologic pathway.

Other medical conditions

A history of adult-onset diabetes mellitus has been associated with increased risk of NHL in some, but not all, studies (Hjalgrim et al, 1997; Cerhan et al, 1997; Wideroff et al, 1997; Zendehdel et al, 2003; Smedby et al, 2006). Likewise, psoriasis (Boffetta et al, 2001; Gelfand et al, 2003) and inflammatory bowel disorders (Mir-Madjlessi et al, 1986; Arseneau et al, 2001; Askling et al, 2005) have occasionally, but not invariably, been associated with increased lymphoma risks. Inflammatory myositis (poly- and dermatomyositis) has also been reported to increase risk of NHL (Hill et al, 2001). However, this risk increase (of lymphomas as well as of malignancies overall) has consistently been observed to be highest around the time of the myositis diagnosis (Hill et al, 2001). Thus, these disorders may occur as paraneoplastic syndromes, and it is not clear if the myositis disorders in themselves confer any elevation in NHL risk.

Other Risk Factors

Ultraviolet light

Numerous studies have described increased risks of malignant lymphomas, including chronic lymphocytic leukemia, following a diagnosis of skin cancer (malignant melanoma, squamous cell carcinoma, and basal cell carcinoma). Conversely, an increased risk of all three forms of skin cancer has been noted following a history of lymphoma (Adami et al, 1995; Frisch and Melbye, 1995; Levi et al, 1996; Lens and Newton-Bishop, 2005). These observations, along with parallel time trends in incidence of skin cancer and NHL, gave rise to the formerly popular hypothesis that ultraviolet radiation (UVR) exposure would increase not only the risk of skin cancer, but also of NHL (Zheng et al, 1992; Melbye et al, 1996). However, when investigators recently began to analyze this relationship directly, rather the contrary was observed. In two large case-control studies from Australia and Scandinavia, consistent inverse associations between various measures of frequent UVR exposure and risk of NHL were observed (Hughes et al, 2004; Smedby et al, 2005b). In a large pooled analysis (Kricker et al, 2007), an inverse association between frequent recreational sun exposure and risk of NHL was indicated in 8 out of 10 participating studies, and in the overall results. Possible mechanisms behind an inverse association between UVR and NHL risk include UV-induced systemic immune modulation (Norval, 2001) or photo-activation of vitamin D-production (Holick, 2003). UVR-induced effects on immunity are incompletely known, but appear to include a downregulation of antigen-presenting activity, increased levels of suppressor T-cells, and a shift toward a Th2-type response (Norval, 2001; Aubin, 2003). These observations were previously interpreted as supporting the hypothesis of an increased lymphoma risk with increased sun exposure, but the long-term effects that may be of relevance for lymphoma development are not clear. Indeed, Kanariou et al (2001) have reported that prolonged intense exposure to sunlight may be associated with immunostimulation rather than immunosuppression. Moreover, biologically active vitamin D promotes differentiation and inhibits proliferation of lymphoma cells in vitro (Hickish et al, 1993), suggesting that it may have a preventive effect against lymphomagenesis. Results from a prospective cohort study showed a nonsignificantly inverse association between multiple determinants of vitamin D exposure (including dietary intake, skin pigmentation, and geographic residence) and NHL risk (Giovannucci et al, 2006).

Hair dyes

The evidence for an association between use of hair dyes and the risk of NHL is not convincing. Compounds in hair dyes may be mutagenic and carcinogenic in laboratory experiments (Ames et al, 1975) and some products have indeed been removed from the market over the past 20 years. Experimental work, however, has indicated that usual concentrations of incriminated compounds do not have this effect (Bracher et al, 1990). The epidemiologic literature on this topic is mixed. Several large studies have not documented an increased risk, whereas others, mostly small, showed a positive association (Cantor et al, 1988; Zahm et al, 1992; Grodstein et al, 1994; Correa et al, 2000; Holly et al, 1998; Zhang et al, 2004a; Benavente et al, 2005). Studies that differentiate between products have suggested a possible association with the use of black hair products, whereas others have been null (Thun et al, 1994; Holly et al, 1998). In the case-control study by Holly et al (1998), comprising more than 700 cases and 1600 controls, the only association found was for men using semipermanent hair dyes. In two other large case-control studies (Zhang et al, 2004a; de Sanjosé et al, 2006), a small increased risk of NHL was noted predominantly in relation to hair dye use before 1980.

CONCLUSION

For several decades the incidence of NHL has increased more rapidly than that of almost any other cancer. Reasons for the increase of most NHL subtypes are obscure since strong, well-established risk factors such as immunosuppression, autoimmunity, and certain infectious agents explain at most only a small fraction of the cases.

Other possible risk associations with particular food products, medications, pesticides, and hair dyes also do not satisfactorily explain the increase.

The worldwide nature of the increase in NHL indicates that we should be looking for a ubiquitous exposure that has a modest or weak association with NHL. Furthermore, the strong connection between immune modulation and NHL risk suggests that we should focus on factors that influence immune modulation. Another intriguing possibility that deserves more attention is whether the pool of individuals susceptible to developing NHL has steadily increased during more recent decades, as survival after severe illness has improved with better treatment regimens. The relevance of such a scenario would, of course, require that subjects who previously would have had a higher risk of dying at a young age be immunologically different from other persons.

Recent evaluations of epidemiologic patterns of NHL according to histologic subtype have documented clear differences among the different NHL subtypes, which strongly suggests that to some extent they may also have different risk factor profiles. A number of very large NHL case-control studies have been initiated in recent years that allow for subtype analyses. These initiatives have already led to an increase in our understanding of some of the factors involved in the NHL pathogenesis and shown that associations often differ according to NHL subtype. More questions still remain than answers in relation to the etiology of NHL, but the number of research groups dedicated to NHL research has never been higher or more productive, which gives hope that our understanding of NHL may greatly improve in the coming years.

REFERENCES

Aboulafia DM, Pantanowitz L, Dezube BJ. AIDS-related non-Hodgkin lymphoma: still a problem in the era of HAART. AIDS Read 2004;14:605–17.

Adami J, Frisch M, Glimelius B, Yuen J, Melbye M. Evidence of an association between non-Hodgkin's lymphoma and skin cancer. Br Med J 1995;310:1491–95.

Adami J, Glimelius B, Cnattingius S, Ekbom A, Zahm SH, Linet M, et al. Maternal and peri-natal factors associated with non-Hodgkin's lymphoma among children. Int J Cancer 1996;65:774–77.

Adami J, Nyrén O, Bergström R, Ekbom A, McLaughlin JK, Hogman C, et al. Blood transfusion and non-Hodgkin lymphoma: lack of association. Ann Intern Med 1997a; 127:365–71.

Adami HO, Tsaih S, Lambe M, Hsieh C, Adami J, Trichopoulos D, et al. Pregnancy and risk of non-Hodgkin's lymphoma: a prospective study. Int J Cancer 1997b;70:155–58.

Ambinder RF, Lemas MV, Moore S, Yang J, Fabian D, Krone C. Epstein-Barr virus and lymphoma. Cancer Treat Res 1999;99:27–45.

Ambinder RF. Epstein-Barr virus-associated lymphoproliferative disorders. Rev Clin Exp Hematol 2003;7:362–74.

Ames BN, Kammen HO, Yamasaki E. Hair dyes are mutagenic: identification of a variety of mutagenic ingredients. Proc Natl Acad Sci USA 1975;72:2423–27.

Andreone P, Gramenzi A, Lorenzini S, Biselli M, Cursaro C, Pileri S, et al. Posttransplantation lymphoproliferative disorders. Arch Intern Med 2003;163:1997–2004.

Arseneau KO, Stukenborg GJ, Connors AF, Jr., Cominelli F. The incidence of lymphoid and myeloid malignancies among hospitalized Crohn's disease patients. Inflamm Bowel Dis 2001;7:106–12.

Askling J, Ekbom A. Risk of non-Hodgkin's lymphoma following tuberculosis. Br J Cancer 2001;84:113–15.

Askling J, Linet M, Gridley G, Halstensen TS, Ekstrom K, Ekbom A. Cancer incidence in a population-based cohort of individuals hospitalized with celiac disease or dermatitis herpetiformis. Gastroenterology 2002;123: 1428–35.

Askling J, Brandt L, Lapidus A, Karlen P, Bjorkholm M, Lofberg R, et al. Risk of haematopoietic cancer in patients with inflammatory bowel disease. Gut 2005;54:617–22.

Aubin, F. Mechanisms involved in ultraviolet light-induced immunosuppression. Eur J Dermatol 2003;13:515–23.

Baecklund E, Iliadou A, Askling J, Ekbom A, Backlin C, Granath F, et al. Association of chronic inflammation, not its treatment, with increased lymphoma risk in rheumatoid arthritis. Arthritis Rheum 2006;54:692–701.

Banks PM. Changes in diagnosis of non-Hodgkin's lymphomas over time. Cancer Res 1992;52:5453s–5455s.

Becker N, Deeg E, Nieters A. Population-based study on lymphoma in Germany: rationale, study design and first results. Leuk Res 2004; 28:713–24.

Beiderbeck AB, Holly EA, Sturkenboom MC, Coebergh JW, Stricker BH, Leufkens HG. Prescription medications associated with a decreased risk of non-Hodgkin's lymphoma. Am J Epidemiol 2003b;157:510–6.

Beiderbeck AB, Holly EA, Sturkenboom MC, Coebergh JW, Stricker BH, Leufkens HG. No increased risk of non-Hodgkin's lymphoma with steroids, estrogens and psychotropics (Netherlands). Cancer Causes Control 2003a;14:639–44.

Bell DA, Liu Y, Cortopassi GA. Occurrence of bcl-2 oncogene translocation with increased frequency in the peripheral blood of heavy smokers. J Natl Cancer Inst 1995; 87(3): 223–224.

Benavente Y, Garcia N, Domingo-Domenech E, Alvaro T, Font R, Zhang Y et al.Regular use of hair dyes and risk of lymphoma in Spain. Int J Epidemiol 2005;34:1118–22.

Bernard SM, Cartwright RA, Bird CC, Richards ID, Lauder I, Roberts BE. Aetiologic factors in lymphoid malignancies: a case-control epidemiological study. Leuk Res 1984;8:681–9.

Bernatsky S, Boivin JF, Joseph L, Rajan R, Zoma A, Manzi S, et al. An international cohort study of cancer in systemic lupus erythematosus. Arthritis Rheum 2005a;52:1481–90.

Bernatsky S, Ramsey-Goldman R, Rajan R, Boivin J-F, Joseph L, Lachance S, et al. Non-Hodgkin's lymphoma in systemic lupus erythematosus. Ann Rheum Dis 2005b;64: 1507–9.

Bernstein L, Ross RK. Prior medication use and health history as risk factors for non-hodgkin's lymphoma: preliminary results from a case-control study in Los Angeles County. Cancer Res 1992;52:5510S–5515S.

Besson H, Brennan P, Becker N, Nieters A, De Sanjose S, Font R, et al. Tobacco smoking, alcohol drinking and non-Hodgkin's lymphoma. A European multicenter case-control study (Epilymph). Int J Cancer 2006;119: 901–8.

Biggar RJ, Frisch M, Engels EA, Goedert JJ. The risk of T-cell lymphomas in persons with AIDS. J Acquir Immune Defic Syndr 2001;26: 371–76.

Boffetta P, Gridley G, Lindelof B. Cancer risk in a population-based cohort of patients hospitalized for psoriasis in Sweden. J Invest Dermatol 2001;117:1531–37.

Boice JD Jr. Radiation and non-Hodgkin's lymphoma. Cancer Res 1992;52:5489S–5491sS.

Bracher M, Fallelr C, Grotsch W, Marshall R, Spengler J. Studies on the potential mutagenicity of p-phenylenediamine in oxidative hairdye mixtures. Mutat Res 1990;241:313–23.

Brandt L, Kristofferson U, Olsson H, Mitelman F. Relation between occupational exposure to organic solvents and chromosome aberrations in non-Hodgkin's lymphoma. Eur J Haematol 1989;42:298–302.

Breslin P, Kang HK, Lee Y, Burt V, Shepard BM. Proportionate mortality study of US Army and US Marine Corps veterans of the Vietnam War. J Occup Med 1988;30:412–19.

Brown LM, Gibson R, Burmeister LF, Schuman LM, Everett GD, Blair A. Alcohol consumption and risk of leukemia, non-Hodgkin's lymphoma, and multiple myeloma. Leuk Res 1992;16:979–84.

Cantor KP, Blair A, Everett G, VanLier S, Burmeister L, Dick FR, et al. Hair dye use and risk of leukemia and lymphoma. Am J Public Health 1988;78:570–71.

Cartwright RA, McKinney PA, O'Brien C, Richards ID, Roberts B, Lauder I, et al. Non-Hodgkin's lymphoma: case control epidemiological study in Yorkshire. Leuk Res 1988; 12:81–88.

Catassi C, Fabiani E, Corrao G, Barbato M, De Renzo A, Carella AM, et al. Risk of non-Hodgkin lymphoma in celiac disease. JAMA 2002;287:1413–19.

Cerhan JR, Cantor KP, Williamson K, Lynch CF, Torner JC, Burmeister LF. Cancer mortality among Iowa farmers: recent results, time trends, and lifestyle factors (United States). Cancer Causes Control 1998;9:311–19.

Cerhan JR, Wallace RB, Folsom AR, Potter JD, Sellers TA, Zheng W, et al. Medical history risk factors for non-Hodgkin's lymphoma in older women. J Natl Cancer Inst 1997;89: 314–18.

Cerhan JR, Habermann TM, Vachon CM, Putnam SD, Zheng W, Potter JD, et al. Menstrual and reproductive factors and risk of non-Hodgkin lymphoma: the Iowa women's health study (United States). Cancer Cause Control 2002a;13:131–36.

Cerhan JR, Vachon CM, Habermann TM, Ansell SM, Witzig TE, Kurtin PJ, et al. Hormone replacement therapy and risk of non-Hodgkin lymphoma and chronic lymphocytic leukemia. Cancer Epidemiol Biomarkers Prev 2002b;11:1466–71.

Cerhan JR, Bernstein L, Severson RK, Davis S, Colt JS, Blair A, et al. Anthropometrics, physical activity, related medical conditions, and the risk of non-Hodgkin lymphoma. Cancer Cause Control 2005;16:1203–14.

Cerroni L, Zochling N, Putz B, Kerl H. Infection by Borrelia burgdorferi and cutaneous B-cell lymphoma. J Cutan Pathol 1997;24:457–61.

Chan AC, Ho JW, Chiang AK, Srivastava G. Phenotypic and cytotoxic characteristics of peripheral T-cell and NK-cell lymphomas in relation to Epstein-Barr virus association. Histopathology 1999;34(1):16–24

Chang ET, Smedby KE, Zhang SM, Hjalgrim H, Melbye M, Ost A, et al. Alcohol intake and risk of non_hodgkin lymphoma in men and women. Cancer Cause Control 2004;15: 1067–76.

Chang ET, Hjalgrim H, Smedby KE, Akerman M, Tani E, Johnsen HE, et al. Body mass index and risk of malignant lymphoma in Scandinavian men and women. J Natl Cancer Inst 2005a;97:210–18.

Chang ET, Smedby KE, Zhang SM, Hjalgrim H, Melbye M, Ost A, et al. Dietary factors and risk of non-Hodgkin lymphoma in men and women. Cancer Epidemiol Biomarkers Prev 2005d;14:512–20.

Chang ET, Smedby KE, Hjalgrim H, Schollkopf C, Porwit-MacDonald A, Sundstrom C, et al. Medication use and risk of non-Hodgkin's lymphoma. Am J Epidemiol 2005c;162:965–74.

Chang ET, Smedby KE, Hjalgrim H, Porwit-MacDonald A, Roos G, Glimelius B, et al. Family history of hematopoietic malignancy and risk of lymphoma. J Natl Cancer Inst 2005b;97:1466–74.

Chiu BCH, Cerhan JR, Folsom AR, Sellers TA, Kushi LH, Wallace RB, et al. Diet and risk of non-Hodgkin lymphoma in older women. JAMA 1996;275:1315–21.

Chiu BCH, Cerhan JR, Gapstur SM, Sellers TA, Zheng W, Lutz CT, et al. Alcohol consumption and non-Hodgkin lymphoma in a cohort of older women. Br J Cancer 1999;80:1476–82.

Chiu BC, Weisenburger D D, Zahm SH, Cantor KP, Gapstur SM, Holmes F, et al. Agricultural pesticide use, familial cancer, and risk of non-Hodgkin lymphoma. Cancer Epidemiol Biomarkers Prev 2004;13:525–31.

Chow EJ, Holly EA. Blood transfusions and non-Hodgkin's lymphoma. Epidemiol Rev 2002;24:269–79.

Correa A, Jackson L, Mohan A, Perry H, Helzlsouer K. Use of hair dyes, hematopoietic neoplasms, and lymphomas: a literature review. II. Lymphomas and multiple myeloma. Cancer Invest 2000;18:467–79.

Cross AJ, Ward MH, Schenk M, Kulldorff M, Cozen W, Davis S, et al. Meat and meat-mutagen intake and risk of non-Hodgkin lymphoma: results from a NCI-SEER case-control study. Carcinogenesis 2006;27:293–97.

D'Amore F, Hasle H, Hansen KS. Occupational exposures and non-Hodgkin's lymphoma. Hematol Rev 1992;6:183–99.

De Re V, De Vita S, Marzotto A, Rupolo M, Gloghini A, Pivetta B, et al. Sequence analysis of the immunoglobulin antigen receptor of hepatitis C virus-associated non-Hodgkin lymphomas suggests that the malignant cells are derived from the rheumatoid factor-producing cells that occur mainly in type II cryoglobulinemia. Blood 2000;96:3578–84.

De Sanjosé S, Benavente Y, Nieters A, Foretova L, Maynadié M, Cocco PL, et al. Association between personal hair dyes and lymphoid neoplasms in Europé. Am J Epidemiol 2006; 164:47–55.

De Stefani E, Fierro L, Barrios E, Ronco A. Tobacco, alcohol, diet and risk of non-Hodgkin's lymphoma: a case-control study in Uruguay. Leuk Res 1998;22:445–52.

Devesa SS, Fears T. Non-Hodgkin's lymphoma time trends: United States and international data. Cancer Res 1992;52:5432S–5440S.

Doody MM, Linet MS, Glass AG, Friedman GD, Pottern LM, Boice JD Jr, et al. Leukemia, lymphoma, and multiple myeloma following selected medical conditions. Cancer Causes Control 1992;3:449–56.

Eltom MA, Jemal A, Mbulaiteye SM, Devesa SS, Biggar RJ. Trends in Kaposi's sarcoma and non-Hodgkin's lymphoma incidence in the United States from 1973 through 1998. J Natl Can Inst 2002;94:1204–10.

Engels EA, Pfeiffer RM, Goedert JJ, Virgo P, McNeel TS, Scoppa SM, et al. Trends in cancer risk among people with AIDS in the United States 1980–2002. AIDS 2006;20: 1645–54.

Epstein MA, Achong BG, Barr YM. Virus particles in cultured lymphoblasts from Burkitt lymphoma. Lancet 1964;1:702–3.

Ferlay J, Bray F, Pisani P, Parkin DM. GLOBOCAN 2002: Cancer Incidence, Mortality and Prevalence Worldwide. IARC CancerBase No. 5. version 2.0, IARCPress, Lyon, 2004.

Fernberg P, Odenbro A, Bellocco R, Bofetta P, Pawitan Y, Adami J. Tobacco use, body mass index and the risk of malignant lymphomas—a nationwide cohort study in Sweden. Int J Cancer 2006;118:2298–302.

Ferreri J, Guidoboni M, Ponzoni M, De Conciliis C, Dell'Oro S, Fleischhauer K, et al. Evidence for an association between Clamydia psittaci ad ocular adnexal lymphomas. J Natl Cancer Inst 2004;96:586–94.

Ferreri J, Ponzoni M, Guidoboni M, De Conciliis C, Resti AG, Mazzi B, et al. Regression of ocular adnexal lymphoma after Chlamydia psittaci-eradicating antibiotic therapy. J Clin Oncol 2005;23:5067–73.

Filipovich AH, Mathur A, Kamat D, Shapiro RS. Primary immunodeficiencies: genetic risk factors for lymphoma. Cancer Res 1992;52: 5465S–5467S.

Fortuny J, de Sanjose S, Becker N, Maynadie M, Cocco PL, Staines A, et al. Statin use and risk

of lymphoid neoplasms: results from the European case-control study EPILYMPH. Cancer Epidemiol Biomarkers Prev 2006; 15:921–25.

Franceschi S, Serraino D, Bidoli E, Talamini R, Tirelli U, Carbone A, et al. The epidemiology of non-Hodgkin's lymphoma in the northeast of Italy: a hospital-based case-control study. Leuk Res 1989;13:465–72.

Freedman DM, Cantor KP, Ward MH, Helzlsouer KJ. A case-control study of nitrate in drinking water and non-Hodgkin's lymphoma in Minnesota. Arch Environ Health 2000;55:326–29.

Freedman DS, Tolbert PE, Coates R, Brann EA, Kjeldsberg CR. Relation of cigarette smoking to non-Hodgkin's lymphoma among middle-aged men. Am J Epidemiol 1998;148:833–41.

Frisch M, Biggar RJ, Goedert JJ. Human papillomavirus–associated cancers in patients with human immunodeficiency virus infection and acquired immunodeficiency syndrome. J Natl Cancer Inst 2000;92:1500–10.

Frisch M, Melbye M. New primaries after squamous cell skin cancer. Am J Epidemiol 1995;141:916–22.

Garry VF, Nelson RL, Whorton EP, Wiencke JK. Chromosomal aberrations and sister- chromatid exchanges in tool and die workers. Mutat Res 1989;225:1–9.

Gelfand JM, Berlin J, Van Voorhees A, Margolis DJ. Lymphoma rates are low but increased in patients with psoriasis: results from a population-based cohort study in the United Kingdom. Arch Dermatol 2003;139:1425–29.

Giordano TP, Henderson L, Landgren O, Chiao EY, Kramer JR, El-Serag H, et al. Risk of non-Hodgkin lymphoma and lymphoproliferative precursor diseases in US veterans with hepatitis C virus. JAMA 2007;297: 2010–17.

Giovannucci E, et al. Prospective study of predictors of vitamin D status and cancer incidence and mortality in men. J Natl Cancer Inst 2006;90:451–59.

Gisbert JP, Garcia-Buey L, Pajares JM, Moreno-Otero R. Prevalence of hepatitis c virus infection in B-cell non-Hodgkin's lymphoma: systematic review and metaanalysis. Gastroenterology 2003;125:1723–32.

Goedert JJ, Cote TR, Virgo P, Scoppa SM, Kingma DW, Gail MH, et al. Spectrum of AIDS-associated malignant disorders. Lancet 1998;351:1833–39.

Goodlad JR, Davidson MM, Hollowood K, Batstone P, Ho-Yen DO. Borrelia burgdorferi-associated cutaneous marginal zone lymphoma: a clinicopathological study of two cases illustrating the temporal progression of B.

burgdorferi-associated B-cell proliferation in the skin. Histopathology 2000a;37:501–8.

Goodlad JR, Davidson MM, Hollowood K, Ling C, MacKenzie C, Christie I, et al. Primary cutaneous B-cell lymphoma and Borrelia burgdorferi infection in patients from the Highlands of Scotland. Am J Surg Pathol 2000b;24:1279–85.

Green PH, Fleischauer AT, Bhagat G, Goyal R, Jabri B, Neugut AI. Risk of malignancy in patients with celiac disease. Am J Med 2003; 115:191–95.

Grodstein F, Hennekens CH, Colditz GA, Hunter DJ, Stampfer MJ. A prospective study of permanent hair dye use and hematopoietic cancer. J Nat Cancer Inst 1994;86: 1466–70.

Gronbaek K, D'Amore F, Schmidt K. Autoimmune phenomena in non-Hodgkin's lymphoma. Leuk Lymphoma 1995;18:311–16.

Groves FD, Linet MS, Travis LB, Devesa SS. Cancer surveillance series: non-Hodgkin's lymphoma incidence by histologic subtype in the United States from 1978 through 1995. J Natl Cancer Inst 2000;92:1240–51.

Grulich AE, Vajdic CM, Kaldor JM et al. Birth order, atopy, and risk of non-Hodgkin lymphoma. J Natl Cancer Inst 2005;97:587–94.

Guidoboni M, Ferreri AJ, Ponzoni M, Doglioni C, Dolcetti R. Infectious agents in mucosa-associated lymphoid tissue-type lymphomas: pathogenic role and therapeutic perspectives. Clin Lymphoma Myeloma 2006;6:289–300.

Hartge P, Devesa SS. Quantification of the impact of known risk factors on time trends in non-Hodgkin's lymphoma incidence. Cancer Res 1992;52:5566S–5569S.

Hartge P, Devesa SS, Fraumeni JF Jr. Hodgkin's and non-Hodgkin's lymphomas. Cancer Surv 1994;19–20:423–53.

Herrinton LJ, Friedman GD. Cigarette smoking and risk of non-Hodgkin's lymphoma subtypes. Cancer Epidemiol Biomarkers Prev 1998;7:25–28.

Hervonen K, Vornanen M, Kautiainen H, Collin P, Reunala T. Lymphoma in patients with dermatitis herpetiformis and their first-degree relatives. Br J Dermatol 2005;152:82–86.

Hickish T, Cunningham D, Colston K, Millar BC, Sandle J, Mackay AG, et al. The effect of 1,25-dihydroxyvitamin D3 on lymphoma cell lines and expression of vitamin D receptor in lymphoma. Br J Cancer 1993;68:668–72.

Hill CL, Zhang Y, Sigurgeirsson B, Pukkala E, Mellemkjaer L, Airio A, et al. Frequency of specific cancer types in dermatomyositis and polymyositis: a population-based study. Lancet 2001;357:96–100.

Hjalgrim H, Frisch M, Ekbom A, Kyvik KO, Melbye M, Green A. Cancer and diabetes—a follow-up study of two population-based cohorts of diabetic patients. J Intern Med 1997;241:471–75.

Hjalgrim H, Frisch M, Begtrup K, Melbye M. Recent increase in the incidence of Non-Hodgkin's lymphoma among young men and women in Denmark. Br J Cancer 1996;73: 951–54.

Hjalgrim H, Edgren G, Rostgaard K, Reilly M, NamTran T, Titlestad KE, et al. The occurrence of cancer in blood transfusion recipients. Manuscript submitted 2006a.

Hjalgrim H, Friborg J, Melbye M. The epidemiology of Epstein-Barr virus and its association with malignant disease. In: A Arvin, G Campadielli-Fiume, E Mocarski, P Moore, B Roizman, R Whitley, K Yamanishi. Human Herpesviruses: Biology, Therapy and Immunoprophylaxis. Cambridge University Press, Cambridge, 2006b

Holick, M. F. Vitamin D: A millenium perspective. J Cell Biochem 2003;88:296–307.

Holly EA, Lele C. Non-Hodgkin's lymphoma in HIV-positive and HIV-negative homosexual men in the San Francisco Bay Area: allergies, prior medication use, and sexual practices. J Acquir Immune Defic Syndr Hum Retrovirol 1997;15:211–22.

Holly EA, Lele C, Bracci PM. Hair-color products and risk for non-Hodgkin's lymphoma: a population-based study in the San Francisco Bay Area. Am J Public Health 1998; 88:1767–73.

Holly EA, Lele C, Bracci PM, McGrath MS. Case-control study of non-Hodgkin's lymphoma among women and heterosexual men in the San Francisco Bay Area, California. Am J Epidemiol 1999;150:375–89.

Holm LE, Blomgren H, Lowhagen T. Cancer risks in patients with chronic lymphocytic thyroiditis. N Engl J Med 1985;312:601–4.

Holmes GK, Prior P, Lane MR, Pope D, Allan RN. Malignancy in coeliac disease—effect of a gluten free diet. Gut 1989;30:333–38.

Hughes AM, Armstrong BK, Vajdic CM, Turner J, Grulich AE, Fritschi,L, et al. Sun exposure may protect against non-Hodgkin lymphoma: A case-control study. Int J Cancer 2004;112: 865–71.

Huh J, Cho K, Heo DS, Kim JE, Kim CW. Detection of Epstein-Barr virus in Korean peripheral T-cell lymphoma. Am J Hematol 1999;60:205–14.

International Agency for Research on Cancer. Epstein-Barr Virus and Kaposi's Sarcoma Herpesvirus/Herpesvirus 8. Monographs on the Evaluation of Carcinogenic Risks to Humans. Lyon, IARC, 1997.

Ioannidis JP, Vassiliou VA, Moutsopoulos HM. Long-term risk of mortality and lymphoproliferative disease and predictive classification of primary Sjogren's syndrome. Arthritis Rheum 2002;46:741–47.

Iwata H, Matsuo K, Hara S, Takeuchi K, Aoyama T, Murashige N, et al. Use of hydroxy-methyl-glutaryl coenzyme A reductase inhibitors is associated with risk of lymphoid malignancies. Cancer Sci 2006;97: 133–38.

Jaffe ES, H. N., Stein H, Vardiman JW (eds.) Pathology and genetics of tumours of hematopoietic and lymphoid tissues. Lyon: IARC Press, 2001.

Judde JG, Lacoste V, Briere J, Kassa-Kelembho E, Clyti E, Couppie P, et al. Monoclonality or oligoclonality of human herpesvirus 8 terminal repeat sequences in Kaposi's sarcoma and other diseases. J Natl Cancer Inst 2000; 92:729–36.

Kanariou M, Petridou E, Vrachnou E, Trichopoulos D. Lymphocyte alterations after prolonged sunlight exposure. Journal of Epidemiology and Biostatistics 2001;6:463–65.

Kato I, Koenig KL, Shore RE, Baptiste MS, Lillquist PP, Frizzera G, et al. Use of anti-inflammatory and non-narcotic analgesic drugs and risk of non-Hodgkin's lymphoma (NHL) (United States). Cancer Causes Control 2002;13:965–74.

Kelemen LE, Cerhan JR, Lim U, Davis S, Cozen W, Schenk M, et al. Vegetables, fruit, and antioxidant-related nutrients and risk of non-Hodgkin lymphoma: a National Cancer Institute Surveillance, Epidemiology, and End Results population-based case-control study. Am J Clin Nutr 2006;83:1401–10.

Khuder SA, Mutgi AB, Schaub EA, Tano BD. Meta-analysis of Hodgkin's disease among farmers. Scand J Work Environ Health 1999; 25:436–41.

Kirsch IR, Lipkowitz S. A measure of genomic instability and its relevance to lymphoma-genesis. Cancer Res 1992;52:5545S–5546S.

Kricker A, Armstrong BK, Hughes A-M, Goumas C, Smedby KE, Zheng T, et al. Personal sun exposure and risk of non-Hodgkin lymphoma. A pooled analysis from the Inter Lymph Consortium. Int J Cancer 2007 [E pub Aug 20]

Kusters JG, van Vliet AH, Kuipers EJ. Pathogenesis of Helicobacter pylori infection. Clin Microbiol Rev 2006;19:449–90.

La Vecchia C, Negri E, Franceschi S. Medical history and the risk of non-Hodgkin's lymphomas. Cancer Epidemiol Biomarkers Prev 1992;1:533–36.

Lamm SH, Engel A, Byrd DM. Non-Hodgkin lymphoma abd benzene exposure: a systematic literature review. Chem Biol Interact 2005;153–54:231–37.

Lecuit M, Abachin E, Martin A, Poyart C, Pochart P, Suarez F, et al. Immunoproliferative small intestinal disease associated with Campylobacter jejuni. N Eng J Med 2004;350: 239–48.

Lee E, Burnett CA, Lalich N, Cameron LL, Sestito JP. Proportionate mortality of crop and livestock farmers in the United States, 1984–1993. Am J Ind Med 2002;410–20.

Lens, M. B., Newton-Bishop, J. A. An association between cutaneous melanoma and non-Hodgkin's lymphoma: pooled analysis of published data with a review. Ann Oncol 2005;16:460–65.

Levi F, Randimbison L, Te VC, La Vecchia C. Non-Hodgkin's lymphomas, chronic lymphocytic leukaemias and skin cancers. Br J Cancer 1996;74:1847–50.

Manns A, Hisada M, La Grenade L. Human T-lymphotropic virus type I infection. Lancet 1999;353:1951–58.

Melbye M, Adami HO, Hjalgrim H, Glimelius B. Ultraviolet light and non-Hodgkin's lymphoma. Acta Oncol 1996;35:655–57.

Melbye M, Smedby KE, Lehtinen T, Rostgaard K, Glimelius B, Munksgaard L, et al. Atopy and risk of non-Hodgkin lymphoma. J Natl Cancer Inst 2007;99:158–66.

Mir-Madjlessi SH, Farmer RG, Easley KA, Beck GJ. Colorectal and extracolonic malignancy in ulcerative colitis. Cancer 1986;58:1569–74.

Moore P. The emergence of Kaposi's sarcoma-associated herpesvirus (human herpesvirus 8). N Engl J Med 2000;343:1411–13.

Morton LM, Hartge P, Holford TR, Holly EA, Chiu BC, Vineis P, et al. Cigarette smoking and risk of non-Hodgkin lymphoma: a pooled analysis from the International Lymphoma Epidemiology Consortium (interlymph). Cancer Epidemiol Biomarkers Prev 2005a;14: 925–33.

Morton LM, Zheng T, Holford TR, Holly EA, Chiu BC, Constantini AS, et al. Alcohol consumption and risk of non-Hodgkin lymphoma: a pooled analysis. Lancet Oncol 2005b;6:469–76.

Morton LM, Schenk M, Hein DW, Davis S, Zahm SH, Cozen W, et al. Genetic variation in N acetyltransferase 1 (NAT1) and 2 (NAT2) and risk of non-Hodgkin lymphoma. Pharmacogenet Genomics 2006a;16:537–45.

Morton LM, Wang SS, Devesa SS, Hartge P, Weisenburger DD, Linet MS. Lymphoma incidence patterns by WHO subtype in the United States, 1992–2001. Blood 2006b;107: 265–76.

Mueller NE. Hodgkin's disease. In: Schottenfeld D, Fraumeni J Jr (Eds): Cancer Epidemiology and Prevention. Oxford, Oxford University Press, 1996, pp 893–919.

Nava VE, Jaffe ES. The pathology of NK-cell lymphomas and leukemias. Adv Anat Pathol 2005;12(1):27–34.

Navarro WH, Kaplan LD. AIDS-related lymphoproliferative disease. Blood 2006;107:13–20.

Negri E, Little D, Boiocchi M, La Vecchia C, Franceschi S. B-cell non-Hodgkin's lymphoma and hepatitis C virus infection: a systematic review. Int J Cancer 2004;111:1–8.

Nelson RA, Levine AM, Marks G, Bernstein L. Alcohol, tobacco and recreational drug use and the risk of non-Hodgkin's lymphoma. Br J Cancer 1997;76:1532–37.

Nelson RA, Levine AM, Bernstein L. Reproductive factors and risk of intermediate- or high-grade B-cell non-Hodgkin's lymphoma in women. J Clin Oncol 2001;19:1381–87.

Norval, M. Effects of solar radiation on the human immune system. J Photochem Photobiol B 2001;63:28–40.

Obrams GI, O'Conor G. Time trends and pathological classification: a summary. Cancer Res 1992;52:5570s

O'Brien TR, Decoufle P, Boyle CA. Non-Hodgkin's lymphoma in a cohort of Vietnam veterans. Am J Public Health 1991;81:758–60.

Opelz G, Dohler B. Lymphomas after solid organ transplantation: a collaborative transplant study report. Am J Transplant 2004;4:222–30.

Pallesen G, Hamilton Dutoit SJ. The association of Epstein-Barr virus (EBV) with T cell lymphoproliferations and Hodgkin's disease: two new developments in the EBV field. Adv Cancer Res 1993;62:179–238.

Paltiel O, Schmit T, Adler B, Rachmilevitz EA, Polliack A, Cohen A, et al. The incidence of lymphoma in first-degree relatives of patients with Hodgkin disease and non-Hodgkin lymphoma: results and limitations of a registry-linked study. Cancer 2000;88:2357–66.

Pan SY, Mao Y, Ugnat AM, Canadian Cancer Registries Epidemiology Research Group. Physical activity, obesity, energy intake, and the risk of non-Hodgkin's lymphoma: a population-based case-control study. Am J Epidemiol 2005;162:1162–73.

Poiesz BJ, Papsidero LD, Ehrlich G, Sherman M, Dube S, Poiesz M, et al. Prevalence of HTLV-I-associated T-cell lymphoma. Am J Hematol 2001;66:32–38.

Purdue MP, Bassani DG, Klar NS, Sloan M, Kreiger N, the Canadian Cancer Registries Epidemiology Research Group. Dietary factors and risk of non-Hodgkin lymphoma by histologic subtype: a case-control study. Cancer Epidemiol Biomarkers Prev 2004;13:1665–76.

Quintana PJ, Delfino RJ, Korrick S, Ziogas A, Kutz FW, Jones EL, et. al. Adipose tissue levels of organochlorine pesticides and polychlorinated biphenyls and risk of non-Hodgkin's lymphoma. Environ Health Perspect 2004;112:854–61.

Roman E, Ansell P, Bull D. Leukaemia and non-Hodgkin's lymphoma in children and young adults: are prenatal and neonatal factors important determinants of disease? Br J Cancer 1997;76:406–15.

Ron E. Ionizing radiation and cancer risk: evidence from epidemiology. Radiat Res 1998;150:S30–S41.

Rothman N, Skibola CF, Wang SS, Morgan G, Lan Q, Smith MT, et al. Genetic variation in TNF and IL10 and risk of non-Hodgkin lymphoma: a report from the InterLymph Consortium. Lancet Oncol 2006;7:27–38.

Sandin S, Hjalgrim H, Glimelius B, Rostgaard K, Pukkala E, Askling J. Incidence of non-Hodgkin lymphomas in Sweden, Denmark, and Finland—an epidemic that was. Cancer Epidemiol Biomarkers Prev 2006;15:1295–300.

Savitz DA, Andrews KW. Review of epidemiologic evidence on benzene and lymphatic and hematopoietic cancers. Am J Ind Med 1997;31:287–95.

Scherr PA, Mueller NE. Non-Hodgkin's lymphomas. In: Schottenfeld D, Fraumeni JF Jr (Eds): Cancer Epidemiology and Prevention. Oxford and New York, Oxford University Press, 1996, pp 920–45.

Schroeder JC, Olshan AF, Baric R, Dent GA, Weinberg CR, Yount B, et al. Agricultural risk factors for t(14;18) subtypes of non-Hodgkin's lymphoma. Epidemiology 2001;12:701–9.

Schroeder JC, Olshan AF, Baric R, Dent GA, Weinberg CR, Yount B, et al. A case-control study of tobacco use and other non-occupational risk factors for t(14;18) subtypes of non-Hodgkin's lymphoma (Unitd States). Cancer Cause Control 2002;13:159–68.

Schuler F, Hirt C, Dolken G. Chromosomal translocation t(14;18) in healthy individuals. Semin Cancer Biol 2003;13(3):203–9.

Schuz J, Kaatsch P, Kaletsch U, Meinert R, Michaelis J. Association of childhood cancer with factors related to pregnancy and birth. Int J Epidemiol 1999;28:631–39.

Tatham L, Tolbert P, Kjeldsberg C. Occupational risk factors for subgroups of non-Hodgkin's lymphoma. Epidemiology 1997;8:551.

Schollkopf C, Smedby KE, Hjalgrim H, Rostgaard K, Gadeberg O, Roos G, et al. Cigarette smoking and risk of non-Hodgkin lymphoma—a population-based case-control study. Cancer Epidemiol Biomarkers Prev 2005;14:1791–96.

Selby WS, Gallagher ND. Malignancy in a 19-year experience of adult celiac disease. Dig Dis Sci 1979;24:684–88.

Sigurgeirsson B, Agnarsson BA, Lindelof B. Risk of lymphoma in patients with dermatitis herpetiformis. Br Med J 1994;308:13–15.

Skibola CF, Curry JD, Nieters, A. Genetic susceptibility to lymphoma. Haematologica 2007; 92:960–69.

Smedby KE, Hjalgrim H, Melbye M, Torrang A, Rostgaard K, Munksgaard L, et al. Ultraviolet radiation exposure and risk of malignant lymphomas. J Natl Cancer Inst 2005b; 97:199–209.

Smedby KE, Akerman M, Hildebrand H, Glimelius B, Ekbom A, Askling J. Malignant lymphomas in coeliac disease: evidence of increased risks for lymphoma types other than enteropathy-type T cell lymphoma. Gut 2005a;54:54–59.

Smedby KE, Hjalgrim H, Askling J, Chang ET, Gregersen H, Porwit-MacDonald A, et al. Autoimmune and chronic inflammatory disorders and risk of non-Hodgkin lymphoma by subtype. J Natl Cancer Inst 2006;98: 51–60.

Talamini R, Polesel J, Montella M, Dal Maso L, Crovatto M, Crispo A, et al. Food groups and risk of non-Hodgkin lymphoma: a multicenter, case-control study in Italy. Int J Cancer 2006;118:11:2871–76.

Tavani A, La Vecchia C, Franceschi S, Serraino D, Carbone A. Medical history and risk of Hodgkin's and non-Hodgkin's lymphoma. Eur J Cancer Prev 2000a;9:59–64.

Tavani A, La Vecchia C, Gallus S, Lagiou P, Trichopoulos D, Levi F, et al. Red meat intake and cancer risk: a study in Italy. Int J Cancer 2000b;86:425–28.

Tavani A, Pregnolato A, Negri E, Franceschi S, Serraino D, Carbone A, et al. Diet and risk of lymphoid neoplasms and soft tissue sarcomas. Nutr Cancer 1997;27:256–60.

Theander E, Henriksson G, Ljungberg O, Mandl T, Manthorpe R, Jacobsson LT. Lymphoma and other malignancies in primary sjogren's syndrome A cohort study on cancer incidence and lymphoma predictors. Ann Rheum Dis 2006;65:796–803.

Thun MJ, Altekruse SF, Namboodiri MM, Calle EE, Myers DG, Heath CW Jr. Hair dye use and risk of fatal cancers in US women. J Natl Cancer Inst 1994;86:210–15.

Vineis P, D'Amore F. The role of occupational exposure and immunodeficiency in B-cell malignancies. Working Group on the Epidemiology of Hematolymphopoietic Malignancies in Italy. Epidemiology 1992;3:266–70.

Voulgarelis M, Dafni UG, Isenberg DA, Moutsopoulos HM. Malignant lymphoma in primary Sjogren's syndrome: a multicenter, retrospective, clinical study by the European Concerted Action on Sjogren's Syndrome. Arthritis Rheum 1999;42:1765–72.

Ward MH, Zahm SH, Weisenburger DD, Gridley G, Cantor KP, Saal RC, et al. Dietary factors and non-Hodgkin's lymphoma in Nebraska (United States). Cancer Causes Control 1994;5:422–32.

Ward MH, Cerhan JR, Colt JS, Hartge P. Risk of non-Hodgkin lymphoma and nitrate and nitrite from drinking water and diet. Epidemiology 2006;17:375–82.

Waterhouse D, Carman WJ, Schottenfeld D, Gridley G, McLean S. Cancer incidence in the rural community of Tecumseh, Michigan: a pattern of increased lymphopoietic neoplasms. Cancer 1996;77:763–70.

Weiss LM, Jaffe ES, Liu XF, Chen YY, Shibata D, Medeiros LJ. Detection and localization of Epstein-Barr viral genomes in angioimmunoblastic lymphadenopathy and angioimmunoblastic lymphadenopathy-like lymphoma. Blood 1992;79(7):1789–95.

Wideroff L, Gridley G, Mellemkjaer L, Chow WH, Linet M, Keehn S. Cancer incidence in a population-based cohort of patients hospitalized with diabetes mellitus in Denmark. J Natl Cancer Inst 1997;89:1360–65.

Wiernik PH, Wang SQ, Hu XP, Marino P, Paietta E. Age of onset evidence for anticipation in familial non-Hodgkin's lymphoma. Br J Haematol 2000;108:72–79.

Willemze R, Kerl H, Sterry W, Berti E, Cerroni L, Chimenti S, et al. EORTC classification for primary cutaneous lymphomas: a proposal from the Cutaneous Lymphoma Study Group of the European Organization for Research and Treatment of Cancer. Blood 1997;90:354–71.

Willet EV, Smith AG, Dovey GJ, Morgan GJ, Parker J, Roman E. Tobacco and alcohol consumption and the risk of non-Hodgkin lymphoma. Cancer Cause Control 2004;15: 771–80.

Willet EV, Skibola CF, Adamson P, Skibola DR, Morgan GJ, Smith MT, et al. Non-Hodgkin lymphoma, obesity and energy homeostasis polymorphisms. Br J Cancer 2005;93:811–16.

Wolfe F. Inflammatory activity, but not methotrexate or prednisone use predicts non-Hodgkin's lymphoma in rheumatoid arthritis: a 25-year study of 1,767 RA patients [abstract]. 41 (suppl 9),Arthritis Rheum 1998;41(9):188.

Wood GS, Kamath NV, Guitart J, Heald P, Kohler S, Smoller BR, et al. Absence of Borrelia burgdorferi DNA in cutaneous B-cell lymphomas from the United States. J Cutan Pathol 2001;28:502–7.

Wood C, Harrington W. AIDS and associated malignancies. Cell Res 2005;15:947–52

Zahm SH, Hoffman-Goetz L, Dosemeci M, Cantor KP, Blair A. Occupational physical activity and non-Hodgkin's lymphoma. Med Sci Sports Exerc 1999;31:566–71.

Zahm SH, Weisenburger DD, Babbitt PA, Saal RC, Vaught JB, Blair A. Use of hair coloring products and the risk of lymphoma, multiple myeloma, and chronic lymphocytic leukemia. Am J Public Health 1992;82:990–97.

Zahm SH, Weisenburger DD, Holmes FF, Cantor KP, Blair A. Tobacco and non-Hodgkin's lymphoma: combined analysis of three case-control studies (United States). Cancer Causes Control 1997;8:159–66.

Zahm SH, Weisenburger DD, Saal RC, Vaught JB, Babbitt PA, Blair A. The role of agricultural pesticide use in the development of non-Hodgkin's lymphoma in women. Arch Environ Health 1993;48:353–58.

Zendehdel K, Nyren O, Ostenson CG, Adami HO, Ekbom A, Ye W. Cancer incidence in patients with type 1 diabetes mellitus: a population-based cohort study in Sweden. J Natl Cancer Inst 2003;95:1797–800.

Zhang S, Hunter DJ, Rosner BA, Colditz GA, Fuchs CS, Speizer FE, et al. Dietary fat and protein in relation to risk of non-Hodgkin's lymphoma among women. J Natl Cancer Inst 1999;91:1751–58.

Zhang Y, Holford TR, Leaderer B, Boyle P, Zahm SH, Flynn S, et al. Hair-coloring product use and risk of non-Hodgkin's lymphoma: a population-based case-control study in Connecticut. Am J Epidemiol 2004a;159:148–54.

Zhang Y, Holford TR, Leaderer B, Boyle P, Zahm SH, Owens PH, et al. Blood transfusion and risk of non-Hodgkin's lymphoma in Connecticut women. Am J Epidemiol 2004b;160:325–30.

Zhang Y, Holford TR, Leaderer B, Zahm SH, Boyle P, Morton LM, et al. Prior medical conditions and medication use and risk of non-Hodgkin lymphoma in Connecticut United States women. Cancer Causes Control 2004c;15:419–28.

Zhang T, Mayne ST, Boyle P, Holford TR, Liu WL, Flannery J. Epidemiology of non-Hodgkin lymphoma in Connecticut. 1935–1988. Cancer 1992;70:840–49.

Zheng T, Blair A, Zhang Y, Weisenburger DD, Zahm SH. Occupation and risk of non-Hodgkin's lymphoma and chronic lymphocytic leukemia. J Occup Environ Med 2002;44:469–74.

Zheng T, Holford TR, Leaderer B, Zhang Y, Zahm SH, Flynn S, et al. Diet and nutrient intakes and risk of non-Hodgkin's lymphoma in Connecticut women. Am J Epidemiol 2004;159:454–66.

28

Leukemias

ELENI PETRIDOU, APOSTOLOS POURTSIDIS,
AND DIMITRIOS TRICHOPOULOS

During the early twentieth century discovery of the viral etiology of leukemia in animal species generated a lot of optimism that this situation would apply also to humans. Though the etiology remains largely unknown, childhood leukemia, perhaps the most emotionally charged of all malignancies, is now effectively treated in more than 80% of cases in developed countries. This is indeed one of the biggest successes in contemporary therapeutic oncology.

The atomic bomb explosions in Hiroshima and Nagasaki provided a sad opportunity to study in detail the important role of ionizing radiation in the causation of leukemia. Hence, for the general public, leukemia has been closely linked to radiation, whether ionizing or nonionizing. Fortunately, ionizing radiation is currently under such strict control that only a small proportion of leukemia cases can be attributed to this exposure.

Etiologic research on leukemia is hindered by the fact that no candidate virus has been identified, with the exception of human T-cell lymphotropic virus 1 (HTLV-1)

for a rare form of leukemia. This makes it difficult to undertake informative seroepidemiologic studies. Moreover, there are no biomarkers of radiation exposure that can be used in epidemiologic research. Last, but not least, it is extremely cumbersome to evaluate hypotheses linking herd immunity to childhood leukemia with traditional epidemiologic designs, because herd immunity as an exposure variable is difficult to operationalize.

Leukemia has become distinguished from the other malignancies as a disease that is much more amenable to treatment than to prevention. Nevertheless, this chapter focuses on the potential for prevention of leukemia by examining what little we know and how much we do not know about the causes of this disease in humans.

CLINICAL SYNOPSIS

Subgroups

Leukemias comprise a heterogeneous group of acute and chronic myelogenous and lymphocytic malignancies originating in different cells of the hematopoietic system. In modern classifications, numerous subtypes of leukemia are defined on the basis of cell lineage, maturational stage, and genotype. The four major forms of leukemia are: acute lymphocytic leukemia (ALL); acute myeloid leukemia (AML); chronic lymphocytic leukemia (CLL), which can be considered as a non-Hodgkin's lymphoma; and chronic myeloid leukemia (CML). Acute leukemias affect both adults and children, whereas chronic leukemias predominantly occur among adults. Specifically, figures of the various subtypes for children versus adults are as follows: acute lymphocytic leukemia: 80% versus 14%; acute myeloid: 15% versus 32%; chronic lymphocytic: 1% versus 36%; and chronic myeloid: 4% versus 18%.

Symptoms

Acute leukemia often appears abruptly, and practically all organs and tissues may be affected. Predominant symptoms, caused by anemia, thrombocytopenia, neutropenia, and a deteriorated immune response, are fatigue, malaise, easy bruisability, fever, and infections. In contrast, the onset of chronic leukemia is often gradual, and the disease may be accidentally discovered when a blood count is obtained. In chronic lymphocytic leukemia enlarged lymph nodes are an early sign, whereas a left upper-abdominal mass due to splenomegaly is common in chronic myeloic leukemia.

Diagnosis

Besides routine tests and bone marrow examination, cytochemistry, immunophenotyping, and cytogenetics play important roles in the diagnostic process, and are key to diagnosis, classification, treatment, and prognosis.

Treatment

Acute leukemias are currently treated predominantly with a combination of chemotherapeutic agents. Clinical trials contribute to the continuing improvement of chemotherapy regimens. Some patients with chronic lymphatic leukemia survive for many years without treatment, progress slowly, frequently managed by watchful follow-up, and eventually succumb to unrelated diseases, whereas others have a rapidly fatal disease despite aggressive therapy. Currently the only chance for cure of chronic myelogenous leukemia is through allogeneic bone marrow transplantation. This results in the ablation of the Philadelphia positive clone of cells and thus arrest of the disease. However, the recent discovery of the drug imatinib, a tyrosine kinase inhibitor, has revolutionized treatment for CML. Imatinib directly targets the product of the *BCR-ABL* fusion gene on the Philadelphia chromosome reducing the amount of abnormal protein produced by the chromosomal translocation, thereby controlling disease progression.

Prognosis

Worldwide leukemia accounts for some 300 000 new cases and 222 000 deaths annually. This rather high (74%) deaths/new cases ratio reflects the poor prognosis of the disease in many parts of the world, where the rather complex treatment regimes required are not available. Around 2000, the overall 5-year relative survival for patients with all leukemias—clinically and prognostically a heterogeneous group— was around 44% in the United States and Western Europe but significantly lower (29%) in Eastern European countries. Because an excess mortality continues well beyond 5 years after diagnosis, long-term cure proportions are more than 10 percentage points lower than the 5-year survival proportions. European data for the main subtypes of leukemia cases diagnosed in the late 1980s according to the International Classification of Diseases (ICD) show a substantial variation of the 5-year survival across countries.

Progress

Dramatic progress has taken place, notably in the treatment of childhood leukemia. In the United States, the 5-year relative survival for leukemia overall increased from

14% in the early sixties to ~48% by year 2000. Statistics for patients of all ages do not adequately reflect this progress and survival rates differ considerably by type of leukemia, age at diagnosis, gender, and race. For instance, on the eve of the new millenium overall survival rates were 65 % for ALL (> 88% among children under 5 years of age); 74% for CLL; 20% for AML (> 50% among children under 15); and ~40% for CML. Collaborative randomized trials indicate that treatment efficacy has continued to improve, chiefly through a more optimal use of regimens comprising combined chemotherapeutics and improvement of supportive care.

DESCRIPTIVE EPIDEMIOLOGY

The classification of leukemias is complex and it has changed over the years. The vast majority of the epidemiologic literature, however, whether descriptive or analytic, has relied on the traditional classification into acute myeloid leukemia (AML), chronic myeloid leukemia (CML), acute lymphoid leukemia (ALL), and chronic lymphoid leukemia (CLL).

Leukemias are moderately common and cases of leukemia account for ~3% of all cancers in both developed and developing countries (Parkin et al, 2005). The sixfold variation in incidence around the world is more limited than that of most other malignancies, with highest incidence rates noted in North America and Australia/New Zealand. The low rates reported in sub-Saharan Africa, however, probably represent, to some extent, failure of diagnosis. Although leukemias share some common etiologic factors, notably ionizing radiation, the descriptive epidemiology of the various types of the disease is not identical. Thus, CLL is uncommon in Southeast Asia, whereas the incidence of ALL is very low in Africa.

The age incidence of the disease is overall bimodal, with an early peak in childhood and a subsequent gradual rise (Figs. 28–1 and 28–2). The early peak is almost exclusively accounted for by ALL, whereas CLL

is predominantly a disease of the elderly. The risk of myeloid leukemia, either acute or chronic, increases monotonically with age, but the age gradient is somewhat lower than that of lymphoid leukemia. AML rates are highest in the first 2 years of life and subsequently decrease to a nadir at approximately the age of 9 years, followed by a slow increase during the adolescent years (Smith et al, 2005). Incidence rates are usually higher in males (56%) than in females and in most populations are higher among whites than among blacks (Parkin et al, 2005).

Among children, leukemia is the most common form of malignancy, representing about one-third of all forms of childhood cancer in white populations. Acute lymphoid leukemia is by far the most common subtype of leukemia among children under 19 years of age, being responsible, at least in white populations, for more than three out of four leukemia cases. The early peak of childhood ALL (2 to 5 years) may have been a relatively recent phenomenon. First noticed in the United Kingdom in the early twentieth century, it was documented in Japan in the 1960s, later on in other developed countries, whereas it is still absent in most of the developing world (Ross, 2003). This pattern may be accounted for by postponement of development of herd immunity for several agents because of improvements in hygienic conditions and reduction of sibship size (Smith et al, 1998; Petridou et al, 2001).

Figures 28–3 and 28–4 demonstrate the variability of overall leukemia incidence rates around the world. In interpreting these figures, it should be kept in mind that overall leukemia rates depend heavily on adult cases. Three inferences can be drawn from these figures. First, international variability is less evident for leukemia than for other cancer sites; second, the incidence among males is slightly higher than that among females; and, third, and more subtle, there is an intriguing correspondence between body stature and leukemia risk. The third of these inferences, and perhaps even the second, has been attributed by

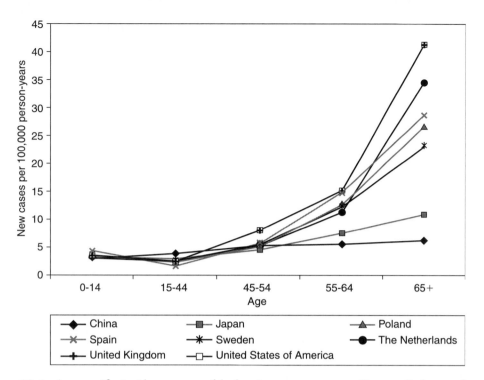

Figure 28–1. Age-specific incidence rates of leukemia among women. (*Source*: Ferlay et al, 2004)

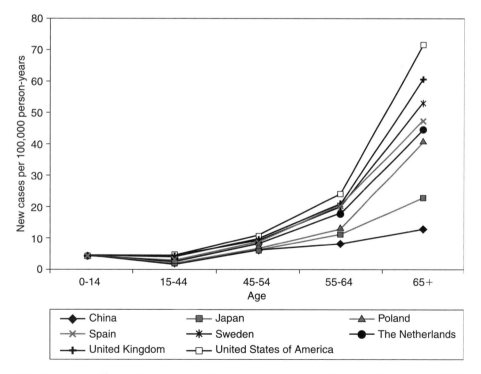

Figure 28–2. Age-specific incidence rates of leukemia among men. (*Source*: Ferlay et al, 2004)

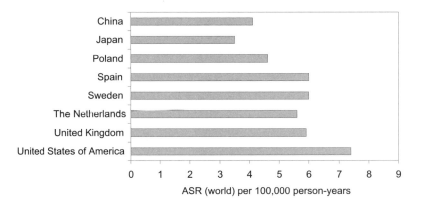

Figure 28–3. Age-standardized (to the world population) incidence rates of leukemia among women. (*Source*: Ferlay et al, 2004)

some authors on the presumably higher number of available stem cells in the bone marrow of taller individuals (Trichopoulos and Lipworth, 1995).

Mortality from leukemias in general and childhood leukemia in particular has decreased over time, mostly due to therapeutic improvements. Indeed, the reduction in fatality of childhood leukemia may be the single most important therapeutic accomplishment in cancer treatment. The real incidence trends over time of various subtypes of leukemia have not been conclusively documented. Data from most registries indicate a slightly increasing trend, which is less evident, or even absent, in long-established and well-functioning registries such as that of Nordic countries

(Hjalgrim et al, 2003a). Several explanations have been advanced to explain these trends, including the following:

1. The increasing trends are artificial due to better diagnostic tools and improved registration procedures.
2. The increasing trends are real on account of more widespread exposure to environmental factors that could increase the incidence of leukemia. Several such factors have been contemplated, including extreme low-frequency electric and magnetic fields (International Commission for Non-Ionizing Radiation Protection Standing Committee of the Epidemiologic Literature on EMF and Health 2001), various chemicals in the envi-

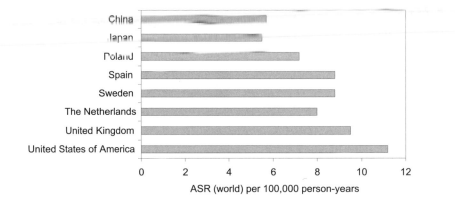

Figure 28–4. Age-standardized (to the world population) incidence rates of leukemia among men. (*Source*: Ferlay et al, 2004)

ronment (WHO, 2005), and changing prevalence of selected perinatal factors (Schuz et al, 1999).

3. The increasing trends are real on account of factors that are largely endogenous, including body size (Trichopoulos and Lipworth, 1995) and, for childhood leukemia, the later development of herd immunity (Petridou et al, 1993; Petridou et al, 2000) and the higher birth weight (Cnattingius et al, 1995a; Hjalgrim et al, 2003b).

GENETIC AND MOLECULAR EPIDEMIOLOGY

Inherited Susceptibility

Genetic factors probably play a role given the occurence of familial cases, the high concordance in monozygotic twins, the frequent association of leukemia cases with constitutional karyotypic aberrations, and the presence of leukemia in the spectrum of genetic instability syndromes. Acute leukemia of both the lymphoid and myeloid type among children is associated strongly with Down's syndrome, and the association has been attributed to the presence of the additional chromosome 21 (trisomy 21). Children with Down's syndrome are about 20 times more likely to develop either ALL or AML than are other children. Down's syndrome is also associated with transient leukemia-a leukemia-like condition within the first month of life, which resolves on its own without the use of chemotherapy (Cnattingius et al, 1995b).

Three rare syndromes characterized by inherited chromosomal instability—Bloom's syndrome (Yankiwski et al, 2000), Fanconi's anemia, and ataxia-telangiectasia—are also associated with childhood leukemia. Several other genetic disorders (neurofibromatosis, Wiscott-Aldrich Syndrome, Klinefelter syndrome) also carry an increased risk of developing leukemia, but these disorders more commonly lead to non-Hodgkin's lymphoma (Gaynon et al, 2003). There is also evidence linking immunodeficiency diseases with acute leukemia and other forms of leukemia (Gatti and Good, 1971).

Among identical twins, concordance of ALL of childhood is high (about 20%), possibly because they share the same placenta. It is thought that a genetic change during fetal life is shared by both fetuses. In contrast, fraternal (not identical) twins and other siblings have only slightly increased chances of concordantly developing leukemia (Buckley et al, 1996). Familial clustering has been reported mostly with respect to adult leukemia, especially CLL and AML (Yuille et al, 2000). Childhood leukemia represents an occasional manifestation of the Li-Fraumeni syndrome (Kleihues et al, 1997). Associations of various leukemia forms with certain antigens of the human leukocyte antigen (HLA) system have been reported, but the observed patterns have not been entirely consistent (Taylor et al, 2002). Molecular rearrangements in 11q23, the mixed lineage leukemia (MLL) gene, are far more common in infant leukemia than in leukemia of older children or adults. They have been attributed to mutations during pregnancy (Eguchi et al, 2003).

Somatic Events

Cytogenetic analyses in AML generate similar results in adults and children. In contrast, cytogenetic findings differ markedly between children and adults with ALL. Figure 28–5 shows major molecular subsets of acute lymphoblastic leukemia—that is, the type of leukemia that has been extensively investigated in this context. Hyperdiploidy (> 50 chromosomes) is the most frequent cytogenetic aberration in childhood ALL, comprising one-fourth of all cases, but it is only a small subgroup in adult ALL (6% of all cases) (Greaves and Wiemels, 2003). By contrast, hypodiploidy (< 46 chromosomes) is found in approximately 5% of both pediatric and adult ALL patients (Harrison et al, 2004).

Structural abnormalities also occur in ALL. They are limited to the leukemic cells, a finding consistent with the presumed clonal nature of the disease. A good example for age-dependent incidence of genetic aberrations is the most frequent aberration in pediatric ALL, which is t(12;21) or its

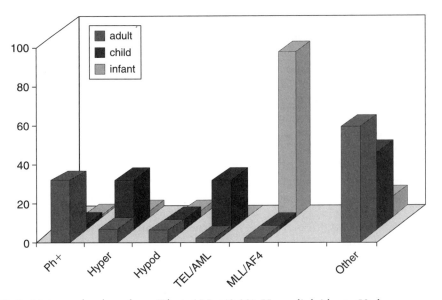

Figure 28–5. Major molecular subsets {Ph + ALL: t(9;22), Hyperdiploidy : > 50 chromosomes, Hypodiploidy : < 46 chromosomes, TEL/AML 1 : t(12;21), MLL/AF4 : t(4;11), other : t(1;19), t(8;14), t(14;11), etc} of acute lymphoblastic leukaemia in infants (<1 year old), children (2–10 years old) and adults.

molecular counterpart *TEL/AML1*. It is predominant in precursor-B-cell ALL in patients 2 to 5 years of age but very rare in adolescents or adults (Aguiar et al, 1996); and it is associated with excellent prognosis (Loh and Rubnitz, 2002). These cytogenetic changes are generally considered disease manifestations rather than constitutional abnormalities, although many of them occur at sites of known oncogenes. Thus, B-cell ALL has been reported to be linked with immunoglobulin genes, whereas T-cell ALL has been frequently associated with genes coding for the T-cell antigen receptor (Raimondi et al, 1988; Hogge, 1994). A translocation between chromosomes 4 and 11 appears to be associated with a mutation of the *MLL*. Particularly common in infant leukemia, this mutation predicts an almost fivefold increased risk of adverse outcomes (Pui et al, 2002).

Among adults with acute lymphoid leukemia, the frequency of hyperdiploidy is considerably lower than that among children with this form of leukemia. By contrast, adult cases of ALL display the Philadelphia

chromosome (the hallmark of CML) in a proportion that may exceed 20%, whereas this cytogenetic finding is rarely evident among children (Greaves, 2002). The CLL in Philadelphia chromosome–positive adults is generally of the B lineage and rarely, if ever, of the T lineage (Schiffer, 1997a).

Karyotypic abnormalities in adult AML are frequent and are considered manifestation of the underlying disease processes. Deletions in chromosomes 5 and 7, abnormalities in chromosomes 11 and 16, and translocations between chromosomes 8 and 21, 15 and 17, 9 and 11, 6 and 9, as well as between 9 and 22, are fairly common and have been found to be related to both morphology and prognosis (Schiffer, 1997b). Over 80% of cases of childhood AML show cytogenetic abnormalities and it is possible that ultimately all cases will be shown to possess a defect (Olney et al, 2003).

In adult CLL, trisomy 12 is a common abnormality, whereas structural abnormalities frequently involve chromosome 13q at the site of the Retinoblastoma suppressor gene (Chiorazzi et al, 2005). Cytogenetic abnormalities are more common in CLL of the B lineage and several cases have been described with juxtaposition of the *BCL-1* gene and the hemoglobulin heavy chain gene (Rai and Keating, 1997). Cytogenetic lesions are occasionally found in the leukemic clone early in the course of the disease but more appear as the disease progresses. Patients showing 13q14 abnormalities have a relatively benign disease. In contrast, the presence of trisomy 12 is associated with atypical morphology and progressive disease, whereas deletions of bands 11q22-q23 are associated with extensive lymph node involvement and aggressive disease (Döhner et al, 2000; Dighiero, 2005).

In CML, the typical cytogenetic abnormality, found in 90% to 95% of patients, is the Philadelphia chromosome, which results from a reciprocal translocation following a break on chromosome 9 at band q34.1 and on chromosome 22 at band q11.21 (Melo et al, 2003). Mosaicism with respect to the Philadelphia chromosome is occasionally observed in the early stages of CML. The key molecular events surrounding the formation of the Philadelphia chromosome have now been largely elucidated. They involve a reciprocal translocation that leads to the juxtaposition of parts of two specific genes: The gene on chromosome 9 is the *C-ABL* proto-oncogene, whereas the gene on chromosome 22 originates from the breakage cluster region (*BCR*). The new fusion gene, which is created through the translocation (*BCR/C-ABL*), has a protein product with unique properties that plays a central role in both the genesis and the treatment of CML (Wetzler, 2005). Some patients may have complex translocations (designated as variant translocations) involving three, four, or five chromosomes (usually including chromosomes 9 and 22). However, the molecular consequences of these changes appear similar to those resulting from the typical t(9;22). It is worth noting that the fusion gene *BCR/C-ABL* can be detected even in the minority of cases of typical CML that lack the Philadelphia

chromosome (Verfaillie, 1998; Farhi and Rosenthal, 2000).

RISK FACTORS

Tobacco

No clear evidence of any tobacco-related excess risk has been found for lymphoid leukemia/lymphoma (IARC, 2004). Most studies examining the association between tobacco smoking and myeloid leukemia, however, have indicated a positive association of moderate strength, with a relative risk among heavier smokers rarely exceeding 2. Although some studies have not documented an association (Adami et al, 1998), the weight of evidence points to tobacco smoking as one of the few established causes of myeloid leukemia, with population-attributable fractions of around 20% in population groups with a high prevalence of smoking.

Support for a causal relationship of smoking with myeloid leukemia is provided by the finding of known leukaemogens in tobacco smoke. The evidence for an association between smoking and leukemia, and perhaps the exposure–response pattern describing the corresponding association, is stronger for chronic than for acute forms of the disease (Doll et al, 1994b). The effect of parental smoking on the risk of leukemia in the offspring during adulthood has been investigated in a few studies, but the results are inconclusive (Brondum et al, 1999). There is also no convincing evidence that smoking during pregnancy increases the risk of childhood leukemia in the offspring (Pang et al, 2003; Mucci et al, 2004).

Diet

In a major report commissioned by the World Cancer Research Fund and the American Institute for Cancer Research (American Institute for Cancer Research, 1997), leukemia was one of the few malignancies for which the dietary evidence was considered too limited to allow any conclusions. It has recently been reported, however, that women who before and during pregnancy eat more vegetables, fruit, and generally what is considered to be a healthy diet, may have a lower risk of giving birth to a child who develops leukemia (Jensen et al, 2004; Petridou et al, 2005).

Alcohol

Alcohol consumption is a variable routinely used in epidemiologic investigations. Thus, occasional associations with one or another form of leukemia would be bound to emerge by chance alone. Overall, there is little evidence that alcohol intake increases the risk of leukemia of any form. There have been intriguing reports indicating that alcohol consumption during pregnancy may increase the risk of infant leukemia or AML during childhood (van Duijn et al, 1994), but the weight of evidence is that there is no association between paternal alcool consumption and childhood leukemia (Shu et al, 1996).

Reproductive and Perinatal Factors

Little attention has been given to the study of reproductive characteristics of subjects themselves in relation to adult leukemia. In contrast, many studies have explored the relation of maternal and perinatal factors in relation to acute childhood leukemia. Perhaps the most consistent finding has been a positive association between birth weight and childhood leukemia (MacMahon and Newill, 1962; Daling et al, 1984; Robison et al, 1987). A meta-analysis of 18 epidemiologic studies of the association between birth weight and childhood leukemia was consistent with an exposure–response relation with ALL risk increasing approximately 14% per 1000-g increase in birth weight (Hjalgrim et al, 2003b). Other findings, less consistently reported, are positive associations of childhood leukemia with maternal age (Reynolds et al, 2002), viral infections during pregnancy (Naumburg et al 2002a), postpartum asphyxia and use of supplementary oxygen (Naumburg et al, 2002b), maternal anemia during the index pregnancy (Petridou et al, 2000), and previous maternal fetal loss (Cnattingius et al, 1995a; Yeazel et al, 1995; Petridou et al, 1997b; Ross et al, 1997; Ross, 2003).

Hormones

It has been reported that administration of growth hormone (GH) to children may increase leukemia risk, although the association is rather weak and may be concentrated among children who are at high risk of the disease on account of factors such as Fanconi's anemia, previous irradiation, or chemotherapy (Nishi et al, 1999; Alter BP, 2004). Because the effect of growth hormone is mediated through the insulin-like growth factor (IGF) system, a link of IGF-1 to childhood leukemia has been postulated and supporting evidence has been reported (Ross et al, 1996; Petridou et al, 2000). However, a recent review suggests that the incidence of leukemia in GH-treated patients may not differ from that in the general population (Mohammadian and Sadeghi-Nejad, 2003). Moreover, there is no suggestion of an increased risk of relapse for children with ALL treated for GH deficiency (Statement from the Growth Hormone Research Society, 2001). It has recently been reported that among children circulating adiponectin is inversely associated with risk for AML but not with acute ALL (Petridou et al, 2006).

Anthropometric Measures

An intriguing association between height and acute lymphoblastic leukemia in children has been reported (Broomhall et al, 1983), which may have to be considered in conjuction with the positive association of childhood leukemia with birth weight. The constellation of these findings may reflect an underlying positive association between number of stem cells and leukemia risk.

Infections

HTLV-1

Human T-cell leukemia/lymphoma virus 1 (HTLV-1) is responsible for a small fraction of cases of adult leukemia around the world and for a negligible fraction among cases of childhood leukemia. This refers to documented etiology. Furthermore, there is considerable evidence that, directly or indirectly, other infectious agents may cause a substantial fraction, perhaps a majority, of leukemia cases. The most powerful argument for an infectious etiology of leukemia stems from an established role of infectious agents in many animal species. At the molecular level, the agents responsible for animal leukemia and related hematologic cancers have been retroviruses. This has directed efforts to identify a human leukemogenic agent of this nature.

In the early 1980s such an agent, human T-cell leukemia/lymphoma virus 1 (HTLV-1), was identified and convincingly linked to the rare adult T-cell leukemia/lymphoma, a disease common in southern Japan but also present in the Caribbean region and some places in Africa (Stuver et al, 1993). This virus causes a latent persistent infection in blood T lymphocytes, which in a minority of infected individuals leads to adult T-cell leukemia/lymphoma. It is highly cell associated, and transmission through transfusion depends on cellular blood components. Human T-cell leukemia/lymphoma virus 1 is transmitted perinatally, possibly via breast-feeding, sexually with higher efficiency from men to women than the reverse, and through intravenous drug use (Gessain, 1999). A constant descriptive finding is that the prevalence of antibodies to HTLV-1 increases continuously with age among women, whereas it reaches a plateau among men at around age 50.

Human T-cell leukemia/lymphoma virus 1 has also been linked to a rare form of myelopathy, the tropical spastic paraparesis. In addition to HTLV-1, HTLV-2 has occasionally been associated with a T-cell variant of hairy cell leukemia and perhaps with other forms of leukemia, although this virus is generally believed to be clinically benign in comparison to HTLV-1 (Murphy, 1993; Gessain, 1999).

Clustering

Contagious infections caused by agents with high infectivity and high pathogenicity, for example measles, frequently generate time clustering. Place clustering can be caused by contagious agents with modest or limited infectivity and pathogenicity as well as by noninfectious agents, for example chemical pollutants. Contagious agents with limited infectivity and pathogenicity are more likely than noninfectious agents to migrate across geographic regions. Therefore, moving place clusters (that is, time-place clustering) are taken as a powerful indication of causality involving an infectious agent (MacMahon and Trichopoulos, 1996).

Many clusters, particularly of childhood leukemia cases, have been described over time, but their investigation has not been particularly fruitful because of difficulties in statistical documentation and limitations in laboratory tools—that is, inability to specify in advance the target outcome, namely, a predefined biomarker. Nevertheless, justifiably or not, the many reports of leukemia clusters have strengthened the perception that infectious agents may be responsible, at least in part, for the etiology of leukemia, and of childhood leukemia in particular (Birch et al, 2000). Data from the National Registry of Childhood Tumours, (which covers the entire childhood population of the UK) showed that the rates of ALL peaked slightly in 1976 and 1990, just after influenza epidemics (Kroll et al, 2006).

Infections and childhood leukemia

The vast majority of cases of childhood leukemia are of unknown etiology. Evidence from animal studies and the occurrence of childhood leukemia during a period when the immune system is rapidly evolving—in conjunction with the role that infectious agents play in the modulation of this evolution—led several investigators to postulate that one or more common infections in genetically susceptible or environmentally conditioned individuals may play a role in the pathogenesis of childhood leukemia (Buffler et al, 2005).

The epidemiologic evidence supporting an infectious etiology of childhood leukemia consists of:

1. studies that, as indicated, have suggested time-place clustering of cases of childhood leukemia (MacMahon, 1992);

2. investigations indicating a decreasing risk of childhood leukemia with birth order, presumably because later-born children are infected earlier in life via their older siblings (Perrillat et al, 2002);

3. reports suggesting that childhood leukemia is associated with delayed establishment of herd immunity (Petridou et al, 1993; Jourdan-Da Silva et al, 2004); and,

4. investigations involving population mixing as a pattern that underlies temporal or spatial excesses of childhood leukemia (Kinlen and Balkwill, 2001; Kinlen and Doll, 2004; Wartenberg et al, 2004).

Researchers who have focused on the possible infectious origins of childhood leukemia have developed different hypotheses, with common elements (Petridou et al, 1993; Smith, 1997). According to the core hypothesis, acute lymphoblastic leukemia is a disease of affluent societies characterized by a rare response to one or more fairly common infections. It postulates that, for most common infections, the biological norm is to be encountered very early in life through the mother or other siblings. In most contemporary societies, however, exposure density of infants and toddlers to infections has been greatly reduced by improvements in hygiene and changing sociodemographic conditions (O' Connor SM and Boneva RS, 2007).

Lack of early exposure may leave the immune system unmodulated, so that late infections with common microorganisms confront an inappropriately programmed immune system and may trigger a strong immune response and subsequent clonal expansion (Petridou et al, 2001). Kinlen (1995) has suggested that a specific virus or viruses may be involved, whereas others have thought that timing of infections rather than antigenic specificity is the crucial factor (Petridou et al, 1993; Smith, 1997; Gilham et al, 2005). A study of unusual design provided some support for the latter hypothesis (Petridou et al, 2001).

Physical Activity

There have been no important studies exploring the relationship, if any, of physical activity with the risk of leukemia of any type.

Ionizing Radiation

Ionizing radiation is one of the few established causes of acute leukemia and CML, whereas there is little evidence for involvement of ionizing radiation in the causation of CLL, now considered a non-Hodgkin's lymphoma. Because ionizing radiation has initiating properties in the carcinogenic process, there should be no safe threshold. In empirical research, however, it has been difficult to document an effect of very low levels of ionizing radiation on leukemia risk.

Exposure to ionizing radiation is measured in Grays (Gy); 1 Gy equals 100 rads. Absorbed dose, on the other hand, is measured in Sieverts (Sv); 1 Sv equals 100 rems. For ionizing radiation with high penetration potential and, therefore, low linear energy transfer (LET), such as x-rays and gamma rays, 1 Gy equals 1 Sv.

It is widely accepted that the exposure–response curve for leukemia risk in relation to ionizing radiation is adequately approximated by a straight line, except at very high exposures, at which cell killing distorts the linear pattern. Many studies have evaluated the relative risk (usually at 1 Sv or 100 rems) as well as the average excess absolute risk (usually per 10 000 person-years/Sv). The estimates vary, depending on a number of factors, including the type of radiation (low or high LET), localized or whole body radiation, and so on. For whole-body low-LET exposure, as among the survivors of the nuclear explosions in Hiroshima and Nagasaki, the relative risk of AML at 1 Sv has been estimated as 4.4, with 95% confidence intervals ranging from 3.2 to 5.6. For more localized low-LET exposures the relative risks have been mostly, but not always, lower.

Figure 28–6 summarizes the dose–risk relation for the three main types of leuke-

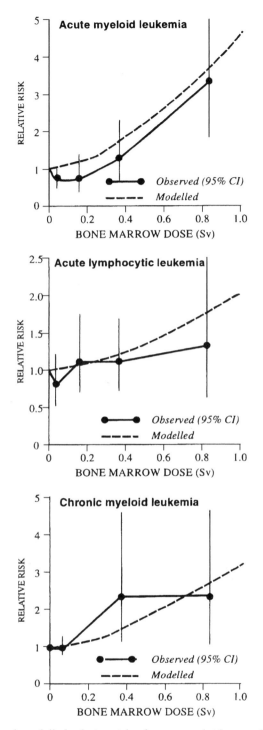

Figure 28–6. Observed and modelled relative risk of acute myeloid, acute lymphocytic and chronic myeloid leukemia in a combined analysis of data for the Japanese atomic bomb survivors, women treated for cervical cancer, and patients treated for ankylosing spondylitis. The values are specific to an attained age of 50 years, after exposure at 25 years, and depict the dose-response at doses less than 1 Sv.

mia. For high-LET exposures, such as those from alpha rays, relative risks in excess of 10 have been reported. Since high-LET ionizing radiation cannot penetrate the skin, such exposures have occurred in unusual situations, notably after intentional intake of Thorotrast, an alpha-particle-emitting radiographic contrast medium (United Nations Scientific Committee on the Effects of Atomic Radiation, 1993, 2000).

Modification of the effect of low-LET ionizing radiation on leukemia risk by age at exposure and follow-up time has been reported. Following a latency of a few years, the relative risk reaches a maximum after 5 to 10 years and declines rapidly thereafter. The relative risk is also higher when age at exposure is less than 20 years, although the excess absolute risk is higher among older individuals. This is because the baseline risk (among unexposed individuals) generally increases with age and therefore is already high during the crucial 5 to 10 years following the exposure.

Susceptibility to the leukemogenic effects of ionizing radiation is highest during intrauterine life, when even low doses of diagnostic radiation have been reported to cause small increases in childhood leukemia risk (MacMahon, 1962; Naumburg et al, 2001). There is also evidence that the incidence of infant leukemia increased following intrauterine exposure to ionizing radiation from the Chernobyl accident (Petridou et al, 1996; Moysich et al, 2002). Within Germany, however, there was no concomitant geographic variation between fallout pattern and incidence of infant leukemia (Michaelis et al, 1997; Petridou 1997a). By contrast, paternal preconception exposure to low-level ionizing radiation, such as that experienced by workers in nuclear plants, does not appear to increase the risk of childhood leukemia in their offspring (Doll et al, 1994a; Petridou et al, 1996 ; Buka I et al, 2007).

Extreme low-frequency electric and magnetic fields (ELF-EMF) generated by electric currents at frequencies of 50Hz to 60 Hz have been intensively studied during the past 20 years in relation to malignancies of various forms. Magnetic fields have received more attention because electric fields do not penetrate physical structures, although in empirical research it is difficult to distinguish the effects of the former from those of the latter. Epidemiologic studies have mostly focused on brain tumors and various forms of leukemia, possibly because so little is known about the etiology of these malignancies (Buka I et al, 2007). There is now a gradually developing consensus that little evidence links ELF-EMF to brain tumors among children or adults or to leukemia among adults.

For childhood leukemia, however, data are less clear-cut. Neither electric nor magnetic fields have the potential to initiate the process of carcinogenesis, but a promotional role of magnetic fields cannot be confidently ruled out. The epidemiologic evidence is also equivocal (Ahlbom et al, 2004; Kheifets and Shimkhada, 2005). On the one hand, two major studies undertaken in the United States by Linet et al (1997) and in the United Kingdom by the UK Childhood Cancer Study Investigators (1999) have generated reassuringly null results. On the other hand, sophisticated meta-analyses (International Commission for non-Ionizing Radiation Protection Stading Committee, 2001; Angelillo and Villari, 1999) have indicated a statistically significant excess risk of childhood leukemia at high levels of exposure to ELF-EMF. Lastly, a population-based case-control study from Japan based on weekly measured magnetic fields in the child's bedroom showed an increased risk above 0.4 μT magnetic fields level for ALL only, whereas for AML, no elevated risk was observed. (Kabuto et al, 2006).

On balance, the lack of a sound theoretical basis for the carcinogenic potential of ELF-EMF, the absence of convincing experimental evidence in laboratory animals, and the inconclusive epidemiologic data should be interpreted as indicating that a role for ELF-EMF in the etiology of childhood leukemia is unlikely but not impossible.

Occupation

The study of the association between exposure to occupational factors and leukemia risk is hindered by the fact that available occupational groups may not be large enough for the documentation of an association, particularly if the association is limited to only a few of the leukemia subtypes. Chronic lymphoid leukemia, for example, appears to be less dependent than other forms of leukemia on environmental influences.

Occupational exposure to ionizing radiation

Radiologists and medical x-ray workers were found to be at increased risk of leukemia in the earlier decades of the twentieth century (Matanoski et al, 1984). However, studies of these categories of workers during the past few decades, when protective measures were instituted and adhered to, have generated mostly null results.

Nuclear workers are a heterogeneous group, and the heterogeneity may well reflect variable exposure to ionizing radiation, which, however, rarely exceeds 50 mSv (5 rems). Null studies are as common as those reporting slightly positive results, although among the latter, the relative risk estimates rarely reach 2 and are frequently nonsignificant. Given the initiating carcinogenic properties of ionizing radiation and thus the lack of a safety threshold, the observed small excess leukemia risk among nuclear workers in some studies appears plausible, particularly when protective measures have not been strictly adhered to (Kendall et al, 1992).

A retrospective cohort study was coordinated by the WHO's International Agency for Research on Cancer to estimate the risk of cancer death, including leukemia, after low-level exposure to high-energy photon (gamma-ray) radiation in a worldwide population of over 400 000 nuclear industry workers in 15 countries (Cardis et al, 2005). The excess relative risk for leukemia excluding chronic lymphocytic leukemia was 1.93 per Sv but barely significant. Thus,

only a small proportion of cancer deaths, including leukemia deaths, would be expected to occur from low-dose chronic exposures to x- and gamma-ray radiation among current nuclear workers.

Uranium miners are heavily exposed to radon decay products that largely emit alpha particles. Not unexpectedly, given the high LET characteristics of alpha particles, no excess leukemia risk has been documented. Moreover, no elevation in risk has been found among radium-dial workers. Notwithstanding the absence of adequate empirical evidence, some borderline elevation of leukemia risk among these workers should not be confidently excluded.

Occupational exposure to nonionizing radiation

Several occupations involve exposures to extreme low-frequency electric and magnetic fields, as well as to higher-frequency but nonionizing electromagnetic radiation. Such occupations are radio and television work, electrician, electric utility work, power line work, and several other categories. Of these nonionizing exposures, ELF-EMF have been most extensively investigated for carcinogenicity and particularly for leukemogenesis (IARC, 2002). In contrast to residential ELF-EMF exposures, however, occupational exposures are no less likely to be related to electric than to magnetic fields. This is because obstacles, including walls, do not always separate the source of exposure from the exposed individuals in occupational settings, as they do in residential settings, since they block electric but not magnetic fields.

Many studies and meta-analyses have been undertaken, and a marginal risk increase of about 25% may represent a fair summary of the evidence (NRPB, 2003). The increment has been smaller in cohort studies than in case-control investigations, and there have been conflicting results with respect to the leukemia outcome subtype. The collective evidence does not support a link between nonionizing electric and magnetic fields or higher-frequency electromagnetic radiation, on the one hand,

and adult leukemia of any type, on the other. This biomedically questionable hypothesis, however, cannot be definitely refuted, because conclusive empirical evidence for a null association is very difficult to obtain (Ahlbom et al, 2004).

Occupational exposure to benzene
Benzene has been conclusively linked to leukemia. Initial reports referred to acute leukemia, particularly AML, but also to other forms of the disease, including erythroleukemia and myelodysplastic syndromes, which have been linked to benzene exposures (Hayes et al, 2001). In some studies, exposure–response relations have been reported, with exposure measured in terms of benzene levels or duration of exposure (Lynge et al, 1997). Nevertheless, at the population level, occupations account for only a small fraction of total benzene exposure, with cigarette smoking, automobile exhaust, and consumer products being responsible for most of the benzene exposure. Occupations that have been associated with benzene exposure include shoe, leather, and rubber industry work, refinery occupations, printing, and painting (Yaris et al, 2004). As in many occupational studies, it has not been easy to attribute conclusively all or part of the excess risk to benzene, other solvents, or other compounds (Siemiatycki et al, 2004). There is also evidence for an association between childhood leukemia and paternal exposure to solvents including benzene, carbon tetrachloride, and hydrocarbons as well as to paints and pigments (Colt and Blair, 1998 , Buka I et al, 2007).

Other occupational exposures
An excess leukemia risk has occasionally been reported among plastics workers involved in the processing of styrene monomers and butadiene, as well as among workers exposed to pesticides, but the evidence remains inconclusive (Cole et al, 1993; Dich et al, 1997). Exposure to ethylene oxide and to diesel exhausts, handling of antineoplastic drugs, and certain occupations—including embalming, pathology, metal and foundry work, barbering and hairdressing, dry cleaning, and underground mining—have also been reported to be at increased risk of leukemia (Ward et al, 1997; Kipen, 2005). The elevated risk in barbers and hairdressers is noteworthy, as nonoccupational use of hair dyes has not been associated with the disease. Farmers have also been found to be at increased risk of leukemia, but the evidence does not allow distinction between late development of herd immunity, viral exposures, and exposure to insecticides, herbicides, and fungicides as the responsible agent(s).

Parental occupation
Several parental occupations, notably those involving exposure to pesticides, have been linked to childhood leukemia but the evidence is inconclusive (Zahm and Ward, 1998; Feychting et al, 2001). Some of the common limitations of these studies are small case numbers, exposure misclassification, and recall bias. Children of fathers working in the Shellafield nuclear plant in the United Kingdom were reported to be at increased risk of childhood leukemia, but a series of subsequent investigations did not support the initial suggestive finding (Doll et al, 1994a).

Medical Conditions and Treatment

Diagnostic radiation
Prenatal diagnostic x-rays, particularly during the last trimester of pregnancy, imparting exposures to the embryo of 1 to 2 rads (10–20 mGy), have been linked to ALL, although the relative risk is probably no higher than about 1.5. Among children and adults, there is no conclusive evidence that diagnostic radiography increases leukemia risk to a demonstrable extent (Boice et al, 1981; Shu et al, 2002). Nevertheless, it has been argued that diagnostic radiography in developed countries may be responsible for about 1% of all leukemia cases (Evans et al, 1986).

Therapeutic radiation
Exposure to ionizing radiation is higher in radiotherapy than in diagnostic radiation.

Studies of patients with ankylosing spondylitis who were treated with x-rays have documented an increased incidence of AML and CML (Darby et al, 1987). Increases in AML and CML have also been demonstrated among women with cancer of the uterine cervix or the endometrium or with benign gynecologic conditions treated with x-rays, although the risk increment was modest. Among patients with Hodgkin's disease, those treated with radiotherapy alone have shown little evidence of an increase in the AML risk. In contrast, those treated with both radiotherapy and chemotherapy have shown a substantial increase in this risk, which indicates a causal interaction at the molecular level (Andrieu et al, 1990).

Also, evidence derived from studies of patients with non-Hodgkin's lymphoma indicates that total-body irradiation with low doses of radiation increases the risk of AML substantially more than partial-body high-dose irradiation (Lavey et al, 1990). It is possible that much higher exposures to ionizing radiation, like those following atomic bomb explosions, do not convey a proportionally increased leukemia risk because of the killing of susceptible cells (Yoshimoto, 1990). Finally, an increased risk of leukemia has been seen among children who have received therapeutic radiation for tinea capitis and enlarged thymus but, interestingly, not among children treated with radiotherapy alone for malignancies.

Chemotherapy agents

Cancer chemotherapeutic agents, in particular alkylating drugs such as cyclophosphamide and melphalane, which require no metabolic transformation for their action, have been shown to cause secondary leukemia, particularly AML. The relative risk of secondary AML is high when alkylating agents are used to treat hematopoietic malignancies (Swerdlow et al, 1992), moderately high when they are used to treat solid tumors (Kaldor et al, 1990), and modestly elevated when they are used to treat non-malignant conditions such as psoriasis or rheumatoid arthritis (Lee et al, 1991).

Other drugs

Several other drugs have been implicated in the etiology of leukemia, but the evidence is inconclusive. Among them, chloramphenicol, pregnancy- or delivery-related analgesics, tranquilizers, anesthetics, and immunesuppressive agents have received the most attention. Reports that neonatal injection of vitamin K may increase the childhood leukemia risk have not been corroborated (Klebanoff et al, 1993; Petridou et al, 1997b). No association has been found between childhood leukemia and use of oral contraceptives before and antibiotics during the index pregnancy.

Vaccinations

Earlier reports that bacille Calmette-Guérin vaccination reduces the risk of childhood leukemia have not been supported by subsequent investigations. No association was found with infant vaccinations or vaccination during the index pregnancy.

Bone marrow transplantation

Secondary leukemia has been reported after bone marrow transplatation, mostly arising in donor cells (Witherspoon et al, 1989; Marolleau et al, 1993; Matsuyama et al, 2000). The multitude of interventions that accompany bone marrow transplantation makes it difficult to identify the factor that is more likely to be involved in secondary leukemogenesis. In this context, the possibility that chronic antigenic stimulation may play a role, particularly in chronic lymphoid leukemogenesis, should also be considered.

CONCLUSION

There has been considerable progress in treating leukemia, particularly childhood leukemia, and in determining the molecular processes that characterize the various forms of the disease. In contrast, limited progress has been made in identifying the causes of leukemia. We have only been able to dismiss a major causal role of nonionizing radiation, specific occupations, and common lifestyle variables. An environmental chemical might be responsible for one or more forms of leukemia, but it is unlikely that such a factor(s) could explain more than a small fraction of leukemia cases. It seems more likely that an unidentified virus or another biological agent underlies the occurrence of many, even most, cases of leukemia, particularly childhood leukemia.

Another possibility is that leukemia, at least childhood leukemia, represents an unusual response to growth and immuno-stimulating factors or processes against a background of delayed establishment of herd immunity. These factors or processes would not have to be specific, and this makes their identification through epidemiologic investigations of traditional design difficult and challenging.

REFERENCES

Adami J, Nyrén O, Bergström R, Ekbom A, Engholm G, Englund A, et al. Smoking and the risk of leukemia, lymphoma, and multiple myeloma (Sweden). Cancer Causes Control 1998;9:49–56.

Aguiar RC, Sohal J, van Rhee F, Carapeti M, Franklin IM, Goldstone AH, et al. TEL-AML1 fusion in acute lymphoblastic leukaemia of adults. M.R.C Adult Leukaemia Working Party. Br J Haematol 1996;95:673–77.

Ahlbom A, Green A, Kheifets L, Savitz D, Swerdlow A.ICNIRP (International Commission for Non-Ionizing Radiation Protection) Standing Committee on Epidemiology): Epidemiology of Health Effects of Radiofrequency Exposure. Environ Health Perspect 2004;112;1741–54.

Alter BP. Growth hormone and the risk of malignancy. Pediatr Blood and Cancer 2004 ; 43 ; 534–35.

American Institute for Cancer Research. Food, Nutrition and the Prevention of Cancer: A Global Perspective. Washington, DC, American Institute for Cancer Research, 1997, pp 1–670.

Andrieu JM, Ifrah N, Payen C, Fermanian J, Coscas Y, Flandrin G. Increased risk of secondary acute nonlymphocytic leukemia after extended-field radiation therapy combined with MOPP chemotherapy for Hodgkin's disease. J Clin Oncol 1990;8:1148–54.

Angelillo IF, Villari P. Residential exposure to electromagnetic fields and childhood leu-

kaemia: a meta-analysis. Bull World Health Org 1999;77:906–15.

Birch JM, Alexander FE, Blair V, Eden OB, Taylor GM, McNally RJQ. Space—time clustering patterns in childhood leukemia support role for infection. Br J Cancer 2000;82:1571–76.

Boice JD, Monson RR, Rosenstein M. Cancer mortality in women after repeated fluoroscopic examinations of the chest. J Natl Cancer Inst 1981;66:863–67.

Brondum J, Shu XO, Steinbuch M, Severson RK, Potter JD, Robison LL. Parental cigarette smoking and the risk of acute leukemia in children. Cancer 1999;85:1380–88.

Broomhall J, May R, Lilleyman JS, Milner RDG. Height and lymphoblastic leukemia. Arch Dis Child 1983;58:300–1.

Buckley JD, Buckley CM, Breslow NE, Draper GJ, Roberson PK, Mack TM. Concordance for childhood cancer in twins. Med Pediatr Oncol 1996;26:223–29.

Buffler PA, Kwan ML, Reynolds p, Urayama K. Environmental and Genetic Risk Factors for Childhood Leukemia: Appraising the Evidence. Cancer Investigation 2005 ; 1:60–75.Buka I, Koranteng S, Vargas ARO. Trends in Childhood Cancer incidence : Review of Enviromental Linkages. Pediatr Clin N Am 2007 ; 54 : 177–203.

Cardis E, Vrijheid M, Blettner M, Gilbert E, Hakama M, C Hill, et al. Risk of cancer after low doses of ionising radiation: retrospective cohort study in 15 countries. BMJ 2005; 331:77.

Chiorazzi N, Rai KR, and Ferrarini M. Chronic lymphocytic leukemia. N Engl J Med 2005;352:804–15.

Cnattingius S, Zack MM, Ekbom A, Gunnarskog J, Kreuger A, Linet M, et al. Prenatal and neonatal risk factors for childhood lymphatic leukemia. J Natl Cancer Inst 1995a;87:908–14.

Cnattingius S, Zack M, Ekbom A, Gunnarskog J, Linet M, Adami HO. Prenatal and neonatal risk factors for childhood myeloid leukemia. Cancer Epidemiol Biomarkers Prev 1995b;4:441–45.

Cole P, Delzell E, Acquavella J. Exposure to butadiene and lymphatic and hematopoietic cancer. Epidemiology 1993;4:96–103.

Colt JS, Blair A. Parental occupational exposures and risk of childhood cancer. Environ Health Perspect 1998;106(S3):909–25.

Daling JR, Starzyk P, Olshan AF, Weiss NS. Birth weight and the incidence of childhood cancer. J Natl Cancer Inst 1984;72:1039–41.

Darby SC, Doll R, Gill SK, Smith PG. Long term mortality after a single treatment course with X-rays in patients treated for ankylosing spondylitis. Br J Cancer 1987;55:179–90.

Dich J, Zahm SH, Hanberg A, Adami H. Pesticides and cancer. Cancer Causes Control 1997;8:420–43.

Dighiero G. CLL Biology and prognosis. Hematology. Am Soc Hematol Educ Program 2005;278–84.

Doll R, Evans HJ, Darby SC. Paternal exposure not to blame. Nature 1994a;367:678–80.

Doll R, Peto R, Wheatley K, Gray R, Sutherland I. Mortality in relation to smoking: 40 years' observations on male British doctors. Br Med J 1994b;309:901–11.

Döhner H, Stilgenbauer S, Benner A, Leupolt E, Kröber A, Bullinger L, et al. Genomic aberrations and survival in chronic lymphocytic leukemia. N Engl J Med 2000;343: 1910–16.

Eguchi M, Eguchi-Ishimae M, Greaves MF. The role of the MLL gene in infant leukemia. Int J Hematol 2003;78:390–401.

Evans JS, Wennberg JE, McNeil BJ. The influence of diagnostic radiography on the incidence of breast cancer and leukemia. N Engl J Med 1986;315:810–15.

Farhi DC, Rosenthal NS. Acute lymphoblastic leukemia. Clin Lab Med 2000;20:17–28.

Ferlay J, Bray F, Pisani P, Parkin DM. GLOBOCAN 2000: Cancer Incidence, Mortality and Prevalence Worldwide. International Agency for Research on Cancer, Lyon, 2001.

Feychting M, Plato N, Nise G, Ahlbom A. Paternal occupational exposures and childhood cancer. Environ Health Perspect 2001;109: 193–96.

Gatti RA, Good RA. Occurrence of malignancy on immunodeficiency diseases. A literature review. Cancer 1971;28:89–98.

Gaynon PS, Angiolillo AL, Franklin JL, Reaman GH. Childhood acute lymphoblastic leukemia In: Kufe DW, Pollock RE, Weischselbaum RR, Bast RC, Gansler TS, Holland JF, Frei E (Eds): Cancer Medicine, 6th ed. Hamilton, Ontario, BC Decker Inc. 2003, pp 2307–16.

Gessain A. Lymphoproliferative associated with human T-cell leukemia/lymphoma virus type I and type II. In: Degos L, Linch D, Lowenberg B (Eds): Text of Malignant Haematology Martin Dunitz Ltd 1999, pp 227–47.

Gilham C, Peto J, Simpson J, Roman E, Eden T, Greaves MF, Alexander FE, for the UKCCS Investigators. Day care in infancy and risk of childhood acute lymphoblastic leukaemia: findings from UK case-control study. BMJ 2005;330:1294.

Greaves MF. Science, medicine, and the future: Childhood leukaemia. BMJ 2002;324:283–87.

Greaves MF, Wiemels J. Origins of chromosome translocations in childhood leukaemia. Nat Rev Cancer 2003;3:639–49.

Harrison CJ, Moorman AV, Broadfield ZJ, Cheung KL, Harris RL, Jalali GR, et al. Three distinct subgroups of hypodiploidy in acute lymphoblastic leukaemia. Br J Haematol 2004;125:552–59.

Hayes RB, Songnian Y, Dosemeci M, Linet M. Benzene and lymphohematopoietic malignancies in humans. Am J Ind Med 2001;40: 117–26.

Hjalgrim LL, Rostgaard K, Schmiegelow K, Soderhall S, Kolmannskog S, Vettenranta K, et al. Age- and sex-specific incidence of childhood leukemia by immunophenotype in the Nordic countries. J Natl Cancer Inst 2003a; 95:1539–44.

Hjalgrim LL, Westergaard K, Rostgaard K, Schmiegelow K, Melbye M, Hjalgrim H, et al. Birth weight as a risk factor for childhood leukemia: a meta-analysis of 18 epidemiologic studies. Am J Epidemiol 2003b;158: 724–35.

Hogge DE. Cytogenetics and oncogenes in leukemia. Curr Opin Oncol 1994;6:3–13.

International Agency for Research on Cancer (IARC). Non-ionizing radiation, part 1: Static and extremely low-frequency (ELF) electric and magnetic fields. Lyon, France: International Agency for Research on Cancer, 2002.

International Agency for Research on Cancer (IARC). Tobacco Smoke and Involuntary Smoking. Lyon, France: IARC Monographs on the Evaluation of Carcinogenic Risks to Humans, 2004.

International Commission for non-Ionizing Radiation Protection (ICNIRP) Stading Committee on Epidemiology : Ahlbom A, Cardis E, Green A, Linet M, Savitz D, and Swerdlow A. Review of the Epidemiologic Literature on EMF and Health. Environ Health Perspect 2001 ; 109(suppl 6) : 911–33.

Jensen CD, Block G, Buffler P, Ma X, Selvin S, Month S. Maternal dietary risk factors in childhood acute lymphoblastic leukemia (United States). Cancer Causes Control 2004;15:559–70.

Jourdan-Da Silva N, Perel Y, Mechinaud F, Plouvier E, Gandemer V, Lutz P, et al. Infectious diseases in the first year of life, perinatal characteristics and childhood acute leukaemia. Br J Cancer 2004;90:139–45.

Kabuto M, Nitta H, Yamamoto S, Yamaguchi N, Akiba S, Honda Y, et al. Childhood leukemia and magnetic fields in Japan: A case-control study of childhood leukemia and residential power-frequency magnetic fields in Japan. Int JCancer 2006;119:643–50.

Kaldor JM, Day NE, Pettersson F, Clarke EA, Pedersen D, Mehnert W, et al. Leukemia following chemotherapy for ovarian cancer. N Engl J Med 1990;322:1–6.

Kendall GM, Muirhead CR, MacGibbon BH, O'Hagan JA, Conquest AJ, Goodill AA, et al. Mortality and occupational exposure to radiation: first analysis of the National Registry for Radiation Workers. Br Med J 1992;304:220–25.

Kheifets L, Shimkhada R. Childhood Leukemia and EMF: Review of the Epidemiologic Evidence. Bioelectromagnetics 2005;Suppl 7: S51–S59.

Kinlen LJ. Epidemiological evidence for an infective basis in childhood leukaemia. Br J Cancer 1995;71:1–5.

Kinlen LJ, Balkwill A. Infective cause of childhood leukaemia and wartime population mixing in Orkney and Shetland, UK. Lancet 2001;357:858.

Kinlen L, Doll R. Population mixing and childhood leukaemia: Fallon and other US clusters. Br J Cancer 2004;91:1–3.

Kipen H. Leukemia. In: Levy BS, Wagner GR, Rest KM et al. (Eds): Preventing Occupational Disease and Injury, 2nd ed. Washington DC: American Public Health Association, 2005, pp 310–12.

Klebanoff MA, Read JS, Mills JL, Shiono PH. The risk of childhood cancer after neonatal exposure to vitamin K. N Engl J Med 1993;329:905–8.

Kleihues P, Schauble B, zur Hausen A, Esteve J, Ohgaki H. Tumors associated with P53 germline mutations: a synopsis of 91 families. Am J Pathol 1997;150:1–13.

Kroll ME, Draper GJ, Stiller CA, Murphy MFG. Childhood Leukemia Incidence in Britain, 1974–2000: Time Trends and Possible Relation to Influenza Epidemics. J Natl Cancer Inst 2006;98:417–20.

Lavey RS, Eby NL, Prosnitz LR. Impact on second malignancy risk of the combined use of radiation and chemotherapy for lymphomas. Cancer 1990;66:80–88.

Lee K, Baglin TP, Marcus RE.Therapy-related leukaemia in Wegener's granulomatosis. Clin Lab Haematol 1991;13:207–9.

Linet MS, Hatch EE, Kleinerman RA, Robison LL, Kaune WT, Friedman DR, et al. Residential exposure to magnetic fields and acute lymphoblastic leukemia in children. N Engl J Med 1997;337:1–7.

Loh ML, Rubnitz JE. TEL/AML1-positive pediatric leukemia: prognostic significance and therapeutic approaches. Curr Opin Hematol 2002;9:345–52.

Lynge E, Anttila A, Hemminki K. Organic solvents and cancer. Cancer Causes Control 1997;8:406–19.

MacMahon B. Prenatal x-ray exposure and childhood cancer. J Natl Cancer Inst 1962; 28:1173–91.

MacMahon B. Is acute lymphoblastic leukemia in children virus related? Am J Epidemiol 1992;136:916–24.

MacMahon B, Newill VA. Birth characteristics of children dying of malignant neoplasms. J Natl Cancer Inst 1962;28:231–44.

MacMahon B, Trichopoulos D. Epidemiology: Principles and Methods, 2nd ed. Boston, Little, Brown, 1996.

Marolleau JP, Brice P, Morel P, Gisselbrecht C. Secondary acute myeloid leukemia after autologous bone marrow transplantation for malignant lymphomas. J Clin Oncol 1993;11:590–91.

Matanoski GM, Sartwell P, Elliott E, Tonascia J, Sternberg A. Cancer risks in radiologists and radiation workers. In: Boice JD Jr, Fraumeni JF Jr (Eds): Radiation Carcinogenesis: Epidemiology and Biological Significance. New York, Raven Press, 1984, pp 83–96.

Matsuyama T, Horibe K, Kato K, Kojima SS. Bone marrow transplantation for children with acute myelogenous leukaemia in the first complete remission. Eur J Cancer 2000;36:368–75.

Melo JV, Hughes TP, Apperley JF. Chronic Myeloid Leukemia. Hematology Am Soc Hematol Educ Program 2003;132–52.

Michaelis J, Kaletsch U, Burkart W, Grosche B. Infant leukaemia after the Chernobyl accident. Nature 1997;387:246.

Mohammadian S, Sadeghi-Nejad A. Current State of Growth Hormone Therapy. Int J Endocrinol Metab 2003;2:71–83.

Moysich KB, Menezes RJ, Michalek AM. Chernobyl-related ionising radiation radiation exposure and cancer risk: an epidemiological review. Lancet Oncol 2002;3:269–79.

Mucci LA, Granath F, Cnattingius S. Maternal smoking and childhood leukemia and lymphoma risk among 1,440,542 Swedish children. Cancer Epidemiol Biomarkers Prev 2004;13:1528–33.

Murphy EL. HTLV-II-related disease. Lancet 1993;341:888.

Naumburg E, Bellocco R, Cnattingius S, Jonzon A, Ekbom, A. Perinatal exposure to infection and risk of childhood leukemia. Med Pediatr Oncol 2002a;38:391–97.

Naumburg E, Bellocco R, Cnattingius S, Jonzon A, Ekbom A. Supplementary oxygen and risk of childhood leukemia. Acta Paediatr 2002b;91:1328–33.

Naumburg E, Bellocco R, Cnattingius S, Hall P, Boice JR, Ekbom A. Intrauterine exposure to diagnostic x-ray and risk of childhood leukemia subtype. Radiat Res 2001;156: 718–23.

National Radiological Protection Board (NRPB). Health effects from radiofrequency electromagnetic fields. Chilton, United Kingdom: National Radiological Protection Board, 2003.

Nishi Y, Tanaka T, Takano K, Fujieda K, Igarashi Y, Hanew K, et al. Recent status in the occurrence of leukemia in growth hormone–treated patients in Japan. GH Treatment Study Committee of the Foundation for Growth Science, Japan. J Clin Endocrinol Metab 1999;84:1961–65.

O' Connor SM and Boneva RS. Infectious Etiologies of childhood leukemia: Plausibility and challenges to proof. Environ Health Perspect 2007 ; 115:146–50.

Olney HJ, Gozzetti A, Rowley JD. Chromosomal Abnormalities in childhood Hematologic Malignant Diseases. In: Nathan DG, Oskin SH, et al. (Eds): Haematology of Infancy and Childhood, 6ᵗʰ ed. ()Saunders 2003, pp 1101–25.

Pang D, McNally R, Birch JM. Parental smoking and childhood cancer: results from the United Kingdom Childhood Cancer Study. Br J Cancer 2003;88:373–81.

Parkin DM, Bray F, Ferlay J, Pisani P. Global cancer statistics 2002. CA Cancer J 2005; 55:74–108.

Perrillat F, Clavel J, Auclerc MF, Baruchel A, Leverger A, Nelken B, et al. Day-care, early common infections and childhood acute leukaemia: a multicentre French case–control study. Br J Cancer 2002;86:1064–69.

Petridou E, Dalamaga M, Mentis A, Skalkidou A, Moustaki M, Karpathios T, et al. Evidence supporting the infectious aetiology of childhood leukemia: the role of low herd immunity. Cancer Causes Control 2001;12: 645–52.

Petridou E, Kassimos D, Kalmanti M, Kosmidou H, Haidas S, Flytzani V, et al. Age of exposure to infections and childhood leukemia risk. Br Med J 1993;307:774.

Petridou E, Ntouvelis E, Dessypris N, Terzidis A, Trichopoulos D and the Childhood Hematology-Oncology Group. Maternal diet and acute lymphoblastic leukemia in young children. Cancer Epidemiol Biomarkers Prev 2005;14:1935–39.

Petridou E, Mantzoros CS, Dessypris N, Dikalioti SK, Trichopoulos D and the Childhood Hematology Oncology Group. Adiponectin in relation to childhood myeloblastic leukaemia. Br J Cancer 2006;94:156–60.

Petridou E, Skalkidou A, Dessypris N, Moustaki M, Mantzoros C, Spanos E, et al. Endogenous risk factors for childhood leukemia in relation to the IGF system (Greece). The Childhood Haematologists-Oncologists Group. Cancer Causes Control 2000;11: 765–71.

Petridou E, Trichopoulos D, Dessypris N, Flytzani V, Haidas S, Kalmanti M, et al. Infant leukaemia after in utero exposure to radiation from Chernobyl. Nature 1996;382: 352–53.

Petridou E, Trichopoulos D, Dessypris N, Flytzani V, Haidas S, Kalmanti M, et al. Infant leukaemia after the Chernobyl accident [letter]. Nature 1997a;387:246.

Petridou E, Trichopoulos D, Kalapothaki V, Pourtsidis A, Kogevinas M, Kalmanti M, et al. The risk profile of childhood leukaemia in Greece: a nationwide case-control study. Br J Cancer 1997b;76:1241–47.

Pui CH, Gaynon PS, Boyett JM, Chessells JM, Baruchel A, Kamps W, et al. Outcome of treatment in childhood acute lymphoblastic leukaemia with rearrangements of the 11q23 chromosomal region. Lancet 2002;359: 1909–15.

Rai KR, Keating MJ. Chronic lympocytic leukemia. In: Holland JF, Bast RC, Morton DL, Frei E, Kufe DW, Weichsetbaum RR (Eds): Cancer Medicine, 4th ed. Baltimore, Williams & Wilkins, 1997, pp 2697–2718.

Raimondi SC, Behm FG, Roberson PK, Pui CH, Rivera GK, Murphy SB, et al. Cytogenetics of childhood T-cell leukemia. Blood 1988; 72:1560.

Reynolds P, Von Behren J, Elkin EP. Birth characteristics and leukemia in young children. Am J Epidemiol 2002;155:603–13.

Robison LL, Codd M, Gunderson P, Neglia JP, Smithson WA, King FL. Birth weight as a risk factor for childhood acute lymphoblastic leukemia. Pediatr Hematol Oncol 1987;4: 63–72.

Ross JA, Perentesis JP, Robison LL, Davies SM. Big babies and infant leukemia: a role for insulin-like growth factor-1? Cancer Causes Control 1996;7:553.

Ross JA, Potter JD, Shu XO, Reaman GH, Lampkin B, Robison LL. Evaluating the relationships among maternal reproductive history, birth characteristics, and infant leukemia: a report from the Children's Cancer Group. Ann Epidemiol 1997;7:172–79.

Ross JA. Etiology of infant leukemia: observations and future directions. Am Soc Clin Oncol 2003;3:243–49.

Schiffer CA. Acute lymphocytic leukemia in adults. In: Holland JF, Bast RC, Morton DL, Frei E, Kufe DW, Weichsetbaum RR (Eds): Cancer Medicine, 4th ed. Baltimore, Williams & Wilkins, 1997a, pp 2667–80.

Schiffer CA. Acute myeloid leukemia in adults. In: Holland JF, Bast RC, Morton DL, Frei E, Kufe DW, Weichsetbaum RR (Eds): Cancer Medicine, 4th ed. Baltimore, Williams & Wilkins, 1997b, pp 2617–49.

Schuz J, Kaatsch P, Kaletsch U, Meinert R, Michaelis J. Association of childhood cancer with factors related to pregnancy and birth. Int J Epidemiol 1999;28:631–39.

Shu XO, Ross JA, Pendergrass TW, Reaman GH, Lampkin B, Robison LL. Parental alcohol consumption, cigarette smoking, and risk of infant leukemia: a childrens cancer group study. J Natl Cancer Inst 1996;88:24–31.

Shu XO, Potter JD, Linet MS, Richard K, Severson RK, Han D, et al. Diagnostic x-rays and ultrasound exposure and risk of childhood acute lymphoblastic leukemia by immunophenotype. Cancer Epidemiol Biomarkers Prev 2002;11:177–85.

Siemiatycki J, Richardson L, Straif K, Latreille B, Lakhani R, Campbell S, et al. Listing occupational carcinogens. Environ Health Perspect 2004;112:1447–59.

Smith M. Considerations on a possible viral etiology for B-precursor acute lymphoblastic leukemia of childhood. J Immunother 1997; 20:89–100.

Smith MA, Lynn A, Ries G, Gurney JG, Ross JA. SEER Pediatric Monograph, NCI, 2005.

Smith MA, Simon R, Strickler HD, McQuillan G, Ries LA, Linet MS. Evidence that childhood acute lymphoblastic leukemia is associated with an infectious agent linked to hygiene conditions. Cancer Causes Control 1998;9:285–98.

Statement from the Growth Hormone Research Society. Critical evaluation of the safety of recombinant human growth hormone administration. J Clin Endocrinol Metab 2001;86:1868–70.

Stuver SO, Tachibana N, Okayama A, Shioiri S, Tsunetoshi Y, Tsuda K, et al. Heterosexual transmission of human T-cell leukemia/lymphoma virus type I among married couples in southwestern Japan: an initial report from the Miyazaki Cohort Study. Infect Dis 1993;167:57–65.

Swerdlow AJ, Douglas AJ, Hudson GV, Hudson BV, Bennett MH, MacLennan KA. Risk of second primary cancers after Hodgkin's disease by type of treatment: analysis of 2846 patients in the British National Lymphoma Investigation. Br Med J 1992;304: 1137–43.

Taylor GM, Dearden S, Ravetto R, Ayres M, Watson P, Hussain A, et al. Genetic susceptibility to childhood common acute lymphoblastic leukemia is associated with polymorphic peptide-binding pocket profiles in, HLA-DRB1*0201. Hu Mol Genet 2002; 11:1585–97.

Trichopoulos D, Lipworth L. Is the cancer causation simpler than we thought, but more intractable? Epidemiology 1995;6:423–24.

UK Childhood Cancer Study Investigators. Exposure to power-frequency magnetic fields and the risk of childhood cancer. Lancet 1999;354:1925–31.

United Nations Scientific Committee on the Effects of Atomic Radiation. Sources and Effects of Ionizing Radiation. Report to the General Assembly. United Nations Sales Pub. No. E. 94 IX.2. New York, United Nations, 1993.

United Nations Scientific Committee on the Effect of Atomic Radiation. Sources and effects of ionizing radiation. UNSCEAR 2000 Report to the General Assembly, with Scientific Annexes, volume II: Effects. New York, United Nations Publications, 2000.

van Duijn CM, van Steensel-Moll HA, Coebergh JW, van Zanen GE. Risk factors for childhood acute non-lymphocytic leukemia: an association with maternal alcohol consumption during pregnancy? Cancer Epidemiol Biomarkers Prev 1994;3:457–60.

Verfaillie CM. Biology of chronic myelogenous leukemia. Hematol Oncol Clin North Am 1998;12:1–29.

Ward E, Burnett C, Ruder A, Davis-King K. Industries and cancer. Cancer Causes Control 1997; 8:356–70.

Wartenberg D, Schneider D, Brown S. Childhood leukemia incidence and the population mixing hypothesis in US SEER data. Br J Cancer 2004;90:1771–76.

Wetzler M. Chronic Myeloid Leukemia. In: Chang AE, Ganz PA, Hayes DA, Kinsella T, Pass HI, Schiller JH, Stone RM, Strecher V (Eds): Oncology : An evidence-based Approach. Springer publ, 2005, pp 1220–30.

WHO, 2005. Effects of air pollution on children's health and development : A review of the evidence.

Witherspoon RP, Fisher LD, Schoch G, Martin P, Sullivan KM, Sanders J, et al. Secondary cancers after bone marrow transplantation for leukemia or aplastic anemia. N Engl J Med 1989;321:784–89.

Yankiwski V, Marciniak RA, Guarente L, Neff NF. Nuclear structure in normal and bloom syndrome cells. Proc Natl Acad Sci USA 2000;97:5214–19.

Yaris F, Dikici M, Akbulut T, Yaris E, Sabuncu H. Story of benzene and Leukemia : Epidemiologic Approach of Muzaffer Aksoy. J Occup Health 2004;46:244–47.

Yeazel MW, Buckley JD, Woods WG, Ruccione K, Robison LL. History of maternal fetal loss and increased risk of childhood acute leukemia at an early age. A report from the Childrens Cancer Group. Cancer 1995;75:1718–27.

Yoshimoto Y. Cancer risk among children of atomic bomb survivors. A review of RERF epidemiologic studies. Radiation Effects

Research Foundation. JAMA 1990;264:596–600.

Yuille MR, Matutes E, Marossy A, Hilditch B, Catovsky D, Houlston RS. Familial chronic lymphocytic leukaemia: a survey and review of published studies. Br J Haematol 2000; 109:794–99.

Zahm SH, Ward MH. Pesticides and childhood cancer. Environ Health Perspect 1998; Supp1.3:893–908.

Epilogue

The epidemiologic search for cancer causes has been conducted in earnest for barely 50 years. This book documents the striking success that the field has had in establishing these causes for many cancer sites—lung, breast, stomach, colorectal, liver, cervical, endometrial, and skin cancers, for instance— although there are sites for which we still have few definitively established causes, including leukemias, lymphomas, and pancreas and brain cancers. It is natural to ask whether we have reached an age of "diminishing returns," during which ever greater efforts will be made to establish weaker and less prevalent risk factors for less common cancer sites.

If the past is prologue to the future, then the pace of new discoveries in the past decade suggests that we are in a golden age of epidemiologic inquiry into the causes of cancer. Table E–1 lists factors that have been generally accepted in the past 20 years as highly probable causes of certain specific cancers. Table E–2 is perhaps an equally important list of exposures that recent research has shown are probably not major

causes of the cancers listed, although previous research had suggested associations. Many of these findings have been pinned down since the early 1990s, suggesting that the pace of epidemiologic discovery is accelerating.

In the last 5 years the completion of the Human Genome Project, the discovery that much of common genetic variation can be captured by genotyping a subset of all variants through the information from the International HapMap Project, and the technological developments that have made it possible to measure > 500 000 Single Nucleotide Polymorphisms in a single assay, have all combined to permit us to search genome-wide for common variants associated with specific cancers. This offers genetic epidemiologists the prospect of discovering major common genetic variants that account for inherited predisposition to specific cancers in the next 5 years. Initial successes in 2006 established a locus for prostate cancer that may account for over 30% of prostate cancer risk in Caucasians and a larger proportion in men of African

Table E–1. Risk factors for specific cancers accepted as causal since the beginning of the 1980s

Risk factor	Cancer
Helicobacter pylori infection	Stomach
HPV infection	Cervix
HBV, HCV infection	Liver
Passive smoking	Lung
Postmenopausal hormones	Breast, Endometrium
Tubal ligation (protective)	Ovary
Physical activity (protective)	Colorectum
Obesity	Kidney, Breast (postmenopausal), Esophagus (adenocarcinoma)
Smoking	Pancreas
Smoking	Liver
Reflux symptoms	Esophagus (adenocarcinoma)
Inherited genetic variants in 8q24	Prostate
Several genetic variants	Breast

HPV, human papillomavirus; HBV, hepatitis B virus; HCV, hepatitis C virus.

ancestry. Further findings for prostate cancer, breast and colorectal cancer, have been reported in 2007. Finding these genetic variants will permit us to assess gene–environment interactions with the real genetic risks well measured, instead of using the weak surrogate of family history. Understanding the physiological role of these genes should open up much new understanding of mechanisms of specific cancers. Whether this understanding leads directly

Table E–2. Some selected hypothesized risk factors accepted as probably not major causes of the listed cancers, based on epidemiologic research since the beginning of the 1980s

Risk factor	Cancer
HSV II infection	Cervix
PCBs and DDT	Breast
Dietary fat	Breast
Coffee	Pancreas
Reserpine (an antihypertensive)	Breast
Saccharine	Bladder
Cell phone use	Brain

HSV II, herpes simplex virus II; PCBs, polychlorinated biphenyls; DDT, dichlorodiphenyltrichloroethane.

to preventive advice, chemoprevention, and/or therapies, only time will tell.

It is interesting then, that epidemiology is far from universally accepted as a successful science. The pages of our journals are full of thoughtful, self-critical analyses of our methods and their limitations. Occasionally these doubts receive a public airing. Almost everybody, epidemiologists and critics alike, accepts that the problems stem not only from the application of epidemiologic methods, but also from the fact that much of our work takes place under the spotlight of public scrutiny. Thus, it is inevitable that a single prominent "positive" study of a prevalent exposure will receive more publicity than several "negative" (and perhaps better-designed) studies of the same association.

When the first positive study of an association receives wide press attention, the association sometimes becomes accepted wisdom. Then one or more subsequent negative studies will be publicized as "overturning" this wisdom. The attention our studies receive is a mixed blessing. It is certainly nice to be noticed, but if we all agree that it is rare for a single epidemiologic study to be definitive, then do most studies deserve any public notice at all? The answer, of course, is "no", but in an age in which the public is interested in the causes of disease, especially cancer, and thus buys the newspapers, watches the TV stations, and monitor the internet sites that publicize the latest findings, would we really prefer to be ignored and have our findings go completely unheeded? Probably not. Yet it does behoove us to be self-critical, and pay more attention to the process of communicating our results to the public and policy makers.

In the Epilogue to the first edition we asked "whether readers of a second edition of this textbook will find much new information in 5 or 10 years time. We feel optimistic about continued progress and expect the book to become quite rapidly out-of-date." This second edition has been necessary in part because of new findings and the need to update the text. We are equally confident that a third edition will be necessary in another 5 to 10 years.

There are several reasons for our continued optimism:

- Our understanding of study design and methods for limiting bias in epidemiologic studies continues to improve. Overall study quality has improved, and average sample sizes have increased.
- Prospective studies are able to provide larger numbers of cases of common cancers than was previously possible and are beginning to provide data on less common cancer sites.
- The recognition that single studies are often underpowered, particularly for assessment of effect modification, has led the continued formation of Consortia to permit analysis of pooled primary data to increase power. This also helps provide the most definitive evidence available at an earlier stage, eliminating some of the back-and-forth in the literature that can contribute to confusion.
- Many cancer sites have been understudied. If lymphoma or brain cancer had received the attention that has been given to more common cancers such as breast and colorectal cancer, for instance, we would probably know more about their causes.
- Newer methods of exposure assessment are becoming available. Better analytic techniques are reducing the amount of specimen required to measure nutrients and exogenous chemicals in blood and other tissues, and are decreasing the random laboratory error in these measurements.

- The availability of catalogues of common between-person genetic variation make it possible to define the genetic variants responsible for much of the inherited component of risk of specific cancers, at least for those sites for which adequate numbers of samples from cases have been assembled.
- Newer methods of cancer definition are being validated. Entities that look similar under the microscope may have different etiologic factors, and molecular techniques may help separate entities that have previously been lumped together.

For all these reasons, we feel that epidemiology still has much to offer the field of cancer research. Whether our best days are ahead of us or behind us remains to be seen, but the substantial fractions of prostate, breast, brain, lymphoma, leukemia, and other cancers that remain unexplained indicate that we still have much work to do. Our recent track record in explaining mysteries such as the decline in stomach cancer incidence (Chapter 10) the increase in adenocarcinoma of the esophagus (Chapters 9), and recent changes in breast cancer incidence (Chapter 16), should give us confidence in our approach and methods. We can be proud of recent achievements in our field. Any individual study result may be less than certain, but of one thing we can be sure—the field of cancer epidemiology has much more to contribute.

Index

Note: Page numbers followed by *f* and *t* indicate figures and tables respectively.